Pharmacology for
NURSE ANESTHESIOLOGY

Edited by

Richard G. Ouellette, MEd, CRNA
Staff Anesthetist
Wesley Long Community Hospital
Moses Cone Health System
Greensboro, North Carolina

Joseph Anthony Joyce, BS, CRNA
Staff Anesthetist
Wesley Long Community Hospital
Moses Cone Health System
Greensboro, North Carolina

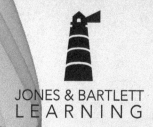

JONES & BARTLETT
LEARNING

World Headquarters
Jones & Bartlett Learning
40 Tall Pine Drive
Sudbury, MA 01776
978-443-5000
info@jblearning.com
www.jblearning.com

Jones & Bartlett Learning Canada
6339 Ormindale Way
Mississauga, Ontario L5V 1J2
Canada

Jones & Bartlett Learning International
Barb House, Barb Mews
London W6 7PA
United Kingdom

Jones & Bartlett Learning books and products are available through most bookstores and online booksellers. To contact Jones & Bartlett Learning directly, call 800-832-0034, fax 978-443-8000, or visit our website, www.jblearning.com.

Substantial discounts on bulk quantities of Jones & Bartlett Learning publications are available to corporations, professional associations, and other qualified organizations. For details and specific discount information, contact the special sales department at Jones & Bartlett Learning via the above contact information or send an email to specialsales@jblearning.com.

The authors, editor, and publisher have made every effort to provide accurate information. However, they are not responsible for errors, omissions, or for any outcomes related to the use of the contents of this book and take no responsibility for the use of the products and procedures described. Treatments and side effects described in this book may not be applicable to all people; likewise, some people may require a dose or experience a side effect that is not described herein. Drugs and medical devices are discussed that may have limited availability controlled by the Food and Drug Administration (FDA) for use only in a research study or clinical trial. Research, clinical practice, and government regulations often change the accepted standard in this field. When consideration is being given to use of any drug in the clinical setting, the health care provider or reader is responsible for determining FDA status of the drug, reading the package insert, and reviewing prescribing information for the most up-to-date recommendations on dose, precautions, and contraindications, and determining the appropriate usage for the product. This is especially important in the case of drugs that are new or seldom used.

Production Credits:

Publisher: Kevin Sullivan
Acquisitions Editor: Amy Sibley
Associate Editor: Patricia Donnelly
Editorial Assistant: Rachel Shuster
Associate Production Editor: Katie Spiegel
Marketing Manager: Rebecca Wasley

V.P., Manufacturing and Inventory Control: Therese Connell
Composition: Arlene Apone
Cover Design: Anne Spencer
Cover Image: © Bella D/Shutterstock, Inc.
Printing and Binding: Courier Stoughton
Cover Printing: Courier Stoughton

Library of Congress Cataloging-in-Publication Data
Ouellette, Richard G.
  Pharmacology for nurse anesthesiology / Richard G. Ouellette, Joseph Anthony Joyce.
     p. ; cm.
  Includes bibliographical references and index.
  ISBN 978-0-7637-8607-6
  1. Pharmacology. 2. Nurse anesthetists. I. Joyce, Joseph Anthony. II. Title.
  [DNLM: 1. Anesthetics—pharmacology—Nurses' Instruction. 2. Drug Therapy—nursing. 3. Nurse Anesthetists. QV 81 O93p 2011]
  RM300.O94 2011
  615'.1—dc22
                          2009054074

6048

Printed in the United States of America
14 13   10 9 8 7 6 5 4 3 2

Dedication

This book is dedicated to the memory of John F. Garde, MS, CRNA,
"Clinician, educator, administrator, mentor, and friend."

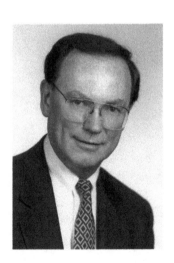

Contents

Foreword: Pharmacology for the Nurse Anesthetist.. xiii

Contributors xv

SECTION I   **General Pharmacologic Concepts** 1

Chapter 1   **Pharmacokinetics: The Study of Drug Disposition** 3
Objectives   3
Introduction   3
Pharmacokinetics   3
Routes of Administration   3
Solubility   5
Absorption, Distribution, Metabolism, and Elimination   7
Mathematical Modeling   10
Dosing Calculations   14
Key Points   15
Chapter Questions   15
References   15

Chapter 2   **Pharmacodynamics: Study of Drug Action** 17
Objectives   17
Introduction   17
Receptor Theory   17
Receptor Interactions   19
Receptor Regulation   22
Receptor Types   23
Non–Receptor-Mediated Effects   25
Mechanisms of General Anesthesia   25
Key Points   26
Chapter Questions   26
References   26

Chapter 3   **Cultural, Environmental, and Genetic Influences on Drug Therapy** 27
               Objectives   27
               Introduction   27
               Historic Perspective   27
               Cultural and Environmental Influences   28
               Genetic Influences   33
               Conclusion   35
               Key Points   35
               Chapter Questions   35
               References   35

SECTION II   **Pharmacology of Anesthetic Practice** 39

Chapter 4   **Anesthetic Induction Agents** 41
               Objectives   41
               Introduction   41
               Barbiturates   41
               Etomidate   44
               Ketamine   45
               Propofol   48
               Key Points   50
               Chapter Questions   50
               References   50

Chapter 5   **Benzodiazepines** 53
               Objectives   53
               Introduction   53
               Mechanism of Action   53
               Clinical Pharmacology   53
               Clinical Uses and Indications   55
               Side Effects and Contraindications   55
               Drug Interactions, Guidelines, and Precautions   56
               Dosages, Administration, and Practical Aspects   57
               Key Points   58
               Chapter Questions   59
               References   59

Chapter 6   **Opioid Agonists, Antagonists, and Agonist-Antagonists** 61
               Objectives   61
               Introduction   61
               History of the Use of Opioids   61
               Mechanisms of Action   61
               Clinical Pharmacology   62
               Clinical Uses and Indications   64
               Comparative Pharmacology of Other Drugs in Class   65
               Adverse Effects and Contraindications   69
               Drug Interactions   70
               Guidelines and Precautions   70
               Practical Aspects of Drug Administration (Applications in the Operating Room)   72
               Key Points   73
               Chapter Questions   73
               References   74

Chapter 7   **Nonopioid Analgesics and Their Role in Anesthesia Practice**..................................77
Objectives 77
Introduction 77
Epidemiology and Etiology 77
Pathophysiology 77
Mechanisms of Pain 78
Cyclooxygenase Inhibitors 78
Cyclooxygenase Enzymes 79
Classification of NSAIDs 79
Side Effects of Nonselective and COX-2 NSAIDs 86
Ketamine 87
Dextromethorphan 89
Centrally Acting α_2 Agonists 89
Key Points 91
Chapter Questions 91
References 91

Chapter 8   **Neuromuscular Blocking Drugs** 95
Objectives 95
Introduction 95
Mechanisms of Action 95
Clinical Pharmacology (Prototype: Rocuronium) 99
Metabolism 101
Elimination 103
Clinical Uses and Indications 103
Side Effects and Contraindications 106
Drug Interactions 110
Guidelines and Precautions 111
Dosage and Administration 112
Practical Aspects of Drug Administration 113
Key Points 114
Chapter Questions 114
References 114

Chapter 9   **Pharmacology of Local Analgesics**...119
Objectives 119
Introduction 119
Mechanisms of Action 119
Clinical Pharmacology 121
Commonly Used Local Anesthetic Agents 125
Systemic Administration 128
Toxicity 129
Systemic Local Anesthetic Toxicity 130
Summary 133
Key Points 133
Chapter Questions 133
References 133

Chapter 10   **Anticholinergics**..139
Objectives 139
Introduction 139
Parasympathetic Mechanism of Action 139

Muscarinic Receptors   139
Muscarinic Receptor Antagonists   142
Key Points   146
Chapter Questions   146
References   147

Chapter 11   **Anticholinesterases** **149**
Objectives   149
Introduction   149
Mechanism of Action   149
Myasthenia Gravis   150
Alzheimer's Dementia   150
Clinical Pharmacology   151
On the Horizon   156
Train-of-Four   156
Key Points   157
Chapter Questions   157
References   157

Chapter 12   **Inhalation Anesthesia** **159**
Objectives   159
Introduction   159
Historical Context of Inhalation Anesthetics   159
Pharmacokinetic Issues: Uptake and Distribution   164
Uptake of Inhaled Anesthetics   166
Pharmacodynamics and Inhaled Anesthetics   169
Modern Inhaled Anesthetics   171
Impact of Inhaled Anesthetics by System   173
Other Issues Related to Inhaled Anesthetics   180
Key Points   181
Chapter Questions   182
References   182

SECTION III   **General Pharmacology** **191**
Chapter 13   **Antibiotics** **193**
Objectives   193
Introduction   193
General Principles   193
Pharmacokinetic and Pharmacodynamic Principles   194
Antibiotic Selection and Specific Antibiotic Classes   195
β-Lactam Compounds   196
Aminoglycosides   201
Macrolides   203
Tetracyclines   205
Clindamycin   206
Vancomycin   207
Fluoroquinolones   208
Metronidazole   208
Practical Aspects of Antibiotic Use   209
Key Points   213
Chapter Questions   214
References   214

Chapter 14   **Antiemetic Drugs and Therapies.** **215**
Objectives   215
Introduction   215
Physiology of Emesis   216
Selective Serotonin Receptor Antagonists   216
Corticosteroids   219
Butyrophenones   219
Benzamides   220
Phenothiazines   220
Antihistamines (H_1 Receptor Antagonists)   221
Anticholinergics   223
Neurokinin-1 Receptor Antagonists   223
Miscellaneous Drugs and Therapies   224
Anesthetic Techniques for Preventing PONV   225
Conclusion   226
Key Points   226
Chapter Questions   227
References   227

Chapter 15   **Prophylaxis for Aspiration Pneumonitis.** **231**
Objectives   231
Introduction   231
Interventions for the Prevention of AP   236
Summary and Anesthesia Implications   252
Conclusions   252
Key Points   253
Chapter Questions   253
Answers and Discussion   254
Acknowledgments   254
References   254

Chapter 16   **Diuretics** **257**
Objectives   257
Introduction   257
Anatomy and Physiology Associated with Urine Formation   257
Diuretic Agents   258
Anesthetic Implications   265
Key Points   266
Chapter Questions   266
References   266

Chapter 17   **Antihypertensive Drugs** **269**
Objectives   269
Introduction   269
Mechanisms of Action of Antihypertensive Drugs   269
Anesthetic Management of Acute Perioperative Hypertension   294
Key Points   299
Chapter Questions   299
References   299

Chapter 18   **Steroids** **303**
Objectives   303
Introduction   303
Clinical Pharmacology   304
Side Effects and Contraindications   305

Drug Interactions   306
Practical Aspects of Drug Administration   306
Clinical Uses and Indications   307
Comparative Pharmacology of Other Drugs in Class   308
Dosage and Administration   309
Key Points   311
Chapter Questions   311
Answers and Discussion   312
References   312

Chapter 19   Herbal and Dietary Supplements **315**
Objectives   315
Introduction   315
Historical Perspective   315
Legislative Intervention   315
Anesthesia Implications   316
Preoperative Assessment   316
Commonly Used Dietary Supplements   316
Summary   321
Key Points   321
Chapter Questions   322
References   322

Chapter 20   α- and β-Adrenergic Receptor Agonists and Antagonists **323**
Objectives   323
Introduction   323
Catecholamines   323
Types of Adrenergic Receptors   324
Caution in α- and β-Adrenergic Drug Usage in Geriatric Populations   340
Key Points   340
Chapter Questions   342
References   342

Chapter 21   Drug Therapy Associated With Autocoids **347**
Objectives   347
Introduction   347
Histamine Agonists and Antagonists   347
Bradykinin Agonist and Antagonist   353
Serotonin Agonist and Antagonist   354
Prostaglandins   356
Conclusion   361
Key Points   361
Chapter Questions   362
References   362

Chapter 22   Anticoagulants and Their Reversal **367**
Objectives   367
Introduction   367
Cascade Model of Coagulation   367
Cell-Based Model of Coagulation   368
Direct and Indirect Thrombin Inhibitors   369
Conclusion   383
Key Points   383
Chapter Questions   383
References   383

Chapter 23 **Antiarrhythmics** 385
Objectives 385
Introduction 385
Muscarinic Receptor Antagonists 386
β-Adrenergic Receptor Antagonists 388
Calcium Channel Antagonists 390
Sodium Channel Blockers 391
Amiodarone (Cordarone, Pacerone) 393
Adenosine (Adenocard) 396
Vasopressin (Antidiuretic Hormone, Arginine Vasopressin) 397
Magnesium 397
Summary 398
Key Points 398
Chapter Questions 398
Answers and Discussion 399
References 399

SECTION IV **Pharmacologic Management of Disease: Anesthetic Considerations** 403

Chapter 24 **Malignant Hyperthermia: Dantrolene** 405
Objectives 405
Malignant Hyperthermia 405
Conditions and Disorders in the Differential Diagnosis of MH 407
Tests for Diagnosing MH Susceptibility 407
Anesthesia for the MH-Susceptible Individual 408
Pharmacologic Intervention 408
Summary 413
Key Points 413
Chapter Questions 413
References 414

Chapter 25 **Pharmacology of Asthma: Anesthesia Implications** 417
Objectives 417
Introduction 417
Origins 417
Incidence 418
Pathophysiology 418
Signs and Symptoms: Preanesthesia Evaluation 420
Differential Diagnosis 422
Pharmacologic Intervention: Management and Control of Disease 422
Practical Aspects: Surgery and Asthma 428
Summary 432
Key Points 432
Chapter Questions 433
References 433

Chapter 26 **Immune System and Anesthesia: Pharmacologic Implications** 437
Objectives 437
Introduction 437
Review of Normal Immune Function 437
Drugs Used in the Perioperative Setting 438
Anesthetic Technique and Immune System Responses 441
Summary 441
Key Points 442
Chapter Questions 442
References 442

Chapter 27 **Pharmacologic Considerations in Obstetric Anesthesia Practice** 445
Objectives   445
Introduction   445
Physiologic Changes of Pregnancy   445
Pathophysiologic Conditions in Pregnancy and Postpartum   446
Pharmacology of Drugs Used in Obstetric Anesthesia Practice   448
Key Points   452
Chapter Questions   453
References   453

Chapter 28 **Psychiatric Disorders and Their Pharmacologic Management** 457
Objectives   457
Introduction   457
Etiology and Pathophysiology of Common Psychiatric Disorders   457
Pharmacologic Management of Psychiatric Disorders   460
Anesthesia Considerations in the Patient Treated for Mental Illness   475
Anesthesia Considerations in Patients Having ECT   476
Key Points   477
Chapter Questions   477
References   478

Chapter 29 **Pharmacology of Congestive Heart Failure** 481
Objectives   481
Epidemiology   481
Etiology and Pathophysiology   481
Classification   482
Treatment   483
Anesthesia Implications   493
Key Points   493
Chapter Questions   494
References   494

SECTION V **Drug Interactions** 499

Chapter 30 **Drugs Interactions of Relevance to the Anesthetist** 501
Objectives   501
Introduction   501
Drugs Used for Anesthetic Management and Interactions Pertinent to Anesthesia   501
Drugs Pertinent to Anesthesia That Induce or Inhibit Metabolism of Drugs   506
Antihypertensive Drug Interactions Pertinent to Anesthesia   507
Psychopharmacologic Agent Interactions Pertinent to Anesthesia   508
Warfarin (Coumadin) Drug Interactions Pertinent to Anesthesia   511
Drug Interactions Pertinent to Anesthesia That Affect Drug Absorption   511
Drug Interactions Pertinent to Anesthesia That Affect Drug Distribution   512
Cardiac Drug Interactions Pertinent to Anesthesia   512
Beta-Blocking Drug Interactions Pertinent to Anesthesia   513
Antibiotic Drug Interactions Pertinent to Anesthesia   514
Miscellaneous Drug Interactions Pertinent to Anesthesia   515
Summary   516
Key Points   516
Chapter Questions   516
References   518

Index 521

Foreword: Pharmacology for the Nurse Anesthetist

In 1990 I was hired as Director of Accreditation for the Council on Accreditation of Nurse Anesthesia Educational Programs. Later, I also assumed responsibility as Director of Education for the American Association of Nurse Anesthetists. During the 12 years I served as Director I was awarded the Helen Lamb Outstanding Educator Award and earned a doctoral degree; however, these honors do not provide any information about my interest in pharmacology or my professional involvement in the anesthetic and adjunct drugs used by nurse anesthetists.

My first introduction to the administration of an anesthetic drug was during my first job as a registered nurse. I was working in the delivery room at a local hospital where all mothers received some sort of inhalation analgesia or anesthesia for delivery, which was a common practice in the late 1950s and early 1960s. This meant that a nurse anesthetist was called for every delivery.

The Head Nurse Anesthetist at our hospital was a single woman who lived nearby in the School of Nursing's student residence. Because of her close proximity to the hospital and dedication to service, she was available within a few minutes to provide anesthesia care at any time of the day or night. I recall many times when she would be in demand in both the delivery room and operating room at the same time. When this happened, she would have me or another delivery room nurse administer ether analgesia to the mother. We were warned to only administer the vapor intermittently and to never open the vaporizer on the anesthesia machine above a certain level that she had predetermined. Fortunately, our patients never lost consciousness as a result of her instruction and ether's slow onset of action.

By 1968 I had graduated from anesthesia school with an awareness of how lucky we had been as untrained nurses to administer ether analgesia to patients without any complications. It was also apparent to me that the delivery of anesthesia had changed considerably in a short time,

making me wonder what other changes might be on the horizon. In the years that followed graduation from anesthesia school, I taught pharmacology classes to student nurse anesthetists in the classroom and helped them to apply pharmacologic principles in the clinical area. Teaching pharmacology was a wonderful opportunity for me to monitor the development of a myriad of drugs that were introduced to alleviate or abolish the pain and suffering of patients requiring anesthesia care.

In my opinion, *Pharmacology for the Nurse Anesthetist* represents how far nurse anesthesia has come as a profession over the years. When I began practice as a nurse anesthetist there were very few anesthesia books available to me. A pharmacology book edited by individuals such as Richard Ouellette and Joseph Joyce would have been welcomed enthusiastically by me and my students!

As an untrained nurse administering ether analgesia to laboring patients, I could not have envisioned such an important publication written by a group of anesthesia scholars that deals with basic pharmacology, specific drugs, and the pharmacologic management of disease in anesthesia practice. Readers of this book will find that it is an important addition to their personal library as well as a great reference for teachers and students of anesthesia. I encourage you to read the book and to benefit from the knowledge it provides.

Betty J. Horton, PhD, CRNA
Director of Education and Accreditation (Retired)
American Association of Nurse Anesthetists and
Council on Accreditation of Nurse Anesthesia
Educational Programs

Contributors

Steve Alves, PhD, CRNA
Coordinator, Nurse Anesthesia Program
Northeastern University
School of Nursing
Boston, Massachusetts

Penelope S. Benedik, PhD, CRNA, RRT
Staff CRNA
Brazos Anesthesiology Associates
Bryan, Texas

Gregory Bozimowski, MS, CRNA
Assistant Professor
University of Detroit Mercy
Graduate Program of Nurse Anesthesiology
Detroit, Michigan

Courtney Brown, MSN, CRNA
Clinical Education Coordinator, Nurse Anesthesia Program
Wake Forest University
Baptist Medical Center
Winston-Salem, North Carolina

Nancy Bruton-Maree, MS, CRNA
Program Director
Raleigh School of Nurse Anesthesia
The University of North Carolina at Greensboro
Raleigh, North Carolina

Reamer Bushardt, PharmD, RPh, PA-C
Associate Professor and Director
Division of Physician Assistant Studies
Medical University of South Carolina
Charleston, South Carolina

Anthony Chipas, PhD, CRNA
Division Director, Anesthesia for Nurses
Medical University of South Carolina
Charleston, South Carolina

Ronald M. Dick, PhD, RPh
Professor and Director of Science and Technology
Barry University
Miami Shores, Florida

Colleen Dunwoody, MS, RN-BC
Advanced Practice Nurse, Pain Management
University of Pittsburgh Medical Center Presbyterian
Pittsburgh, Pennsylvania

Sass Elisha, EdD, CRNA
Assistant Director
Kaiser Permanente School of Anesthesia
Pasadena, California

Timothy Finn, MS, CRNA
University of Chicago Medical Center
Department of Anesthesia and Critical Care
Chicago, Illinois

Mark Gabot, MSN, CRNA
Staff Nurse Anesthetist
Kaiser Permanente Medical Center
Fontana, California

Sarah E. Giron, MS, CRNA
Senior Staff Nurse Anesthetist
University of California, Los Angeles
Los Angeles, California

Clifford Gonzales, MSN, CRNA
Clinical Instructor
Wake Forest University
Baptist Medical Center
Winston-Salem, North Carolina

Charles A. Griffis, PhD, CRNA
Assistant Clinical Professor
Department of Anesthesiology
University of California, Los Angeles
Los Angeles, California

Richard Henker, PhD, RN, CRNA, FAAN
Associate Professor
University of Pittsburgh
School of Nursing
Pittsburgh, Pennsylvania

Joseph Anthony Joyce, BS, CRNA
Staff Anesthetist
Wesley Long Community Hospital
Moses Cone Health System
Greensboro, North Carolina

Mary C. Karlet, PhD, CRNA
Chair, Department of Nurse Anesthesia
Samford University
Birmingham, Alabama

Mark A. Kossick, DNSc, CRNA, APN
Professor
School of Nursing
Western Carolina University
Cullowhee, North Carolina

Michael Kremer, PhD, CRNA, FAAN
Associate Professor
Director, Nurse Anesthesia Program
Rush University
College of Nursing
Chicago, Illinois

Lynn L. Lebeck, PhD, CRNA
Director, Anesthesia Program
University of Michigan–Flint
Hurley Medical Center
Flint, Michigan

Lillia Loriz, PhD, ARNP
Director, School of Nursing
University of North Florida
Jacksonville, Florida

Russell R. Lynn, MSN, APN, CRNA
Associate Program Director
School of Nursing
University of Pennsylvania
Philadelphia, Pennsylvania

Kiran Macha, MBBS, MPH
Clinical Research Coordinator, Nurse Anesthetist Program
School of Nursing
University of North Florida
Jacksonville, Florida

Erica J. McCall, MSN, CRNA
Senior Staff Anesthetist
UCLA Medical Center
Los Angeles, California

John P. McDonough, EdD, CRNA
Professor and Director, Nurse Anesthetist Program
School of Nursing
University of North Florida
Jacksonville, Florida

John McFadden, PhD, CRNA
Associate Dean, College of Health Sciences
Barry University
Miami Shores, Florida

Debra R. Merritt, MSN, CRNA
Women's Hospital
Greensboro, North Carolina

John M. O'Donnell, DrPH, MSN, RN, CRNA
Director and Instructor, Nurse Anesthesia Program
University of Pittsburgh
School of Nursing
Pittsburgh, Pennsylvania

Richard G. Ouellette, MEd, CRNA
Staff Anesthetist
Wesley Long Community Hospital
Moses Cone Health System
Greensboro, North Carolina

Sandra M. Ouellette, MEd, CRNA, FAAN
President, R&S Ouellette, Inc.
Winston-Salem, North Carolina

Michael Rieker, DNP, CRNA
Director, Nurse Anesthesia Program
Wake Forest University Baptist Medical Center
Winston-Salem, North Carolina

Allan Schwartz, DDS, CRNA
Dentist-Certified Registered Nurse Anesthetist
ProDental, affiliate of Heartland Dental Care
Columbia, Missouri

Henry C. Talley, PhD, CRNA, APRN
Director, CRNA Program
College of Nursing
Michigan State University
East Lansing, Michigan

Nancy L. Tierney, DMP, CRNA
Program Director
Charleston Area Medical Center School of
    Nurse Anesthesia
Charleston, West Virginia

Priscilla P. Walkup, DMP, CRNA
Senior Instructor
Charleston Area Medical Center School of
    Nurse Anesthesia
Charleston, West Virginia

William A. White, Jr., DMP, CRNA
Instructor
Charleston Area Medical Center School of
    Nurse Anesthesia
Charleston, West Virginia

Terry C. Wicks, MHS, BSN, CRNA
Catawba Valley Medical Center
Hickory, North Carolina

General
Pharmacologic
Concepts

Pharmacokinetics: The Study of Drug Disposition

Ronald M. Dick, PhD, RPh

Objectives

After completing this chapter, the reader should be able to

- Describe the role pharmacokinetics plays in determining drug movement between body tissues.
- Determine how various disease states affect the pharmacokinetic parameters of a drug.
- Calculate specific pharmacokinetic parameters such as volume of distribution, clearance, and half-life.
- Explain the differences between phase I and phase II metabolism.
- Describe how drug dosing regimens can be altered to maintain safe therapeutic drug levels.

Introduction

The word "pharmacology" is derived from the Greek word *Pharmakon* and the suffix *-logia* and is defined as the science or study of drugs.[1] As far back as recorded history, and undoubtedly before that, humans have used plant and animal materials to treat various ailments and disorders.[2] Studies have shown that humans are not alone in the use of natural substances to treat various disorders. Other primates, specifically gorillas and chimpanzees, have been observed ingesting certain plants in what is thought to be a self-treatment for intestinal parasites.[3,4] Indeed, even less-advanced animal species such as some arthropods and fish have been shown to collect materials from plants or other animals to use in their own chemical defense against predators.[4] Considering these findings, pharmacology may well be one of the oldest applied sciences known.

Pharmacology, like all other areas of science, comprises a series of basic principles and concepts that form the foundation of the science. The most basic of these principles arises from the chemical sciences. One could even argue that pharmacology is really just an applied chemical science because all drugs are chemical substances and the biologic systems on which they interact are nothing but a series of chemical molecules and reactions. These chemical principles are useful for describing how a drug interacts at the molecular level with various enzymes, receptors, and tissues throughout the body. These interactions form the basis for two important areas of study in pharmacology: pharmacokinetics and pharmacodynamics. In very simplistic terms, pharmacokinetics explains the effect of the body on a drug, whereas pharmacodynamics explains the effect of a drug on the body.[5] Combined, these areas help explain how a drug molecule moves through the body, elicits its effect at a specific site, and is subsequently inactivated and removed from the body. Understanding these key concepts is critical to the modern delivery of anesthesia. In a sense, today's anesthesia provider is a practicing clinical pharmacologist[6] whose daily practice involves the administration of drugs and the monitoring of his or her patient for effects.

Pharmacokinetics

One of the more important aspects of pharmacology deals with how drug molecules are handled by the body from the initial administration to the final elimination of the agent. It is the understanding of these principles and their mechanisms that allow the determination of various properties of specific drug molecules such as half-life, onset and duration of effects, and drug dosing, among many others. Together these concepts and principles form the basis of pharmacokinetics, which incorporates mathematical models to help explain and predict how a drug is handled by the body.

Routes of Administration

Drugs are administered to patients in several different ways depending on many different factors, such as available formulations, need for immediate action, patient compliance and convenience, and the ability to get the drug to the site of action. In an outpatient environment, noninvasive routes (oral, topical) are usually preferred if possible, whereas in an inpatient setting, all routes of drug administration are common. In an operating room environment, administration of drugs by various parenteral and inhalational routes is more common. All routes of administration have specific advantages and disadvantages and must be considered based on patient needs and availability of dose forms.

Oral

Of all drug doses administered, drugs given by the oral route far outnumber any other route. This is mainly due to the noninvasive nature of the oral route and relatively good patient compliance. This is the route of choice for any drug that needs to be administered frequently or over an extended period of time. However, not all drugs can be given orally. Some drugs are not absorbed well after oral administration or are destroyed by stomach acid or enzymatic activity in the gastrointestinal (GI) tract. Other drugs are very irritating to the GI tract or may cause localized reactions that preclude their oral use. In addition, some drugs may need to be administered so frequently because of rapid elimination that oral dosing is just not practical. Compounds to be administered orally are usually produced in a tablet or capsule dose form that dissolves in the stomach or small intestine and is absorbed across GI membranes.

Topical

Many drugs are administered to the outer layers of the skin in dose forms that include creams, ointments, drops, powders, sprays, and transdermal patches. The topical route is most often used to treat a local disorder of the skin, eyes, and ears. However, drugs can also be applied to mucosal membranes such as the throat and vagina to treat localized disorders. Absorption of drug molecules across the skin is limited with most drugs; however, some drugs are absorbed into the general systemic circulation, allowing the use of the topical route to treat various systemic disorders. Transdermal patches and some creams/ointments are the most common means of supplying systemic therapy by the topical route.

Inhalational

Gaseous, volatile, and aerosolized compounds can be administered by inhalation. Although gaseous and volatile agents penetrate completely to the alveoli for absorption into the body, most aerosols are composed of particles that are too large to penetrate all the way to the alveoli. These drugs are therefore primarily used for localized therapy of airway and bronchial tissue.

Rectal

Rectal administration is particularly useful for patients that are unconscious or experiencing severe nausea and vomiting. The rectum comprises the last 6 inches of the large intestine and is usually devoid of stool. Solid dosage forms inserted into the rectum tend to be pulled back up into the lower regions of the large intestine. One of the primary functions of the large intestine is to remove excess water from the stool, and therefore the region contains an unpredictable volume of water in which to solubilize a drug for absorption. This makes rectal administration for systemic absorption unpredictable. However, because of the local blood flow, drugs absorbed rectally and through the lower portion of the large intestines do not travel to the liver before traveling back to the heart and thus avoid problems associated with first-pass metabolism.

Parenteral

Intravenous

This is the most common means of supplying a drug directly into the general systemic circulation. There is no absorptive phase with this route because the drug is supplied directly into the systemic circulation through an accessible vein. Drugs can be given rapidly (intravenous [IV] push) or more slowly (infusion). Local irritation of the vein in the region of administration is possible with some drugs. This can usually be mitigated by slower administration, thus allowing the drug to mix and dilute in the local venous blood as it is being injected.

Intra-arterial

This route is typically used to provide a drug to a specific target tissue in high concentration before it has a chance to dilute in the general circulation. Common uses are in chemotherapy and diagnostics. The arterial walls are not usually as sensitive as the veins, and so fewer local irritations are reported.

Epidural

This route is most commonly used to supply local anesthetic agents for pain relief during childbirth. The injection is made in a localized region inside the bony spine but external to the dura mater that surrounds the spinal cord.

Subcutaneous

Administration by this route is useful to provide a constant and relatively slow absorption of a drug. However, only nonirritating agents can be given by this route because localized irritation can lead to localized tissue necrosis. In addition, only relatively small volumes can be administered subcutaneously without excessive localized pain on injection. Some compounds and solid dose forms can be given as a depot injection, thus prolonging the duration of action of the supplied agent.

Intramuscular

Like the subcutaneous route, only nonirritating substances should be administered by this route. Irritating substances cause increased injection site pain and can cause localized necrosis. Although larger volumes can be injected intramuscularly than subcutaneously, the total volume at any one site is limited to approximately 5 mL to avoid excessive injection pain. Absorption into the general circulation is faster following intramuscular injection than after subcutaneous administration for most compounds. Depot injections, where the drug is usually prepared in oil, can be administered via this route to provide a slow absorption of the agent over a prolonged period, thus providing long-term therapy with fewer doses.

Solubility

To understand how a drug molecule can enter the body and move into different tissues, knowledge of that drug's physical properties is necessary. Drug molecules are chemical compounds and as such may be charged, uncharged, acidic, basic, or neutral structures. They may be gases, liquids, or solids at room temperature and thus require different dosage forms and routes for administration to a patient. These characteristics are critical in drug development and how the drug enters and interacts in the body.

One of the most important physical characteristics of a drug molecule is its solubility in various materials. Solubility of a drug affects drug dosage form design decisions and how the drug moves through various body tissues once administered. Most drug molecules cross tissue membranes by simple lipid diffusion. To enter a tissue, the drug must be able to move across cellular membranes that are composed of a lipid bilayer. To enter this hydrophobic layer, a drug molecule must have at least some lipid solubility or it cannot enter the cellular membrane and thus

cannot cross biologic membranes by diffusion. However, if the drug is too lipid soluble it will not be able to move out of the membrane once it enters. The ratio of a drug's lipid solubility to water solubility at equilibrium is known as the oil-to-water partition coefficient, which is used as a predictor of how well a drug will cross biologic membranes to reach target tissues. Usually, the oil that is used for solubility determinations is octanol, an eight-carbon alcohol. Octanol is used because its oil solubility characteristics are very close to that of biologic membranes.[7,8] Although water is often used for the aqueous solubility measurement, an aqueous buffer solution similar in makeup to extracellular fluid may be used instead. Therefore the standard oil-to-water partition coefficient may also be seen as an octanol-to-water or octanol-to-buffer partition coefficient. The larger the value of this partition coefficient, the greater the lipid solubility of the drug.

Although the oil-to-water partition coefficient helps determine how well a drug molecule can cross biologic membranes, some drugs cross membranes by specialized transport molecules in the membrane. An example of this is the transport of the amino acids, which are charged molecules at physiologic pH. Because they are charged, they are not very lipid soluble and will not cross membranes by simple lipid diffusion. These transport molecules are proteins and are present in membranes to allow the movement of some compounds into or out of cells that do not cross easily by simple diffusion. Some drug molecules can use these specialized carriers to cross membranes and enter tissues even if the drug molecules cannot cross the membranes by lipid diffusion.

A different form of partition coefficient is used to describe the solubility of gases and volatile agents that are administered in gaseous mixtures. This is referred to as the blood-to-gas partition coefficient. Gases and volatile agents administered in air are administered to a patient via the inhalational route. For these compounds to cross the alveolar membranes and into the blood, they must possess some lipid solubility characteristics and some degree of blood solubility. However, unlike an oil-to-water partition coefficient, which is based on the concentration of the agent in each component, when discussing the partitioning of a gaseous or volatile molecule the partial pressure of the agent in each component is used. Therefore the blood-to-gas partition coefficient is the partial pressure of the gas or volatile agent in the blood divided by the partial pressure of the gas or volatile agent in the gas at the alveoli (P_A) once equilibrium has been reached. Partial pressures of the gases and volatile agents is similar (although not exactly the same) to concentrations of nongaseous molecules. Gases or volatile agents move from a region of higher partial pressure to a region of lower partial pressure. Therefore the higher initial partial pressure of a gas or volatile agent being inhalationally administered at the alveoli is the driving force for movement of the molecules into the blood until equilibrium is reached.

Another form of partition coefficient is occasionally used to discuss the relative solubility of a drug in a tissue compared with the blood. This is known as the tissue-to-blood partition coefficient and is specific for the tissue being examined. These values are useful in determining what specific tissues a drug enters and to what extent. However, these values cannot be used to determine effect. Some drugs may only enter a tissue to a small extent compared with other agents but may still produce greater effects.

Many drug molecules are either weak acids or weak bases and as such may be charged at physiologic pH. These molecules will not cross biologic membranes by diffusion when they are in their charged form. However, as weak acids or bases they exist in a ratio of charged to uncharged molecules that is dependent on the pH of their environment and their specific acid or base character. An acidic group on a molecule is one that can give up a proton (H^+) and becomes charged once the proton has been removed from the molecule. A basic group on a molecule is one that can accept a proton and becomes charged once that proton binds to the molecule. Every acidic or basic group on a molecule has a particular propensity to gain or lose these protons determined by the relative hydrogen ion concentration in their environment. The pH where an acid or base exists 50% in the ionized form and 50% in the un-ionized form is known as the pK_a, or $-\log(K_a)$, where K_a is the acid dissociation constant. Every acidic or basic molecule has a specific pK_a value that is experimentally determined. From this pK_a it is possible to determine the relative ratio of charged to uncharged molecules that exists at a specific pH. The equation used to determine this is known as the Henderson-Hasselbalch equation,[9]

$$pH = pK_a + \log \frac{[UP]}{[P]} \; ,$$

where pH is the pH of the solution containing the drug (usually a physiologic pH if the drug is in the body), pK_a is the specific pK_a of the acidic or basic drug, [UP] is the concentration of the unprotonated form of the acid or base, and [P] is the concentration of the protonated form. It is important to remember that an acidic compound is charged when it is unprotonated and uncharged in the protonated form. A basic compound is uncharged in the unprotonated

form and charged when protonated. By using this equation for a known acidic or basic compound, it is possible to determine the relative ratio of charged to uncharged molecules at a specific pH. Knowing this ratio provides information concerning how highly ionized (charged) the compound may be in the body. This is important because the ionized form does not normally cross membranes, and the higher the ratio of ionized to un-ionized, the slower the compound is to cross into tissues to exert its effect. An example of this is the local anesthetic lidocaine, which is a weak base with a $pK_a = 7.9$. At physiologic pH (7.4), the un-ionized-to-ionized ratio can be calculated as follows:

$$pH = pK_a + \log \frac{[UP]}{[P]}$$

$$7.4 = 7.9 + \log \frac{[UP]}{[P]}$$

$$-0.50 = \log \frac{[UP]}{[P]}$$

$$antilog(-0.50) = \frac{[UP]}{[P]}$$

$$0.32 = \frac{[UP]}{[P]}$$

Because the unprotonated (UP) form of a base is the un-ionized form and the protonated form (P) is the ionized form, this example demonstrates that at equilibrium there are approximately 32 un-ionized molecules of lidocaine for every 100 ionized molecules at pH 7.4. As the un-ionized molecules move across membranes in the body, a new equilibrium occurs among the remaining molecules to maintain the same ratio. Therefore even though there are ionized molecules present that cannot cross membranes initially, with time they will convert to un-ionized molecules and will be able to cross. Examination of another local anesthetic with a higher pK_a such as procaine, which has a pK_a of 8.9 at pH 7.4, the equilibrium ratio of approximately 32 un-ionized molecules is present for every 1000 ionized molecules. Because there are 10 times more ionized molecules in this case, it would be expected that procaine would exhibit a slower onset than lidocaine because it takes longer for the ionized molecules to be converted to the un-ionized form that can cross the cell membranes. These examples provide insight into how acidic or basic molecules can cross membranes by simple diffusion and how pK_a values of a molecule can influence the rate of onset of a drug's action.

Absorption, Distribution, Metabolism, and Elimination

Absorption

In biologic systems, drug absorption is considered to be the movement of drug molecules across membranes and into the bloodstream. Except for routes of administration that place the drug directly into the bloodstream (i.e., IV), all administered drugs have some absorptive phase if they need to enter the blood to reach a nonlocal site of action. Each route of administration or specific drug compound may have certain nuances associated with absorption, thereby requiring different dosage formulations to facilitate absorption.

The rate of absorption of drug molecules across membranes by passive diffusion is described by Fick's Law:

$$\text{Diffusion Rate} = \frac{(\Delta C)(\text{Membrane Area})(\text{Drug Solubility})}{\text{Membrane Thickness } \sqrt{\text{Drug Molecular Weight}}},$$

where the rate of diffusion across a specific membrane depends on the concentration (or partial pressure for a gaseous or volatile agent) differential or gradient across the membrane, the area of the membrane over which the drug may be absorbed, the solubility of the drug in the membrane, the thickness of the membrane, and the molecular weight of the drug, which is related to the size of the drug molecule. Therefore having a large difference in drug concentration from one side of the membrane to the other increases the diffusion rate, as does a large membrane area for absorption and a drug that is easily soluble into the membrane. However, thicker membranes or large molecules decrease the rate of diffusion.

Oral Drug Absorption

Most common oral dose forms are swallowed and rely on the stomach and/or small intestines for absorption. Solid dosage forms (i.e., tablets and capsules) must first undergo dissolution, which is the process by which the solid dosage form breaks down into individual molecules or very small absorbable particles. Liquid dose forms usually do not require this step unless they contain small suspended particles that need to dissolve further. Most drugs dissolve into their absorbable particles in the stomach; however, the acidic environment of the stomach may destroy acid labile substances. These drugs require a different dose form, usually composed of an enteric coating, which protects the drug from the stomach acidity and allows transport to the small intestines where the dose form then dissolves.

Once a drug has dissolved into individual molecules or very small particles, it may be absorbed across membranes and into the bloodstream. This process is driven by passive diffusion through the cellular membranes unless a specific carrier exists to carry the drug molecules across the membranes. Because passive diffusion requires the drug molecule to be in a lipid-soluble form, the ionization state of a weakly acidic or basic drug becomes important. Although most drugs are best absorbed in the small intestines, some drugs, especially weakly acidic drugs, are absorbed in the stomach. This again can be explained by the Henderson-Hasselbalch equation because in the acidic environment of the stomach, acidic drugs tend to exist more in their un-ionized form and are therefore better absorbed. Weakly basic drugs exist mainly in their ionized form in the acidic stomach contents and are therefore not well absorbed. In the small intestines, bicarbonate secreted with bile raises the pH of the GI contents and causes weakly basic drugs to convert more to their un-ionized, more lipid-soluble form, thereby facilitating their absorption from the small intestine. In addition, the small intestine wall is composed of small protrusions called microvilli that greatly increase the surface area for absorption of most compounds.

Although lipid solubility plays an important role in the rate of drug absorption across the small intestine, large octanol-to-buffer partition coefficients actually impede absorption. This is because the small intestine wall is covered with a more water-soluble polysaccharide layer known as the glycocalyx layer. This layer coats the epithelial cells of the small intestine and keeps very lipid-soluble compounds from crossing to the epithelial cells, thus limiting absorption. However, a certain degree of lipid solubility is required to cross the epithelial membranes by diffusion once the drug penetrates the glycocalyx layer. Highly lipid-soluble drugs may also bind to fats in the GI tract and can then be absorbed by epithelial endocytosis rather than passive diffusion.

Distribution

Once a drug is absorbed into the bloodstream it is transported throughout the body and may cross into tissues, where it may act. This is known as drug distribution. In the plasma some drugs bind to varying degrees to proteins located in the bloodstream. The two most common proteins to which drug molecules bind are plasma albumin and α_1-acid glycoproteins. These protein molecules are very large and have many sites on their structure to which drug molecules may attach. The binding to these sites is usually fairly weak, and the drug molecules attach and detach readily. Although some drug molecules do not bind to plasma proteins to any appreciable extent, others are highly protein bound. An example of this is the anticoagulant drug warfarin, which is approximately 99% bound to plasma proteins.[10] Because only the free, unbound drug is available to cross membranes into tissues, a large amount of drug in the plasma that is bound to plasma proteins is unavailable to act. However, this protein binding is an equilibrium type of interaction, and as free drug leaves the plasma and moves into tissues, a new equilibrium maintains the relative bound-to-unbound ratio. Therefore the plasma protein binding can act as a depot or reservoir of drug, which can slowly supply additional free drug into the plasma as the free drug concentration decreases due to distribution into tissues or elimination.

Distribution of drug molecules into tissues from the bloodstream again depends on mechanisms of absorption. To enter a tissue there needs to be a specific transport protein capable of moving the drug into the tissue, or the drug may enter the tissue by endocytotic mechanisms or passive diffusion. Because the bloodstream is primarily an aqueous medium, lipophilic molecules are not very soluble and tend to cross lipid-soluble membranes into tissues readily by passive diffusion. The driving forces for diffusional distribution into a tissue are the relative solubility of the compound in a particular tissue, the concentration gradient, and the rate of blood flow to the particular tissue. A tissue that receives a high blood flow can absorb a drug faster because more drug molecules are being presented to this tissue per unit time than a tissue that receives a slower blood flow. This explains why the highly lipophilic anesthetic agents have short onset times. The brain has a high proportion of lipid, and thus lipophilic molecules readily cross from the bloodstream into the brain. In addition, the brain receives approximately 15% of cardiac output, which allows a large percentage of the anesthetic molecules in the plasma to be presented to the brain for absorption.

Like other processes, drug distribution into a tissue eventually reaches an equilibrium between the tissue concentration and plasma concentration. As the plasma concentration of the drug decreases due to elimination or distribution into other tissues, the equilibrium reached in some tissue shifts and the drug now begins to move back into the plasma to reestablish the equilibrium relationship. The movement of a drug from one tissue to another as equilibrium shifts in the body is known as redistribution and is the reason some of the highly lipophilic anesthetics exit the brain quickly and redistribute to body fat where they are more soluble, leading to a short duration of action.

Metabolism

Many drug molecules are converted in the body into other chemical compounds by a process known as metabolism or biotransformation. These processes normally produce more polar, water-soluble compounds, which are easier for the body to eliminate. Occasionally, however, a metabolic process may convert a drug molecule into a less polar compound that is more difficult to eliminate from the body. Unless this metabolite is further metabolized into a polar metabolite, it can build up and lead to potential toxicities. Drugs metabolized to less polar forms thus rarely make it to market. Although all tissues have the capability of metabolizing some drug molecules, the liver is the primary organ of metabolism in the body. Other important metabolizing tissues include the lung, kidney, skin, and epithelial cells of the GI tract. In addition, some metabolic reactions occur in the plasma. Drug metabolism is broken down into two types or phases of reactions based on how the compound is metabolized.

Phase I Metabolism

This type of metabolism involves primarily oxidation-reduction reactions and occurs mainly in hepatocytes by mixed function oxidase enzyme systems located on the smooth endoplasmic reticulum. These enzyme systems are linked to heme proteins and are referred to as the cytochrome P-450 system (CYPs). This is actually a family of enzymes, each of which may be responsible for the metabolism of different drug molecules. Although there are more than 50 known CYP enzymes, six are responsible for more than 90% of drug metabolism: CYP1A2, CYP2C9, CYP2C19, CYP2D6, CYP3A4, and CYP3A5.[11] The most common types of chemical reactions that occur by phase I metabolism are hydroxylation, oxidation, reduction, and hydrolysis. Some drug molecules undergo multiple phase I metabolic conversions. More polar metabolites may now enter the bloodstream and be removed from the body by the kidneys, or they may enter the biliary fluid and be excreted in bile. Some compounds may also be further metabolized by other enzyme systems. Because phase I metabolism is enzymatic, it is possible to saturate the ability of the enzymes to metabolize a particular compound. This can occur when too much of a single compound is administered or when multiple agents are administered that use the same enzymes for metabolism. This results in a buildup of the drug molecule and an increased half-life of the compound, potentially leading to toxicity. Some drugs or environmental exposures such as smoking may increase the number of active enzymes, a process known as induction. In this case, because there are more enzymes present to metabolize a particular compound, any compound that depends on the induced system for biotransformation is converted more rapidly, resulting in a shorter half-life. Other drugs can inhibit these enzymes, leading to an increased half-life of any compound that is normally metabolized by the inhibited enzyme system.

Phase II Metabolism

These reactions are often referred to as synthetic reactions because large polar compounds are attached to the molecule being metabolized. Although some drug molecules may undergo phase II metabolism as the primary method of biotransformation, often a drug molecule that has already been biotransformed by a phase I metabolic reaction may be further metabolized by a phase II reaction (Figure 1-1). The attachment of large polar groups to the molecule greatly increases the compound's water solubility, making elimination by renal or biliary routes easy. In hepatocytes the enzymes responsible for phase II metabolism are located in the cytoplasm and on the smooth endoplasmic reticulum. The most common type of reaction is glucuronic acid conjugation, where a sugar group known as uridine diphosphoglucuronic acid (UDPGA) is attached to the drug molecule. Sugar groups are very water soluble, and the attachment of UDPGA greatly increases the water solubility of the molecule. Another common phase II metabolic process is the attachment of the tripeptide glutathione, which through several steps finally produces a mercapturic acid derivative of the drug molecule that can then be excreted. Other synthetic reactions include sulfate, glycine and glutamine conjugations, and acylation reactions. For many drug molecules phase II reactions are the most important means of inactivating a drug molecule and allowing it to be removed from the body.

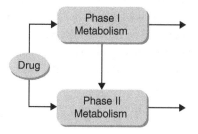

Figure 1-1 Metabolism of a drug molecule by either phase I or phase II metabolism. Many drugs that undergo phase I metabolism may be further metabolized by additional phase I or phase II reactions before being excreted.

First-Pass Metabolism

Drugs administered orally for absorption from the GI tract into the body are subject to a particular metabolic effect known as the first-pass effect. When a drug is absorbed across the GI membranes, it enters the hepatic portal system, which carries the drug molecules directly to the liver. If the drug is highly metabolized by the liver and exhibits a high extraction ratio, then a large percentage of the drug molecules may be destroyed (metabolized) before entering the general systemic circulation. Some drugs (e.g., lidocaine) are so highly metabolized that only a small portion of the absorbed drug reaches the general systemic circulation. The term "bioavailability" is used to help quantify the amounts of a drug that reach the general systemic circulation after absorption and is most commonly used to express the percentage of an oral drug that reaches the general systemic circulation. Bioavailability (F) is determined by dividing the amount of drug reaching the general systemic circulation (Amt_{oral}) by the amount entering the circulation after an IV dose of the same amount (Amt_{IV}) as was given orally:

$$F = \frac{Amt_{oral}}{Amt_{IV}}.$$

When the drug is given intravenously, there is no first-pass effect because the drug does not go directly to the liver before mixing throughout the circulation. Therefore the amount reaching the general systemic circulation is the most that a given dose can achieve. If the same dose given orally demonstrates the same amount entering the general systemic circulation as the IV dose, then the calculated bioavailability value would be 1.0, which means that no first-pass metabolism occurred. In reality, however, this is rarely the case because some of the oral drug is usually lost either due to some first-pass metabolism or failure of the dose to be completely absorbed. Lidocaine, if given orally, has a bioavailability of only 30%.[12]

Esterases

The body possesses many different enzymes that can split ester molecules. In the plasma an enzyme known as plasma esterase or pseudocholinesterase is responsible for metabolizing and inactivating many ester drug molecules, such as succinylcholine, etomidate, and procaine, among others. Other locations of esterases in the body are in cholinergic neuron synapses (acetylcholinesterase), on red blood cells, and in many other cells, including hepatocytes.

Metabolism in Other Tissues

As previously discussed, most tissues possess the ability to metabolize some drug molecules. The importance of a specific tissue on the overall metabolism of a particular compound varies with the compound, the tissue blood flow, and its penetration into the metabolizing tissue. The lung receives a high blood flow and is therefore good at metabolizing some drug molecules. One of the important lung metabolic reactions involves the conversion of angiotensin I to angiotensin II by angiotensin-converting enzyme. This enzyme is the target of the angiotensin-converting enzyme inhibitors such as captopril. Other tissues are also capable of some drug metabolic reactions, which are usually secondary to liver metabolism.

Elimination

Drug elimination encompasses all processes by which a specific drug molecule is removed from the body. Metabolizing a drug molecule into a different form, whether the new form is active or not, is one type of drug elimination. Although the metabolite molecule may still be present, it is not the same chemical, and therefore the original drug molecule is no longer present in the body. In addition to drug metabolism, drug excretion comprises the remainder of normal drug elimination mechanisms. The primary excretory organ in the body is the kidney, and kidney blood flow and drug protein binding are important in determining the rate of drug elimination by renal mechanisms. Drug molecules of molecular weights up to approximately 5000 amu are freely filtered at the glomerulus of the renal nephron. Protein molecules, such as albumin, are normally excluded from the filtrate by their large size. However, because only free drug can be filtered at the glomerulus, plasma proteins play an important role in the filtration mechanism. Drugs that are highly protein bound are not as readily filtered. The structure of the filtration pores also plays a role in filtration selectivity. Because of negatively charged groups located inside the filtration pores, positively charged molecules are attracted to the pores and are more easily filtered, whereas negatively charged molecules, especially large molecules, are repulsed and are not filtered as readily. In addition to glomerular filtration, another mechanism by which drug molecules may enter the renal tubule is known as secretion and occurs primarily in the proximal tubule. Transport carrier molecules in this region move drug molecules by active transport from the blood into the proximal tubule. Examples of molecules secreted at the proximal tubule by specific carriers include organic acids, organic bases, and conjugated metabolites.

Another important process that plays a role in drug excretion in the kidney is the reabsorption process. This occurs primarily in the proximal and distal regions of the nephron and occurs mainly by the movement of lipid-soluble drugs as they cross out of the renal tubular fluid back into the bloodstream by simple diffusion. Total renal excretion of a specific compound therefore is the amount filtered plus the amount secreted minus the amount reabsorbed. Because renal tubular fluid is an aqueous medium, polar water-soluble molecules will be retained in the fluid best. Also, because the pH of urinary fluid is usually in the range of 5–8, most weak acids and weak bases are somewhat ionized and thus easily excreted. Urinary acidifiers can be used to more fully ionize weakly basic drugs and enhance their excretion rate. Conversely, urinary alkalinizers enhance the elimination rate of weak acidic drugs.

Biliary excretion is another important mechanism of drug elimination. Active transport carriers in liver cells can secrete drug molecules and metabolites directly into bile. These molecules are then excreted into the GI tract where the molecules usually are eliminated in the fecal material. However, some glucuronide conjugates of drug molecules can undergo cleavage by enzymes produced by intestinal microorganisms. The attached glucuronide group is removed, thus releasing the original drug molecule. If this molecule is reabsorbed into the body, the duration of effect of the drug may be increased. This process is known as enterohepatic recycling and can greatly increase the effective half-life of the drug.

Lung excretion is mainly limited to the gaseous and volatile anesthetics. Most of these agents are almost entirely eliminated by lung excretion, with some being metabolized to a small extent.

Other excretion routes, including breast milk and sweat, are not significant means of drug excretion. Many different drugs may enter breast milk, but it is a small amount compared with other excretion mechanisms. Where it is important, however, is in the exposure of the infant to these molecules via the breast milk. Mothers must be aware that almost all drugs they take will be present to some degree in breast milk, and their child may be affected by exposure to those compounds.

Mathematical Modeling

Many of the pharmacokinetic concepts just discussed can be quantitatively approximated by using mathematical models. These models are designed based on specific characteristics of individual drug molecules and the rates at which the various absorption, distribution, metabolism, and elimination processes in the body occur. Fortunately, most drugs can be adequately described through two basic models, known as the one-compartment and the two-compartment models.

In a one-compartment model (Figure 1-2) the entire body is viewed as a single compartment where the drug freely and evenly distributes to all tissues. Therefore the central compartment (also known as the plasma compartment) has a drug concentration equal to the drug concentration at the tissue site where the drug elicits its effects. The initial entry of the drug into the central compartment depends on the method of drug administration. Except for administrative techniques by which the drug is directly injected into the bloodstream (e.g., IV or intra-arterial), all other means of drug administration require drug molecules to cross cellular membranes to gain access to the central compartment and then be transported throughout the body. This initial movement from the site of administration into the central compartment is known as the absorptive phase, and the rate (k_a) of this movement can be quantitated. Drug molecules are then transported throughout the body and cross into other tissues where they may elicit their effects. The key to the one-compartment model is that once equilibrium is reached, the drug concentration at the site of action is approximately the same as in the plasma. Therefore if a plasma sample is taken and the drug concentration determined, that concentration would be the same as at the site of action of the drug. All drug molecules, no matter how they are administered, must be eliminated. This elimination can again be characterized by a rate (k_e) that takes into account the summation of rates for all routes of elimination for the particular drug (e.g., metabolism and excretion). Drugs well characterized by the one-compartment model are often small molecules and/or highly water-soluble molecules that tend to distribute through the body following total body water.

The two-compartment model (Figure 1-3) is similar in concept to a one-compartment model with the addition of a second compartment. Drugs that follow a

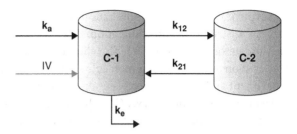

Figure 1-3 Two-compartment model illustrating entry of drug by absorption (k_a) or direct injection (i.e., IV) into the central compartment (C-1), distribution (k_{12}) into the tissue compartment (C-2), redistribution (k_{21}) from the tissue compartment back into the central compartment, and elimination from the central compartment (k_e).

two-compartment model do not demonstrate similar concentrations between the central compartment and the site of drug action at steady state. To adjust for these differences, consideration must be given to the rate of the drug moving into the tissue compartment from the central compartment (k_{12}) where the drug acts and the rate of back movement from the tissue to the central compartment (k_{21}). Many drugs can be characterized by two-compartment modeling. Although some drugs seem to follow more complex models (e.g., three- or four-compartment models), their behavior can often be adequately approximated by the two-compartment model.

The rates of drug movement for compartment models are determined experimentally from serial plasma samples (Figure 1-4). When administered by IV injection, there is

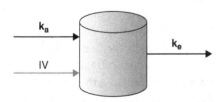

Figure 1-2 One-compartment model illustrating entry of drug by absorption (k_a) or direct injection (i.e., IV) and elimination from the body (k_e).

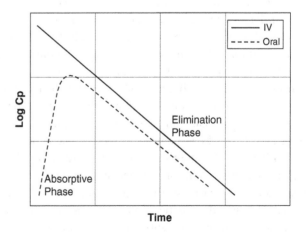

Figure 1-4 Comparison of oral and IV log (plasma concentration) versus time curves for the same drug. Elimination is via first-order kinetics. Note the lack of an absorptive phase with the IV dosing route and the same elimination rate by both routes.

no absorptive phase, and the only rate processes demonstrated are distribution and elimination. Of greatest interest is the rate of elimination (k_e). The elimination process begins as soon as the first drug molecule enters the central compartment and therefore is present during all phases of the plasma concentration curve. Once absorption (if any) is complete and the drug has reached steady-state distribution between tissue compartments and the central compartment, the steady decrease in the plasma concentration (Cp) seen with time is entirely due to elimination. Mathematically,

$$k_e = \frac{-d\mathrm{Cp}}{dt} \text{, and}$$

$$k_e = \frac{-\Delta \mathrm{Cp}}{\Delta t} \; .$$

From this, the elimination rate constant for a drug can be determined.

In the human body, the elimination of drugs, whether by metabolism or excretion of unchanged drug molecules, is normally a first-order rate process. First-order rate kinetics is best understood as being dependent on the concentration of the agent being eliminated. As the concentration of the drug in the plasma decreases, less drug is available at the site of metabolism or excretion, and thus as the concentration decreases, the amount being eliminated is also decreasing. This change in the amount of drug being eliminated per unit time follows a logarithmic decline, and therefore the elimination of a drug following first-order kinetics is a logarithmic rate. Occasionally, another type of rate process is seen during elimination. This is known as a zero-order rate process and is seen when the metabolism or excretion processes become saturated. In this case the concentration of the drug is unrelated to the amount of the agent being eliminated. This occurs when the drug concentration is so high that all available metabolic enzymes or transport mechanisms are eliminating as many drug molecules as they can and altering the drug concentration does not change how many molecules can be eliminated per unit time. Therefore in zero-order elimination kinetics, a constant amount or number of drug molecules are eliminated per unit time. This is not a logarithmic decline as seen in first-order kinetics but is instead a linear elimination. Luckily, most therapeutic drug concentrations never reach saturation (zero-order) kinetics and are instead eliminated by first-order rate processes. Even if a drug concentration did reach levels high enough to saturate the normal elimination processes, as the concentration decreases it would move back into normal first-order rate elimination.

The elimination rate for a specific drug is not always the same in all patients. Factors, such as age, disease state, and genetics, can alter a patient's elimination rate of a specific agent. Fortunately, however, most drugs whose elimination rate is fairly consistent among individuals can be used to determine average elimination rates. These rates can then be used in other calculations to obtain commonly disseminated pharmacokinetic parameters for a specific drug.

Elimination Half-life

One of the most common pharmacokinetic parameters is the elimination half-life ($t_{1/2}$). Assuming the elimination rate is a first-order process, the elimination half-life can be calculated by

$$t_{1/2} = \frac{\ln 2}{k_e} \; .$$

In this equation, ln is the natural log required due to the logarithmic nature of first-order elimination kinetics and the value "2" refers to the change in the concentration by a factor of two (one-half). This equation can be further simplified by substituting the value of the natural log of 2, which is 0.693

$$t_{1/2} = \frac{0.693}{k_e} \; .$$

The elimination half-life is widely available for every marketed drug; however, published values for some drugs have a wide range of half-lives due to patient variability. It is important to remember that if a drug is eliminated primarily through liver metabolism, any hepatic disorder that diminishes the metabolic capacity of the liver may cause an increased half-life for that agent in a patient. The same holds for a patient with decreased renal function taking a drug that is primarily eliminated by renal excretion. In addition, some drug interactions are known to alter the half-life of some drugs. This is most commonly seen with drugs that induce liver metabolic enzymes (e.g., phenobarbital, rifampin, carbamazepine) or inhibit the metabolic enzymes (e.g., cimetidine, ciprofloxacin, isoniazid).[13]

Another common term associated with half-life is the half-life of effect. Some drugs (e.g., diazepam) are converted into metabolites in the body, which have the same effect as the parent compound. Looking at the half-life of the original compound only can then give a false idea of the duration of effects. Therefore the half-life of effect is used to encompass all possible active metabolites of the parent compound that may prolong the duration of the parent drug and thus provide a more accurate handle of the half-life of the expected effects, not just of the parent drug.

Volume of Distribution

The volume of distribution (Vd) is often referred to as the apparent volume of distribution because it is not necessarily a true volume but is instead a theoretical (apparent) volume of plasma in which the drug is dissolved. The values for the volume of distribution of a drug do not necessarily relate to the plasma volume. If a drug stays in the plasma compartment (e.g., heparin), then the volume of distribution is directly related to the plasma volume. However, if the drug leaves the plasma compartment to concentrate to a large extent in tissues, then the volume of distribution can be very large. This is because the amount of drug remaining in the plasma is small and its concentration is low, causing the apparent volume of distribution to appear very large. Apparent volumes of distribution for some drugs (e.g., propranolol) can reach hundreds of liters in a 70-kg patient. Values are commonly presented in liters per kilogram to allow for different patients. Obviously, their body volume is not that large. The main advantage of volume of distribution values is that they are useful to determine quickly whether the drug stays in the plasma, follows total body water, or concentrates in body tissues. For a one-compartment model, the apparent volume of distribution can be calculated from the dose of the drug (D_0) and the plasma concentration of the drug at time 0 (Cp_0):

$$Vd = \frac{D_0}{Cp_0} .$$

Although the initial dose of the drug is easy to obtain, the plasma concentration at time 0 is more difficult. It is impossible to actually sample the plasma compartment at time 0 even if the drug was given intravenously because a certain period of time is required for the drug to evenly disperse throughout the plasma compartment. Starting a serial plasma sample curve of drug concentration versus time at approximately 5 minutes allows time for initial mixing and can be used to back-extrapolate to time 0 to obtain the value. The volume of distribution is even more difficult to calculate for multicompartment models.[14] The volume of distribution can also be obtained from the clearance of a drug (see below).

Clearance

In pharmacokinetics, clearance is used to quantitate the rate by which a drug is removed from the body. Plasma clearance (Cl) is the volume of plasma that is *entirely* cleared of the drug per unit time, thereby giving clearance units of volume/time. Based on the definition, if 50% of a drug is removed from a given quantity of plasma from a particular organ, then that organ has only cleared 100% of the drug from half the volume of plasma. Total body clearance values are easily calculated from the elimination rate constant and volume of distribution for a specific drug:

$$Cl = k_e Vd .$$

Because a drug may be metabolized or excreted by multiple tissues in the body, each tissue has its own clearance rate that is calculated from each tissue's elimination rate constant for the drug. Therefore the sum of all these individual drug clearance values equals total body clearance:

$$Cl_{total} = Cl_{hepatic} + Cl_{renal} + Cl_{lung} + Cl \cdots .$$

As with other related pharmacokinetic parameters, the clearance of a drug is altered in cases of various disease states that affect the elimination rate of the drug. So, for example, if a drug is cleared to a large extent by the liver and the patient experiences hepatic insufficiency, the total body clearance of the drug decreases and the drug would tend to accumulate in the body. To maintain the proper drug concentration for effect may then require a dosage adjustment to lower the drug plasma concentration.

Drug Dosing

Determining proper drug dosages is critical to proper patient care and is one of the major advantages of understanding concepts such as drug clearance. Nowhere are these concepts more important than in anesthesia, where the drugs used to induce an anesthetized state are very toxic with little room for dosage errors.

Therapeutic Window

All drugs exhibit some concentration at their site of action at which the desired therapeutic effect is initially produced. In addition, most if not all drugs also demonstrate the initiation of side effects or toxicities at some specific concentration in a particular tissue. The sites of the desired therapeutic effects may or may not be the same site that produces the undesirable effects. If the undesirable effects are relatively minor and can be tolerated, they are usually referred to as side effects of the drug. However, some effects are intolerable or potentially life threatening and are referred to as toxicities. These concepts are actually pharmacodynamic principles because they are related to the effect of the drug on the body. However, the concept is important to introduce at this point because the basis for proper patient dosing requires maintaining a therapeutic drug concentration while avoiding toxic concentrations. Because the plasma concentration is the only drug concentration readily accessible in the body, most therapeutic and toxic concentrations are based on the plasma concentration. Unfortunately, not all drugs elicit their tissue effects based directly on the tissue concentration. Other drugs (e.g., lithium carbonate) have well-defined therapeutic windows with strong relationships between the plasma concentration and the therapeutic and toxic concentrations. For drugs that exhibit a correlation between plasma concentration and effects, the goal of proper dosing is to keep the patient's plasma drug concentration above the minimum therapeutic concentration (Cp_{ther}) and below the plasma concentration associated with toxicity (Cp_{tox}) (Figure 1-5). Related to this idea is the therapeutic index or therapeutic ratio. The therapeutic index (TI) is the ratio of the toxic dose (D_{tox}) to the therapeutic dose (D_{ther})[15]:

$$TI = \frac{D_{tox}}{D_{ther}}.$$

Therefore drugs with large TI values are safer than drugs with smaller values. For example, diazepam, a fairly safe drug with a wide therapeutic window, has a TI greater than 100, whereas digoxin, which has a narrow therapeutic window, has a TI of approximately 2.[15] A new form of IV desflurane under study has a reported TI of approximately 3 in rats,[16] demonstrating the need for great care in its administration.

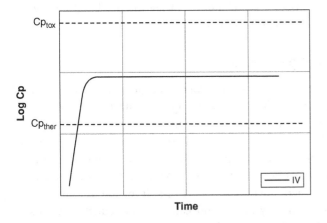

Figure 1-5 Graph illustrating the therapeutic window for a particular drug. Note the drug administered by IV infusion maintaining a safe plasma concentration above the minimum therapeutic concentration and below the toxic plasma concentration.

Dosing Calculations

To properly administer therapeutic drug doses requires that the purpose and method of drug administration are determined. It is a simple matter to determine the required dose of a drug that is to be administered in a single dose. It is more difficult and patient specific to determine dosing regimens for repeated IV dosing or IV infusions while trying to keep the patient's plasma concentration within the therapeutic window.

Intravenous Infusion Dosing

The goal when supplying a drug by IV infusion is to supply the exact amount of drug that is being eliminated by the patient to keep the patient's plasma concentration steady (steady state). The truth is that any dose supplied by IV infusion will meet this goal. Different infusion rates alter only the maintained plasma concentration as long as the drug concentration stays within first-order kinetics. This is because as the plasma concentration increases, first-order elimination states that a larger amount of the drug is removed per unit time. To calculate the infusion rate (k_{in}) (mg/min) required for IV infusion administration, only the steady-state plasma concentration (Cp_{ss}) (mg/mL) desired and the clearance of the drug (mL/min) are required:

$$K_{in} = CP_{ss}\, Cl.$$

However, using this approach requires approximately five drug half-lives to reach 95% of the eventual steady-state plasma concentration when administering a drug by continuous IV infusion. Therefore it may take a considerable period of time before steady state is achieved for drugs with long half-lives. A loading dose can be used to push the patient's plasma concentration to the eventual steady-state level more rapidly. The loading dose (D_{load}) (mg) is calculated from the volume of distribution of the drug in the patient (mL) and the steady-state plasma concentration desired to be reached (mg/mL):

$$D_{load} = Vd\, Cp_{ss}.$$

When the planned continuous IV infusion is preceded with a properly calculated loading dose, the desired steady-state plasma concentration will be reached immediately and then maintained for as long as the IV infusion is continued. However, if a new plasma steady state is desired in the patient, just changing the infusion rate will again take approximately five drug half-lives to reach the new steady state.

Intermittent Dosing

It is possible to maintain a patient's plasma drug concentration within the therapeutic window by supplying the drug in individual doses. This may even be preferred, especially for outpatient care. However, the drug being administered must have a reasonably long half-life to avoid requiring dosing intervals to be so short that they would require the patient to disrupt normal sleep periods if at all possible. Dosing should not be shorter than 6-hour intervals and should preferably be given every 12 or 24 hours to enhance patient compliance, especially if the drug is being self-administered. [17] Drugs to be dosed intermittently must have a therapeutic window wide enough to ensure that during the period between doses the plasma drug concentration does not fall below the minimum therapeutic concentration. Also, the plasma drug concentration cannot rise above the minimum toxic concentration when the dose is administered. Intermittent dosing can be accomplished by repeated IV dosing; however, the most common route is via oral administration. As in IV infusion dosing, without a loading dose it takes approximately five half-lives of the drug to reach 95% of the steady-state level in the plasma. The difference with repeated dosing is that no single steady-state concentration is reached. With each dose administered, the plasma level increases as the dose enters the plasma. The concentration then decreases at a rate based on the elimination rate of the drug until the next dose is administered. This creates a plasma concentration curve with peaks when the drug is given and troughs that bottom out just before the next dose is administered. Once steady state is reached, as long as neither the dose nor the dosing interval is changed, all peaks and troughs will occur at equal plasma concentrations. An average between the peak and trough concentrations is known as the average steady state. Although it is possible to calculate the required doses and dosing interval to reach a desired plasma concentration,[18] this information is usually supplied by the manufacturer and is rarely calculated today.

Key Points

- Routes of Drug Administration
- Drug Absorption, Distribution, Metabolism, and Elimination
- Pharmacokinetic Modeling
- Therapeutic Window
- Drug Half-life
- Volume of Distribution
- Clearance
- Drug Dosing

Chapter Questions

1. Explain what effect lowering the stomach pH would have on the ionized state of an acidic drug in the stomach.
2. What effect will increasing plasma protein binding of a drug have on the drug's ability to cross membranes into tissues?
3. Explain why doubling the dose of a constant IV infusion does not double the patient's plasma concentration of the drug.
4. What determines whether a drug can be modeled by a one-compartment model or a more complex multicompartment model?
5. What chemical characteristics increase and decrease the ability of a drug molecule to cross membranes?

References

1. *Mosby's Medical Dictionary*, 8th ed. St. Louis, MO: Mosby; 2008.
2. Vallance P, Smart TG. The future of pharmacology. *Br J Pharmacol*. 2006;147(Suppl 1):S304–S307.
3. Krief S, Hladik CM, Haxaire C. Ethnomedicinal and bioactive properties of plants ingested by wild chimpanzees in Uganda. *J Ethnopharmacol*. 2005;101:1–15.
4. Huffman MA. Animal self-medication and ethno-medicine: exploration and exploitation of the medicinal properties of plants. *Proc Nutr Soc*. 2003;62:371–381.
5. Stoelting RK, Hillier SC. Pharmacokinetics and pharmacodynamics of injected and inhaled drugs. In: Stoelting RK, Hillier SC, eds. *Pharmacology and Physiology in Anesthetic Practice*, 4th ed. Philadelphia: Lippincott Williams & Wilkins; 2006:3–41.
6. Fallacaro MD. Forward. In: Kier LB, Dowd CS, eds. *The Chemistry of Drugs for Nurse Anesthetists*. Park Ridge, IL: AANA Publishing; 2004.
7. Block JH. Physiochemical properties in relation to biological action. In: Block JH, Beale JM Jr, eds. *Wilson and Gisvold's Textbook of Organic Medicinal and Pharmaceutical Chemistry*, 11th ed. Philadelphia: Lippincott Williams & Wilkins; 2003:3–42.
8. Weindlmayr-Goettel M, Gilly H, Sipos E, Steinbereithner K. Lipid solubility of pancuronium and vecuronium

determined by n-octanol/water partitioning. *Br J Anaesth.* 1993;70:579–580.

9. Katzung BG. Introduction. In: Katzung BG, Masters SB, Trevor AJ, eds. *Basic and Clinical Pharmacology*, 11th ed. New York: McGraw-Hill; 2009:1–13.

10. Armstrong AW, Golan DE. Pharmacology of hemostasis and thrombosis. In: Golan DE, et al., eds. *Principles of Pharmacology: The Pathophysiologic Basis of Drug Therapy.* Philadelphia: Lippincott Williams & Wilkins; 2005: 335–356.

11. Lynch T, Price A. The effect of cytochrome P450 metabolism on drug response, interactions, and adverse effects. *Am Fam Physician.* 2007;76:391–396.

12. Ritschel WA, Elconin H, Alcorn GJ, Denson DD. First-pass elimination of lidocaine in the rabbit after peroral and rectal route of administration. *Biopharm Drug Dispos.* 1985;6:281–290.

13. Kharasch ED. Principles of drug biotransformation. In: Evers AS, Maze M, eds. *Anesthetic Pharmacology: Physiologic Principles and Clinical Practice.* Philadelphia: Churchill Livingstone; 2004:59–78.

14. Buxton IOL. Pharmacokinetics and pharmacodynamics: the dynamics of drug absorption, distribution, action, and elimination. In: Brunton LL, Lazo JS, Parker KL, eds. *Goodman & Gilman's The Pharmacological Basis of Therapeutics*, 11th ed. New York: McGraw-Hill; 2006:1–39.

15. Becker DE. Drug therapy in dental practice: general principles part 2—pharmacodynamic considerations. *Anesth Prog.* 2007;54:19–24.

16. Zapata-Sudo G, Abrao MA, Trachez MM, Sudo RT. Anesthetic and hemodynamic effects of desflurane lipid emulsion. *Anesthesiology.* 2005;103:A693.

17. Greenberg RN. Overview of patient compliance with medication dosing: a literature review. *Clin Ther.* 1984;6(5):592-599.

18. LaMattina JC, Golan DE. Pharmacokinetics. In: Golan DE, et al., eds. *Principles of Pharmacology: The Pathophysiologic Basis of Drug Therapy.* Philadelphia: Lippincott Williams & Wilkins; 2005:27–43.

2
Pharmacodynamics: The Study of Drug Action

Ronald M. Dick, PhD, RPh

Introduction

The branch of pharmacology that relates drug concentration to biologic effect is known as pharmacodynamics. Major goals of this area of study are determining the proper dose to administer to elicit the desired effect while avoiding toxicity. Although pharmacokinetics can be used to determine dosing requirements necessary to maintain a particular drug concentration, it is the relationship between drug concentration and effect that ultimately decides appropriate dosing. The ultimate goal is to maintain a drug concentration within the proper therapeutic window thereby avoiding toxicity while providing an adequate concentration of the drug to provide the desired effect.

Most drug effects are induced by the interaction of a drug molecule with specific molecular structures in the body known as receptors.[1] However, some drug effects are non–receptor mediated and are caused by the particular physical or chemical properties of the drug molecule. To firmly grasp the concepts of how effects, both desired and deleterious, are induced in the body by a drug molecule requires an understanding of where and how these molecules interact.

Receptor Theory

The idea that drug molecules interact at specific sites in the body is not new. The initial idea of materials within the body to which administered drugs interact has been attributed to the work of Langley and Ehrlich in the late 1800s and early 1900s.[2] Proof of the receptor concept lagged

behind theory, and it would take the introduction of the β-adrenergic antagonist, propranolol, in 1965 to provide the data necessary to completely convince the scientific community that receptors truly exist. Since then, specific molecular targets of action have been identified for nearly all drugs, and evidence for the receptor theory continues to grow. However, a few drugs, such as osmotic laxatives, do not appear to require receptor interactions to provide their effects. Another class of compounds of particular interest, the general anesthetics, apparently exhibit such a wide array of effects that some in the scientific community still do not subscribe to the idea that a receptor-mediated response is necessary for action, even though multiple receptor interactions have been identified.[3]

The basic concept of drug–receptor interactions can be described by the "lock and key" model in which a receptor structure (the lock) has a region with a particular shaped pocket at which an appropriately shaped molecule (the key) can interact (Figure 2-1). The substance that interacts at the receptor binding site is known as a ligand. It is important to remember that receptors evolved over the ages to provide particular functions within the body. Although a particular drug may be identified as interacting with a particular receptor, the reason that a receptor exists is to interact with some normal endogenous ligand or common environmental material. Therefore drug molecules that interact at receptors either mimic or inhibit normal body compounds. In addition, because both receptors and the compounds with which they interact are chemical entities, they behave according to chemical principles. Receptors themselves are normally characterized as protein structures, either a single protein or a complex comprised

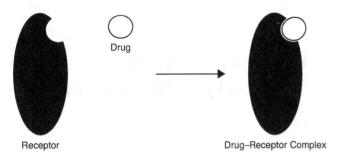

Figure 2-1 "Lock and key" representation of drug–receptor binding.

of multiple protein subunits. The binding site on the receptor complex where the ligand interacts may only be a small portion of the molecule. The interaction of a drug molecule with its receptor can be represented in the manner shown in Figure 2-2, where D is the drug concentration, R is the free receptor concentration, and DR is the concentration of receptor molecules occupied by drug molecules. The interaction of the ligand at its binding site on the receptor complex is governed by two important concepts: affinity and intrinsic activity.

Affinity is best described as how well a particular compound is drawn into and held at the binding site. A relative affinity constant can be determined from the relationship outlined in Figure 2-2. At equilibrium, the dissociation constant (K_D) of a drug–receptor complex is equal to k_{off}/k_{on}. The equilibrium affinity constant (K_A) is the reciprocal of the equilibrium dissociation constant ($1/K_D$). Therefore the smaller the equilibrium dissociation constant is, the greater the affinity of the drug for the receptor. This is useful when examining how well different drugs bind to a specific receptor complex. To understand how individual molecules, such as drug molecules, move around a receptor zone, it is important to remember that these molecules are present in a mix of other molecules and move in a random manner driven by Brownian motion. The interaction of a molecule, whether it is a drug molecule or the normal receptor ligand, with its receptor is primarily a matter of chance. The likelihood that a particular type of compound will interact at a given receptor is based on the number of molecules (concentration) located near the receptor site. The greater the concentration, the more likely it is that the

random motion of a particular molecule will bring it close enough to a receptor site to interact. If a molecule is able to interact with the receptor site, it is said to have affinity for that site. The stronger it interacts, the greater its affinity for that receptor site.

The concept of interaction at the receptor site is based mainly on the ligand's shape and chemical makeup. The receptor site may have particular chemical functional groups that interact at specific places. For example, a positively charged group at a specific location within the binding pocket may interact with a negatively charged region on a ligand, thus increasing the binding force between the two compounds and increasing the affinity. Most ligands bind very briefly with the receptor site and then are knocked out of the site by collisions with other molecules that are jostling around in the surrounding area. Therefore even a drug with high affinity may only interact with a receptor zone briefly. However, if the concentration of the ligand molecules in the surrounding area is high, the likelihood of continued receptor–ligand interaction increases. This idea is critical to understanding drug action. The greater the drug concentration at a receptor zone, the more likely it is that a drug molecule will be occupying the receptor site at any given time. As the drug concentration goes down, the percentage of time the receptor is occupied also decreases.

The other important factor governing how a ligand interacts at a receptor zone is known as intrinsic activity. Whereas affinity describes how well a particular compound interacts with the binding site of a receptor complex, intrinsic activity is used to describe the effect the ligand has when it interacts with a receptor site. A ligand may have good affinity, but if it has no intrinsic activity it will elicit no response when it binds to the receptor zone. On the other hand, a ligand that has good intrinsic activity will elicit a strong response at the receptor zone if it also has good affinity. But if the affinity of the compound for the receptor site is low, even a high level of intrinsic activity will not elicit much of a response.

The response generated from a receptor interaction can be plotted against the dose of a drug to produce the classic dose–response curve known so well in pharmacology (Figure 2-3). In a typical dose–response curve, the dose of the drug is assumed to be proportional to the concentration of the drug at the receptor zone. Data for dose–response curves depend on the effect of the drug being examined. An appropriate response to the drug is chosen, and different drug doses are plotted against the response generated. One example is changes in muscle strength when different doses of a particular muscle stimulant are administered. At low doses, little response is observed. However, at some

$$D + R \underset{k_{off}}{\overset{k_{on}}{\rightleftarrows}} DR$$

Figure 2-2 Drug–receptor formation showing the rate of drug binding and release from the receptor.

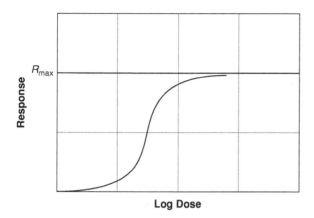

Figure 2-3 Log dose–response curve. R_{max} is the maximal response.

particular dose, the response begins to increase suddenly. This is because a certain number of receptors need to be occupied before a response is observed. Once a critical number of receptors are occupied, increasing the dose increases the response. However, this increase in response is not linear but is instead logarithmic.

Dose–response curves are normally plotted as the log of the dose on the x axis versus the linear response on the y axis. In this type of plot, the log of the dose is directly proportional to the response and is seen as a straight line through the middle range of the plot. This represents the most appropriate dose range to produce the observed effect. As the dose increases further, the curve again loses its logarithmic relationship between dose and response. Every response has a maximum, and as this maximal response is neared, increases in occupied receptors produce less and less of an increase in response. At some point the response reaches its maximum, and no further increases in drug dose produce a greater effect. This does not mean that all available receptors have been occupied, just that the tissue is unable to produce a greater response. In fact, the number of receptors that are occupied when the response becomes maximal may only be a small percentage of available receptors. This apparent excess of receptors seen at most receptor zones allows small concentrations of a ligand to elicit a graded response.

Receptor Interactions

The ways in which ligands interact with receptors vary greatly among different compounds and receptors. Most receptors are large, complex protein structures that are held in a particular shape or conformation based on their

specific environment. Proteins are made up of amino acids, and some amino acids are affected by the pH of the micro-environment surrounding the compound. If the local pH changes slightly, certain amino acids within the receptor protein may become charged (or uncharged). This change can cause the protein complex to alter its conformation and thereby alter the shape of a ligand binding zone on the protein. This could either enhance or diminish the ability of a specific ligand to bind to the zone. This concept illustrates the importance of the microenvironment surrounding the receptor protein. Just as pH changes may affect the shape of the receptor complex, other compounds that interact with the protein may also alter the receptor protein conformation. These changes in molecular shape may occur at various places within the receptor complex, not only at the receptor binding site. In fact, these conformational changes in the receptor complex explain how most drugs and endogenous ligands elicit their effects upon binding to a receptor site. The interaction of the ligand at the specific binding site causes some conformational change in the receptor complex, thereby altering the function of the protein complex.

Proteins have many functions within the body, including enzymes, channels, and transporters. If a particular receptor zone is located on one of these proteins, the normal effect of that specific protein may be altered by the induced conformational change. Therefore an enzyme whose normal conformation does not allow it to interact with its substrate may be activated when a specific ligand binds to a receptor site. Or, conversely, an enzyme that is normally active may be shut off when a specific ligand interacts at a receptor zone on the molecule. The same idea can be applied to other protein structures such as channel proteins or transport proteins. These may also be activated or inactivated by ligand interactions at specific receptor zones. In the body this provides a means of controlling normal function and allows the organism a means to fine tune its biologic processes based on specific needs. The discovery that exogenous compounds interact at specific receptor sites and can be used to alter biologic function has led to major changes in the ways that new drugs are designed. Determining the specific functions of a compound in the body, such as an enzyme, and then designing a chemical compound that can interact with the substance provides a means to alter various biologic processes.

There are several different ways in which drug molecules may interact with complex protein molecules in the body. It is through these different mechanisms that the ability to control various biologic processes has been developed.

Agonists and Antagonists

For every receptor in the body, there is an endogenous compound that is believed to be able to act. Sometimes, however, the receptor is identified by actions of an exogenous compound before the normal endogenous ligand is identified. Such has been the case in the discovery of the benzodiazepine receptor and the search for an endogenous ligand.[4,5] Many compounds have been identified in the body that appear to act on this receptor zone (the endozepines, for *endo*genous benzodia*zepines*), but none has been conclusively proven to be secreted specifically to interact at this receptor zone.[6,7] The interaction of compounds with the receptor zone has been based on the way in which they interact with the receptor complex and the results of their interactions. These interactions can be roughly classified as receptor agonists and receptor antagonists.

Receptor Agonists

The interaction of a ligand with a receptor zone that invokes some functional change in the receptor complex is an example of an agonist reaction. Most drug molecules that elicit an agonistic effect mimic the effects of an endogenous compound at the receptor. The strength of binding to the receptor and the overall effect elicited depend on the compound's affinity and intrinsic activity. To be a good agonist at a specific receptor site requires good affinity and good intrinsic activity. When an exogenous molecule interacts with a specific receptor, it blocks the body's endogenous ligand from interacting with the receptor for as long as the exogenous compound occupies the receptor. Usually, however, exogenous agonists are given to increase the normal agonistic stimulation of the receptor and blocking the endogenous agonist is of no consequence. Drugs with good receptor affinity but intrinsic activity that is less than the normal endogenous agonist are termed partial agonists because their response at the receptor is less than the endogenous agonist or less than a particular response from an exogenously administered standard agonist (Figure 2-4). An example of a partial agonist is the action of buprenorphine at the opioid μ-receptor where its agonist effect is less than morphine. Some drugs have been classified as superagonists, which are compounds that elicit greater effects at the specific receptor zone than the defining receptor agonist. Fentanyl is an example of a superagonist, being approximately 100 times more potent at opioid μ-receptors than morphine.

Other types of agonists are the physiologic agonists, which are compounds that produce the same bodily effects but through an entirely different receptor system and

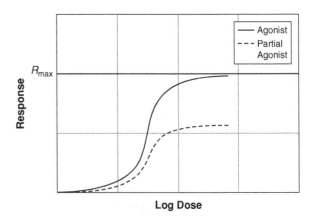

Figure 2-4 Comparison of full and partial agonists.

mechanism. An example of physiologic agonists is the anesthetic effect of ketamine, which acts at *N*-methyl-D-aspartate (NMDA) receptors, and the effect of propofol, which acts at the γ-aminobutyric acid (GABA)$_A$ receptor complex. Both agents produce a loss of consciousness but act at different receptor sites. Other agonistic drugs may not be able to elicit a specific response on their own but instead require the action of multiple compounds to produce an effect. These types of agonist drugs are often referred to as coagonists because more than one is required for effect. An example of coagonists is the stimulation of some NMDA receptors that require binding of both glycine and glutamate.

Agonist drugs are also characterized on their selectivity. Selective agonists act primarily at only one specific receptor zone, whereas nonselective agonists may act at many different receptor types. An example involves the β-adrenergic agonist isoproterenol, which stimulates both β$_1$ and β$_2$ receptors, and albuterol, which is considered a selective β$_2$ agonist.

Receptor Antagonists

Some drugs produce their effects by interaction at the receptor complex, but instead of stimulating the receptor or mimicking the normal endogenous ligand for that receptor, they block or decrease agonist interaction at the receptor zone. This causes a loss of the effect that is normally produced by the receptor agonist. Although many drug molecules have been designed with this type of function, there are only a few known instances of endogenous compounds capable of this form of receptor interaction. The most common type of antagonism produced by drug molecules is referred to as competitive antagonism (Figure 2-5), in which the antagonist interacts at the same receptor site as the normal agonist. The antagonist therefore must possess affinity to allow it to interact with the receptor site.

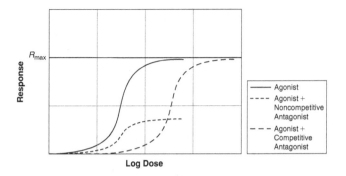

Figure 2-5 Comparison of responses generated following administration of a competitive antagonist or noncompetitive antagonist.

However, the antagonist does not appreciably stimulate the receptor and thus has little to no intrinsic activity. Interaction of compounds with the receptor site on molecules is based on the law of mass action, which in this case means that the more molecules in the area around the receptor that can bind to a receptor (greater concentration), the greater the likelihood that the receptor will be occupied by one of the molecules at any given time. If molecules of an antagonist are added to the area around the receptor where there are already agonist molecules, then the more molecules of antagonist present, the greater the likelihood that an antagonist molecule will be bound to the receptor at any given time. If the antagonist concentration is increased even further, it becomes even less likely that an agonist molecule can "compete" for receptor binding (Figure 2-6).

What makes competitive antagonism particularly interesting is that a competitive antagonist can be used to decrease the normal effects at a particular receptor zone and then an agonist that acts at that specific site can later be added to compete away the added competitive antagonist. This is the principle used often in anesthesia with neuromuscular

blocking drugs. A neuromuscular blocking drug, such as vecuronium, which is a competitive antagonist at the neuromuscular nicotinic receptor site, acts to block the normal endogenous agonist, acetylcholine, from binding to the receptor. The effect of the competitive antagonist can be decreased by increasing the agonist at the receptor, and drugs such as neostigmine are administered to decrease the metabolism of acetylcholine, allowing more of it to exist around the receptor zone and thus reversing the effect of the administered neuromuscular blocker.[8]

Another important type of receptor antagonism, referred to as noncompetitive antagonism (see Figure 2-5), can actually occur by two different mechanisms. The first mechanism is seen by compounds that bind irreversibly or for such a long time as to be effectively irreversible. Once a receptor site has been occupied by an irreversible agent, no concentration of agonist molecules around the site will allow the site to be reclaimed by an agonist. In effect, it appears as if the receptor has been removed from the system. If many receptors on a particular tissue are irreversibly inhibited, then the maximal response of the tissue to the agonist will be decreased because there are not enough noninhibited receptors remaining to elicit a maximal response, even if all were stimulated with an agonist. Once the receptors have become inhibited by the irreversible antagonist, even if the antagonist concentration in the area around the receptor zone decreases, the effect of antagonism will continue. This type of antagonism can be demonstrated through the administration of phenoxybenzamine, an irreversible inhibitor of α-adrenergic receptors.

The second way in which noncompetitive antagonism can occur is when a compound interacts with the receptor complex at a different binding site from the agonist site, called the allosteric site. If the binding of the antagonist

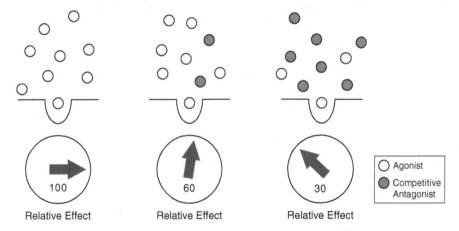

Figure 2-6 Representation of decreasing receptor effect as the concentration of a competitive antagonist increases around a receptor zone.

molecule to its binding site causes a conformational change in the receptor complex, that may alter the conformation of the binding site of the normal agonist. If this occurs, the agonist may no longer be able to bind to its site and elicit its effect. As seen with irreversible antagonism, increasing the concentration of the agonist molecule will not increase the effect because the binding site is unavailable, thus making this type of inhibition noncompetitive and therefore decreasing the maximal response of the tissue to its normal agonist. However, unlike irreversible antagonism, the binding to the allosteric site is not necessarily irreversible, and as the concentration of the allosteric antagonist decreases, the receptor complex may return to its previous conformation and again function normally.

An example of allosteric inhibition is the decrease in affinity of glycine at the glycine receptor complex when strychnine binds to an allosteric site. In certain neuronal pathways in the spinal cord, glycine receptors act with glycine to inhibit the pathway. The binding of strychnine to its allosteric site decreases the affinity of glycine for its binding site, thus diminishing the glycine-based inhibition of the pathway. Therefore the action of strychnine increases the stimulation of the pathway, leading to convulsions.[9]

Related to the concept of allosteric inhibition is the opposite, or allosteric potentiation. This is not a form of antagonism but actually appears more like a form of agonism. In allosteric potentiation a compound acts at an allosteric site and enhances the affinity of the normal agonist at its binding site. The classic example of this is the way the benzodiazepines and some anesthetics act at allosteric sites on the $GABA_A$ complex to increase the affinity of GABA for its binding site. Because GABA causes an inhibitory response through the $GABA_A$ complex, increasing the affinity of GABA causes a greater degree of inhibition.[10]

Inverse agonists are another group of compounds that produce effects that appear as if an antagonist has been delivered to a receptor zone. However, unlike other antagonists, the effect of these compounds can be reversed by the addition of a competitive antagonist. To understand the action of the inverse agonists, the concept of a receptor and its associated effector (e.g., enzyme, ion channel) as existing in an on or off state based on whether the receptor site is occupied with an agonist or not needs to be modified. Many ion channels are not completely open or closed without their receptor agonist present. In such a state, some ions pass through the channel normally because it is neither fully open nor fully closed. An agonist will cause the channel to either open or close more than normal. An inverse agonist produces the opposite effect. If an agonist opens an ion channel more than seen at rest, then an inverse agonist

closes the channel more than at rest. Receptors that act this way are classified as constitutive receptors and are capable of wide-ranging effects. As the concept of constitutive receptor activity has been more broadly accepted, it has become apparent that many drugs once thought to be competitive antagonists should now be classified as inverse agonists.[11]

Two other types of receptor antagonism are based in part on agonistic effects. As discussed, some agonist drugs may exhibit less agonistic effects than the normal endogenous agonist or some drugs used as the reference standard. These drugs appear to have less intrinsic activity at the receptor site. Therefore they are labeled partial agonists. However, while they occupy the receptor site, they are keeping the normal agonist from interacting with the receptor. If the normal agonist possesses more intrinsic activity, then as long as the partial agonist is present on the receptor, less effect is seen than if the normal agonist were interacting with the receptor. In effect, it appears as if an antagonist is interacting at the receptor. Therefore these drugs are frequently referred to as partial agonists/antagonists. The final type of antagonist to be presented is also a type of agonist. However, in this case the compounds act as agonists at one type of receptor and antagonists at other receptors. These compounds are referred to as agonist/antagonists. One example of such a compound is the analgesic nalbuphine, which acts as an antagonist at opioid μ-receptors and as an agonist at opioid κ-receptors.[12]

Receptor Regulation

As discussed, most receptors are proteins and as such are synthesized by protein synthesis mechanisms inside the cell nucleus and cell body. After synthesis, these receptor molecules may be functional on their own or may require further assembly with other components, such as other protein subunits, to produce a functional receptor complex. The receptor proteins may be stored in an inactive form inside the cell or in the cell membrane until needed. The number of active receptors present appears to be controlled and can be increased or decreased as needed by the cell. A common experiment to demonstrate this regulation is the destruction of a nerve leading to a receptor zone on the surface of a muscle cell. Normally, the receptors on the muscle cell receive signals to initiate muscle contraction from the release of the neurotransmitter, acetylcholine, from the presynaptic neuron. If this neuron leading to the receptor zone is destroyed, no acetylcholine is present at the receptor zone. The cell, in an apparent attempt to sense the missing acetylcholine, increases the number of acetylcholine receptors on the surface of the receptor zone. This is termed up-regulation and is seen whenever a normally present receptor agonist decreases at a receptor zone below some point. After up-regulation, a cell becomes hypersensitive to the receptor agonist. Any sudden release or application of a receptor agonist to a highly up-regulated zone can lead to overstimulation and potential cell injury or death.

Cells can also regulate the number of receptors in the other direction. If a receptor zone is experiencing excessive stimulation from an agonist, it can decrease the number of available receptors. If the receptors were located on the cell membrane, these receptors may be internalized and stored for future use or destroyed. This process of decreasing the number of available receptors is termed down-regulation. The administration of many compounds over a long period of time can lead to down-regulation of some receptors. If the administered agent is suddenly discontinued, there may be inadequate receptor stimulation, which can lead to problems. For this reason many drugs that have been provided to a patient for a prolonged period should not be suddenly discontinued but should instead be tapered off over a period of several days to allow the patient's receptor sites and systems to adjust to the lack of the previously supplied compound. A special related condition, known as physiologic tolerance, can be seen with the administration of some drugs. In this situation administration of a drug may lead to physiologic changes in the number of receptors to the compound (down-regulation). As the number of receptors decreases, larger doses of the drug may be required to elicit the same effect. The exact cause of tolerance development to various drugs is still unclear, however, and morphine, which frequently causes tolerance, does not appear to do so by simply down-regulating receptors.[13,14]

Receptor Types

As more and more receptors have been discovered in the body, it has become clear that most drug effects are due to some type of receptor interaction. When drug receptors were first identified, major research efforts were made into identifying specific receptors to known therapeutic agents. With the current ability to decipher large sections of the genetic code, receptors have been identified before an endogenous ligand has been located. This has led to an explosion in the number of known receptor types and subtypes in recent years, the importance of which will be under study for many years. Some identified receptor subtypes differ only in a few amino acids in their overall protein structure, which may

prove inconsequential. In addition, individual variations and population genetic differences provide other modified receptors in some people (see Chapter 3). Most specific receptors fall into one of several broad classes of receptors based on their structure and general mechanism of action.

Ligand-Gated Ion Channels

Cellular membranes are studded with many different types of ion channels. Some ion channels, such as the inward rectifier potassium channel, are permanently open, thereby providing a means for ion conductance across the membrane based entirely on concentration and electrical gradients. Other ion channels may be voltage gated, opening and closing in response to particular cellular voltage differentials, such as voltage-gated sodium and potassium channels. Another group of ion channels are controlled by a chemical receptor zone that interacts with specific ligand molecules (Figure 2-7). These ligand-gated ion channels (also known as ionophores) are formed from multiple (usually five) protein subunits that span the entire cellular membrane in their active state. The protein subunits surround a central ion passageway or pore through which specific ions can pass. Many different forms of ligand-gated ion channels exist; however, all appear to be developmentally related and are structurally similar. The pore may be normally open or normally closed, with the action of a ligand binding to an associated location on the structure forcing the pore into the opposite state. The ligand binding site may be intracellular, extracellular, or located within the channel and may require more than one molecule of ligand to bind to different binding sites on the complex to fully activate the channel.

Of the different varieties of ligand-gated ion channels known, most are activated by specific neurotransmitters (e.g., acetylcholine, glycine, GABA, glutamic acid, serotonin)

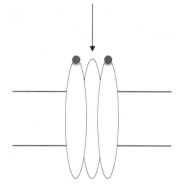

Figure 2-7 Cross-sectional diagram of ligand-gated ion channel embedded in cell membrane. The channel is in the open state with two molecules of ligand bound to extracellular receptor sites.

binding to extracellular binding sites. Different varieties also gate different ions (e.g., sodium, potassium, calcium, or chloride). One specific example is the neuromuscular nicotinic acetylcholine receptor[1] located on skeletal muscle at the neuromuscular junction. Acetylcholine released from somatic cholinergic nerve terminals at the synapse binds to two receptor sites on the nicotinic receptor on the postsynaptic membrane, stimulating an allosteric change in the pentameric receptor complex that opens the ion channel and allows sodium ions to enter the cell from the extracellular fluid. This initiates a local depolarization, which can then lead to the initiation of muscle contraction.

Metabophores

Metabophores are transmembrane receptors that are composed of an external binding site and an internal enzymatic component. Interaction of an extracellular ligand to the binding site causes a modification of the intracellular component of the protein that then initiates one of several known metabolic conversions of intracellular compounds, such as the direct conversion of GTP to cGMP. This then acts as a second messenger inside the cell, triggering additional biochemical processes (Figure 2-8).

G-Protein Coupled Receptors

This class of receptor is responsible for detecting specific extracellular ligands and initiating an intracellular response. In some ways these receptors are similar to metabophores in that they may control biochemical pathways inside the cell in response to an external signal. However, the mechanism by which these receptor complexes act is quite different and considerably more complex. A metabophore directly links some enzymatic function to the ligand interaction, whereas the G-protein coupled receptor complex initiates a series of changes that may eventually lead to control of a specific enzyme. The G-protein coupled receptor family is the most common type of receptor structure found on cell membranes. They comprise a large transmembrane protein with

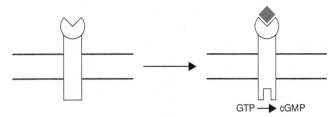

Figure 2-8 Example metabophoric receptor embedded in cell membrane. Binding of the receptor agonist activates the intracellular enzymatic domain, producing cGMP from GTP.

seven transmembrane loops. The extracellular region forms the binding site for the specific ligand.

Many drugs, hormones, neurotransmitters, and other signaling compounds act as ligands at specific G-protein coupled receptors. The intracellular side of the transmembrane protein is linked to the G-protein complex. When a ligand binds to the extracellular binding site, a conformational change occurs that triggers the substitution of GTP on the G-protein in place of GDP. This then activates the G-protein complex, allowing the separation of the G-protein from the transmembrane protein. The G-protein can then migrate and interact with various effector macromolecules, leading to their activation or inhibition. The G-protein then undergoes hydrolysis, converting the GTP to GDP and deactivating the effector molecule. The G-protein complex then recombines with the transmembrane protein in preparation for another round of activation.

Many internal effectors such as ion channels and enzymes (e.g., phospholipase C, adenylyl cyclase, phosphodiesterase) have been shown to be activated or inhibited by variants of the G-protein subunits, leading to a wide range of intracellular effects (Figure 2-9). An example of G-protein coupled receptors are the β-adrenergic receptors that, when stimulated by a β-adrenergic agonist, initiate the activation of adenylyl cyclase, allowing the intracellular production of cAMP, which acts as an intracellular second messenger capable of initiating other biochemical changes within the cell.[15]

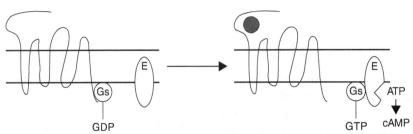

Figure 2-9 G-Protein coupled receptor example. The binding of a specific ligand to the seven-transmembrane loop protein initiates the activation of the G-protein complex (Gs = G stimulatory protein) by allowing GTP substitution for GDP. The G-protein then migrates to interact with effector molecules (E), here represented as adenylyl cyclase, which then catalyzes the conversion of ATP to cAMP, a cellular second messenger.

Intracellular Receptors

Although all receptors discussed to this point have been associated with the cell membrane, there are some receptors located inside the cell. This should not really be surprising given the wide variety and number of processes that occur inside a cell. Many intracellular biochemical reactions are controlled by the concentration of their products or reactants acting on the enzymes responsible for the reaction. Locating the binding sites that provide control of specific enzymes and developing drugs that can interact at those binding sites is a common goal of new drug design.

One class of intracellular receptors has been fairly well characterized. These are the steroid receptors.[16] Most steroid molecules are very lipid soluble and easily cross the cell membrane and enter the cell via passive diffusion. Once inside the cell, the steroid molecule binds to a specific inactive protein complex. The binding of the steroid to the complex causes an attached inactivating protein to dissociate from the complex. The activated complex is then transported into the nucleus of the cell where it usually forms a dimer with another activated receptor complex. This dimer then binds to specific regions of the nucleic DNA and can increase or decrease transcription of specific genes into RNA for translation into proteins. Unlike receptor-mediated ion channel interactions, which are nearly instantaneous in response, steroid receptor–induced effects are slower to begin and tend to last longer due to the lag time for protein synthesis.

Transporters

Although very small compounds can cross cell membranes via water pores and lipid-soluble agents can cross membranes by passive membrane diffusion, many molecules are either too large or not lipid soluble enough to enter cells by these mechanisms. The movement of these molecules across membranes involves the use of various transport proteins. These transporters may or may not require energy to move select molecules from one side of the membrane to the other. Many different types of transporter protein have been characterized. Some are very selective for the compounds that can be transported and others less so. Several transporter proteins have become the targets of drug therapy, especially the neurotransmitter reuptake proteins.[17] One specific example involves the serotonin selective reuptake inhibitors, such as fluoxetine. These agents act on a transport protein known as SERT which is found on serotonin nerve terminals and is responsible for serotonin reuptake back into the nerve terminal. Inhibition of serotonin reuptake leads to altered function of serotonergic neurons and is commonly used to treat depression. Due

to their function, many other transport proteins are now or will become targets for drug therapy.

Non–Receptor-Mediated Effects

Although receptor-mediated effects account for most of the actions known to be elicited by current drugs, a few agents produce their therapeutic effects without receptor interactions. Most agents that do not rely on receptors for effect seem to instead rely on their physical or chemical properties to alter normal body function. Consider the use of dextran 70 as a plasma expander. It is used primarily because of its osmotic properties and relatively slow elimination. Another example is the use of ammonium chloride to decrease the pH of urine. This is occasionally useful to enhance the elimination rate of some basic compounds and is based entirely on the acid-base chemistry of the compounds in urinary fluid.

Mechanisms of General Anesthesia

For many years the inhalational general anesthetic agents were believed to produce anesthesia entirely due to their high degree of lipid solubility and alteration of cellular membrane function (Meyer-Overton rule, Mullins hypothesis). This suggested a mechanism that was due to the physical properties of the agents and not a receptor-mediated function. Like other areas of science (i.e., physics), a single unified theory explaining the action of all anesthetics was particularly attractive. Additional research has unfortunately complicated the picture. Current theories place increasing importance on evidence of receptor interactions as the primary mechanism of the general anesthetic agents, both inhalational and parenteral. Although lipid solubility of the agents is undoubtedly important, it may be more related to getting the agents to their required site of action than actual effect. The general anesthetics appear to elicit their primary effects by increasing inhibitory signals or decreasing excitatory signals in the brain and/or spinal cord. Examples of agents that appear to increase inhibitory pathways are the agents that act on the $GABA_A$ ionophoric complex. This ligand-gated ion channel opens in response to GABA, allowing chloride ions to enter the cell. The increasing negative charge due to the chloride ions lowers the local intracellular voltage (hyperpolarized), making the cell more resistant to depolarization. Many of the general anesthetic agents (e.g., the barbiturates, propofol, etomidate, isoflurane, desflurane, and sevoflurane) all appear to act, in large part, by binding to the $GABA_A$ receptor complex at specific sites and causing an allosteric potentiation of GABA binding to its receptor site. This causes increased inhibitory activity believed to induce an anesthetized state. Other general anesthetic agents (e.g., nitrous oxide, xenon, ketamine) appear to act to decrease excitatory signaling through NMDA glutamate receptors and nicotinic acetylcholine receptors in the brain or spinal cord.

The exact mechanism of the general anesthetics is still unclear. It is believed to be more likely due to a variety of causes linked to physical properties and multiple receptor zone effects.

Key Points

- Drug–Receptor Theory
- Agonists and Antagonists
- Receptor Types
- Receptor Location and Function
- Mechanisms of General Anesthetics

Chapter Questions

1. Explain how different types of drug–receptor interactions can elicit physiologic effects.
2. How can drug-induced allosteric changes affect receptor activity?
3. Why does doubling the dose of a drug not double the response even if the original and doubled doses are in the "linear" range of the log dose–response curve?
4. In what ways are metabotropic and G-protein coupled receptors similar? How do they differ?
5. Explain the concept of receptor antagonism and how this relates to neuromuscular blockade?

References

1. Simon JB, Golan DE. Drug-receptor interactions. In: Golan DE, et al., eds. *Principles of Pharmacology: The Pathophysiologic Basis of Drug Therapy*. Philadelphia: Lippincott Williams & Wilkins; 2005:3–16.
2. Maehle AH. "Receptive substances": John Newport Langley (1852–1925) and his path to a receptor theory of drug action. *Med History*. 2004;48:153–174.
3. Eger EI II, Eisenkraft JB, Weiskopf RB. Mechanisms of inhaled anesthetic actions. In: Eger EI II, ed., *The Pharmacology of Inhaled Anesthetics*. San Francisco: EI Eiger; 2002:32–42.
4. Mullen KD, Martin JV, Mendelson WB, Bassett ML, Jones EA. Could an endogenous benzodiazepine ligand contribute to hepatic encephalopathy? *Lancet*. 1988;1:457–459.
5. Pélissolo A. The benzodiazepine receptor: the enigma of the endogenous ligand. *Encephale*. 1995;21:133–140.
6. Cortelli P, Avalione R, Baraldi M, et al. Endozepines in recurrent stupor. *Sleep Med Rev*. 2005;9:477–487.
7. Baraldi M, Avalione R, Corsi L, Venturini I, Baraldi C, Zeneroli ML. Natural endogenous ligands for benzodiazepine receptors in hepatic encephalopathy. *Metab Brain Dis*. 2009;24:81–93.
8. Bevan JC, Collins L, Fowler C, et al. Early and late reversal of rocuronium and vecuronium with neostigmine in adults and children. *Anesth Analg*. 1999;89:333–339.
9. Burnham WM. Antiseizure drugs (anticonvulsants). In: Kalant H, Roschlau WHE, eds. *Principles of Medical Pharmacology*, 5th ed. Philadelphia: B.C. Decker; 1989: 203–213.
10. Stoelting RK, Hillier SC. Benzodiazepines. In: Stoelting RK, Hillier SC, eds. *Pharmacology and Physiology in Anesthetic Practice*, 4th ed. Philadelphia: Lippincott Williams & Wilkins; 2006:140–154.
11. Greasley PJ, Clapham JC. Inverse agonism or neutral antagonism at G-protein coupled receptors: a medicinal chemistry challenge worth pursuing? *Eur J Pharmacol*. 2006; 553:1–9.
12. Gutstein HB, Akil H. Opioid analgesics. In: Brunton LL, Lazo JS, Parker KL, eds. *Goodman & Gilman's The Pharmacological Basis of Therapeutics*, 11th ed. New York: McGraw-Hill; 2006:547–590.
13. He L, Fong J, von Zastrow M, Whistler JL. Regulation of opioid receptor trafficking and morphine tolerance by receptor oligomerization. *Cell*. 2002;108:271–282.
14. Lüscher C. Drugs of abuse. In: Katzung BG, Masters SB, Trevor AJ, eds. *Basic and Clinical Pharmacology*, 11th ed. New York: McGraw-Hill; 2009:553–568.
15. Hemmings HC, Girault JA. Signal transduction mechanisms: receptor-effector coupling. In: Evers AS, Maze M, eds. *Anesthetic Pharmacology: Physiologic Principles and Clinical Practice*. Philadelphia: Churchill Livingstone; 2004: 21–39.
16. von Zastrow M, Bourne HR. Drug receptors & pharmacodynamics. In: Katzung BG, Masters SB, Trevor AJ, eds. *Basic and Clinical Pharmacology*, 11th ed. New York: McGraw-Hill; 2009:15–35.
17. Giacomini KM, Sugiyama Y. Membrane transporters and drug response. In: Brunton LL, Lazo JS, Parker KL, eds. *Goodman & Gilman's the Pharmacological Basis of Therapeutics*, 11th ed. New York: McGraw-Hill; 2006:41–70.

3

Objectives

After completing this chapter, the reader should be able to

- Describe the impact of culture, environment, and genetic variations on drug responses between individuals.
- Identify known and possible factors that influence the cytochrome P-450 system.
- Relate basic genetic concepts to the nurse anesthetist's pharmacology practice.
- Summarize the effect of common genetic polymorphisms on drug target proteins, drug metabolizing enzymes, and other biochemical systems that influence pharmacotherapy.
- Devise a clinically relevant strategy for assessing factors that may affect an individual's response to drugs.

Cultural, Environmental, and Genetic Influences on Drug Therapy

John McFadden, PhD, CRNA

Introduction

Clinical pharmacology requires that healthcare providers make decisions about issues such as drug dosages, timing, and monitoring for intended and unintended effects. This need led to the development of standardized drug doses, dosing intervals, therapeutic blood concentrations, and lists of frequent adverse effects and complications. Using these standardized tools is helpful for all healthcare providers. It is well recognized, however, that responses to drugs vary between individuals.

Unpredictable differences in both pharmacodynamics and pharmacokinetics pose many challenges in clinical pharmacology decision making, particularly for anesthesia providers. Most medications administered during anesthesia are administered through inhalation or intravenous routes. These routes typically provide for a short time interval until both intended effects and adverse effects are observed. Opportunities for monitoring serum concentrations are limited because of time constraints. Additionally, many agents used to create and maintain an anesthetized state carry a high risk of a variety of life-threatening effects, such as apnea, bradycardia, vasodilation, and/or changes in intracranial pressure. The time intervals between onset, effect, observable physical manifestations of the effect, and deleterious outcomes can be very brief. Hence, there is a need for every anesthesia provider to be able to predict, evaluate, deduce, and react to individual drug responses with both speed and accuracy. Strategies to help better predict interindividual response differences to drugs should lead to safer anesthesia care, a primary objective for all anesthesia providers.

Historic Perspective

Understanding the basic principles of pharmacodynamics and pharmacokinetics is imperative for anesthesia providers. Because the science behind these concepts is evolutionary, practitioners must be dedicated to engaging in lifelong learning. Consider how the trial-and-error approach to drug therapy has been pervasive in the history of health care. Choosing a dose of medication and then being prepared to either administer additional doses or counteract the drug's effect has been a pervasive theme in numerous healthcare specialties. The recognition that the therapeutic window of many drugs is very small, especially those used in anesthesia, has supported the need to identify those indicators that may influence whether a drug dose is efficacious or toxic.

Reasons for variations in drug responses between people have been postulated for more than two centuries. Factors such as age, body weight, allergies, cigarette smoking, and the impact of concurrent medication use are examples of the many influences that have been assessed by practitioners from the mid-1800s through today (Table 3-1). During the past several decades research has supported the need to consider these cultural and environmental factors, as well as other possible determinants. The combined influence of these factors is sometimes referred to as "ethnic pharmacology" or "ethnopharmacology." The term ethnopharmacology more accurately refers to the study of a culture's traditional use of plants for medicinal purposes.

The idea that genetics may impact a person's response to a drug is also traced back to the 1800s though the works of scientists such as Francis Galton, Archibald E. Garrod,

Table 3-1 Common Factors Attributed to Variable Drug Responses

Identified differences in anatomy and physiology
Existing pathologic conditions
Known or suspected allergies
Age
Gender
Body habitus/weight
Concurrent medication/herbal drug use (drug–drug interactions)
Exposure to environmental chemicals
Dietary habits, including alcohol intake
Cigarette smoking
Genetics
Ethnic and cultural practices

and J. B. S. Haldane.[1–3] This spirit of investigation continued through the 20th century and is ongoing today. For example, in the 1950s Kalow identified that some patients undergoing electroconvulsive therapy experienced a longer than expected effect from intravenously administered succinylcholine. This led to the idea that individual differences in the amount of plasma cholinesterase exist as a result of genetics.[4,5] Likewise, in 1960 Denborough and Lovell wrote of a family's experiences with anesthetic complications as a result of an unidentified inherited metabolic disorder.[6] This is now called malignant hyperthermia and further supports the understanding that genetics influences drug responses. Through the work of countless clinicians and scientists, a blending of two sciences—genetics and pharmacology—led to the development of the term "pharmacogenetics." The mapping of the human genome and further understanding of how people's gene variations affect how they respond to a drug resulted in the broader term "pharmacogenomics." These terms, however, are frequently used interchangeably in clinical practice today.

Today's practitioners recognize that differences between an individual's responses to an administered drug are both complex and multifactorial. A growing body of evidence is adding to the list of modifiers that lead to the interindividual variations to a given dose of a drug. Researchers continue to uncover the impact of cultural, environmental, and genetic influences on drug choice, dose requirements, and outcomes.

Cultural and Environmental Influences

Consider an individual's exposure to things like air, water, and food as exogenous substances. A person's geographic environment, food and beverage preferences, and other habits and behaviors may result in exposure to some substances more or less than others. When these nonindigenous chemical substances, referred to as xenobiotics, make contact with and enter the body, they are viewed as foreign materials. The body subsequently initiates strategies to modify, degrade, and eventually eliminate these foreign substances, calling on many of the enzymatic systems that have been developed over human evolution. In fact, these systems developed as a result of exogenous substance exposure. Repeated exposure to some substances over time may result in a variety of anatomic and physiologic changes. This includes changes to the drug targets, or the biochemical systems that absorb, distribute, metabolize, or eliminate the drugs. In some cases the body evolves to tolerate these non-naturally occurring substances.

Several biochemical systems, commonly divided into phase I and phase II reactions (see Chapter 1), are known to react with drugs in an attempt to eliminate them from the body. Examples include the cytochrome P-450 monooxygenase system, the flavin-containing monooxygenase system, the sulfotransferase system, alcohol and aldehyde dehydrogenase systems, the esterases and amidases for hydrolysis, the amino acid N-acyl transferases for acetylation, and the monoamine oxidase systems.

The cytochrome P-450 system is one of the most recognized and important metabolizing pathways. This collection of metabolizing microsomal enzymes act upon chemicals that enter the body through food, environment, or medications. In humans there are currently 50 known functionally active enzymes. These enzymes are labeled with the abbreviation "CYP." Based on their amino acid sequence, they are then identified by family using an Arabic numeral, followed by a subfamily classification using a letter, followed by another Arabic number to distinguish different isoforms within the subfamily.[7] For example, CYP1A2 is involved in the metabolism of caffeine, ondansetron, and theophylline. Another common enzyme, CYP3A4, is involved in the metabolism of dexamethasone, fentanyl, and oxycodone. It is supposed that the vast majority of drug oxidation involves six CYP enzymes: CYP1A2, CYP2C9, CYP2C19, CYP2D6, CYP2E1, and CYP3A4.[8] A gene encodes the instruction for the construction of each of the CYP enzymes. The gene that correlates with the enzyme carries the same label but is identified by italics, for example, *CYP1A2* or *CYP3A4*.

The CYP enzymes are influenced by a variety of factors, including exposure to some of the chemicals they metabolize. Some chemical substances stimulate this enzymatic system to metabolize quicker; others inhibit it. A drug therefore may undergo an enzymatic process more quickly or more slowly. If the originally ingested parent drug compound is responsible for exerting its effect on a target, midazolam for example, and that parent drug compound is more rapidly metabolized, less drug will be available to exert an effect. A higher dosage of that drug will be required for the intended effect. What if the ingested drug is a prodrug—that is, a compound that is inactive (or minimally active) but is metabolized into active metabolites that exert its intended pharmacologic effects? If the parent compound is metabolized more rapidly into the active metabolite, codeine for example, more of the active drug metabolite will be available quickly and could lead to a toxic effect. Among other factors, diet and nutrition are both implicated as modulators of this enzymatic system.

Dietary Influences

Until recently foods were rarely considered ingested "chemicals" that could affect the body. One exception recognized by nurses for several decades are those foods rich in vitamin K, such as green leafy vegetables, like spinach or kale. It is common knowledge that this particular food–drug interaction has the potential to alter the effectiveness of the drug Coumadin. More recently, however, the rise in popularity of various herbal remedies to prevent, influence, or treat diseases has increased awareness of the impact food can have on physiologic processes. Drawing along this line of thought, food intake could influence enzymatic activity and therefore influence the body's reactions to a drug, as suggested by the work of Parke and Ioannides.[9,10]

One food substance that has received attention for possible health effects is the phytochemical. Phytochemicals, or phytonutrients, are naturally occurring chemicals in plants that are consumed as food. Long used for medicinal purposes, it has been suggested that some phytochemicals may contribute to health by acting as antioxidants or exhibiting anti-inflammatory effects. Some examples of phytochemicals include lutein, found in leafy green vegetables, beta-carotene found in carrots and pumpkins, and lycopene found in tomatoes. An example of a phytochemical from the Pacific yew tree used in the manufacturing of a medication is the antineoplastic agent paclitaxel (Taxol).

Evidence has emerged that phytochemicals influence the cytochrome P-450 metabolic processes. Cruciferous vegetables, such as broccoli, Brussels sprouts, and cauliflower, have been shown to induce or stimulate the cytochrome P-450 enzyme CYP1A2, thereby increasing the rate of phase I biochemical processes (Table 3-2).[11–13] In vitro studies suggest that cruciferous vegetables also contain other classes of chemicals that both stimulate and inhibit various cytochrome P-450 enzymes.[14,15] The effects of vegetables in the Apiaceae family, like carrots and celery, have been shown to decrease cytochrome P-450 enzyme activity.[11]

Grapefruit juice has long been identified as a beverage that interferes with the first-pass metabolism and transportation of many drugs, including felodipine, saquinavir, midazolam, and erythromycin.[16–19] It is theorized that the compounds in grapefruit juice inhibit the intestinal cytochrome P-450 enzyme activity but facilitate drug absorption. Combined, these actions lead to an increased plasma drug level. Several studies have demonstrated prolongation of this effect lasting several days.[20–22]

Other common foods like potatoes, tomatoes, and eggplants—all high in solanaceous glycoalkaloids—may pose problems for certain drugs, including those used during an anesthetic.[23] Solanaceous glycoalkaloids reportedly inhibit both acetylcholinesterase and butyrylcholinesterase (plasma cholinesterase). As little as one serving of mashed potatoes increases serum solanaceous glycoalkaloid levels. This impacts the metabolism of many chemicals, including cocaine, ester-type local anesthetics, neuromuscular blocking agents, and esmolol. Ethnic groups who traditionally consume high quantities of these foods (e.g., those from Turkey, Morocco, and Middle Eastern regions where eggplant is a dietary staple) may very well be at risk for altered responses to these drugs. Again, additional research is needed.

Alcohol Consumption

Much has been written about the effect that drinking alcoholic beverages has on various medications and health in general. Alcohol consumption is fairly common, and the frequency of alcohol ingestion appears to vary between groups. In 2006 the Centers for Disease Control and Prevention, an agency of the U.S. Department of Health and Human Services, reported that more than 60% of adults in households surveyed consumed alcohol in the past year; 20% of current drinkers report having five or more drinks

Table 3-2 Examples of Cruciferous Vegetables

Bok choy
Broccoli
Cabbage
Cauliflower
Collard greens
Kale
Radish
Wasabi
Watercress

on at least 1 day in the past year.[24] Some groups contain a higher percentage of alcohol consumers, although outliers certainly exist on both ends of the spectrum, making generalizations difficult at best. Non-Hispanic whites and males between the ages of 18 and 44 are reported to be the heaviest users. Adult males are two times more likely to binge drink than adult women. Evidence that the impact of alcohol consumption poses a particularly concerning public health impact on Native Americans and Alaska Native populations exists.[25,26] From an international perspective, the prevalence of alcohol abuse and dependence among Europeans is even higher than in the United States.[27]

Acute alcohol intoxication poses a different set of problems than chronic alcohol use. Changes in sensorium create psychomotor impairments and can lead to a higher risk of injury, vomiting, delayed gastric emptying, and decisional incapacity. An elevated blood alcohol level is known to cause an increased sensitivity to other drugs because of its additive depressant effects.

Chronic alcohol consumption, associated with alcohol use disorder, is frequently accompanied by concurrent illnesses.[28,29] These may include pathology of the nervous, cardiovascular, gastrointestinal, and renal systems. Alcohol-associated hepatic disease raises additional concerns for the anesthesia provider. Long-term alcohol abuse has also been linked to an altered immune response, resulting in a significantly increased risk of postoperative infection, prolonged stays in the intensive care unit, and prolonged stays in the hospital.[30]

Drinking alcohol is known to induce a number of anatomic and physiologic consequences. For example, if the patient is hypoalbuminemic and/or has impaired hepatic blood flow, drug distribution and metabolism will be impaired. As a result, the duration of neuromuscular blocking agents may be prolonged. Additionally, drinking alcohol may modulate synaptic and extrasynaptic γ-aminobutyric acid (GABA) receptors in the thalamus.[31] Chronic alcohol consumption is known to proliferate the membranes of the endoplasmic reticulum, accelerate ethanol metabolism, and boost the production of acetaldehyde.[32] Table 3-3 provides a description of the effects of alcohol consumption on some frequently prescribed medications. Because chronic alcohol use is known to induce the CYP enzymes, particularly CYP2E1, dose requirements for many of the drugs used during an anesthetic may need to be increased, including propofol, barbiturates, opioids, and the minimum alveolar concentration (MAC) of inhalation agents. Ironically, just as alcohol and liver disease affect the CYP enzymes, the CYP enzymes appear to have a role in the origin of several liver diseases. CYP metabolism of some parent compounds to their toxic metabolites, like acetaminophen and halothane, provokes hepatotoxicity.[33]

Smoking

The Centers for Disease Control and Prevention tracks and provides statistics on tobacco use in the United States. It is estimated that more than 20% of Americans are current cigarette smokers. Some ethnic and geographic groups engage in smoking more than others. The rate of tobacco product use among Native American and Alaska Native tribes is significantly higher than in the general U.S. population. Some Native American and Alaska Native tribes have use rates as high as 40%. Likewise, age is also a factor: The prevalence of smoking among U.S. teenagers is higher than adults.[34]

There are clinical anesthesia implications of engaging in cigarette smoking that extend beyond the usual known health risks. These effects are influenced by the length of time an individual has smoked, the makeup of the cigarettes smoked, and how the smoker inhales. The compounds associated with both the particulate and gaseous components of cigarette smoke, including benzene, polyphenols, arsenic, carbon monoxide, and polycyclic aromatic hydrocarbons (PAHs), influence the activities of the enzymes in the CYP system. PAHs are also derived from some environmental pollutants and charbroiled meats. Many of these substances, particularly the PAHs, induce certain enzymes, specifically CYP1A1, CYP1A2, and CYP2E1.[35] As a result the drugs or substrates that are metabolized by those affected enzymes are metabolized more quickly in smokers.[36] Smokers therefore require higher doses of some drugs, for example, theophylline and morphine. Table 3-3 describes the effects of cigarette smoking on many commonly prescribed medications.

It is commonly known among anesthesia providers that smoking is a risk reducer for postoperative nausea and vomiting.[37] The benefit hardly extends beyond this example. PAHs and their metabolites are unfortunately also known to induce DNA mutations, contributing to the potential development of cancer.

Several drugs germane to the practice of anesthesiology are impacted by the effects of cigarette smoke, including neuromuscular blocking agents (increased dose needed), opioids (increased dose needed), and some sedatives (increased dose needed).[38] Some of the evidence, however, remains conflicting; differing conclusions point to the need for continued inquiry into this clinically relevant topic.

Table 3-3 Potential Interactions Between Cigarette Smoking, Alcohol Consumption, and Frequently Prescribed Medications

Product	Effects of Cigarette Smoking	Effects of Alcohol Consumption
Lipitor		Possible liver damage
Hydrocodone/APAP	Decreased analgesic effect	Increased CNS depression
Toprol-XL	Decreased drug effect	Increased drowsiness/dizziness
Norvasc		Increased drowsiness/dizziness and decreased BP
Amoxicillin		
Synthroid		
Nexium		
Lexapro		Not recommended
Albuterol		
Singular		
Lisinopril		Decreased BP and increased adverse effects
Ambien	Decreased sedation	Increased drowsiness
Zyrtec	Theoretical	Increased drowsiness/dizziness
Prevacid		Decreased medication effect and increased acid production
Zoloft		Not recommended
Warfarin	Increased clearance	Increased anticlotting effect
Advair	Decreased drug effect	Not recommended
Furosemide		Increased adverse effects of alcohol
Fosamax	Not recommended	Not recommended
Protonix		
Azithromax		
Effexor XR		Increased adverse effects
Zocor		Possible liver damage
Plavix	Theoretical	Increased bleeding possibility
Oxycodone/APAP	Decreased analgesic effect	Increased CNS depression
Vytorin		Possible liver damage
Cephalexin		
Diovan		Decreased BP and increased adverse effects
Metformin		Inhibits alcohol metabolism
Atenolol	Decreased drug effect	Increased drowsiness/dizziness
Prednisone		Can damage stomach
Levaquin		
Lotrel		Decreased BP and increased adverse effects
Zetia		Increased dizziness
Seroquel		Increased drowsiness and adverse effects
Wellbutrin XL	Theoretical	Increased risk of seizures
Celebrex		Increased risk of GI bleed
Avandia		Increased risk of hypoglycemia
Hydrochlorothiazide		Increased adverse effects
Actos		Increased risk of hypoglycemia
Diovan HCT		Decreased BP and increased adverse effects
Premarin	Anti-estrogen effects	

(continues)

Table 3-3 Potential Interactions Between Cigarette Smoking, Alcohol Consumption, and Frequently Prescribed Medications *(continued)*

Product	Effects of Cigarette Smoking	Effects of Alcohol Consumption
Altace		Decreased BP and increased adverse effects
Crestor		Possible liver damage
Coreg	Decreased drug effect	Increased drowsiness/dizziness
Flomax		Increased dizziness
Actonel	Not recommended	Not recommended
Nasonex	Decreased drug effect	
Risperdal		Increased drowsiness and adverse effects
Yasmin 28	Increased adverse effects	Slow alcohol elimination
Lantus	Decreased absorption	Increased risk of hypoglycemia
Viagra		
Tricor		Possible liver damage
Alprazolam	Decreased sedation	Increased CNS depression
Cozaar		Decreased BP and increased adverse effects
Digitek		
Ibuprofen		Increased risk of GI bleed
Trazodone		Increased CNS depression
Cymbalta	Theoretical	Possible liver damage
Codeine/APAP	Decreased analgesic effect	Increased CNS depression
Triamterene and hydrochlorothiazide	Theoretical	Increased adverse effects
Paroxetine	Theoretical	Increased CNS depression
Adderall XR		Not recommended
Clonazepam	Decreased sedation	Increased CNS depression
Omnicef		
Aricept		Increased drowsiness/dizziness
Fluoxetine		Increased CNS depression
Propoxyphene/APAP	Increased doses needed	Increased CNS depression
Gabapentin		Increased adverse effects
Fexofenadine		
Valtrex		
Concerta		Not recommended
Ortho-Tri-Cyclen Lo	Increased adverse effects	Slow alcohol elimination
Aciphex		
Clonidine		
Topamax		Increased drowsiness/sedation
Xalatan		Increased adverse effects
Lorazepam	Decreased sedation	Increased CNS depression

BP, blood pressure; CNS, central nervous system; GI, gastrointestinal.

Source: Smith RG. An appraisal of potential drug interactions in cigarette smokers and alcohol drinkers. *J Am Podiatr Med Assoc.* 2009;99:81-88. Reprinted with permission from American Podiatric Medical Association.

Herbal Preparations

Much has been written about the interaction between prescribed medications and consumed herbal preparations. These interactions are significant because it is estimated that more than 46% of the U.S. population uses at least one prescription medication per month, and more than 20% uses three or more prescription medications per month.[39] Because many of the herbal preparations marketed as preventive or therapeutic agents contain phytochemicals, they have potential impact on many of the cytochrome P-450 enzymes. St. John's wort, for example, has been implicated in causing a decrease in the therapeutic plasma levels of the immunosuppressant cyclosporine, the protease inhibitor indinavir, the antiretroviral drug nevirapine, and oral contraceptives, to name a few.[40-44]

Clearly, science supports the existence of a relationship between variations in drug responses and such cultural practices as food preferences and intake, use of herbal preparations, alcohol use, and cigarette smoking. In fact, exposure to any number of environmental chemical compounds over time has the potential to influence the biochemical processes of the body. Fortunately, researchers are continuously identifying inhibitors and inducers so the challenge of optimizing drug doses for therapy is becoming less reliant on probability and chance.

Genetic Influences

Technologic advancements in genomics have enhanced our understanding of many areas of health care. The answers to many important clinical questions have been expanded to include the genetic basis of disease etiology and treatment. A basic understanding of genetics is now expected of those pursuing a study of healthcare sciences. Although a thorough explanation of genetics is beyond the scope of this text, it is important to provide an overview of some key definitions to understand the basis of some interindividual differences to drug responses.

Basic Genetic Concepts

A gene is the basic unit of inheritance that is responsible for a trait or characteristic. In essence, genes behave as the "instruction manuals" for an organism's body, encoding the directives that define its unique features and characteristics. The complete set of these instructions for making an organism—a "master instruction manual"—is called its genome. Found in the nucleus of every cell, there is estimated to be somewhere around 30,000 genes in every human being.

Genes are made of molecules of DNA. DNA is known for its twisted ladder shape, called the double helix. This double helix is built with a sugar–phosphate backbone along which are arranged pairs of four nitrogenous bases, or nucleotides: adenine, which pairs with thymine, and cytosine, which pairs with guanine (A, T, C, and G). Human genomes contain more than 3 billion DNA base pairs. The base pairs combine in various combinations, known as the DNA sequence, which serve as the directives for the cell to synthesize proteins. Proteins are produced from amino acids. It is these proteins that provide for the structure of cells and enzymes for biochemical processes. The proteins enable each cell in the body to perform a specific function.

DNA is packaged in storage units known as chromosomes. A chromosome is a physically separate molecule of DNA. Each human cell is organized into two sets of 23 chromosomes, for a total of 46 chromosomes. Of these 46 chromosomes, 44 are autosomes and 2 are sex chromosomes. One set of chromosomes is provided by the maternal side and one set of the chromosomes is provided by the paternal side of the offspring. It is this passing of chromosomes from parent to child, which eventually yields traits, that is the basis of heredity. Our genes, therefore, encode the instructions that delineate our unique identity.

Genetic Variations

Humans possess obvious and not so obvious genetic variations, from hair color to blood type. The unique genetic makeup of a cell or individual is its genotype. The outward appearance or physical expression of a genotype is known as a phenotype. These genotypic variations are the consequence of the small mutations in DNA sequence that occur in all organisms. These mutations may occur during the process of DNA replication and are spontaneous.

Mutations provide the human species—in fact, all species—with an opportunity for adaptation to new environments ("survival of the fittest" concept). If a variation exists in greater than 1% of the population, it is labeled a polymorphism. Variations that exist in less than 1% of the population are termed mutations. An allelomorph—commonly known as an allele—is the word for any one of the alternative forms of a gene. The normal expression of a gene is known as the wild-type allele. Mutant alleles occur because of an alteration of the wild-type allele.

A DNA polymorphism that is caused by a single nucleotide alteration—such as A (adenine) replacing one of the other three nucleotide letters (C, G, or T)—is called a single nucleotide polymorphism, or SNP. SNPs occur in the human population more than 1% of the time and help identify a person's predisposition to a variety of diseases. They also are the basis for the interindividual differences in drug responses because they may alter the drug's pharmacodynamics or pharmacokinetics. Categorizing SNPs, their impact on drug responses, and then being able to identify an individual's SNPs would allow healthcare providers to better predict a person's responses to a drug.

Making the Clinical Connection

Is it possible to correlate a phenotype with a person's underlying genotype in hopes of identifying variant drug responses or diseases? The answer is complex and remains not fully answerable. Genotyping is certainly more accurate than using race, ethnic groups, or other phenotypes to project a drug response. Some genetic polymorphisms, however, are more frequently expressed within a group of people with a commonality, like gender or geographic origin. Identifying gender is fairly easy; geographic origin is not so easy. Commonly, we refer to a group of people with a shared origin as a "race" or "ethnic group." Race and ethnicity, however, are challenging labels to apply, especially given our heterogeneous and mobile society. Therefore self-identified race or ethnicity is not consistently predictive. As a result, phenotypic expressions may provide clues but not certainty regarding underlying genetic variations. Nonetheless, some polymorphisms are more common in some groups of people than in others.

Polymorphisms occur in drug target proteins and target pathways, in drug-metabolizing enzymes, and in unrelated physiologic variances that coincidentally influence pharmacodynamics and/or pharmacokinetics. Polymorphisms in the genes specifically for drug-metabolizing enzymes have been identified and are somewhat common. Some polymorphisms result in greater enzyme activity, whereas others result in greatly reduced or no enzyme activity. Also,

some enzyme activity appears to be "polymorphically distributed." Depending on their genes, a percentage of the population demonstrates reduced enzyme activity and is categorized as poor metabolizers. Another percentage of the population with normal enzyme activity is categorized as extensive metabolizers. And yet another percentage of the population with increased enzyme activity is termed ultra-extensive or ultra-rapid metabolizers.

These distributions have been found to vary between ethnic groups and are enzyme dependent (Table 3-4). For example, several variants of the CYP2C19 enzyme have been identified. This particular enzyme is involved with the metabolism of many drugs, including the proton pump inhibitor omeprazole. One variant, CYP2C19*17, which is associated with ultra-extensive metabolizers, appears relatively common in three ethnic groups: Swedes, Ethiopians, and Chinese (at 18%, 18%, and 4% frequencies, respectively). This is believed to result in 40% lower omeprazole concentrations for people in these groups.[45]

Another example is the CYP2D6 enzyme, which is involved in the metabolism of approximately 25% of all drugs, including beta-blockers, amide local anesthetics, antiemetics, and opioids. It is estimated that approximately 10% of European whites have the variant allele associated with being a poor metabolizer. For the clinician managing pain, this translates into a percentage of that population who fail to adequately convert codeine to morphine. Thus these individuals receive inadequate analgesia from the standard dose of codeine.[46,47]

The possible genetic factors influencing drug responses are limitless. In 2004 Liem and colleagues[48] provided empirical support for something most anesthesia practitioners suspected: Individuals with natural red hair, an expression of a mutation of the melanocortin-1 receptor gene, required a statistically significant higher minimum alveolar concentration of inhalation anesthetic compared with individuals with dark hair. Some studies even suggest that gender is a factor: Gan and his associates[49] found that

Table 3-4 Outcome of Genetic Disposition on Enzyme Activity and Drug Response

Genetic Disposition	Rate of Metabolism	Outcome of Standard Dose of an *Active* Drug	Outcome of Standard Dose of a *Pro*-Drug
Poor metabolizer (PM)	Slower than "normal"	Slower metabolism increases risk of overdose, side effects	Insufficient active metabolites to create an effect; underdose; pro-drug accumulates and may cause side effects
Extensive metabolizer (EM)	"Normal"	Expected drug effect	Expected drug effect
Ultra-extensive/ rapid metabolizer (UM)	Faster than "normal"	Rapid metabolism of drug necessitates higher than standard dose to achieve intended effect	Active metabolites produced quickly; rapid effect could increase risk of side effects

men had significantly longer recovery times than women after general anesthesia with propofol.

Conclusion

Clearly, current science supports a wide array of factors that clinicians must consider in making decisions that involve clinical pharmacology. The traditional approach of simply basing doses and expected outcomes on limited variables like age, weight, hepatic function, and renal function are no longer defendable. A growing body of evidence substantiates the influences of variable factors like culture and environmental issues as well as genes, which remain constant throughout life. Pharmacogenetic information will continue to expand. Healthcare providers, particularly CRNAs, must possess a working knowledge of genetics and be able to apply it to clinical practice. This expanding and evolving area also underscores the importance for every CRNA to establish an evidence-based practice, engaging in continued self-development and lifelong learning. This will help to reduce the risk involved with medication administration and enhance patient safety initiatives. It is a professional imperative that every patient deserves.

Key Points

- Many factors contribute to interindividual variations in drug responses observed, including culture, environment, and genetics.
- Exposure to xenobiotics may result in changes to drug targets or the biochemical systems that absorb, distribute, metabolize, or eliminate the drugs.
- The CYP enzymes are influenced by a variety of factors, including exposure to some of the chemicals that they metabolize.
- Humans possess obvious and not so obvious genetic variations. These genotypic variations are the consequence of the small mutations in the DNA sequence that occur in all organisms. Mutations provide the human species with an opportunity for adaptation to new environments.
- Some genetic polymorphisms are more frequently expressed within a group of people who share a commonality. Polymorphisms occur in drug target proteins and target pathways, in drug-metabolizing enzymes, and in unrelated physiologic variances that coincidentally influence pharmacodynamics and/or pharmacokinetics.

Chapter Questions

1. What factors are currently believed to contribute to interindividual variations to a given dose of a drug?
2. How do cultural practices and behaviors, such as dietary preferences or cigarette smoking, influence drug pathways and drug-metabolizing enzymes?
3. What association exists between an individual's genotype and phenotype?
4. Which genetic polymorphisms are associated with a specific ethnic or racial group?
5. How do interindividual variations to drug responses affect the practice of anesthesiology?

References

1. Garrod AE. *Inborn Errors of Metabolism*. London: Frowde, Hodder & Stoughton; 1909.
2. Galton F. *Hereditary Genius: An Inquiry Into Its Laws and Consequences*. London: MacMillan; 1869.
3. Haldane JBS. Disease and evolution. *Ric Sci Supp A*. 1949; 19:68–76.
4. Kalow W. Familial incidence of low pseudocholinesterase. *Lancet*. 1956;2:576.
5. Kalow W, Gunn DR. The relationship between dose of succinylcholine and duration of apnea in man. *J Pharm Exp Ther*. 1957;120:203.
6. Denborough MA, Lovell RR. Anaesthetic deaths in a family. *Lancet*. 1960;2:45.
7. Wilkinson GR. Pharmacokinetics. In: Hardman JG, Limbird LE, eds. *Goodman & Gilman's The Pharmacological Basis of Therapeutics*, 3rd ed. New York: McGraw-Hill; 2001:3–29.
8. Tanaka E. Clinically important pharmacokinetic drug-drug interactions: role of cytochrome P450 enzymes. *J Clin Pharm Ther*. 1998;23:403–416.
9. Park DV, Ioannides C. The role of nutrition in toxicology. *Drug Metab Rev*. 1994;26:739–765.
10. Park DV, Ioannides C. Drug-phytochemical interactions. *Inflammopharmacology*. 2003;11:7–42.
11. Lampe JW, King IB, Li S, et al. Brassica vegetables increase and apiaceous vegetables decrease cytochrome P450 1A2 activity in humans: changes in caffeine metabolite ratios in response to controlled vegetable diets. *Carcinogenesis*. 2000;21:1157–1162.
12. Visiten K, Poulsen HE, Loft S. Foreign compound metabolism capacity in man measured from metabolites of dietary caffeine. *Carcinogenesis*. 1992;13:1561–1568.

13. Vang O, Frandsen H, Hansen KT, Sorensen JN, Sorensen H, Andersen O. Biochemical effects of dietary intakes of different broccoli samples. I. Differential modulation of cytochrome P-450 activities in rat liver, kidney, and colon. *Metabolism.* 2001;50:1123–1129.

14. Maheo K, Morel F, Lanquet S, et al. Inhibition of cytochrome P-450 and induction of glutathione S-transferases by sulphoraphane in primary human and rat hepatocytes. *Cancer Res.* 1997;57:3649–3652.

15. Nakajima M, Yoshida R, Shimada N, Yamazaki H, Yokoi TL. Inhibition and inactivation of human cytochrome P450 isoforms by phenethyl isothiocyanate. *Drug Metab Disp.* 2001;29:1110–1113.

16. Bailey DG, Malcolm J, Arnold O, Spence JD. Grapefruit juice–drug interactions. *Br J Clin Pharmacol.* 1998;6:101–110.

17. Kupferschmidt HH, Ha HR, Ziegler WH, Meier PJ, Krahenbuhl S. Interaction between grapefruit juice and midazolam in humans. *Clin Pharmacol Ther.* 1995;58:20–28.

18. Kupferschmidt HH, Fattinger KE, Ha HR, Follath F, Krahenbuhl S. Grapefruit juice enhances the bioavailability of the HIV protease inhibitor saquinavir in man. *Br J Clin Pharmacol.* 1998;45:355–359.

19. Kanazawa S, Ohkubo T, Sugawara K. The effects of grapefruit juice on the pharmacokinetics of erythromycin. *Eur J Clin Pharmacol.* 2001;56:799–803.

20. Lundahl J, Regårdh CG, Edgar B, Johnson G. Relationship between the time of intake of grapefruit juice and its effect on pharmacokinetics and pharmacodynamics of felodipine in healthy subjects. *Eur J Clin Pharmacol.* 1995;49:61–67.

21. Lilja JJ, Kivistö KT, Neuvonen PJ. Duration of effect of grapefruit juice on the pharmacokinetics of the CYP3A4 substrate simvastatin. *Clin Pharmacol Ther.* 2000;68:384–390.

22. Takanaga H, Ohnishi A, Murakami H, et al. Relationship between time after intake of grapefruit juice and the effect on pharmacokinetics and pharmacodynamics of nisoldipine in healthy subjects. *Clin Pharmacol Ther.* 2000;67:201–214.

23. McGehee DS, Krasowski MD, Fund DL, Wilson B, Gronert GA, Moss J. Cholinesterase inhibition by potato glycoalkaloids slows mivacurium metabolism. *Anesthesiology.* 2000;93:510–519.

24. Centers for Disease Control and Prevention. Health, United States, 2008, tables 68 and 69. Available at: http://www.cdc.gov/nchs/data/hus/hus08. Accessed August 21, 2009.

25. Szlemko WJ, Wood JW, Thurman PJ. Native Americans and alcohol: past, present, and future. *J Gen Psychol.* 2006;133:435–451.

26. Centers for Disease Control and Prevention. MMWR: attributable deaths and years of potential life lost among American Indian and Alaska Natives—Unites States, 2001–2005.

Available at: http://www.cdc.gov/mmwr/preview/mmwrhtml/mm5734a3.htm. Accessed August 21, 2009.

27. Bloomfield K, Stockwell T, Gmel G, Rehn N. International comparisons of alcohol consumption. *Alcohol Res Health.* 2003;27:95–109.

28. Tonnesen H. The alcohol patient and surgery. *Alcohol Alcohol.* 1999;34:148–152.

29. Tonnesen H. Alcohol abuse and postoperative morbidity. *Dan Med Bull.* 2003;50:129–160.

30. Lau A, von Dossow V, Sander M, MacGuill M, Lanske N, Spies C. Alcohol use disorder and perioperative immune dysfunction. *Anesth Analg.* 2009;108:916–920.

31. Jia F, Chandra D, Homanics GE, Harrison NL. Ethanol modulates synaptic and extrasynaptic $GABA_A$ receptors in the thalamus. *J Pharmacol Exp Ther.* 2008;326:475–482.

32. Konishi M, Ishii H. Role of microsomal enzymes in development of alcoholic liver diseases. *J Gastroenterol Hepatol.* 2007;22(Suppl 1):S7–S10.

33. Villeneuve JP, Pichette V. Cytochrome P450 and liver diseases. *Curr Drug Metab.* 2004;5:273–282.

34. Centers for Disease Prevention and Health Promotion. Chronic disease prevention and health promotion, tobacco use: targeting the nation's leading killer, at a glance 2009. Available at: http://www.cdc.gov/nccdphp/publications/aag/osh.htm. Accessed August 9, 2009.

35. Zevin S, Benowitz NL. Drug interactions with tobacco smoking: an update. *Clin Pharmacokinet.* 1999;36:425–438.

36. Smith RG. An appraisal of potential drug interactions in cigarette smokers and alcohol drinkers. *J Am Podiatr Med Assoc.* 2009;99:81–88.

37. Chimbira W, Sweeney BP. The effect of smoking on postoperative nausea and vomiting. *Anaesthesia.* 2000;55:540–544.

38. Sweeney BP, Graying M. Smoking and anaesthesia: the pharmacological implications. *Anaesthesia.* 2009;64:179–186.

39. Centers for Disease Control and Prevention. Health, United States, 2008, table 98. Available at: http://www.cdc.gov/nchs/data/hus/hus08.pdf. Accessed August 26, 2009.

40. Barone GW, Curley BJ, Ketel BL, Lightfoot ML, Abul-Ezz SR. Drug interaction between St. John's wort and cyclosporine. *Ann Pharmacother.* 2000;34:1013–1016.

41. Ruschitzka F, Meier PJ, Turina M, Lüscher TF, Noll G. Acute heart transplant rejection due to St. John's wort. *Lancet.* 2000;355:548–549.

42. Piscitelli SC, Burstein AH, Chaitt D, Alfaro RM, Falloon J. Indinavir concentrations and St. John's wort. *Lancet.* 2000;355:547–548.

43. de Maat MM, Hoetelmans RM, Mathôt RA, et al. Drug interaction between St. John's wort and nevirapine. *AIDS.* 2001;15:420–421.

44. Yue QY, Bergquist C, Gerdén B. Safety of St. John's wort (*Hypericum perforatum*). *Lancet.* 2000;355:576–577.

45. Sim SC, Risinger C, Dahl ML, et al. A common novel *CYP2C19* gene variant causes ultrarapid drug metabolism relevant for the drug response to proton pump inhibitors and antidepressants. *Clin Pharmacol Ther.* 2006;79:103–113.

46. Caraco Y, Sheller J, Wood, AJ. Impact of ethnic origin and quinidine coadministration on codeine's disposition and pharmacodynamics effects. *J Pharm Exp Ther.* 1999;290:413–422.

47. Zwisler ST, Enggaard TP, Noehr-Jensen L, et al. The hypoalgesic effect of oxycodone in human experimental pain models in relation to the CYP2D6 oxidation polymorphism. *Basic Clin Pharmacol Toxicol.* 2009;104:335–344.

48. Liem EB, Lin CM, Suleman MI, et al. Anesthetic requirement is increased in redheads. *Anesthesiology.* 2004;101:279–283.

49. Gan TJ, Glass PS, Sigl J, et al. Women emerge from general anesthesia with propofol/alfentanil/nitrous oxide faster than men. *Anesthesiology.* 1999;90:1283–1287.

Pharmacology of Anesthetic Practice

Anesthetic Induction Agents

Russell R. Lynn, MSN, APN, CRNA

Introduction

In this chapter we focus on the pharmacologic properties of currently available anesthetic induction agents. The paradigm of intravenous (IV) anesthesia has shifted from one of primarily an agent to achieve induction of general anesthesia to that of total IV anesthesia. Total IV anesthesia has gained significant attention with the development of IV agents with rapid onset and ultra-short duration. In addition to these pharmacodynamic changes, the advent of advanced delivery systems with increasingly technologic systems and continuous electroencephalogram monitoring has placed a great deal of attention on these agents as well as the need for research and development of new agents with enhanced pharmacodynamic properties to allow nurse anesthetists to provide greater flexibility in providing anesthesia.

Barbiturates

The hallmark barbiturate agent is sodium thiopental, which was introduced into clinical practice in 1934. Another agent in this class is methohexital, which was developed and introduced into practice in 1957.[1] Barbiturates are derived from barbituric acid, which lacks central nervous system (CNS) activity. Structural alterations at number 2 and 5 carbon position allow barbiturates to take on a sedative-hypnotic action. Additional substitutions of branched chains rather than straight chains at the number 5 carbon position result in greater hypnotic activity. Substitution of a methyl radical at the number 5 carbon position produces a convulsant property, as seen with methohexital, whereas a phenol group at the number 5 carbon produces enhanced anticonvulsant properties, as seen with phenobarbital. Thiobarbiturates are formed when sulfur is substituted at the number 2 carbon position. This substitution increases lipid solubility and is associated with an enhanced hypnotic potency, a rapid onset, and short duration of action, such as seen with thiopental when compared with pentobarbital, which has an oxygen molecule substitution at the number 2 carbon position.[2]

Barbiturates exert their sedative-hypnotic effect in the CNS by interacting with the inhibitory neurotransmitter system, principally acting with γ-aminobutyric acid (GABA) on the $GABA_a$ receptor. GABA is the primary inhibitory neurotransmitter found within the CNS. When this agonist interacts with the $GABA_a$ receptor, it increases the duration of the chloride channel opening, allowing for a greater influx of chloride ions into the cell and creating a state of hyperpolarization, thereby inhibiting a subsequent action potential. Several medications, including etomidate and propofol, activate the $GABA_a$ receptors on different areas, essentially causing the same reaction: hyperpolarization of the cell membrane.[3] The ability of barbiturates to depress the reticular activating system, which is associated with human ability to maintain wakefulness, may be associated with its ability to decrease the rate of GABA neurotransmitter dissociation away from its $GABA_A$ receptor.[3] Barbiturates also exert a depressant effect on the sympathetic nervous system (SNS) ganglia. Although this effect does not decrease nerve conduction, it may explain the decrease in systemic blood pressure after IV administration of barbiturates.[3]

Pharmacokinetics

The desired pharmacologic effect of an IV anesthetic is to produce a level of sedation that progresses to hypnosis and unconsciousness as a result of a predictable dose. This effect is achieved after a rapid IV bolus is administered and plasma concentrations reach equilibrium with the brain within about 30 seconds (thiopental and methohexital) and is a reflection of rapid perfusion to CNS tissue. Factors that impact reaching this equilibrium quickly are cardiac output, blood volume, lipid solubility, protein binding, and the degree of ionization.[2–4,6] Of these factors, lipid solubility is the primary determinant of distribution. However, tissue perfusion remains an important determinant with regard to delivery and distribution of barbiturates in the body. As an example, alterations in perfusion such as seen in a hypovolemic patient accentuate delivery of barbiturates to CNS tissue located in the brain while further diminishing blood flow to skeletal muscle and adipose tissue, thus increasing drug concentration at the effect site (i.e., brain) while decreasing redistribution of the drug away from active CNS tissue, leading to profound cerebral and cardiovascular depression.[2,3,6]

Protein binding and lipid solubility are similar in barbiturates and are determined in large part by the amount of non-ionized drug available in active form because the ionized drug remains insoluble in lipid tissue. Thiopental is highly lipid soluble and is highly protein bound (72–86% bound to albumin). This does not appear to be altered with changes in serum pH between 7.35 and 7.5. Decreases in available protein for drug binding lead to exaggerated drug effects. Conditions such as uremia, liver cirrhosis, or hypoalbuminemia may lead to decreased protein binding and more free drug, ultimately leading to drug sensitivity or exaggerated clinical effects.

After a single IV bolus dose of barbiturate, redistribution to the muscle and adipose compartments leads to rapid reawakening. Within 30 to 40 seconds, the CNS tissues receive approximately 10% of the administered dose, and then concentrations decrease over the subsequent 5 minutes to one-half of the peak concentration due to redistribution. This redistribution occurs quickly because of the high lipid solubility of barbiturates in the CNS and the rate of cerebral perfusion.

Skeletal muscle tissue is an area in which barbiturates are redistributed because of this compartment's perfusion. Equilibrium between the plasma and skeletal muscle compartments is reached within 15 minutes after an initial IV bolus dose.[4] This point illustrates the importance of a decreased dose when there is a state of poor perfusion to the skeletal muscle compartment, as seen in the hypovolemic state or in conditions where there is a decreased amount of lean muscle mass, such as seen in the elderly population.[5–7]

The adipose compartment continues to have rising levels of thiopental 30 minutes after injection.[4] Because thiopental's fat-to-blood partition coefficient is 11, thiopental will continue to move into the fat compartment until the fat compartment is 11 times more saturated than the plasma compartment.[2] This only emphasizes the significance of perfusion to the site of redistribution. This compartment serves as a reservoir to additional doses of highly lipid-soluble barbiturates, slowing awakening with repeated doses and illustrating that doses should be calculated based on lean body mass.[5,6]

Metabolism

Redistribution away from CNS active tissue and not metabolism accounts for the cessation of hypnotic effects and rapid awakening associated with the use of barbiturates. The initial step to cause pharmacologic inactivation of barbiturate acids occur with side chain oxidation at the number 5 carbon position, which yields carbonic acid and hydroxyl thiopental, a water-soluble compound with little CNS activity. The principal method and site for thiopental metabolism is oxidation of the substitution at the number 5 carbon position, desulfuration at the number 2 carbon, and finally hydrolytic opening of the barbituric ring.[2] This primarily occurs within the endoplasmic reticulum of the hepatocytes. It should be noted that although hepatic dysfunction may slow redistribution, significant hepatic dysfunction must be present to cause prolonged duration of action as a result of decreased metabolism.[2,3] Metabolism of thiopental occurs slowly at a rate of 10% to 24% per hour.[5]

Because methohexital is less lipid soluble than thiopental, more drug remains in the plasma and is exposed to hepatic metabolic processes, resulting in a three- to four-fold increase in the metabolic rate when compared with thiopental. Oxidation of methohexital's side chain results in the creation of inactive metabolites. It should be noted that early awakening from methohexital, like thiopental, is a direct result of redistribution away from CNS active tissue and is not a result of its elevated rate of metabolism, as seen with methohexital. This elevated metabolic rate, however, is reflected in earlier return to psychomotor baseline function because less methohexital will be available to become sequestered in the adipose compartment, leading to prolonged dissipation or distribution from adipose compartment back into plasma compartment. Therefore hepatic clearance of methohexital is more dependent on cardiac output and hepatic perfusion than hepatic clearance of thiopental.[2,5]

Excretion

Even though all barbiturates are filtered by renal glomeruli, their high degree of protein binding allows for significant reabsorption with less than 1% of the administered dose excreted unchanged in the urine.[2]

Clinical Uses

Barbiturates are primarily used for their hypnotic properties and clinically used to induce general anesthesia. Additional clinical uses for barbiturates are the treatment of elevated intracranial pressure (ICP) and seizures. Barbiturates do not possess analgesic properties, and it is thought that these agents may actually lower the pain threshold, producing a state of antianalgesia. Although barbiturates produce unreliable sedation in the presence of pain, the concept of antianalgesia remains questionable.[2,8]

Induction doses of barbiturates cause a dose-dependent reduction in systemic blood pressure along with elevations of heart rate. The reduction in arterial pressure is related to a reduced output from the medullary vasomotor center, leading to vasodilatation of peripheral vessels and a reduced venous return to the right atrium. A central vagolytic effect is the most likely cause of the elevation in heart rate. Despite these changes, cardiac output is usually maintained by increased myocardial contractility as a compensatory baroreceptor reflex. Caution should be exercised in the absence of an adequate baroreceptor response, such as seen in patients with hypovolemia or congestive heart failure, because there may be profound reductions of both arterial blood pressure and cardiac output due to unopposed peripheral venous vasodilatation. Patients whose chronic hypertension is poorly controlled may experience wide swings in arterial blood pressure during induction if there is not a reduction in dosage. Therefore varied cardiovascular responses are possible with a barbiturate induction depending on volume status, baseline autonomic tone, and preexisting cardiovascular status.[9]

An anesthetic induction with barbiturates causes a depressed ventilatory response to hypercarbia or hypoxemia as a result of central depression of the medullary ventilatory centers. These agents may also lead to upper airway obstruction and apnea. Barbiturates do not completely obtund airway reflexes; therefore asthmatic patients may develop bronchospasm or the lightly anesthetized patient may develop laryngospasm with the introduction of the laryngoscope before achieving an appropriate level of anesthetic.

Barbiturates cause cerebral vasoconstriction, resulting in a reduction of cerebral blood flow and hence a reduced ICP. This reduction of ICP exceeds the decline in arterial pressure, thus maintaining cerebral perfusion pressure (cerebral perfusion pressure is equal to mean arterial pressure minus ICP or central venous pressure, whichever value is greater). Further protection of cerebral tissue by barbiturates is achieved through their ability to cause a reduction in cerebral metabolic oxygen requirements ($CMRO_2$) by up to 50% of normal.[9] This effect may offer protection during transient focal ischemic events but shows little benefit to global ischemia, such as those seen after cardiac arrest. Barbiturates do not cause muscle relaxation and in fact in the case of methohexital may actually induce involuntary skeletal muscle contractions.[9]

Barbiturates are contraindicated in patients who have inducible porphyrias. Although anaphylactic and anaphylactoid reactions are very rare,[7–9] sulfur-containing thiobarbiturates evoke mast cell–mediated histamine release, whereas oxybarbiturates do not.[9]

Barbiturates actions are potentiated by other centrally acting nervous system depressants such as ethanol or opioids.[9] Treatment of extravasations of barbiturates includes

Table 4-1 Comparison of Methohexital Versus Thiopental

Agent	Volume of Distribution (L/kg)	Protein Binding	Onset of Action	Duration of Action (min)	Elimination (h)	Clearance (mL/kg/min)
Methohexital	1.9–2.2	73%	IV 30–40 seconds	5–7	1.5–5	9.3–12.1
			Rectal 8–10 min			
Thiopental	1.7–2.5	72–86%	IV 60 seconds	10–30	3–8	1.6–4.3
			Rectal 5–11 min			

Source: From References 7 and 8.

Table 4-2 Barbiturate Agent Dose Range

Agent	Induction Dose (mg/kg)	Maintenance Dose
Methohexital	1–1.5	20–40 mg/4–7 min
Thiopental	3–5	50–100 mg PRN

PRN, as needed.

Source: From References 7–9.

administration of procaine 1% and the local application of heat to relieve pain and enhance vasodilatation.[7] Although there has not been an established treatment plan for the inadvertent intra-arterial injection of barbiturates, there is weak support in the literature for several interventions such as administration of a sympathetic block to the affected area if possible, immediate heparinization to prevent thrombus formation, and infiltration of an α-adrenergic blocking agent into the vasospastic area.[7]

Barbiturates should not be mixed with succinylcholine or other medications with an acidotic pH because precipitation will occur. It should also be noted that thiopental has a pH of 10.5 to 11, which will inhibit bacterial growth.[7]

No clinically significant activity is noted at the neuromuscular junction that results in relaxation of skeletal muscle. Because barbiturates have a rapid onset, they may be used in the treatment of grand mal seizures. However, since the advent of benzodiazepines with greater specificity in terms of site of action, benzodiazepines have become a better choice in the treatment of grand mal seizures.

Etomidate

Etomidate is a carboxylated imidazole-containing compound introduced to clinical practice in the United States in 1983 as an induction agent.[10] Etomidate is chemically unlike other induction agents in that its structure contains an imidazole nucleus that renders etomidate water soluble at acidic pH, but at physiologic pH it undergoes an intermolecular rearrangement resulting in a closed-ring structure that enhances lipid solubility.[2,3] Etomidate appears to exert its inhibitory effect at the GABA$_a$ receptor, binding to a specific site or sites and thereby enhancing its affinity for the inhibitory neurotransmitter GABA. Etomidate lacks the ability to modulate other ligand-gated ion channels.[2,10] Etomidate's predominant structure is isomer R(+), and this structure accounts for its anesthetic properties. Etomidate exerts a disinhibitory effect on the subcortical structures that suppress extrapyramidal motor activities,

which account for 30% to 60% of the incidence of myoclonus on induction.[9,11] This myoclonus side effect can be reduced or eliminated by the coadministration of a small dose of an opioid or a benzodiazepine.[3,10,12]

Pharmacokinetics

A combination of very high lipid solubility and a large fraction of non-ionized (99%) drug at physiologic pH accounts for etomidate's very rapid onset of action. Etomidate can reach peak brain concentration within 1 minute after IV injection. Approximately 76% of injected drug is protein bound primarily to albumin.[2,10] The rapid awakening after a single IV bolus dose is primarily due to redistribution of the active drug to neurologically inactive sites.[2,9] Prompt full recovery is the result of rapid metabolism that primarily occurs by hydrolysis of the ethyl side chain to carboxylic acid, a water-soluble inactive compound. Hepatic microsomal enzymes along with plasma esterases are responsible for this rapid metabolism. Less than 3% of the administered drug is recovered unchanged in the urine, whereas 85% of the inactive metabolite is found in the urine and 13% found in bile. Etomidate clearance is five times faster than thiopental.[2,9,10] Etomidate has a distribution half-life of 2.6 ± 1.3 minutes, a volume of distribution of 4.5 ± 2.2 L/kg, and an elimination half-life of 4.6 ± 2.6 hours.[10]

Clinical Uses

Etomidate may be used as an alternative to thiopental or propofol to induce general anesthesia when hemodynamic stability is critical. Etomidate should not be used for prolonged sedation because it suppresses adrenal function and has been associated with increased mortality when used in this fashion. The induction dose of etomidate is 0.2 to 0.4 mg/kg IV and reaches brain concentrations within 1 minute, producing unconsciousness.[2,3,9,10] It should be noted that etomidate does not provide analgesia, and therefore coadministration of a potent analgesic agent such as an opioid should be considered to avoid the hyperdynamic response associated with a direct laryngoscopy and intubation of the trachea. Postoperative nausea and vomiting have also been associated with etomidate.[2,3,9] Awakening after a single bolus dose of etomidate is quicker when compared with barbiturates and is attributed to etomidate's faster metabolism and lack of sequestration in the adipose compartment, resulting in a lower cumulative effect.[2,10] The primary restricting factor for widespread use of etomidate as an induction agent is its ability to suppress adrenocortical function even after a single bolus dose.[3,9,10]

Side Effects

Central Nervous System

Similar to barbiturates, etomidate is a vasoconstrictor and decreases cerebral blood flow by 35%, thus reducing ICP. Etomidate also decreases $CMRO_2$ demand by 45%. Because etomidate has minimal effects on hemodynamic values, cerebral perfusion pressure is maintained. Electroencephalographic patterns are similar to those caused by thiopental with the exception of increased beta activity, which may produce convulsion-like electroencephalographic patterns in focal epileptic patients. Therefore one should exercise caution when administering etomidate to focal epileptic patients. Conversely, etomidate does possess an anticonvulsant property having been used to terminate status epileptics.[3,9,10]

Cardiovascular

Etomidate is relatively cardiovascular stable and produces very minimal effects even in the presence of cardiovascular disease.[3,9,10,12] In fact, etomidate is considered the induction agent of choice for patients with cardiovascular disease or in situations where preserving a normal arterial blood pressure is paramount because etomidate may possess minimal α-adrenergic agonist properties, allowing for hemodynamic stability on induction.[2,3,10,13] Etomidate, however, should be used with extreme caution when administering to an acutely hypovolemic patient because sudden and profound hypotension may occur. Etomidate does not cause a release of histamine or decreased renal or hepatic blood flow.[3,10,12] Accidental intra-arterial injection has not been shown to produce any transient or long-term complications.[10]

Respiration

Although apnea is a possibility (usually associated with rapid administration), ventilatory suppression is less dramatic when compared with barbiturates. These effects on ventilation are transient and usually last between 3 and 5 minutes but could be exaggerated by the coadministration of opioids, benzodiazepines, or inhalational agents. Most patients induced with etomidate exhibit a decreased tidal volume with a compensatory increase in frequency.[2,13]

Allergy

The occurrence of an anaphylactic response is very rare with etomidate. However, during the induction phase it can be difficult to separate which agent administered may be responsible for producing the anaphylactic response because muscle relaxants are much more likely to cause a histamine release.[2]

Adrenal Suppression

Etomidate inhibits steroidogenesis by reducing the conversion of cholesterol to cortisol by suppression of 11-β-hydroxylase and 17-α-hydroxylase, the enzymes responsible for this conversion.[3,14] Adrenal suppression appears to be at the level of the adrenal cortex and occurs within 30 minutes of administering a single dose; it may last between 5 and 24 hours, resulting in diminished cortisol and aldosterone levels.[14–17] In specific patient subpopulations, such as in those with sepsis, who would greatly benefit from an intact and fully functional adrenal system, careful consideration should be given to the appropriateness of selection of induction agent.[17] Consideration with regard to steroid supplementation is also appropriate should the benefits of etomidate outweigh the risks of other induction agents because morbidity and mortality are increased in septic patients who receive as little as a one-time intubating dose of etomidate.[14,16–22] The literature remains controversial with regard to the use of etomidate with impending sepsis, and until the clinical significance of short-term adrenal suppression is clearly understood, the use of etomidate will be questioned.[16–22]

■ Ketamine

In 1970 the development and introduction of ketamine into clinical practice raised the expectation that the community achieved a monoanesthetic agent: One agent to provide amnesia, analgesia, and immobility was at hand. Ketamine is chemically similar to phencyclidine with a structure that contains a chiral center at the C_2 carbon of the cyclohexanone ring where two optical isomers exist: left-sided S(+) ketamine and right-sided S(−) ketamine. Ketamine is commercially available in a racemic mixture containing both optical isomers and the preservative benzethonium chloride.[23–24] Its pK_a is 7.5, and ketamine's lipid solubility is 10 times that of thiopental.[23–25] Ketamine provides rapid onset of action and short duration of action, achieving peak plasma concentrations within 1 minute after IV administration and within 5 minutes after intramuscular (IM) injection. Because ketamine is not highly protein bound, it is able to leave the blood rapidly initially to areas with high perfusion such as the brain, where peak plasma concentrations can be four to five times higher than plasma concentrations. Ketamine's significant lipid solubility allows for rapid transfer across the blood–brain barrier.[2] Ketamine causes increased cerebral blood flow and elevated cardiac output, which also leads to further speed of its cerebral effects. Initial awakening is related to redistribution to nonactive compartments.[9]

Ketamine produces a "dissociative" state of anesthesia described as an electrical and physiologic dissociation between the thalamoneocortical and limbic systems.[25] This produces a state characterized as cataleptic: Although the patient appears to be awake, they are unaware of the environment. Their eyes remain open with intact corneal and light reflexes and a slow nystagmic gaze.[24,25] Hypertonus and involuntary movements may be present. Ketamine produces profound analgesia and amnesia.[24] Biotransformation of ketamine occurs in the liver and produces several metabolites. The initial pathway involves the N-demethylation by cytochrome P-450 into norketamine. Norketamine has been shown to be an active metabolite and one-fifth to one-third as potent as ketamine in animal models.[26] This active metabolite may act to prolong ketamine's analgesia effects. Norketamine further undergoes hydroxylation and conjugation into inactive soluble compounds that are excreted in the urine.[23] Less than 4% of ketamine is recovered unchanged in urine, whereas less than 5% is found unchanged in fecal excretion. This indicates that most ketamine undergoes biotransformation.

Clinical Application

Ketamine has been shown to have several clinical indications. Anesthesia is induced when ketamine is administered intravenously at a dose range of 1 to 2 mg/kg or intramuscularly at 4 to 8 mg/kg. A loss of consciousness is seen within 30 to 60 seconds after IV administration or 2 to 4 minutes after IM administration. A return to consciousness is seen between 10 and 20 minutes after initial administration; however, a complete return to awareness may take an additional 60 to 90 minutes. Ketamine has been shown to produce retrograde amnesia. The unconsciousness associated with ketamine induction is accompanied by near-normal pharyngeal and laryngeal reflexes along with an increased production of salivary secretions. The inclusion of an antisialagogue should be considered as part of the preoperative medication regimen to reduce this excessive salivary secretion that may lead to coughing and laryngospasm. Glycopyrrolate may be a more desirable antisialagogue instead of those that can cross the blood–brain barrier such as atropine or scopolamine, because these agents may worsen ketamine-induced emergence delirium.[2]

Ketamine interacts with multiple binding sites throughout the body including N-methyl-D-aspartate (NMDA) along with non-NMDA glutamate receptors, nicotinic and muscarinic cholinergic receptors, monoaminergic receptors, and finally opioid receptors enabling the compound to have several clinical effects.[24] In addition to these receptors, ketamine also interacts with voltage-dependent ion channels, including sodium and calcium. Ketamine's inhibition of the sodium channels accounts for its mild local anesthetic effects, whereas its inhibition of the calcium channel reflects its ability to cause cerebral vasodilatation, enabling the compound to have several clinical effects.[24]

Ketamine has several other clinical applications when administered at subanesthetic dose ranges. Its ability to provide intense analgesia and amnesia allows ketamine to be used as an adjunct agent for painful procedures of short duration, such as dressing changes and debridement of tissue for the burn patient. Tolerance may develop with multiple exposures over a short time interval.[24] Ketamine has also been shown to improve postoperative analgesia and functional outcome when incorporated as part of a multimodal analgesic regimen.[26] Because of ketamine's rapid onset when administered intramuscularly, it has been a useful agent when inducing the difficult to manage patient, such as the mentally challenged or intoxicated patient requiring induction of anesthesia. Additionally, the induction of patients who are acutely hypovolemic has been safely accomplished using ketamine, taking advantage of the drug's ability to stimulate the SNS, thereby avoiding hypotension on induction.[23–25,27–29] Ketamine used as an induction agent also significantly conserves core body temperature during the first hour of anesthesia by avoiding peripheral vasodilatation and the shunting of core body heat to the periphery.[30]

Side Effects

Central Nervous System

Ketamine produces various side effects within the CNS that are considerably different from other IV induction agents. Ketamine at induction doses is capable of increasing cerebral blood flow as much as 60% as a result of significant decreases in cerebral vascular resistance.[31] Patients with intracranial pathology have been considered at risk for elevation in ICP when ketamine is administered. However, several studies involving both animals and humans have demonstrated no elevation of ICP when ventilations were mechanically controlled and ketamine was administered in dose ranges of 0.5 to 5 mg/kg.[32–35] These results suggest that ketamine can be safely administered to anesthetized patients who are mechanically ventilated without adverse effects due to alterations in cerebral hemodynamics. Traditional dogma identified ketamine as an agent that would cause elevations in $CMRO_2$. However, evidence shows that this may not be valid.[23]

Ketamine's antagonistic effect at the NMDA receptors may suggest the compound plays a neuroprotective role because activation of these receptors has been implicated as a source of cerebral ischemic damage.[23,27,28] Ketamine has been found to increase the cortical amplitude of somatosensory evoked potentials. However, visual and auditory evoked potentials are decreased by ketamine.[36]

Cardiovascular

Although ketamine has a direct negative inotropic effect on the myocardium, this effect is often overshadowed by its SNS stimulation. The SNS stimulation is not completely understood, and two theories are offered. First, because there are elevated circulating catecholamines after ketamine administration, it is thought that a central inhibition of catecholamine reuptake at the postganglionic nerve ending occurs. Second, ketamine may cause a direct agonistic effect on the SNS outflow of catecholamine. Both theories result in an elevation of hemodynamic parameters.[23] Systemic and pulmonary pressures, heart rate, cardiac output, cardiac workload, and myocardial oxygen requirements are all elevated after ketamine administration.[37] Arterial blood pressure in adults typically rises within 3 to 5 minutes of administration by 20 to 40 mm Hg and returns to predrug readings within 10 to 20 minutes. These effects can be blunted by the preadministration of a benzodiazepine, a short-acting α or β blocking agent, or coadministration of a potent inhalational agent.[23] Critically ill patients may exhibit an unexpected decrease in blood pressure when ketamine is administered if there is an inability of the sympathetic response to overshadow the direct negative myocardial effects associated with ketamine administration.[25–27]

Ketamine's effect on the cardiac rhythm appears to be inconsistent as ketamine may actually reverse digitalis-induced dysrhythmias. However, two case reports by Cabbabe and Behhanane (1985) discuss patients sedated with ketamine developing dysrhythmias when infiltration of local anesthetics containing epinephrine occurred.[23]

Respiration

Ketamine's effect on ventilation is minimal unless given in a rapid bolus or coadministered with opioids, which may lead to apnea. There is a dose-related shift to the right of the CO_2 response curve, but no changes in its slope are observed. Upper airway reflexes remain intact. Ketamine increases the production of salivary and tracheobronchial secretions, often requiring protection of the lungs from aspirate, and may require the addition of an antisialagogue to the preoperative medication regimen. Ketamine is a potent bronchial dilator and has been successfully used to decrease airway resistance in the face of bronchospasm and status asthmaticus.[38] The likely cause of this positive side effect is related to the elevation in circulating catecholamine levels.[23,38] Ketamine also produces as much as a 40% elevation in pulmonary vascular resistance and thereby increases the right ventricular workload by as much as 20%. There is also an intrapulmonary shunt as a result of this increased pulmonary resistance.[25]

General

Ketamine rarely causes an allergic reaction and is not associated with histamine liberation. Ketamine may also cause an irreversible inhibition of platelet aggregation similar to that seen with aspirin.[23] Ketamine appears to enhance nondepolarizing muscle relaxants by possibly interfering with calcium ion binding.[2] There may also be a prolonged duration of apnea associated with succinylcholine administration, reflecting inhibition of plasma cholinesterase activity.[2] Seizures have been described by Hirshmann et al. (1982) when ketamine is administered to patients receiving aminophylline infusions.[2] It appears that the combination of aminophylline and ketamine may lower the seizure threshold.[2]

Ketamine causes an increase in uterine tone and intensity of contraction in the first trimester but arguably has variable effects on uterine tone and contractility at term.[25] However, when compared with thiopental induction, ketamine provides rapid induction, greater analgesia and amnesia, and comparable incidences of unpleasant emergence delirium; fetal mortality was lower with ketamine. The induction of the maternal patient with ketamine provides better fetal umbilical pH, larger base excess, and less neonatal hypotension.[25]

Emergence phenomena with ketamine have an occurrence rate of between 5% and 30% and are described as sensations of floating, vivid dreams, and hallucinations. It is more commonly seen in female patients over 16 years of age who have received large doses of ketamine and whose operative time is short. The administration of a benzodiazepine has been shown to significantly decrease the occurrence of emergence delirium.[23] No evidence exists that emergence in a quiet area has any impact on emergence delirium.[2]

Propofol

Propofol, a nonbarbiturate sedative-hypnotic anesthetic agent, was approved by the U.S. Food and Drug Administration for clinical practice in 1989.[39] Propofol (2,6-diisopropylphenol) is available as a 1% solution for IV use. Because of its low water solubility, it requires a lipid vehicle and is prepared in an emulsion of 10% soybean oil as the oil phase, 2.25% glycerol, and 1.2% purified egg lecithin as the emulsification agent.[40] Propofol, unlike previous induction agents, is not a chiral compound.

Propofol exerts its sedative-hypnotic characteristics predominantly on the $GABA_a$ receptors with no effect noted on the ligand-gated ion channels. Because GABA is the predominant inhibitory neurotransmitter within the CNS, activation permits the increase of chloride transmembrane conduction, allowing for hyperpolarization to occur. This hyperpolarization of the postsynaptic cell membrane results in an inhibition of the neuron.

Administration of propofol as a rapid IV bolus in a dose range of 1.5 to 2.5 mg/kg (equally potent as thiopental 4–5 mg/kg or methohexital 1.5 mg/kg) causes unconsciousness within 30 seconds. However, a unique characteristic of propofol is that it produces a more complete and rapid reawakening compared with other IV induction agents. After the initial bolus, there is rapid redistribution of propofol away from effect sites (brain) to other less well-perfused tissues (muscle), which accounts for the rapid decline in plasma levels and reawakening. Propofol's metabolic clearance exceeds that of hepatic blood flow, indicating an extrahepatic pathway associated with propofol metabolism.[39,40]

Hepatic metabolism of propofol is extensive and rapid, resulting in an inactive water-soluble sulfate and glucuronic acid metabolites with renal clearance.[41] Cytochrome P-450 hydroxylation of propofol into 4-hydroxypropofol, an active metabolite one-third as potent as propofol, may occur. This active metabolite then undergoes glucuronidation or sulfation into a water-soluble inactive substance.[41] Although controversial, pulmonary uptake and elimination may also be responsible for extrahepatic metabolism of propofol.[42] Propofol can be altered in pulmonary tissue to form 2,6-diisopropyl-1,4 quinol and may impact the initial availability of propofol because it appears that significant amounts of propofol are involved with first-pass pulmonary uptake and then released back into the systemic circulation.[41–43]

Renal elimination plays a paramount role in the elimination of propofol.[41] Although rapid redistribution and metabolism are responsible for propofol's characteristic rapid reawakening, there appears to be no evidence that hepatic or renal dysfunction impacts this. Propofol does cross into fetal circulation but appears to be rapidly cleared in the neonate.[43] Although propofol is present in breast milk 4 to 8 hours in concentrations ranging from 0.12 to 0.97 mg/mL after an induction dose of propofol, the effects on the neonate would be negligible.[43]

Since its introduction into clinical practice in 1989, propofol has become the drug of choice for many aspects of anesthesia. One such aspect is when a rapid return of neurologic function is warranted, such as ambulatory surgery where a timely discharge from the postanesthesia care unit is important.[39]

Induction of general anesthesia with propofol is achieved with an IV dose of 1.5 to 2.5 mg/kg, producing unconsciousness in 30 seconds. Pediatric patients require a larger induction dose of propofol on a milligram per kilogram basis due to their larger volume of distribution and an elevated clearance rate.[39] Propofol level found in colostrum after a single induction dose is similar to that of thiopental, and neonate ingestion should be avoided for 4 to 8 hours after propofol administration.[44] Geriatric patients require careful consideration and generally require a reduced induction dose (reduced by 25–50%) due to a smaller central volume of distribution and a reduced clearance rate.[39–45] Others[46] suggest that alternatives to propofol be considered for induction of patients over 50 years of age to avoid significant hypotension after induction. Adachi et al. suggested the consideration of a patient's cardiac output in addition to age and weight before calculating an induction dose of propofol.[45] Patients with an elevated cardiac output may require a larger dose of propofol to achieve a hypnotic state.[45] The use of propofol as an induction agent for patients with hypotension, decreased cardiac output, or hemorrhagic shock requires a significant reduction in the induction dose and absolute careful titration to desired effects to avoid profound hypotension and cardiovascular collapse.[47–51] Standard induction dose should be reduced by 36% to 43%[47] or by as much as 50%[45] for the hemorrhagic patient undergoing vigorous resuscitation or up to 80% to 90% reductions for patients undergoing initial fluid resuscitation.[48] Several factors appear to support this dose reduction: increased peak plasma levels of propofol seen in hemorrhagic shock, reduction of cardiac output leading to a slower redistribution of propofol away from active sites, and slower metabolism leading to more active drug.[49] Coadministration of premedicants such as fentanyl or midazolam has been shown to have an additive effect on reducing systemic blood pressure when given with a propofol induction.[51] Maintenance of general anesthesia with a propofol infusion at rates between 100 and 300 mcg/kg/min can be accomplished with the addition of an opioid to provide analgesia.[39] General anesthesia maintained by propofol infusion is associated with less postoperative nausea and vomiting and minimal residual sedation effects.[39]

Propofol has become the agent of choice for sedation given its short context-sensitivity half-time and prompt recovery without residual sedation.[52] Typical infusion rates range from 25 to 100 mcg/kg/min to produce reliable amnesia effects.[39] The addition of midazolam and/or an opioid may provide a combination useful for monitored anesthesia care requiring deeper sedation along with an analgesic component. Propofol infusions have been used in the intensive care arena to provide sedation for mechanically ventilated patients, including postoperative patients recovering from cardiac or neurosurgery or head injuries. Propofol's ability to control the stress response and anticonvulsive and amnesic properties are desirable in this patient population.[39] Propofol infusion syndrome has been described as an unexplained tachycardia, metabolic acidosis with myocardial dysfunction, and possibly rhabdomyolysis in patients receiving a propofol infusion.[53] This has been seen in both pediatric and adult populations and usually with infusion rates greater than 75 mg/kg/min for a duration greater than 24 hours; however, cases have been reported with short-term infusions for surgical anesthesia.[33,39,54] Propofol infusions with unexplained tachycardia should prompt providers to conduct laboratory evaluations for metabolic acidosis and serum lactate concentrations. Early stages of metabolic acidosis can be resolved by discontinuance of the propofol infusion; however, progressive cardiogenic shock should be treated more aggressively.[53,54]

Propofol's antiemetic properties, although not clearly understood, appear to be exerted in the subcortical center, possibly providing a direct depressant effect on the vomiting center.[55] Nevertheless, the occurrence of postoperative nausea and vomiting is decreased when propofol is used regardless of the technique and even when administered at subtherapeutic doses of 10- to 15-mg boluses.[55] Induction and maintenance with propofol is more effective in preventing postoperative nausea and vomiting when compared with ondansetron.[56]

Propofol has an anticonvulsant property that is exerted on the GABA-mediated presynaptic and postsynaptic neuron by its inhibition of chloride ion channels. Doses greater than 1 mg/kg have been demonstrated to decrease seizure duration.[57]

Side Effects

Central Nervous System

Propofol decreases cerebral blood flow, ICP, and $CMRO_2$.[39,58] Large doses of propofol may decrease arterial blood pressure enough to alter cerebral perfusion pressure.[39,58,59]

Propofol does not alter cerebral vascular autoregulation responses to blood flow or $PaCO_2$.[60] Sedation with propofol for patients produces similar electroencephalographic changes seen with thiopental and at high doses induces burst suppression.[39] Spinal cord function monitoring such as cortical somatosensory evoked potentials are not significantly altered by propofol administration.[39,61]

Cardiovascular

Propofol at comparable thiopental doses produces a greater decrease in systemic blood pressure, cardiac output, and systemic vascular resistance. These changes are primarily due to the relaxation of vascular smooth muscle caused by propofol inhibition of the SNS.[39,45,46,48–50,62] Propofol also exhibits a negative inotropic effect that may be caused by decreasing intracellular calcium availability.[39,62] Hypotension after propofol induction may be substantially exacerbated in the geriatric population and in those patients with hypovolemia or left ventricular dysfunction. Adequate fluid resuscitation is suggested before administration of a markedly reduced dose of propofol for induction.[39,45–50] There may be a depression of the baroreceptor reflex associated with propofol. Bradycardia and asystole have been reported after induction of anesthesia with propofol. These dysrhythmias have occurred despite prophylaxis or treatment with anticholinergics; in fact, responsiveness to atropine is attenuated, suggesting that propofol suppresses the SNS, allowing for parasympathetic system dominance.[63] Treatment of propofol-induced bradycardia or asystole may require a β agonist such as isoproterenol.[39,62]

Lungs

Propofol causes a dose-dependent depression of ventilations, leading to apnea in 25% to 35% of patients who receive an induction dose.[63] Whereas a sedative infusion will result in depression of tidal volume and respiratory rate, ventilatory responses to hypoxia and hypercarbia suggesting supplemental oxygen should always be applied.[39,63] Hypoxic pulmonary vasoconstriction remains intact with propofol administration.[63]

Propofol strongly supports bacterial growth; however, its solvent appears to have some bactericidal and bacteriostatic properties. Nevertheless, there have been reports of postsurgical infections manifested by temperature elevations associated with the administration of propofol.[39,64] Because of these incidences, it is recommended that aseptic techniques be instituted when handling propofol that include the disinfecting of the rubber stopper or ampule neck with 70% isopropyl alcohol. The entire contents of the ampule or vial should be drawn into a sterile syringe and used promptly. Any opened but unused propofol should be discarded within 6 hours of opening. Propofol infusion tubing should be discarded every 12 hours.[39,64]

Pain on Injection

The incidence of pain on injection associated with propofol ranges from 78% to 90% in adults during induction of general anesthesia and is more common with injection sites in the dorsum of the hand.[40,65,66] Several methods to alleviate this pain have been noted in the literature. Although the manufacturer suggests that nothing should be added to this mediation, lidocaine of different volumes and concentrations have been added to the same syringe containing propofol in clinical practice. This may alter the stability of the propofol and result in the appearance of an oily surface layer and the coalescence of oil droplets, which may lead to changes in the macroscopic appearance. These oil droplets may coalesce to a size large enough to occlude peripheral capillaries. Intravenous administration of droplets larger than 5 μm in diameter may pose a risk of pulmonary embolism.[40] Masaki et al.[40] reported finding oil droplets larger than 5 μm after adding 20 to 40 mg of lidocaine to 200 mg of propofol. Alternative methods may involve placing a tourniquet proximally to the IV site and administering lidocaine via the IV line and then removing the tourniquet and administering the propofol via the same IV site with superb efficacy.[67] Alternative approaches have included pretreatment with remifentanil[67] or ketamine 100 mcg/kg,[66] which have both shown positive results in decreasing pain associated with the injection of propofol.

Key Points

- Chemical Structures of Anesthesia Induction Agents
- Pharmacodynamics of Anesthesia Induction Agents
- Pharmacokinetics of Anesthesia Induction Agents
- Indications, Dosage, and Common Side Effects of Anesthesia Induction Agents

Chapter Questions

1. Are providers satisfied with the currently available induction agents?

2. With further research will we achieve a monoanesthetic agent capable of providing amnesia, analgesia, and lack of movement without impacting ventilation or cardiac status?

3. How will dexmedetomidine impact the induction of general anesthesia?

4. How will uncovering an individual's metabolic profile impact our selection of and dosing of an induction agent?

5. How will an aging population impact research into future induction agents?

6. What impact will the growing amount of noninvasive procedures have on development of future induction agents?

7. What impact will the growth of ambulatory surgery centers have on the development of future induction agents?

8. How will this future research be funded?

References

1. Hudson RJ, Stanski DR, Burch PG. Pharmacokinetics of methohexital and thiopental in surgical patients *Anesthesiology*. 1983,59:215–219.

2. Stoelting RK, Hiller SC. *Pharmacology and Physiology in Anesthetic Practice*, 4th ed. Philadelphia: Lippincott Williams & Wilkins; 2006.

3. Barash PG, Cullen BF, Stoelting RK. *Clinical Anesthesia*, 5th ed. Philadelphia: Lippincott Williams & Wilkins; 2006.

4. Saidman LJ, Eger EL. The effect of thiopental metabolism on duration of anesthesia. *Anesthesiology*. 1966;27:118–126.

5. Mark LC, Brand I, Kamuyssi S, et al. Thiopental metabolism by human liver in vivo and in vitro. *Nature*. 1965;206:1117–1119.

6. Homer TD, Stanski DR. The effects on increasing age on thiopental. *Anesthesiology*. 1985;62:714–724.

7. *Drug information online: Anesthetics, Barbiturate (Systemic)*. Available at: www.drugs.com/mmx/thiopental-sodium.html. Accessed June 20, 2009.

8. Kitahata LM, Saberksi L. Are barbiturates hyperanalgesic *J Anesthesiol*. 1992;77:1059–1061.

9. Morgan GE, Mikhail MS, Murray MJ. *Clinical Anesthesiology*, 4th ed. New York: McGraw-Hill; 2006.

10. Giese JL, Stanley TH. Etomidate: a new intravenous anesthetic induction agent. *Pharmacotherapy*. 1983;3:251–257.

11. Tomlin SL, Jenkins A, Lieb WR, et al. Stereoselective effects of etomidate optical isomers on gamma-aminobutyric acid type A receptors in animals. *Anesthesiology*. 1998;88:707–718.

12. Huter L, Schreiber T, Gugel M, Schwarzkopf K. Low-dose intravenous midazolam reduces etomidate-induced myo-clonus: a prospective, randomized study in patients undergoing elective cardioversion. *Anesth Analg.* 2007;105:1290–1302.

13. Gooding JM, Weng JT, Smith RA, Berninger GT, Kirby RR. Cardiovascular and pulmonary responses following etomidate induction of anesthesia in patients with demonstrated cardiac disease. *Anesth Analg.* 1979;58:40–42.

14. Sarkar M, Laussen PC, Zurakowski D, Shukla A, Kussman B, Odegard K. Hemodynamic responses to etomidate on induction of anesthesia in pediatric patients. *Anesth Analg.* 2005;101:645–650.

15. Zed PJ, Abu-Laban RB, Harrison DW. Intubating conditions and hemodynamic effects of etomidate for rapid sequence intubation in the emergency department: an observational cohort study. *Acad Emerg Med.* 2006;13:378–383.

16. Fragen RJ, Shanks CA, Molteni A, Avram MJ. Effects of etomidate on hormonal responses to surgical stress. *Anesthesiology.* 1984;61:652–656.

17. Nestor NB, Burton JH. ED use of etomidate for rapid sequence induction. *Am J Emerg Med.* 2008;26:946–950.

18. Heldreth AN, Mejia VA, Maxwell RA, Smith PW, Dart BW, Barker DE. Adrenal suppression following a single dose of etomidate for rapid sequence induction: a prospective randomized study. *J Trauma.* 2008;65:573–579.

19. Ray DC, McKeown DW. Effect of induction agent on vasopressor and steroid use, and outcome in patients with septic shock. *Crit Care.* 2007;11:1–8.

20. Zed PJ, Mabasa VH, Slavik RS, Abu-Laban RB. Etomidate for rapid sequence intubation in the emergency department: is adrenal suppression a concern? *Can J Emerg Med.* 2006;8:347–350.

21. Tekwani KL, Watts HF, Rzechula KH, Sweis RT, Kulstad EB. A prospective observational study of the effect of etomidate on septic patients mortality and length of stay. *Acad Emerg Med.* 2009;16:11–14.

22. Sprung CL, Annane D, Keh D, et al. Hydrocortisone therapy for patients with septic shock. *N Engl J Med.* 2008;358:111–124.

23. Reich DL, Silvay G. Ketamine: an update on the first twenty-five years of clinical experience. *Can J Anaesth.* 1989;36:186–197.

24. Kohrs R, Durieux ME. Ketamine: teaching an old drug new tricks. *Anesth Analg.* 1998;87:1186–1193.

25. White PF, Way WL, Trevor AJ. Ketamine—its pharmacology and therapeutic uses. *Anesthesiology.* 1982;56:119–136.

26. Nenigauz C, Guignard B, Fletcher D, Sessler DI, Dupont X, Chauvin M. Interoperative small dose ketamine enhances analgesia after outpatient knee arthroscopy. *Anesth Analg.* 2001;93:606–612.

27. Himmelseher S, Durieux ME. Revising a dogma: ketamine of patients with neurological injury? *Anesth Analg.* 2005;101:524–534.

28. Kirota K, Lambert DG. Ketamine: its mechanisms of action and unusual clinical uses. *Br J Anaesth.* 1996;77:441–444.

29. Morris C, Perris A, Klein J, Mahoney P. Anaesthesia in haemodynamically compromised emergency patients: does ketamine represent the best choice of induction agent? *Anaesthesia.* 2009;64:532–539.

30. Ikeda T, Kazama T, Sessler D, et al. Induction of anesthesia with ketamine reduces the magnitude of redistribution hypothermia. *Anesth Analg.* 2001;93:934–938.

31. Takeshita H, Okuda Y, Sari A. The effects of ketamine on cerebral circulation and metabolism in man. *Anesthesiology.* 1972;36:69–75.

32. Pfenninger E, Dick W, Ahnefeld FW. The influence of ketamine on both normal and raised ICP of artificially ventilated animals. *Eur J Anaesth.* 1985;2:297–307.

33. Friesen RH, Thieme PE, Honda AT, et al. Changes in anterior fontanel pressure in preterm neonates receiving isoflurane, halothane, fentanyl, or ketamine. *Anesth Analg.* 1987;66:431–434.

34. Mayberg TS, Lam AM, Matta BF, et al. Ketamine does not increase cerebral blood flow velocity or intracranial pressure during isoflurane/nitrous oxide anesthesia in patients undergoing craniotomy. *Anesth Analg.* 1995;81:84–89.

35. Albanese J, Arnaud S, Ray M, et al. Ketamine decreases intracranial pressure and electroencephalographic activity in traumatic brain injury patients during propofol sedation. *Anesthesiology.* 1997;87:1328–1334.

36. Schubert A, Licine MG, Lineberry PJ. The effects of ketamine on human somatosensory evoked potentials and its modification by nitrous oxide. *Anesthesiology.* 1990;72:33–39.

37. Tweed WA, Minuck MS, Mymin D. Circulatory response to ketamine anesthesia. *Anesthesiology.* 1972;37:613–619.

38. Sarma VJ. Use of ketamine in severe asthma. *Acta Anaesth Scand.* 1992;36:106–107.

39. Smith I, White PF, Nathanson M, Gouldson R. Propofol: an update on its clinical use. *Anesthesiology.* 1994;81:1005–1043.

40. Masaki Y, Tanaka M, Nishikawa T. Physiochemical compatibility of propofol-lidocaine mixture. *Anesth Analg.* 2003;97:1646–1651.

41. Takizawa D, Hiraoka H, Goto F, Yamamoto K, Horiuchi R. Human kidneys play an important role in the elimination of propofol. *Anesthesiology.* 2005;102:327–330.

42. Kuipers JA, Boer F, Olieman W, Burm AG, Bovill J. First pass lung uptake and pulmonary clearance of propofol. *Anesthesiology.* 1999;91:1780–1787.

43. Pawidowica AL, Fornol E, Mardarowicz M. The role of human lung in biotransformation of propofol. *Anesthesiology.* 2000;93:922–997.

44. Dailland P, Cockshott ID, Lirzin JD, et al. Intravenous propofol during cesarean section: placental transfer, concentrations in breast milk, and neonatal effects. *Anesthesiology.* 1989;71:827–834.

45. Adachi Y, Watanabe K, Higuchi H, Satoh T. The determinants of propofol induction of anesthesia dose. *Anesth Analg.* 2001;92:656–661.

46. Reich DL, Hossain S, Krol M, et al. Predictors of hypotension after induction of general anesthesia. *Anesth Analg.* 2005; 101:622–628.

47. Gurese E, Sungurtekin H, Tomatir E, Dogan II. Assessing propofol induction of anesthesia dose using bispectral index analysis. *Anesth Analg.* 2004;98:128–131.

48. Shafer S. Shock values. *Anesthesiology.* 2004;101:567–568.

49. Johnson K, Egan T, Kern SE, White JL, McJames SW. The influence of hemorrhagic shock on propofol: a pharmacokinetic and pharmacodynamic analysis. *Anesthesiology.* 2003;99:409–420.

50. Johnson KB, Egan T, Kern SE, McJames SW, Cluff ML, Pace NL. Influence of hemorrhagic shock followed by crystalloid resuscitation on propofol. *Anesthesiology.* 2004;101:647–659.

51. Olmos M, Ballester JA, Vidarte MA, Elizalde JL, Escobar A. The combined effect of age and premedication on the propofol requirements for induction by target controlled infusion. *Anesth Analg.* 2000;90:1157–1161.

52. Bryson HM, Fulton BR, Fauld D. Propofol: update on its use in anesthesia conscious sedation. *Drugs.* 1995;50:513–559.

53. Cravens GT, Packer DL, Johnson ME. Incidence of propofol infusion syndrome during noninvasive radiofrequency ablation for atrial flutter or fibrillation. *Anesthesiology.* 2007;106:1134–1138.

54. Burro BK, Johnson ME, Packer DL. Metabolic acidosis associated with propofol in the absence of other factors. 1995;50:513–559.

55. Borgeat A, Wilder-Smith OHG, Suter PM. The nonhypnotic therapeutic applications of propofol. *Anesthesiology.* 1994;84:642–656.

56. Gan TJ, Ginsberg B, Grant BS. Double-blinded, randomized comparison of ondansetron and intraoperative propofol to prevent post operative nausea and vomiting. *Anesthesiology.* 1996;85:1036–1042.

57. Avramov MN, Husain MM, White PF. The comparative effects of methohexital, propofol, and etomidate for electroconvulsive therapy. *Anesth Analg.* 1995;81:596–602.

58. Kaisti KK, Langsjo JW, Aalto S. Effects of sevoflurane, propofol, and adjunct nitrous oxide on regional cerebral blood flow, oxygen consumption, and blood volume in humans. *Anesthesiology.* 2003;99:603–613.

59. Giard R, Moumdjian R, Boudreault D. The effect of propofol sedation on intracranial pressure of patients with space occupying lesion. *Anesth Analg.* 2004;99:573–577.

60. Strebel S, Kaufmann M, Guardiola PM, Schafer HG. Cerebral vaso-motor responsiveness to carbon dioxide is preserved during propofol and midazolam anesthesia in humans. *Anesth Analg.* 1994;78:884–888.

61. Boisseau N, Madany M, Staccini P. Comparison of the effects of sevoflurane and propofol on cortical somatosensory evoked potentials. *Br J Anaesth.* 2002;88:785–789.

62. Robinson BJ, Ebert TJ, O'Brien TJ. Mechanisms whereby propofol mediates peripheral vasodilatation in humans. Sympathetic inhibition or direct vascular relaxation? *Anesthesiology.* 1997;86:64–72.

63. Bouillon T, Bruhn J, Radu-Radulescu L, et al. Mixed effects modeling of the intrinsic ventilatory depressant potency of propofol in the non steady state. *Anesthesiology.* 2004; 100:240–250.

64. Kuehnert MJ, Webb RM, Fochimsen EM, et al. *Staphylococcus aureus* blood stream infections among patients undergoing electroconvulsive therapy traced to breaks in infection control and possible extrinsic contamination by propofol. *Anesth Analg.* 1997;85:420–425.

65. Masaki Y, Tanaka M, Nishikawa T. Changes in propofol concentration in a propofol lidocaine 9:1 volume mixture. *Anesth Analg.* 2000;90:989–892.

66. Koo SW, Cho SJ, Kim YK, Ham KD, Hwang JH. Small dose ketamine reduces the pain of propofol injection. *Anesth Analg.* 2006;103:1444–1447.

67. Aouda MT, Siddik-Sayyid SM, Al-Alami AA, Barabka AS. Multimodal analgesia to prevent propofol induced pain: pretreatment with remifentanil and lidocaine versus remifentanil or lidocaine alone. *Anesth Analg.* 2007;104: 1540–1543.

Benzodiazepines

Steve Alves, PhD, CRNA
Timothy Finn, MS, CRNA

Objectives

After completing this chapter, the reader should be able to

- Describe the mechanism of action of benzodiazepines.
- Contrast the application, benefits, and disadvantages of various specialized approaches to administering benzodiazepines.
- Discuss drug interactions of benzodiazepines with opioids.
- List three side effects of benzodiazepines in adults.

Introduction

Benzodiazepines represent a class of drugs that possess varying degrees of anxiolysis, sedation, and anticonvulsant actions; spinal cord–mediated skeletal muscle relaxation; and amnestic properties. Benzodiazepines are an ideal drug for treating and managing anxiety, insomnia, seizure disorders, and muscle spasms and as a premedication for surgical, invasive interventional radiography, and dental procedures. Since their discovery and development in the 1950s and early 1960s, benzodiazepines have become the mainstay for reducing anxiety and providing sedation in the preanesthetic care of patients. First developed by an Austrian chemist, Leo Sternbach, chlordiazepoxide (Librium) was patented as the first in a series of benzodiazepines introduced in the 1960s through the 1980s.[1] Benzodiazepines are categorized as short acting, intermediate acting, or long acting, depending on their individual elimination half-life. The most commonly used benzodiazepines in clinical anesthesia care are midazolam (Versed), lorazepam (Ativan), and diazepam (Valium). The therapeutic uses, routes of administration, and pharmacologic aspects of benzodiazepines that are marketed in the United States are summarized in Table 5-1.

Mechanism of Action

Structurally, benzodiazepines consist of a benzene ring fused to a seven-member diazepine ring. Diazepine is a seven-member heterocyclic compound with two nitrogen atoms. All benzodiazepines in clinical use have the capacity to promote the binding of the major inhibitory neurotransmitter γ-aminobutyric acid (GABA) to the $GABA_a$ subtype of GABA receptors. GABA receptors exist as multisubunit, ligand-gated chloride channels, thereby enhancing the GABA-induced ionic currents through these channels.[2] The chloride channels are held open for an extended period of time, resulting in a hyperpolarization of the postsynaptic cell membrane and making the cells less excitable. They attach themselves only to the α subunits of GABA receptors located in the cerebral cortex, cerebellar cortex, and thalamus.[3]

Clinical Pharmacology

Benzodiazepines can be absorbed orally, intramuscularly, intravenously, intranasally, and rectally to produce their effects. Upon intravenous (IV) injection of a single dose, they are readily circulated to the brain, affecting the $GABA_a$ receptor sites within seconds.[3] After attaching to the receptor sites, they eventually become terminated by a process of redistribution to tissues. Diazepam, midazolam, and lorazepam are all absorbed in the gastrointestinal tract when given orally. Peak plasma levels are achieved in about 1 to 2 hours. Intramuscular injections of lorazepam and midazolam are well absorbed and usually take 30 to 90 minutes for peak plasma levels to be achieved.

Midazolam, lorazepam, and diazepam are all lipid soluble. Midazolam is stored as water soluble, but at physiologic pH it closes its imidazole ring, making it highly lipid soluble. Imidazole is an organic compound with the formula $C_3H_4N_2$. This aromatic heterocyclic is classified as an

Table 5-1 Drug and Trade Names, Routes of Administration, Therapeutic Uses, and $t_{1/2}$ β of Benzodiazepines

Drug (Trade Name)	Routes of Administration	Therapeutic Uses	$t_{1/2}$ β (h)
Alprazolam (Xanax)	Oral	Anxiety disorders, agoraphobia	12–15
Chlordiazepoxide (Librium)	Oral, IM, IV	Anxiety disorders, management of alcohol withdrawal, anesthetic premedication	8–18
Clonazepam (Klonopin)	Oral	Seizure disorders, adjunctive treatment in acute mania, certain movement disorders	18.7–39
Clorazepate (Tranxene)	Oral	Anxiety disorders, seizure disorders	2.4–3
Diazepam (Valium)	Oral, IM, IV, rectal	Anxiety disorders, status epilepticus, skeletal muscle relaxation, anesthetic premedication	36–50
Estazolam (Prosom)	Oral	Insomnia	14–15
Flurazepam (Dalmane)	Oral	Insomnia	2–3
Lorazepam (Ativan)	Oral, IM, IV	Anxiety disorders, preanesthetic medication	10–22
Midazolam (Versed)	IM, IV	Preanesthetic, intraoperative medication	1.7–2.6
Oxazepam (Serax)	Oral	Anxiety disorders	3–21
Prazapam (Centrax)	Oral	Anxiety disorders	63–72
Quazepam (Doral)	Oral	Insomnia	25–41
Temazepam (Restoril)	Oral	Insomnia	10–21
Triazolam (Halcion)	Oral	Insomnia	2–3
Eszopiclone (Lunesta)	Oral	Insomnia	6–8
Zaleplon (Sonata)	Oral	Insomnia	1–2
Zolpidem (Ambien)	Oral	Insomnia	2–3
Benzodiazepine Receptor Antagonist			
Flumazenil (Romazicon)	IM, IV	Reversal of benzodiazepine agonists	0.7–1.3

IM, intramuscular; IV, intravenous.

alkaloid. Despite similar volumes of distributions (1.0–1.5 L/kg) and similar percentage of protein binding (96–98%) of all three, midazolam is a far superior benzodiazepine to be used in the anesthesia clinical setting due to its high clearance level (6–8 mL/kg/min) compared with diazepam or lorazepam (0.2–1.0 mL/kg/min). The percentage protein binding for all three are all similar at 96% to 98%.[2,3]

Benzodiazepines are metabolized by the liver, specifically by the cytochrome P-450 enzyme induction system.

It is important to understand that some benzodiazepines may have active metabolites, whereas others do not. Midazolam has active metabolites that are quickly conjugated and exhibit no secondary effects after metabolism, whereas diazepam does have active metabolites that can still produce some sedative effects, resulting in an elimination half-life up to 20 hours.

After a single-dose injection, benzodiazepines have multiple effects on the body systems. In the central nervous system they cause a reduction in the cerebral oxygen metabolism and cerebral blood flow.[3] Benzodiazepines appear to have some cerebral protection against hypoxia and are useful as anticonvulsants for seizure activity. They produce a mild muscle relaxant effect within the spinal cord.

Benzodiazepines have little effect on the cardiovascular system. Cardiac output is not altered. Changes in blood pressure are due to changes in the systemic vascular resistance.[4] Midazolam is known to produce more of a decrease in blood pressure than diazepam. Benzodiazepines have been used successfully in patients with congestive heart failure where their cardiac output is maintained.

Benzodiazepines can be used successfully in patients with a history of chronic obstructive pulmonary disease but should be monitored because of an increase in $PaCO_2$ levels, causing respiratory depression. Respiratory depression is commonly observed in patients with some form of respiratory disease, and ventilation should be monitored in all patients. Caution must be used when administering benzodiazepines with narcotics due to their synergistic effect. Airway assistance with supplemental oxygen may be required. Benzodiazepines can also depress the swallowing reflex and decrease upper airway activity, making an individual more susceptible to pulmonary aspiration.[3]

Benzodiazepines undergo hepatic metabolism by cytochrome P-450 enzymes. Vigilance must be used in patients with cirrhosis or liver disease. Metabolism can be affected, resulting in prolonged half-lives and metabolites. Patients with a history of alcohol abuse may require higher doses of benzodiazepines. Hepatic clearance of midazolam is five times greater than that of lorazepam or diazepam. Cytochrome P-450 enzymes are altered by certain drugs that can slow metabolism, including cimetidine, erythromycin, calcium channel blockers, heparin, and antifungal drugs.[5] Benzodiazepines are eliminated through the renal system. The volume of distribution, half-life, and clearance are unaffected in patients with renal insufficiency.[3] Patients with renal failure may experience prolonged sedation due to an accumulation of some metabolites.

Clinical Uses and Indications

When given preoperatively, benzodiazepines produce both sedative and anxiolytic effects. Antegrade amnesia is produced usually upon injection and can last until the recovery period. Midazolam is the prominent benzodiazepine given preoperatively; however, diazepam and lorazepam produce similar effects. Benzodiazepines are an excellent choice in

the pediatric population. When administered orally about 15 minutes before entering the operating room, pediatric patients sometimes tolerate the separation from their parents and the induction process well.[6]

Benzodiazepines can be used as induction drugs but not on a routine basis due to the amount administered for induction and the time it takes for induction to occur. Consideration must be used for the postoperative recovery when administering benzodiazepines. They are used for induction when hemodynamic states (i.e., cardiac output) are to be preserved. They can reduce the minimum alveolar concentration of volatile agents as much as 30%.[5]

Nonbenzodiazepine Hypnotic Drugs

Three nonbenzodiazepine hypnotics have been approved by the U.S. Food and Drug Administration (FDA) for the treatment of insomnia: zolpidem (Ambien), zaleplon (Sonata), and eszopiclone (Lunesta).[2] These drugs are only used for the treatment of insomnia, and their mechanism of action is not fully understood. It is believed that they act on GABA receptors similar to benzodiazepines but have a rapid onset and short duration of action. They provide a hypnotic state but lack any anxiolysis or anticonvulsant properties. They do impair memory and performance of tasks and therefore must be used with caution. Table 5-1 provides a summary of the nonbenzodiazepine hypnotic drugs.

Benzodiazepine Antagonist

Flumazenil (Romazicon) is the only known antagonist approved by the FDA that inhibits the effects of benzodiazepines. Flumazenil competitively inhibits the activity at the benzodiazepine recognition site on the GABA/benzodiazepine receptor complex. When injected, flumazenil helps to reverse, partially or completely, the sedative effects of benzodiazepines.[2] Caution must be used when administering flumazenil because the half-life of benzodiazepines can last longer than the half-life of flumazenil, leading to a state of resedation. Patients should be monitored closely for respiratory depression and resedation.

Side Effects and Contraindications

When administered appropriately, benzodiazepines have a high margin of safety, especially when compared with other IV induction agents (i.e., barbiturates and propofol). Benzodiazepines are relatively free of allergic effects and do not appear to suppress the adrenal gland.[2] The most significant concern with midazolam is respiratory depression, especially with patients at risk. Respiratory-depressant effects of midazolam are greater than lorazepam and diazepam at equipotent doses.[4] In addition, the respiratory-depressant effects of all benzodiazepines are amplified in the presence of opioids and other sedative agents and in patients with severe pulmonary disease.

The major side effects of lorazepam and diazepam, along with respiratory depression, are venous irritation and the risk of thrombophlebitis, problems related to aqueous insolubility and the requisite solvent.[4] At the time of peak concentration in plasma, hypnotic doses of benzodiazepines can be expected to cause varying degrees of lightheadedness, lassitude, increased reaction time, motor incoordination, impairment of mental and motor functions, confusion, and antegrade amnesia.[2] Other less common side effects of benzodiazepines are weakness, headache, blurred vision, vertigo, nausea and vomiting, epigastric distress, and diarrhea. Finally, cognition appears to be affected less than motor performance.[2,4]

Drug Interactions, Guidelines, and Precautions

Benzodiazepines have synergistic sedative effects with other central nervous system depressants, including inhalational and IV anesthetics, opiates, and α_2 agonists. Benzodiazepines have the capacity to reduce anesthetic requirements for both inhalation anesthetics[4] and IV anesthetics, such as propofol[7,8] and thiopental. There is a synergistic interaction of midazolam and fentanyl for induction of anesthesia, and it is also reported that midazolam potentiates the respiratory effects of alfentanil.[4] However, the analgesic action of opiates in the rat model is reduced in the presence of benzodiazepines.[9] Further evidence that benzodiazepines inhibit the analgesic effects of opioids is when flumazenil, a benzodiazepine antagonist, enhances the postoperative analgesic properties of morphine, reduces morphine requirements, and decreases the sedative, emetic, and cardiopulmonary-depressant effects of morphine in patients who have received benzodiazepines after surgery.[10,11] Studies of α_2 agonists, such as dexmedetomidine, have shown synergistic sedative effects while reversing the cardiovascular depressant effects of benzodiazepines in rats.[12]

Individual benzodiazepines may have different interactions with certain drugs. Depending on their metabolic pathway, benzodiazepines can be roughly divided into two groups.[13] The largest group consists of those that are metabolized by cytochrome P-450 enzymes and possess significant potential for interactions with other drugs. The other group comprises those that are metabolized through glucuronidation, such as lorazepam, oxazepam, and temazepam, and generally have few drug interactions. Many drugs, including oral contraceptives, some antibiotics, antidepressants, and antifungal agents, inhibit cytochrome P-450 enzymes in the liver. These drugs reduce the rate of elimination of the benzodiazepines that are metabolized by cytochrome P-450, leading to possibly excessive accumulation and increased side effects. Conversely, drugs that induce cytochrome P-450 enzymes, such as St. John's wort, the antibiotic rifampicin, and the anticonvulsants carbamazepine and phenytoin, accelerate elimination of many benzodiazepines and decrease their action.[14] Taking benzodiazepines with alcohol, opioids, and other central nervous system depressants potentiates their action and thus often results in increased sedation, impaired motor coordination, suppressed breathing, and other adverse effects that may potentially be lethal.[14]

Pregnancy and Newborns

The FDA categorizes benzodiazepines as either Category D or X, which means potential for harm in the unborn has been demonstrated.[15] Therefore benzodiazepines taken during pregnancy have adverse effects on the infant. Abrupt withdrawal in benzodiazepine-dependent pregnant women may result in spontaneous abortions and provoke suicidal ideation.[16] Exposure to benzodiazepines during pregnancy has been associated with a slightly increased risk of cleft palate in newborns (from 0.06% to 0.07%), a controversial conclusion because some studies find no association between benzodiazepines and cleft palate.[17]

Benzodiazepine use by expectant mothers shortly before the delivery may result in floppy infant syndrome, with the newborns suffering from hypotonia, hypothermia, lethargy, and breathing and feeding difficulties.[18] Cases of neonatal withdrawal syndrome have been described in infants chronically exposed to benzodiazepines in utero. This syndrome may be difficult to recognize as it starts several days after delivery—for example, as late as 21 days with chlordiazepoxide. The symptoms include tremors, hypertonia, hyperreflexia, hyperactivity, and vomiting and may last for up to 3 to 6 months.[18] Tapering down the dose during pregnancy may lessen its severity. If used in pregnancy, those benzodiazepines with a better and longer safety record, such as diazepam or chlordiazepoxide, are recommended over potentially more harmful benzodiazepines, such as alprazolam or triazolam, and using the lowest effective dose for the shortest period of time minimizes the risks to the unborn child.[19]

The literature concerning the safety of benzodiazepines in pregnancy is unclear and controversial.[20] Initial concerns regarding benzodiazepines in pregnancy began with findings in animals that did not necessarily cross over to humans. Conflicting findings have been found in newborns exposed to benzodiazepines.[20] Neurodevelopmental disorders and clinical symptoms are commonly found in newborns exposed to benzodiazepines in utero.[21]

Benzodiazepine-exposed newborns have a low birth weight but catch up at an early age; however, smaller head circumferences found in newborns exposed to benzodiazepines persist. Other adverse effects of benzodiazepines taken during pregnancy are deviating neurodevelopmental and clinical symptoms, including craniofacial anomalies, delayed development of pincer grasp, and deviations in muscle tone and pattern of movements. Motor impairments in infants are impeded for up to 1 year after birth. Gross motor development impairments take 18 months to return to normal, but fine motor function impairments persist.[21] In addition to the smaller head circumference found in benzodiazepine-exposed infants, mental retardation, functional deficits, long-lasting behavioral anomalies, and lower intelligence occur.

Older Adults

Adverse effects of benzodiazepines are increased in older adults. The long-term effects of benzodiazepines and benzodiazepine dependence in the elderly can resemble dementia, depression, or anxiety syndromes. Adverse effects on cognition can be mistaken for the effects of old age. Benzodiazepines should be prescribed to the elderly only with caution and for a short period at low doses. The short-acting drugs, such as oxazepam, alprazolam, and triazolam, are more beneficial because of their rapid elimination half-lives.[2] The association of a past history of benzodiazepine use and cognitive decline is unclear, with some studies reporting a lower risk of cognitive decline in former users, some finding no association, and some indicating an increased risk of cognitive decline.[22]

Dosages, Administration, and Practical Aspects

Because benzodiazepines possess sedative, hypnotic, anxiolytic, anticonvulsant, muscle relaxant, and amnesic actions, they are extremely useful in a variety of indications such as alcohol dependence, seizures, anxiety, panic, agitation, and insomnia.[23] Benzodiazepines are well tolerated and are generally safe and effective drugs in the short term for a wide range of conditions. Tolerance can develop to

their effects, and there is also a risk of dependence and a withdrawal syndrome when discontinued. These factors, combined with other possible secondary effects after prolonged use such as psychomotor, cognitive, or memory impairments, limit their long-term applicability.[24]

Midazolam, lorazepam, and diazepam may be administered for preoperative sedation, induction, and maintenance of general anesthesia; conscious sedation for invasive procedures; or for postoperative sedation of patients in critical care units. Table 5-2 provides dosage suggestions for the use of diazepam, midazolam, and lorazepam in premedication, sedation, and induction of anesthesia. The dose–response relationship of these drugs varies considerably among patients and during different clinical circumstances.[4] It is therefore important to carefully titrate these drugs to the desired level of sedation in patients to prevent inadequate or excessive sedation and unwanted side effects. It is also critical that the dosing of benzodiazepines is decreased in the presence of other drugs with sedative and cardiopulmonary-depressant effects, such as opioids, other sedative-hypnotics, antipsychotics, and general anesthetics. In addition, patients receiving benzodiazepines for postoperative sedation may have increasing dose requirements of the first 24 to 36 hours as the patient emerges from the residual sedative effects of general anesthesia and surgery.[4] Therefore dose requirements for benzodiazepines to maintain constant levels of sedation may decrease.

Benzodiazepines are often prescribed for a wide variety of conditions. They are very useful in intensive care to sedate patients receiving mechanical ventilation or for those in extreme distress and high-level anxiety. Again, caution is exercised in these situations, because the risk of respiratory depression is always a concern. Clearly, precautions should be used in relation to benzodiazepine

Table 5-2 Use, Routes, and Dosages of Diazepam, Midazolam, and Lorazepam in Premedication, Sedation, and Induction of Anesthesia

Drug	Use	Route	Dosage (mg/kg)
Diazepam	Premedication	Oral	0.2–0.5
	Sedation	IV	0.04–0.2
	Induction	IV	0.3–0.6
Midazolam	Premedication	IM	0.07–0.15
	Sedation	IV	0.01–0.1
	Induction	IV	0.1–0.4
Lorazepam	Premedication	Oral	0.05
		IM	0.03–0.05
	Sedation	IV	0.03–0.04

IM, intramuscular.

overdose, and appropriate treatment (including flumazenil) should be readily available.

Benzodiazepines are an extremely effective premedication given before surgery. They provide both anxiety relief and produce amnesia, which can be useful to reduce the patient's memory of any unpleasant experiences from the procedure. Midazolam is the most commonly used agent for this because of its strong sedative actions and fast recovery times as well as its water solubility, which will reduce pain upon injection. However, if marked amnesic properties are desired in a given situation, lorazepam, with its prolonged half-life, is a more effective drug choice. Finally, benzodiazepines are well known for their strong muscle-relaxing properties and can be useful in the treatment of muscle spasms. However, in the long term, tolerance develops and the muscle-relaxant properties of benzodiazepines become less effective.[4]

Procedural Sedation in Children

Procedural sedation in children is clearly a common practice that has emerged over the past 20 years, especially with newer drugs (i.e., midazolam and propofol). Midazolam is the most common benzodiazepine used for procedural sedation and analgesia and is preferred over the longer acting diazepam.[6] Time to peak effect for midazolam is brief with IV administration (2–3 minutes), and duration is short (45–60 minutes). When IV access is problematic and/or the child is frightened or uncooperative, the intramuscular, oral, intranasal, and rectal routes can also be considered. However, the anesthetist must be mindful of the respiratory-depressive effects of benzodiazepines. Both the oral and the intranasal routes have limitations. The oral route can lead to unreliable concentrations in serum and clinical effect due to first-pass hepatic metabolism. The intranasal route typically has a mucosal irritating effect, which is painful and may produce further anxiety in the child.[6] The mucosal irritation is thought to be a result of the low pH and the presence of the preservative benzyl alcohol, and buffering the solution does not decrease the irritation.[25–27]

Midazolam can be effectively used in children for moderate and deep sedation through careful IV titration and vigilant monitoring for respiratory depression. However, some children need larger dosages than would be typical for adults on a milligram per kilogram basis, and paradoxical responses, such as unexpected agitation and hyperexcitability, are common.[6] Paradoxical reactions, which have been reported in all routes of administration, are characterized as inconsolable crying, combativeness, disorientation, agitation, and restlessness and have been reported in 1% to 15% of children receiving midazolam.[6]

Key Points

- Benzodiazepines affect GABA receptors, leading to hyperpolarization of postsynaptic cell membranes.
- Midazolam is water soluble, but at physiologic pH it closes its imidazole ring, making it highly lipid soluble.
- Flumazenil is the only FDA-approved drug that competitively inhibits the effects of benzodiazepines. Caution must be used when administering flumazenil because the half-life is shorter than the half-life of benzodiazepines.
- Three nonbenzodiazepine drugs used for the treatment of insomnia affect GABA receptors: zolpidem (Ambien), zaleplon (Sonata), and eszopiclone (Lunesta).
- Benzodiazepines have a high margin of safety, are relatively free of allergic effects, and do not appear to suppress the adrenal gland.
- The most significant concern with midazolam is respiratory depression, especially with patients at risk. The respiratory-depressant effects of midazolam are greater than lorazepam and diazepam at equipotent doses.
- Benzodiazepines have synergistic sedative effects with other central nervous system depressants, including inhalational and IV anesthetics, opiates, and α_2 agonists.
- Benzodiazepines are categorized as either Category D or X by the FDA, meaning potential for harm in the unborn has been demonstrated.
- Benzodiazepine use by expectant mothers shortly before delivery may result in floppy infant syndrome, with the newborns suffering from hypotonia, hypothermia, lethargy, and breathing and feeding difficulties.
- Neurodevelopmental disorders and clinical symptoms are commonly found in newborns exposed to benzodiazepines in utero. Benzodiazepine-exposed newborns have a low birth weight but catch up at an early age. Smaller head circumferences found in newborns exposed to benzodiazepines appear to persist. Other adverse effects of benzodiazepines taken during pregnancy are deviating neurodevelopmental and clinical symptoms, including craniofacial anomalies, a slightly increased risk of cleft palate, delayed development of pincer grasp, and deviations in muscle tone and pattern of movements.
- Adverse effects of benzodiazepines are increased in older adults. The long-term effects of benzodiazepines and benzodiazepine dependence in the elderly can resemble dementia, depression, or anxiety

syndromes. Adverse effects on cognition can be mistaken for the effects of old age.

- Midazolam can be effectively used in children for moderate and deep sedation through careful IV titration and vigilant monitoring for respiratory depression.
- Paradoxical reactions, which have been reported in all routes of administration, are characterized as inconsolable crying, combativeness, disorientation, agitation, and restlessness and have been reported in 1% to 15% of children receiving midazolam.

Chapter Questions

1. How are benzodiazepines used in anesthesia practice?
2. How do benzodiazepines differ chemically and in distribution and clearance from other benzodiazepines?
3. What properties make midazolam a highly desirable agent for use in premedication and sedation?
4. How do benzodiazepines interact with other commonly used drugs in anesthetic practice?
5. What are the adverse concerns and practice aspects in the use of benzodiazepines with pregnancy, older adults, and children?

References

1. Sternbach LH. The benzodiazepine story. *J Med Chem.* 1979;22:1–7.
2. Charney DS, Mihic SD, Harris RA. Hypnotics and sedatives. In: Brunton LL, Lazo JS, Parker KL, eds. *Goodman & Gilman's: The Pharmacological Basis of Therapeutics,* 11th ed. New York: McGraw-Hill; 2006:401–427.
3. Stoelting RK, Hillier SC. Benzodiazepines. In: Stoelting RK, Hillier SC, eds. *Pharmacology and Physiology in Anesthetic Practice,* 4th ed. Baltimore: Lippincott Williams & Wilkins; 2006:140–154.
4. Rudolph U, Crestani F, Möhler H, et al. Sedatives, anxiolytics, and amnestics. In: Evers AS, Maze M, eds. *Anesthetic Pharmacology: Physiologic Principles and Clinical Practice.* Philadelphia: Churchill Livingstone; 2004:417–434.
5. Morgan GE, Mikhail MS, Murray MJ. Nonvolatile anesthetic agents. In: Morgan GE, Mikhail MS, Murray MJ, eds. *Clinical Anesthesiology.* New York: McGraw-Hill; 2005:187–192.
6. Krauss B, Green SM. Procedural sedation and analgesia in children. Available at: http://www.thelancet.com. Accessed July 16, 2009.
7. McClune S, McKay AC, Wright PM, Patterson CC, Clarke SJ. Synergistic interaction between midazolam and propofol. *Br J Anaesth.* 1992;69:239–240.
8. Short TG, Chui PT. Propofol and midazolam act synergistically in combination. *Br J Anaesth.* 1991;67:538–539.
9. Daghero AM, Bradley EL, Kissin I. Midazolam antagonizes the analgesic effect of morphine in rats. *Anesth Analg.* 1987;66:940–944.
10. Gross JB, Blouin RT, Zandsberg S, Conrad PF, Häussler J. Effects of flumazenil on ventilatory drive during sedation with midazolam and alfentanil. *Anesthesiology.* 1996;85:710–713.
11. Weinbroum AA, Weisenberg M, Rudick V, Geller V, Niv D. Flumazenil potentiation of postoperative morphine analgesia. *Clin J Pain.* 2000;16:940–944.
12. Bol CJ, Vogelaar JP, Tang JP, Mandema JW. Quantification of pharmacodynamic interaction between dexmedetomidine and midazolam in the rat. *J Pharmacol Exp Ther.* 2000;294:343–347.
13. Chouinard G. Issues in the clinical use of benzodiazepines: potency, withdrawal, and rebound. *J Clin Psychiatry.* 2004;65(Suppl 5):7–12.
14. Longmore M, Scally P, Collier J. *Oxford Handbook of Clinical Specialties,* 6th ed. New York: Oxford University Press; 2003:365–366.
15. Wyatt RJ, Chew RH. *Wyatt's Practical and Psychiatric Practice: Forms and Protocols for Clinical Use,* 3rd ed. Danvers, MA: American Psychiatric Publishing; 2004:195–198.
16. Roach SS, Ford SM. Sedatives and hypnotics. In: Roach SM, ed. *Roach's Introductory to Clinical Pharmacology,* 8th ed. Baltimore: Lippincott Williams & Wilkins; 2006:234–236.
17. Dolovich LR, Addis A, Vaillancourt JM, Power JD, Koren G, Einarson TR. Benzodiazepines use in pregnancy and major malformations or oral cleft: meta-analysis of cohort and case-control studies. *Br Med J.* 1998;317:839–843.
18. Iqbal MM, Sobhan T, Ryals T. Effects of commonly used benzodiazepines on the fetus, the neonate and the nursing infant. *Psych Serv.* 2002;53:39–49.
19. Lal R, Gupta S, Rao R, Kattimani S. Emergency management of substance overdose and withdrawal. Available at: http://www.whoindia.org. Accessed June 6, 2009.
20. McGrath C, Buist A, Norman TR. Treatment of anxiety during pregnancy: effects of psychotropic drug treatment on the developing fetus. *J Drug Saf.* 1999;20:171–186.
21. Koren G. *Medication Safety in Pregnancy and Breastfeeding.* New York: McGraw-Hill; 2007.
22. Verdoux H, Lagnaoui R, Begaud B. Is benzodiazepine use a risk factor for cognitive decline and dementia? A literature review of epidemiological studies. *Psychol Med.* 2005;35: 307–315.
23. Olkkola KT, Ahonen J. Midazolam and other benzodiazepines. In: *Handbook of Experimental Pharmacology.* New York: Springer; 2008:335–360.

24.   Tesar GE. High potency benzodiazepines for short-term management of panic disorders: the U.S experience. *J Clin Psychiatry.* 1990;51:4–7.

25.   Davies F, Waters M. Oral midazolam for conscious sedation of children during minor procedures. *J Accid Emerg Med.* 1998;15:244–248.

26.   Fatovitch DM, Jacobs IG. A randomized, controlled trial of oral midazolam and buffered lidocaine for suturing lacerations in children. *Ann Emerg Med.* 1995;25:209–214.

27.   Connors K, Terndrup TE. Nasal versus oral midazolam for sedation of anxious children undergoing laceration repair. *Ann Emerg Med.* 1994;24:1074–1079.

6

Opioid Agonists, Antagonists, and Agonist-Antagonists

Richard Henker, PhD, RN, CRNA, FAAN
Colleen Dunwoody, MS, RN-BC

Objectives

After completing this chapter, the reader should be able to

- Explain the mechanisms for pain relief provided by opioid agonists and opioid agonist-antagonists.
- Describe the pharmacokinetics and pharmacodynamics for opioid agonists, opioid agonist-antagonists, and opioid antagonists.
- Identify the most common adverse effects of various opioids by mode of delivery.
- Discuss the mechanisms of metabolism and elimination of opioid agonists, opioid agonist-antagonists, and opioid antagonists.
- Summarize the effects of opioids on stress response.

Introduction

In 2002, 42.5 million inpatient surgeries in the United States were performed.[1] Each year 8 million surgeries are performed in 4000 ambulatory care surgery centers across the United States.[2] Management of pain is central to the care of these patients. Although opioids have many adverse effects, they are frequently used to treat postoperative pain. Advances in the management of pain have included a heightened awareness of the need to assess pain each time vital signs are recorded.

History of the Use of Opioids

The use of opium has been documented for over 2 centuries, but the use of opioids for postoperative pain management has only occurred since the 18th century.[3] The first documented cases of the use of opioids for postoperative pain relief were in Scotland in the late 1700s by James Moore and 5 years later by Benjamin Bell. Oral administration of opioids at that time was found to provide inadequate surgical anesthesia, but oral opioids did provide good postoperative pain relief.[3] Administration of subcutaneous morphine was first reported in 1836 by Lafargue, a French physician. The effects of morphine were thought to be mostly local, although Charles Hunter published a paper in the *Medical Times Gazette* in 1858 that reported the systemic effects of subcutaneous injections of morphine. In the early 1900s morphine administered via spinal injections was found to provide pain relief, although this technique did not regain popularity until the 1970s.[3]

Mechanisms of Action

Definition of Pain

Pain is defined by the International Association for the Study of Pain as "an unpleasant sensory and emotional experience associated with actual or potential tissue damage, or described in terms of such damage. While it is unquestionably a sensation in part or parts of the body, it is always unpleasant and therefore, an emotional experience."[4] Two of the often described components of pain are the objective observations of tachycardia and elevated blood pressure that are frequently used as indicators of pain, but there is also the subjective component of pain. Pain is identified through self-report and is best communicated through pain rating scales. Individuals that have difficulty communicating pain include cognitively impaired adults and children, who do not have the necessary cognitive abilities to use a pain scale.[4]

Description of Mechanisms of Pain

Nociception is the process in which painful stimuli are detected, transduced, and transmitted, peripherally and in the central nervous system (CNS).[5] Tissue injury activates the inflammatory process, increasing the peripheral sensitivity of nociceptors due to influx of mediators into the injured tissues. Signals initiated by the nociceptors are carried to the dorsal horn of the spinal cord.[6] Subsequently, output neurons from the dorsal horn cross into the anterior lateral quadrant and ascend the spinal cord via A-δ and C fibers in the spinothalamic tract to the thalamus and then to the primary somatosensory cortex.[7]

Opioid receptors affect the transmission of painful stimuli by opening sodium, calcium, and potassium channels, thus decreasing the firing of action potentials in neurons involved in pain transmission.[8]

Consequences of Pain

Pain associated with inadequate analgesia is known to be related to postoperative complications and prolonged recovery associated with immune system function. Page and colleagues[9] evaluated the effects of surgical stress on tumor metastasis in rats. Rats treated with fentanyl after surgical stress compared with controls were found to have a decrease in tumor retention by 65%. Page and colleagues[9] suggest that natural killer cell activity was found to be decreased in the rats not treated with fentanyl.

Acute pain has also been found to stimulate the neuroendocrine stress response, increasing adrenergic neural activity and plasma catecholamine concentration and sympathetic tone and hypothalamically mediated reflexes.[10] Cardiovascular-related effects associated with the stress response include hypertension and tachycardia. Subsequently, there is an increase in myocardial oxygen demand, causing increased myocardial irritability, which can precipitate myocardial ischemia and infarction. From a respiratory standpoint, pain increases minute ventilation in response to the overall increase in body oxygen consumption and decreases tissue oxygenation.[11] When surgery involves the abdominal or thoracic cavities, respiratory effects can include hypoventilation,[12] decreased tidal volume, ability to cough, and the development of atelectasis.[13] Additional adverse responses to pain include anxiety,[14] sleep disturbance, and depression.[15] Overall, adequate pain control is vital in the profession of nurse anesthesia because the consequences of pain can significantly affect patient outcome.

Clinical Pharmacology

Prototype: Fentanyl

The rapid onset and short duration of fentanyl (*N*-[1-phenethyl-4-piperidyl]) make it an ideal opioid for use during a balanced anesthetic and also for treating patients with acute pain. Fentanyl provides analgesia by stimulating primarily μ receptors.[16] Activation of μ opioid receptors opens potassium channels to inhibit the firing of action potentials in pain pathways throughout the CNS.[8] Fentanyl is 100 times more potent than morphine and is more specific for μ receptors than other opioid receptors.[16]

Although fentanyl has many benefits for patient care, there are also many adverse effects associated with its use. Adverse effects that are more frequently seen in anesthesia applications include respiratory depression, chest rigidity, bradycardia, and sedation. Administration of high doses of fentanyl in opioid-naive patients being treated for acute pain places patients at risk for chest rigidity and respiratory depression. The greatest risk for respiratory depression is 5 to 15 minutes after rapid administration of high doses of fentanyl.[17]

Pharmacokinetics

Fentanyl is a potent opioid agonist: 100 mcg of fentanyl is equivalent to 10 mg of morphine. The distribution time of fentanyl is 1.7 minutes, and the redistribution time is 13 minutes. The volume of distribution for fentanyl is 4 L/kg. The half-life of fentanyl is 219 minutes. Onset is almost immediate, and duration of the effects of fentanyl is 30 minutes to 1 hour. Most of the fentanyl given intravenously is metabolized on first pass in the liver by the cytochrome P-450 (CYP) system, specifically CYP3A4. Seventy-five percent of intravenous (IV) fentanyl is cleared in the urine, mostly as metabolites. Ten percent of the fentanyl that is cleared via the urine is unchanged from the original drug.[17] The chemical structure of fentanyl is shown in Figure 6-1.

Pharmacodynamics

Opioid Receptors

Three different opioid receptors were discovered in the 1970s in different parts of the brain. Fentanyl is known to affect mostly μ opioid receptors with less activation of κ and δ receptors. Specific effects were found to be associated with each receptor. Of the various opioid receptors, the μ_1 and μ_2 subtype of opioid receptors are most related to analgesia.[18] Other effects that are specific to μ receptors include

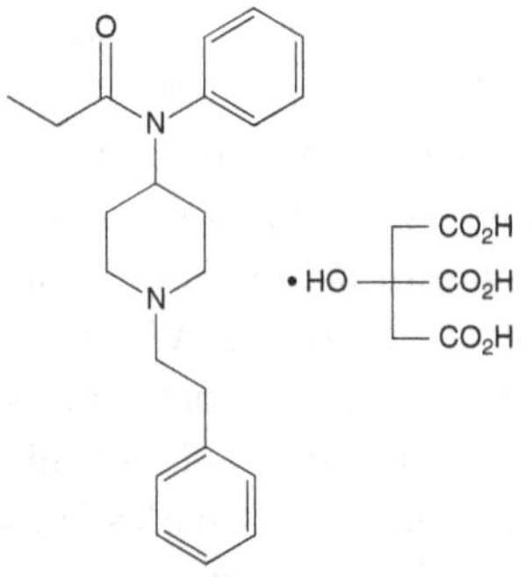

Figure 6-1 Chemical structure of fentanyl.

Source: Figure from: http://dailymed.nlm.nih.gov/dailymed/drugInfo .cfm?id=15172.

respiratory depression, bradycardia, sedation, euphoria, and gastrointestinal (GI) dysmotility, in addition to prolactin and growth hormone release. μ receptors are known to be in the cerebral cortex, amygdala, thalamus, periaqueductal gray matter, hypothalamus, hippocampus thalamus, midbrain, pons, medulla, dorsal horn of the spinal cord, the gut, immune cells, and peripheral tissues.[8] Activation of κ opioid receptors is also associated with analgesia, although the effect on pain is not nearly as strong as activation of μ or δ opioid receptors.[19] Respiratory depression is much less with activation of κ and δ receptors. κ receptors are associated with dysphoria. Although only three types of opioid receptors have been reported here, multiple opioid receptors have been identified.

Genetic Variations in μ Opioid Receptors

The genetic code for the μ opioid receptor (*OPRM1*) is located on chromosome 6q24-q25. Mutations in *OPRM1* are reflected in protein sequences in μ opioid receptors and have been associated with variation in agonist binding.[19] Areas that are likely to show genetic variation are termed single nucleotide polymorphisms (SNPs). These SNPs include the A to G transition at nucleotide 118 (rs1799971) and the C to T transition at nucleotide 17 (rs1799972).[20] Both of these SNPs result in amino acid differences in the proteins that make up the μ opioid receptor. The A118G polymorphism results in an asparagine being replaced by an aspartate, and the C17T polymorphism results in an alanine being replaced by valine. Therefore differences in genotype are reflected in the protein structure and function of μ receptors, potentially influencing the binding of opioids to these receptors.

The frequency of the genetic variants (AG and GG) of A118G occurs in 10.5% to 18.8% of the population, and genetic variants of C17T (CT and TT) occur in 1% to 10% of the population.[19] It should be noted that considerable differences occur by racial and ethnic groups in genotype expression. Crowley and colleagues[21] evaluated OPRM1 polymorphisms in African Americans and found greater numbers of the C17T substitution but fewer A118G substitutions. In studies reported by Chou et al.,[22,23] the incidence of the polymorphisms in Asians having knee arthroplasty and abdominal hysterectomy were reported as 38% and 46%, respectively. Given the high incidence of polymorphisms in various ethnic groups, identification of genetic variants before surgery would provide guidance in administering opioids and preventing complications associated with under- or over-medicating patients.

Clinical implications of μ opioid receptor polymorphisms have been evaluated in substance-dependent populations.

Initial work evaluating μ opioid receptor genotypes, specifically A118G, found an association with substance dependence,[24–27] but a recent meta-analysis including 22 studies involving patients with various types of substance dependence (i.e., heroin, alcohol, opioids, cocaine) found no relationship between the A118G and substance dependence.[28] The incidence of substance dependence in control groups was questioned by the authors of the meta-analysis.

Clinical studies have evaluated the relationship of the A118G genetic variants and postoperative pain. Clinical studies by Chou and colleagues evaluated postoperative pain in knee arthroplasty (*n* = 147),[23] and a second study evaluated postoperative pain after abdominal hysterectomy (*n* = 80).[24] In both studies the amount of morphine used was highest for the GG genotype. Ideally, in the future OPRM1 genotype can be determined before surgery and used as one factor to determine opioid dose.

Age

Age is often provided as rationale for decreased opioid administration in the elderly, although it has been reported that pain in the elderly is often undertreated.[29] The elderly are more likely to have pain due to deteriorating health and undergoing surgery, particularly for procedures such as cataract extraction, diskectomies, joint replacements, coronary artery bypass, transurethral resection of the prostate, and so on. Although the elderly are often undertreated for pain, it should be noted that the elderly are also more likely to undergo changes that require individualized management of pain with opioids. Absorption of medications may be affected by GI abnormalities such as malabsorption or diarrhea. Decreased hepatic function leads to decreased production of protein carriers that allow for increased half-life of opioids. Decreased hepatic function also leads to decreased metabolism of opioids by the CYP system. Increased body fat that occurs with age can also alter the distribution area of opioids, depending on the lipid or water solubility of the opioid. Decreased renal function in the elderly can impact elimination of active metabolites.[30]

It should be noted that although the elderly are thought to be undertreated, Likar and colleagues[31] found decreased pain intensity in the elderly when comparing pain relief by age group. In addition, the elderly group required less rescue pain medication when compared with other groups.

Gender

Some variability in opioid response is attributed to gender. Cepeda and Carr[32] found that women reported greater pain intensity when compared with men in the postanesthesia care unit after having abdominal surgery, and women were found to require significantly more morphine than men to obtain the same pain relief. Anatomic differences in pain sensation by gender were indicated by changes in cerebral blood flow during positron emission tomography.[33] Fillingim and colleagues[34] found pain threshold to be lower in men with the GG variant of the A118A genetic polymorphism. Women with the GG variant of the A118G polymorphism were found to have a higher pain threshold. Minto and colleagues[35] found no gender differences in pharmacodynamics or pharmacokinetics with standardized administration of remifentanil. Considerable controversy remains regarding response to opioids by gender.

Alcohol

The effects of chronic alcohol use have been reported to increase the requirement of opioids for treatment of pain. Lemmens and colleagues[36] reported that increased amounts of alfentanil were required in subjects taking in moderate amounts of alcohol on a daily basis. Decreased sensitivity of the CNS increases the requirement of opioids in patients taking in alcohol on a daily basis. The cross-tolerance between alcohol and opioids suggests that patients with a history of alcohol intake require greater amounts of opioids.[36]

Metabolism and Elimination

Many drugs are metabolized either by phase I or phase II metabolism in the liver. Opioids such as fentanyl, alfentanil, sufentanil, and methadone are metabolized by phase I metabolism using the CYP system in the liver. Opioids such as hydromorphone and meperidine are broken down by phase II metabolism that includes glucuronidation, sulfation, glutathione conjugation, acetylation, and methylation.[37] Genotypes of the CYP system can alter the impact of metabolism of some opioids. Five predominant polymorphisms of the CYP2D6 alter the biotransformation of codeine, oxycodone, hydrocodone, dextropropoxyphene, and methadone. The most affected opioid is codeine, but hydrocodone, oxycodone, and methadone may also be slightly affected by genotype.[38] Fentanyl is affected the least of all the opioids by the genetic variability in the CYP system and thus one of the reasons fentanyl is a good choice for analgesia during the perioperative period.

After phase I or II metabolism, most opioids are eliminated via the urine. Drugs such as fentanyl are cleared in the urine mostly as metabolites, although 10% of the fentanyl is cleared via the urine unchanged from the original drug when given intravenously.[17] Two percent of sufentanil is cleared unchanged in the urine.

The CYP system is also involved in the metabolism of antiemetics that may be used to treat opioid-induced nausea. Candiotti and colleagues[39] compared poor metabolizers, intermediate metabolizers, extensive metabolizers, and ultrarapid metabolizers in terms of the incidence of nausea and vomiting. The ultrarapid metabolizers had the highest percentage of nausea and vomiting. Janicki and colleagues[40] also found the greatest incidence of nausea and vomiting in ultrarapid metabolizers.

Clinical Uses and Indications

Adjunct to General Anesthesia and Suppression of Stress Response

Although it seems as though opioids have considerable adverse effects, the benefit of opioids is not only the relief of pain but also the reduction of the stress response. Fentanyl is often used to blunt the stress response during induction and surgical procedures. Exogenous opioids reduce the production of adrenocorticotropic hormone and subsequently cortisol. Stress response due to surgery is associated with hemodynamic instability and metabolic catabolism. High doses of fentanyl are known to be effective at blunting the stress response, particularly for major procedures such as cardiac surgery. Fentanyl is often the drug of choice for high-dose opioids due to the release of histamine and active metabolites associated with morphine.[30] Other opioids such as sufentanil are used as an adjunct to general anesthesia.

Postoperative Pain Relief

Acute pain in postoperative patients is due to a variety of factors. Patients undergoing orthopedic procedures experience both incisional pain of the skin and bone pain that is attributed to stretching of nociceptors as well as microfractures that occur with bone fractures.[41] In addition, the production of mediators such as prostaglandins associated with the inflammatory response in the surrounding soft tissue and the development of muscle spasm contribute to the development of pain with fractures.[41] Various physiologic and psychological factors often make it difficult to predict the pain response. Pain is best assessed in postoperative patients by subjective response.[29]

Postoperative pain is frequently treated on an as-needed basis. Although this method seems to provide opioids to postoperative patients at an appropriate time, the as-needed regimen leads to the frequent development of breakthrough pain.[29] If patients do not request pain medication with the initial increase in pain, the pain becomes moderate to severe and is more difficult to treat. Regularly scheduled opioid administration provides fewer peaks and valleys in terms of pain relief. Patients are less likely to have breakthrough pain if opioids are provided on a regular schedule.[29]

Premedication

Opioids not only provide analgesia, but they also have sedative effects. The opioid-induced sedation that often occurs in opioid-naive patients can be useful as a premedication. Use of benzodiazepines as premedication in elderly patients is sometimes associated with decreased cognitive abilities and confusion postoperatively.[42] Use of opioids such as fentanyl for sedation may be a more optimal choice in the elderly.

Methods of Administration

Determination of method of opioid administration depends on type of pain and opioids required. If a patient has acute pain associated with surgery, IV, intrathecal, or epidural administration may be the best method of providing opioids. Chronic cancer pain may be best treated with fentanyl patches that provide pain medication via a transdermal route. When providing anesthesia for patients with a fentanyl patch, leaving the patch in place and giving additional fentanyl provide more effective pain relief. Removal of the fentanyl patch decreases the amount of fentanyl provided to the patient, although a reservoir of fentanyl will continue to be provided to a patient in the skin.

Preemptive Analgesia

Giving opioids "upfront" is a common practice of nurse anesthetists that occurs before incision after induction. This form of preemptive analgesia prevents the firing of action potentials to transmit pain and decreases the sensitization of the CNS to pain impulses. Ideally, preemptive analgesia decreases the amount of moderate and severe postoperative pain that is more difficult to treat; therefore preemptive opioids are beneficial in preventing pain.

Multimodal Analgesia

Benefits of using opioids with nonsteroidal anti-inflammatory drugs (NSAIDs), cyclooxygenase-2 inhibitors, and acetaminophen are improved pain relief and decreased adverse effects when compared with using opioids alone. Pain intensity has been found to be less with the use of NSAIDs with opioids

at 24 hours when compared with opioids alone.[43] Opioid sparing was reported by Elia and colleagues[43] to be 15% when using multimodal therapy. Other benefits reported with the use of multimodal therapy include decreased sedation, decreased postoperative nausea and vomiting (PONV), and early ambulation.[43] One of the risks associated with multimodal therapy with NSAIDs is increased bleeding and risk of renal failure.[44] Although studies published by Scott Reuben in this area are no longer considered credible, there is evidence that there are advantages to the use of multimodal therapy.[45]

Comparative Pharmacology of Other Drugs in Class

Equianalgesia

An equianalgesic table provides a mathematical guide to compare opioid analgesics between oral and parenteral routes and/or between different opioids (Table 6-1). These tables are often estimates based on single-dose parenteral trials but can be useful to determine the dose and route of administration of a different opioid that provides approximately equivalent pain relief. Considerable variability in analgesic response exists between individuals, so when the patient experiences insufficient analgesia or excessive adverse effects (ADEs) from one opioid, it is useful to switch to another. Factors such as tolerance and cross-tolerance, pharmacokinetic and pharmacodynamic variability, use of adjunctive analgesics, and other CNS-active medications may affect the patient's response to opioid medications. There is incomplete cross-tolerance between opioids. This means that switching a patient from one opioid to another apparently equivalent opioid may be an overestimate because the tolerance that the patient developed to the first opioid may not be the same for the second. Demographic factors such as age, gender, and ethnicity as well as renal function and the type of pain also influence patient response to opioids.

Several rules may be applied to the use of an equianalgesic table:

- Always use the same table to reduce errors and facilitate memorization.
- Start conservatively and titrate to effect.
- Provide rescue doses to cover analgesic gaps and breakthrough pain.
- Calculate doses based on 24-hour usage during which pain has been reasonably well controlled.

Table 6-1 Equianalgesic Chart: Approximate Equivalent Doses of Opioids for Moderate to Severe Pain

Equianalgesic Chart: Approximate equivalent doses of opioids for moderate to severe pain.

ANALGESIC	PARENTERAL (IM, SC, IV) ROUTE[1,2] (mg)	PO ROUTE[1] (mg)	COMMENTS
MU OPIOID AGONISTS			
MORPHINE	10	30	Standard for comparison. Multiple routes of administration. Available in immediate-release and controlled-release formulations. Active metabolite M6G can accumulate with repeated dosing in renal failure.
CODEINE	130	200 NR	IM has unpredictable absorption and high side effect profile; used PO for mild to moderate pain; usually compounded with nonopioid (e.g., Tylenol #3).
FENTANYL	100 µg/h parenterally and transdermally ≅ 4 mg/h morphine parenterally; 1 µg/h transdermally ≅ 2 mg/24 h morphine PO	—	Short half-life, but at steady state, slow elimination from tissues can lead to a prolonged half-life (up to 12 h). Start opioid-naive patients on no more than 25 µg/h transdermally. Transdermal fentanyl NR for acute pain management. Available by oral transmucosal route.
HYDROMORPHONE (Dilaudid)	1.5	7.5	Useful alternative to morphine. No evidence that metabolites are clinically relevant; shorter duration than morphine. Available in high-potency parenteral formulation (10 mg/mL) useful for SC infusion; 3 mg rectal ≅ 650 mg aspirin PO. With repeated dosing (e.g., PCA), it is more likely that 2–3 mg parenteral hydromorphone = 10 mg parenteral morphine.

-------------------------------- **fold here** ------------------------------

ANALGESIC	PARENTERAL (IM, SC, IV) ROUTE (mg)	PO ROUTE (mg)	COMMENTS
LEVORPHANOL (Levo-Dromoran)	2	4	Longer acting than morphine when given repeatedly. Long half-life can lead to accumulation within 2–3 days of repeated dosing.
MEPERIDINE	75	300 NR	No longer preferred as a first-line opioid for the management of acute or chronic pain due to potential toxicity from accumulation of metabolite, normeperidine. Normeperidine has 15- to 20-h half-life and is not reversed by naloxone. NR in elderly or patients with impaired renal function; NR by continuous IV infusion.
METHADONE (Dolophine)	10	20	Longer acting than morphine when given repeatedly. Long half-life can lead to delayed toxicity from accumulation within 3–5 days. Start PO dosing on PRN schedule; in opioid-tolerant patients converted to methadone, start with 10–25% of equianalgesic dose.
OXYCODONE	—	20	Used for moderate pain when combined with a nonopioid (e.g., Percocet, Tylox). Available as single entity in immediate-release and controlled-release formulations (e.g., OxyContin); can be used like PO morphine for severe pain.
OXYMORPHONE (Numorphan)	1	10 rectal	Used for moderate to severe pain. No PO formulation.

(Continued.)

[1] Duration of analgesia is dose dependent; the higher the dose, usually the longer the duration.

[2] IV boluses may be used to produce analgesia that lasts approximately as long as IM or SC doses. However, of all routes of administration, IV produces the highest peak concentration of the drug, and the peak concentration is associated with the highest level of toxicity, e.g., sedation. To decrease the peak effect and lower the level of toxicity, IV boluses may be administered more slowly, e.g., 10 mg of morphine over a 15-minute period or smaller doses may be administered more often, e.g., 5 mg of morphine every 1–1.5 hours.

FDA = Food and Drug Administration; NR = not recommended; ≅ roughly equal to.

- Reduce the 24-hour total by at least 25% to account for incomplete cross-tolerance when switching opioids and then calculate the interval dose. This does not apply when changing the route of administration only.
- When making a recommendation as a consultant, include your calculations in the communication to the requesting healthcare provider (HCP).
- When converting to methadone, consult a methadone conversion resource and consider the patient's opioid tolerance.
- Ongoing, diligent assessment is necessary after conversion with the option for liberal titration and adjustment.

Morphine

Morphine is the gold standard of opioids and is available worldwide for pain relief. All other opioids are compared with morphine. Morphine is available in a variety of preparations that can be used parenterally, orally, intrathecally, and as epidural preparations. Glucuronidation of morphine leads to the development of morphine-3-glucuronide and morphine-6-glucuronide by phase II metabolism.[30] Morphine-3-glucuronide does not provide analgesia and makes up 60% of all morphine metabolites; morphine-6-glucuronide (M6G) is an active metabolite

Table 6-1 Equianalgesic Chart: Approximate Equivalent Doses of Opioids for Moderate to Severe Pain *(continued)*

Equianalgesic Chart: Approximate equivalent doses of opioids for moderate to severe pain. (cont'd)

ANALGESIC	PARENTERAL (IM, SC, IV) ROUTE[1],[2] (mg)	PO ROUTE[1] (mg)	COMMENTS
AGONIST-ANTAGONIST OPIOIDS:	Not recommended for severe, escalating pain. If used in combination with mu agonists, may reverse analgesia and precipitate withdrawal in opioid-dependent patients.		
BUPRENORPHINE (Buprenex)	0.4	—	Not readily reversed by naloxone; NR for laboring patients.
BUTORPHANOL (Stadol)	2	—	Available in nasal spray.
DEZOCINE (Dalgan)	10	—	
NALBUPHINE (Nubain)	10	—	
PENTAZOCINE (Talwin)	60	180	

Selected References For more complete information and additional references, see: Pasero C, Portenoy RK, McCaffery M. Opioid analgesics. pp. 161-299. In: McCaffery M, Pasero C: **Pain Clinical Manual**, St. Louis, 1999, Mosby, pp. 241-243.

American Pain Society (APS): **Principles of analgesic use in the treatment of acute and cancer pain**, ed. 3, Glenview, IL, 1992, APS.
Lawlor P, Turner K, Hanson J, et al: Dose ratio between morphine and hydromorphone in patients with cancer pain: a retrospective study, **Pain** 72(1,2):79-85, 1997.
Manfredi PL, Borsook D, Chandler SW, et al: Intravenous methadone for cancer pain unrelieved by morphine and hydromorphone: clinical observations, **Pain** 70:99-101, 1997.
Portenoy RK: Opioid analgesics. In Portenoy RK, Kanner RM, editors: **Pain management: theory and practice**, Philadelphia, 1996, FA Davis Company, pp. 249-276.

Equianalgesic Chart

Approximate equivalent doses of PO nonopioids and opioids for mild to moderate pain

ANALGESIC	PO DOSAGE (MG)
Nonopioids	
Acetaminophen	650
Aspirin (ASA)	650
Opioids[†]	
Codeine	32–60
Hydrocodone[††]	5
Meperidine (Demerol)	50
Oxycodone[†††]	3–5
Propoxyphene (Darvon)	65–100

[†] Often combined with acetaminophen; avoid exceeding maximum total daily dose of acetaminophen (4000 mg/day).

[††] Combined with acetaminophen, e.g., Vicodin, Lortab.

[†††] Combined with acetaminophen, e.g., Percocet, Tylox. Also available alone as controlled-release OxyContin and immediate-release formulations.

A Guide to Using Equianalgesic Charts

- Equianalgesic means approximately the same pain relief.
- The equianalgesic chart is a guideline. Doses and intervals between doses are titrated according to the individual's response.
- The equianalgesic chart is helpful when switching from one drug to another, or switching from one route of administration to another.
- Dosages in the equianalgesic chart for moderate to severe pain are not necessarily starting doses. The doses suggest a ratio for comparing the analgesia of one drug to another.
- For elderly patients, initially reduce the recommended adult opioid dose for moderate to severe pain by 25% to 50%.
- The longer the patient has been receiving opioids, the more conservative the starting doses of a **new** opioid.

Selected References: For more complete information and additional references, see: McCaffery M, Portenoy RK: Nonopioids: Acetaminophen and nonsteroidal antiinflammatory drugs. pp. 129-160. In: McCaffery M, Pasero C: **Pain: Clinical Manual**, St. Louis, 1999, Mosby, p. 133.

American Pain Society (APS): **Principles of analgesic use in the treatment of acute pain and cancer pain,** ed. 3, Glenview, IL, APS, 1992.
Kaiko R, Lacouture P, Hopf K, et al: Analgesic efficacy of controlled-release (CR) oxycodone and CR morphine. **Clin Pharmacol Ther** 59:130, 1996.

■ From McCaffery M, Pasero C: **Pain: Clinical Manual**, Copyright©, 1999, Mosby.

Source: For more complete information and additional references, see: McCaffery M, Portenoy RK: Nonopioids: Acetaminophen and nonsteroidal antiinflammatory drugs. pp. 129-160. In: McCaffery M, Pasero C: *Pain: Clinical Manual*, St. Louis, 1999, Mosby, p. 133. American Pain Society (APS): *Principles of analgesic use in the treatment of acute pain and cancer pain*, ed. 3, Glenview, IL, APS, 1992. Kaiko R, Lacouture P, Hopf K, et al: Analgesic efficacy of controlled-release (CR) oxycodone and CR morphine. *Clin Pharmacol Ther* 59:130, 1996. From McCaffery M, Pasero C: *Pain: Clinical Manual*, © 1999, Mosby.

that makes up 10% of all morphine metabolites, and it does provide analgesia. Binding of M6G to μ opioid receptors is 4 times less than that of morphine, and binding of M6G to κ receptors is 20 times less than morphine. Patients with renal failure are at risk for increased levels of active metabolites. Hydromorphone should be considered as an intermediate opioid in patients with decreased renal function. The chemical structure of morphine is shown in Figure 6-2.

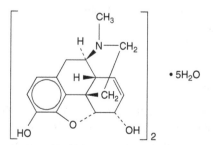

Figure 6-2 Chemical structure of morphine.

Source: Figure from: http://dailymed.nlm.nih.gov/dailymed/drugInfo.cfm?id=8115.

Alfentanil

Alfentanil is a synthetic opioid that is a phenylpiperidine derivative. Alfentanil has a rapid onset. In addition to analgesia, alfentanil is used to blunt the stress response during surgical procedures. Duration after IV administration for alfentanil is 30 to 60 minutes, with a half-life in adults of 83 to 97 minutes.[37] The chemical structure of alfentanil is shown in Figure 6-3.

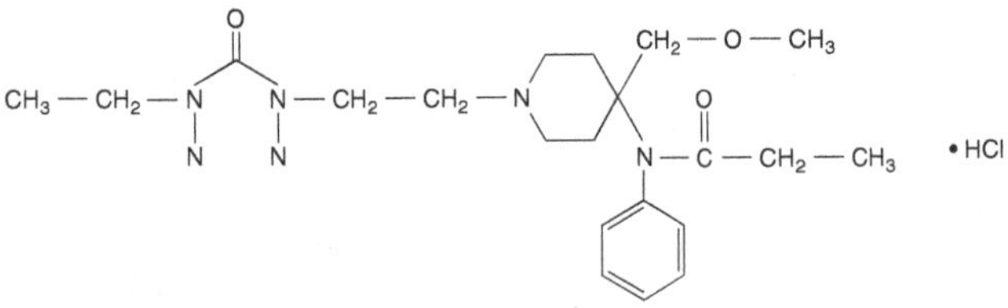

Figure 6-3 Chemical structure of alfentanil.

Source: Figure from: http://dailymed.nlm.nih.gov/dailymed/drugInfo .cfm?id=6884.

Sufentanil

This synthetic opioid is a phenylpiperidine derivative that is 10 times more potent than fentanyl. Sufentanil administered at 8 mcg/kg provides general anesthesia and is frequently used in high doses for cardiac and major surgical procedures. One of the adverse effects of concern with the administration of sufentanil is rigidity in the chest with high doses.[17] The chemical structure of sufentanil is shown in Figure 6-4.

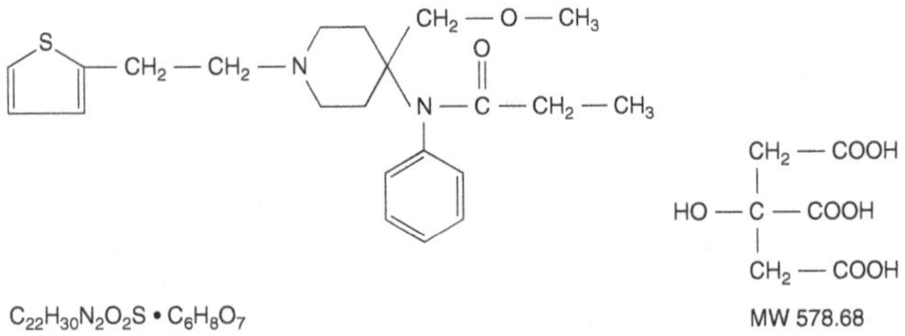

Figure 6-4 Chemical structure of sufentanil.

Source: Figure from: http://dailymed.nlm.nih.gov/dailymed/drugInfo .cfm?id=1055#nlm34088-5.

Remifentanil

Remifentanil has a rapid onset and a short duration of action that can be used for a variety of surgical procedures. Because of the short duration of action, this medication is given as an infusion. Boluses of remifentanil can lead to respiratory muscle rigidity and apnea. Break down of remifentanil occurs by hydrolysis of the propanoic acid-methyl ester linkages.[17] Esterases that break down remifentanil are from tissue and blood. Remifentanil is not broken down by plasma cholinesterase; therefore atypical pseudocholinesterase deficiency does not affect metabolism of remifentanil.[17] Renal and hepatic disease states do not affect the breakdown of remifentanil. The chemical structure of remifentanil is shown in Figure 6-5.

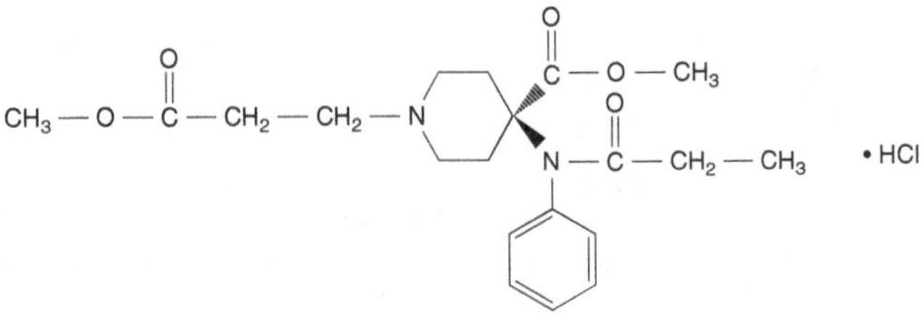

Figure 6-5 Chemical structure of remifentanil.

Source: Figure from: http://dailymed.nlm.nih.gov/dailymed/drugInfo .cfm?id=5250.

Hydromorphone

This intermediate-acting semisynthetic opioid is particularly useful for treating moderate and severe pain. Onset of IV hydromorphone is 5 minutes, with a duration of 4 to 5 hours in opioid-naive patients and 3 to 4 hours in patients that have developed tolerance to opioids.[17,29] The advantage of the use of hydromorphone over morphine is the lack of active metabolites that build up in patients with renal failure. The active metabolite M6G is increased in patients with renal failure. The chemical structure of hydromorphone is shown in Figure 6-6.

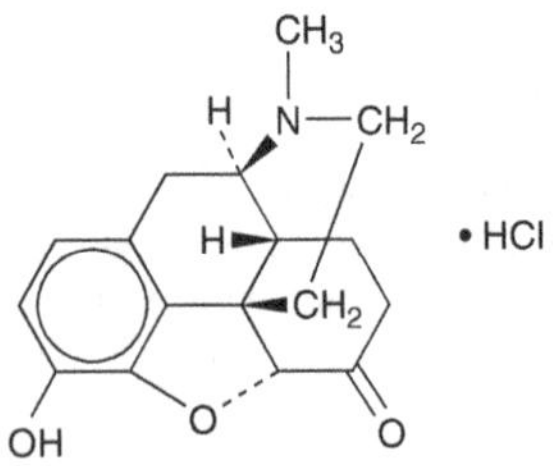

Figure 6-6 Chemical structure of hydromorphone.

Source: Figure from: http://dailymed.nlm.nih.gov/dailymed/drugInfo .cfm?id=6833.

Meperidine

Meperidine is a synthetic opioid in the phenylpiperidine group. Although meperidine has been used frequently to provide analgesia in the past, its use has decreased substantially due to the increased awareness of the risk for toxicity related to the metabolite normeperidine.[4] Increased levels of normeperidine have been associated with the development of seizures.[4] The American Pain Society recommends not using meperidine in patients with sickle cell disease, CNS disorders, and renal disease processes or in children.[4] In addition, meperidine has been found to have untoward adverse effects in patients taking monoamine oxidase inhibitors. The combination of monoamine oxidase inhibitors and meperidine has led to severe respiratory depression, coma, cyanosis, and hypotension.[17]

Adverse Effects and Contraindications

Opioid-Induced Sedation

Approximately 20% to 60% of patients receiving opioids after surgery are severely sedated.[46–48] Exacerbating the situation, clinical practice often involves targeting a level of sedation as a surrogate for pain relief with the assumption that a sedated patient is without pain. This occurs despite findings from a study by Lentschener and colleagues[47] in which 58% of the most sedated patients were found to have moderate to severe pain compared with 18% of patients in the less-sedated group. Nonetheless, opioids are well known to cause sedation, but the underlying mechanisms regarding opioid-induced sedation are still not fully understood. Clinically, it has been noted that respiratory depression is most likely to occur in sedated patients, although little research has been done on the association between opioid-induced sedation and opioid-induced respiratory depression.[49]

Consciousness is associated with increased activity in the reticular activating system mediated by catecholamines, whereas sleep is a restorative process associated with increased production of serotonin. Opioids are known to increase the amount of time animals sleep.[50] It has been reported that the characteristics of sleep in animals given opioids are altered when compared with controls. Slow wave sleep and rapid-eye-movement sleep were found to be decreased in animals given opioids. In studies of humans,[49] results regarding electroencephalographic analysis in patients receiving moderate doses of opioid were not conclusive. In general, Young-McCaughan and Miaskowski[49] state that little is known regarding the mechanisms associated with the development of opioid-induced sedation.

Opioid-Induced Respiratory Depression

Respiratory depression induced by the administration of opioids is clinically well established. Patients that are opioid-naive being treated for acute pain are most likely to experience respiratory depression.[4] Although the adverse respiratory effects of opioids are well established both clinically and academically, the underlying physiology of this phenomenon is only partly understood, despite the fact that these compounds have been used therapeutically for thousands of years. Several authors[51,52] note that opioid-induced respiratory depression can be attributed to direct opioid stimulation of opioid receptors on the brainstem. Respiratory depression is classically attributed to stimulation of μ_2 opioid receptors, although the exact mechanism has yet to be described. However, studies have extended our knowledge base and indicate that opioid-induced respiratory depression may be the result of cumulative effects on cortical areas and in central and peripheral chemoreceptors in addition to the previously mentioned brainstem receptors.[53,54] The roles of cortical areas and chemoreceptors in opioid-induced respiratory depression are yet to be fully described and serve to pose more questions in regard to an adverse effect of opioids that is very familiar but poorly understood.

Table 6-2 Opioid Pharmacology

	Fentanyl	Remifentanil	Morphine	Hydromorphone	Methadone
Onset	Almost immediate	Almost immediate	5–10 min	5 min	10–20 min
Duration	0.5–1 h	5–10 min	4 h	4–5 h	
Half-life	2–4 h	10–20 min	2–4 h	2–3 h	8–59 h
Protein binding	80–85%	70%	30–35%	8–19%	85–90%
Metabolism	Phase I metabolism via CYP3A4	Hydrolysis of ester linkages from nonspecific tissue and blood esterases	Primarily phase II metabolism via glucuronic acid	Primarily phase II metabolism via glucuronic acid	Phase I metabolism via CYP3A4, CYP2B6, and CYP2C19

Source: From references 17, 31, and 39.

Gastrointestinal Effects of Opioids

Opioid receptors are not only present in the CNS but are present in the GI tract as well. Activation of these receptors affects GI function in a number of different ways. Overall, opioids decrease gastric motility, gastric emptying, and peristalsis. Frequent GI problems associated with opioid administration include nausea, constipation, fecal impaction, and potentially obstruction. Biliary spasm is known to occur with all opioids.

Nausea

PONV is still a major concern of patients having surgery. Twenty percent to 30% of patients undergoing surgery experience PONV.[55] Nausea is a subjective phenomenon of an unpleasant, wavelike sensation experienced in the back of the throat and/or epigastrium. Stimulation of serotonin, histamine, and dopamine receptors in the chemoreceptor trigger zone in the medulla are thought to be associated with the mechanisms for PONV. Risk factors for the development of PONV include four different categories: specific factors, anesthetic risk factors, surgical risk factors, and type of surgery (Table 6-3).[56]

Constipation

Constipation is a frequent adverse effect that occurs with opioid use. Tolerance to opioids does not develop in regard to constipation. According to the American Pain Society,[4] there is no one laxative that is better than another in the treatment of constipation due to opioid use.

Other Common Effects of Opioids

Opioids depress the cough reflex by direct effect on the cough center in the medulla. Use of opioids to suppress the cough reflex is common for procedures that involve the upper airway, although at the same time it decreases protection of the airway.

Drug Interactions

One of the consequences of combining drugs such as opioids and benzodiazepines is a synergistic effect on opioid-induced sedation and opioid-induced respiratory depression. The combination of opioids and benzodiazepines has also been found to lower blood pressure, systemic vascular resistance, and cardiac index. In addition, the combination of opioids with hypnotics such as propofol has also been found to decrease blood pressure.

Table 6-3 Risk Factors for Postoperative Nausea and Vomiting

Patient-specific factors
Female gender
Nonsmoking
History of PONV
Anesthetic risk factors
Volatile anesthetics
Nitrous oxide
Intraoperative and postoperative opioids
Surgical risk factors
Duration of surgery
Type of surgery
Laparoscopic
Laparotomy
Breast
Strabismus
Plastic surgery
Maxillofacial
Gynecologic
Abdominal
Neurologic
Ophthalmologic
Urologic

Source: From reference 58.

Guidelines and Precautions

Preoperative Assessment

One of the keys to pain management during the perioperative period is identification of those factors that will help determine opioid requirements during surgery. Amount of opioid used before surgery impacts the amount of opioid used during surgery. Opioid-naive patients are more sensitive to opioids and are more likely to have adverse effects such as opioid-induced sedation and respiratory depression. Gender may play a role in opioid requirements. Length of incision and type of surgery are also thought to play a role in opioid requirements.[57] Renal and liver function also impact metabolism and elimination of opioids. See Table 6-4 for complete dosage and indications of opioids.

Partial Agonists, Agonist-Antagonists, and Antagonists

Use of opioids that have antagonist effects on μ and κ receptors can be useful in the management of pain. However, clinicians need to be aware that substituting these

Table 6-4 Opioid Dosage and Administration

	Dose	Indications	Side Effects
Fentanyl	Low dose (2 mcg/kg)	Minor painful procedures.	Opioid-naive patients at risk for respiratory depression.
	Moderate dose (2–20 mcg/kg)	Major surgical procedures to reduce stress response.	Likely to cause respiratory depression. Patients need to be monitored postoperatively for respiratory depression.
	High dose (20–50 mcg/kg)	Cardiac or neurosurgical procedures requiring decrease in stress response.	Respiratory depression likely. Rigidity of respiratory muscles more likely.
Remifentanil	0.1–1.0 mcg/kg/min	Major surgical procedures requiring a decrease in stress response.	Respiratory depression likely. Rigidity of respiratory muscles more likely.
Sufentanil	1–2 mcg/kg	Major surgical procedures requiring a decrease in stress response.	Respiratory depression likely. Rigidity of respiratory muscles more likely.
Alfentanil	8–20 mcg/kg	Major surgical procedures requiring a decrease in stress response.	Alfentanil is more likely to cause hypotension than fentanyl. Respiratory depression likely.
Hydromorphone	0.2–0.6 mg/kg	Intermediate-acting opioid that can be used intraoperatively but also postoperatively.	Respiratory depression likely in opioid-naive patients.
Morphine	2.5–5 mg/kg	Intermediate-acting opioid that can be used intraoperatively but also postoperatively.	Active metabolite M6G contributes to analgesia, particularly in patients with renal disease.
Methadone	2.5–10 mg	Detoxification for opioid addiction. Can also be used for treatment of acute pain.	Respiratory depression likely. Can cause prolonged Q-T interval.

medications for long-term use of μ receptor agonists can lead to withdrawal symptoms. Agonist-antagonist medications can also lead to confusion and hallucinations, particularly in the elderly and those with decreased renal function.[4] The analgesic effects of agonist-antagonist medications are limited compared with μ opioid agonists.

Nalbuphine

Nalbuphine is a synthetic opioid agonist-antagonist that has strong κ agonist binding and is a μ receptor antagonist. κ agonist activity provides analgesia with less risk of respiratory depression. The recommended IV dose is 10 mg for a 70-kg adult. Onset of nalbuphine is 2 to 3 minutes with a duration of analgesic activity of 3 to 6 hours. The chemical structure of nalbuphine is shown in Figure 6-7.

Buprenorphine

Buprenorphine is a partial agonist that provides analgesia and can lead to respiratory depression, but there is little euphoria associated with its use. Peak effects of buprenorphine occur in 15 minutes and last up to 6 hours.[17] When given to patients that have been receiving μ opioid agonists, buprenorphine can act as an antagonist and lead to opioid withdrawal symptoms. Buprenorphine is often used in drug rehabilitation settings for opioid addiction alone or in combination with naloxone.[4] The chemical structure of buprenorphine is shown in Figure 6-8.

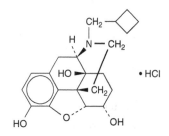

Figure 6-7 Chemical structure of nalbuphine.

Source: Figure from: http://dailymed.nlm.nih.gov/dailymed/drugInfo.cfm?id=5573.

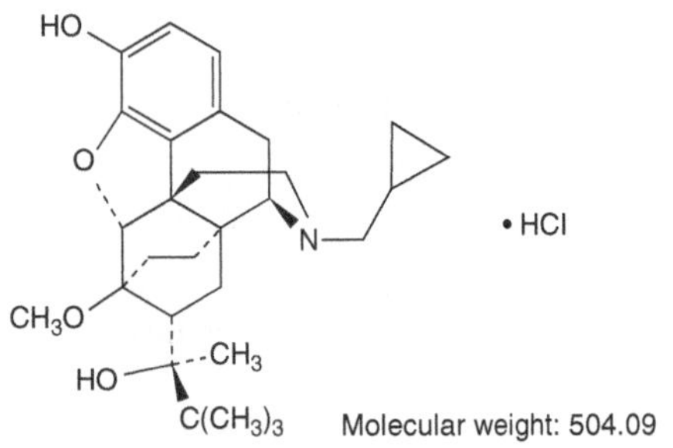

Figure 6-8 Chemical structure of buprenorphine.

Source: Figure from: http://dailymed.nlm.nih.gov/dailymed/drugInfo.cfm?id=5889.

Naloxone

Naloxone is an opioid antagonist that is frequently used for patients with respiratory depression or significant sedation. Naloxone has also been used to treat shock in the past. Patients in a stressed state not only produce adrenocorticotropic hormone from proopiomelanocortin, but endogenous opioids such as β-endorphin are also produced from proopiomelanocortin. Naloxone not only blocks exogenous opioids but also endogenous opioids. The μ opioid receptors are most strongly blocked by naloxone, but it does have antagonist effects on other opioid receptors. The average serum half-life of naloxone is 64 minutes; thus one of the concerns with administration is the lack of prolonged effect in patients receiving longer duration opioids.[17] Rapid administration of naloxone can lead to withdrawal symptoms such as seizures, arrhythmias, and severe pain. Naloxone typically is provided as 0.4 mg/mL and should be diluted in 10 mL saline and administered 0.5 mL at a time to prevent the development of severe pain and withdrawal manifestations. Figure 6-9 shows the chemical structure of naloxone.

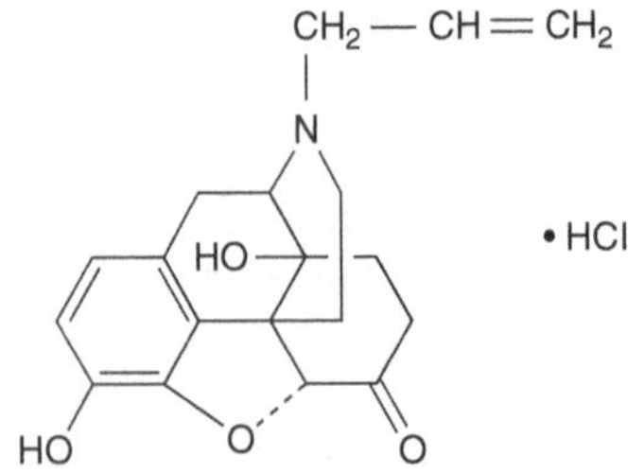

Figure 6-9 Chemical structure of naloxone.

Source: Figure from: http://dailymed.nlm.nih.gov/dailymed/drugInfo.cfm?id=8645.

Practical Aspects of Drug Administration (Applications in the Operating Room)

Although pain is defined as a subjective response to injury, anesthesia providers are unable to elicit a pain score from patients under the effects of general anesthesia. Heart rate and blood pressure are often used as indicators of stress response due to pain, although there are many pitfalls associated with using these clinical signs. Heart rate and blood pressure are not good indicators of pain in patients receiving beta-blockers and so pain may be undertreated. Patients with tourniquet pain or a full bladder may be overtreated with opioids when using heart rate and blood pressure as indicators of adequate analgesia.

Constriction of the pupils is another physiologic indicator of response to opioids that can be used under general anesthesia.[58] Opioids directly affect the Edinger-Westphal nucleus of the occulomotor nerve. Stimulation of this nucleus causes a parasympathetic response with resultant miotic changes in the pupil. These pupillary changes have been associated with opioid levels in humans.[58] Clinically, constricted pupils provide an indication of greater plasma opioid levels. This assessment can be used in conjunction with other clinical signs to assess response to opioids.

Respiratory rate also provides an indicator of pain and response to opioids. The clinician should consider the impact of other conditions on respiratory rate, but hyperpnea is often associated with pain. Respiratory rate can be used as an indicator for the titration of opioids while the patient continues under the effects of anesthesia. A respiratory rate of greater than 20 breaths per minute is an indication for additional opioids. A respiratory rate of less than 12 breaths per minute is an indication that the patient has received more than adequate amounts of opioid.

Pain rating scales are often used as indicators of pain before and after surgery. Although these scales are often helpful in assessing pain, they are affected by a patient's past history. A pain scale rating of 8 before surgery may not be the same as an 8 after surgery. Scales vary depending on a patient's experience with various types of pain.

When transferring care, communication of pain and treatment of pain should include pain scores, treatments, and those treatments that have been more successful. It is also important to identify the amount of opioid and other treatments a patient was receiving before surgery. Opioid requirements as noted earlier in this chapter vary based on previous opioid requirements.

Opiate Tolerance, Physical Dependence, and Addiction

Tolerance is defined by the American Pain Society[4] as a "state of adaptation in which exposure to a drug induces changes that result in a diminution of one or more of the drug's effects over time." It should be noted that tolerance may lead to greater doses of opioids to provide analgesia; therefore no upper limit is provided for dosage of opioids. Tolerance to opioid-induced adverse effects can be beneficial. Tolerance to opioid-induced adverse effects of respiratory depression and sedation occurs more quickly than analgesia. Unfortunately, tolerance to some adverse effects, such as constipation, does not occur.

Physical dependence is defined by the American Pain Society[4] as the "state of adaptation that is manifested by drug class specific withdrawal syndrome that can be produced by abrupt cessation, rapid dose reduction, decreasing blood level of the drug, and/or administration of an antagonist." The most effective way to decrease physical dependence is to gradually decrease the dose of the opioid.[29] If a patient continues to use opioids even though the disease process has diminished, this is considered physical dependence. Physical dependence on an opioid should not be confused with addiction.

Addiction is defined by the American Pain Society[4] as a "primary, chronic, neurobiologic disease, with genetic, psychosocial, and environmental factors influencing its development and manifestations. It is characterized by behaviors that include one or more of the following: impaired control over drug use, compulsive use, continued use despite harm, and craving." Addiction is associated with overuse of an opioid. Additional behaviors that have been noted with addiction are irritability, apathy, anxiety, or depression. Addiction affects other aspects of an individual's life, such as legal, economic, or social aspects.[4]

Key Points

- Intraoperative opioids not only provide anesthesia but also blunt the stress response during surgery.

- Opioids are likely to cause respiratory depression when given rapidly to opioid-naive patients.

- The development of PONV is often associated with the administration of opioids.

- Postoperative opioids are best given on a scheduled basis to prevent breakthrough pain.

- Morphine metabolite M6G provides analgesia, and higher levels of this metabolite are present in patients with renal failure.

- Response to opioids may depend on a variety of factors that should be considered such as age, gender, genotype, type of surgery, and previous opioid use.

Chapter Questions

Conversion Example

Ms. Anders has advanced uterine cancer. Her abdominal pain is well controlled with 40 mg OxyContin every 12 hours and occasional (three to four times a week) oxycodone 10 mg for breakthrough pain. She has developed a bowel obstruction that requires surgery. She will be allowed to consume nothing by mouth (NPO) for at least 24 hours after surgery.

A conversion from oral oxycodone 80 mg (24-hour intake) to IV fentanyl is needed. Because Ms. Anders uses a maximum of four doses of oxycodone 10 mg/wk, it will not be added to her 24-hour total intake of 80 mg. Perform the following math to elicit the conversion:

1. Calculate the 24-hour total dose: oxycodone 80 mg/ 24 hours.

2. Set up the simple proportion equation:

$$\frac{\text{Oxycodone 20 mg}}{\text{Fentanyl 100 mcg/h}} = \frac{\text{(current dose) oxycodone 80 mg}}{\text{(planned dose) fentanyl} \times \text{mg IV}} = 400 \text{ mcg/h}$$

3. Reduce dose by 25% to account for incomplete cross-tolerance = 300 mcg/h.

4. Some practitioners recommend reducing the dose by an additional 25% when both the opioid and the route are being changed; therefore the dose would be 200 mcg/h.

The rescue (breakthrough) dose varies from 10% to 25% of the 24-hour total dose. Ms. Anders should be assessed frequently for both pain and adverse effects and the doses adjusted accordingly.

References

1. Centers for Disease Control and Prevention. Fast stats A to Z. National Center for Health Statistics. Available at: http://www.cdc.gov/nchs/fastats/insurg.htm. Accessed July 15, 2009.

2. Federated Ambulatory Surgery Association. *Frequently asked questions.* Available at: http://ascassociation.org/faqs/faqaboutascs/. Accessed August 15, 2009.

3. Hamilton GR, Baskett TF. In the arms of Morpheus: the development of morphine for postoperative pain relief. *Can J Anaesth.* 2000;47:367–374.

4. American Pain Society. *Principles of Analgesic Use in the Treatment of Acute Pain and Cancer Pain.* Glenview IL: American Pain Society; 2008.

5. McCleskey EW, Gold MS. Ion channels of nociception. *Annu Rev Physiol.* 1999;61:835–856.

6. Schaible HG, Richter F. Pathophysiology of pain. *Langenb Arch Surg.* 2004;389:237–243.

7. Treede RD, Kenshalo DR, Gracely RH, Jones AK. The cortical representation of pain. *Pain.* 1999;79:105–111.

8. Minami M, Satoh M. Molecular biology of the opioid receptors: structures, functions and distributions. *Neurosci Res.* 1995;23:121–145.

9. Page GG, Blakely WP, Ben-Eliyahu S. Evidence that postoperative pain is a mediator of the tumor-promoting effects of surgery in rats. *Pain.* 2001;90:191–199.

10. Halter JB, Pflug AE, Porte D Jr. Mechanism of plasma catecholamine increases during surgical stress in man. *J Clin Endocrinol Metabol.* 1977;45:936–944.

11. Akca O, Melischek M, Scheck T, et al. Postoperative pain and subcutaneous oxygen tension. *Lancet.* 1999;354:41–42.

12. Brooks-Brunn JA. Predictors of postoperative pulmonary complications following abdominal surgery. *Chest.* 1997;111: 564–571.

13. Puntillo K, Weiss SJ. Pain: its mediators and associated morbidity in critically ill cardiovascular surgical patients. *Nurs Res.* 1994;43:31–36.

14. Rhudy JL, Meagher MW. Fear and anxiety: divergent effects on human pain thresholds. *Pain.* 2000;84:65–75.

15. Eisendrath SJ. Psychiatric aspects of chronic pain. *Neurology.* 1995;45(12 Suppl 9), S26–S34.

16. Jaffe JH, Martin WR. Opioid analgesics and antagonists. In: Rall TW, Nies AS, Taylor P, eds. *Goodman and Gilman's The Pharmacological Basis of Therapeutics,* 4th ed. New York: Pergamon Press; 1990:485–521.

17. National Library of Medicine Daily Med. Available at: http://dailymed.nlm.nih.gov/dailymed/about.cfm. Accessed August 15, 2009.

18. Han W, Ide S, Sora I, Yamamoto H, Ikeda K. A possible genetic mechanism underlying individual and interstrain differences in opioid actions: focus on the mu opioid receptor gene. *Annals of the New York Academy of Sciences.* 2004;1025: 370–375.

19. Lotsch J, Geisslinger G. Are mu-opioid receptor polymorphisms important for clinical opioid therapy? *Trends Mol Med.* 2005;11:82–89.

20. Bond C, LaForge KS, Tian M, et al. Single-nucleotide polymorphism in the human mu opioid receptor gene alters beta-endorphin binding and activity: possible implications for opiate addiction. *Proc Nal Acad Sci USA.* 1998; 95:9608–9613.

21. Crowley JJ, Oslin DW, Patkar AA, et al. A genetic association study of the mu opioid receptor and severe opioid dependence. *Psychiatr Genet.* 2003;13:169–173.

22. Chou WY, Wang CH, Liu PH, et al. Human opioid receptor A118G polymorphism affects intravenous patient-controlled analgesia morphine consumption after total abdominal hysterectomy [see comment]. *Anesthesiology.* 2006;105:334–337.

23. Chou WY, Yang LC, Lu HF, et al. Association of mu-opioid receptor gene polymorphism (A118G) with variations in morphine consumption for analgesia after total knee arthroplasty. *Acta Anaesth Scand.* 2006;50:787–792.

24. Becker A, Grecksch G, Kraus J, et al. Rewarding effects of ethanol and cocaine in mu opioid receptor-deficient mice. *Naunyn Schmied Arch Pharmacol.* 2002;365:296–302.

25. Berrendero F, Kieffer BL, Maldonado R. Attenuation of nicotine-induced antinociception, rewarding effects, and dependence in mu-opioid receptor knock-out mice. *J Neurosci.* 2002;22:10935–10940.

26. Ray LA, Hutchison KE. A polymorphism of the mu-opioid receptor gene (OPRM1) and sensitivity to the effects of alcohol in humans. *Alcohol Clin Exp Res.* 2004;28:1789–1795.

27. Roberts AJ, McDonald JS, Heyser CJ, et al. mu-Opioid receptor knockout mice do not self-administer alcohol. *J Pharmacol Exp Ther.* 2000;293:1002–1008.

28. Arias A, Feinn R, Kranzler HR. Association of an Asn40Asp (A118G) polymorphism in the mu-opioid receptor gene with substance dependence: a meta-analysis. *Drug Alcohol Depend.* 2006;83:262–268.

29. McCaffery M, Pasero C. *Pain: Clinical Manual.* Philadelphia: Mosby; 1999.

30. van Dorp EL, Romberg R, Sarton E, et al. Morphine-6-glucuronide: morphine's successor for postoperative pain relief? *Anesth Analg.* 2006;102:1789–1797.

31. Likar R, Vadlau EM, Breschan C, et al. Comparable analgesic efficacy of transdermal buprenorphine in patients over and under 65 years of age. *Clin J Pain.* 2008;24:536–543.

32. Cepeda MS, Carr DB. Women experience more pain and require more morphine than men to achieve a similar degree of analgesia. *Anesth Analg.* 2003;97:1464–1468.

33. Paulson PE, Minoshima S, Morrow TJ, Casey KL. Gender differences in pain perception and patterns of cerebral activation during noxious heat stimulation in humans. *Pain*. 1998;76:223–229.

34. Fillingim RB, Kaplan L, Staud R, et al. The A118G single nucleotide polymorphism of the mu-opioid receptor gene (OPRM1) is associated with pressure pain sensitivity in humans. *J Pain*. 2005;6:159–167.

35. Minto CF, Schnider TW, Egan TD, et al. Influence of age and gender on the pharmacokinetics and pharmacodynamics of remifentanil. I. Model development. *Anesthesiology*. 1997;86:10–23.

36. Lemmens HJ, Bovill JG, Hennis PJ, Gladines MP, Burm AG. Alcohol consumption alters the pharmacodynamics of alfentanil. *Anesthesiology*. 1989;71:669–674.

37. Donnelly AJ, Baughman VL, Gonzales JP, Golembiewski J, Tomsik EA. *Anesthesiology & Critical Care Drug Handbook*, 8th ed. Hudson, OH: Lexi-Comp; 2008.

38. Lotsch J, Skarke C, Liefhold J, Geisslinger G. Genetic predictors of the clinical response to opioid analgesics: clinical utility and future perspectives. *Clin Pharmacokinet*. 2004; 43:983–1013.

39. Candiotti KA, Birnbach DJ, Lubarsky DA, et al. The impact of pharmacogenomics on postoperative nausea and vomiting: do CYP2D6 allele copy number and polymorphisms affect the success or failure of ondansetron prophylaxis? *Anesthesiology*. 2005;102:543–549.

40. Janicki PK, Schuler HG, Jarzembowski TM, Rossi M II. Prevention of postoperative nausea and vomiting with granisetron and dolasetron in relation to CYP2D6 genotype [see comment]. *Anesth Analg*. 2006;102:1127–1133.

41. Haegerstam GA. Pathophysiology of bone pain: a review. *Acta Orthop Scand*. 2001;72:308–317.

42. Jacobs JR, Reves JG, Marty J, White WD, Bai SA, Smith LR. Aging increases pharmacodynamic sensitivity to the hypnotic effects of midazolam. *Anesth Analg*. 1995;80:143–148.

43. Elia N, Lysakowski C, Tramer MR. Does multimodal analgesia with acetaminophen, nonsteroidal antiinflammatory drugs, or selective cyclooxygenase-2 inhibitors and patient-controlled analgesia morphine offer advantages over morphine alone? Meta-analyses of randomized trials. *Anesthesiology*. 2005;103:1296–1304.

44. Kranke P, Morin AM, Roewer N, et al. Patients' global evaluation of analgesia and safety of injected parecoxib for postoperative pain: a quantitative systematic review. *Anesth Analg*. 2004;99:797–806.

45. Shafer SL. Notice of retraction. [Retraction of Basran S, Frumento RJ, Cohen A, et al. *Anesth Analg*. 2006 Jul;103:15–20.] *Anesth Analg*. 2009;108:1953.

46. Aubrun F, Monsel S, Langeron O, Coriat P, Riou B. Postoperative titration of intravenous morphine. *Eur J Anaesth*. 2001;18:159–165.

47. Lentschener C, Tostivint P, White PF, et al. Opioid-induced sedation in the postanesthesia care unit does not insure adequate pain relief: a case-control study. *Anesth Analg*. 2007;105:1143–1147.

48. Paqueron X, Lumbroso A, Mergoni P, et al. Is morphine-induced sedation synonymous with analgesia during intravenous morphine titration? *Br J Anaesth*. 2002;89:697–701.

49. Young-McCaughan S, Miaskowski C. Definition of and mechanism for opioid-induced sedation. *Pain Manage Nurs*. 2001; 2:84–97.

50. Furst S. Brain monoamines are involved in the sedative effects of opiates and neuroleptics. *Progr Clin Biol Res*. 1990; 328:311–314.

51. Takeda S, Eriksson LI, Yamamoto Y, Joensen H, Onimaru H, Lindahl SG. Opioid action on respiratory neuron activity of the isolated respiratory network in newborn rats. *Anesthesiology*. 2001;95:740–749.

52. Takita K, Herlenius EA, Lindahl SG, Yamamoto Y. Actions of opioids on respiratory activity via activation of brainstem mu-, delta- and kappa-receptors: an in vitro study. *Brain Res*. 1997;778:233–241.

53. Cashman JN, Dolin SJ. Respiratory and haemodynamic effects of acute postoperative pain management: evidence from published data. *Br J Anaesth*. 2004;93:212–223.

54. Pattinson KT. Opioids and the control of respiration. *Br J Anaesth*. 2008;100:747–758.

55. Tramer MR. A rational approach to the control of postoperative nausea and vomiting: evidence from systematic reviews. Part II. Recommendations for prevention and treatment, and research agenda. *Acta Anaesth Scand*. 2001;45:14–19.

56. Gan TJ, Meyer TA, Apfel CC, et al. Society for ambulatory anesthesia guidelines for the management of postoperative nausea and vomiting [see comment]. *Anesth Analg*. 2007;105:1615–1628.

57. Janssen KJ, Kalkman CJ, Grobbee DE, et al. The risk of severe postoperative pain: modification and validation of a clinical prediction rule. *Anesth Analg*. 2008;107:1330–1339.

58. Schmidt H, Lotsch J. Pharmacokinetic-pharmacodynamic modeling of the miotic effects of dihydrocodeine in humans. *Eur J Clin Pharmacol*. 2007;63:1045–1054.

Objectives

After completing this chapter, the reader should be able to

- Review the World Health Organization analgesic ladder.
- Describe the role of nonopioid analgesics in anesthesia practice.
- Discuss the analgesic properties of ketamine.
- Review the properties of nonsteroidal analgesics in the context of the perioperative period.
- Describe appropriate perioperative utilization of centrally acting α_2 agonists.

7

Nonopioid Analgesics and Their Role in Anesthesia Practice

Michael Kremer, PhD, CRNA, FAAN

Introduction

The International Association for the Study of Pain describes pain as "an unpleasant sensory and emotional experience associated with actual or potential tissue damage, or described in terms of such damage."[1] Pain is an unpleasant subjective experience that results from interaction of the ascending and descending nervous systems that involves biochemical, physiologic, psychological, and neocortical processes. Pain can affect every aspect of life, including sleep, thought processes, emotions, and activities of daily living. Because there are no reliable objective markers for pain, only patients can describe the intensity and quality of their pain.[2]

Pain is the most frequent symptom that prompts visits to healthcare providers.[1] Patients often do not obtain satisfactory pain relief, leading to pain assessment as "the fifth vital sign." The Joint Commission mandates the involvement of patients in the assessment and treatment of their pain.[3]

Epidemiology and Etiology

Most people experience pain at some point during their lives. In some cases pain may be mild to moderate, intermittent, and easily managed, with minimal effects on the activities of daily living. Pain may also be chronic, severe or disabling, all consuming, and resistant to treatment.[2] When acute pain related to surgery is imposed on chronic pain, the anesthesia provider is challenged to provide adequate analgesia.

According to the American Pain Foundation, greater than 50 million individuals in the United States suffer from chronic pain, and an additional 25 million experience acute pain from injury or surgery. About 20% of adults, primarily women and the elderly, experience chronic pain such as back pain, headache, and joint pain.[4]

The prevalence for different types of pain includes moderate intensity back pain in 10% to 15% of the adult population, migraine headaches in 25 million individuals, and other types of headaches in 90% of Americans. Pain due to fibromyalgia affects 4 million Americans. Cancer is often associated with both acute and chronic pain. Some 70% of patients diagnosed with cancer experience significant pain.[4]

Pathophysiology

The pathophysiology of pain provides a basis for understanding the mechanisms of action for opioid and nonopioid analgesics. The types of pain that have been described include nociceptive, inflammatory, neuropathic, and functional. Nociceptive pain is transient and related to a noxious stimulus at receptors that are located in cutaneous tissue, bone, muscle, connective tissue, vessels, and viscera. Nociceptors may be classified as thermal, chemical, or mechanical. The nociceptive system includes receptors in the periphery to the spinal cord, brainstem, and cerebral cortex where the perception of pain occurs. The nociceptive system is an essential physiologic function that prevents additional tissue damage due to the autonomic withdrawal reflex. When tissue damage ensues despite the nociceptive response, inflammatory pain follows. The physiologic response shifts from responding to painful stimuli to protection of injured tissue. The inflammatory response contributes to pain hypersensitivity that prevents contact with or movement of the injured area until healing is complete, reducing further tissue damage.[2]

Neuropathic pain is spontaneous in nature and includes hypersensitivity to pain associated with damage to or pathologic changes in the peripheral nervous system, as in diabetic peripheral neuropathy, HIV/AIDS, polyneuropathy, postherpetic neuralgia, and pain originating in the central nervous system (CNS) from spinal cord injury, multiple sclerosis, and stroke. Functional pain is pain sensitivity due to an abnormal processing or function of the CNS related to normal stimuli. Fibromyalgia and irritable bowel syndrome manifest this abnormal sensitivity or hyperresponsiveness.[5]

Mechanisms of Pain

The mechanisms of nociceptive pain are clearly elucidated and provide a basis for understanding other types of pain. After stimulation of nociceptors, tissue injury causes the release of substances, including bradykinin, serotonin, potassium, histamine, prostaglandins, and substance P, that may further sensitize and/or activate nociceptors. Nociceptor activation produces action potentials that via transduction are transmitted along myelinated A-δ fibers and unmyelinated C fibers to the spinal cord. The A-δ fibers are responsible for initial fast, sharp pain and release excitatory amino acids that activate α-amino-3-hydroxy-5-methylisoxazole-4-propionic acid receptors in the dorsal horn. The C fibers produce secondary pain that is described as dull, aching, burning, and diffuse. These nerve fibers synapse in the dorsal horn of the spinal cord, where multiple neurotransmitters, including glutamate, substance P, and calcitonin gene–related peptide, are released. Transmission of pain signal occurs along the spinal cord extending to the thalamus, which acts as the pain relay center to the cortex, where pain is perceived.[2]

Pain modulation, or inhibition of nociceptive impulses, occurs through multiple processes. Gate control theory posits that pain modulation occurs at the dorsal horn.[6] The brain processes a finite number of signals simultaneously. Other sensory stimuli at nociceptors may alter pain perception. This explains the mechanism of action for counterirritants and transcutaneous electrical nerve simulation in pain management.[7,8]

Pain modulation also occurs through other complex processes. The endogenous opiate system, consisting of

endorphins (enkephalins, dynorphins, and β-endorphins), interacts with μ, δ, and κ receptors throughout the CNS to inhibit pain impulses and alter perceptions of pain. The CNS also includes inhibitory descending pathways from the brain that can blunt pain transmission in the dorsal horn. Neurotransmitters that are involved in this descending system include endogenous opioids, serotonin, norepinephrine, γ-aminobutyric acid, and neurotensin. The perception of pain involves nociceptive stimulation and physiologic and psychological input that contribute to the perception of pain. Therefore cognitive behavioral treatments such as distraction, relaxation, and guided imagery can reduce the perception of pain through alteration of pain processing in the cortex.[2]

Normally, a balance exists between excitatory and inhibitory neurotransmission. Changes in this balance can occur peripherally and centrally that result in the exaggerated responses and sensitization that are seen in inflammatory, neuropathic, or functional chronic pain. Pain in these settings may occur with or without a stimulus. Pain may arise from a stimulus that is not typically associated with pain (allodynia), such as a light touch in a patient with neuropathic pain. Hyperalgesia is an exaggerated and/or prolonged pain response to a stimulus that is associated with pain and can occur due to increased sensitivity in the CNS.[9,10]

This brief review of the physiologic mechanisms of pain provides a background for the study of nonopioid analgesics. Drugs in this category are of interest to anesthesia providers, because these drugs decrease minimal alveolar concentration (MAC) requirements, have opioid-sparing properties, facilitate more rapid recovery from anesthesia, prolong postoperative analgesia, and potentially can increase patient satisfaction with their anesthetic experience.

The analgesic ladder of the World Health Organization demonstrates the gradations in pharmacologic pain management options. Figure 7-1 displays this model and provides a foundation for analgesic management, including the use of nonopioid analgesics and adjuvant drugs such as tricyclic antidepressants or anticonvulsants.

Cyclooxygenase Inhibitors

Cyclooxygenase (COX) catalyzes the syntheses of prostaglandins from arachidonic acid.[11,12] Prostaglandins mediate physiologic processes, including inflammatory responses, maintenance of renal perfusion, and platelet aggregation (Figure 7-2). Nonsteroidal anti-inflammatory drugs

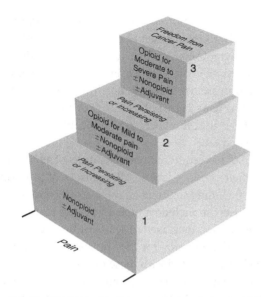

Figure 7-1 The World Health Organization analgesic ladder.

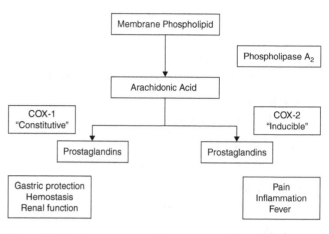

Figure 7-2 Cyclooxygenase pathways.
Source: From Gilron, Milne, Hong (2003).

(NSAIDs) block the action of COX enzymes and inhibit the generation of prostaglandin mediators. The resulting therapeutic effects include analgesia and anti-inflammatory properties with the potential side effects of gastric ulceration, decreased renal perfusion, and bleeding.[13]

Cyclooxygenase Enzymes

COX activity is associated with the isoenzymes, constitutively expressed as COX-1 and inflammatorily induced COX-2. COX-1 can be found in gastric mucosa, renal parenchyma, and platelets and is up-regulated slightly in response to inflammatory hormones. This enzyme is involved in platelet aggregation, maintenance of gastrointestinal mucosal integrity, and renal function. COX-2 is inducible and is expressed at injury sites, such as the brain and kidneys, and mediates inflammation, fever, pain, and carcinogenesis. COX-2 has no protective role in the tissues where it resides. COX-2 expression facilitates oncogenic processes, such as tumor invasion, angiogenesis, and metastasis. Transient COX-2 up-regulation in the spinal cord related to surgical inflammation may be important in central sensitization.[14] Inflammation results in up-regulation of COX-2 expression by 10- to 20-fold.[15]

NSAID-mediated suppression of prostaglandins and thromboxanes, which play homeostatic roles in the stomach (prostaglandin E_2 and prostaglandin I_2), kidneys (prostaglandin E_2), and platelets (thromboxane A_2 and prostaglandin I_2), is believed to be the mechanism responsible for the major adverse effects of NSAIDs. Inhibition of prostaglandin synthesis is thought to be the mechanism responsible for NSAID-induced bronchospasm and osteogenesis suppression.[13]

Characteristics of the NSAIDs include:

- Decreased activation and sensitization of peripheral nociceptors
- Attenuation of the inflammatory response
- Absence of dependence or addiction potential
- Synergistic effect with opioids
- Preemptive analgesic effects, e.g., decreased neuronal sensitization
- Absence of respiratory depression
- Minimal nausea and vomiting compared with opioids
- Long duration of action
- Less dose variability compared with opioids
- No papillary changes
- No effects on cognition[11]

Classification of NSAIDs

NSAID is an inclusive term that denotes a range of drugs that have analgesic, anti-inflammatory, and antipyretic effects. These drugs can be categorized as conventional nonspecific inhibitors of both COX isoforms (ibuprofen, naproxen, aspirin, acetaminophen, ketorolac) and COX-2 selective inhibitors (celecoxib, rofecoxib, valdecoxib, parecoxib). All NSAIDs and COX-2 inhibitors exhibit ceiling effects. Exceeding the ceiling effect dose increases the risk of drug-induced toxicity. COX-1 inhibition is responsible for many of the adverse effects associated with conventional NSAIDs.[13]

The chemical classification of NSAIDs is as follows:

Carboxylic acids
- Acetylated: aspirin
- Nonacetylated: sodium salicylamide, diflusinal

Acetic acids
- Indomethacin, tolmetin

Propionic acids
- Ibuprofen, naproxen, fenoprofen, ketoprofen

Enolic acids
- Phenylbutazone, piroxicam

Pyrrolopyrrole
- Ketorolac[13]

Conventional NSAIDs possess many desirable features described in Table 7-1. It is believed that COX-1 mediates physiologic function and COX-2 is involved in pathophysiologic processes. Therefore selective COX-2 enzyme inhibitors were developed to treat inducible inflammatory symptoms and related pain. COX-2 inhibitors largely have improved side effect profiles compared with conventional NSAIDs.[13] There have been significant risk-to-benefit considerations with some of the COX-2 enzyme inhibitors. Table 7-2 lists the potential adverse effects produced by NSAIDs.

In 2004 Merck announced a voluntary withdrawal of rofecoxib (Vioxx) from the U.S. and worldwide markets due to safety concerns regarding increased risk of myocardial infarctions and cerebrovascular accidents in patients taking rofecoxib. Rofecoxib was approved by the U.S. Food and Drug Administration (FDA) in 1999 for relief of the signs and symptoms of osteoarthritis and rheumatoid arthritis, to manage acute pain in adults, and to treat menstrual symptoms. At this writing the FDA is determining if the risk of cardiovascular events (myocardial infarction, cerebrovascular accident, death) may be increased in patients receiving celecoxib (Celebrex). In 2005 the FDA asked Pfizer to voluntarily remove valdecoxib (Bextra) from the market.[15]

The FDA has requested manufacturers of all NSAIDs to change their product labels. All sponsors of prescription NSAIDs, including celecoxib, have been asked to revise the package insert to include a boxed warning that highlights the potential for increased risk of cardiovascular events along with the potential for life-threatening gastrointestinal bleeding associated with these drugs.[15]

Controversy has also surrounded research findings reported on some COX-2 drugs. Twenty-one articles and abstracts published over a 15-year period, many of which reported research on perioperative analgesia involving COX-2 inhibitors, were identified as fraudulent and were retracted.[16]

Conventional NSAIDs

The properties of nonspecific inhibitors of COX-1 and COX-2 are well known. These traditional NSAIDs, such as ibuprofen, reduce swelling, soreness, and minor pain. They may be used to treat pain after minor surgical procedures or combined with opioids for treatment after major surgery and during home recovery. Combining NSAIDs with opioids can provide optimal pain relief with fewer side effects, such as nausea, drowsiness, and constipation. Many oral opioids are combined with acetaminophen, so it is important to limit the daily dose of this drug given its effects on the liver.[17] Acetaminophen toxicity is a leading cause of acute liver failure. Doses exceeding the package-recommended 4 g/day have been associated with severe liver damage.[18]

Table 7-1 Characteristics of Nonsteroidal Anti-inflammatory Drugs

Decreased activation and sensitization of peripheral nociceptors
Attenuation of the inflammatory response
Absence of dependence or addiction potential
Synergistic effect with opioids
Preemptive analgesic effects, e.g., decreased neuronal sensitization
Absence of respiratory depression
Minimal nausea and vomiting compared with opioids
Long duration of action
Less dose variability compared with opioids
No papillary changes
No effects on cognition

Source: From reference 11.

Table 7-2 Potential Adverse Effects Produced by Nonsteroidal Anti-inflammatory Drugs

Inhibition of platelet aggregation
Gastric ulceration
Renal dysfunction
Hepatocellular injury
Asthma exacerbation
Allergic reactions
Tinnitus
Urticaria

Source: From reference 11.

Aspirin (Acetylsalicylic Acid)

Aspirin is a salicylate that produces analgesia and irreversible acetylation of the COX enzyme, with decreased synthesis and release of prostaglandins. Aspirin is a weak inhibitor of renal prostaglandin synthesis and is unlikely to produce clinically relevant effects at doses less than the anti-inflammatory range. The leukotriene pathway remains intact when aspirin is ingested. Aspirin does not interact with opioid receptors and has little effect on the release of histamine or serotonin. Aspirin is quickly hydrolyzed to salicylic acid, which has no acetylation capacity but inhibits prostaglandin synthesis by a nonacetylation mechanism.[13]

Aspirin is rapidly absorbed from the small bowel and to a lesser extent from the stomach. The absorption rate for aspirin is related to the dissolution rate of the administered tablet and gastric emptying time. If gastric pH is high, aspirin is more ionized and the rate of absorption is decreased. The presence of food also delays absorption of aspirin from the gastrointestinal tract. There is no evidence that sodium bicarbonate given with aspirin (buffered aspirin) has a faster onset of action, greater peak intensity, or longer analgesic effect.[13]

Once aspirin is absorbed into the systemic circulation, it is rapidly hydrolyzed in the liver to salicylic acid. Because of this rapid hydrolysis, plasma aspirin concentrations are rarely more than 20 mcg/mL. Aspirin is pharmacologically active and does not require hydrolysis to salicylic acid for its effects. Metabolism of salicylic acid also occurs in the liver, where it is conjugated with glycine to form salicyluric acid. Salicyluric acid is excreted in the urine along with free salicylic acid. Renal excretion of free salicylic acid varies: from up to 85% of the ingested drug when the urine is alkaline to as low as 5% in acidic urine. Plasma concentrations of salicylic acid are increased with renal dysfunction characterized by decreased glomerular filtration rate or decreased secretory activity in the proximal tubules. The elimination half-time for aspirin is 15 to 20 minutes and for salicylic acid is 2 to 3 hours.[13]

Aspirin is more frequently administered for the following indications: (1) analgesia for low-intensity pain associated with headache and musculoskeletal disorders, (2) antipyretic, and (3) antiplatelet drug to prevent myocardial infarction and certain forms of ischemic stroke.[19,20]

The analgesic activity of aspirin is limited to a small dose range, below which there is little effect and above which an increase in dose results in toxicity with little increase in analgesia. The antipyretic effects of aspirin result from its prevention of pyrogen-induced release of prostaglandins in the CNS, including the hypothalamus.[13]

The antiplatelet effect of low-dose aspirin (75–325 mg/day) is due to irreversible acetylation of platelet COX-1 by nonhydrolyzed aspirin with failure to generate thromboxane resulting. Thromboxane is a potent inducer of platelet release and aggregation. The inhibitory effect occurs rapidly, before aspirin appearing in the systemic circulation, likely due to the acetylation of platelet prostaglandin synthase in the portal circulation. A daily aspirin maintenance dose of 40 mg causes complete inhibition of platelet COX-1 demonstrated by more than 95% decrease in serum thromboxane concentrations.[20]

The major adverse side effects of aspirin are related to gastrointestinal tract dysfunction and inhibition of platelet function. Other side effects include CNS stimulation, hepatic and renal dysfunction, metabolic alterations, uterine effects, and allergic reactions.[20–22]

Acetaminophen

Acetaminophen is widely used for its analgesic and antipyretic properties. This drug is available in a number of over-the-counter and prescription products. Acetaminophen is not considered a true NSAID because it lacks significant anti-inflammatory effects. In oral doses of 325 to 650 mg every 4 to 6 hours, acetaminophen is an alternative to aspirin as an analgesic and antipyretic, especially in pediatric patients and those for who salicylates are not recommended (e.g., peptic ulcer disease) or in whom prolongation of bleeding time would be problematic. Unlike salicylates, acetaminophen does not produce gastric irritation, change platelet aggregation, or antagonize the effects of uricosuric drugs. The anti-inflammatory effects of acetaminophen are weak related to the modest peripheral inhibitory effects of prostaglandin synthesis produced by this drug. Strong central inhibition of prostaglandin synthesis provides analgesic and antipyretic effects.[13]

The systemic absorption of acetaminophen is almost complete after oral administration, and significant binding to serum proteins does not occur. Acetaminophen is converted via conjugation and hydroxylation in the liver to inactive metabolites with small amounts of drug excreted unchanged.[13]

It has been estimated that lowered consumption of acetaminophen could lessen the incidence of end-stage renal disease by 8% to 10%. The acetaminophen metabolite *p*-aminophenol is nephrotoxic. The long-term renal toxicity of NSAIDs may be caused by ongoing inhibition of prostaglandin synthesis, resulting in medullary ischemia.[23]

Hepatic necrosis and death may follow a single dose of acetaminophen greater than 15 g. In otherwise healthy adults, hepatic toxicity can occur when daily acetaminophen doses exceed 4 g and at lower daily doses in the presence of alcohol abuse. High acetaminophen doses result in the formation of N-acetyl-p-benzoquinone, which is thought to be responsible for hepatotoxicity. This metabolite is normally scavenged by glutathione, an intracellular antioxidant. With an overdose, glutathione stores are exhausted, allowing the toxic reactive metabolite to accumulate and bind to hepatocytes. Acetylcysteine is an antioxidant that substitutes for glutathione as a scavenger and is effective in preventing liver damage from acetaminophen when given within 8 hours after an acetaminophen overdose.[2]

Other Anti-inflammatory Agents

Diflunisal is a fluorinated salicylic acid derivative that differs chemically from salicylates but has analgesic, antipyretic, and anti-inflammatory effects. Antiarthritic effects are prominent, and antipyretic action is not clinically useful. The most frequent side effects of this drug are nausea, vomiting, and gastrointestinal irritation. The effect of diflunisal on platelet function and bleeding time is dose related but compared with aspirin is reversible. Acute interstitial nephritis may occur, and transient increases in plasma concentrations of transaminases may occur.[13]

Indomethacin is a methylated indole derivative with analgesic, antipyretic, and anti-inflammatory properties equivalent to those of salicylates. This drug is one of the most potent COX inhibitors available. Its anti-inflammatory effects are useful in the management of patients with arthritis. Indomethacin is the drug of choice in treating ankylosing spondylitis and may be considered for the initial treatment of Reiter syndrome. Indomethacin provides anti-inflammatory effects that are comparable with those produced by colchicine when treating gouty arthritis. Neonatal cardiac failure related to patent ductus arteriosus may be treated with one dose of indomethacin, demonstrating the ability of this drug to selectively inhibit the synthesis of prostaglandins. Severe adverse effects limit the usefulness of indomethacin: Gastrointestinal disturbances and severe frontal headaches are common. Indomethacin inhibits platelet aggregation. Allergic reactions may occur, and cross-sensitivity with salicylates is likely. Liver function tests may become abnormal, and patients with preexisting renal disease may experience an exacerbation. Neutropenia, thrombocytopenia, and aplastic anemia are rare.[13]

Sulindac is a substituted analogue of indomethacin and has similar analgesic, antipyretic, and anti-inflammatory effects. The parent drug is an inactive prodrug but is reduced in vivo to the sulfide form, which is responsible for the pharmacologic effects. The active metabolite is cleared slowly from the plasma, with an elimination half-time of about 16 hours. Side effects include inhibition of platelet aggregation, gastrointestinal irritation, renal dysfunction, and altered liver function tests. It has been suggested that because sulindac does not affect the renal synthesis of prostaglandins to the extent that other NSAIDs do, it may be the preferred drug in patients with renal disease or impaired renal perfusion.[25]

Tolmetin is an analgesic, antipyretic, and anti-inflammatory drug that, like salicylates, causes gastric irritation and prolongs bleeding time. It is more potent than salicylates and less potent than indomethacin or phenylbutazone. After oral administration, absorption is rapid with extensive plasma protein binding. Most of tolmetin is inactivated by decarboxylation.[13]

Propionic Acid Derivatives

Ibuprofen, naproxen, and diclofenac are nonsteroidal propionic acid derivatives with prominent analgesic, antipyretic, and anti-inflammatory effects, reflecting inhibition of prostaglandin synthesis. Propionic acid derivatives are comparable with salicylates in treating osteoarthritis, rheumatoid arthritis, and acute gouty arthritis. Naproxen is unique because its longer elimination half-time makes twice-daily administration effective.[13]

Ibuprofen is principally eliminated by metabolism to hydroxyl or carboxyl conjugates, with less than 1% of the drug appearing unchanged in the urine. Naproxen is metabolized by dealkylation to cytochrome P-450, and less than 10% is eliminated unchanged in the urine. Diclofenac is eliminated by metabolism to glucuronide, hydroxyl, and sulphate conjugates followed by excretion in the urine and bile. Gastrointestinal irritation and mucosal ulceration are less severe than the irritation that sometimes accompanies salicylates. Platelet function is changed, but the duration of COX inhibition varies with the specific drug. Inhibition of prostaglandin synthesis may exacerbate renal dysfunction in patients with preexisting renal dysfunction in whom prostaglandins are important for maintaining renal blood flow.[13]

Phenylbutazone is an effective anti-inflammatory drug that is useful to treat acute gout and rheumatoid arthritis. Acute exacerbations of these conditions respond well to phenylbutazone. Phenylbutazone is an effective alternative to colchicine in acute gout, providing control in 85% of patients within 24 to 36 hours. Because of its toxicity, this drug should not be given for more than 7 days. Phenylbutazone is rapidly absorbed from the gastrointestinal tract. Plasma protein binding is 98%. Metabolism of this drug is extensive and involves glucuronidation and hydroxylation of the phenyl rings on the butyl side chain. Significant side effects of phenylbutazone are frequent and include anemia and agranulocytosis. Nausea, vomiting, epigastric discomfort, and skin rashes are frequent. Phenylbutazone displaces drugs, including warfarin, oral hypoglycemics, and sulfonamides, from protein binding sites. Increased bleeding may occur when phenylbutazone and warfarin or aspirin are coadministered.[13]

Piroxicam differs chemically from other NSAIDs but produces similar pharmacologic effects. Like salicylates, this drug inhibits prostaglandin synthesis. Administration of 20 mg in a single dose or in divided doses provides prolonged effects. Extensive protein binding (99%) may displace other drugs, such as aspirin or oral anticoagulants, from albumin binding sites.[13]

Ketorolac

Ketorolac is an NSAID with potent analgesic effects and moderate anti-inflammatory activity when given intramuscularly or intravenously.[26] This drug is useful for postoperative analgesia as the sole drug, in less painful ambulatory procedures, and to supplement opioids. Ketorolac potentiates the antinociceptive actions of opioids. In contrast with dose-dependent analgesic effects of opioids, ketorolac and other NSAIDs have a ceiling effect with respect to postoperative analgesia.[27] Using ketorolac as the only intraoperative analgesic may be associated with an increased incidence of purposeful movement on surgical incision.[28] Ketorolac 30 mg intramuscularly produces analgesia that is equivalent to morphine 10 mg or meperidine 100 mg. An important benefit of ketorolac-induced analgesia is the absence of ventilatory or cardiac depression. Ketorolac has little or no effect on biliary tract dynamics, making this drug useful for analgesia when spasm of the biliary tract is undesirable.[29]

After intramuscular injection, maximum plasma concentrations of ketorolac are attained within 45 to 60 minutes, and the elimination half-time is about 5 hours.[30] Protein binding is greater than 99%, and the clearance of this drug is less than that of opioids. Clearance is further decreased in the elderly, and the ketorolac dose for geriatric patients should be less than that given to younger patients. Ketorolac is metabolized principally by glucuronic acid conjugation.[13]

Similar to other NSAIDs, ketorolac inhibits platelet thromboxane production and platelet aggregation by reversible inhibition of prostaglandin synthetase. The modest prolongation of bleeding time and decreased platelet aggregation that result last until the drug is eliminated from the body.[13]

Life-threatening bronchospasm may follow the administration of ketorolac to patients with nasal polyposis, asthma, and aspirin sensitivity.[31] Cross-tolerance between aspirin and other NSAIDs is common. Although the molecular structures of these drugs are very different, they all share the common mechanism of COX inhibition. Ketorolac appears to have little potential for producing renal toxicity when adequate fluid balance is maintained and renal function does not depend on prostaglandins. Modest increases in plasma concentrations of liver transaminases may occur in some patients treated with ketorolac. Gastrointestinal irritation and perforation, nausea, sedation, and peripheral edema may accompany the administration of this NSAID.[13]

Ketorolac, like other NSAIDs, has antipyretic, anti-inflammatory, and analgesic actions. This drug is chemically related to indomethacin and tolmetin. Ketorolac inhibits COX, leading to decreased formation of the precursors of prostaglandins and thromboxanes from arachidonic acid. Decreased prostaglandin synthesis accounts for therapeutic and adverse effects of NSAIDs. Analgesia is produced via peripheral action where blockade of pain impulse generation occurs due to decreased prostaglandin activity.[32]

Like other NSAIDs, ketorolac may cause gastrointestinal ulceration and bleeding. These effects likely result from ketorolac-induced reduction of prostaglandin synthesis, which produces a protective effect on the gastric mucosa. Ketorolac may cause renal toxicity (e.g., sodium and fluid retention, decreased renal perfusion, and decreased renal function), probably by inhibiting the synthesis of renal prostaglandins, which are directly involved in the maintenance of renal hemodynamics and sodium and fluid balance. Renal prostaglandins are especially important in maintaining renal function in the presence of generalized vasoconstriction or volume depletion.[32]

The onset of action for ketorolac is dose dependent and ranges from 30 minutes to 1 hour. Peak plasma concentrations after a single dose of ketorolac are shown in Table 7-3.

The time to peak effect for intramuscular or intravenous (IV) ketorolac is 1 to 2 hours. Oral ketorolac achieves its peak effect in 2 to 3 hours. The duration of action for parenteral ketorolac is 4 to 6 hours (see www.ketorolac.org). The usual adult prescribing limits for ketorolac in patients who are ages 16 to 64 years and weigh at least 50 kg with normal renal function are 120 mg daily by parenteral administration, not to exceed 5 days. Patients who weigh less than 50 kg and/or patients with renal function impairment and the elderly should not have more than ketorolac 60 mg/day. In patients up to 16 years of age, the safety and

Table 7-3 Peak Plasma Concentrations of Ketorolac

| Route | Dose (mg) | Concentration | |
		mcg/mL	μmol/L
Intramuscular	15	1.14 ± 0.32	3.03 ± 0.85
	30	2.42 ± 0.68	6.44 ± 1.81
	60	4.5 ± 1.27	11.97 ± 3.38
Intravenous	15	2.47 ± 0.51	6.57 ± 1.36
	30	4.65 ± 0.96	12.37 ± 2.55
Oral	10	0.87 ± 0.22	2.31 ± 0.58

Source: From reference 32.

efficacy of ketorolac have not been established. Doses of 1 mg/kg of body weight are suggested by the manufacturer.[32]

Ketorolac is indicated for short-term management of moderately severe acute pain that would otherwise require treatment with an opioid. This drug is commonly used to relieve postoperative pain. Oral ketorolac can be used to continue therapy after initial injectable administration. Because the risk of gastrointestinal bleeding and other severe adverse effects increases with the duration of treatment, ketorolac should not be administered by any route or combination of routes for greater than 5 days.[32]

A more recent route for the administration of ketorolac is intra-articular. Findings from one study on patients who underwent shoulder surgery indicated that a combination of intra-articular ropivacaine, morphine, and ketorolac followed by intermittent injections of ropivacaine as needed provided improved analgesia, less morphine consumption, and improved patient satisfaction compared with the control group. Subjects in the treatment group in this study who received IV ketorolac consumed less morphine and were more satisfied with their treatment than patients in the control group.[33]

The benefits of preoperative ketorolac related to preemptive analgesia have been studied, with some articles reporting lower postoperative pain scores in patients who received preoperative or intraoperative ketorolac.[34,35] Clinicians caring for surgical patients are increasingly using multimodal analgesia to treat postoperative pain.

Before ketorolac is used perioperatively, its platelet aggregation-inhibiting activity, which increases the risk of bleeding, needs to be considered. Postoperative hematomas and other signs of wound bleeding have been reported in patients who received ketorolac. One recommendation is to not give ketorolac before major surgery to prevent postoperative pain or to administer ketorolac intraoperatively when control of bleeding is critical.[32]

COX-2–Specific Inhibitors

Selective COX-2–specific enzyme inhibitors have analgesic efficacy comparable with that of conventional anti-inflammatory drugs.[11] These drugs lack effects on platelets at therapeutic doses and may be associated with decreased gastrointestinal side effects in patients with arthritis, compared with the nonspecific NSAIDs. The risk of acute myocardial infarction and cerebrovascular accident may be increased in patients treated chronically with selective COX-2–specific enzyme inhibitors. The analgesic effects provided by these drugs may not be superior to those provided by historically older drugs.[13]

Celecoxib was the first selective COX-2 inhibitor that became available in 1998. This drug is recommended to treat pain and inflammation associated with osteoarthritis and rheumatoid arthritis. For patients with osteoarthritis, an initial dose of 200 mg/day is recommended. In patients with rheumatoid arthritis, a dose of 100 to 200 mg twice daily is recommended.[13]

Rofecoxib has been used to treat acute pain associated with surgery, starting with a loading dose of 50 mg followed by 25 mg/day. Treatment of dental pain with rofecoxib 50 mg produces analgesia similar to naproxen or ibuprofen. A single daily dose of 12.5 to 25 mg is recommended for patients with osteoarthritis. However, the increased risk of myocardial infarctions and cerebrovascular accidents associated with this drug resulted in the withdrawal of this drug from the market in 2004.[15]

Valdecoxib 40 mg may be administered 1 hour preoperatively for relief of postoperative pain and an additional 40 mg postoperatively if needed. The recommended dose for osteoarthritis and rheumatoid arthritis is 10 mg/day. A twice-daily dose of 20 mg or a once-daily dose of 40 mg is recommended to treat pain associated with primary dysmenorrhea.[13]

Parecoxib is the only COX-2–specific inhibitor available in parenteral form. For postoperative pain relief, parecoxib 40 mg is given 1 hour preoperatively followed by an additional 40 mg postoperatively if needed. Parecoxib is a prodrug that is converted in vivo to valdecoxib.[36]

Selective COX-2 inhibitors differ from nonspecific NSAIDs in that they are all highly lipophilic, neutral, nonacidic molecules with limited solubility in aqueous media. Celecoxib is a sulfonamide that is extensively distributed into tissues. Metabolism is by cytochrome P-450 enzymes to hydroxyl, carboxylic acid, and glucuronide derivatives with only 2% of the drug excreted unchanged by the kidneys. Rofecoxib is a sulfone that is not as well distributed in tissues and is metabolized primarily by cytosolic reduction in the liver, and less than 1% appears unchanged in the urine.

Parecoxib is a parenterally administered inactive prodrug that undergoes rapid amide hydrolysis in vivo to the pharmacologically active COX-2 inhibitor valdecoxib.[36] Valdecoxib is metabolized to 1-hydroxyvaldecoxib by hepatic cytochrome P-450 enzymes. Because both parecoxib and valdecoxib inhibit cytochrome P-450, there is potential for these COX-2 inhibitors to inhibit metabolism of other drugs.[36]

The perceived beneficial effects of COX-2 inhibitors have resulted in use of these drugs for conditions associated with inflammation and pain. COX-2 inhibitors are useful to treat patients experiencing pain due to osteoarthritis, rheumatoid arthritis, acute gout, and dysmenorrhea. Most adverse effects of NSAIDs are in patients receiving these drugs chronically for the treatment of arthritis. Pain associated with musculoskeletal conditions is effectively treated with COX-2 inhibitors. Acute postoperative pain associated with major orthopedic surgery and arthroscopy is responsive to COX-2 inhibitors, and the lack of antiplatelet effects allows these drugs to be continued throughout the perioperative period. The efficacy of COX-2 inhibitors has been demonstrated for relief of dental pain.[11]

NSAIDs are commonly used for postoperative pain management.[37] NSAIDs demonstrate a ceiling effect when used for postoperative analgesia, versus the dose-dependent analgesic effects of opioids (Figure 7-3). It is thought that NSAIDs reduce postoperative pain through suppression of COX-mediated production of prostaglandin E_2, which is believed to be the primary inflammatory prostaglandin that directly activates and up-regulates the sensitivity of peripheral nociceptors to cause pain. Prostaglandins are known to cross the blood–brain barrier and have a role in spinal nociception, which supports a spinal analgesic mechanism of NSAIDs. Opioid requirements for postoperative pain management are decreased by up to 50% by NSAIDs.[38] COX-2 is constitutively expressed in the brain and spinal cord and is up-regulated after persistent noxious inputs so that spinal COX-2 inhibition may be important for decreasing postinjury hyperalgesia.[13]

The postoperative analgesia produced by COX-2 inhibitors is similar to that yielded by conventional nonselective NSAIDs.[12] The advantage of COX-2 inhibitors versus nonselective NSAIDs is the lack of effects on platelet function and bleeding.[38] COX-2 inhibitors may be acceptable for administration to patients with histories of gastritis or gastric ulcers who cannot receive conventional NSAIDs. COX-2 inhibitors may be a safer alternative to nonselective NSAIDs because these drugs are well-tolerated by patients with asthma.[39]

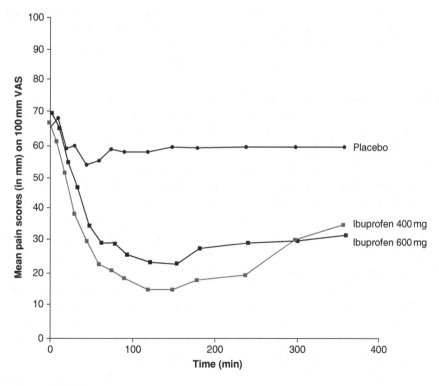

Figure 7-3 The ceiling effects of NSAIDs.

Source: Available at: http://img.medscape.com/fullsize/migrated/574/279/574249.gif.

Side Effects of Nonselective and COX-2 NSAIDs

NSAID-induced gastrointestinal toxicity accounts for up to 30% of gastric ulcers.[40] Concomitant therapy with histamine-2 receptor antagonists, proton pump inhibitors, or misoprostol decreases the incidence of gastrointestinal ulcers associated with NSAIDs.[41] Because prostaglandins help maintain gastrointestinal mucosal integrity and because only COX-1 is present in the gastrointestinal tract, it is believed that gastrointestinal toxicity produced by nonselective NSAIDs is primarily due to inhibition of COX-1 activity. Prostaglandins normally protect the gastrointestinal mucosa from damage by maintaining mucosal blood flow and increasing mucosal secretion of mucus and bicarbonate. Blockade of COX-1 activity by NSAIDs decreases prostaglandin synthesis and lowers gastrointestinal mucosal blood flow and secretion of mucus and bicarbonate. The incidence of gastrointestinal side effects (gastric and duodenal ulcers) is decreased by about 50% in patients treated with selective COX-2 inhibitors.[42]

Platelet aggregation and hemostasis require platelets to generate thromboxane A_2 from prostaglandins. Because platelets do not contain COX-2, all synthesis of thromboxane A_2 in platelets is mediated by COX-1. Conventional nonspecific NSAIDs inhibit COX-1 and impair platelet aggregation. Patients on anticoagulants should be monitored when receiving nonspecific NSAIDs, especially aspirin, which has irreversible effects on platelets. COX-2 inhibitors do not appear to have significant interactions with anticoagulant drugs. Preoperative NSAID therapy significantly increases intraoperative and postoperative blood loss in children undergoing tonsillectomy.[43] COX-2 inhibitors do not affect platelet aggregation, bleeding time, or postoperative blood loss. Thrombotic events occur more frequently in patients treated with COX-2 inhibitors compared with traditional NSAIDs. Aspirin in doses of 75 to 325 mg daily induces irreversible inactivation of platelet COX that lasts for the life of the platelet, which is 7 to 10 days.[20]

The risk of a thrombotic episode or myocardial infarction might be increased in patients on COX-2 inhibitors.[44] This may reflect COX-2 inhibitor selective suppression of prostaglandin I_2 (vasoprotective) without affecting thromboxane A_2 (procoagulant).[45] Increased risk of myocardial infarction and cerebrovascular accident in patients treated with rofecoxib for 18 months or longer resulted in the withdrawal of this drug from the market in 2004. There may be an increased incidence of congestive heart failure in patients treated with COX-2 inhibitors.[13]

Prostaglandins modulate systemic pressure due to their effects on vascular tone in arteriolar smooth muscle and control of extracellular fluid volume. Prostaglandins offset the response to vasoconstrictor hormones and influence sodium balance due to their natriuretic effects. NSAIDs may interfere with pharmacologic control of systemic hypertension, although the average effects of these drugs on blood pressure is usually small.[46]

NSAIDs do not affect renal function in healthy patients. When renal toxicity occurs, it is likely due to NSAID-induced inhibition of prostaglandin synthesis, which leads to renal medullary ischemia. Prostaglandins are involved in the autoregulation of renal blood flow and glomerular filtration, and they influence the transport of ions and water. Tubulointerstitial nephritis caused by NSAIDs (analgesic nephropathy) has been associated with chronic ingestion of phenacetin, which was withdrawn from the market for this reason. Acetaminophen is a phenacetin metabolite that has been associated with an increased incidence of end-stage renal disease. It has been estimated that decreased consumption of acetaminophen could lower the incidence of end-stage renal disease by 8% to 10%. Factors that influence NSAID-induced nephrotoxicity include hypovolemia, preexisting renal disease, congestive heart failure, sepsis, combination with other potentially nephrotoxic drugs or radiographic contrast material, diabetes mellitus, and cirrhosis.[47]

Nonselective NSAIDs interfere with the production of vasodilating prostaglandins and may result in decreased glomerular filtration rate and sodium retention, which manifest as systemic hypertension and edema. The nephrotoxic potential of NSAIDs is increased in patients who require prostaglandins for renal vasodilation. Prerenal azotemia reflecting decreased renal perfusion is the most frequent pattern of renal injury related to the use of NSAIDs. Elderly patients treated with NSAIDs are at increased risk for nephrotoxicity. Hyperchloremic metabolic acidosis, often associated with hyperkalemia, is an effect of NSAIDs, especially in patients with preexisting renal disease. The renal and cardiovascular effects of COX-2 inhibitors are similar to those of conventional NSAIDs. There is evidence that preoperative administration of ketorolac to well-hydrated patients anesthetized with sevoflurane does not produce glomerular or tubular dysfunction.[48] Postoperative acute renal failure has been observed in an otherwise healthy patient who was taking ibuprofen preoperatively.[49]

Increases in the plasma concentrations of liver transaminases may accompany treatment with NSAIDs. Rare cases of severe hepatic dysfunction with jaundice and hepatic failure may occur during NSAID therapy.[13]

Sulfonamide hypersensitivity is a contraindication to treatment with celecoxib and valdecoxib. COX-2 inhibitors should not be administered to patients who have experienced asthma, urticaria, or allergic-type reactions to aspirin. Patients who have respiratory sensitivity to aspirin often develop dose-dependent reactions to aspirin or COX-1, whereas COX-2 inhibitors are usually well tolerated in these patients.[13]

NSAIDs may trigger bronchoconstriction in susceptible asthmatic patients through blockage of COX-mediated conversion of arachidonic acid to prostaglandins, especially prostaglandin E_2, which is a potent anti-inflammatory substance. This inhibition of prostaglandin production results in shunting of arachidonic acid toward the lipoxygenase pathway and production of bronchoconstrictor and proinflammatory leukotrienes.[13]

Drug-induced meningitis has been reported after administration of ibuprofen and H_2 receptor antagonists.[50] Signs and symptoms often appear within a few hours after drug ingestion but may be delayed for weeks. Beyond the typical features of meningitis, there may be periorbital edema, conjunctivitis, hypotension, parotitis, pancreatitis, fatigue, and seizures. Fever is a common feature of drug-induced meningitis. Recovery should occur when the drug is discontinued.

NSAIDs may impair bone healing to the extent that these drugs are not recommended for patients undergoing spinal fusion surgery. Earlier suggestions that COX-2 inhibitors did not interfere with bone healing have not been validated.[51]

The most common interaction in this drug category is between oral anticoagulants and NSAIDs, with increased risk of gastrointestinal hemorrhage resulting. Concurrent administration of NSAIDs, including COX-2 inhibitors and aspirin, increases the risk of gastrointestinal ulceration. COX-2 inhibitors may increase the plasma concentrations of warfarin, which emphasizes the need to monitor anticoagulant therapy. When NSAIDs and potassium-sparing diuretics are combined, there is an increased risk of hyperkalemia. NSAID-induced decreases in renal function may decrease the clearance of digoxin, lithium, and aminoglycoside antibiotics. NSAIDs may interfere with the antihypertensive actions of beta-blockers, diuretics, and angiotensin-converting enzyme inhibitors. Plasma lithium concentrations may be increased in patients treated with COX-2 inhibitors.[13]

Ketamine

Ketamine is a phencyclidine derivative that produces dissociation between the thalamocortical and limbic systems.[52] Dissociative anesthesia is similar to a cataleptic state, wherein the eyes remain open with a slow nystagmic gaze. Despite not communicating, the patient may be awake. Variable degrees of hypertonus and purposeful muscle movements may occur independently of surgical stimulation. The patient experiences amnesia and intense analgesia. Ketamine produces profound analgesia at subanesthetic doses.[13]

Ketamine is water soluble and resembles phencyclidine in its structure. There are two optical isomers of ketamine, S(+) and R(−) ketamine. S(+) ketamine produces more intense analgesia, more rapid metabolism, less salivation, and a lower incidence of emergence reactions than R(−) ketamine.[53] The analgesic potency of S(+) ketamine is greater than racemic ketamine as well as R(−) ketamine. Ketamine isomers produce less fatigue and cognitive impairment than equianalgesic small-dose racemic ketamine.[54]

Ketamine has noncompetitive binding to the phencyclidine recognition site on the N-methyl-D-aspartate (NMDA) receptors. Ketamine may exert effects at other sites, including opioid receptors, monoaminergic receptors, muscarinic receptors, and voltage-sensitive sodium and L-type calcium channels.[55] The inflammatory mediators produced locally by compression of nerve roots can activate neutrophils that then adhere to blood vessels and impede blood flow. Ketamine suppresses production of inflammatory mediators by neutrophils and improves blood flow. Direct inhibition of cytokines may also contribute to the analgesic effects of ketamine.[56]

NMDA receptors are members of the glutamate receptor family. These ligand-gated ion channels are unique because channel activation requires binding of the excitatory neurotransmitter glutamate with glycine.[52] Ketamine inhibits NMDA receptor activation by glutamate, decreases presynaptic release of glutamate, and potentiates the effects of γ-aminobutyric acid. The interaction with phencyclidine binding sites is stereoselective, with the S(+) isomer of ketamine having the greatest affinity.[13]

Ketamine interacts with μ, δ, and κ opioid receptors. Ketamine may be antagonist at μ receptors and an agonist at κ* receptors. Ketamine is also active at the σ receptor, although this receptor is not classified as an opioid receptor and the interaction with ketamine is weak.[57] Ketamine also interacts with voltage-gated sodium channels, sharing a binding site with local anesthetics.[55]

The pharmacokinetic properties of ketamine are similar to those of thiopental, with a rapid onset of action, short duration of action, and high lipid solubility. Ketamine has a pK of 7.5 at physiologic pH. Peak plasma concentrations of ketamine occur within 1 minute after IV injection and 5 minutes after intramuscular administration. Ketamine does not have significant protein binding and leaves the blood rapidly to be distributed into tissues. The extreme lipid solubility of ketamine ensures its rapid transfer across the blood–brain barrier. Subsequently, ketamine is redistributed from the brain and other highly perfused tissues to less well-perfused tissues. Ketamine has a high hepatic clearance rate of 1 L/min and a volume of distribution of 3 L/kg, which results in an elimination half-time of 2 to 3 hours.[13]

Ketamine is metabolized extensively by the hepatic microsomal enzymes. An important metabolic pathway is demethylation of ketamine by cytochrome P-450 enzymes to form norketamine.[58] This active metabolite may contribute to prolonged effects of ketamine, such as analgesia, especially with repeated doses or continuous IV infusion. Norketamine is eventually hydroxylated and then conjugated to form more water-soluble and inactive glucuronide metabolites that are excreted by the kidneys. Chronic administration of ketamine stimulates activity of the enzymes responsible for its metabolism. Accelerated ketamine metabolism as a result of enzyme induction may explain tolerance to the analgesia effects of ketamine that occurs in patients who receive repeated doses of this drug. Tolerance may develop in burn patients who receive more than two short-interval exposures to ketamine.[59] Development of tolerance is also thought to be related to ketamine dependence.[58]

Ketamine is a unique drug that provides intense analgesia at subanesthetic doses and produces prompt induction of anesthesia when administered intravenously at higher doses. Inclusion of an antisialagogue in the preoperative medication is recommended to decrease the likelihood of coughing and laryngospasm due to ketamine-induced secretions. Glycopyrrolate may be preferable because belladonna alkaloids easily cross the blood–brain barrier and could increase the incidence of emergence delirium.[13]

Intense analgesia can be attained with subanesthetic doses of ketamine, ranging from 0.2 to 0.5 mg/kg intravenously.[60] Plasma concentrations of ketamine that produce analgesia are lower after oral versus intramuscular administration, possibly reflective of a higher norketamine concentration related to hepatic first-pass metabolism that occurs after oral administration. Analgesia is believed to be greater for somatic than for visceral pain. The analgesic effects of ketamine are due to its activity in the thalamic and limbic systems, which interpret nociceptive feedback. Small doses of ketamine are useful adjuncts to opioid analgesia.[61]

Spinal cord sensitization is responsible for the pain that occurs with touching or moving an injured body part. The development of spinal cord sensitization involves activation of NMDA receptors, located in the dorsal horn of the spinal cord. NMDA receptors are excitatory amino acid receptors important in processing and modulating painful stimuli.[62] Excitatory amino acids, especially glutamate, act at NMDA receptors and are important in spinal nociceptive pathways. Inhibition of spinal NMDA receptors by drugs such as ketamine, magnesium, and dextromethorphan is useful in the management of postoperative pain and has opioid-sparing properties. The affinity of S(+) ketamine for NMDA receptors is four times greater than its R(−) isomer, and the analgesic potency of S(+) ketamine is two times greater than that of racemic ketamine. Analgesia can be produced by ketamine during labor without related depression of the neonate.[63,64] Neonatal neurobehavioral scores of infants born by vaginal delivery with ketamine analgesia are lower than those for infants born with epidural anesthesia but higher than the scores in infants delivered with general anesthesia.[65] Postoperative sedation and analgesia after pediatric cardiac surgery can be produced by continuous ketamine infusions at rates of 1 to 2 mg/kg/h.

Ketamine is the only injected anesthetic that stimulates the cardiovascular system and produces emergence delirium. Ketamine increases cerebral blood flow and cerebral metabolic oxygen requirements.[66] Ketamine is a potent cerebral vasodilator that can increase cerebral blood flow by 60% in a normocapnic patient.[67] This drug is contraindicated in patients with increased intracranial pressure.

Ketamine produces cardiovascular effects similar to those provided by sympathetic nervous system stimulation. Direct stimulation of the CNS leading to increased sympathetic nervous system outflow is the likely mechanism for the cardiovascular stimulation produced by ketamine.[68] Plasma concentration of epinephrine and norepinephrine increases within 2 minutes after ketamine administration and returns to control levels 15 minutes later.[69]

Ketamine does not produce significant respiratory depression. The ventilatory response to carbon dioxide remains constant during ketamine anesthesia. Breathing frequency may decrease for 2 to 3 minutes after ketamine administration. Apnea can occur if ketamine is administered rapidly intravenously or when combined with opioids. Upper airway muscle tone is well maintained, and upper airway reflexes remain intact after the administration of ketamine.[70] Ketamine has bronchodilatory effects and has been used to treat bronchospasm and status asthmaticus.[71] The mechanism by which ketamine produces airway relaxation is not clear, although increased concentration of circulating catecholamines, inhibition of catecholamine uptake, voltage-sensitive calcium channel block, and inhibition of postsynaptic nicotinic or muscarinic receptors have all been posited to contribute.[72]

Ketamine does not provoke histamine release and has rarely been associated with allergic reactions.[73] Tests of hepatic and renal function are not altered by ketamine.[13]

Emergence from ketamine anesthesia may be associated with visual, auditory, proprioceptive, and confusional illusions, which may progress to delirium. Cortical blindness may transiently occur. Dreams and hallucinations, often with morbid content and experienced in bright color, can occur for up to 24 hours after ketamine administration. Emergence delirium is likely related to depression of the inferior colliculus and medial geniculate nucleus by ketamine, which causes misinterpretation of auditory and visual stimuli.[58] Loss of sensation in the skin and musculoskeletal systems interferes with the perception of gravity and produces sensations of bodily detachment or floating in space. The incidence of emergence delirium after ketamine ranges from 5% to 30%.[58] The factors that are associated with an increased occurrence of emergence delirium include age younger than 15 years, female gender, IV ketamine doses greater than 2 mg/kg, and a history of personality problems or frequent dreaming.[58]

Benzodiazepines are the most effective agents for prevention of emergence delirium in patients who receive ketamine. Midazolam prevents emergence delirium after ketamine more effectively than diazepam.[74,75]

Dextromethorphan

Dextromethorphan, a *d*-isomer of levorphanol, is a low-affinity NMDA antagonist commonly found in over-the-counter cough suppressants. It is equipotent with codeine as an antitussive and does not have analgesic or physical dependence properties. Dextromethorphan rarely produces sedation or gastrointestinal disturbances. Its euphoric effects account for the abuse potential associated with dextromethorphan. The signs and symptoms of excessive intake of dextromethorphan include systemic hypertension, tachycardia, somnolence, agitation, slurred speech, ataxia, diaphoresis, skeletal muscle rigidity, seizures, coma, and decreased core body temperature. Hepatotoxicity must be considered when dextromethorphan with acetaminophen is ingested in excessive quantities.[13]

Centrally Acting α_2 Agonists

α_2-Adrenergic agonists provide clinical effects through binding to α_2 receptors, which have three subtypes: α_{2A}, α_{2B}, and α_{2C}. α_{2A} receptors mediate sedation, analgesia, and sympatholysis. α_{2B} receptors mediate vasoconstriction and possibly antishivering effects. α_{2C} activation may be linked to the startle response.[13]

The highest concentration of α_2 receptors is in the pontine locus ceruleus, which provides sympathetic nervous innervation of the forebrain, and is a modulator of vigilance. The sedative effects of α_2 agonists reflect inhibition of the nucleus.[76] Clonidine stimulates α_2-adrenergic inhibitory neurons in the medullary vasomotor center. Decreased sympathetic nervous system outflow from the CNS to peripheral tissues results. Manifestation of decreased sympathetic nervous system outflow include peripheral vasodilation and decreased systemic blood pressure, heart rate, and cardiac output. The ability of clonidine to modify the function of potassium channels in the CNS (cell membranes become hyperpolarized) may be the mechanism that accounts for decreased MAC requirements related to clonidine and more selective α_2-adrenergic agonists (e.g., dexmedetomidine). α_2 receptors on blood vessels mediate vasoconstriction, and on peripheral sympathetic nervous system nerve endings inhibit norepinephrine release. Neuraxial clonidine inhibits the release of spinal substance P and nociceptive neuron firing related to noxious stimulation.[13]

The quality of sedation associated with α_2-agonists differs from the sedation produced by drugs such as midazolam and propofol that act on γ-aminobutyric acid receptors.[77] Dexmedetomidine acts on α_2 receptors and produces sedation through decreasing sympathetic nervous system activity and the level of arousal. The result is a sedated patient who can be awakened easily.[13]

Clonidine is a centrally acting selective partial α_2 adrenergic agonist (200:1 α_2 to α_1) that acts as an antihypertensive agent because it decreases sympathetic nervous system output from the CNS. Clonidine is especially effective for treatment of patients with severe hypertension or rennin-dependent disease. The usual adult daily dose is 0.2 to 0.3 mg orally. The availability of a transdermal clonidine patch designed for weekly administration is useful for surgical patients transiently unable to ingest oral medications.[13]

Clonidine and dexmedetomidine, centrally acting α-adrenergic agonists, provide sedation, decrease anesthetic requirements, and foster perioperative hemodynamic stability (e.g., attenuation of blood pressure and heart rate responses to surgical stimulation) as well as sympathoadrenal stability. Also, α_2 receptors in the spinal cord modulate pain pathways, which results in analgesia. Common use of clonidine as an anesthetic adjuvant and provision of postoperative sedation without ventilatory depression have been limited due to its half-life of 6 to 10 hours. Dexmedetomidine has a half-time of 2 to 3 hours and is more potent than clonidine at α_2 receptors.[78]

Clonidine

Neuraxial administration of preservative-free clonidine (150–450 mcg) yields dose-dependent analgesia without respiratory depression, pruritus, nausea and vomiting, or delayed gastric emptying.[79,80] Urinary retention, a common complication of epidural opioids, is uncommon when epidural clonidine is used to provide postoperative analgesia. Activation of postsynaptic α_2 receptors in the substantia gelatinosa of the spinal cord is the mechanism presumed to produce analgesia when clonidine is administered. Clonidine and morphine, when used together as neuraxial analgesics, do not exhibit cross-tolerance.[81] Hypotension, sedation, and dryness of the mouth can accompany neuraxial clonidine. When clonidine 1 mcg/kg is added to lidocaine used for IV regional anesthesia, postoperative analgesia is enhanced. IV regional administration of clonidine 1 mcg/kg relieves sympathetically mediated pain.[82]

Clonidine 5 mcg/kg as an oral premedicant blunts reflex tachycardia associated with direct laryngoscopy, decreases intraoperative lability of blood pressure and heart rate, decreases plasma catecholamine concentrations, and decreases MAC requirements.[83,84] The same preanesthetic clonidine dose enhances the postoperative analgesia produced by intrathecal morphine with tetracaine, without increasing the intensity of the morphine-related side effects.[85]

Clonidine 75 to 150 mcg added to solutions containing tetracaine or bupivacaine for subarachnoid block prolongs the duration of sensory and motor blockade.[85] Clonidine 150 mcg added to intrathecal bupivacaine prolongs the anesthetic and analgesic effects of this drug without causing unwanted side effects.[86] Clonidine 150 to 200 mcg by mouth 1 to 1.5 hours before a subarachnoid block with lidocaine or tetracaine results in significant prolongation of sensory block.[87] However, clonidine premedication increases the incidence of clinically significant bradycardia and hypotension. Clonidine 0.5 mcg/kg added to a 1% mepivacaine-containing solution increases the duration of axillary blocks.[88]

Clonidine is absorbed rapidly after oral dosing and reaches peak plasma concentrations within 60 to 90 minutes. The elimination half-time of clonidine is between 9 and 12 hours. Approximately 50% of clonidine is metabolized in the liver, and the rest is excreted unchanged in the urine. The duration of hypotension after a single oral dose is about 8 hours. The transdermal route requires about 48 hours to produce therapeutic plasma concentrations.[13]

The decrease in systolic blood pressure associated with clonidine is greater than the decrease in diastolic pressure. There is minimal effect on the systemic vascular resistance when clonidine is taken chronically, and cardiac output, which decreases initially, returns to near predrug levels.[13]

α_2 agonists have minimal respiratory depressant effects, and these drugs do not potentiate the ventilatory depressant effects of opioids.[89] Simultaneous IV administration of clonidine and fentanyl may lead to accumulation of fentanyl, which increases the risk for respiratory depression.[90]

The most common side effects related to clonidine are sedation and xerostomia. Given the agonist effect on postsynaptic α_2 receptors in the CNS, nearly 50% decreases in MAC requirements are observed in patients pretreated with clonidine.[91]

Abrupt discontinuation of clonidine antihypertensive therapy can provoke rebound hypertension as soon as 8 hours and as late as 36 hours after the last dose. Rebound hypertension is most likely to occur in patients who receive more than 1.2 mg of clonidine daily. Hypertension is due to a more than 100% increase in circulating catecholamines and intense peripheral vasoconstriction.[92] Symptoms of clonidine withdrawal include nervousness, diaphoresis, headache, abdominal pain, and tachycardia. β-Adrenergic blockade may exaggerate the magnitude of rebound hypertension through blocking the β_2 vasodilating effects of catecholamines with unopposed α vasoconstriction.[93] Rebound hypertension can usually be controlled by reinstitution of clonidine therapy or providing a vasodilator such as hydralazine or sodium nitroprusside.[13]

Dexmedetomidine

Dexmedetomidine is a highly selective, specific, and potent α_2-adrenergic agonist, with 1620:1 α_2-to-α_1 activity.[94] Dexmedetomidine is a dextroisomer and pharmacologically active element of medetomidine, which has been used historically in veterinary practice for its hypnotic, sedative, and analgesic effects. When compared with clonidine, dexmedetomidine is 7 to 10 times more selective for α_2 receptors and has a shorter duration of action than clonidine. Dexmedetomidine is considered a full agonist at the α_2 receptor, whereas clonidine is a partial agonist with a ratio of α_2-to-α_1 activity of 220:1.[94] Atipamezole is a selective α_2 receptor antagonist that rapidly reverses the sedative and cardiovascular effects of IV dexmedetomidine.[95]

The elimination half-time of dexmedetomidine is 2 to 3 hours compared with 6 to 10 hours for clonidine. Dexmedetomidine is highly protein bound and is subject to extensive hepatic metabolism. The methyl and glucuronide conjugates are excreted by the kidneys. Dexmedetomidine has weak inhibitory properties on the cytochrome P-450 enzyme systems that could manifest as increased plasma concentrations of opioids administered during anesthesia.[96]

Pretreatment with dexmedetomidine attenuates hemodynamic responses to tracheal intubation, decreases plasma catecholamine concentrations during anesthesia, decreases MAC requirements, and increases the likelihood of hypotension.[78] Dexmedetomidine decreases MAC for volatile agents in animals by more than 90% compared with 25% to 40% for clonidine.[97] Dexmedetomidine produces marked dose-dependent sedation and analgesia with mild respiratory depression. Dexmedetomidine in high doses (loading dose of 1 mcg/kg followed by 5–10 mcg/kg/h intravenously) produces total IV anesthesia without concomitant respiratory depression.[98] Maintenance of adequate minute ventilation is useful in patients with upper airway pathology. Dexmedetomidine effectively blunts the cardiostimulatory and postanesthetic delirium effects of ketamine.[99] When dexmedetomidine 0.5 mcg/kg is added to lidocaine used for IV regional anesthesia, the quality of anesthesia and postoperative analgesia are improved without additional side effects.[100] Severe bradycardia may follow the administration of dexmedetomidine, and cardiac arrest has been reported in a patient receiving a dexmedetomidine infusion as a supplement to general anesthesia. Dexmedetomidine should be used cautiously in patients with low left ventricular ejection fractions.[101]

Dexmedetomidine is useful for sedation of postoperative patients in the critical care environment, especially when controlled ventilation is required. Compared with remifentanil, dexmedetomidine infusions do not result in clinically significant respiratory depression, and the sedation produced is similar to natural sleep.[102] After tracheal extubation, patients sedated with dexmedetomidine breathe spontaneously and appear to be calm.[101] Both clonidine and dexmedetomidine can be used in critical care to prevent drug withdrawal symptoms after long-term sedation with benzodiazepines. Because of its sympatholytic and vagomimetic actions, dexmedetomidine may be associated with systemic hypotension and bradycardia. The availability of a specific dexmedetomidine antagonist, atipamezole, may be useful.

Key Points

- The WHO analgesic ladder demonstrates a foundational role for nonopioid analgesics in the treatment of acute and chronic pain.
- Opioid-sparing properties of non-narcotic analgesics may decrease the incidence of postoperative nausea and vomiting and decrease MAC requirements.
- The intense analgesia produced by ketamine contributes significantly to opioid-sparing.
- Nonsteroidal anti-inflammatory agents attenuate the inflammatory response associated with the arachidonic acid cascade, initiated by surgical trauma.
- Centrally acting α_2 agonists administered in conjunction with local anesthetics or administered systemically reduce MAC requirements and produce sedation and analgesia without respiratory depression.

Chapter Questions

1. When considering analgesic regimens for acute and chronic pain, describe the role of nonopioid analgesics as conceptualized in the analgesic ladder of the World Health Organization.
2. What are some limitations associated with acetaminophen when this medication is used chronically to treat pain?
3. Describe controversies associated with research on COX-2 inhibitors.
4. At which receptor sites does ketamine exert its analgesic effects? What is the dose range of this drug that is associated with analgesia versus anesthesia?
5. What is the analgesic potency of ketorolac relative to morphine? List the limitations to the use of ketamine in the perioperative setting.
6. Describe some of the risks and benefits associated with dexmedetomidine when this drug is used in the perioperative setting.

References

1. International Association for the Study of Pain. IASP pain definition. Available at: http://www.iasp-pain.org. Accessed June 7, 2009.
2. O'Neil CK. Pain management. In: Burns MA, Wells BG, Schwinghammer TL, et al., eds. *Pharmacotherapy Principles and Practice*. New York: McGraw-Hill; 2008:487–501.
3. The Joint Commission. *The Joint Commission urges patients to "speak up" about pain*. Available at http://www.jointcommission.org/NewsRoom/NewsReleases/nr_pain_management.htm. Accessed June 7, 2009.
4. American Pain Foundation. Pain facts and figures. Available at: http://www.painfoundation.org/page.asp?file=Newsroom/PainFacts.htm. Accessed June 7, 2009.
5. Bradesi S. Role of the central immune system in function disorders. Available at: http://www.giresearch.org/site/gi-research/iffgd-research-awards/2007/immune-system. Accessed June 11, 2009.
6. DeLeo J. Basic science of pain. *J Bone Joint Surg.* 2006;88:58–62.
7. Nakama-Kitamura M. The role of contextual cues on counterirritation in the development process of analgesic tolerance to morphine. *Life Sci.* 2002;72:531–540.
8. Walsh D, Howe T, Johnson M, Sluka K. Transcutaneous electrical nerve stimulation for acute pain. *Cochrane Database Syst Rev.* 2009;Apr 15(2):CD006142.
9. Sandkühler J. Models and mechanisms of hyperalgesia and allodynia. *Physiol Rev.* 2009;89:707–758.

10. Gajraj N. Cyclooxygenase-2 inhibitors. *Anesth Analg.* 2003;96: 1720–1738.

11. Gilron I, Milne B, Hong M. Cyclooxygenase-2 inhibitors in postoperative pain management: current evidence and future directions. *Anesthesiology.* 2003;99:1198–1208.

12. Stoelting R, Hillier S. *Pharmacology and Physiology in Anesthetic Practice*, 4th ed. Philadelphia: Lippincott Williams & Wilkins; 2006.

13. Dolan S, Kelly J, Huan M, et al. Transient up-regulation of spinal cyclooxygenase-2 and neuronal nitric oxide synthase following surgical inflammation. *Anesthesiology.* 2003; 98:170–180.

14. COX-2 selective (includes Bextra, Celebrex, and Vioxx) and non-selective non-steroidal anti-inflammatory drugs (NSAIDs). Available at: http://www.fda.gov/Drugs/DrugSafety/Postmarket DrugSafetyInformationforPatientsandProviders/ucm103420 .htm. Accessed June 17, 2009.

15. Shafer S. Tattered threads. *Anesth Analg.* 2009;108:1361–1363.

16. Pain medications after surgery. Available at: http://www.mayo clinic.com/health/pain-medications/PN00060/METHOD= print. Accessed June 17, 2009.

17. Bami: acetaminophen (Tylenol) toxicity is leading cause of acute liver failure. Available at: http://www.bami.uswordpress/ 2009/0June 01/acetaminophen-tylenol-is-leading-cause-of-acute-liver-failure/. Accessed June 17, 2009.

18. Patrono C. Aspirin as an antiplatelet drug. *N Engl J Med.* 1994;330:1287–1294.

19. Schror K. Antiplatelet drugs: a comparative review. *Drugs.* 1995;50:7–28.

20. Settipane G. Adverse reactions to aspirin and related drugs. *Arch Intern Med.* 1981;141:328–332.

21. Williard J, Lange R, Hills L. The use of aspirin in ischemic heart disease. *N Engl J Med.* 1992;327:175–181.

22. Perenger T, Whelton P, Klag M. Risk of kidney failure associated with the use of acetaminophen, aspirin, and nonsteroidal anti-inflammatory drugs. *N Engl J Med.* 1994;331:1675–1679.

23. Smilkstein M, Knapp G, Kulig K, Rumack B. Efficacy of oral *N*-acetylcysteine in the treatment of acetaminophen overdose. *N Engl J Med.* 1988;319:1557–1562.

24. Ciabattoni G, Boss A, Patrignani P, et al. Effects of sulindac on renal and extrarenal eicosanoid synthesis. *Clin Pharmacol Ther.* 1987;41:380–383.

25. Kenny G. Ketorolac trometamo—a new non-opioid analgesic. *Br J Anaesth.* 1990;65:445–447.

26. O'Hara D, Fragen R, Kinzer M, Pemberton D. Ketorolac tromethamine as compared with morphine sulfate for treatment of postoperative pain. *Clin Pharmacol Ther.* 1987; 41:556–561.

27. Ding Y, Friedman, B, White P. Use of ketorolac and fentanyl during outpatient gynecologic surgery. *Anesth Analg.* 1993;77:205–210.

28. Krimmer H, Bullingham, R, Lloyd J, Bruch H. Effects on biliary tract pressure in human of intravenous ketorolac tromethamine compared with morphine and placebo. *Anesth Analg.* 1992;75:204–207.

29. Jung D, Mroszcak E, Bynum L. Pharmacokinetics of ketorolac tromethamine in human after intravenous, intramuscular and oral administration. *Eur J Clin Pharmacol.* 1988; 35:423–425.

30. Haddow G, Riley E, Isaacs R, et al. Ketorolac, nasal polyposis and bronchial asthma: a cause for concern. *Anesth Analg.* 1993;76:420–422.

31. Ketorolac tromethamine. Available at: http://ketorolac.org/. Accessed June 17, 2009.

32. Axelsoon K, Gupta A, Johanson E, et al. Intraarticular administration of ketorolac, morphone and ropivacaine combined with intraarticular patient-controlled regional analgesia for pain relief after shoulder surgery: a randomized, double-blind study. *Anesth Analg.* 2008;106: 328–333.

33. Al-Samsam T, Chelly J. Is the administration of ketorolac associated with preemptive analgesia? *Anesthesiology.* 2001; 94:599–603.

34. Dorr L, Raya J, Long W, Boutary M, Sirianni L. Multimodal analgesia without parenteral narcotics for total knee arthroplasty. *J Arthroplasty.* 2008;23:502–508.

35. Ibrahim A, Park S, Feldman J, et al. Effects of parecoxib, a parenteral COX-2-specific inhibitor on the pharmacokinetics and pharmacodynamics of propofol. *Anesthesiology.* 2002;96:88–95.

36. White P, Kehlet H, Liu S. Perioperative analgesia: what do we still know? *Anesth Analg.* 2009;108:1364–1367.

37. Kharasch E. Perioperative COX-2 inhibitors: knowledge and challenges. *Anesth Analg.* 2004;98:1–3.

38. McCrory C, Lindahl S. Cyclooxygenase inhibition for postoperative analgesia. *Anesth Analg.* 2002;95:169–176.

39. Laine L. Nonsteroidal anti-inflammatory drug gastropathy. *Gastrointest Endosc Clin North Am.* 1996;6:489–504.

40. Rostom A, Wells G, Tugwell P, et al. The prevention of chronic NSAID-induced upper gastrointestinal toxicity: A Cochrane collaboration metaanalysis of randomized controlled trials. *J Rheumatol.* 2000;27:2203–2214.

41. Bombardier C. An evidence-based evaluation of the gastrointestinal safety of coxibs. *Am J Cardiol.* 2002;89:3–9.

42. Marret E, Flahault A, Samama C, et al. Effects of postoperative, nonsteroidal antiinflammatory drugs on bleeding risk

after tonsillectomy: Meta-analysis of randomized, controlled trials. *Anesthesiology.* 2003;98:1497–1502.

43. Mukherjee D, Nissen S, Topol E. Risk of cardiovascular events associated with selective COX-2 inhibitors. *JAMA.* 2001;286:954–959.

44. FitzGerald G. Coxibs and cardiovascular disease. *N Engl J Med.* 2004;351:1709–1711.

45. Gurwitz Z, Avorn J, Bohn R, et al. Initiation of antihypertensive treatment during nonsteroidal anti-inflammatory drug therapy. *JAMA.* 1994;272:781–786.

46. Perneger T, Whelton P, Klag M. Risk of kidney failure associated with the use of acetaminophen, aspirin and nonsteroidal anti-inflammatory drugs. *N Engl J Med.* 1994;331:1675–1679.

47. Laisalmi M, Teppo A, Koivusalo A. The effect of ketorolac and sevoflurane anesthesia on renal glomerular and tubular function. *Anesth Analg.* 2001;93:1210–1213.

48. Sivarajan M, Wasse L. Perioperative acute renal failure associated with preoperative intake of ibuprofen. *Anesthesiology.* 1997;86:1390–1392.

49. Burke D, Wildsmith J. Meningitis after spinal anesthesia. *Br J Anaesth.* 1997;78:635–636.

50. Mamusa S, Burton J, Groat J, et al. Ibuprofen-associated pure white-cell aplasia. *N Engl J Med.* 1986;31:624–625.

51. Kohrs R, Durieux M. Ketamine: teaching an old drug new tricks. *Anesth Analg.* 1998;87:1186–1193.

52. Kienbaum P, Heuter T, Paviakovic G, et al. S(+)-ketamine increases muscle sympathetic activity and maintains the neural response to hypotensive challenges in humans. *Anesthesiology.* 2001;94:252–258.

53. Pfenninger E, Durieux M, Himmelsehr S. Cognitive impairment after small-dose ketamine isomers in comparison to equianalgesic racemic ketamine in human volunteers. *Anesthesiology.* 2002;97:357–366.

54. Wagner L, Gingrich K, Kulli J, et al. Ketamine blockage of voltage-gated sodium channels: evidence for a shared receptor site with local anesthetics. *Anesthesiology.* 2001;95:1406–1413.

55. Weigand M, Schmidt H, Zhao Q, et al. Ketamine modulates the stimulated adhesion molecule expression on human neutrophils in vitro. *Anesth Analg.* 2000;90:206–212.

56. Hurstveit O, Maurset A, Oye I. Interactions of the chiral forms of ketamine with opioid, phencyclidine and muscarinic receptors. *Pharmacol Toxicol.* 1995;77:355–359.

57. White P, Way W, Trevor A. Ketamine: its pharmacology and therapeutic uses. *Anesthesiology.* 1982;56:119–136.

58. Demling R, Ellerbee S, Jarrett F. Ketamine anesthesia for tangential excision of burn eschar: a burn unit procedure. *J Trauma.* 1978;18:269–270.

59. Himmelseher S, Durieux M. Ketamine for perioperative pain management. *Anesthesiology.* 2005;102:211–220.

60. Subramaniam K, Balachundar S, Steinbrook R. Ketamine as adjuvant analgesic to opioids: a quantitative and qualitative systematic review. *Anesth Analg.* 2004;99:482–495.

61. Liu H-T, Hollmann M, Liu W-H, et al. Modulation of NMDA receptor function by ketamine and magnesium: Part I. *Anesth Analg.* 2001;92:1173–1181.

62. Akamatsu T, Bonica J, Rhemet R. Experiences with the use of ketamine for parturition. I. Primary anesthetic for vagina delivery. *Anesth Analg.* 1974;53:284–287.

63. Janeczko G, El-Etr A, Youngest S. Low-dose ketamine anesthesia for obstetrical delivery. *Anesth Analg.* 1974;53:828–831.

64. Hodgkinson K, Marx G, Kim S, et al. Neonatal neurobehavioral tests following vaginal delivery under ketamine, thiopental and extradural anesthesia. *Anesth Analg.* 1977;56:548–553.

65. Reich D, Silvay G. Ketamine: an update on the first twenty-five years of clinical experience. *Can J Anaesth.* 1989;36:186–197.

66. Takeshita H, Okuda Y, Sari A. The effects of ketamine on cerebral circulation and metabolism in man. *Anesthesiology.* 1972;36:69–75.

67. Wong D, Jenkins L. An experimental study of the mechanism of action of ketamine on the central nervous system. *Can Anaesth Soc J.* 1974;21:57–67.

68. Baraka A, Harrison T, Kachachi T. Catecholamine levels after ketamine anesthesia in man. *Anesth Analg.* 1973;52:198–200.

69. Taylor T, Towey R. Depression of laryngeal reflexes during ketamine anesthesia. *Br Med J.* 1971;2:688–689.

70. Sarma V. Use of ketamine in acute severe asthma. *Acta Anaesth Scand.* 1992;36:106–107.

71. Hirota K, Lambert D. Ketamine: its mechanism(s) of action and unusual clinical uses. *Br J Anaesth.* 1996;77:441–444.

72. Laxenaire M, Moneret-Vautrin D, Vervloet D. The French experience of anaphylactoid reactions. *Int Anesth Clin.* 1985;23:145–160.

73. Cartwright P, Pingel S. Midazolam and diazepam in ketamine anesthesia. *Anaesthesia.* 1984;59:439–442.

74. Toft P, Romer U. Comparison of midazolam and diazepam to supplement total intravenous anesthesia with ketamine for endoscopy. *Can J Anaesth.* 1987;34:466–469.

75. Nelson L, Lu J, Guo T, et al. The alpha$_2$ adrenoreceptor agonist dexmedetomidine converges on an endogenous sleep-promoting pathway to exert its sedative effects. *Anesthesiology.* 2003;98:428–436.

76. Shelly M. Dexmedetomidine: a real innovation or more of the same? *Br J Anaesth.* 2001;87:677–678.

77. Kamibiyashi T, Maze M. Clinical uses of alpha$_2$-adrenergic agonists. *Anesthesiology*. 2000;93:1345–1349.

78. Asai T, McBeth C, Stewart J. Effect of clonidine on gastric emptying of liquids. *Br J Anaesth*. 1997;78:28–33.

79. Eisenach J, DeKock M, Klimscha W. Alpha$_2$-adrenergic agonists for regional anesthesia: a clinical review of clonidine (1984–1995). *Anesthesiology*. 1996;85:655–674.

80. Milne B, Cervenko F, Jhamandas K, et al. Local clonidine: analgesia and effect on opiate withdrawal in the rat. *Anesthesiology*. 1985;62:34–38.

81. Reuben S, Steinberg R, Klatt J, et al. Intravenous regional anesthesia using lidocaine and clonidine. *Anesthesiology*. 1999; 91:654–658.

82. Aantaa R, Maakola M, Kallio A, et al. Reduction of the minimum alveolar concentration of isoflurane by dexmedetomidine. *Anesthesiology*. 1997;86:1055–1060.

83. Quintin L, Bouilloc X, Butin E, et al. Clonidine for major vascular surgery in hypertensive patients: a double-blind, controlled, randomized study. *Anesth Analg*. 1996;83:687–695.

84. Goyagi T, Makoto T, Nishikawa T. Oral clonidine enhances the pressor response to ephedrine during spinal anesthesia. *Anesth Analg*. 1998;87:1336–1339.

85. Strebel S, Gurzeler J, Schneider M, et al. Small-dose intrathecal clonidine and isobaric bupivacaine for orthopedic surgery: a dose-response study. *Anesth Analg*. 2004;99: 1231–1238.

86. Liu S, Chiu A, Neal J, et al. Oral clonidine prolongs lidocaine spinal anesthesia in human volunteers. *Anesthesiology*. 1995;82:1353–1359.

87. Singelyn F, Gouverneur J, Robert A. A minimum dose of clonidine added to mepivacaine prolongs the duration of anesthesia and analgesia after axillary brachial plexus block. *Anesth Analg*. 1996;83:1046–1050.

88. Bailey P, Sperry R, Johnson G, et al. Respiratory effects of clonidine alone and combined with morphine in humans. *Anesthesiology*. 1991;74:43–48.

89. Bernard J, Lagarde D, Souron R. Balanced postoperative analgesia: effect of intravenous clonidine on blood gases and pharmacokinetics of intravenous fentanyl. *Anesth Analg*. 1994;79:1126–1131.

90. Ghigone M, Calvillo O, Quintin L. Anesthesia and hypertension: the effect of clonidine on perioperative hemodynamics and isoflurane requirements. *Anesthesiology*. 1987;67:3–10.

91. Husserl F, Messerli F. Adverse effects of antihypertensive drugs. *Drugs*. 1981;22:188–210.

92. Stiff J, Harris D. Clonidine withdrawal complicated by amitriptyline therapy. *Anesthesiology*. 1983;59:73–74.

93. Sandler A. The role of clonidine and alpha$_2$-agonists for postoperative analgesia. *Can J Anaesth*. 1996;43:1191–1194.

94. Sheinin H, Aantaa R, Anttila M, et al. Reversal of the sedative and sympatholytic effects of dexmedetomidine with a specific alpha$_2$ adrenoreceptor antagonist atipamezole. A pharmacodynamic and kinetic study in healthy volunteers. *Anesthesiology*. 1998;89:574–584.

95. Buhrer M, Mappes A, Lauber R, et al. Dexmedetomidine decreases thiopental dose requirement and alters distribution pharmacokinetics. *Anesthesiology*. 1994;80:1216–1221.

96. Segal I, Vickery R, Walton J, Doze V, Maze M. Dexmedetomidine diminishes halothane anesthetic requirements in rats through a postsynaptic alpha$_2$ adrenergic receptor. *Anesthesiology*. 1988;69:818–823.

97. Ramsay M, Luterman D. Dexmedetomidine as a total intravenous anesthetic agent. *Anesthesiology*. 2004;101:787–790.

98. Levanen J, Makela M, Scheinin H. Dexmedetomidine premedication attenuates ketamine-induced cardiostimulatory effects and postanesthetic delirium. *Anesthesiology*. 1995;82:1117–1125.

99. Memis D, Turan A, Karamanhoglu B, et al. Adding dexmedetomidine to lidocaine for intravenous regional anesthesia. *Anesth Analg*. 2004;98:835–840.

100. Kremer M. Response to Rich J: Dexmedetomidine as a sole sedating agent with local anesthesia in a high-risk patient for axillofemoral bypass graft: a case report. *AANA J*. 2006;73:5.

101. Hsu Y, Cortinez, L, Robertson K, et al. Dexmedetomidine pharmacodynamics. Part I. Crossover comparison of the respiratory effects of dexmedetomidine and remifentanil in healthy volunteers. *Anesthesiology*. 2004;101:1066–1076.

102. Venn R, Bradshaw C, Spencer R, et al. Preliminary UK experience of dexmedetomidine, a novel agent for postoperative sedation in the intensive care unit. *Anaesthesia*. 1999;54:1136–1142.

Objectives

After completing this chapter, the reader should be able to

- Describe the normal physiology of the neuromuscular junction.
- Explain the role of acetylcholine (ACh) and the nicotinic ACh receptor in muscle contraction.
- Describe the function of muscle relaxant medications and contrast the mechanisms of action of aminosteroidal, benzylisoquinoline, and depolarizing relaxants.
- Formulate an anesthetic plan that incorporates a neuromuscular blocker, accounting for how the attributes of the drug fit with the proposed surgery.
- Contrast the application, benefits, and disadvantages of various specialized approaches to administration of nondepolarizers, including the priming dose, defasciculating dose, and rapid sequence induction.
- Devise a plan for monitoring the effects of the neuromuscular blocker during various phases of the surgery.
- Contrast the expected findings, error rate, and application of various modes of peripheral nerve stimulator monitoring.
- Describe the issue of postoperative residual relaxation and discuss a plan for minimizing the occurrence of it.

Introduction

Neuromuscular blocking drugs (NMBs) are a mainstay of modern anesthesia practice. In fact, a great many advances in surgery and anesthesia care would not have been possible if not for the ability, afforded by neuromuscular paralysis, to produce reliable immobility and profound muscle relaxation. The development of neuromuscular relaxants is inextricably linked to the progression of anesthesia care itself, with a rapid rate of advancement of each noted after the middle of the 20th century. The history of muscle relaxants is traced back to precivilized South American bushmen. Observations from 17th century explorers described these hunters using extracts from certain plants to induce paralysis in prey by "poisoning" the tips of arrows with the substance. Interestingly, the hunters had developed an adequately sophisticated understanding of the alkaloids they were using to know that they themselves would not be similarly affected by eating the "poisoned" quarry. The

8

Neuromuscular Blocking Drugs

Michael Rieker, DNP, CRNA

paralyzing substance, curarine, was extracted from a number of plants, but the subtype, which came from the chondrodendron tomentosum plant and which was typically packed into bamboo tubes, came to be known as *d*-tubocurarine and then as the shorter term, curare.[1] Curare was first commonly used in medicine in the 1940s to prevent injury in patients undergoing electroconvulsive therapy. Later, muscle relaxants were used to facilitate surgery and tracheal intubation.

The development of muscle relaxants is ongoing in search of an ideal agent. Thus far, the success of a particular class of agents (such as in reducing organ-dependent elimination) has been tempered by attendant side effects (such as histamine release). There may not be a single ideal agent, because a given characteristic (such as short duration of action) may be beneficial in some but not all applications of the drug. Nonetheless, some characteristics that would describe the ideal agent have not yet been provided among the available agents (Box 8-1). Although some argue the semantics of different labels for the drugs that impair neuromuscular function, for the purpose of this chapter the terms "neuromuscular blockers," "paralytics," and "muscle relaxants" are used interchangeably.

Mechanisms of Action

A useful understanding of the pharmacology of neuromuscular blockers must first follow an understanding of neuromuscular physiology. Skeletal muscle receives innervation from motor nerves (α motor neurons) that arise from cell bodies in the ventral horn of spinal gray matter. The nerve terminal manufactures acetylcholine (ACh) from acetate and choline. The acetate is supplied by acetyl coenzyme A from the mitochondria, and choline is derived from dietary intake and liver production. The enzyme choline acetyl-

transferase combines the acetate and choline into ACh. The neurotransmitter is then stored in vesicles, called *quanta*.

Motor End Plate

The interaction between nerve and muscle occurs at the neuromuscular junction (NMJ), where the nerve axon terminates in close approximation to an area on the muscle fiber known as the *motor end plate*. Close to the terminus, the motor neuron branches into multiple fibers that innervate individual muscle fibers. The motor nerve plus the innervated muscle fibers are known as a motor unit. The ratio of nerve fibers to muscle fibers varies between motor units, depending on the complexity of movement controlled by the unit. The ratio varies from one nerve fiber controlling one or two muscle fibers for very fine movements to over 1:1000 for gross movement areas, with the average ratio being approximately 1:100.

The motor end plate contains gyri, or folds of the sarcolemma, which are populated by nicotinic cholinergic receptors (nAChRs). These receptors tend to be concentrated on the "shoulders" of the junctional folds, placing them in close approximation to the "active zones" of the motor nerve terminal, from where the vesicles of ACh are opened into the synaptic cleft (Figure 8-1). As a wave of depolarization propagates down the motor nerve axon and reaches the nerve terminal, sodium and potassium flux depolarizes the terminal of the nerve. Fast calcium channels open, quickly increasing the intracellular calcium level in the nerve terminal. This rise in calcium causes the vesicles of ACh to fuse with the nerve membrane and to release the transmitter into the synaptic cleft. Each vesicle contains approximately 5000 to 10,000 molecules of ACh, and 200 to 400 vesicles are released with each depolarization.[2]

Because of the complimentary structures of the nerve terminal and the motor end plate, the synaptic cleft of the NMJ is very small, approximately 20 to 50 nm in width.[3] As a result, ACh released from the nerve reaches the muscle quickly, where it interacts with nAChRs. After ACh is released by the nerve to interact with receptors on the muscle, the enzyme acetylcholinesterase, located in proximity to the nAChRs (Figure 8-2), hydrolyzes the neurotransmitter, and the choline and acetate are taken up into the nerve terminal where they can be recycled into new ACh (Figure 8-3). Being in close proximity to the nAChR, the acetylcholinesterase is responsible for the discreteness of the effects of ACh released from the motor nerves. The ACh is inactivated before it is able to leave the NMJ and cause effects elsewhere. However, to facilitate recovery from NMBs, acetylcholinesterase is intentionally inhibited to make ACh more abundant and therefore more

Box 8-1 Characteristics of the Ideal Neuromuscular Blocker

- Rapid, predictable onset of effects within one circulation time to facilitate rapid securing of the airway.

- Absence of histamine release, influence on heart rate, bronchial tone, or other side effects.

- Metabolism that is not organ dependent; does not demonstrate variability due to age, body mass index, disease state, or other factors; and does not result in active metabolites.

- Nondepolarizing, so administration does not cause myalgia or increase intracranial, intragastric, or intraocular pressures.

- Lack of histamine release or other systemic side effects.

- Adaptable to long cases, without cumulative effects.

- Predictable depth of blockade at known per-kilogram doses to obviate the need for peripheral nerve stimulator monitoring.

- Availability of a reversal agent that may be used at any time after neuromuscular blockade (such as in the case of failed airway) and that does not cause significant side effects.

- Ability to be reversed quickly and completely without residual effects.

- Absence of placental transfer, when administered to a parturient patient.

- Nonantigenic; not a trigger for malignant hyperthermia.

- Organ-independent metabolism without active metabolites.

- The ability to produce hypnosis and/or amnesia during the interval of muscle relaxation. (Note: This attribute would preclude the occurrence of awareness during paralysis; however, it would probably not be compatible with the points about placental transfer or standard per-kilogram dosing.)

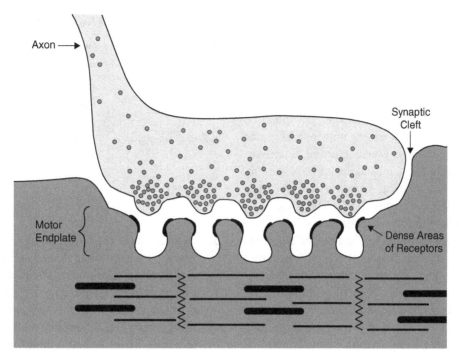

Figure 8-1 Neuromuscular junction.

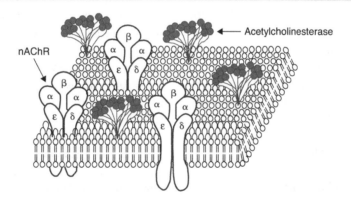

Figure 8-2 Muscle membrane.

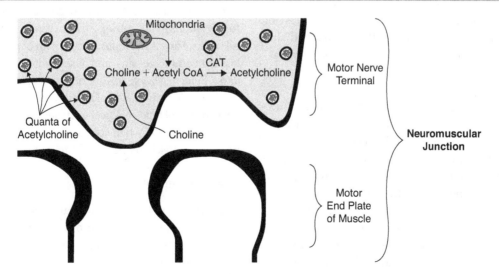

Figure 8-3 Acetylcholine manufacturer.

competitive in stimulating the nAChR over the muscle relaxants present. Therefore the primary side effects of this reversal relate to widespread systemic effects of ACh.

Receptors of the NMJ

The myofibril cell membrane is a typical phospholipid bilayer. The nAChR is a ligand-gated, ionotropic receptor traversing the cell membrane. When activated, this channel allows the egress of potassium and the influx of sodium. Small, random releases of small amounts of ACh occur constantly, producing miniature end-plate potentials. However, in response to a full depolarization of the nerve and normal quantal release of ACh, when a sufficient quantity of receptors is activated, the motor end plate becomes depolarized. When the muscle membrane becomes depolarized from its normal resting potential to the threshold potential, this depolarization spreads out from the motor end plate to initiate contraction of the entire muscle cell. Depending on the strength of the neural stimulus, some or all fibers of the muscle contract.

There are numerous types of nAChR besides those found in the NMJ. Numerous distinct neuronal-type nAChR are found in the central nervous system and on autonomic ganglia. In the normal adult state, the receptors present in the NMJ are of a limited subtype, but conditions that impair neuronal stimulation to the NMJ precipitate the proliferation of alternate types of receptors with different response characteristics to agonists. The typical nAChR consists of five subcomponents, designated β (beta), δ (delta), ε (epsilon), and two α (alpha) subunits (Figure 8-2).

Mechanisms of Receptor Involvement

Neuromuscular blockers are classified structurally as aminosteroids (having a nucleus of four fused rings) or benzylisoquinolines, if they are of the nondepolarizing type. A third class with a distinct structure is simply classified according to mechanism, the depolarizing muscle relaxants (Table 8-1).

Because of structural similarities with ACh, neuromuscular blockers can occupy the α subunits of the nAChR receptor, namely by binding with the receptor at the quaternary ammonium group of the muscle relaxant. Because activation of the receptor requires agonists occupying both α subunits, NMBs binding with these α subunits prevents their occupation by ACh, in what is the primary mechanism of action of nondepolarizing NMBs. The AChR can be activated to open the channel only when *both* α subunits are occupied by an agonist, such as ACh or succinylcholine. This fact serves as the basis for the primary mechanism of action of NMBs. Nondepolarizing NMBs must

Table 8-1 Classification of Neuromuscular Blockers

Classification	Specific Agents
Aminosteroid	Rocuronium
	Vecuronium
	Pipecuronium
	Pancuronium
Benzylisoquinoline	Atracurium
	Cisatracurium
	Doxacurium
Depolarizing	Succinylcholine

occupy only one of the two α subunits of a given receptor to prevent the activation of that receptor.

In addition to the postsynaptic nAChR, there are presynaptic cholinergic receptors on the motor nerve terminal. These receptors have a slightly different structure, containing three α and two β subunits only; thus they more resemble the neuronal-type ACh receptors found elsewhere in the body. When activated, these receptors serve to facilitate and augment the release of ACh by stimulating mobilization of ACh in the motor nerve terminal.[4] This point is important in making distinctions between the pharmacology of different classes of NMBs. The presynaptic nAChRs are thought to stimulate mobilization of ACh and increase the quantal release of the transmitter in response to frequent activation of the neuromuscular unit. This mechanism would explain posttetanic facilitation, an increase in the strength of muscle contraction after an intense, repetitive electrical stimulus to the nerve. It also explains the phenomenon of "fade," a decrease in strength of responses to more slowly repetitive stimuli, resulting from effects of NMBs on the presynaptic receptors.[5] The varying affinity of the presynaptic nAChR for different classes of NMBs has been a common explanation for variations in fade observed between the classes of muscle relaxants. Fade is most observable with benzylisoquinolines, less with aminosteroids, and absent with depolarizing relaxants.[6] Evidence suggests that other receptors and mediators (such as adenosine) also play a role in ACh release and the observation of fade.[7,8] However, in any case it is apparent that a synergism exists when concurrently administering nondepolarizing muscle relaxants of different classes (Table 8-2).

Depolarizing Relaxants

Depolarizing muscle relaxants are a special class of drug with the unique mechanism of acting as an agonist at the nAChR. Succinylcholine is the only agent in this class currently in use. Succinylcholine is comprised of two molecules of ACh linked at the acetate methyl group. Because of the structural similarity to endogenous ACh, succinylcholine

Table 8-2 Mechanism of Action of Neuromuscular Blocking Drugs

1. Occupation of at least one α subunit of postsynaptic nAChRs to prevent activation of those receptors (primary mechanism of nondepolarizing NMBs)

2. Occupation of at least one α subunit of presynaptic nAChRs to reduce ACh release from motor nerve terminal (secondary mechanism of steroidal NMBs; more pronounced in benzyl-isoquinoline-type drugs)

3. Occupation and activation of both α subunits of postsynaptic nAChRs, with prolonged depolarization of the motor end plate, which prevents further transmission of neuromuscular impulses (mechanism of depolarizing type of NMB, namely succinylcholine)

4. Open channel blockade; lodging of a molecule inside the open channel of the nAChR, blocking further ion flow (occurs mostly with deep block/high concentration of acetylcholine or relaxant molecules)

acts as an agonist at the nAChR. However, succinylcholine is hydrolyzed by plasma cholinesterase in a reaction that is slower than that by which acetylcholinesterase metabolizes ACh. As a result of this relatively slowed metabolism, succinylcholine remains in the NMJ longer, alternately depolarizing various nAChR in the junction. The initial depolarization of the motor end plate triggers voltage-gated channels on the muscle tissue adjacent to the NMJ, causing a brief contraction of all muscles that are stimulated by the succinylcholine. There is also a second, time-limited gate on the muscle, and these two gates must operate sequentially to produce a muscle contraction. Because succinylcholine lingers in the NMJ longer than ACh does, the junction remains depolarized for a few minutes until the succinylcholine is metabolized. Because the initial voltage-gated channels in the NMJ are never "reset," the required sequential activation of ion channels outside the NMJ cannot occur. Therefore after the brief initial contraction of muscles (known as *fasciculations*), the muscles affected by succinylcholine remain flaccid and insensitive to efferent neural input until the succinylcholine is metabolized.

Clinical Pharmacology (Prototype: Rocuronium)

Pharmacokinetics

Muscle relaxants are large molecules with a quaternary ammonium structure, which is a permanently charged group consisting of a nitrogen atom surrounded by four alkyl groups (Figure 8-4). As a result muscle relaxants exhibit a low volume of distribution. Their water-soluble nature limits passage into the brain (rendering them devoid of effects on cognition) and across the placenta (allowing their safe use during pregnancy and cesarean delivery). They are poorly absorbed from the gastrointestinal tract, explaining why historic use of curare to immobilize prey did not cause paralysis in the people who then consumed the meat of the captured animals. As a result these drugs have relatively uncomplicated pharmacokinetics; however, patient characteristics such as body mass index, gender, age, and ethnicity influence the observed pharmacology.[9]

Rocuronium is an aminosteroidal muscle relaxant of intermediate duration. In the evolution of NMBs, rocuronium is the latest successful drug in the quest for a rapid onset, intermediate-acting drug with a benign side effect profile. Dosed at 0.6 mg/kg, or two times the ED_{95}, rocuronium has an onset of 1 to 2 minutes. Rocuronium has a lower potency than other common steroidal nondepolarizers. Because it is dosed at a greater milligram mass, the onset is faster, as there are more molecules present to occupy sites on the nicotinic receptors. This onset allows intubation relatively quickly.[10] Because of its short onset, rocuronium is also useful for rapid sequence intubation. When dosed at four times the ED_{95}, or 1.2 mg/kg, rocuronium has an onset of less than 1 minute, which can facilitate a rapid sequence (without ventilation) or modified rapid sequence (with low-pressure ventilation) intubation without oxygen desaturation in most patients.[11,12]

When there is desire to avoid a depolarizing relaxant and when the duration of rocuronium will not contraindicate this use, rocuronium provides similar quality of relaxation at a slightly longer onset interval than succinylcholine.[13] Some research has found rocuronium to provide acceptable intubation conditions 60 seconds after a dose of 0.6 mg/kg.[14] However, others found rocuronium at 0.6 mg/kg to provide less optimal intubating conditions than succinylcholine at 60 seconds after dosing. Sluga et al. found under these conditions that onset was faster and intubating conditions were superior among patients receiving succinylcholine 1 mg/kg as compared with those receiving rocuronium 0.6 mg/kg for rapid sequence induction.[15]

Other researchers also found a lesser quality of relaxation of the larynx after rocuronium compared with succinylcholine, particularly when a lower dose of rocuronium is

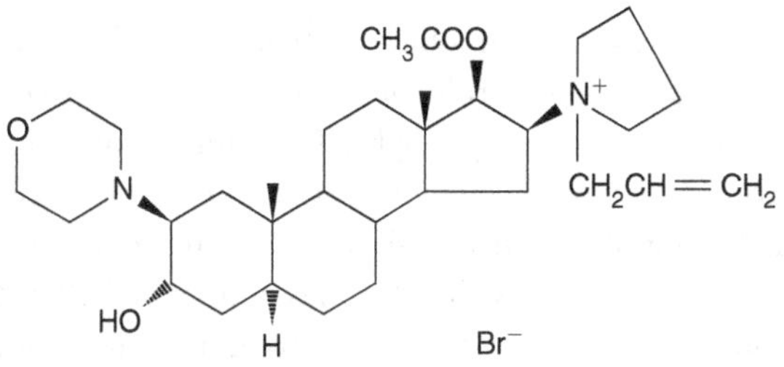

Figure 8-4 Rocuronium structure.

used.[16,17] Nonetheless, due to concerns about the side effects of succinylcholine such as myalgias, potassium and histamine release, and bradycardia, practitioners may prefer to use rocuronium to facilitate rapid sequence induction, if the trade-off of a longer duration of action does not controvert its use. In this case, dosing at 1.2 mg/kg provided the best chance of achieving adequate conditions quickly.

Effect of Cardiac Output

The onset of rocuronium can be altered by changes in the cardiac output. Ephedrine has been demonstrated to speed the onset of rocuronium, due to the increase in cardiac output.[18,19] Conversely, a low cardiac output, such as may be induced by β-adrenergic blockers, will slow the onset of muscle relaxation after rocuronium.[20,21] To varying degrees these effects are most likely also present with other muscle relaxants.

Effect of Organ Disease

Because steroidal-type nondepolarizers undergo some hepatic metabolism and rely on renal excretion, severe hepatic or renal disease may prolong the effects of these relaxants. However, rocuronium demonstrates only modest prolongation in recovery in patients with liver disease.[22] Liver disease influences other classes of NMB drugs only to the extent that, when severe, it can reduce the amount of plasma cholinesterase available to metabolize succinylcholine. The benzylisoquinoline compounds atracurium and cisatracurium are independent of influence by the liver or kidneys, except to the extent that the metabolite laudanosine can accumulate in the presence of renal failure and prolonged infusions of those drugs. Typically not a concern in the context of perioperative administration, laudanosine is a central nervous system stimulant that can induce seizures at high accumulated levels. Changes in plasma protein levels could theoretically influence the pharmacokinetic attributes of NMBs by reducing the volume of distribution. In practice, changes in levels of α_1-acid glycoprotein, for example, create little clinical alteration in rocuronium characteristics.

Patient Characteristics

When administered to obese patients, the duration of action is significantly prolonged when dosing rocuronium according to actual body weight. The duration of action of rocuronium has been demonstrated to exceed twice the normal amount, when dosed according to actual weight in obese patients. It is therefore recommended that dosage should be based on ideal body weight.[23] An exception to this recommendation is with succinylcholine, wherein a

clinically insignificant prolongation of duration may outweigh the threat of inadequate intubating conditions in a challenging airway situation.[24] This consideration would favor dosing succinylcholine based on actual body weight, when the patient situation dictates.

Patient age influences the pharmacokinetic profile of muscle relaxants, with shorter onset but prolonged recovery time noted in infants compared with adults. Dosed at 1.5 times the ED_{95} to infants, rocuronium demonstrates a similar recovery time as it does at two times ED_{95} in adults.[25] Different study designs with different relaxants yield varying observations regarding the pharmacokinetics of these drugs in infants. The combination of a larger volume of distribution, immature NMJ, and immature hepatic metabolism may be responsible for the variability in response in infants. Children have the highest dose required for NMBs, based on age. Elderly patients exhibit a normal to increased duration of action of relaxants. Gender influences the response to some muscle relaxants, with female patients demonstrating a 20% to 30% reduction in required dose of rocuronium (but not cisatracurium) compared with male patients.[26,27]

Pharmacodynamics

The basic pharmacodynamics of NMBs were discussed already, namely the competitive occupation of at least one α subunit of the nAChR, preventing activation by ACh. The notable exception is succinylcholine, which acts as an agonist at the nAChR. If one bears in mind that succinylcholine acts as an *agonist* at the nicotinic receptor (as opposed to thinking of it as an *antagonist* of neuromuscular function), the dissimilarities from other NMBs become more apparent. For example, succinylcholine acts as an antagonist to nondepolarizing relaxants. Pretreatment with a nondepolarizer before administration of succinylcholine requires a larger dose of succinylcholine to be used.

Sensitivity of Different Muscle Groups

All NMBs first affect small and rapidly moving muscle units. Therefore neuromuscular blockade is apparent around the eyes or fingers before affecting other parts of the body. When the priming technique is used, the first sign of clinical effects indeed is often the patient's complaint of diplopia, because the extraocular muscles exhibit weakness before other areas. The diaphragm and larynx are more resistant to the effects of NMBs than are other areas, such as the hand. Thus there is a disparity between monitoring information at the hand and the level of relaxation of the larynx and diaphragm. During surgical maintenance, this disparity may lead to patient movement, if relaxants are dosed strictly according to the twitch response at the hand. It is not uncommon for patients to appear "flat" in their response to a peripheral nerve stimulator (PNS) at the hand, whereas abdominal muscle tone or diaphragmatic movement is present. In cases where strict akinesia must be maintained, it may be necessary to dose the NMB at levels deeper than what can be monitored by the traditional train-of-four. In these cases the posttetanic count is a useful mode of monitoring. The disparity between sensitivity to relaxants at the diaphragm and the adductor pollicis creates challenges during maintenance, but this also represents a margin of safety on emergence, whereby any given level of blockade observed at the hand can be assumed to be less at the diaphragm.

Cardiovascular Effects

Some neuromuscular blockers have the ability to stimulate or inhibit cardiovascular receptors. Pancuronium is most associated with cardiovascular stimulation through its ability to block cardiac muscarinic receptors and elevate the heart rate. The degree of heart rate change is inverse to the preexisting rate, with the greatest increase observed in patients with a slow heart rate. This effect had made pancuronium an attractive choice as part of high-dose opioid techniques, when the opposing heart rate effects of opioids and pancuronium can counterbalance each other. Rocuronium sometimes exhibits a similar but more modest effect on the heart rate, particularly in pediatric patients.

Rarely, succinylcholine may mimic ACh at autonomic ganglia, causing cardiovascular stimulation characterized by tachycardia. More commonly, the cardiovascular effects of succinylcholine result from stimulation of muscarinic receptors, leading to bradycardia. This effect is more prevalent after a repeat dose of succinylcholine than it is after a single dose. Succinylcholine, as well as atracurium, may cause histamine release, leading to flushing, hypotension, and rebound tachycardia.

Confounding Factors

A number of physiologic and pharmacologic factors may alter the pharmacodynamics of muscle relaxants. This may occur by altering the availability of ACh receptors (myasthenia gravis or burn injury), interfering with the role of ions in the NMJ or the sarcomere (calcium channel blockers and magnesium), causing direct blockade of the ion channel (antibiotics), and other mechanisms. Box 8-2 outlines some factors that alter the pharmacodynamics of relaxants.

Box 8-2 Factors That Alter the Pharmacodynamics of Relaxants

Potentiate effects of relaxants

- Acetylcholine (in excessive amounts desensitizes the receptors)
- Acidosis
- Antibiotics (particularly polymyxin, aminoglycosides, clindamycin)
- Calcium channel blockers
- Furosemide
- Guillain-Barré disease
- Hypothermia
- Local anesthetics
- Magnesium sulfate
- Multiple sclerosis
- Muscular dystrophies
- Myasthenia gravis (nondepolarizers)
- Myasthenic syndrome (all relaxants)
- Volatile anesthetics

Cause resistance to relaxants

- Burn injury (however, causes potassium release with succinylcholine)
- Denervation (however, causes potassium release with succinylcholine)
- Myasthenia gravis (succinylcholine)

Metabolism

Neuromuscular blockers undergo metabolism by various means, characteristic of the class of drug. Ten percent to 30% of aminosteroid relaxants undergo metabolism by hepatic microsomal enzymes, with the remainder of drug excreted unchanged in the bile or urine. Benzylisoquinolines, in contrast, bear the principal advantage of metabolism that does not depend on hepatic or renal function.

Metabolism of Nondepolarizers

Pancuronium is excreted unchanged in the urine in proportions of 80% of the administered dose, causing concern when using this drug in the presence of impaired renal function, due to prolongation of effects. Pancuronium may exhibit at least a doubling of its effect in the presence of renal failure. On the other hand, rocuronium, with a renal excretion fraction closer to 20%, is more easily managed in the administration to patients with renal disease, although it may demonstrate more variability in duration of action in patients with renal failure.[28,29] Advancing age prolongs the metabolism of nondepolarizers[30] and introduces variability in the duration of action of these drugs by approximately 15 to 20 minutes.[31] When using cisatracurium, both of these effects are lessened to an amount that has little clinical significance in most cases.

Because of organ-independent metabolism, the benzylisoquinolines, atracurium and cisatracurium, are most desirable in elderly patients or in those with renal insufficiency. These drugs primarily undergo ester hydrolysis in the plasma by nonspecific esterases (distinct from plasma cholinesterase, which metabolizes succinylcholine). Their metabolism is also secondarily carried out by enzymatic Hoffman elimination, which depends on blood pH for degradation (higher pH promotes breakdown).[32] Changes in temperature also influence the metabolism of atracurium and its *cis* isomer; however, within the context of the physiologic pH and temperature range, appreciable clinical changes in the duration of atracurium and cisatracurium are unlikely to be noticeable.[33]

Metabolism of Succinylcholine

Succinylcholine undergoes metabolism by breakdown of the ester linkage in the middle of the molecule by plasma cholinesterase, also known as pseudocholinesterase. This enzyme is distinct from acetylcholinesterase, which breaks ACh into acetate and choline; however, the natural substrate of plasma cholinesterase is not known. Plasma cholinesterase is formed in the liver and is very efficient at degrading succinylcholine. In fact, most of the administered dose of succinylcholine is degraded before it reaches the NMJ, a fact that explains why the drug is typically dosed at three to four times the ED_{95}.[34] When a shorter duration of succinylcholine is desired, a more modest dose of 0.3 to 0.5 mg/kg may be used, but administration should be followed by a rapid flush of intravenous fluid to help promote distribution of the drug to the effect site, before significant degradation in the plasma can occur. Although plasma cholinesterase is formed in the liver, it is not until significant levels of liver failure occur that a deficiency of plasma cholinesterase is appreciated clinically.

Genetic variants in the expression of the gene for plasma cholinesterase can influence the activity of the enzyme on the metabolism of succinylcholine. Although there are numerous isoforms, they can be summarized as "normal," "heterozygous atypical," and "homozygous atypical." Plasma cholinesterase activity is measured by the ability of the local anesthetic dibucaine to inhibit the activity of the enzyme. In the normal condition, dibucaine inhibits 80% of the activity of plasma cholinesterase. Plasma cholinesterase that is not responsive to the effects of dibucaine is also less effective at metabolizing succinylcholine. The dibucaine number, then, indicates the percent inhibition of the enzyme by dibucaine, and that number is proportional to the effectiveness of the enzyme at metabolizing succinylcholine (Table 8-3). A dibucaine number of 80 or higher is normal. A dibucaine number of 60 would represent an individual who is heterozygous atypical (incidence around 1 in 500). This person would exhibit a prolongation of effects of succinylcholine up to an hour in duration. A dibucaine number of 20 to 40 would represent homozygous atypical (incidence around 1 in 3000). This person would exhibit a significant prolongation of succinylcholine, which could persist for 4 to 6 hours.

In the case of prolonged relaxation from succinylcholine resulting from deficiencies in plasma cholinesterase, supportive treatment with controlled ventilation and sedation should be used until spontaneous recovery occurs. Reversal should *not* be attempted with an acetylcholinesterase inhibitor, as may be used in the case of phase II block. Acetylcholinesterase inhibitors also inhibit plasma cholinesterase and further complicate the problem. Purified human plasma cholinesterase provides another option in managing this complication, as the succinylcholine could be reversed by administration of this compound.[35] Because of multiple genotypes that may code for abnormalities of the plasma cholinesterase enzyme, a range of findings in dibucaine number and the corresponding duration of succinylcholine may be found. For example, the rare Es genotype demonstrates approximately 8 hours' duration of succinylcholine effects.

Table 8-3 Interpretation of the Dibucaine Number

Dibucaine Number	Interpretation	Expected Duration of Succinylcholine
80	Normal	5–8 min
40–60	Heterozygous atypical	30–60 min
20	Homozygous atypical	4–6 h

Elimination

Neuromuscular blockers are eliminated either unchanged in the urine or bile or as metabolites after degradation by hepatic microsomal enzyme. Pediatric patients tend to demonstrate a faster elimination, whereas older patients may demonstrate prolonged elimination. Changes in cardiac output, decreased muscle mass, and increased body fat, as well as declining hepatic and renal function, can alter the pharmacokinetics of NMBs in the elderly.[36] Atracurium and cisatracurium are particularly suited for administration to renal patients, because the active forms do not depend on renal elimination.

Clinical Uses and Indications

Neuromuscular blockers may serve one or many purposes in surgery: facilitating endotracheal intubation, patient positioning or surgical exposure, preventing patient movement from reflexes or subconscious responses to surgical stimulation, and, in some cases, facilitating placement of other airway devices. Some have found that light muscle relaxation facilitates placement of the laryngeal mask airway and prevents possible laryngospasm or biting that may occur with its placement.[37] To treat laryngospasm unresponsive to positive airway pressure, succinylcholine may be administered by various routes: intramuscular (4 mg/kg), intravenous (as low as 0.1 mg/kg), or intralingual or intraosseous (in the absence of an intravenous line).[38] The use of neuromuscular blockers should be dictated by the requirements of the anesthetic and surgical plan. During intra-abdominal surgery, relaxation of the abdominal musculature facilitates surgical exposure, and absence of diaphragmatic movement may aid the surgeon's ability to perform the procedure. Relaxants may facilitate specific surgical procedures, such as allowing abdominal insufflation during laparoscopic cases or preventing movement when even slight movement may disrupt the surgery, such as in ophthalmologic or neurosurgery. However, many surgical procedures can be performed without the use of muscle relaxation. In these cases relaxants may be used initially to facilitate intubation and patient positioning but then allowed to dissipate, without redosing during the case.

In surgeries requiring relaxed muscles for surgical exposure or where patient movement would be deleterious, consistent redosing or a continuous infusion of NMBs may be used. Muscle relaxants are sometimes used to provide safety during brief procedures, such as electroconvulsive therapy. In that case succinylcholine is commonly used to provide a short duration of relaxation during the brief procedure, so the patient is not injured during tonic-clonic seizure movement. Considering the potential for residual relaxation postoperatively, it is advisable to use NMBs only when indicated and to allow ample time for their spontaneous decrement before the desired time of extubation. The choice of relaxant should be based on a number of considerations about the situation of intended use (Box 8-3).

Peripheral Nerve Stimulator Monitoring

The most common method of monitoring the onset, effect, and duration of NMBs is through the use of a PNS. Delivering electrical current across a motor nerve, a PNS can provide an assessment of the NMJ by the observed response of the target muscle group. The most common sites for PNS monitoring are the ulnar nerve (Table 8-4), the temporal branch of the facial nerve (Table 8-5), and the common peroneal nerve (Table 8-6). Major limitations to the sites are disparities between peripheral responsiveness to NMBs in comparison with the diaphragm and larynx and general lack of sensitivity to indicate low levels of relaxation.

The ulnar nerve is the site most commonly used due to ease of access and lack of stray muscle stimulation. Blockade at this site occurs slightly after onset of blockade at the larynx and diaphragm, but the final depth of block appears greater upon stimulation of the ulnar nerve in comparison with that at the diaphragm. This difference in depth of block may lead one to underdose the relaxant, based on the response at the hand, whereas the patient retains the

---

Box 8-3 Considerations in Selecting a Particular Neuromuscular Blocker

- Duration of action (short, intermediate, or long acting) is matched with desired duration of effect.
- Drug is not contraindicated, due to patient sensitivities (succinylcholine in burn patients, etc.).
- Mechanism of metabolism and elimination are amenable to patient's comorbidities.
- Any common side effects (pancuronium, heart rate elevation; atracurium, histamine release) are not contraindicated by the patient's comorbidities.
- Choice is cost-effective for the intended volume/duration used.

Table 8-4 Neuromuscular Monitoring Sites on the Arm

Nerve	Muscle	Response	Advantage	Disadvantage
Ulnar	Adductor pollicis	Adduction of thumb	More sensitive to relaxant; useful for recovery	*Under*estimates *onset* but *over*estimates *depth* of block at the diaphragm
	Hypothenar eminence muscles	Flexion of fifth finger	Responses similar to larynx and diaphragm	15–20% more resistant to non-depolarizing relaxants than adductor pollicis

Table 8-6 Neuromuscular Monitoring Sites on the Foot

Nerve	Muscle	Response	Advantage	Disadvantage
Posterior tibial	Flexor hallucis brevis	Plantar flexion of the great toe	Less sensitive than ulnar nerve Can better monitor deep block	Slower onset than ulnar nerve Less useful for intubation Lower sensitivity may obscure residual relaxation
Common peroneal	Extensor hallucis longus	Dorsiflexion of the great toe		

ability to breathe, cough, or produce other movements. However, this site is useful for monitoring recovery from relaxation, because the level of remaining relaxation at the diaphragm and larynx is less than that apparent at the hand. The response to PNS of the facial nerve more closely resembles the actual timing and depth of blockade at the central structures of most concern (the diaphragm and larynx). The main disadvantage of this site is that the electrical current may circumvent the NMJ and cause direct stimulation of the adjacent muscles, inappropriately suggesting a need for additional muscle relaxant.

Once the monitoring site has been determined, the most common modes of peripheral nerve stimulation are outlined in Figure 8-5. The single-twitch mode is most useful for monitoring onset, when complete neuromuscular blockade is indicated by near-total disappearance of the twitch response. Of all the PNS modes the train-of-four (TOF) is probably the most commonly used, mainly because this single mode has application to onset, maintenance, and recovery of neuromuscular blockade. When this mode is used for maintenance, the number of responses to TOF stimulation is correlated with the degree of blockade (Table 8-7). When all four twitches have returned during recovery, the remaining fade (or decrease in twitch height) from the first to the

fourth twitch can be correlated with small amounts of residual blockade. This measurement is called the TOF ratio.

Because it is difficult for the human hand or eye to interpret subtle amounts of fade from the first to the fourth twitch, the double-burst stimulation mode was developed. Consisting of two sets of grouped stimuli that appear as just two responses, the double burst provides a stronger twitch response, the interpretation of which is not degraded by the distraction of two intervening twitches, as in the TOF. The double-burst stimulation does improve sensitivity in detecting residual fade, albeit only modestly. In one study the sensitivity to detect a TOF ratio of 0.9 was improved only from 11% with the TOF mode to 14% with double-burst stimulation.[39] Even at deeper levels of blockade, anesthetists have been found unable to detect fade through observation of the PNS response. Research has shown that fade becomes difficult to detect once the TOF ratio exceeds 0.4.[40] Clearly, this level of blockade indicates a significant level of relaxation, suggesting that anesthetists would have a low likelihood of identifying when the TOF ratio reaches the 0.9 level, which is a desirable indication of safe extubation.

Table 8-7 demonstrates the principles of interpretation of the TOF, single-twitch, and posttetanic count modes and

Table 8-5 Neuromuscular Monitoring Sites on the Face

Nerve	Muscle	Response	Advantage	Disadvantage
Facial temporal	Corrugator supercilii	Eyebrow twitch	Less sensitive; use for onset	Muscle stimulation possible
Facial zygomatic	Orbicularis oculi	Eyelid squint	Correlates well with diaphragm Useful to monitor deep levels of block Onset and recovery faster than ulnar nerve Easy access	Stray stimulation possible in other branches of nerve

Table 8-7 Relationships Between Various PNS Modes

Approximate Receptors Blocked (%)	TOF Count	T_4/T_1 TOF Ratio	Single-Twitch Depression	Posttetanic Count
0	4	1.0	0	
25	4	0.75	0	
50	4	0.5	0	
< 75	4	0.25	0	
75	3	0	75	
80	2	0	80	
90	1	0	90	
> 92	0	0	100	
100	0	0	100	10
100+	0	0	100	5
100++	0	0	100	0

the relationships between those modes. When neuromuscular blockade is complete, additional NMBs administered to the patient serve to prolong the duration of the block (indicated by the notation "100+" in Table 8-7). Note that Table 8-7 presents *conceptual* information to demonstrate

relationships. The specific presentation of fade of twitch response varies with the individual neuromuscular blocker used and with various patient factors. Also note that fade, as indicated by the TOF ratio, is more evident on recovery than during onset of neuromuscular block.

Mode	Characteristics	Main Uses	Interpretation
Single Twitch	0.2 ms in duration	Onset / Monitor depolarizing block	Divide twitch height by height of control twitch prior to relaxation. Depression of twitch relates to degree of block from 75–95%.
Train-of-Four	4 stimuli 500 ms apart	Onset, maintenance, recovery, extubation (ratio) / No potentiation (frequent use OK)	1. Count responses to determine block of 75–95% ($\times$/4 response). 2. Compare height of fourth to first twitch ("T_4/T_1 or TOF ratio") > 0.9 = adequate pulmonary function for extubation.
Double-Burst Stimulation	3 rapid stimuli, followed in 750 ms by 2 or 3 more (depending on device)	Extubation (easier to evaluate fade clinically than TOF) / More sensitive than TOF, less painful than tetany	Equal twitch height corresponds to $T_4/T_1 > 0.7$. No discernable fade = no significant block.
Tetany 50 Hz	0.2-μs pulse width, repeated every 20 ms	Extubation (fade within 5 seconds indicates residual block)	5-second sustained response (no fade) suggests ready for extubation (not necessarily complete reversal). Indicates muscle strength equivalent to 5-second head lift.
Tetany 100 Hz	0.2-μs pulse width, repeated every 10 ms	Extubation (more sensitive, but less specific than 50 Hz; can cause fade in absence of relaxant)	
Post-tetanic count	50 Hz tetanus $\times$ 5 sec, then 3 sec pause, then single twitch every 1 sec	Predict recovery time (deep block) / Maintain deep block / Verify stimulator function/leads	Number of twitches correlates inversely with time required for return of single twitch. 1 twitch = ~10 min (longer for pancuronium). 10 twitches = imminent return of first twitch on TOF. When TOF = 0/4, PTC can rule out stimulator malfunction by eliciting a response.

Figure 8-5 Peripheral nerve stimulator modes.

Tetanic stimulation (0.2-ms stimuli repeated every 10 or 20 μs) adds sensitivity to the detection of low levels of relaxation.[41] The desired observation is the presence of a strong motor response that does not diminish during a sustained tetanic stimulus of 5-seconds duration. However, tetanic stimulation is not as sensitive as acceleromyometry in detecting very low levels of residual relaxation, and it comes with unique side effects. Tetanic stimulation is painful, and thus it may introduce a noxious stimulus to patients during emergence, when it is often more desirable to reduce stimulation and discomfort. The repetitive stimulation of the motor nerve by the tetanic stimulus also increases mobilization of ACh. This effect of causing posttetanic facilitation is useful in monitoring deep levels of blockade but may produce a false-positive result in subsequent stimulation techniques on the same nerve for up to 5 minutes. Thus a TOF test performed shortly after tetanic stimuli may demonstrate an artificially elevated TOF ratio. In particular, 100-Hz tetany provides more sensitivity than 50 Hz, but the more vigorous stimulation alters ACh mobilization so much that prolonged stimulation at 100 Hz can deplete ACh release and cause fade, even in the absence of muscle relaxants.[42]

Side Effects and Contraindications

Neuromuscular blockers are contraindicated in patients with hypersensitivity to the intended agent or in patients for whom artificial pulmonary ventilation or adequate sedation cannot be provided. However, in a life-threatening situation, such as is encountered in trauma anesthesia, the need for an effective anesthetic may supersede the requirement for sedation. Other contraindications stem from particular side effects of the specific agents.

Depolarizing Relaxants

Unique pharmacokinetic qualities and organ-independent metabolism have created a niche for succinylcholine. In spite of some significant side effects, succinylcholine maintains an advantage over other available relaxants when a fast onset and/or a very short duration are required. The characteristic fasciculations caused by succinylcholine cause adverse rises in intragastric, intracranial, and intraocular pressure. However, succinylcholine also increases lower esophageal sphincter pressure. Because of its unique mechanism of causing generalized muscle contractions, succinylcholine causes complications in patients with myotonia, those who cannot tolerate the increase in serum

potassium that accompanies the widespread release of potassium from muscle cells, and those who have proliferation of extrajunctional ACh receptors.

Myalgia

The widespread fasciculations caused by succinylcholine have been inculpated in the occurrence of general muscle pain, or *myalgia*, which can follow succinylcholine use. Myalgia occurs in a wide range of reported incidence, and the evidence is equivocal as to whether there is an exclusive causal relationship between fasciculations and myalgias. Myalgia can occur after anesthetics where succinylcholine is not used, and there is a lower incidence of myalgia in patients who received a larger dose of succinylcholine. Nonetheless, there is a widespread belief confirmed by some research that inhibiting fasciculations can reduce the incidence or severity of myalgia in patients receiving succinylcholine.[43] Some methods used are preadministration of a defasciculating dose of a nondepolarizer (10% of the usual intubating dose), lidocaine, nonsteroidal anti-inflammatory drugs, or a "self-taming" dose of succinylcholine (10 mg).

Cardiovascular Effects

Succinylcholine, being structured as two linked molecules of ACh (Figure 8-6), has the potential to activate various ACh receptors outside of the NMJ. As a result, diverse cardiovascular effects are more common after succinylcholine than after nondepolarizing relaxants. Ventricular and nodal dysrhythmias and histamine release are potential side effects of succinylcholine. Bradycardia may also result, particularly after a repeat bolus dose of the drug.

Malignant Hyperthermia

Succinylcholine has two potentially lethal side effects, one of which is triggering malignant hyperthermia. Succinylcholine

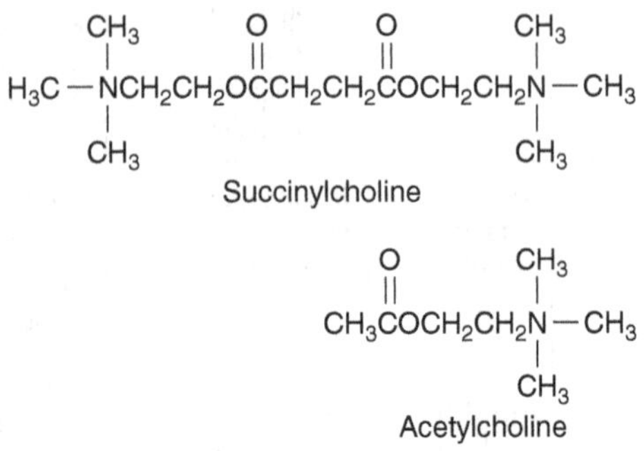

Figure 8-6 Succinylcholine.

is a more potent trigger than the volatile agents and should not be administered to patients with known or associated (familial history) susceptibility to malignant hyperthermia. Masseter muscle rigidity sometimes results as an idiosyncratic reaction to succinylcholine administration. A 1994 study found a 60% incidence of malignant hyperthermia susceptibility among patients who exhibited masseter muscle rigidity after succinylcholine.[44] Because there is not an absolute correlation between masseter muscle rigidity and malignant hyperthermia, some suggest that no further action needs to be taken after masseter spasm other than monitoring closely for malignant hyperthermia. However, conservative management of the patient with masseter muscle spasm after succinylcholine includes consideration of discontinuing the anesthetic and surgery immediately or proceeding with the anesthetic using non–malignant hyperthermia-triggering agents and close intraoperative and postoperative monitoring for incipient signs of malignant hyperthermia.

Hyperkalemia

Because of the widespread depolarization of muscles, serum potassium rises after succinylcholine administration by approximately 0.5 mEq/L.[45] This may present a contraindication to the use of succinylcholine if it would be detrimental for the patient's preexisting potassium level to rise by this amount. Pretreatment with magnesium or a small amount of nondepolarizing relaxant can reduce the potassium release.[46] When administering a nondepolarizer before succinylcholine for pretreatment against potassium release or fasciculations, it should be noted that the two drugs act as antagonists in their effects at the nAChR. Therefore the dose of succinylcholine is typically increased to 1.5 mg/kg after a nondepolarizer (except pancuronium, which partially inhibits plasma cholinesterase and balances its antagonistic effect on succinylcholine).

Because the serum potassium rises slightly, it would seem intuitive to avoid succinylcholine in patients with renal failure; however, the scientific literature does not support a universal contraindication in this situation. As with all patients, the practitioner must be mindful of the preexisting potassium level.[47] Much more concerning is the potassium release that occurs after succinylcholine in conditions of reduced neural influence to the NMJ.

In conditions of reduced neural input, additional ACh receptors proliferate. Because it is most uncharacteristic to find nAChRs outside of the NMJ, they are collectively referred to as "extrajunctional receptors"; however, it should be noted that these receptors are of various morphologies,

and they exist both within and outside of the NMJ (Figure 8-7). Normal neural stimulation of the NMJ suppresses the formation of extrajunctional receptors, and their creation can be considered a type of up-regulation in its absence. The reduction in neural input can come from a wide range of conditions: physical damage to the motor nerve, higher level damage to the upper motor neuron, muscular dystrophies, immobility, burns, chemical denervation with long-term muscle relaxants, and numerous others[48] (Box 8-4).

Some extrajunctional receptors resemble an immature form of nAChR, where the ϵ subunit is replaced by a γ subunit. Others, such as the α-7 nAChR, are entirely distinct in subtype composition from normal receptors (Figure 8-8). One detrimental characteristic of the extrajunctional receptors is that they spread outside of the NMJ, so that acetylcholine release no longer causes a discrete response localized to the junction. Instead, these channels open along a wider range of muscle membrane, releasing potassium into the extracellular fluid. Because of different morphologies of these receptors, they are also more sensitive to agonists. Channel opening is more persistent, so that a greater efflux of potassium occurs when they are stimulated. At the same time they pose resistance to antagonists, such that PNS

Box 8-4 Potential Causes of Extrajunctional Receptor Formation

- Upper motor neuron/lower motor neuron lesion
- Multiple sclerosis
- Guillain-Barré disease
- Amyotrophic lateral sclerosis
- Muscular dystrophies
- Cerebrovascular accident
- Infection with *C. botulinum/C. tetani*
- Sepsis (causes motor demyelinating neuropathy)
- Burns (exceeding ~9% body surface area)
- Chemical denervation (chronic/intensive care unit use of NMBs, magnesium)
- Ischemia induced by peripheral vascular disease
- Renal failure
- Diabetes
- Immobility

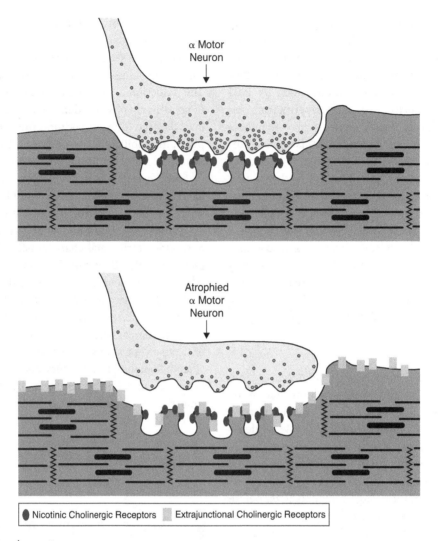

Figure 8-7 Extrajunctional receptors.

monitoring on a hemiplegic arm, for example, would demonstrate a falsely high degree of neuromuscular function compared with the rest of the body.

In the presence of conditions that give rise to extrajunctional receptors, administration of succinylcholine may rapidly lead to hyperkalemia, possibly resulting in cardiac arrest. In acute situations, such as a burn injury, succinylcholine use should not result in a hyperkalemic response within the first few hours after the injury. Conventional approaches suggest that precautions should be taken to avoid succinylcholine beginning 24 hours after the burn, spinal cord injury, or other precipitating event. In the case of a condition that resolves, the potential for hyperkalemia with succinylcholine should be considered for at least 6 months after resolution of the condition. Pretreatment with a nondepolarizer cannot prevent the potassium

release that occurs from succinylcholine in the presence of extrajunctional receptors.

Because of the incidence of congenital neuromuscular disease that gives rise to extrajunctional receptors but which may not be diagnosed for the first few years of life, the use of succinylcholine in children is cautioned. In 1993 the package insert for succinylcholine began carrying the warning that in the pediatric population the drug "should be reserved for emergency intubation or instances where immediate securing of the airway is necessary" due to the potential for undiagnosed skeletal muscle myopathy that may result in a hyperkalemic response. At the same time, succinylcholine remains the fastest means of resolving a severe laryngospasm or securing an airway in an emergency situation, giving rise to the maxim about succinylcholine in pediatric anesthesia: "Always have it; never use it."

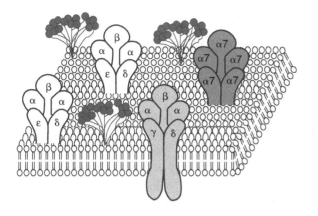

Figure 8-8 Abnormal receptors.

Phase II Block

A unique complication of succinylcholine can occur in the form of a distinctly characterized clinical blockade that resembles not a depolarizing block but a nondepolarizing block. Tachyphylaxis usually heralds the onset of this complication, and the typical lack of fade, posttetanic potentiation, and reversibility of the depolarizing block are replaced by the observed presence of these factors. Because the clinical manifestations of the depolarizing block now take on characteristics of a nondepolarizing block, the complication is sometimes called "dual block" or, more technically, "phase II block" (Figure 8-9). Resulting primarily from multiple or excessive doses of succinylcholine that exceed approximately 2 mg/kg, aspects of phase II block begin to be observable even at very modest doses of succinylcholine.[49]

Myotonia

Myotonia encompasses multiple disease states characterized by abnormality in repolarization of muscles. These diseases are generally caused by autoantibodies against or mutation of potassium, sodium, or chloride channels. Abnormalities in activation of these channels lead to inhibition of repolarization, enhanced transmitter release, and hyperexcitability of muscle contraction. Patients with neuromyotonia (Isaac's syndrome or continuous muscle fiber activity syndrome), myotonic dystrophy (Steinert's disease), myotonia congenita (Thomsen's disease), paramyotonia congenita, periodic hyperkalemic paralysis, and others may be subject to prolonged sustained muscle contraction (~5 minutes) after succinylcholine.

Intraocular Pressure

A particular side effect of succinylcholine is a transient increase in intraocular pressure that follows its administration. This results because the extraocular muscles are multiply innervated and thus respond to the agonism of succinylcholine at multiple points. Though transient (a useful mnemonic is that the increase is "8 mm Hg for 8 minutes"), it may be particularly detrimental in patients with open eye injuries in whom rapid sequence induction may be indicated. There is evidence that the increase in pressure can be attenuated by various premedicants such as lidocaine, sufentanil, and dexmedetomidine.[50,51] However, with the acceptability of using rocuronium to provide relaxation as part of a rapid sequence induction, the

	Non-depolarizing Block and Phase II Depolarizing Block	Phase I Depolarizing Block
Response to Repetitive Stimulation	Fade	Decreased amplitude without fade
Posttetanic Potentiation	Yes	No
Reversible with Acetylcholinesterase Inhibitors	Yes	No

Figure 8-9 Block types.

concern about succinylcholine in this scenario is becoming less clinically relevant.

Nondepolarizing Relaxants

Containing a quaternary ammonium compound, nondepolarizing relaxants have a low volume of distribution and a low incidence of side effects. They cross the placenta and blood–brain barrier in minute amounts and cause no appreciable effect on cerebral function or on the fetus when administered to pregnant patients. Among aminosteroids, the steroidal structure does not imply that nondepolarizing relaxants produce a hormonal function, and in fact they do not.

Histamine Release

The most notable side effects of the currently used nondepolarizers are histamine release from atracurium and an increase in heart rate from pancuronium. The benzylisoquinolines in general are most associated with histamine release, and this is the most detrimental side effect of atracurium. A significant improvement on this drug came in the form of a purification of the *cis-* enantiomer, cisatracurium. Not only does it demonstrate no histamine release,[52] but cisatracurium is more than twice as potent as atracurium, and the lower dose requirement further reduces the potential for laudanosine accumulation. Although histamine release is low at moderate doses and with slow administration of atracurium, the potential for complications related to it make atracurium a less favorable choice in the presence of asthma, carcinoid syndrome, and other diseases sensitive to histamine.

Anaphylactic Reactions

Anaphylaxis and anaphylactoid reactions are common after exposure to muscle relaxants. Results from a 2-year survey in which 789 cases were reported indicated NMBs were the most common cause, responsible for almost 60%, or 306 cases. Rocuronium was implicated in 132 patients (over 40%) and succinylcholine in 69 (over 20%). Cross-reactivity between NMBs is also noted in 75% of anaphylaxis cases.[53] Other surveys found succinylcholine to have the highest propensity to cause anaphylactic reactions. Skin-prick sensitivity to muscle relaxants has been found to be as high as 10%, an incidence that does not correlate with the observed incidence of anaphylaxis among surgical patients receiving NMBs.[54] Patients may be sensitive to muscle relaxants even without prior exposure, as they may have been exposed to the quaternary ammonium structure in other common compounds.

Other Side Effects

Older generation relaxants such as pancuronium are most prone to side effects such as prolongation in renal disease, tachycardia from muscarinic blockade, and postoperative residual relaxation.[55] Later-developed relaxants such as rocuronium and cisatracurium are to a great degree free from significant side effects. Rocuronium can cause pain on injection, a problem when "priming" or otherwise administering the drug before inducing sedation or hypnosis. This injection pain can be reduced by alkalinizing the rocuronium solution.[56,57] At the same time, because rocuronium is delivered in an acidic medium, care should be taken not to mix it with alkaline medications (such as barbiturates) in the same syringe or to administer them concurrently in the same intravenous line to prevent salt formation.

Drug Interactions

The duration of effect of muscle relaxants may be altered by the presence of other medications. Because elimination of steroidal muscle relaxants is partially due to metabolism by the cytochrome P-450 system, drugs that induce microsomal enzymes (such as hydantoins or barbiturates) can attenuate these muscle relaxants by increasing their degradation. For example, the duration of rocuronium is decreased significantly in patients taking phenytoin due to induction of hepatic enzymes. This effect has been demonstrated to become active with vecuronium after 1 week's duration of administration of phenytoin.[58] However, in the presence of acute administration of phenytoin, muscle relaxation may be augmented.[59] Similar findings are present with exposure to acute versus chronic phenobarbital.[60] Common pharmacodynamic alterations of muscle relaxants involve medications that interfere with ACh production or calcium influx into the motor nerve terminal. Calcium channel blockers such as verapamil, which block the L-subtype (slow) calcium channels on the motor nerve terminal, are synergistic with nondepolarizing relaxants. Blockade of these channels hinders calcium influx, which is required to initiate ACh release from the nerve. Because these drugs do not influence the fast calcium channels, they *augment* the neuromuscular blockade but do not directly alter the pharmacodynamics of NMBs.

Volatile anesthetics also interfere with calcium transport, and they directly block presynaptic ACh receptors, potentiating muscle relaxants. This effect can be seen with any volatile anesthetic but has been shown to be particularly exaggerated with desflurane. In a prospective study of

57 patients, desflurane was shown to prolong the duration of a single bolus dose of rocuronium (0.9 mg/kg). The time to return to 5% of control twitch height in the presence of sevoflurane was 59 minutes, under propofol anesthesia was 51 minutes, and under desflurane anesthesia was 90 minutes.[61] This study did not use a large sample size, and the use of the volatile anesthetics at equipotent MAC doses (but therefore different concentrations due to potency differences) may explain the disparity in effects on the NMJ between agents. Indeed, the potency issue may explain why previous studies failed to find a significant prolongation of muscle relaxants in the presence of more potent volatile anesthetics, such as isoflurane.

Muscle relaxants may create drug interactions with other relaxants. The duration of action can be prolonged when structurally different nondepolarizing blocking agents are given concurrently. Historically, a combination of pancuronium with curare or metocurine produced a drug with greater potency, which could therefore be dosed at a lower level, reducing the side effects of both drugs involved. With more contemporary agents a synergistic effect has been demonstrated when an intubating dose of rocuronium is followed by a maintenance dose of cisatracurium.[62] A nondepolarizer that follows succinylcholine often demonstrates a reduced time to onset. This has been noted with atracurium and cisatracurium.

Because succinylcholine is metabolized by plasma cholinesterase, drugs that influence the activity of that enzyme may impair metabolism of succinylcholine. Metoclopramide, pancuronium, oral contraceptives, neostigmine, and echothiophate are all known to impair plasma cholinesterase.[63–65] Prolonged use of muscle relaxants (such as in the intensive care unit) can induce a chemical denervation and give rise to extrajunctional receptors and the potential for hyperkalemia after succinylcholine. The concomitant administration of muscle relaxants and corticosteroids has been associated with development of myopathy. This potential should be considered when receiving such a patient to surgery or when consulting on muscle relaxant use in the intensive care unit.

Guidelines and Precautions

Residual Relaxation

Although popular contemporary NMBs such as rocuronium demonstrate a short duration of action, the incidence of residual relaxation is high.[39] This incidence exists regardless of the use of pharmacologic reversal or conservative dosing and monitoring of the NMBs. The anesthetist can reasonably expect that a significant number of patients treated with NMBs will arrive in the post-anesthesia care unit with residual effects of the relaxants. Fortunately, in most patients the effects of residual relaxation do not become clinically relevant. Subclinical relaxation postoperatively contributes to pharyngeal dysfunction, reduced hypoxemic drive, and puts some patients at risk for respiratory compromise if hypothermia, hypercarbia, or other forms of respiratory embarrassment result.[66–69]

Factors such as advanced age, abdominal or chest surgery, or administration of respiratory depressant medications may compound an otherwise inconspicuous effect of residual relaxation and create a clinically significant complication. Methods to reduce the incidence of residual relaxation include using relaxants with a shorter duration (rocuronium) or faster recovery index (cisatracurium), dosing based on ED_{95} instead of the typical intubating dose, maintaining a lighter level of paralysis where appropriate (TOF 2–3 of 4), and relying on nonrelaxant drugs to maintain akinesis (opioids, hypnotics).

Monitoring for Reversal

The currently used techniques of monitoring for the purpose of reversing the effects of NMBs are grossly inadequate in their efficacy. To determine small amounts of residual relaxation, traditional peripheral nerve stimulation has a high specificity but a very low sensitivity for identifying low levels of relaxation.[39] It has been demonstrated that most anesthetists cannot detect tactile fade when the TOF ratio is greater than 0.4.[70] This is concerning, because in the presence of even limited degrees of residual neuromuscular block, impairment of laryngeal reflexes and hypoxic drive may exist.[71,72] Considering the potential complications of residual relaxation, as well as the inherent flaws in monitoring accuracy, a TOF ratio of 0.9 or greater should be considered the goal for reversal before extubation. However, it is noteworthy that some muscle weakness persists in patients after longer surgeries, even if the TOF ratio shows minimal fade (TOF ratio = 0.9).[73]

More accurate and objective means of neuromuscular monitoring will improve providers' ability to recognize and distinguish subtleties in the level of a patient's degree of blockade. Mechanomyography is the gold standard of neuromuscular monitoring; however, the technology has not been adapted to move from the laboratory to a device practically suited for intraoperative use. Accelerometry is a reasonable substitution for mechanomyography, providing a good correlation with mechanomyography but with a wider variability of results and a slightly slower indication of recovery.[74,75] Compounding the problem of inadequate monitoring, the current means of reversing neuromuscular blockade through inhibition of acetylcholinesterase frequently does not completely reverse the block. There is great promise in the development of new reversal agents, such as γ-cyclodextrin, to vastly improve the efficacy of reversal and probably also to obviate the need to monitor as closely during recovery. Normal indications during peripheral nerve stimulation of various agents are discussed below.

Acetylcholinesterase inhibitor reversal agents can augment spontaneous recovery from NMBs, but their efficacy is limited. Research has shown that 30% to 40% of patients will fail to demonstrate a TOF ratio of greater than 0.9 after surgery, even when neostigmine reversal is carried out[76] and even when reversal is effected at a moderate level of spontaneous reversal.[77] The presence of at least three twitches is advisable before attempting augmentation of reversal with anticholinesterase agents.[78] This is particularly of concern in patients with comorbidities or threat of respiratory insufficiency. Sugammadex, the anticipated γ-cyclodextrin reversal drug for steroidal muscle relaxants, promises to alleviate many of these concerns about residual relaxation due to its highly effective reversal of rocuronium blockade.[79,80]

Dosage and Administration

When administering a relaxant, a variety of dosing schemes may be used. The anesthetist should be familiar with both the ED_{95} and the recommended intubating dose of relaxants. Whereas the ED_{95} provides adequate intubating conditions in almost all patients, more commonly a multiple of the ED_{95} is used. The intubating dose is typically two to four times the ED_{95}. Using a supraeffective dose such as this increases the speed of onset, but it also prolongs the duration of action. There is value in facilitating intubation quickly, in terms of aspiration risk, potential difficulties with mask ventilation, and general speed and efficiency of surgical operations. However, at the same time the potential for residual relaxation exists, and use of more modest doses of relaxants may lessen the potential for complications from this, particularly when the surgical case is brief. For maintenance dosing, 10% to 20% of the intubating dose is repeated as needed as indicated by clinical indications or neuromuscular monitoring. For the patient who is already intubated or in whom the speed of onset is less crucial, the ED_{95} dose is a useful dose to induce relaxation. See Table 8-8 for a comparison of pharmacokinetics of different agents.

When the need for relaxation will be prolonged, NMBs may be administered by infusion. This approach can maintain a constant level of pharmacologic effect and allow less frequent dosing once a steady state has been achieved. The

Table 8-8 Comparison of Pharmacokinetics of Different Agents

	ED_{95} (mg/kg)	Intubating Dose (mg/kg)	Onset (min)	25% Recovery (min)	Degree of Hepatic Metabolism	Prolongation by Renal Failure
Aminosteroids						
Rocuronium	0.3	0.6–1.2	1–2	20–45	Medium	Slight
Vecuronium	0.06	0.1	3	40	Medium	Slight
Pancuronium	0.06	0.1	3–6	60–90	High	Yes
Pipecuronium	0.05	0.1	2–4	90	High	Yes
Benzylisoquinolines						
Atracurium	0.25	0.5	2–3	40	None	None
Cisatracurium	0.05	0.2	2–3	45–60	None	None
Doxacurium	0.025	0.07	4–6	100–120	High	Yes
Depolarizing						
Succinylcholine	0.5	1	0.5	5–7	None	None

pharmacokinetics of cisatracurium facilitates its administration by infusion. Upon return of neuromuscular response after the initial loading or intubation dose, the infusion should be initiated at 3 mcg/kg/min to stop the quick decrement that characterizes the recovery slope of cisatracurium. Once the return of twitches has been halted, the infusion is titrated to clinical effect, typically in a narrow range of 1 to 2 mcg/kg/min. Rocuronium can also be administered by infusion readily at a dosage range of 5 to 15 mcg/kg/min, as can vecuronium at a range of 0.3 to 1 mcg/kg/min. However, cisatracurium is well suited to infusion administration due to its rapid decrement after discontinuation, which exceeds the decrement speed of rocuronium or vecuronium.[81]

Practical Aspects of Drug Administration

Priming Concept

Nondepolarizing NMBs act as competitive antagonists with ACh at the nAChR. Because the receptor requires activation of both α subunits to activate it, muscle relaxants hold a statistical advantage, because it requires only one molecule of relaxant to block a given receptor, whereas it requires two molecules of ACh to activate it. However, there is a physiologic margin of safety in that a large number of receptors must be blocked (around 75%) before significant clinical effects occur. This phenomenon is responsible for a number of important pharmacologic considerations when using NMBs. The first is that because a large number of receptors can be occupied before clinical effects become apparent, there is a delay in onset of the agents (particularly nondepolarizers), until a sufficient number of receptors are blocked.

Lower potency agents that require a larger mass administration tend to demonstrate a faster onset than agents of higher potency, because the higher molecular load occupies the requisite number of receptors more quickly.

Administration of a small dose of a nondepolarizer can also be used to saturate a number of receptors while remaining subclinical in neuromuscular effects. This dose, typically 10% of the calculated intubating dose, serves to prime the system with drug. The result is that the remainder of the drug, when administered, has only a smaller number of receptors remaining to be blocked, and thus the speed of onset after this dose is significantly increased (onset in 30 seconds, vs. 60 without priming).[82,83] The priming dose technique is illustrated in Figure 8-10. Because of interpatient variability, some patients become distressed by diplopia (due to sensitivity of the extraocular muscles) or mild dyspnea that occurs after a priming dose. Compromise in pharyngeal function may theoretically also increase the potential for aspiration as a result of a priming dose. A reasonable alternative is to use a larger dose of rocuronium (1.5 mg/kg) to effect a fast onset, if there is concern about side effects of using the priming technique.[84]

Regardless of how the muscle relaxant was administered during the procedure, the downside of the priming concept is observable upon emergence, when enough receptors become free from the relaxant for the patient to regain gross function, whereas up to 75% of the receptors may remain blocked. The priming theory therefore is a useful benefit to the anesthetist on induction of muscle relaxation, but on emergence it practically defines the clinical concept of residual relaxation. Anesthetists must remain aware that a significant number of receptors may remain blocked even though patients are able to demonstrate fairly robust motor strength.

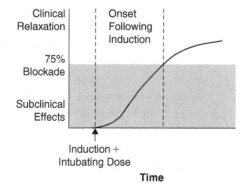

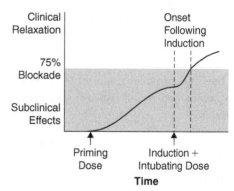

Figure 8-10 Priming dose.

Key Points

- Neuromuscular blockers act primarily by occupying ACh receptors in the NMJ. By acting either as agonists that prevent "resetting" or as antagonists that prevent activation of the receptors, they impair neuromuscular function.

- Relaxants are relatively free from side effects, due to their ionized nature, which prevents distribution to the brain, and their lack of activity on smooth muscle.

- Aminosteroidal relaxants are associated with the least side effects but are metabolized by various proportions of hepatic, biliary, and renal functions.

- Benzylisoquinoline relaxants are most associated with histamine release, but they are metabolized by factors in the blood and do not directly rely on organ systems for metabolism.

- The choice of relaxant is made with consideration of the onset and duration required, the needs of the surgical team, and how the side effect profile of the drug will mesh with the patient's state of health.

- Succinylcholine is the only depolarizing relaxant in use. Although it bears significant potential side effects, it remains the fastest acting and shortest duration relaxant available.

- Side effects of succinylcholine include myalgia and increases in the serum potassium level. Pretreatment with a small dose of a nondepolarizer may help attenuate some of the side effects of succinylcholine.

- Appropriate peripheral nerve monitoring requires determination of the mode most appropriate for the drug in use. It also requires an understanding of how to dose the relaxant vis-à-vis the indication observed on nerve stimulator monitoring.

- The single-twitch mode is very appropriate for succinylcholine, but TOF provides the most information about onset, maintenance, and recovery when using nondepolarizers.

- Peripheral nerve stimulator monitoring is an inexact science at best, fraught with significant error in the determination of residual relaxation.

- Alternative modes, such as double-burst stimulation, and alternate measurements, such as accelerometry, improve the sensitivity of peripheral nerve monitoring to detect residual relaxation.

Chapter Questions

1. If ACh is released from the motor nerve terminal with every muscle contraction, why does all this ACh not cause bradycardia?
2. If the delay in onset of a muscle relaxant is disadvantageous, what would be potential reasons not to just administer the relaxant a few minutes before the induction drug?
3. If a patient has a dibucaine number of 20, what drugs other than succinylcholine will be prolonged?
4. After propofol administration to a morbidly obese, malignant hyperthermia–susceptible patient, the anesthetist is unable to ventilate and cannot open the patient's mouth adequately to intubate. The saturation is falling precipitously and rocuronium is not available. Should succinylcholine be used?
5. During abdominal surgery the surgeon complains that the patient's muscles are "tight" and requests that more relaxant be given. TOF at the adductor pollicis shows no twitches. Is it appropriate to give additional relaxant?
6. If there are equal numbers of ACh and nondepolarizer molecules present in the NMJ, which is more likely to exert its respective effect?
7. Why would muscle relaxants of different classes by synergistic?
8. What is the optimal relaxant for a patient with renal failure (serum potassium 6 mEq/L) who is undergoing a short procedure? What is the second choice?

References

1. Felter HW, Lloyd JU. *King's American Dispensatory*, vol. 2, 18th ed. Cincinnati, OH: Ohio Valley Company; 1898.
2. Murphy GS, Szokol JW. Monitoring neuromuscular blockade. *Int Anesthesiol Clin.* 2004;42:25–40.
3. Howard JF, Jr. Structure and function of the neuromuscular junction. In: Stalberg E, ed. *Clinical Neurophysiology of Disorders of Muscle: Handbook of Clinical Neurophysiology*, vol. 2. St. Louis, MO: Elsevier Health Sciences; 2003:31.
4. Bowman WC, Prior C, Marshall IG. Presynaptic receptors in the neuromuscular junction. *Ann N Y Acad Sci.* 1990;604: 69–81.
5. Takagi S, Adachi YU, Saubermann AJ, Vizi ES. Presynaptic inhibitory effects of rocuronium and SZ1677 on [3H] acetylcholine release from the mouse hemidiaphragm preparation. *Neurochem Int.* 2002;40:655–659.

6. Jonsson M, Dabrowski M, Gurley DA, et al. Activation and inhibition of human muscular and neuronal nicotinic acetylcholine receptors by succinylcholine. *Anesthesiology.* 2006; 104:724–733.

7. Lorenzo SD, Veggetti M, Muchnic S, Losavio A. Presynaptic inhibition of spontaneous acetylcholine release induced by adenosine at mouse neuromuscular junction. *Br J Pharmacol.* 2004;142:113–245.

8. Santafé MM, Salon I, Garcia N, et al. Modulation of ACh release by presynaptic muscarinic autoreceptors in the neuromuscular junction of the newborn and adult rat. *Eur J Neurosci.* 2003;17:119–127.

9. Dahaba AA, Perelman SI, Moskowitz DM, et al. Geographic regional differences in rocuronium bromide dose-response relation and time course of action: an overlooked factor in determining recommended dosage. *Anesthesiology.* 2006;104:950.

10. Bhatt SB, Amann A, Nigrovic V. Onset-potency relationship of nondepolarizing muscle relaxants: a reexamination using simulations. *Can J Physiol Pharmacol.* 2007;85:774–782.

11. Woolf RL, Crawform MW, Choo SM. Dose-response of rocuronium bromide in children anesthetized with propofol: a comparison with succinylcholine. *Anesthesiology.* 1997;87: 1368–1372.

12. Karcioglu O. Dilemma in rapid sequence intubation: succinylcholine vs. rocuronium. *Internet J Emerg Intens Care Med.* 2003;7:9.

13. Perry JJ, Lee JS, Sillberg VA, Wells GA. Rocuronium versus succinylcholine for rapid sequence induction intubation. *Cochrane Database Syst Rev.* 2003;CD002788.

14. Larsen PB, Hansen EG, Jacobsen LS, et al. Intubation conditions after rocuronium or succinylcholine for rapid sequence induction with alfentanil and propofol in the emergency patient. *Eur J Anaesthesiol.* 2005;22:748–753.

15. Sluga M, Ummenhofer W, Studer W, Siegemund M, Marsch SC. Rocuronium versus succinylcholine for rapid sequence induction of anesthesia and endotracheal intubation: a prospective, randomized trial in emergent cases. *Anesth Analg.* 2005;101:1356–1361.

16. Wright PM. Onset and duration of rocuronium and succinylcholine at the adductor pollicis and laryngeal adductor muscles in anesthetized humans. *Anesthesiology.* 1994;81:1110–1115.

17. Karcioglu O, Arnold J, Topacoglu H, Ozucelik, DN, Kiran S, Sonmez N. Succinylcholine or rocuronium? A meta-analysis of the effects on intubation conditions. *Int J Clin Pract.* 2006; 60:1638–1646.

18. Han DW. Significance of the injection timing of ephedrine to reduce the onset time of rocuronium. *Anaesthesia.* 2008;63:856.

19. Leykin Y, Pellis T, Gullo A. Effects of ephedrine on intubating conditions following priming with rocuronium. *Acta Anaesth Scand.* 2005;49:792–797.

20. Szmuk PP The onset time of rocuronium is slowed by esmolol and accelerated by ephedrine. *Anesth Analg.* 2000;90: 1217–1219.

21. Ezri TT. Changes in onset time of rocuronium in patients pretreated with ephedrine and esmolol—the role of cardiac output. *Acta Anaesth Scand.* 2003;47:1067.

22. Magorian T, Wood P, Caldwell J, et al. The pharmacokinetics and neuromuscular effects of Rocuronium bromide in patients with liver disease. *Anest Analg.* 1995;80:754–759.

23. Leykin Y, Pellis T, Lucca M, Lomangino G, Marzano B, Gullo A. The pharmacodynamic effects of rocuronium when dosed according to real body weight or ideal body weight in morbidly obese patients. *Anesth Analg.* 2004;99:1086–1089.

24. Lemmens HJM, Brodsky JB. The dose of succinylcholine in morbid obesity. *Anesth Analg.* 2006;102:438–442.

25. Rapp HJ, Altenmueller CA, Waschke C. Neuromuscular recovery following rocuronium bromide single dose in infants. *Paediatr Anaesth.* 2004;14:329–335.

26. Ueno K. Gender differences in pharmacokinetics of anesthetics. *Masui.* 2009; 58:51–58.

27. Adamus M, Gabrhelik T, Marek O. Influence of gender on the course of neuromuscular block following a single bolus dose of cisatracurium or rocuronium. *Eur J Anaesth.* 2008;25:589.

28. Robertson EN, Driessen JJ, Vogt M, De Boer H, Scheffer GJ. Pharmacodynamics of rocuronium 0.3 mg kg(−1) in adult patients with and without renal failure. *Eur J Anaesth.* 2005;22:929–932.

29. Kocabas S, Yedicocuklu D, Askar FZ. The neuromuscular effects of 0.6 mg kg(−1) rocuronium in elderly and young adults with or without renal failure. *Eur J Anaesth.* 2008;25:940–946.

30. Puhringer FK, Heier T, Dodgson M, et al. Double-blind comparison of the variability in spontaneous recovery of cisatracurium- and vecuronium-induced neuromuscular block in adult and elderly patients. *Acta Anaesth Scand.* 2002;46:364.

31. Arain SR, Kern S, Ficke DJ, Ebert TJ. Variability of duration of action of neuromuscular-blocking drugs in elderly patients. *Acta Anaesth Scand.* 2005;49:312–315.

32. Welch RM. The in vitro degradation of cisatracurium, the R, cis-R'-isomer of atracurium, in human and rat plasma. *Clin Pharmacol Ther.* 1995;58:132.

33. Cammu G, Coddens J, Hendrickx J, Deloof T. Dose requirements of infusions of cisatracurium or rocuronium during hypothermic cardiopulmonary bypass. *Br J Anaesth.* 2000;84:587–590.

34. Kopman AF, Klewicka MM, Neuman GG. An alternate method for estimating the dose-response relationships of neuromuscular blocking drugs. *Anesth Analg.* 2000;90:1191–1197.

35. Kalow W. The relation of plasma cholinesterases to response to clinical doses of succinylcholine. *Can J Anaesth.* 2008;55: 860–868.

36. Cope TM, Hunter JM. Selecting neuromuscular-blocking drugs for elderly patients. *Drugs Aging*. 2003;20:125–140.

37. Sastry SG, Lemmens HJ. The intubating laryngeal mask airway: rocuronium improves endotracheal intubating conditions and success rate. *J Clin Anesth*. 2005;17:163–166.

38. Al-alami A, Zestos MM, Baraka AS. Pediatric laryngospasm: prevention and treatment. *Curr Opin Anaesth*. 2009;22:388–395.

39. Debaene B, Plaud B, Dilly M, Donati F. Residual paralysis in the PACU after a single intubating dose of nondepolarizing muscle relaxant with an intermediate duration of action. *Anesthesiology*. 2003;98:1042–1048.

40. Kopman AF. Antagonism of profound cisatracurium and rocuronium block: the role of objective assessment of neuromuscular function. *J Clin Anesth*. 2005;17:30.

41. Samet A, Capron F, Alla F, Meistelman C, Fuchs-Buder T. Single acceleromyographic train-of-four, 100-Hertz tetanus or double-burst stimulation: which test performs better to detect residual paralysis? *Anesthesiology*. 2005;102:51.

42. Hudes E, Lee KC. Clinical use of peripheral nerve stimulators in anaesthesia. *Can J Anaesth*. 1987;34:525.

43. Schreiber JU, Lysakowski C, Fuchs-Buder T, Tramer MR. Prevention of succinylcholine-induced fasciculation and myalgia: a meta-analysis of randomized trials. *Anesthesiology*. 2005;103:877–884.

44. O'Flynn RP, Shutack JG, Rosenberg H, Fletcher JE. Masseter muscle rigidity and malignant hyperthermia susceptibility in pediatric patients. An update on management and diagnosis. *Anesthesiology*. 1994;80:1228.

45. Yentis SM. Suxamethonium and hyperkalaemia. *Anaesth Intens Care*. 1990;18:92–101.

46. Hernandez-Palazon J, Noguera-Velasco J, Falcon-Arana LF, et al. Precurarization with rocuronium prevents fasciculations and biochemical changes after succinylcholine administration. *Rev Esp Anestesiol Reanim*. 2004;51:184–189.

47. Thapa S, Brull SJ. Succinylcholine-induced hyperkalemia in patients with renal failure: an old question revisited. *Anesth Analg*. 2000;91:237–241.

48. Martyn JA, Richtsfeld, M. Succinylcholine-induced hyperkalemia in acquired pathologic states: etiologic factors and molecular mechanisms. *Anesthesiology*. 2006;04:158–169.

49. Naguib M, Lien CA, Aker J, Eliazo R. Posttetanic potentiation and fade in the response to tetanic and train-of-four stimulation during succinylcholine-induced block. *Anesth Analg*. 2004, 98:1686–1691.

50. Moeini HA, Soltani HA, Gholami AR, Masoudpour H. The effect of lidocaine and sufentanil in preventing intraocular pressure increase due to succinylcholine and endotracheal intubation. *Eur J Anaesth*. 2006;23:739.

51. Mowafi HA, Aldossary N, Ismail SA, Alqahtani J. Effect of dexmedetomidine premedication on the intraocular pressure changes after succinylcholine and intubation. *Br J Anaesth*. 2008;100:485–489.

52. Vershuta D, Kozlov I, Ermolenko A, Ilnitsky V. Histamine-induced hemodynamic changes after vecuronium, rocuronium, and cisatracurium during cardiac surgery: 9AP7-6. *Eur J Anaesth*. 2007;24:124.

53. Mertes PM, Laxenaire M, Alla F. Anaphylactic and anaphylactoid reactions occurring during anesthesia in France in 1999–2000. *Anesthesiology*. 2003;99:536–545.

54. Harper NJN, Dixon T, Dugue P, et al. Suspected anaphylactic reactions associated with anaesthesia. *Anaesthesia*. 2009;64:199.

55. Naguib M, Kopman AF, Ensor JE. Neuromuscular monitoring and postoperative residual curarisation: a meta-analysis. *Br J Anaesth*. 2007;98:302–316.

56. Mencke T, Schreiber JU, Knoll H, et al. Women report more pain on injection of a precurarization dose of rocuronium: a randomized, prospective, placebo-controlled trial. *Acta Anaesth Scand*. 2004;48:1245–1248.

57. Han DW, Koo BN, Choi SH, et al. Neutralized rocuronium (pH 7.4) before administration prevents injection pain in awake patients: a randomized prospective trial. *J Clin Anesth*. 2007;19:418.

58. Platt PR, Thackray NM. Phenytoin-induced resistance to vecuronium. *Anaesth Intens Care*. 1993;21:185–191.

59. Kim JU, Lee YK, Lee YM, Yang HO, Han SM, Yang HS. The effect of phenytoin on rocuronium-induced neuromuscular block in the rat phrenic nerve-hemidiaphragm preparation. The effect of phenytoin on rocuronium-induced neuromuscular block in the rat phrenic nerve-hemidiaphragm preparation. *J Neurosurg Anesthesiol*. 2005;17:149.

60. Braga Ade F, de Barcelos CC, Braga FS, et al. Phenobarbital influence on neuromuscular block produced by rocuronium in rats. *Acta Cir Bras*. 2008;23:343–347.

61. Maidatsi PG, Zaralidou AT, Gorgias NK, Amaniti EN, Karakoulas KA, Giala MM. Rocuronium duration of action under sevoflurane, desflurane or propofol anaesthesia. *Eur J Anaesth*. 2004;21:781–786.

62. Breslin DS, Jiao K, Habib AS, Schultz J, Gan TJ. Pharmacodynamic interactions between cisatracurium and rocuronium. *Anesth Analg*. 2004;98:107–110.

63. Monteiro JN, Hingorani MC. Effect of metoclopramide premedication on the depolarizing block of suxamethonium chloride. *J Anaesth Clin Pharm*. 1993;9:35–37.

64. Symington MJ, Mirakhur RK, Kumar N. Neostigmine but not edrophonium prolongs the action of mivacurium. *Can J Anaesth*. 1996;43:1220–1223.

65. Whittaker M, Charlier AR, Ramaswamy S. Changes in plasma cholinesterase isoenzymes due to oral contraceptives. *J Reprod Fertil*. 1971;26:373–375.

66. Herbstreit F, Peters J, Eikermann M. Impaired upper airway integrity by residual neuromuscular blockade: increased airway collapsibility and blunted genioglossus muscle activity in response to negative pharyngeal pressure. *Anesthesiology.* 2009;110:1253–1267.

67. Eriksson LI. Reduced hypoxic chemosensitivity in partially paralysed man. A new property of muscle relaxants? *Acta Anaesth Scand.* 1996;40:520–523.

68. Hemmerling TM, Michaud G, Trager G, Donati F. Simultaneous determination of neuromuscular blockade at the adducting and abducting laryngeal muscles using phonomyography. *Anesth Analg.* 2004;98:1729–1733.

69. Sakuraba S, Kuwana S, Eriksson LI, et al. Effects of neuromuscular blocking agents on central respiratory chemosensitivity in newborn rats. *Biol Res.* 2005;38:225–233.

70. Kopman AF, Kopman DJ, Ng J, Zank LM. Antagonism of profound cisatracurium and rocuronium block: the role of objective assessment of neuromuscular function. *J Clin Anesth.* 2005;17:30–35.

71. Eikermann M The predisposition to inspiratory upper airway collapse during partial neuromuscular blockade. *Am J Respir Crit Care Med.* 2007;175:9.

72. Jonsson M, Kim C, Yamamoto Y, Runold M, Lindahl SGE, Eriksson LI. Atracurium and vecuronium block nicotine-induced carotid body chemoreceptor responses. *Acta Anaesth Scand.* 2002;46:488–494.

73. Eikermann M, Gerwig M, Hasselmann C, Fiedler G, Peters J. Impaired neuromuscular transmission after recovery of the train-of-four ratio. *Acta Anaesth Scand.* 2007;51:226–234.

74. Capron F, Alla F, Hottier C, Meistelman C, Fuchs-Buder T. Can acceleromyography detect low levels of residual paralysis? A probability approach to detect a mechanomyographic TOF ratio of 0.9. *Anesthesiology.* 2004;100:1119–1124.

75. Capron F, Fortier LP, Racine S, Donati F. Tactile fade detection with hand or wrist stimulation using train-of-four, double-burst stimulation, 50-hertz tetanus, 100-hertz tetanus, and acceleromyography. *Anesth Analg.* 2006;102:1578–1584.

76. Cammu G, DeWitte J, DeVeylder J, et al. Postoperative residual paralysis in outpatients versus inpatients. *Anesth Analg.* 2006;102:426–429.

77. Murphy GS, Szokol JW, Marymount JH, et al. Residual paralysis at the time of tracheal extubation. *Anesth Analg.* 2005;100:1840–1845.

78. Kirkegaard H, Heier T, Caldwell JE. Efficacy of tactile-guided reversal from cisatracurium-induced neuromuscular block. *Anesthesiology.* 2002;96:45–50.

79. Epemolu O, Bom A, Hope F, Mason R. Reversal of neuromuscular blockade and simultaneous increase in plasma rocuronium concentration after the intravenous infusion of the novel reversal agent Org 25969. *Anesthesiology.* 2003;99:632.

80. White PF, Tufanogullari B, Sacan O, et al. The effect of residual neuromuscular blockade on the speed of reversal with sugammadex. *Anesth Analg.* 2009;108:846.

81. Jellish WS, Brody M, Sawicki K, Slogoff S. Recovery from neuromuscular blockade after either bolus and prolonged infusions of cisatracurium or rocuronium using either isoflurane or propofol-based anesthetics. *Anesth Analg.* 2000;91:1250–1255.

82. Schmidt J, Irouschek A, Muenster T, Hemmering TM, Albrecht S. A priming technique accelerates onset of neuromuscular blockade at the laryngeal adductor muscles. *Can J Anaesth.* 2005;52:50–54.

83. Griffith KE. Priming with rocuronium accelerates the onset of neuromuscular blockade. *J Clin Anesthesiol.* 1997;9:204.

84. Han TH, Martyn JA. Onset and effectiveness of rocuronium for rapid onset of paralysis in patients with major burns: priming or large bolus. *Br J Anaesth.* 2009;102:55–60.

Pharmacology of Local Analgesics

Terry C. Wicks, MHS, BSN, CRNA

Introduction

Local anesthetic drugs are used to block the transmission of sensory and motor signals along neuronal pathways and are among the most commonly administered anesthesia agents in current clinical practice. The ability of local anesthetic drugs to interrupt afferent transmission along nociceptive pathways, while often preserving a degree of sensory, motor, and proprioceptive function, renders their clinical administration attractive in a variety of clinical circumstances.

Local anesthetics are injected intravascularly to reduce the pain of the intravenous (IV) administration of irritating drugs, and they are injected locally into tissues to reduce the pain of incision. They can be injected into the subarachnoid or epidural spaces or adjacent to a nerve plexus to produce regional anesthesia. Notably, preemptive interruption in pain transmission may limit sensitization of pain pathways at the tissue, spinal cord, and cortical levels, decreasing the probability of transforming an acute pain experience into a chronic one. To maximize the clinical effectiveness of local anesthetics while minimizing the probability of local anesthetic toxicity, clinicians should thoroughly understand the pharmacology of local anesthetic drugs.

Mechanisms of Action

Sodium Channel Blockade

Excitable cells maintain an electrochemical gradient of positively charged particles across the semipermeable membrane that separates the interior and exterior of the cell. This gradient is maintained by the enzyme sodium-potassium ATPase, which transports three sodium ions out of the cell while simultaneously transporting two potassium ions into the cell. Transmembrane sodium channels open briefly when excitable cells are stimulated. Depolarization occurs with the passage of sodium ions through ion-specific channels down the electrochemical gradient, reducing the transmembrane electrochemical potential. Local anesthetics exert their pharmacologic effects by virtue of their ability to bind to receptors within or near specific ion channels and prevent the conformational changes that permit the flow of positively charged ions through those channels. Although altering the flow of sodium ions through transmembrane channels is the principal desired effect of local anesthetic agents, these drugs also alter the transmembrane conductance of both potassium and calcium ions, leading to predictable, and sometimes undesirable, clinical effects.

Sodium channels in the closed-resting (nonconducting) state have a low affinity for local anesthetics, whereas open channels (conducting) and closed-inactive (nonconducting) channels have relatively higher affinities for local anesthetics. The reduction of transmembrane conductance of sodium ions at low rates of depolarization is referred to as *tonic blockade.* This is believed to be due to binding of local anesthetics to receptors in the closed resting state. When the sodium channel is in either the open state or the closed-inactivate state after activation, local anesthetic molecules have an increased access to the sodium channel binding site, and additional degrees of sodium channel blockade develop. Increased blockade of sodium channel conductance due to the binding of local anesthetic molecules to activated open sodium channels is referred to as *phasic* or *use-dependent* blockade.[1]

Potassium Channel Blockade

In addition to blocking sodium channels, virtually all local anesthetics reversibly engage and block voltage-gated potassium channels. Exploring the effects of local anesthetics at potassium channels may offer insights into their local anesthetic effects as well as their propensity for disrupting normal cardiac function. Binding of local anesthetics to potassium channels in myelinated nerve fibers, including those in the dorsal root ganglia and the dorsal horns, may contribute to conduction blockade by delaying repolarization of these neurons and increasing their refractory period.[2,3]

Potassium channel blockade by local anesthetics appears to be concentration, voltage, and frequency dependent and is characterized by a degree of stereoselectivity. Some species of potassium channels are more highly blocked by R(+) stereoisomers than by S(−) isomers. For example, bupivacaine blockade of potassium channels appears to be more stereospecific than bupivacaine blockade of sodium channels. Racemic bupivacaine is three times more potent at blocking cardiovascular sarcolemmal K_{ATP} channels than is either levobupivacaine or ropivacaine, and levobupivacaine is a slightly more potent blocker of cardiovascular sarcolemmal K_{ATP} channels than is ropivacaine. Although the underlying mechanism of this stereospecificity is uncertain, it may be a reflection of a longer residence time of the dextrorotary isomer at the potassium channel receptor.[4]

The degree of potassium (and sodium) channel blockade parallels the individual local anesthetic's lipid solubility and potency. Further, the intensity of cardiac myocyte potassium channel blockade is enhanced under conditions of stress, hypoxia, and acidosis and leads to prolongation of the action potential duration and worsening of the cardiotoxic effects of bupivacaine.[5] The differences in the effects of local anesthetic racemates at potassium channels may offer clues into the differential cardiotoxicity of S(−) and R(+) local anesthetic enantiomers, despite very little clinical difference in their ability to block peripheral nerve transmission.

Calcium Channel Blockade

The transmission of nociceptive information is a complex phenomenon, and the transmission of pain signals can be altered by interfering with ion transport in sodium, potassium, and calcium channels. Some calcium channel blocking drugs, such as verapamil, have been shown to exhibit mild local anesthetic effects, whereas others, such as nifedipine and nicardipine, have been shown to prolong the duration of action of injected bupivacaine without possessing their own intrinsic local anesthetic effects.[6] Blockade of several calcium channel subtypes at the level of the spinal cord has been shown to modulate pain transmission and may contribute to the development of neuraxial local anesthetic effects.[7–9]

In cardiac and smooth muscle cells, extracellular calcium influx through calcium ion–specific channels is an important component of normal muscle contraction. Local anesthetic drugs can influence calcium channel activity and exert important physiologic effects beyond pain transmission. Examples of these effects include decreased calcium ion movement and concentration within cardiac muscle by inhibiting the transport of calcium by the sarcoplasmic reticulum. This is particularly important within the myocardium where local anesthetic effects on calcium transport can result in decreased myocardial contractility and decreased peak twitch tension.[10]

G-Protein Coupled Receptors

G-protein (guanine nucleotide binding protein) coupled receptors are transmembrane protein complexes that communicate the presence of extracellular ligands to intracellular enzyme- and protein-producing systems. Ligand binding to the extracellular domain of the receptor results in the dissociation of the G-protein from the intracellular portion of the receptor and the subsequent activation of a variety of second messenger systems. In essence, G-proteins act as "molecular switches" involved in the regulation of a multitude of intracellular processes. A number of anesthetic agents, including local anesthetics, opiates, and volatile inhalation agents, influence the activity of G-proteins and G-protein coupled receptors, leading to a variety of generally beneficial effects that include bronchodilation, anti-inflammatory effects, and antithrombotic effects.[11–13] The anti-inflammatory and antithrombotic effects of local anesthetics are particularly interesting because they appear to occur at very low concentrations, depend on the duration of local anesthetic exposure, and do not appear to interfere with normal immunity or coagulation.[14] Because of the wide variety of G-protein coupled receptor subtypes and functions, local anesthetic effects on these receptors may very well vary from one local anesthetic to another. Finally, the duration of exposure and concentration of a particular local anesthetic may influence the effects on the G-protein receptor complex even within the same subspecies of receptor.[15]

In summary, although the ability of local anesthetics to block sodium channel activation in peripheral nerves is a well-understood mechanism of anesthetic action, studies are just beginning to reveal more complex mechanisms by which local anesthetics alter the behavior of other ion channels and can modulate other physiologic processes. Local anesthetics interact with a wide variety of ligand- and voltage-gated channels, including potassium, calcium, and G-protein coupled receptors; Na^+/K^+ ATPase and Ca^{++}/Mg^{++} ATPase enzyme systems; and other transmembrane protein receptors.[1] Finally, in addition to sodium and potassium channel blockade, the production of spinal or epidural anesthesia may involve the modulation of N-methyl-D-aspartate and α-amino-3-hydroxy-5-methyl-4-isoxazolepropionic acid (AMPA) receptors.[16]

Clinical Pharmacology

Pharmacokinetics

In contrast to administering therapeutic agents to achieve systemic effects, anesthesia providers typically administer local anesthetics to produce the local, compartmental, or regional drug effects with the implicit intention of avoiding or at least minimizing their systemic effects. To consistently limit the undesirable systemic effects of local anesthetics, it is important to be familiar with the principles and factors that govern the pharmacokinetic behavior of these agents.

Absorption

To achieve the desired clinical anesthetic effects, local anesthetic drugs are intentionally deposited in close anatomic proximity to their target nerve tissues. This approach is intended to limit the volume and dose of any particular agent that is required to achieve the desired therapeutic effect. After injection, the factors that govern drug absorption influence local anesthetic penetration of nerve tissues and, subsequently, the systemic absorption of the local anesthetic agent. Drug penetration is influenced by the size and shape of the molecule, its lipid solubility, the degree to which it is ionized, and the extent to which it can be bound to serum or tissue proteins.[17] In the case of local anesthetic drugs, increasing molecular size correlates closely with lipid solubility, nerve-blocking potency, protein binding, and duration of action.[18]

Neuronal Penetration, pH, and pK*a*

Local anesthetics must migrate through the phospholipid cellular membrane to reach receptor binding sites that lie in close proximity to the sodium channel on the interior portion of the cell membrane. As salts of weak bases, local anesthetics in solution can exist as either charged or uncharged forms. The neutral or uncharged (lipophilic) form of local anesthetics passes most easily through the cell membrane, whereas the protonated (hydrophilic), or positively charged, form most effectively binds to the receptor and subsequently blocks the sodium channel.

Initially, the degree to which local anesthetics are ionized is directly affected by the pH of their carrier solutions and, subsequently, the extracellular fluid. The pK_a of a local anesthetic is the pH at which the drug is 50% ionized; that is, half of the molecules are charged and half are uncharged. Lowering the pH increases the proportion of ionized local anesthetic molecules and reduces the ability of local anesthetics to penetrate cell membranes. After penetration into the nerve cell membrane, the lower pH of the intracellular fluid shifts the ionization balance toward the ionized moiety and favors local anesthetic binding to the sodium channel receptor.[1]

In the case of lidocaine it has been well established that raising the pH of epinephrine-containing solutions by adding sodium bicarbonate hastens the onset of the anesthetic effects. Commercially prepared solutions of lidocaine compounded with epinephrine typically have a low pH (4.5), and as a result essentially 100% of the local anesthetic drug is in the protonated, or charged, form. By raising the pH of the solution toward the pK_a (7.8) of lidocaine, a greater proportion of the lidocaine molecules become unionized, more lipid soluble, and more easily able to penetrate the cell membrane phospholipid bilayer, thus hastening the onset of the drug action.[19,20] This property holds true for many other local anesthetics, including both amides and esters.[21] Conversely, there is experimental evidence that adding sodium bicarbonate to solutions that do not contain epinephrine (and do not have a significantly acidic pH) may shorten the duration of blockade without significantly hastening the onset of local anesthetic effects.[22]

Distribution

Local anesthetics that are injected into peripheral tissues eventually appear in the systemic circulation before being distributed to other well-perfused tissues. Peak serum levels of local anesthetics correlate closely with the dosage of drug injected, the region into which the local anesthetic is injected, and the drug's rate of clearance.[23] Because of the vascularity of surrounding tissues, intercostal, caudal, and epidural blocks are associated with the highest peak serum levels, whereas plexus blocks and femoral-sciatic nerve blocks typically produce lower peak serum levels. It follows that local cutaneous infiltration results in the lowest peak serum concentrations.[18]

A common clinical practice is to add epinephrine (1:200,000 to 1:400,000) to local anesthetic solutions to prolong their duration of action and to reduce peak serum concentrations after systemic absorption of the drug. Injection of local anesthetics containing epinephrine causes vasoconstriction of epineurial vessels and allows for more intense concentration of local anesthetic within the deep nerve fibers before absorption of the drug into surrounding tissues.[24] Absorption of local anesthetic by the myelin-rich matrix of the nerve, combined with constriction of perineurial vessels, retards the redistribution of local anesthetic drug away from the nerve fibers and prolongs the duration of action of the local anesthetic.[25] Adding epinephrine to local anesthetic solutions also reduces the risk of local anesthetic toxicity by providing a marker for the intravascular injection of local anesthetics.

After their eventual absorption into the serum, local anesthetics are redistributed to organs with rich blood flow (i.e., the liver, kidneys, lungs, and brain). A portion of the local anesthetic mass is protein bound in the serum. The principal serum protein to which local anesthetics are bound is α_1-acid glycoprotein, which may be reduced during pregnancy. Cardiac output, regional blood flow, and capillary permeability and age, weight, and gender influence the time course of redistribution to peripheral tissues. Eventually, the local anesthetic undergoes metabolism. Esters for the most part are metabolized in the plasma, and amides are metabolized in the liver.[17,26]

Concomitant administration of general anesthesia alters the pharmacokinetic behavior of local anesthetics. Potent inhalation anesthetics have the effect of reducing the steady-state volume of distribution and clearance of local anesthetics (in effect doubling their serum concentrations) but do not appear to significantly affect local anesthetic protein binding.[27] Similar effects on local anesthetic disposition occur with the coadministration of IV anesthetics.[28,29]

Distribution in the Subarachnoid Space

Injection of local anesthetics into the subarachnoid space adds additional complexity to the description of local anesthetic disposition because of the anatomically unique character of the subarachnoid space. As with peripheral blockade, neuronal exposure and absorption determines which physiologic functions will be affected by the spinal injection of local anesthetics.[30] After injection of local anesthetics into the subarachnoid space, uptake by intradural tissues is confined to those tissues in close proximity

to the cerebrospinal fluid (CSF) in which the drug is dissolved. The concentration of the local anesthetic within those tissues is proportional to the concentration of that drug in the surrounding CSF. Drug concentration is also influenced by tissue blood flow and the degree of neural tissue myelination. A small portion of the drug is absorbed directly through the pia mater, whereas the majority of the drug finds its way to deeper neuronal tissues of the spinal cord by traveling along the extensions of the subarachnoid space accompanying nutrient blood vessels.[31]

The three-dimensional exposure of the nerve roots as they pass through the CSF strongly suggests that this is the principal site of action of drugs administered in the subarachnoid space. The distribution of local anesthetics within the subarachnoid space determines the extent of spinal anesthesia produced by a given dose of intrathecal local anesthetic. The temperature and baricity of the drug, coupled with the patient's position, are the principal factors determining the distribution of local anesthetics within the subarachnoid space. Local anesthetics stored at room temperature are generally hyperbaric in nature, whereas at body temperature they become hypobaric.[32] Local anesthetics injected into the subarachnoid space begin to sink into the CSF until their temperature rises to the CSF temperature. At body temperature the local anesthetics become less dense and rise in the CSF.

It has been suggested that one avenue for preventing an undesirable cephalad spread of local anesthetics is to warm them to their isobaric temperature before administration, although in practical terms this may seem somewhat cumbersome.[33] During the regression phase of spinal anesthesia, a significant portion of the local anesthetic agent is absorbed into the epidural space, through the dura mater, down a concentration gradient. From there it is absorbed by epidural vessels. A small portion is also absorbed by the vessels supplying the pia mater and spinal cord. Highly lipid-soluble drugs will be more densely concentrated in the lipid-rich myelin tissues and less readily absorbed than less lipid-soluble drugs. Ultimately, the duration of spinal anesthesia is a reflection of the concentration of the drug at its site of action and its subsequent vascular absorption from that site of action.[31]

Metabolism

After absorption, ester-linked local anesthetics are metabolized to pharmacologically inactive metabolites by plasma cholinesterase. Because of the widespread distribution of plasma cholinesterase, ester-linked local anesthetics are rapidly cleared from the plasma. For example, the in vitro half-life of 2-chloroprocaine in maternal and fetal plasma ranges from 11.2 to 15.4 seconds, respectively, whereas the mean half-life after epidural injection is approximately 3.1 minutes.[34] The esters procaine and tetracaine are metabolized more slowly than 2-chloroprocaine. Although the primary metabolic pathway for esters involves metabolism by plasma cholinesterase, a small fraction nonetheless is transported to the liver where it is metabolized. Unlike other esters, cocaine is predominantly metabolized in the liver by hepatic cholinesterase, with a smaller fraction being metabolized in the serum. Finally, para-aminobenzoic acid, a common intermediary product of ester-linked local anesthetic metabolism, may be responsible for allergic reactions to ester-linked local anesthetics in some patients.[23]

In contrast to ester-linked local anesthetics, amide-linked agents are transported to the liver where they are metabolized by hepatic cytochrome P-450 enzymes. Although the metabolic pathways vary somewhat from one amide to another, typically the initial metabolism involves conversion of the local anesthetic to an amino carboxylic acid before eventual *N*-dealkylation and subsequent hydrolysis of the drug.[17] As a consequence of their obligatory hepatic metabolism, amide local anesthetics possess longer elimination half-lives than ester-linked local anesthetics. It follows that for amides the risk of the systemic accumulation of unmetabolized drug and systemic toxicity reactions are increased when compared with ester-linked local anesthetics.[23]

Differential Blockade

Clinical experience has shown that various neural modalities have differential susceptibility to the effects of local anesthetics. During epidural anesthesia, for example, temperature discrimination is one of the first sensory modalities to be lost, whereas pressure sense is one of the last to be diminished. In the case of neuraxial anesthesia, early blockade of myelinated preganglionic sympathetic B fibers results in decreased sympathetic tone, systemic vascular resistance, and venous return. The ensuing decline in systemic blood pressure is one of the earliest clinical signs of the onset of anesthetic action. A-α and A-β fibers are comparatively resistant to the effects of local anesthetics, and as a result when using dilute solutions of local anesthetics, nociception can often be reduced or extinguished while preserving proprioceptive and motor function.

In general, larger fibers tend to be more resistant to blockade than smaller fibers and require a longer length of the nerve fiber to be exposed to local anesthetic for blockade to occur (Table 9-1). This is true particularly for myelinated fibers, because the distances between nodes increase with fiber size. It is widely accepted that for myelinated fibers impulse propagation must fail in three consecutive nodes before signal transmission fails. It is important to remember that the concentration of the local anesthetic at the site of action determines the relative number of individual sodium channels blocked and that as the concentration of local anesthetics is lowered, the length of nerve fiber that needs be exposed to the local anesthetic to block signal propagation is increased.[35] Unmyelinated fibers are believed to be less susceptible to blockade than are myelinated fibers. For example, myelinated A-δ fibers (fast-pin prick pain) in some experimental preparations were more easily blocked than smaller unmyelinated C fibers (slow burning pain).[36] Further, experience has shown that highly lipid-soluble amide local anesthetics tend to block sensory fibers more effectively than motor fibers. Ultimately, fiber type, frequency of stimulation, the length of the nerve fiber exposed to the local anesthetic, and local anesthetic potency all influence the degree of block produced.[37]

Clinical Pharmacology (Prototypical) Structure Activity Relationships

Clinically useful local anesthetic drugs share a common structural framework composed of a lipid-soluble aromatic head, an intermediary carbon chain linkage, and a hydrophilic tail (Figure 9-1). Their comparative potency, lipid solubility, and pK_a are a function of the number and types of substituents on the aromatic ring, the character of their intermediary linking structure, and the addition

Table 9-1 Classification of Nerve Fibers, Function, and Ease of Blockade

Classification	Diameter (μm)	Myelination	Function	Appearance of Blockade
A-α A-β	6–22	Yes	Motor and proprioception	Late
A-γ	3–6	Yes	Muscle tone	Intermediate
A-δ	1–4	Yes	Pain, touch, temperature	Intermediate
B	< 3	Yes	Autonomic	Early
C	0.3–1.3	No	Autonomic, pain, temperature	Intermediate

Source: Adapted with permission from Liu SS, Joseph RS Jr. Local anesthetics. In: Barish PG, Cullen BF, Stoelting RK. *Clinical Anesthesia*, 5th ed. Philadelphia: Lippincott Williams & Wilkins; 2006.

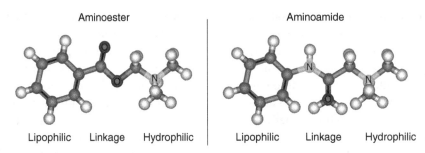

Figure 9-1 Common structural elements of local anesthetics.

of alkyl groups to the amine nitrogen tail. In very broad terms, ester-linked local anesthetics tend to be more potent and have a higher pK_a than amide-linked local anesthetics (Table 9-2).[38] Highly lipid-soluble local anesthetic agents also tend to have greater potency, longer duration of action, and a greater propensity to provoke toxicity. The addition of larger alkyl groups to the aromatic "head" or to the tertiary amine nitrogen convey greater lipid solubility (or more precisely more hydrophobicity) and consequently greater potency. Conversely, greater lipid solubility may prolong the drug's onset of action as a greater proportion of the local anesthetic drug can be absorbed by the surrounding myelin and lipid in nearby tissues before binding to ion channel receptors.[37]

The relative ratio of neutral and ionized forms influences the ability of the drug to penetrate the lipid-rich perineurium encircling the neuron and as a consequence influences

the onset and potency of the drug.[38] Local anesthetics with higher dissociation constants (pK_a) tend to be comparatively more ionized at physiologic pH than those with lower dissociation constants and display a slower onset of action due to reduced solubility of the protonated form in the lipid-rich myelin sheath and cell membrane. This physical chemical trait can be compensated for somewhat by increasing the concentration of the drug administered or by altering the pH of the local anesthetic solution. Lipid solubility also tends to correlate with protein binding and with local anesthetic duration of action.[37] When considering the variables that influence potency, onset of action, and duration, it may be intellectually convenient to consider the structural variables that alter these characteristics individually; however, the structural variations that modify one feature of pharmacokinetic behavior will as a matter of course affect other elements of drug behavior as well (Tables 9-2 and 9-3).

Table 9-2 Physicochemical Properties of Commonly Used Local Anesthetics

	pK_a	Ionized at pH 7.4 (%)	Partition Coefficient (Lipid Solubility)	Relative Potency	Protein Binding (%)
Amides					
Bupivacaine	8.1	83	3420	4	95
Etidocaine	7.7	66	7317	4	94
Lidocaine	7.9	76	366	1	64
Mepivacaine	7.6	61	130	1	77
Prilocaine	7.9	76	129	1	55
Ropivacaine	8.1	83	775	4	94
Esters					
Chloroprocaine	8.7	95	810	4	
Procaine	8.9	97	100	1	6
Tetracaine	8.5	93	5822	16	94

Source: Adapted with permission from Liu SS, Joseph RS Jr. Local anesthetics. In: Barish PG, Cullen BF, Stoelting RK. *Clinical Anesthesia,* 5th ed. Philadelphia: Lippincott Williams & Wilkins; 2006, and Stoelting RK, Hillier SC. Local anesthetics. In: Stoelting RK, Hillier SC. *Pharmacology and Physiology in Anesthetic Practice,* 4th ed. Philadelphia: Lippincott Williams & Wilkins; 2006.

Table 9-3 Comparative Pharmacology of Commonly Used Local Anesthetics

	Maximum Dose (mg)*	Onset	Duration (min)*	Elimination Half-Time (min)
Amides				
Lidocaine	300	Rapid	60–120	96
Etidocaine	300	Slow	240–480	156
Prilocaine	400	Slow	60–120	96
Mepivacaine	300	Slow	90–180	114
Bupivacaine	175	Slow	240–480	210
Levobupivacaine	175	Slow	240–480	156
Ropivacaine	200	Slow	240–480	108
Esters				
Procaine	500	Slow	45–60	9
Chloroprocaine	600	Rapid	30–45	7
Tetracaine	100 (topical)	Slow	60–180	

*For infiltration.

Source: Adapted with permission from: Stoelting RK, Hillier SC. Local anesthetics. In: Stoelting RK, Hillier SC. *Pharmacology and Physiology in Anesthetic Practice,* 4th ed. Philadelphia: Lippincott Williams & Wilkins; 2006.

Chirality, Stereoisomerism, and Stereospecificity

Stereoisomerism is a common characteristic of pharmaceutical agents in general and local anesthetic drugs in particular. Stereoisomerism refers to drugs that have the same chemical formula and arrangement of bonds connecting their atoms yet have differing three-dimensional arrangements of their atoms. When these isomers are structurally stable, can be separated without interconversion, and cannot be made alike by rotating around the axis of a single bond, they are referred to as configurational stereoisomers. Pairs of stereoisomers that are related to one another as mirror images are referred to as enantiomers. Asymmetric substitution of the chiral carbon in local anesthetics possessing a piperidine ring in their hydrophilic "tail" results in the generation of levo- and dextrorotary stereoisomers. Stereoisomers may exhibit similar or differential affinity for receptors and may have very similar or dramatically different effects when bound to particular receptors.[39] Local anesthetic stereoisomers typically have similar lipid solubility, neuronal uptake, and ability to penetrate physiologic membranes. The angular, three-dimensional structure of chiral molecules (in contrast to more planar local anesthetics) influences their binding to ion channel receptors.[40]

Some research and accumulating clinical evidence suggest that stereoisomers appear to exhibit a differential ability to provoke central nervous system (CNS) and cardiovascular system toxicity while not varying significantly in their clinical anesthetic potency. Typically, the R(+) enantiomer exerts the more toxic cardiovascular and CNS effects, and the S(−) enantiomers appear to have a less deleterious effect on intraventricular conduction than either the R(+) enantiomers or racemic mixtures of the same local anesthetic. For example, the degree of cardiac conduction delay is 2.5 times greater with racemic bupivacaine than for levobupivacaine and 4 times greater than for ropivacaine. These local anesthetics have also been shown to provoke a rate-dependent widening of QRS duration, to reduce conduction velocity, and to prolong the ventricular effective refractory period (bupivacaine > levobupivacaine > ropivacaine).[41]

Some studies have suggested differential potency of stereoisomers (dextrorotary isomer > levorotary isomer) at sodium channels during tonic blockade that is enhanced during phasic blockade.[40,42–44] Further, dextrorotary isomers of bupivacaine have been shown to have delayed dissociation from resting inactivated sodium channels. This may account for their very slight (and clinically unimportant) increased potency over the levorotary isomers for sodium channel blockade in peripheral neuronal fibers, a property that would take on increased significance during the more frequent depolarization of the cardiac cycle and may explain, to a degree, the greater cardiotoxicity of dextrorotary isomers of bupivacaine.[44]

Some species of potassium channels have been shown to have significant stereoselectivity for dextrorotary isomers of bupivacaine, and this may also contribute to the cardiotoxicity of dextrorotary local anesthetic isomers.[43] Although there is still much to be learned about the differential pharmacodynamics of dextro- and levo-enantiomers of local anesthetics, there is a substantial likelihood that the use of levo-enantiomer local anesthetics can convey an additional degree of cardiovascular patient safety during the delivery of regional anesthesia.

Commonly Used Local Anesthetic Agents

Ester Local Anesthetics

Procaine has been used in clinical anesthesia practice since early in the 20th century, and it is the prototypical ester-linked local anesthetic (Figure 9-2).[45] Because of procaine's pK_a (8.9), it is 97% ionized at physiologic pH and has a relatively slow onset of action when used for

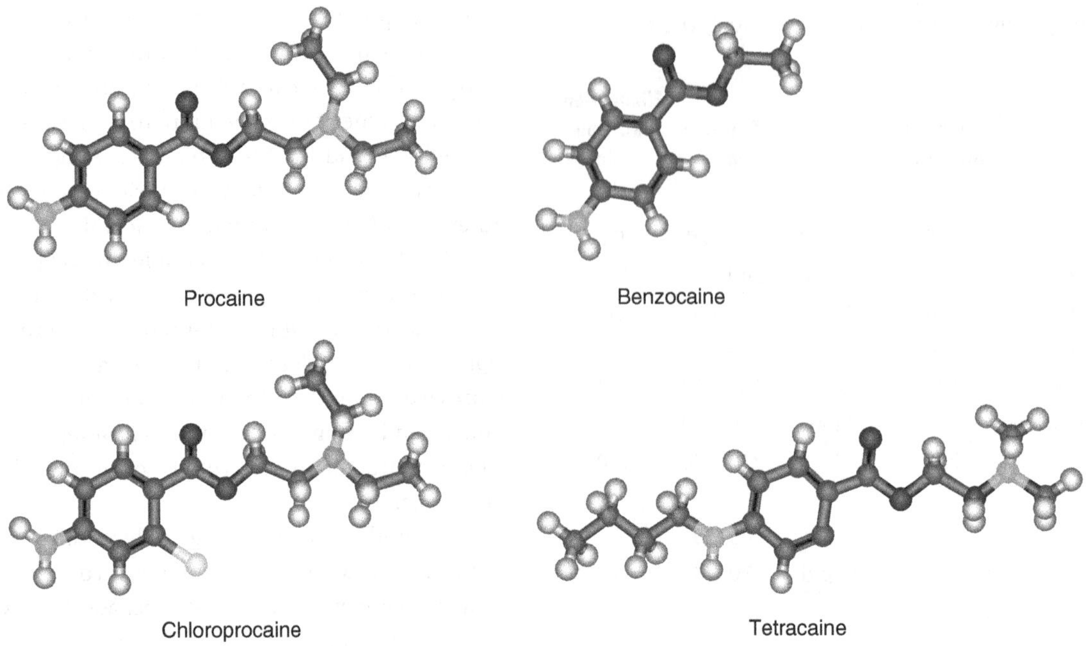

Procaine

Benzocaine

Chloroprocaine

Tetracaine

Figure 9-2 Ester local anesthetics.

infiltration.[23] Its slow onset combined with a short duration of action (45–60 minutes) limit its clinical utility, and its current clinical application is primarily confined to spinal anesthesia. When administered for spinal anesthesia, a 10% solution has a rapid onset of action and a short duration of action. Procaine is rapidly metabolized by serum cholinesterase and has an elimination half-time of under 10 minutes.[37]

Chloroprocaine differs from procaine only in the addition of a chlorine atom to its lipid-soluble benzene ring. It is four times more potent than procaine and has a shorter serum elimination half-time than procaine. Like procaine, the relatively high pK_a of chloroprocaine results in the drug being 95% ionized at pH 7.4. Although intuitively it would seem that chloroprocaine would have a slow onset of action because of its high pK_a, this property is offset by the clinical administration of the drug in 2% to 3% concentrations. Chloroprocaine's rapid onset of action and short duration of action make it an attractive agent for use in peripheral nerve blocks and for epidural anesthetics of short duration. The addition of epinephrine to solutions of chloroprocaine helps to limit peak serum concentrations after plexus or epidural administration and prolongs the duration of action.[23,37] Preservative-free solutions of chloroprocaine are hyperbaric and can be used for short-duration spinal anesthesia. The distribution of block and the duration of action for spinal chloroprocaine are dose dependent (30–60 mg). Currently, however, this remains an off-label use of the drug.[46,47]

Tetracaine is 16 times more potent than procaine and 4 times more potent than chloroprocaine. Although occasionally used in combination with other agents for peripheral nerve blocks or in 2% solutions for topical anesthesia, tetracaine's principal use is in spinal anesthesia where it is administered in 0.5% solutions. Dextrose can be added to tetracaine to increase its baricity; conversely, the drug can be diluted with preservative-free sterile water to render it hypobaric. Tetracaine has the longest duration of action of the ester local anesthetics, and the addition of epinephrine to spinal anesthetic solutions can produce spinal anesthesia lasting 6 or more hours. The addition of fentanyl 10 to 20 mcg to tetracaine spinal anesthesia enhances the quality of the block significantly.[23,37]

Benzocaine is used primarily for topical anesthesia where its onset is very rapid and its clinical effects last for 30 to 60 minutes. Because of its very low pK_a (3.5), it is completely un-ionized at physiologic pH and readily penetrates mucous membranes. Excessive administration of benzocaine can lead to the development of methemoglobinemia. Methemoglobinemia is the result of oxidation of hemoglobin, and central cyanosis occurs when methemoglobin levels exceed 15%. Methylene blue 1 to 2 mg/kg over 5 minutes (maximum dose, 7–8 mg/kg) reverses methemoglobinemia, but the patient should be monitored for the reoccurrence of symptoms.[23,37]

Amide Local Anesthetics

Lidocaine is one of the most frequently administered local anesthetics and, among the amide local anesthetics, is one of the least likely to provoke CNS and cardiovascular system toxicity (Figure 9-3). Because of its therapeutic margin of safety, lidocaine has been used for an extensive variety of clinical anesthetic applications, including topical (4%), infiltration (0.5–1.0%), IV regional (0.25–0.5%), peripheral nerve block (1–2%), epidural (1.5–2%), and spinal (1.5–5%) anesthesia. The onset of action for virtually all applications of lidocaine is rapid, whereas the duration of blockade is of intermediate duration and is somewhat dose dependent. The maximum recommended dose for lidocaine is 300 mg for plain solutions and 500 mg for solutions containing epinephrine. The pK_a of lidocaine is 7.9, and therefore at physiologic pH it is about 76% ionized and its elimination half-time is slightly over 90 minutes.[23,37] Despite its historic track record of clinical safety, lidocaine can be myotoxic and neurotoxic, especially when used in higher concentrations (see Toxicity below). This has been particularly troubling when lidocaine has been administered for spinal anesthesia, because transient neurologic symptoms are not uncommon and catastrophic cauda equina syndrome can occur.[48]

Prilocaine is an amide-linked local anesthetic that pharmacodynamically and pharmacokinetically resembles lidocaine, with similar clinical applications. The pK_a and degree of ionization are 7.9 and 76%, respectively, and like lidocaine, its elimination half-time is about 1.6 hours. Also like lidocaine, it can be used for infiltration (0.5–1%), IV regional anesthesia (0.25–0.5%), peripheral nerve block (1.5–2%), and epidural anesthesia (2–3%). Like benzocaine and lidocaine, prilocaine can cause methemoglobinemia. The maximum recommended dose is 600 mg.[23,37]

Etidocaine is a highly lipid-soluble, long-acting amide local anesthetic with a rapid onset of action. Its low degree of ionization (66%) reflects its pK_a of 7.7, which is closer to physiologic pH than either lidocaine or prilocaine. It is less likely to provoke CNS or cardiovascular toxicity than other long-acting local anesthetics. Etidocaine can be used for infiltration (0.5%), peripheral nerve block (0.5–1.0%), or epidural anesthesia (1.0–1.5%). The maximum recommended dose is 300 mg for plain solutions and 400 mg for solutions containing epinephrine. The elimination half-time for etidocaine is approximately 2.6 hours.[23,37]

Mepivacaine is similar to lidocaine in most of its clinical applications. The pK_a of mepivacaine (7.6) is slightly lower than that of lidocaine (7.9), so it is somewhat less ionized than lidocaine at physiologic pH. Both drugs, however, are characterized by a rapid onset of action, whereas mepivacaine is noted for its extended duration of action, especially when used for peripheral nerve block or epidural anesthesia. Mepivacaine may be used for infiltration (0.5–1.0%), peripheral nerve block (1–1.5%), spinal anesthesia (2–4%), and epidural blockade (1.5–2%). Mepivacaine possesses a slightly longer elimination half-time compared with lidocaine (1.9 h vs. 1.6 h) and is also slightly more potent for provoking CNS toxicity. The maximum recommended dose of mepivacaine is 400 mg for plain solutions and 500 mg for those containing epinephrine. Mepivacaine is closely related to both ropivacaine and bupivacaine in its chemical structure (Figure 9-4).[23,37]

Ropivacaine was the first local anesthetic levo-enantiomer marketed for clinical use in the United States. Ropivacaine is slightly less potent than bupivacaine and is marketed in 0.2%, 0.5%, and 1.0% solutions. Its onset of action for infiltration is rapid (0.2–0.5%), and its duration of action for virtually all clinical applications is prolonged (6–8 h). The onset for peripheral nerve block is slow (0.5–1.0%), and for epidural anesthesia its onset is intermediate (0.5–1.0%) in character. Its elimination half-time is approximately 1.9 hours. The pK_a of ropivacaine is identical to bupivacaine (8.1), and it is 83% ionized at physiologic pH.

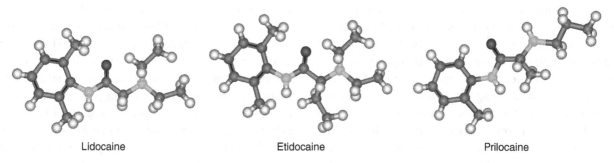

Lidocaine   Etidocaine   Prilocaine

Figure 9-3 Amide local anesthetics lidocaine, etidocaine, and prilocaine.

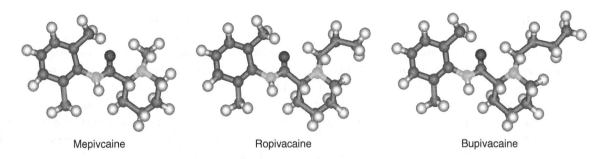

Figure 9-4 Amide local anesthetics mepivacaine, ropivacaine, and bupivacaine.

Ropivacaine is slightly less potent than bupivacaine, and clinically ropivacaine produces a more profound sensory block than motor block.[23,37] Ropivacaine can be used in spinal anesthesia (0.5–0.75%) where it has a relatively rapid onset of action, although it is somewhat less potent and has a shorter duration of action than bupivacaine. Rostral spread of spinal ropivacaine can be improved when hyperbaric solutions rather than plain solutions are used.[49,50] Ropivacaine is noteworthy in that it is less likely than bupivacaine to provoke CNS and cardiovascular system toxicity. This is probably a reflection of a combination of its reduced potency compared with bupivacaine and its formulation as only the levo-enantiomer of the local anesthetic.[51,52]

Bupivacaine is one of the most potent and widely used local anesthetics in clinical use. Its onset of action is rapid for infiltration (0.25%) and for spinal anesthesia (0.5–0.75%), intermediate for peripheral nerve blocks (0.25–0.5%), and slow for epidural anesthesia (0.5–0.75%). Its duration of action is prolonged for virtually all clinical applications. Like ropivacaine, its pK_a is 8.1 and it is 83% ionized at physiologic pH. It is highly tissue protein bound (95%), and its elimination half-time is approximately 3.5 hours. Levobupivacaine has similar physiochemical properties to racemic bupivacaine, although its elimination half-time is somewhat shorter (2.6 vs. 3.5 h).[23,37] In spinal anesthesia, hyperbaric 0.75% bupivacaine produces 1.5 to 2 hours of anesthesia.[53] Because of its lipid solubility and potency, bupivacaine can provide prolonged sensory and motor blockade but is also noteworthy as being the most cardiotoxic of the commonly used local anesthetic agents. Levobupivacaine is less likely to provoke catastrophic toxicity despite sharing virtually all the essential physicochemical and pharmacokinetic properties of bupivacaine and provides nearly identical sensory and motor blockade.

Systemic Administration

Acute Pain Management

In addition to their application for providing local and regional anesthesia, local anesthetics, where systematically administered, may provide some patient groups with both subjective and objective benefits in the perioperative period. In some intra-abdominal surgical procedures infusing low doses of lidocaine during surgery and continuing into the postoperative period has been shown to improve patients' postoperative pain experience. Patients undergoing laparoscopic colectomy were shown to have reduced parenteral opioid requirements, early return of bowel function, reduced postoperative fatigue, and shortened hospital stays when receiving parenteral infusions of lidocaine.[54] Kaba et al.[54] attributed these beneficial effects to the analgesic, anti-hyperalgesic, and anti-inflammatory influence of infused lidocaine on the activity of sodium channels, G-protein couple receptors, and N-methyl-D-aspartate receptors, both peripherally and at the spinal cord level. Similar results were demonstrated for patients undergoing radical prostatectomy and other major abdominal surgeries.[55,56]

Although these results are encouraging for patients undergoing intra-abdominal surgery, they are not necessarily applicable to all patients undergoing major surgery. IV infusions of lidocaine were not found to have a significant analgesic benefit in major orthopedic surgery, underscoring the importance of evaluating the efficacy of this treatment modality for specific surgical populations.[57] For some patients, however, a pain management strategy that includes an IV lidocaine infusion may be advantageous on a number of levels, including its simplicity, reduced dependence on epidural analgesia (which has a number of contraindications and associated risks), relatively low cost, and apparent effectiveness. Additional research is needed to identify those patients most likely to benefit from this treatment and to define the dose that maximizes efficacy while minimizing the risks associated with its administration.[58]

Systemic Administration and Anti-inflammatory Effects

The infusion of low concentrations of local anesthetics has an anti-inflammatory effect that may be beneficial in some clinical settings.[13] Experimental data for some models of acute pulmonary acid injury, inflammatory disease of the gastrointestinal tract, edema due to cutaneous thermal injury, and myocardial ischemia reperfusion injury suggest that the infusion of local anesthetics may reduce or minimize the extent of tissue damage. These anti-inflammatory effects may be the result of inhibiting the release of important inflammatory mediators and free radicals; diminishing the activity of polymorphonuclear granulocytes, macrophages, and monocytes; and reducing the priming of neutrophils by platelet-activating factor.[59,60]

As a cautionary note, local anesthetic effects on inflammation and immunity may not always be beneficial. For example, Kiefer et al. demonstrated in vitro reductions in granulocyte phagocytosis in response to *Staphylococcus aureus* after exposure to bupivacaine and lidocaine in various concentrations. This effect was not demonstrated after ropivacaine administration. Although the implications of these data are not immediately clear, and it is difficult to extrapolate this work directly to clinical practice, it does suggest that for patients with impaired immunity or with active infections, local anesthetic selection could have important implications.[61]

Toxicity

Local anesthetic drugs are useful agents that can convey considerable benefit when administered appropriately. They can also cause tissue damage, permanent neurologic injury, and potentially lethal side effects.

Myotoxicity

High concentrations of local anesthetics have been shown to inhibit myocyte energy production (ATP synthesis) at the mitochondrial level. These effects are the result of the uncoupling of oxidative phosphorylation and the impairment of intracellular enzyme systems. The degree to which these untoward effects occur varies with the lipid solubility (and potency) of the specific local anesthetic. The effect is greatest with bupivacaine, is less so with ropivacaine, and appears to be absent with lidocaine.[62] Although the effects of local anesthetics on myocardial and skeletal muscle energy production vary with lipid solubility, these effects do not necessarily appear to be stereospecific.[63,64]

Conversely, in animal models of myocardial ischemia, there appears to be some protective effect from reperfusion injury when lidocaine is administered before an ischemic event.[60] The underlying mechanism of this effect appears to be related to the ability of lidocaine to limit myocardial leukocyte concentrations in the ischemic area immediately after reperfusion. Additionally, lidocaine may reduce the susceptibility of myocardial cells to hypoxia-induced apoptosis, thereby preventing the extension of the injury into the penumbra of the infarct.

Neurotoxicity

Neurotoxicity associated with administration of local anesthetics is a complex phenomenon that may have numerous components. One mechanism of injury may be related to local anesthetic-mediated elevations of cytoplasmic calcium in susceptible neurons. Lidocaine, at relatively high experimental concentrations, and to a lesser extent bupivacaine cause the release of calcium stores from the endoplasmic reticulum that, in vitro, have been shown to lead to neuronal cell death within 60 minutes of continuous exposure.[65] Normally, sequestration or release of calcium by the endoplasmic reticulum serves as a buffering mechanism that offsets normal increases and decreases in intracellular calcium concentrations. Low concentrations of local anesthetics appear to cause mild and transient increases in intracellular calcium, whereas high concentrations have more deleterious and persistent effects.

Some experimental animal models that mimic the concentrations of local anesthetics that occur during lidocaine spinal anesthesia have demonstrated permanent membrane depolarization and lactate dehydrogenase leakage (suggesting axonal membrane disruption) when local anesthetic exposure lasts longer than 30 minutes.[66] Studies involving other local anesthetics have not produced this type of injury, but it should be emphasized that neuronal injury does occur with local anesthetics other than lidocaine.[67] Several other postulated mechanisms of neuronal injury exist, including activation of caspase enzymes resulting in apoptosis, depolarization of neuronal mitochondria, and interference with mitochondrial respiration. These effects have been shown to occur most notably with local anesthetic concentrations similar to those achieved in poorly distributed lidocaine spinal anesthesia.[68]

Still another postulated mechanism of neuronal injury involves disruption of neuronal membranes by solubilization of membrane lipids by local anesthetics, which at the appropriate concentration and pH self-aggregate and form micelles that possess detergent-like properties. Self-aggregation is possible when compounds possess both lipophilic and hydrophilic components in their structures. The concentrations at which lidocaine, tetracaine, and procaine self-aggregate are very similar to those used in clinical anesthesia, and this detergent-like effect may be an element of some neuronal injuries.[69]

Finally, the route of administration appears to be an important variable in determining the degree of neurotoxicity, particularly with lidocaine.[70] In animal models lidocaine administered in the subarachnoid space frequently results in persistent neurologic impairment. In contrast, epidural doses of lidocaine that produced similar degrees of motor block rarely caused neurologic impairment or histiologic evidence of neural injury, even in 10% concentrations. Clearly, the site of action, distribution of local anesthetic, and opportunity for dilution of the local anesthetic differ for these two techniques. These results highlight the relatively reduced risk of neurotoxicity when local anesthetic drugs are injected into the epidural rather than the subarachnoid space.

Interestingly, adding epinephrine to lidocaine administered into the subarachnoid space has been shown to increase the severity of neuronal injury, whereas neuronal damage has not been shown to occur with intrathecal epinephrine alone.[71] Epinephrine-mediated vasoconstriction may delay the absorption of lidocaine and increase the duration of neuronal exposure to the drug, increasing the risk of neuronal injury.

Transient Neurologic Symptoms

Awareness that temporary pain and dysesthesia in the buttocks and lower extremities may follow spinal anesthesia, particularly when lidocaine has been injected into the subarachnoid space, has become common place. Transient neurologic symptoms (TNS) ordinarily occur within 24 hours of recovery from spinal anesthesia. The pain of TNS occurs with an otherwise normal neurologic exam and without magnetic resonance imaging or electrophysiologic evidence of abnormality. Although the concern about the cause of TNS has justifiably focused on lidocaine neurotoxicity, the potential of other drugs to cause TNS is well documented.[72,73] Nonetheless, the occurrence of TNS after spinal anesthesia with drugs other than lidocaine is significantly less frequent. Prilocaine, for example, has been shown to produce significant neurotoxicity in the laboratory, whereas TNS is a rare clinical event after prilocaine spinal anesthesia.[74]

Intuitively, it may seem logical that reducing the concentration of lidocaine could reduce the incidence of TNS after spinal anesthesia, but this has been clearly demonstrated not to be the case. Either 1% or 2% lidocaine produces an incidence of TNS statistically indistinguishable from that of 5% lidocaine.[75,76] Similarly, altering the baricity or mixing lidocaine with CSF does not reduce the frequency of TNS after spinal anesthesia.

In summary, the risk of TNS after spinal anesthesia with lidocaine is seven times greater than the risk of TNS with bupivacaine, procaine, or prilocaine.[73] It is abundantly clear that the most effective strategy for minimizing the risk of TNS is to avoid the injection of lidocaine into the subarachnoid space.

Cauda Equina Syndrome

Cauda equina syndrome is an unusual but catastrophic clinical complication that can occur after spinal anesthesia. Symptoms include persistent bowel and bladder dysfunction, pain, and loss of sensory and motor function. Local anesthetic neurotoxicity leading to cauda equine syndrome appears to be a function of both the concentration of the local anesthetic and the duration of local anesthetic exposure. Although most commonly associated with lidocaine administered through spinal microcatheters, it has been reported after single-injection lidocaine spinal anesthetics as well. Lidocaine has been shown to induce neuronal mitochondrial apoptosis and neuronal cell death in concentrations commonly occurring with intrathecal administration for spinal anesthesia. Alternatively, at higher intrathecal concentrations, such as those encountered with repeated dosing through intrathecal catheters, neuronal necrosis may be due to interference with neuronal ATP production or other effects.[77]

Although historically the concern regarding neurotoxicity and spinal anesthesia has focused on lidocaine, neurotoxicity can result from the administration of other local anesthetics into the subarachnoid space, including both bupivacaine and ropivacaine. Whereas not all studies have demonstrated a differential neurotoxicity between these three drugs in vitro, clinically cauda equina syndrome occurs much more frequently after lidocaine than with bupivacaine or ropivacaine spinal anesthesia.[78]

Systemic Local Anesthetic Toxicity

In general, the appearance and severity of symptoms of systemic toxicity from local anesthetic overdose follows a consistent and predictable pattern. Although the toxicity of local anesthetic agents tends to parallel their relative potencies and lipid solubility, differences in toxicity exist between the various local anesthetic agents even when administered at equipotent doses. Characteristically, clinical symptoms of CNS toxicity tend to appear before symptoms of cardiovascular toxicity (Table 9-4). This is particularly true when toxicity is due to absorption from a site of deposition or from accumulation during an IV infusion. Interestingly, although general anesthesia may mask the CNS manifestations of local anesthetic toxicity, clinical experience has shown, and research with animal models supports, that even absent general anesthesia, during rapid infusions, or following bolus IV injections, cardiac arrest may occur with few or no symptoms of CNS toxicity preceding cardiac collapse.[79]

CNS Symptoms

The initial symptoms of systemic toxicity are ordinarily characterized by CNS excitability and the sudden onset of seizure activity after IV injection of local anesthetic agents. CNS excitement reflects depression of the CNS inhibitory centers. The onset and severity of CNS toxicity parallel the rate of appearance of the drug in the plasma and the peak serum concentration. It is noteworthy that even relatively small doses of local anesthetics in the cerebral circulation provoke CNS excitation and seizure activity.

Interestingly, Takahashi et al. found that including epinephrine in solutions of lidocaine administered intravenously resulted in a lowering of the serum lidocaine level required to produce seizure activity. They postulated that this was the result of an epinephrine-induced decrease in the fraction of protein-bound lidocaine and an increased delivery of lidocaine to the CNS. This effect was thought to have been the result of increased cardiac output due to the

presence of epinephrine and a resulting decreased volume of distribution for lidocaine.[80]

Commonly, the increased muscle activity associated with seizure activity can be associated with the development of metabolic acidosis. Excitation of the CNS also contributes to the development of cardiac dysrhythmias.[81] Although animal studies suggest that CNS excitement alone does not commonly cause lethal dysrhythmias, it is certainly conceivable that CNS excitement could contribute to the genesis of a lethal cardiac dysrhythmia when coexisting cardiac toxicity is present. CNS symptoms of local anesthetic toxicity occur at lower doses and lower serum levels with bupivacaine than with levobupivacaine or ropivacaine.[51]

Cardiovascular System Symptoms

Impaired Contractility

Toxic serum levels of local anesthetics can impair the contractile function of the myocardium and interrupt the normal transmission of signals through the conduction system of the heart. Conventional wisdom suggests that serum concentrations required to produce cardiovascular toxicity tend to be two- to threefold higher than those required to produce CNS toxicity (as manifested as seizure activity).[18,37] Studies in animal models, however, demonstrate that a significant degree of myocardial depression and a decrease in cardiac output can occur early in local anesthetic toxicity that tends to be masked somewhat by the neuroexcitatory effects of local anesthetic toxicity.[27] Local anesthetic effects on the myocardium include a decrease in the force of contraction, which results in decreased cardiac output, stroke volume, and mean arterial blood pressure.[82]

Decreases in myocardial performance and impaired cardiac conduction reflect the ability of potent local anesthetics to block the normal function of sodium, potassium, and calcium channels and to alter the handling of calcium at the sarcoplasmic reticulum.[83–86] Because of the effects of local anesthetics on excitable cells, it is not surprising that coronary artery disease and preexisting conduction abnormalities may increase the likelihood and severity of the cardiac manifestations of local anesthetic toxicity.[87,88] Studies of bupivacaine's action on intact myocardial cells suggest that bupivacaine may also inhibit the sensitivity of cardiac myofibrils to the inotropic effects of calcium.[89]

Rate Changes and Rhythm Disturbances

As a result of the effects of local anesthetics on the myocardium, patients experiencing local anesthetic toxicity demonstrate decreases in heart rate, myocardial

Table 9-4 Symptoms of Local Anesthetic Toxicity (Lidocaine)

Plasma Concentration (mcg/mL)	Effect/Symptom
1–5	Analgesia
5–10	Circumoral numbness, tinnitus, skeletal muscle twitching, systemic hypotension, myocardial depression
10–15	Seizures, unconsciousness
15–25	Apnea, coma
> 25	Cardiovascular depression

Source: Adapted with permission from: Stoelting RK, Hillier SC. Local anesthetics. In: Stoelting RK, Hillier SC. *Pharmacology and Physiology in Anesthetic Practice,* 4th ed. Philadelphia: Lippincott Williams & Wilkins; 2006.

contractility, coronary blood flow, and myocardial oxygen consumption, as well as varying degrees of heart block (decreased atrial, nodal, and ventricular conduction) and the provocation of a variety of ectopic arrhythmias.[90] In severe local anesthetic toxicity, ectopy and conduction abnormalities result in the development of malignant ventricular rhythms, including ventricular tachycardia, ventricular fibrillation, and asystole. Although the extent of *inotropic* impairment appears to be related to local anesthetic potency, optical isomers of chiral local anesthetics exhibit differential effects with regard to their ability to cause delays within the heart's conduction system. The R(+) isomer of bupivacaine causes significantly more conduction delay than does the S(−) isomer, whereas the racemic formulation is intermediate in its effects on conduction. Ropivacaine causes conduction delays in a fashion similar to bupivacaine. However, ropivacaine concentrations required to produce those effects are as much as fivefold higher than for bupivacaine.[91] Animal model experiments using IV infusions of local anesthetics consistently resulted in death from cardiac dysfunction that was heralded by the rapid onset of ventricular fibrillation or pulseless electrical activity with or without preceding ventricular tachycardia.[92]

Management of Toxicity Reactions

Preventing local anesthetic toxicity is preferable to treating local anesthetic toxicity. All due measures to achieve this goal should be considered before the institution of regional anesthetic blockade (Box 9-1).

In the management of local anesthetic toxicity, as in nearly all anesthetic crises, prior planning, preparation, and swift intervention increase the likelihood of a successful outcome. Immediate recognition of the problem and rapid institution of advanced cardiac life support measures are crucial components of effectively managing local anesthetic toxicity, and some evidence suggests that prior simulation training may contribute to successful treatment outcomes.[93] The key clinical elements of managing local anesthetic toxicity include immediate interventions to provide definitive airway security and ventilation, interrupt seizure activity, and effectively treat cardiac dysrhythmias.

The management of local anesthetic toxicity reactions has undergone significant transformation recently as clinical case reports of the efficacy of lipid emulsion administration have provided compelling support for its use in rescuing patients unresponsive to conventional treatments (Box 9-2).[87,94–96] Although mounting anecdotal evidence

---

Box 9-1 Strategies for Preventing Local Anesthetic Toxicity

- Limit the dosage and concentration of local anesthetic agent to the lowest that will accomplish the desired therapeutic result.
- Administer the local anesthetic in small boluses, allowing for the appearance of subjective and objective symptoms of intravascular injection between doses before proceeding with the next test dose.
- Use long-acting agents for long procedures to limit the need for repeat bolusing.
- Include low concentrations of epinephrine in local anesthetic solutions (1:200,000–1:400,000) to reduce vascular uptake of local anesthetic and as a marker for detecting intravascular injection of local anesthetic, unless specifically contraindicated.
- Administer premedications to raise the seizure threshold.
- Aspirate between injections to reduce the likelihood of accidental intravascular injection.
- Apply all appropriate monitors, such as electrocardiographs, pulse oximetry, and blood pressure, before beginning treatment.

Box 9-2 Management of Local Anesthetic Toxicity Reactions

- Before administering regional anesthesia block, ensure that all resuscitation drugs and equipment are available, including monitors, drugs, airway equipment, suction, crash cart, and additional personnel.
- Administer supplemental oxygen and control the airway as indicated.
- Protect the patient from aspiration and ensure adequate ventilation.
- Administer anticonvulsants to interrupt seizure activity.
- Institute advanced cardiac life support measures if cardiac arrest ensues, and consider cardiopulmonary bypass if available.
- Administer lipid emulsion bolus (1–3 mL/kg 20% lipid emulsion*) followed by a continuous lipid emulsion infusion (0.25–0.5 mL/kg/h†). Repeat bolus two to three times.
- Monitor for recurrence of CNS or cardiovascular system local anesthetic toxicity.

*From reference 98.
†From reference 99.

supports its use, it is worth noting that the administration of lipid emulsion does engender certain risks, among them allergic reactions. Fortunately, in single uses or short-term administration, complications are rare.[97] The precise mechanism by which lipid emulsion facilitates recovery from local anesthetic toxicity remains speculative but may involve the creation of a lipid "sink" that binds the circulating local anesthetic, thereby diverting the local anesthetic drug away from the myocardium (reversing the concentration gradient) and allowing recovery of cardiac performance. In many cases patient response to lipid emulsion administration has been surprisingly prompt.[98–101]

Summary

Local anesthetics exert their principal beneficial effects by virtue of their ability to bind to sodium channel receptors and block the passage of sodium ions through ion-specific transmembrane pores, preventing neuronal depolarization. The potency of local anesthetics in this regard is primarily a reflection of their lipid solubility and the extent of their ionization. The lipid solubility of local anesthetic drugs also correlates with their degree of protein binding, duration of action, and their potential for provoking toxicity reactions. Although interruption of nociceptive neuronal transmission is the principal desired effect of local anesthetics, they also modulate the activity of potassium and calcium channels and influence the behavior of a variety of other cellular messenger systems. Despite the beneficial effects of local anesthetic drugs, they can cause cellular and systemic toxicity, and caution must be exercised in their administration to minimize the risk of patient injury.

Key Points

- The primary mechanism of action for local anesthetic drugs reflects their ability to block sodium channels. Local anesthetics do, however, influence the behavior of other ion channels and second messenger systems as well.
- Lipid solubility is closely correlated with potency and duration of action.
- pK_a correlates closely with onset of action.
- Epinephrine reduces systemic uptake of local anesthetics and prolongs the duration of action of many local anesthetics.
- Ester-linked local anesthetics are metabolized in the serum, whereas amide-linked local anesthetics are metabolized in the liver.
- Clinically useful local anesthetics share a common structural framework composed of a lipid-soluble aromatic head, an intermediary carbon chain linkage, and a hydrophilic tail.
- The uncharged form of the local anesthetic most easily penetrates the neural membrane, whereas the charged form binds to the sodium channel receptor.
- Levorotary local anesthetic enantiomers are less likely to provoke CNS or cardiovascular system toxicity than either dextrorotary enantiomers or racemic mixtures of local anesthetics.
- Local anesthetics can have important clinical effects on ion channels and second messenger systems beyond the realms of local or regional anesthesia.
- Local anesthetics in high concentrations can be toxic to muscle and neural tissues and can cause cell death.
- The severity of systemic toxicity reflects the rate of appearance of local anesthetics in the plasma and the peak plasma level. CNS symptoms usually, but not always, precede cardiovascular symptoms.
- The administration of lipid emulsion, along with prompt advanced cardiac life support measures, has gained increasing acceptance as a first-line component of local anesthetic toxicity management.

Chapter Questions

1. What is the principal mechanism by which local anesthetics produce anesthetic blockade?
2. What influence does lipid solubility have on the pharmacodynamic behavior of local anesthetics?
3. Discuss the influence of pK_a on the onset of action of local anesthetics.
4. How does the linkage in the intermediate carbon chain affect the metabolism of local anesthetics?
5. Discuss three possible mechanisms by which local anesthetics cause neuronal injury.
6. What are the essential elements of preventing and managing local anesthetic toxicity reactions?

References

1. Butterworth JF, Strichartz GR. Molecular mechanisms of local anesthesia: a review. *Anesthesiology.* 1990;72:711–734.
2. Punke MA, Friederich P. Lipophilic and stereospecific interactions of amino-amide local anesthetics with human Kv1.1 channels. *Anesthesiology.* 2008;105:895–904.
3. Komai H, McDowell T. Local anesthetic inhibition of voltage gated potassium currents in rat dorsal root ganglion neurons. *Anesthesiology.* 2001;94:1089–1095.

4. Nau C, Vogel W, Hempelmann G, Brau ME. Stereoselectivity of bupivacaine in local anesthetic-sensitive ion channel of peripheral nerve. *Anesthesiology.* 1999;91:786–795.

5. Kawano T, Oshita S, Takahashi A, et al. Molecular mechanisms of the inhibitory effects of bupivacaine, levobupivacaine and ropivacaine on sarcolemmal adenosine triphosphate-sensitive potassium channels in the cardiovascular system. *Anesthesiology.* 2004;101:390–398.

6. Smith FL, Davis RW, Carter R. Influence of voltage-sensitive Ca^{++} channel drugs on bupivacaine infiltration anesthesia in mice. *Anesthesiology.* 2001;95:1189–1197.

7. Nebe J, Vanegas H, Schaible HG. Spinal application of omega-conotoxin GVIA, an N-type calcium channel antagonist, attenuates enhancement of dorsal spinal neuronal responses caused by intra-articular injection of mustard oil in the rat. *Exp Brain Res.* 1998;120:61–69.

8. Neugebauer V, Vanegas H, Nebe J, Rumenapp P, Schaible HG. Effects of N- and L-type calcium channel antagonists on the responses of nociceptive spinal cord neurons to mechanical stimulation of the normal and the inflamed knee joint. *J Neurophysiol.* 1996;76: 3740–3749.

9. Sluka KA. Blockade of calcium channels can prevent the onset of secondary hyperalgesia and allodynia induced by intradermal injection of capsaicin in rats. *Pain.* 1997;71:157–164.

10. Mio Y, Fukuda N, Kusakari Y, Amaki Y Tanifuji Y, Kurhara S. Comparative effects of bupivacaine and ropivacaine on intracellular calcium transients and tension in ferret ventricular muscle. *Anesthesiology.* 2004;101:888–894.

11. Hollmann MW, Strumper D, Herroeder S, Durieux ME. Receptors, G proteins, and their interactions. *Anesthesiology.* 2005;103:1066–1078.

12. Hollman MW, McIntire WE, Garrison JC, Durieux ME. Inhibition of mammalian Gq protein function by local anesthetics. *Anesthesiology.* 2002;97:1451–1457.

13. Hollman MW, Durieux ME. Local anesthetics and the inflammatory response: a new therapeutic indication? *Anesthesiology.* 2000;93:858–875.

14. Hollmann MW, Herroeder SH, Kurz KS, et al. Time-dependent inhibition of G protein-coupled receptor signaling by local anesthetics. *Anesthesiology.* 2004;100:852–860.

15. Benkwitz C, Garrison JC, Linden J, Durieux ME, Hollmann MW. Lidocaine enhances G_{ai} protein function. *Anesthesiology.* 2003;99:1093–1101.

16. Yanagidate F, Strichartz GR. Bupivacaine inhibits activation of neuronal spinal extracellular receptor-activated kinase through selective effects on ionotropic receptors. *Anesthesiology.* 2006;104:805–814.

17. Buxton ILO. Pharmacokinetics and pharmacodynamics: the dynamics of drug absorption, distribution, action, and elimination. In: Brunton LL, Lazo JS, Parker KL, eds. *Goodman and Gilman's The Pharmacological Basis of Therapeutics,* 11th ed. New York: McGraw-Hill; 2006:1–22.

18. Butterworth J. Clinical pharmacology of local anesthetics. In: Hadzig A, ed. *Textbook of Regional Anesthesia and Acute Pain Management.* New York: McGraw-Hill; 2007:112–115.

19. Catchlove RFH. Potentiation of two different local anesthetics by carbon dioxide. *Br J Anaesth.* 1973;45:471–474.

20. Ritchie JM, Greengard P. On the mode of action of local anesthetics. *Annu Rev Pharmacol.* 1966;6:405–430.

21. Wong K, Strichartz GR, Raymond SA. On the mechanism of potentiation of local anesthetics by bicarbonate buffer: drug structure-activity studies on isolated peripheral nerve. *Anesth Analg.* 1993;76:131–143.

22. Sinnott, CJ, Garfield JM, Thalhammer JG, Strichartz GR. Addition of sodium bicarbonate to lidocaine decreases the duration of peripheral nerve block in the rat. *Anesthesiology.* 2000;93:1045–1052.

23. Stoelting RK, Hillier SC. Local anesthetics. In: Stoelting RK, Hillier SC, eds. *Pharmacology and Physiology in Anesthetic Practice,* 4th ed. Philadelphia: Lippincott Williams & Wilkins; 2006:179–207.

24. Mulroy MF, Norris MC, Spencer LS. Safety steps for epidural injection of local anesthetics: review of the literature and recommendations. *Anesth Analg.* 1997;85:1346–1346.

25. Sinnott CJ, Cogswell LP III, Johnson A, Strichartz GR. On the mechanism by which epinephrine potentiates lidocaine's peripheral nerve block. *Anesthesiology.* 2003;98:181–188.

26. Kuipers JA, Boer F, de Roode A, Olofsen E, Bovill JG, Burm AGL. Modeling population pharmacokinetics of lidocaine. *Anesthesiology.* 2001;94:566–573.

27. Copeland SE, Ladd LA, Gu X, Mather LE. The effects of general anesthesia on whole body and regional pharmacokinetics of local anesthetics at toxic doses. *Anesth Analg.* 2008;106:1440–1449.

28. Mather LE, Runciman WB, Ilsley AH. Anesthesia-induced changes in regional blood flow. Implications for drug disposition. *Reg Anesth.* 1982;7(suppl):S23–S33.

29. Runciman WB, Myburgh J, Upton RN, Mather LE. Effects of anesthesia on drug disposition. In: Feldman SA, Scurr CF, Paton W, eds. *Mechanisms of Action of Drugs in Anaesthetic Practice,* 2nd ed. London: Edward Arnold; 1993:38–128.

30. Green NM. Distribution of local anesthetic solutions within the subarachnoid space. *Anesth Analg.* 1985;64:715–730.

31. Greene NM. Uptake and elimination of local anesthetics during spinal anesthesia. *Anesth Analg.* 1983;62:1013–1024.

32. Horlocker TT, Wedel DJ. Density, specific gravity, and baricity of spinal anesthetic solutions at body temperature. *Anesth Analg.* 1993;76:1015–1018.

33. Heller AR, Zimmerman K, Seele K, Rossel T, Koch T, Litz RJ. Modifying the baricity of local anesthetics for spinal anesthesia by temperature adjustment. *Anesthesiology.* 2006;105:346–353.

34. Kuhnert BR, Kuhnert PM, Philipson EH. The half-life of 2-chloroprocaine. *Anesth Analg.* 1986;65:273–278.

35. Raymond SA, Steffensen SC, Gugino LD, Strichartz GR. The role of length of nerve exposed to local anesthetics in impulse blocking action. *Anesth Analg.* 1989;68:563–570.

36. Gokin AP, Philip B, Strichartz GR. Preferential block of small myelinated sensory and motor fibers by lidocaine. *Anesthesiology.* 2001;95:1441–1454.

37. Liu SS, Joseph RS Jr. Local anesthetics. In: Barish PG, Cullen BF, Stoelting RK, eds. *Clinical Anesthesia,* 5th ed. Philadelphia: Lippincott Williams & Wilkins; 2006:453–471.

38. Strichartz GR, Sanchez V, Arthur R, Chafetz R, Martin D. Fundamental properties of local anesthetics. II. Measured octanol: buffer partition coefficients and pK$_a$ values of clinically used drugs. *Anesth Analg.* 1990;71:158–170.

39. Nau C, Strichartz GR. Drug chirality in anesthesia. *Anesthesiology.* 2002;97:497–502.

40. Lee-Son S, Wang GK, Concus A, Crill E, Strichartz G. Stereoselective inhibition of neuronal sodium channels by local anesthetics. *Anesthesiology.*1992;77:324–335.

41. Mazoit JX, Decaux A, Bouaziz H, Edouard A. Comparative ventricular electrophysiologic effect of racemic bupivacaine, levobupivacaine, and ropivacaine on the isolated rabbit heart. *Anesthesiology.* 2000;93:784–792.

42. Aya AG, La Coussaye JE, Robert E, et al. Comparison of the effects of racemic bupivacaine, levobupivacaine, and ropivacaine on ventricular conduction, refractoriness and wavelength. *Anesthesiology.* 2002;96:641–650.

43. Nau C, Vogel W, Hempelmann G, Brau M. Stereoselectivity of bupivacaine in local anesthetic-sensitive ion channel of peripheral nerve. *Anesthesiology.* 1999;91:786–795.

44. Vladimirov M, Nau C, Mok WM, Strichartz G. Potency of bupivacaine stereoisomers tested in vitro and in vivo. *Anesthesiology.* 2000;93:744–755.

45. Deschner B, Robards C, Somasundaram L, Harrop-Griffiths W. The history of local anesthesia. In: Hadzic A, ed. *Textbook of Regional Anesthesia and Acute Pain Management.* New York: McGraw-Hill; 2007:3–18.

46. Vath J, Kopacz DJ. Spinal 2-chloroprocaine: the effect of added fentanyl. *Anesth Analg.* 2004;98:89–94.

47. Casati A, Fanelli G, Danelli G, et al. Spinal anesthesia with lidocaine or preservative-free 2-chloroprocaine for outpatient knee arthroscopy: a prospective, randomized, double-blind comparison. *Anesth Analg.* 2007;104:959–964.

48. Zaric D, Christiansen C, Pace NL, Punjasawadwong Y. Transient neurologic symptoms after spinal anesthesia with lidocaine versus other local anesthetics: a systematic review of randomized, controlled trials. *Anesth Analg.* 2005;100:1811–1816.

49. Chung CJ, Choi SR, Yeo KW, Park HS, Lee SI, Chin YJ. Hyperbaric spinal ropivacaine for cesarean delivery: a comparison to hyperbaric bupivacaine. *Anesth Analg.* 2001;93:157–161.

50. Khaw KS, Kee W, Wong M, Ng F, Lee A. Spinal ropivacaine for cesarean delivery: a comparison of hyperbaric and plain solutions. *Anesth Analg.* 2002;94:680–685.

51. Nancarrow C, Rutten AJ, Runciman WB, et al. Myocardial and cerebral drug concentrations and the mechanisms of death after fatal intravenous doses of lidocaine, bupivacaine, and ropivacaine in the sheep. *Anesth Analg.* 1989;69:276–283.

52. Graf BM, Abraham I, Eberbach N, Kunst G, Stowe DF, Martin E. Differences in cardiotoxicity of bupivacaine and ropivacaine are the result of physicochemical and stereoselective properties. *Anesthesiology.* 2002;96:1427–1434.

53. Tsai T, Greengrass R. Spinal anesthesia. In: Hadzic A, ed. *Textbook of Regional Anesthesia and Acute Pain Management.* New York: McGraw-Hill; 2007:193–227.

54. Kaba A, Laurent SR, Detroz BJ, et al. Intravenous lidocaine infusion facilitates acute rehabilitation after laparoscopic colectomy. *Anesthesiology.* 2007;106:11–18.

55. Groudine SB, Fisher HAG, Kaufman RP, et al. Intravenous lidocaine speeds the return of bowel function, decreases postoperative pain, and shortens hospital stay in patients undergoing radical retropubic prostatectomy. *Anesth Analg.* 1998;86:235–239.

56. Koppert W, Weigand M, Neumann F, et al. Perioperative intravenous lidocaine has preventive effects on postoperative pain and morphine consumption after major abdominal surgery. *Anesth Analg.* 2004;98:1050–1055.

57. Martin F, Cherif K, Gentili ME, et al. Lack of impact of intravenous lidocaine on analgesia, functional recovery, and nociceptive pain threshold after total hip arthroplasty. *Anesthesiology.* 2008;109:118–123.

58. Omote K. Intravenous lidocaine to treat postoperative pain management novel strategy with a long-established drug. *Anesthesiology.* 2007;106:5–6.

59. Hollmann MW, Gross A, Jelacin N, Durieux ME. Local anesthetic effects on priming and activation of human neutrophils. *Anesthesiology.* 2001;95:113–122.

60. Kaczmarek D, Herzog C, Larmann J, et al. Lidocaine protects from myocardial damage due to ischemia and reperfusion in mice by its antiapoptotic effects. *Anesthesiology.* 2009;110:1041–1049.

61. Kiefer RT, Ploppa A, Krueger WA, et al. Local anesthetics impair human granulocyte phagocytosis activity, oxidative

burst, and CD11b expression in response to *Staphylococcus aureus*. *Anesthesiology*. 2003;98:842–848.

62. Sztark F, Malgat M, Dabadie P Mazat JP. Comparison of the effects of bupivacaine and ropivacaine on heart cell mitochondrial energetics. *Anesthesiology*. 1998;88:1340–1349.

63. Sztark F, Nouette-Gaulain K, Malgat M, Dabadie P, Mazat J. Absence of stereospecific effects of bupivacaine isomers on heart mitochondrial bioenergetics. *Anesthesiology*. 2000;93:4556–4562.

64. Nouette-Gaulain K, Sirvent P, Canal-Raffin M, et al. Effects of intermittent femoral nerve injections of bupivacaine, levobupivacaine, and ropivacaine on mitochondrial energy metabolism and intracellular calcium homeostasis in rat psoas muscle. *Anesthesiology*. 2007;106:1026–1034.

65. Johnson ME, Saenz JA, DaSilva AD, Uhl CB, Gores GJ. Effect of local anesthetic on neuronal cytoplasmic calcium and plasma membrane lysis (necrosis) in a cell culture model. *Anesthesiology*. 2002;97:1466–1476.

66. Kanai Y, Katsuki H, Takasaki M. Lidocaine disrupts axonal membrane of rat sciatic nerve in vitro. *Anesthesiology*. 2000;91:944–948.

67. Malinovsky JM, Charles F, Baudrimont M, et al. Intrathecal ropivacaine in rabbits: pharmacodynamic and neurotoxicologic study. *Anesthesiology*. 2002;97:429–435.

68. Johnson ME, Uhl CB, Spittler KH, Wang H, Gores GJ. Mitochondrial injury and caspase activation by the local anesthetic lidocaine. *Anesthesiology*. 2004;101:1184–1194.

69. Kitagawa N, Oda M, Totoki T. Possible mechanism of irreversible nerve injury caused by local anesthetics. *Anesthesiology*. 2004;100:962–967.

70. Kirihara Y, Saito Y, Sakura S, Hashimoto K, Kishimoto T. Comparative neurotoxicity of intrathecal and epidural lidocaine in rats. *Anesthesiology*. 2003;99:961–968.

71. Hashimoto K, Hampl KF, Nakamura Y, Bollen AW, Feiner J, Drasner K. Epinephrine increases the neurotoxic potential of intrathecally administered lidocaine in the rat. *Anesthesiology*. 2001;94:876–881.

72. Kishimoto T, Bollen AW, Drasner K. Comparative spinal neurotoxicity of prilocaine and lidocaine. *Anesthesiology*. 2002;97:1250–1253.

73. Zaric D, Christiansen C, Pace NL, Punjasawadwong Y. Transient neurologic symptoms after spinal anesthesia with lidocaine versus other local anesthetics: a systematic review of randomized, controlled trials. *Anesth Analg*. 2005;100:1811–1816.

74. Konig W, Ruzick D. Absence of transient radicular irritation after 5000 spinal anaesthetics with prilocaine. *Anaesthesia*. 1997;52:182–183.

75. Tong D, Wong J, Chung F, et al. Prospective study on incidence and functional impact of transient neurologic symptoms

associated with 1% versus 5% hyperbaric lidocaine in short urologic procedures. *Anesthesiology*. 2003;98:485–494.

76. Hampl KF, Schneider MC, Pargger H, Gut J, Drewe J, Drasner K. A similar incidence of transient neurologic symptoms after spinal anesthesia with 2% and 5% lidocaine. *Anesth Analg*. 1996;83:1051–1054.

77. Werdehausen R, Braun S, Essmann F, et al. Lidocaine induces apoptosis via the mitochondrial pathway independently of death receptor signaling. *Anesthesiology*. 2007;107:136–143.

78. Lirk P, Haller I, Colvin HP, et al. In vitro inhibition of mitogen-activated protein kinase pathways protects against bupivacaine and ropivacaine-induced neurotoxicity. *Anesth Analg*. 2008;106:1465–1464.

79. Dony P, Dewindle V, Vanderick B, et al The comparative toxicity of ropivacaine and bupivacaine at equipotent doses. *Anesth Analg*. 2000;91:1489–1492.

80. Takahashi R, Oda Y, Tanaka K, Morishima HO, Inoue K, Asada A. Epinephrine increases the extracellular lidocaine concentration in the brain. *Anesthesiology*. 2006;105:984–989.

81. Ladd LA, Chang DH-T, Wilson KA, Copeland SE, Plummer JL, Mather LE. Effects of CNS site-directed carotid arterial infusions of bupivacaine, levobupivacaine, and ropivacaine in sheep. *Anesthesiology*. 2002;97:418–428.

82. Copeland SE, Ladd LA, Gu X, Mather LE. The effects of general anesthesia on the central nervous and cardiovascular system toxicity of local anesthetics. *Anesth Analg*. 2008;106:1429–1439.

83. Clarkson CW, Hondeghem LM. Mechanism for bupivacaine depression of cardiac conduction: fast block of sodium channels during the action potential with slow recovery from block during diastole. *Anesthesiology*. 1985;62:396–405.

84. Rossner KL, Freese KJ. Bupivacaine inhibition of L-type calcium current in ventricular cardiomyocytes of hamster. *Anesthesiology*. 1997;87:926–934.

85. Lynch C. Depression of myocardial contractility in vitro by bupivacaine, etidocaine, and lidocaine. *Anesth Analg*. 1986;65:551–559.

86. Komai H, Lokuta AJ. Interaction of bupivacaine and tetracaine with the sarcoplasmic reticulum Ca^{2+} release channel of skeletal and cardiac muscles. *Anesthesiology*. 1999;90:835–843.

87. Litz RJ, Roessel T, Heller AR, Stehr SN. Reversal of central nervous system and cardiac toxicity after local anesthetic intoxication by lipid emulsion injection. *Anesth Analg*. 2008;106:1575–1577.

88. Warren JA, Thoma RB, Georgescu A, Shah SJ. Intravenous lipid infusion in the successful resuscitation of local anesthetic-induced cardiovascular collapse after supraclavicular brachial plexus block. *Anesth Analg*. 2008;106:1578–1580.

89. Mio Y, Fukuda N, Kusakari Y, Tanifuji Y, Kurihara S. Bupivacaine attenuates contractility by decreasing sensitivity of myofilaments to Ca^{2+} in rat ventricular muscle. *Anesthesiology.* 2002;97:1168–1177.

90. Tanz RD, Heskett T, Loehning RW, Fairfax CA. Comparative cardiotoxicity of bupivacaine and lidocaine in the isolated perfused mammalian heart. *Anesth Analg.* 1984;63:549–556.

91. Graf BM, Abraham I, Eberbach N, Kunst G, Stowe DF, Martin E. Differences in cardiotoxicity of bupivacaine and ropivacaine are the result of physicochemical and stereoselective properties. *Anesthesiology.* 2002;96:1427–1434.

92. Chang DH, Ladd LA, Wilson KA, Gelgor L, Mather LE. Tolerability of large-dose intravenous levobupivacaine in sheep. *Anesth Analg.* 2000;91:671–679.

93. Smith HM, Jacob AK, Segura LG, Dilger JA, Torsher LC. Simulation education in anesthesia training: a case report of successful resuscitation of bupivacaine-induced cardiac arrest linked to recent simulation training. *Anesth Analg.* 2008;106:1581–1584.

94. Ludot H, Tharin JY, Belouadah M, Mazoit JX, Malinovsky JM. Successful resuscitation after ropivacaine and lidocaine-induced ventricular arrhythmia following posterior lumbar plexus block in a child. *Anesth Analg.* 2008;106:1572–1574.

95. Warren JA, Thoma RB, Georgescu A, Shah SJ. Intravenous lipid infusion in the successful resuscitation of local anesthetic-induced cardiovascular collapse after supraclavicular brachial plexus block. *Anesth Analg.* 2008;106:1578–1580.

96. Rowlingson JC. Lipid rescue: a step forward in patient safety? Likely so! *Anesth Analg.* 2008;106:1333–1336.

97. Brull SJ. Lipid emulsion for the treatment of local anesthetic toxicity: patient safety implications. *Anesth Analg.* 2008;106:1337–1339.

98. Weinberg G. Lipid infusion resuscitation for local anesthetic toxicity: proof of clinical efficacy. *Anesthesiology.* 2006;105:7–8.

99. Rosenblatt MA, Abel M, Fischer GW, Itkovich CJ, Eisenkraft JB. Successful use of 20% lipid emulsion to resuscitate a patient after a presumed bupivacaine-related cardiac arrest. *Anesthesiology.* 2006;105:217–218.

100. Stehr SN, Ziegeler JC, Pexa A, et al. The effects of lipid infusion on myocardial function and bioenergetics in L-bupivacaine toxicity in the isolated rat heart. *Anesth Analg.* 2007;104:186–192.

101. Mazoit JX, Le Guen R, Beloeil H, Benhamou D. Binding of long-lasting local anesthetics to lipid emulsions. *Anesthesiology.* 2009;110:380–386.

Anticholinergics

Mary C. Karlet, PhD, CRNA

Introduction

Anticholinergics are drugs that block muscarinic cholinergic receptors. Nondepolarizing muscle relaxants block nicotinic cholinergic receptors on skeletal muscles at the neuromuscular junction. In this chapter anticholinergics specifically refer to *muscarinic* receptor antagonists, which competitively and reversibly block muscarinic receptors. These receptors are located primarily at parasympathetic nervous system (PNS) target sites, and blockade produces a reversal of many PNS actions.

Parasympathetic Mechanism of Action

The parasympathetic division of the autonomic nervous system is organized for discrete and localized discharge. It consists of preganglionic fibers that originate in the central nervous system (CNS) and postganglionic fibers that innervate specific effector organs, namely smooth muscle, cardiac muscle, and glands. Figure 10-1 highlights the basic organization of the somatic and autonomic nervous systems. Preganglionic fibers of the PNS originate in the midbrain, medulla oblongata, and sacral part of the spinal cord. Postganglionic PNS fibers originate in ganglia that are usually close to or within the innervated organ. In general, the PNS slows the heart rate (chronotropic effect), slows cardiac conduction time (dromotropic effect), stimulates gastrointestinal peristalsis and secretion, protects the retina from excessive light, and empties the urinary bladder and rectum. Table 10-1 outlines the innervated effector organs and clinical effects of parasympathetic nerves.

Muscarinic Receptors

The term "cholinergic" was originally proposed by Henry Dale in 1914 to describe neurons that released acetylcholine (ACh). In addition to being released from motor nerves at the neuromuscular junction, ACh is the neurotransmitter released from all preganglionic autonomic fibers. ACh is also released from postganglionic PNS fibers and a few postganglionic sympathetic fibers. Many neurons within the CNS release ACh at central synapses.

Dale investigated the pharmacologic properties of ACh and its receptors, and based on his studies using the plant alkaloids *Amanita muscaria* and *Nicotiana tabacum*, muscarinic and nicotinic receptors were identified (www.nobelprize.org). Muscarinic receptors are located on glands, smooth muscle, and cardiac muscle innervated by postganglionic fibers of the PNS. Activation of muscarinic receptors in the CNS helps regulate cognition, behavior, sensation, movement, and some autonomic functions. Muscarinic receptors are also located on presynaptic nerve terminals at autonomic nervous system ganglia. Activation of these "autoreceptors" decreases ACh release from presynaptic fibers, resulting in actions potentially paradoxical to end-organ effects.

Muscarinic ACh receptors have been further isolated to five distinct subtypes (M_1–M_5). Most organs, tissues, and

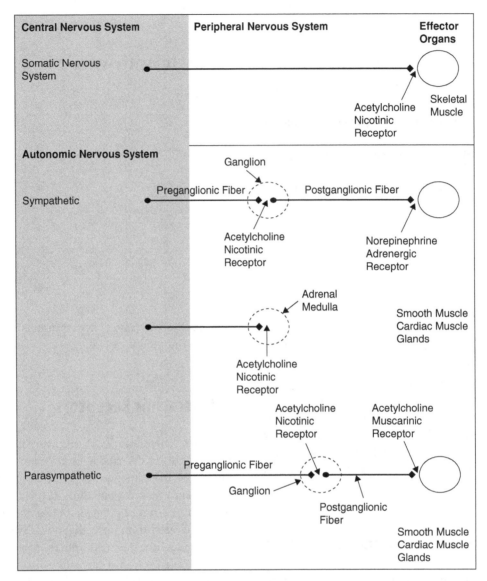

Figure 10-1 Organization of the somatic and autonomic nervous systems.

cells express multiple muscarinic receptor subtypes, but within a given organ one subtype may predominate. For instance, the M_2 receptor is the predominate muscarinic receptor subtype in the heart, whereas bladder contraction is primarily mediated by M_3 receptor subtype activation.[1] Table 10-2 outlines muscarinic receptor subtypes, their primary locations, and their functional effects.

Nicotinic receptors are ligand-gated ion channels (Na^+ and Ca^{2+}) that always produce depolarization and excitation. In contrast, all muscarinic receptors are metabotropic receptors that use G-protein–linked signaling mechanisms to produce excitation or inhibition dependent on the receptor subtype.

M_1, M_3, and M_5 muscarinic receptor subtypes appear to couple to the same G-proteins and signal through similar transduction pathways involving phospholipase C, with the generation of the second messengers diacylglycerol, cyclic AMP, or inositol triphosphate. Likewise, M_2 and M_4 muscarinic receptor subtypes couple through similar G-proteins and signal through similar pathways that lead to decreased cyclic AMP or activation of K^+ channels at the target site. Activation of M_2 and M_4 autoreceptors on preganglionic fibers of the autonomic nervous system is thought to represent a physiologic negative-feedback control mechanism for ACh release at autonomic ganglia.[1–3]

Table 10-1 Effector Organs and Clinical Effects of Parasympathetic Nerves

Parasympathetic Nerve	Effector Organ	Clinical Effect	Cholinergic Receptor Type
Midbrain			
CN III (Edinger-Westphal nerve)	Ciliary muscle in eye	Contraction for near vision	M_2, M_3
Medulla			
CN VII (facial nerve)	Submaxillary and sublingual glands Sphenopalatine ganglia	Enhanced secretion	M_2, M_3
CN IX (glossopharyngeal nerve)	Sphincter of the iris Salivary and lacrimal glands	Pupillary constriction Increased gland secretion	M_2, M_3 M_2, M_3
CN X (vagus nerve)	Esophagus, stomach, intestines	Increased motility and stimulation of secretion	M_2, M_3
	Lungs	Bronchoconstriction Bronchial gland stimulation	M_2, M_3
	Heart	Decreased heart rate Decreased S-A and A-V node conduction velocity Decreased contractile force (atria > ventricles)	$M_2 \gg M_3$
Sacral spinal cord			
Second, third, and fourth sacral spinal cord segments	Bladder	Detrusor muscle contraction; trigone sphincter relaxation	$M_3 > M_2$
	Rectum	Contraction	
	Male sexual organ	Penile erection	M_3

A-V, atrioventricular; CN, cranial nerve; M, muscarinic receptor subtype; S-A, sinoatrial.

Table 10-2 Muscarinic Receptor Subtypes

Muscarinic Receptor Subtypes	Location	Cellular Signal Transduction	Functional Effects
M_1	CNS Autonomic ganglia Glands (gastric and salivary) Lung	Activation of PLC → ↑ IP_3 and ↑ DAG → ↑ Ca^{2+} and PKC; depolarization and excitation	Enhanced cognition; autonomic ganglia depolarization; increased gland secretion; bronchoconstriction
M_2	CNS Smooth muscle (lung) Heart Autonomic nerve terminals	Inhibition of adenyl cyclase, ↓ cAMP; activation of K^+ channels → hyperpolarization and inhibition	↓ HR, ↓ conduction velocity; bronchoconstriction; negative feedback (autoreceptor) reduction of ACh release
M_3	CNS Smooth muscle (bladder, lung) Glands (salivary, mucous) Heart	Activation of PLC → ↑ IP_3 and ↑ DAG → ↑ Ca^{2+} and PKC; depolarization and excitation	Smooth muscle contraction (detrusor contraction and bronchoconstriction); ↑ gland secretion
M_4	CNS	Inhibition of adenyl cyclase, ↓ cAMP; activation of K^+ channels → hyperpolarization and inhibition	Autoreceptor and heteroreceptor-mediated inhibition of transmitter release; analgesia
M_5	Low levels CNS and periphery Predominant in substantia nigra	Activation of PLC → ↑ IP_3 and ↑ DAG → ↑ Ca^{2+} and PKC; depolarization and excitation	Facilitates dopamine release

cAMP, cyclic AMP; DAG, diacylglycerol; HR, heart rate; IP_3, inositol-1,4,5-triphosphate; PKC, protein kinase C; PLC, phospholipase C.

Source: Adapted from Brunton LL, Lazo JS, Parker KL. *Goodman and Gilman's The Pharmacological Basis of Therapeutics,* 11th ed. New York: McGraw-Hill; 2005.

Muscarinic Receptor Antagonists

Muscarinic receptor antagonists that are used in anesthesia practice may be classified as (1) naturally occurring tertiary amine alkaloids of the belladonna plants (atropine and scopolamine), (2) synthetic quaternized congeners of these alkaloids (glycopyrrolate), or (3) synthetic quaternized derivatives administered by inhalation (ipratropium and tiotropium).

Mechanism of Action

Muscarinic receptor antagonists produce their effects by competitively and reversibly binding to muscarinic cholinergic receptors at PNS neuroeffector sites on smooth muscle, cardiac muscle, and gland cells; at other muscarinic receptors in the CNS; and on preganglionic fibers in peripheral autonomic ganglia. The effects of anticholinergic compounds can be overcome if the concentration of ACh at the receptor site is increased sufficiently.

The actions of most anticholinergic agents used in clinical practice have low or no receptor subtype specificity. That is, these drugs do not have selectivity for one receptor subtype over another. Different organs do have different sensitivities to muscarinic receptor antagonism, but the differing anticholinergic actions are mostly quantitative in nature. Because of their nonspecific muscarinic receptor blocking actions, organ-specific effects of anticholinergic drugs used in clinical practice are probably due to their varying membrane permeability (quaternized compounds do not readily cross the blood–brain barrier or other biologic membranes) or to normal baseline target organ parasympathetic tone.[3]

The parasympatholytic effects of anticholinergic agents are dose dependent. Lower doses effectively blunt salivary and bronchial secretion and sweating. With larger doses, the PNS effects on the heart are blocked and the heart rate increases, and the pupils dilate and accommodation of the lens to near vision is inhibited. Still larger doses of anticholinergics are required to inhibit micturition, gastric hydrogen ion secretion, and the tone and motility of the gut.[3] Gastric volume and gastric pH are not affected by standard preoperative doses of anticholinergic drugs. At conventional doses, muscarinic receptor antagonists cause little blockade at nicotinic receptor sites.[3]

Clinical Pharmacology

Central Nervous System

Activation of muscarinic receptors in the CNS generally produces cortical arousal, and they are implicated in the regulation of memory processing. Lipophilic tertiary amines with central anticholinergic actions, such as atropine or scopolamine, result in varying degrees of excitement or depression depending on the dose administered. In the perioperative period, lipophilic antimuscarinics have been associated with an increased incidence of postoperative delirium and memory deficits, especially in the elderly.[4,5] Atropine administered at conventional dosages generally has limited CNS effects. Scopolamine, on the other hand, has prominent CNS depressant effects at low therapeutic doses because it more readily crosses the blood–brain barrier. Quaternary amine compounds, such as glycopyrrolate, produce little or no effect on the CNS because they have limited ability to penetrate the blood–brain barrier.[3]

Some anticholinergics, such as benztropine (Cogentin), are useful adjuncts to levodopa in the treatment of tremors associated with Parkinson's disease. They depress central cholinergic overactivity, which helps balance underactivity of dopaminergic pathways in the substantia nigra. These agents are also used to treat the extrapyramidal side effects associated with some antidopaminergic drugs such as metoclopramide.

Cardiovascular System

Anticholinergic agents reverse PNS effects on the heart by blocking M_2 receptors at the sinoatrial (S-A) and atrioventricular (A-V) nodes, producing an increased heart rate and facilitating A-V nodal conduction.[6] The PR interval is shortened on the electrocardiogram. The increased heart rate may not be tolerated in patients with coronary artery disease because of the associated increased myocardial oxygen demand and decreased oxygen supply.

Transient bradycardia may occur with low or even average atropine, glycopyrrolate, and scopolamine doses. This paradoxical slowing of the heart rate may be the result of blockade of presynaptic ACh autoreceptors with associated augmentation of ACh release at autonomic ganglia, potentially counteracting postsynaptic cholinergic receptor blocking effects at the S-A node. Most vascular beds lack significant parasympathetic innervation, and therefore muscarinic blockers have minimal effects on vascular tone at conventional doses.

The cardiac effects of muscarinic blockers are most evident in young healthy patients with intense vagal tone. At the extremes of ages, infancy and elderly, atropine may have minimal effects in raising the heart rate.

Respiratory Tract

PNS activation produces intense bronchial smooth muscle constriction and copious tracheobronchial secretion by activating M_2 and M_3 muscarinic receptors. Anticholinergics, on the other hand, produce bronchodilation, decrease airway resistance, and blunt vagal-induced hyperresponsiveness. The resulting bronchodilation increases physiologic dead space. These effects are most pronounced with atropine and are more likely to occur with aerosolized forms of anticholinergics. The ability of inhaled anticholinergics to reverse bronchoconstriction is the basis for their effectiveness in treating patients with chronic obstructive pulmonary disease (COPD). Systemically administered anticholinergics produce marked reduction of bronchial mucous secretion and impair mucociliary clearance. In the patient with asthma, mucociliary paralysis can be disadvantageous because inspissation of viscid tracheobronchial secretions can result in mucous plugs, an inability to clear the airways, and dangerous airflow obstruction.[3]

Gastrointestinal Tract and Exocrine Glands

Parasympathetic nerves enhance gastrointestinal motility by facilitating contraction of gastrointestinal smooth muscle. At high doses anticholinergic agents block this effect, resulting in decreased stomach, intestine, and colon motility and tone. At conventional preoperative dosages (atropine, 0.6 mg intravenously; glycopyrrolate, 0.2–0.3 mg intravenously), antimuscarinic drugs relax the lower gastroesophageal sphincter tone and therefore may place the susceptible patient at increased risk for aspiration.[7,8] Anticholinergic agents exert modest antispasmodic action on the gallbladder and bile ducts, but the effect is usually not sufficient to overcome opioid-induced sphincter of Oddi spasm.[3]

Secretions from lacrimal, gastric, pancreatic, intestinal, and salivary glands are diminished with the administration of anticholinergic agents. Salivary and bronchial glands are particularly sensitive to anticholinergic agents, and their administration can completely abolish PNS-induced secretion. Sweat glands normally receive cholinergic sympathetic innervation, and therefore sweat gland secretion is also blocked with anticholinergic drugs.[3] Decreased sweat gland secretion produced by anticholinergics may result in the inability to dissipate heat and result in temperature elevation, especially in young children.[3] Pirenzepine is an anticholinergic agent that appears to have some selectivity for blocking the M_1 receptor in gastric parietal cells, decreasing gastric hydrogen ion secretion.[9]

Eye

PNS activation produces constriction of the pupillary sphincter muscle of the iris and contraction of the ciliary muscles that control lens curvature. Ciliary muscle contraction causes loss of ability to accommodate to far vision.[3] Muscarinic receptor antagonists, on the other hand, dilate the pupil (mydriasis, photophobia) and interfere with near-vision accommodation (cycloplegia).[3] The name "belladonna" stems from the reported use of antimuscarinic plant alkaloids by Italian women to dilate their pupils for visual appeal.[3] Locally applied antimuscarinic eyedrops are used today to produce mydriasis for ophthalmologic procedures. Typical premedicant doses of systemic atropine have little ocular effects. In contrast, scopolamine causes mydriasis and cycloplegia at conventional doses. Of all anticholinergic agents used for preoperative medication, glycopyrrolate has the least effect on the eye.

Genitourinary Tract

Muscarinic activation through the PNS facilitates bladder evacuation by producing detrusor muscle contraction, increased voiding pressure, ureteral peristalsis, and trigone (internal) and external sphincter relaxation.[10] Muscarinic antagonists block PNS effects at the ureters and bladder. These features make anticholinergics useful for treating overactive bladder, ureter spasm, and urinary incontinence. In the surgical patient this may contribute to urinary retention in the postoperative period, a particular concern in the patient with prostate hypertrophy or bladder neck obstruction.

Clinical Uses and Indications

Perioperative uses for anticholinergic agents are summarized in Table 10-3. Different effects of anticholinergic agents used in the perioperative period are summarized in Table 10-4.

Atropine

Atropine is considered the prototypical antimuscarinic agent. Despite lacking specificity for particular muscarinic

Table 10-3 Perioperative Uses of Anticholinergic Agents

- Treatment of bradycardia
- Preoperative medication
- Concomitant use with anticholinesterase agents for reversal of nondepolarizing muscle relaxant–induced skeletal muscle paralysis
- Bronchodilation
- Prevention of motion-induced nausea
- Use for ophthalmic procedures (mydriasis and cycloplegia)
- Antagonism of parietal cell hydrogen ion secretion
- Relaxation of ureteral and biliary smooth muscle

Table 10-4 Comparative Clinical Manifestations of Common Anticholinergic Agents

	Atropine	Scopolamine	Glycopyrrolate
Tachycardia	+++	+	++
Bronchodilation	++	+	++
Sedation	+	+++	0
Antisialagogue effect	++	+++	+++

0, no effect; +, minimal effect; ++ moderate effect; +++ marked effect.

Source: From Morgan GE, Mikhail MS, Murray MJ. *Clinical Anesthesiology,* 4th ed. New York: McGraw-Hill; 2006.

receptor subtypes, atropine has variable dose-related effects on specific organs. Of the anticholinergic drugs used in clinical practice, atropine is the most effective for preventing or treating bradycardia. It is used in the perioperative period to help prevent or treat bradyarrhythmias and restore adequate hemodynamic status, especially in cases of excessive vagal tone. Bradycardia or A-V block may be associated with peritoneal stimulation, the baroreceptor reflex, pressure on the eyeball, extraocular muscle traction, and other vagal-mediated reflex responses. Atropine shortens the PR interval and may lessen an A-V conduction block when vagal overactivity is an etiologic factor.[3]

Preoperative use of atropine or its synthetic analogs for antisialagogue properties is not routine today. However, the ability of anticholinergic agents to reduce secretions in both the lower and upper respiratory tracts make them valuable adjuncts for managing specific patients or specific anesthetic and surgical procedures, including fiberoptic intubation, electroconvulsive treatments, bronchoscopy, and some airway surgeries.[11–13] (Atropine, 0.5 mg intravenously, has been described as useful for treating hiccups after laryngeal mask airway insertion.[14])

Atropine and, alternatively, glycopyrrolate are used in concert with anticholinesterase agents to prevent the parasympathomimetic effects associated with nondepolarizing muscle relaxant reversal with neostigmine, edrophonium, or pyridostigmine at the end of surgery. Because of its more rapid onset of action, atropine is best paired with edrophonium for skeletal muscle relaxant reversal, whereas glycopyrrolate should be used with neostigmine or pyridostigmine because of their similar onset times.[15]

Scopolamine

Scopolamine is a tertiary amine that crosses the blood–brain barrier. The CNS effects are prominent and usually consist of drowsiness and amnesia. A transdermal preparation of scopolamine is effective in protecting against motion-induced nausea and vomiting.[16] Its antiemetic effects are prophylactic. It is much less effective after nausea and vomiting has developed.[3]

Of the antimuscarinic drugs used in anesthesia practice, scopolamine is the most potent antisialagogue. The sedative and antisialagogue effects of scopolamine may be useful adjuncts to some anesthetics. Scopolamine depresses the reticular activating system and has additive effects with opioids, benzodiazepines, and anesthetics.

Scopolamine has pronounced ocular effects and is used in eyedrops for ophthalmic purposes. It should be used with caution as a preoperative medication in patients with glaucoma. Scopolamine has less vagolytic effect on the heart than atropine or glycopyrrolate.

Glycopyrrolate

Glycopyrrolate (Robinul) is a synthetic quaternary ammonium compound that does not readily cross the blood–brain barrier and thus has minimal or no CNS effects. It is a potent antisialagogue and is used in the perioperative period for specific procedures where inhibition of salivary and tracheobronchial secretion is desired without accompanying sedative effects. Glycopyrrolate's vagolytic effect on the heart is similar to the effects of equipotent doses of atropine but with a more delayed onset.[15] Its use in the prevention of perioperative aspiration is limited primarily by its ability to slow gastric emptying at higher doses and the observation that it decreases lower esophageal sphincter tone. It has a slower onset and longer duration of action than atropine and so is best used with neostigmine and pyridostigmine for attenuating the muscarinic effects of skeletal muscle relaxant reversal.

Ipratropium and Tiotropium

Ipratropium (Atrovent) and its derivative tiotropium (Spiriva) are quaternary ammonium compounds that are administered only by inhalation. They work by competitively inhibiting muscarinic receptors in the lung (M_1, M_2, M_3). When inhaled, their actions are restricted almost entirely to the airways. They do not cross the blood–brain barrier and have no effect on heart rate or intraocular pressure.

Tiotropium and ipratropium are indicated for maintenance treatment of bronchospasm associated with COPD, including chronic bronchitis and emphysema. Both agents improve forced expiratory volume and dyspnea when administered to patients with COPD.[17] Unlike systemically administered belladonna alkaloids or their derivatives, ipratropium and tiotropium have the advantage of not inhibiting mucociliary clearance.[17]

Ipratropium is approved by the U.S. Food and Drug Administration for the treatment of common cold rhinorrhea.[17] Ipratropium is also prepared and marketed in combination with β_2-adrenergic agonists, such as an albuterol–ipratropium combination (DuoNeb, Combivent).

Ipratropium and tiotropium have similar qualitative effects. They differ most noticeably in their kinetics. Tiotropium binds to the M_1 and M_3 receptors 100 times longer and with greater affinity than ipratropium, producing a longer duration of action.[17] Dry mouth is the most frequently reported adverse effect for both drugs.[17]

Comparative Pharmacology: Dosage and Administration

Table 10-5 summarizes the packaging and dosages of commonly used anticholinergic agents.

Atropine

Atropine can be administered by the intramuscular (IM) or intravenous (IV) routes. It has an onset time after IV administration of approximately 1 minute and a duration of 30 to 60 minutes. Adult IV or IM doses of 0.4 to 0.6 mg are typical premedicant doses for antisialagogue or vagal blocking effects. Adult doses of 0.5 to 1.0 mg, up to a maximum dose of 3 mg, are used to treat intraoperative bradycardia. Approximately 18% of the drug is excreted unchanged in the urine.

Scopolamine

Scopolamine can be administered via the ophthalmic, oral, transdermal, IM, and IV routes. IV doses of 0.3 to 0.6 mg provide sedation, drying of secretions, and effective protection against motion-induced nausea and vomiting for up to 6 to 8 hours in adults. In pediatric patients, ages 1 to 12 years, 6 mcg/kg can be administered intramuscularly or intravenously every 6 to 8 hours as needed. A 1.5-mg transdermal disk behind the ear, applied at least 4 hours before surgery, can be used to control postoperative nausea and vomiting without intense drying effects or sedation. The transdermal patch is effective for up to 3 days. Scopolamine is metabolized almost completely by the body, and only about 1% is excreted unchanged in the urine.

Glycopyrrolate

Glycopyrrolate can be administered by the oral, IM, or IV routes. IV or IM premedicant doses for glycopyrrolate are 3 to 6 mcg/kg or 0.1 to 0.4 mg in adults. It has an onset after IV administration of 2 to 3 minutes and a duration of approximately 30 to 60 minutes.[15] Nearly 80% of the drug is excreted unchanged in the urine, and elimination is severely impaired in patients with renal failure.[18]

Ipratropium and Tiotropium

Ipratropium bromide is delivered as an aerosolized solution via a metered dose inhaler. The usual dosage of ipratropium inhalation solution is 500 mcg (one unit-dose

Table 10-5 Anticholinergic Agent Packaging and Dosages

Antimuscarinic Agent	Route	Packaging	Dosage

Atropine	IV	0.4 mg/mL, 1 mL
		0.1 mg/mL, 10 mL
		many other dilutions
			Premedicant
			  Adults: 0.4–1.0 mg, IV, IM
			  Children: 10–20 mcg/kg, IV, 30 mcg/kg, oral
			Reverse bradycardia
			  Adults: 0.5–1 mg, IV, up to 3 mg
			  Children: 10–20 mcg/kg

Scopolamine	IV	0.4 mg/mL, 1 mL	Premedicant
			  Adults: 0.3–0.6 mg, IV, IM
			  Children: 6 mcg/kg, IV, IM, subcutaneous
			Transdermal patch: 1.5 mg

Glycopyrrolate	IV	0.2 mg/mL, 1 mL	Premedicant
			  3–6 mcg/kg, IV, IM
			  Adults: 0.1–0.4 mg, IV, IM

Ipratropium	Inhaled	Solution 0.02% in 2.5-mL unit-dose vials (500 mcg unit dose)	500 mcg three to four times per day
Tiotropium	Inhaled	18-mcg capsules for use in HandiHaler inhalation device	18 mcg daily

vial) administered three to four times a day with doses 6 to 8 hours apart. In patients with bronchospasm associated with COPD, significant improvements in pulmonary function occur within 15 to 30 minutes, with maximum responses reached in 30 to 90 minutes. The effects persist for periods of 4 to 5 hours in most patients. Like most inhaled drugs, after administration about 90% of the drug is swallowed and excreted in the feces.[3,17,18]

Tiotropium is delivered as a dry powder by way of a HandiHaler device. Onset of action occurs 30 minutes after inhalation. Peak effects as measured by the maximum increase in forced expiratory volume in 1 second occur in approximately 2 to 3 hours. A typical dosage is 18 mcg. Tiotropium has a longer duration of action than ipratropium, 24 hours, allowing once-daily dosing. Metabolism occurs in the liver, and 7% of the unchanged drug is excreted in the kidney. The elimination half-life is 5 to 6 days. Tiotropium is Pregnancy Category C, and safety and efficacy in children have not been established.[17]

Side Effects and Contraindications

Overdosage from atropine or scopolamine (antimuscarinic agents that cross the blood–brain barrier) can produce a recognizable syndrome called central anticholinergic syndrome. Patients with anticholinergic toxicity exhibit an exaggeration of drug effects, including dry mouth, tachycardia, fever, and impaired vision. Cutaneous flushing (atropine flush) may occur as a compensatory reaction to dissipate heat induced by lack of sweating. CNS manifestations include restlessness, irritability, hallucinations, and unconsciousness. Delayed awakening from anesthesia and ventilatory depression may occur.[19,20] The mnemonic "blind as a bat, red as a beet, mad as a hatter, and dry as a bone" describes key features of the toxicity.

The cholinesterase inhibitor physostigmine, a lipid-soluble tertiary amine that crosses the blood–brain barrier, effectively counteracts the symptoms by increasing the amount of ACh available to compete for muscarinic receptor binding. An initial treatment dose is 15 to 60 mcg/kg. This dose may need to be repeated after 15 to 30 minutes because of the drug's rapid metabolism. Antimuscarinic effects of relaxing bladder smooth muscle can exacerbate urinary retention in susceptible patients, including those with prostate hypertrophy.

Muscarinic receptor blockers normally have little effect on intraocular pressure when administered systemically. Caution is warranted, however, in patients with glaucoma because intraocular pressures can rise in these patients with the administration of muscarinic antagonists, particularly

scopolamine. Glycopyrrolate is predominately excreted unchanged in the kidney and shows impaired clearance in patients with moderate to severe renal disease.

Drug Interactions

Many prescription and over-the-counter drugs used for the treatment of depression, the common cold, overactive bladder, or allergic rhinitis have anticholinergic properties. Certain antipsychotic drugs such as chlorpromazine (Thorazine) and prochlorperazine (Compazine) are relatively potent muscarinic antagonists. Tricyclic antidepressants and some antihistamine drugs can potentiate the effects of antimuscarinics because of their own muscarinic receptor blocking properties. Additive effects with antimuscarinics administered in the perioperative period can result in a substantial anticholinergic load and place patients at risk for toxicity.

Key Points

- There are five muscarinic receptor subtypes, each with specific locations, transduction mechanisms, and effects.

- Most anticholinergic agents in clinical use are not specific for particular receptor subtypes.

- Atropine is the prototypical anticholinergic agent.

- Systemically administered anticholinergic agents increase the heart rate and A-V conduction, inhibit gastrointestinal peristalsis and secretion, produce mydriasis and cycloplegia, and produce smooth muscle relaxation in the urinary bladder and bronchi.

- Caution is warranted when considering administration of antimuscarinic agents in patients with glaucoma.

- Ipratropium and tiotropium have antimuscarinic effects limited to the tracheobronchial airways.

Chapter Questions

1. Describe the organ or tissue location of muscarinic receptors.

2. List the main anticholinergic agents used in anesthesia practice.

3. What are the clinical manifestations of muscarinic receptor blockade?

4. What are the major features of central anticholinergic syndrome?

References

1. Westfall TC, Westfall DP. Neurotransmission: the autonomic and somatic motor nervous systems. In: Brunton LL, Lazo JS, Parker KL, eds. *Goodman and Gilman's The Pharmacological Basis of Therapeutics,* 11th ed. New York: McGraw-Hill; 2005:137–181.

2. Caulfield MP. Muscarinic receptors—characterization, coupling and function. *Pharmacol Ther.* 1993;58:319–379.

3. Brown JH, Taylor P. Muscarinic neurotransmission: the autonomic and somatic motor nervous systems. In: Brunton LL, Lazo JS, Parker KL, eds. *Goodman and Gilman's The Pharmacological Basis of Therapeutics,* 11th ed. New York: McGraw-Hill; 2005:183–200.

4. Bekker AY, Weeks EJ. Cognitive function after anaesthesia in the elderly. *Best Practice Res Clin Anaesth.* 2003;17: 259–272.

5. Silverstein JH, Timberger MB, Reich DL, Uysal S. Central nervous system dysfunction after noncardiac surgery and anesthesia in the elderly. *Anesthesiology.* 2007;106:622–628.

6. Dhein S, van Koppett CJ, Brodde OE. Muscarinic receptors in the mammalian heart. *Pharmacol Res.* 2001;44:161–182.

7. Cotton BR, Smith G. The lower oesophageal sphincter and anaesthesia. *Br J Anaesth.* 1984;56:37–46.

8. Ng A, Smith G. Gastroesophageal reflux and aspiration of gastric contents in anesthetic practice. *Anesth Analg.* 2001; 93:494–513.

9. Lambert DG, Appadu BL. Muscarinic receptor subtypes: do they have a place in clinical anaesthesia? *Br J Anaesth.* 1995; 74:497–499.

10. Fetscher C, Fleichman M, Schmidt M, Krege S, Michel MC. M_3 muscarinic receptors mediate contraction of human urinary bladder. *Br J Pharmacol.* 2002;136:641–643.

11. Brookman CA, Teh HP, Morrison LM. Anticholinergics improve fibreoptic intubating conditions during general anaesthesia. *Can J Anesth.* 1997;44:165–167.

12. Zhengnian D, White PD. Anesthesia for electroconvulsive therapy. *Anesth Analg.* 2002;94:1351–1364.

13. Tait AR, Malviva S. Anesthesia for the child with an upper respiratory tract infection: still a dilemma? *Anesth Analg.* 2005;100:59–65.

14. Kanaya N, Nakayama M, Kanaya J, et al. Atropine for the treatment of hiccup after laryngeal mask insertion. *Anesth Analg.* 2001;93:791–792.

15. Bevan DR, Donati F, Kopman AF. Reversal of neuromuscular blockade. *Anesthesiology.* 1992;77:785–805.

16. Honkavaara P, Saarnivaara I, Klemola UM. Prevention of nausea and vomiting with transdermal hyoscine in adults after middle ear surgery during general anaesthesia. *Br J Anaesth.* 1994;73:763–766.

17. Davis S, Schauer J. Tiotropium. *J Pharm Soc Wisconsin.* 2005; Jan/Feb.

18. Kirvela M, Ali-Melkkila T, Kaila, et al. Pharmacokinetics of glycopyrronium in uraemic patients. *Br J Anaesth.* 1993; 71:437–439.

19. Inoue H, Aizawa H, Takata S, et al. Ipratropium bromide protects against bronchoconstriction during bronchoscopy. *Lung.* 1994;172:293–298.

20. Link J, Papadopoulos G, Dopjans D, Guggenmoos-Holzmann I, Eyrich K. Distinct central anticholinergic syndrome following general anaesthesia. *Eur J Anaesth.* 1997;14:15–23.

Anticholinesterases

Courtney Brown, MSN, CRNA

After completing this chapter, the reader should be able to

- Understand the chemical and structural differences in effects on acetylcholinesterase.
- Differentiate the clinical indications for each of the anticholinesterases discussed.
- Name dosing regimens and combinations with anticholinergics.
- Identify monitoring methods for return of muscular function after neuromuscular blockade.
- Discuss the physiology behind the side effects of anticholinesterases.
- Differentiate the clinical classifications of myasthenia gravis.
- Discuss the newest uses of anticholinesterases aside from as a reversal agent.

Introduction

J. Pal conducted an experiment in 1900 that documented the first intentional reversal of curare poisoning via physostigmine, then found only in its natural plant form from dried ripe seeds of *Physostigma venenosum* or the calabar bean, which grows widely in West Africa.[1] Physostigmine, the first commercially available acetylcholinesterase inhibitor, was chemically synthesized in 1935 by Percy L. Julian. His pioneering research led to the process that made physostigmine and its derivatives readily available for the treatment of glaucoma, myasthenia gravis (MG), and anticholinergic toxic poisoning (as in some nerve agents used in biologic warfare); for the reversal of nondepolarizing neuromuscular blocking drugs; and for treatment of Alzheimer's dementia (AD). Other anticholinesterases were developed, including neostigmine, pyridostigmine, and edrophonium, and in this chapter we compare them pharmacologically with the prototype physostigmine. Echothiophate, an organophosphate, and its implications to anesthesia are also discussed.

Mechanism of Action

All anticholinesterases exert their pharmacologic effects by inhibiting the endogenous enzyme acetylcholinesterase (ACh-E) via differing mechanisms by which these drugs are classified (Table 11-1). A thorough understanding of the physiology of the myoneural junction (see Chapter 8) is inherent to understanding the pharmacologic action of anticholinesterases. The site of action of anticholinesterases can occur both pre- and postsynaptically. Once ACh-E is inhibited, acetylcholine (ACh) builds up within the synaptic cleft of the myoneural junction and competes with nondepolarizing muscle relaxants (NDMRs) for their sites of action on the nicotinic ACh receptor. ACh-E is one of the body's most efficient enzymes. One molecule can rapidly hydrolyze an estimated 300,000 molecules of ACh every minute into the biologic substrates of acetate and choline.[2]

The enzyme itself has an anionic site and an esteratic site that approximates the molecule of ACh (Figure 11-1). Anticholinesterases are classified by which area on the enzyme they exert their effects. Presynaptic effects, such as those associated with edrophonium and physostigmine, initiate ACh release and subsequent desensitization of the motor end plate.[3] Postsynaptic effects, such as those associated with pyridostigmine, neostigmine, and physostigmine, inhibit ACh-E action.[3]

The increased bioavailability of ACh is also responsible for both therapeutic and side effects. Consequently, an overabundance of ACh that would accompany an excessive dose of anticholinesterase also paradoxically increases skeletal muscle weakness through inhibition of the ACh receptor.[4,5] Therefore, because most anticholinesterases rely on hepatic metabolism or renal excretion, patients with renal or hepatic disease are at higher risk for muscarinic side effects and at less risk for *recurarization*, or return of muscle weakness.[6] Contraindications of anticholinesterases include presence of gastric obstruction, urinary tract obstruction, asthma, and peptic ulcers related to the additional muscarinic side effects associated with these drugs.[3]

Table 11-1 Comparative Pharmacokinetics of Anticholinesterases

Drug (Recommended Dosage)	Speed of Onset (min)	Elimination Half-Time (min)	Duration (min)	Site on ACh-E	Principal Site of Action
Physostigmine (0.05 mg/kg)	N/A	40	60	Esteratic	Postsynaptic
Pyridostigmine (0.35 mg/kg)	16	112	76	Esteratic	Postsynaptic
Neostigmine (0.05 mg/kg)	7–10	77	54	Esteratic	Postsynaptic
Edrophonium (0.5 mg/kg)	1–2	110	60	Anionic	Presynaptic

Source: From reference 2: Adapted with permission from Table 9-1 in Stoelting RK, Hillier SC, eds. Anticholinesterase drugs and cholinergic agonists. In: *Pharmacology & Physiology in Anesthetic Practice,* 4th ed. Philadelphia: Lippincott Williams & Wilkins; 2006.

Myasthenia Gravis

MG is a rare, autoimmune neuromuscular disorder (1:5000) in which T-cell–mediated antibodies target the postsynaptic nicotinic receptors of the myoneural junction. The disease commonly initially presents as fatigable weakness characteristically of the ocular muscles resulting in asymmetric ptosis and diplopia. A less common initial presentation involves the oropharyngeal musculature and limb weakness. The disease is characterized by severity of muscular weakness and muscle involvement (Table 11-2). New advances in pathophysiology have found two subtypes of MG. MG with circulating antibodies are seropositive. However, antibodies to muscle-specific tyrosine kinase have been found in patients with seronegative MG.[7] These patients often exhibit thymomas or thymic hyperplasia, although thymectomies have had varying outcomes.[7] Anticholinesterases have been used in this patient setting to increase muscle strength due to the increased bioavailability of ACh at the myoneural junction, mainly pyridostigmine and neostigmine given their longer

duration (Table 11-2).[8] Edrophonium is mainly used in this setting for diagnostic purposes with an 86% (ocular MG) to 95% (generalized MG) sensitivity (see Edrophonium, Clinical Indications and Usage, below), although electrophysiologic and serologic testing are frequently used with less side effects noted.[7] Improved drug regimens include adjuncts to allow for lower anticholinesterase dosages. These patients typically demonstrate resistance to depolarizing agents and sensitivity to NDMRs. Preoperative discussion with the patient should always cover potential postoperative ventilator support.

Alzheimer's Dementia

Nicotinic ACh receptors decrease in number and function in early AD and demonstrate decline even before diagnosis. The hippocampus is typically affected with this phase of the disease, termed mild cognitive impairment. Patients lose the ability to retain new memories. β-Amyloid peptides are

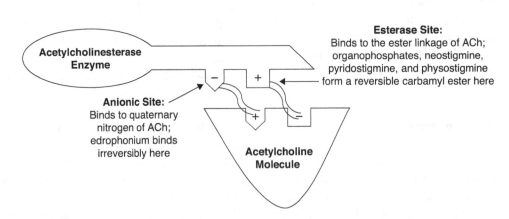

Figure 11-1 Acetylcholinesterase binding site.

Table 11-2 Myasthenia Gravis Foundation of America Clinical Classification

Class	Description	Muscles Involved
I	Ocular	Ocular
II	Mild general	
IIa		Predominately limb/axial muscles
IIb		Predominately oropharyngeal/respiratory muscles
III	Moderate general	
IIIa		Predominately limb/axial muscles
IIIb		Predominately oropharyngeal/respiratory muscles
IV	Severe general	
IVa		Predominately limb/axial muscles
IVb		Predominately oropharyngeal/respiratory muscles
V	Intubation	Generalized

Source: From reference 8. Adapted with permission from Table 1 in Jaretzki A, Barohn R, Ernstoff RM, et al. Myasthenia gravis: Recommendations for clinical research standards. *Neurology.* 2000;55:16–23.

also widely expressed in AD.[9] Given the pathophysiology involving receptors, researchers have been evaluating pharmacologic approaches to improving receptor transmission, including the use of anticholinesterases. Anticholinesterases approved by the U.S. Food and Drug Administration (FDA) in 2008 for the management of AD symptoms are donepezil, rivastigmine, and galantamine. These drugs are not administered by anesthesia providers; thus they are not discussed in detail.

Clinical Pharmacology

Physostigmine (Prototype)

- *Pharmacokinetics:* Physostigmine is the only compound in this drug class that is a tertiary amine, which allows this drug to cross the blood–brain barrier. This property makes this drug useful in the treatment of central anticholinergic syndrome (15–60 µg/kg intravenously). This drug peaks and decreases rapidly during the initial 5 to 10 minutes after injection. The pK_a value is 7.9 and is approximately 75% ionized at physiologic pH.

- *Pharmacodynamics:* Physostigmine forms a carbamyl ester complex at the esteratic site of ACh-E. This

produces reversible inhibition of ACh-E. Once ACh-E is carbamylated, it cannot hydrolyze ACh until this bond dissociates.

- *Metabolism:* This drug is hydrolyzed at the ester linkage. Approximately 90% is metabolized in the liver within 2 minutes of administration.

- *Elimination:* Renal excretion plays a minor role. Most physostigmine binds to high- and low-density lipoproteins in the plasma (29–43%).[3]

Clinical Uses and Indications

Physostigmine was the first anticholinesterase introduced for usage as a reversal agent for muscular paralysis. However, the dosage necessary to achieve reversal is no longer recommended and has limited its utility in this setting. As such, physostigmine is *no longer recommended as a reversal agent* and at plasma levels exceeding 10 µmol/L can directly inhibit variants of the ACh receptor.[4] This effect is reversed at low concentrations, where physostigmine potentiates nicotinic ACh receptor currents.[10] Physostigmine is effective in treating central anticholinergic syndrome (see Chapter 10) in dosages of 15 to 60 µg/kg intravenously as well as reversing somnolent effects of opioids and volatile agents after anesthesia at a dose of 2 mg intravenously. However, this may be accompanied by nausea and vomiting.

Central anticholinergic syndrome is more prevalent in the pediatric and geriatric populations, and this dosage range has been used in both populations.[11] Physostigmine also antagonizes somnolent effects of other drugs, such as tricyclic antidepressants, benzodiazepines, and phenothiazines, and reverses adverse central effects of ketamine (Table 11-3).[3] Physostigmine 2 mg has equivalent analgesic effects as meperidine of 50 mg[12] as well as equivalent reductions of postoperative shivering at a dosage of 40 µg/kg intravenously.

Comparative Pharmacology

Physostigmine is unique among other drugs in its class in the ability to cross the blood–brain barrier through the structural property of tertiary amine. Another unique quality is the rapid metabolism of this drug via ester hydrolysis, whereas the other anticholinesterases primarily are eliminated by renal excretion. Again, physostigmine is not recommended as a reversal to muscle paralysis after nondepolarizing agents. The Interdisciplinary Polyanalgesic Consensus Conference in 2007 identified physostigmine worthy of future study for the use of intrathecal

Table 11-3 Substances Known to Precipitate Central Anticholinergic Syndrome

Anticholinergics	Antispasmodic agents
Atropine	Clidinium
Scopolamine	Propantheline
Antihistamines	**Ophthalmic cycloplegics**
Promethazine	Cyclopentolate
Trimeprazine	Homatropine
Dimenhydrinate	Tropicamide
Antiparkinsonian	**Plants containing anticholinergic alkaloids**
Benztropine	*Atropa belladonna* (deadly night shade)
Biperiden	*Brugmansia* (angel trumpets)
Orphenadrine	*Cestrum nocturnum*
Procyclidine	(night-blooming jessamine)
Tricyclic Antidepressants	*Datura stramonium* (jimson weed)
Amitriptyline	*Hyoscyamus niger* (black henbane)
Butriptyline	*Solanum rostratum*
Clomipramine	(buffalobur nightshade)
Dosulepin	Mandrake (devil's apple)
Doxepin	Astragalus (loco weeds or seeds)
Imipramine	*Lycium barbarum* (matrimony vine)
Lofepramine	
Trimipramine	
Desipramine	
Nortriptyline	
Protriptyline	

administration given the performance of intrathecal neostigmine.[13] Physostigmine has been evaluated and found to protect against apoptosis, or programmed cellular death, in peripheral nerve injury models as a potential cause of neuralgia, or neuropathic pain.[14]

Neostigmine

- *Pharmacokinetics:* Neostigmine is a quaternary ammonium derivative of physostigmine and as such cannot cross the blood–brain barrier or be useful in the treatment of central anticholinergic syndrome. This drug peaks and decreases rapidly during the initial 5 to 10 minutes after injection. It is preserved with methylparaben and propylparaben (preservative-free solutions must be used for the off-label neuraxial administration).

- *Pharmacodynamics:* Neostigmine also forms a carbamyl ester complex with reversible inhibition of ACh-E. Once ACh-E is carbamylated, it cannot hydrolyze ACh until this bond dissociates.

- *Metabolism:* Neostigmine undergoes hydrolysis by cholinesterase and is also metabolized by hepatic enzymes. With anephric patients, or those without renal function, hepatic metabolism accounts for 50% of neostigmine with principal metabolite 3-hydroxyphenyl trimethyl ammonium with 10% the antagonistic properties of neostigmine.

- *Elimination:* Neostigmine is actively secreted into the renal tubules. Renal clearance accounts for 80% of elimination of neostigmine within the first 24 hours: 50% unchanged in urine and 30% as metabolites.

Clinical Uses and Indications

Neostigmine is widely used as a reversal agent after paralysis by nondepolarizing muscle relaxants. Because anticholinesterases can paradoxically cause muscle relaxation at greater than recommended dosages, the use of reversal agents is limited to the time period when a patient is spontaneously recovering from muscle paralysis. There must be evidence that this period is in effect; there must be a twitch present on train-of-four (TOF) assessment to reverse muscle paralysis associated with NDMRs. The dose recommended to reverse effects of neostigmine depends on the degree of paralysis by using TOF (Table 11-5).

Neostigmine and pyridostigmine have been prescribed in the treatment of MG. Because neostigmine is a quaternary ammonium, it does not cross membranes easily. The oral dosage is 30 times the intravenous dosage, with intervals every 2 to 4 hours to maintain muscular strength. However, at these dosages patients on oral neostigmine or pyridostigmine are particularly prone to developing cholinergic crisis (see below), a syndrome manifesting in excessive muscarinic and nicotinic stimulation from ACh.

Neostigmine has also been used in the treatment or prevention of urinary retention and constipation or bowel evacuation. Neostigmine increases gastric motility, but side effects often prohibit continuous usage.[15] When given postoperatively for the prevention of ileus, neostigmine 0.25 to 0.5 mg injected intramuscularly or subcutaneously is recommended (can continue every 4–6 hours over 2–4 days). The same dosage is used for urinary retention, although no more than five injections are recommended along with urinary catheterization as necessary. Neostigmine has also been used to relieve intestinal pseudo-obstruction, although this is off-label usage.[16] Another off-label usage is for bowel evacuation of spinal cord injury patients. The addition of neostigmine 2 mg intramuscularly or subcutaneously combined with glycopyrrolate 0.4 mg significantly ($P < 0.05$) accelerates the evacuation process for spinal cord injury patients from 98 to 74 minutes on average.[16]

Regarding neostigmine and postoperative nausea and vomiting, the literature provides conflicting evidence. In a meta-analysis of 10 randomized, controlled trials, Cheng et al. determined that there was insufficient evidence to conclude that neostigmine increases the risk of postoperative nausea and vomiting.[17] However, this is in direct contrast to a previous meta-analysis by Tramer and Fuchs-Buder that determined that in doses exceeding 2.5 mg, neostigmine increases the risk of postoperative nausea and vomiting.[18] In 2006 Gan reviewed the use of neostigmine as a "well-established" risk factor, citing Tramer and Fuchs-Buder as its only source to make this generic statement. Thus there is not a clear consensus on this topic.[19]

There have been case reports warranting caution with use of neostigmine in cardiac transplant patients. Due to surgical denervation of the heart, some reactions to neostigmine have included asystole,[20] which responded to atropine and epinephrine, to cardiopulmonary arrest, which required extracorporeal membrane oxygenation.[21] Other case reports involve development of a lengthened Q-Tc[22] and complete heart block[23] after reversal of paralysis. Thus in cases of cardiac transplant patients presenting for noncardiac surgery or patients with known lengthened Q-Tc interval, caution should be exercised when administering reversal.

Precautions

The package insert warns that neostigmine should be used with caution in patients with epilepsy, asthma, bradyarrhythmias, recent coronary occlusions, hyperthyroidism, peptic ulcer disease, and vagotonias.[15] Neostigmine should not be used to differentiate myasthenia crisis versus anticholinesterase overdosage (edrophonium is the drug of choice). Again, neostigmine is contraindicated in patients with mechanical intestinal or urinary obstruction and peritonitis.[15]

Comparative Pharmacology

Neostigmine has a slower onset than edrophonium for reversal of muscle paralysis; however, they have a similar duration of action. When combining with the anticholinergic, glycopyrrolate with a dosage of 0.1 mg/kg is typically chosen to match the onset time (2–3 minutes). If atropine is used at a dosage of 10 to 20 mcg/kg, early tachycardia is expected with the difference of onset of atropine versus neostigmine (1 vs. 7 minutes). Late bradycardia may follow as the duration of atropine is half that of neostigmine (30 vs. 60 minutes), potentially necessitating repeat dose. For this same reason it is recommended that the dosage of neostigmine not exceed the maximum of 0.7 mg/kg. Other characteristics known to impede reversal of neuromuscular blockade include aminoglycoside antibiotics, hypothermia, hypercarbia, acidosis,

alkalosis, hypokalemia, hypocalcemia, and hypermagnesemia. In comparison with older adults, neostigmine requires a higher plasma concentration to achieve the same clinical effects demonstrated in infants, children, and young adults.

Neostigmine and pyridostigmine, but not edrophonium, severely depress plasma cholinesterase activity. As such, these drugs should not be used *in the determination* of the ability to reverse a phase II block that may be precipitated by overdosage of succinylcholine versus plasma cholinesterase deficiency (see Chapter 8). In a case report where TOF was not monitored before reversal, administration of neostigmine resulted in 10 hours of ventilator support in a patient with undiagnosed atypical pseudocholinesterase after succinylcholine administration for intubation and vecuronium for maintenance.[5] However, should a phase II block be determined to be potentially reversible by an edrophonium test dose, either neostigmine or edrophonium may be used.

Neostigmine is the only anticholinesterase to be used in the treatment or prevention of acute pain, although this is off-label and must be a preservative-free solution (often comes prepared in methylparaben). The pharmacologic mechanism is derived from inhibition of ACh breakdown in the dorsal horn of the spinal cord or within the meninges.[24] In experimental studies, intrathecal neostigmine of 50 to 100 µg produced postoperative analgesia. However, there is an increased incidence of nausea and vomiting as well as pruritus and prolonged block. The epidural and caudal route is associated with less side effects (dosages of 1–10 µg/kg have been used experimentally)[24]; however, the optimum analgesic dosage has not yet been determined.

There have been case reports of bronchospasm with standard doses of neostigmine. However, this is normally the result of administration to a patient with asthma or reactive airway.[25]

Pyridostigmine

- *Pharmacokinetics:* Pyridostigmine is an analog of neostigmine. As such, it also cannot cross the blood–brain barrier or be useful in the treatment of central anticholinergic syndrome. This drug peaks and decreases rapidly during the initial 5 to 10 minutes after injection.
- *Pharmacodynamics:* Pyridostigmine also forms a carbamyl ester complex with reversible inhibition of ACh-E. Once ACh-E is carbamylated, it cannot hydrolyze ACh until this bond dissociates.
- *Metabolism:* With anephric patients, or those without renal function, hepatic metabolism accounts for 25% of pyridostigmine with principal metabolite

of 3-hydroxy-*N*-methylpyridium, which does not retain antagonistic properties.

- *Elimination:* Renal clearance accounts for 75% of elimination of pyridostigmine with the majority of the drug excreted unchanged.

Clinical Indications and Usage

Pyridostigmine, being closely related to neostigmine, has the same clinical indications of reversal of muscle paralysis after NDMRs and MG. The dosage used for reversal of NDMR is 0.35 mg/kg and like neostigmine is typically combined with glycopyrrolate. At plasma levels of 100 μmol/L, pyridostigmine directly inhibits the ACh receptor, warranting remaining within the recommended dosage.[4]

Comparative Pharmacology

Pyridostigmine has not been tested clinically in the treatment or prevention of chronic pain or central neuraxial blocks. As a treatment for MG, pyridostigmine is dosed every 3 to 6 hours; however, bromide toxicity (pyridostigmine bromide) can manifest as well as cholinergic crisis (see below). Again, pyridostigmine can severely depress plasma cholinesterase activity. As such, these drugs should not be used in the determination of the ability to reverse a phase II block that may be precipitated by overdosage of succinylcholine versus plasma cholinesterase deficiency (see Chapter 8). Of all the anticholinesterases, pyridostigmine has the slowest onset (16 minutes), indicating even greater propensity for early tachycardia associated with combining with atropine for reversal, although tachycardia has also been noted with glycopyrrolate. In comparison with older adults, pyridostigmine requires a higher plasma concentration to achieve the same clinical effects demonstrated in infants, children, and young adults.

Precautions

Pyridostigmine is contraindicated in patients with mechanical intestinal or urinary obstructions. Caution should be used in administration to asthmatic patients. Pyridostigmine, a common drug used in myasthenics, should not be used to distinguish cholinergic crisis, because this drug is typically the precipitating agent of this overdosage syndrome (see Edrophonium Test Dose [Tensilon Test], below).

Cholinergic Crisis

Cholinergic crisis is a toxic syndrome occurring as a result of an overdose in anticholinesterases (as in MG oral treatment) or organophosphates. The effects manifest from excessive ACh at muscarinic receptors as well as nicotinic receptors. Muscarinic effects include miosis, salivation, bradycardia,

wheezing or bronchoconstriction, loss of bladder or bowel control, and abdominal cramps. Nicotinic effects at the myoneural junction include muscle weakness, paralysis, or apnea as a result of desensitization. Central nervous system effects from excess ACh include level of consciousness changes, confusion, seizures, and ventilatory response changes.[26] To remember the effects of cholinergic crisis, the acronym SLUDGEM (salivation, lacrimation, urination, diaphoresis [or defecation], gastrointestinal, emesis, miosis) is used.

Organophosphates is a chemical characteristic of many substances used commercially, including insecticides, herbicides, lubricating oils and hydraulic fluids, and nerve agents used in warfare, such as soman, tabun, sarin, and VX. Physostigmine has been found to be protective if given prophylactically before exposure to organophosphates or nerve agents. It has also been proven useful after exposure when combined with atropine and oxime therapy and is superior to pyridostigmine in this capacity.[3] However, physostigmine is not FDA approved for prophylaxis. The FDA in February 2003 approved pyridostigmine for prophylactic treatment 30 minutes before expected exposure to organophosphates or nerve agents followed by atropine and oxime.[27,28]

The treatment of cholinergic crisis is to use anticholinergics that cross the blood–brain barrier. The Centers for Disease Control and Prevention through the Agency for Toxic Substances and Disease Registry recommends that with severe organophosphate poisoning or nerve gas exposure, adults should receive atropine 2 to 4 mg (or 35–70 μg/kg intravenously every 3–10 minutes until symptoms resolve[2]) and pralidoxime 600 mg intramuscularly for moderate or minimal symptoms, and atropine 6 mg and pralidoxime 1800 mg intramuscularly for severe symptoms (15 mg/kg intravenously over 2 minutes with repeat as necessary after 20 minutes[2]).[29] Oxime drugs such as pralidoxime (at the rate of 50–100 mg/min; usually the total dose does not exceed 1000 mg) reactivate ACh-E, whereas atropine attenuates the muscarinic and central nervous system effects.[29] Pralidoxime is better at counteracting effects at the myoneural junction and autonomic ganglia. Other treatments are selected based on symptoms such as mechanical ventilation and seizure prophylaxis. The pharmacologic treatment of organophosphate poisoning is known as A FLOP (atropine, fluids, oxygen, and pralidoxime).[29]

Edrophonium

- *Pharmacokinetics:* Edrophonium is a quaternary ammonium that lacks a carbamyl group. Edrophonium produces reversible inhibition of ACh-E by forming an electrostatic bond on the anionic site and a hydrogen bond on the esteratic site.

- *Pharmacodynamics:* Once ACh-E and edrophonium form this complex, it cannot hydrolyze ACh until this bond dissociates.

- *Metabolism:* With anephric patients, or those without renal function, hepatic metabolism accounts for 30% of edrophonium, undergoing glucuronidation and forming edrophonium glucuronide, a pharmacologically inactive compound.

- *Elimination:* Edrophonium follows first-order elimination in a two-compartment model. Renal clearance accounts for 75% of elimination of edrophonium. Dosage is not adjusted in anephric patients because elimination of NDMRs is also decreased.

Clinical Indications and Usage

Edrophonium is primarily used as a reversal agent at 0.5 to 1 mg/kg (not to exceed 40 mg); however, edrophonium has specific pharmacokinetic properties that alter how it is used. For reversal, the typical dose is directly related to information solicited from TOF stimulation (Table 11-3). For example, if there is greater than 90% twitch suppression, the dose should be 1 mg/kg (although neostigmine is preferable given greater than 90% suppression) (Table 11-5).

Edrophonium is also useful in determining a phase II block versus plasma cholinesterase deficiency after administration of succinylcholine. When a phase II block is suspected, a test dose of 0.25 mg/kg of edrophonium is administered. If the patient exhibits improvement in muscle strength as evidenced by TOF with this dose, the patient can be reversed with a full dose of either neostigmine or edrophonium. If, however, no improvement is appreciated, then plasma cholinesterase may be present in which anticholinesterase administration may further exacerbate.

Finally, edrophonium has been used to distinguish cardiac dysrhythmias, especially supraventricular in etiology, including those associated with Wolff-Parkinson-White syndrome, by slowing the heart through muscarinic effects of ACh. However, unwanted muscarinic effects should be anticipated, such as bronchospasm, wheezing, and secretions.

Edrophonium Test Dose (Tensilon Test)

Edrophonium is also used to differentiate inadequate anticholinesterase therapy versus cholinergic crisis in the myasthenic patient. Edrophonium 1 mg intravenously may be administered every 1 to 2 minutes up to a maximum of 10 mg (atropine should be immediately available). If improvement occurs, the cause of the muscle weakness is related to inadequate anticholinesterase therapy.[30] If there is increased skeletal weakness, cholinergic crisis is considered (Table 11-4).

Precautions

Because edrophonium is an anticholinesterase used to determine anticholinesterase overdosage versus myasthenic crisis, administration to the patient with anticholinesterase dosage may precipitate emergent intubation after worsened muscular weakness. As such, emergency airway equipment should be immediately available for the Tensilon test.

Edrophonium preparation contains sodium sulfite, which may cause allergic reactions as well as anaphylaxis. Sulfite sensitivity is seen at greater incidence in the asthmatic population. The stopper also contains latex and should be removed rather than punctured for administration to latex-sensitive patients.

Finally, although all anticholinesterases may cause bradycardia and heart blocks if not combined with an anticholinergic, edrophonium has a frequency of more than 10% of arrhythmias to include junctional rhythms, bradycardia, and tachycardia even when combined with an anticholinergic. Of those who develop arrhythmias, 85% had an onset within 2 minutes of administration, with 74% having resolution by 10 minutes after administration with vagal-mediated arrhythmias responsive to atropine.

Comparative Pharmacology

Because edrophonium has the fastest onset (1–2 minutes), it is commonly used in combination with atropine, as in the commercially prepared Enlon Plus™. In contrast, combination with glycopyrrolate with a slower onset may result in early bradycardia and late tachycardia. Edrophonium undergoes conjugation in the liver; thus patients in liver failure warrant further consideration.

Table 11-4 Outcomes of Tensilon Test

Characteristics	Myasthenic Response	Nondiagnostic	Cholinergic Response (Suspect Overdose of Anticholinesterases)
Muscle strength (ocular, dysphonia or dysphagia, dysarthria, respiration, and limb strength)	Increased	No change	Decreased
Fasciculations (eye, facial muscles, or limb muscles)	Absent	Present or absent	Present or absent
Cholinergic symptoms	Absent	Minimal	Severe

As a quaternary ammonium, edrophonium does not cross the blood–brain barrier and is of little use in anticholinergic syndrome. However, it is unique in its diagnostic ability in myasthenic crisis versus inadequate anticholinesterase therapy as well as the differentiation of phase II block versus plasma cholinesterase deficiency. In comparison with younger adults, edrophonium requires a higher plasma concentration to achieve the same effects in the elderly. However, any muscarinic side effects associated with anticholinesterases are milder with edrophonium than with other anticholinesterases.

Echothiophate

- *Pharmacokinetics:* Echothiophate is an organophosphate that forms a stable complex with ACh-E, rendering it inactive on both the esteratic site and the anionic portion. The dosages and concentrations available include 5-mL dropper vials with each drop containing (concentration) 1.5 mg (0.03%), 3 mg (0.06%), 6.25 mg (0.125%), or 12.5 mg (0.25%).
- *Pharmacodynamics:* A topical dose when applied produces long-acting miosis and reduces intraocular pressure by increasing aqueous humor flow.
- *Metabolism:* Once ACh-E and echothiophate form the inactive complex, no metabolism of this complex occurs; it is inert.

Clinical Indications and Usage

Echothiophate is used primarily in the treatment of narrow-angle and wide-angle glaucoma when short-acting anticholinesterases or topical β-adrenergic blockers have failed to reduce intraocular pressure. Maximum effects appear within 4 to 6 hours and last up to 24 hours. However, miosis and decreases in intraocular pressure, which usually lasts 24 to 48 hours, can persist for weeks.

Comparative Pharmacology and Precautions

This drug is the only organophosphate discussed, with long-acting effects related to the irreversible inhibition of ACh-E. There is one side effect for which the anesthetist should be acutely aware: Echothiophate severely depresses plasma cholinesterase and red blood cell esterases. Thus extreme caution should be exercised before administration of succinylcholine. When used in combination with patients on echothiophate therapy, prolonged muscle paralysis and phase II block have been reported. Echothiophate is contraindicated in patients with active uveal inflammation, hypersensitivity, and most closed-angle glaucomas (may increase angle block). Echothiophate is used cautiously in patients with MG because anticholinesterases may have additive effects with ecothiophate therapy. A history of retinal detachment is also a precaution with therapy.

On the Horizon

A newly discovered cholinergic anti-inflammatory pathway has opened research into the use of anticholinesterases for the treatment of septic conditions. Physostigmine (80 µg/kg) was shown to improve survival time from 69 ± 12.3 hours to 131.8 ± 12.6 hours in experimental sepsis in a murine model.[31]

Train-of-Four

TOF nerve stimulation is used to evaluate the degree of surgical muscle paralysis and guides dosing of NDMRs (see Chapter 8). It is recommended that before extubation, full recovery from neuromuscular blockade is achieved (TOF ratio > 0.9). TOF ratios of 0.7 to 0.9 have demonstrated impaired airway reflexes, hypoxia, decreased ventilation, as well as airway obstruction.[32] TOF is also used to determine the timing of reversal administration (Table 11-5) and to detect residual paralysis.

In addition to TOF, other monitoring methods at the anesthetist's disposal give clinical indication of resolution of paralysis that are more reliable than TOF, including double-burst stimulation, 100-Hz tetany, acceleromyographic TOF, and mechanomyographic TOF. Double-burst stimulation and 100-Hz tetany are functions typically included on nerve stimulators. Mechanomyography TOF and acceleromyographic TOF both require a specialized nerve stimulator; mechanomyography is the most reliable but costly. Thus all other methods are frequently compared with this method as a means of assessing reliability. Residual neuromuscular

Table 11-5 Recommended Doses of Neostigmine and Edrophonium According to Train-of-Four

TOF Twitches/4	Fade	Neostigmine Dose (mg/kg)	Edrophonium Dose (mg/kg) Maximum dose: 40 mg
< 2	++++	0.07	1.0
3–4	+++	0.04	0.5
4	++	0.04	0.5
4	+	0.04	0.25

Source: From reference 2. Adapted with permission from Table 9-3 in Stoelting RK, Hillier SC, eds. Anticholinesterase drugs and cholinergic agonists. In: *Pharmacology & Physiology in Anesthetic Practice,* 4th ed. Philadelphia: Lippincott Williams & Wilkins; 2006.

blockade can occur when mechanomyographic TOF yields a fade ratio of less than 0.9. Because TOF does not yield a visual or tactile fade between 0.4 and 0.9, it is an unreliable method for determining if residual paralysis is present. Double-burst stimulation can detect residual paralysis at TOF 0.6 to 0.7, again not meeting the gold standard of 0.9. 100-Hz tetany has had conflicting evidence as to what ratio it determines residual paralysis (range 0.4–0.9).[33,34] Often, the acceleromyography TOF yields a ratio of 1.0 when mechanomyography TOF is 0.9. Thus to determine absence of residual blockade, a ratio of 1.0 is recommended.[33]

Because many institutions do not use acceleromyography-enabled nerve stimulators, the anesthetist should use standard TOF, double-burst stimulation, and clinical indicators to make a judgment that residual paralysis is not present. The anesthetist should factor spontaneous tidal volume, sustained head lift, and negative inspiratory pressure in the decision to extubate. *When in doubt, do not take the tube out.*

Key Points

- Anticholinesterases are used in the reversal of NDMRs; the treatment of MG, glaucoma, anticholinergic toxicity, and organophosphate poisoning; as well as a stimulant for urinary retention and constipation or prevention of postoperative ileus.
- Physostigmine crosses the blood–brain barrier and as such is useful in the treatment of central anticholinergic syndrome, as well as shivering and somnolence associated with other medical treatment.
- Neostigmine, pyridostigmine, and echothiophate therapy depress plasma cholinesterase activity and prolong the duration of succinylcholine. Edrophonium does not depress plasma cholinesterase.
- Edrophonium is a useful medicinal diagnostic in the form of the Tensilon test. It can be used to differentiate anticholinesterase overdosage (cholinergic crisis) versus myasthenic crisis and phase II block versus plasma cholinesterase deficiency after succinylcholine administration.
- Side effects associated with all anticholinesterases are a consequence of the abundance of ACh that results from administration. They can be classified as muscarinic (lacrimation, meiosis, increased secretions, abdominal cramps, blurred vision, bradycardia, bronchoconstriction, sweating, vomiting, urination, defecation, and/or diarrhea) or nicotinic (muscle cramps, fasciculations, hypertension or hypotension, and/or muscle weakness).

Chapter Questions

1. Which anticholinesterases are preferred for the treatment of MG? Why?
2. What are the possible anesthetic implications of administering an anticholinesterase before an NDMR?
3. How does the chemical binding of anticholinesterases affect ACh? How does each anticholinesterase affect ACh-E?
4. What structural property allows physostigmine to cross the blood–brain barrier? Do you know other drugs with this chemical structure?
5. What effect does renal insufficiency have on anticholinesterases? Are all anticholinesterases renally excreted?
6. Can you prophylactically prevent the effect neostigmine has on the denervated heart? How?
7. Which anticholinergic should be combined with which anticholinesterase? Why? What are the effects of the wrong choice in combination?
8. Which anticholinesterases have shown promise in the treatment or prevention of chronic pain? What is the mechanism? Is this FDA approved?
9. Describe how the Tensilon test is used. What syndromes can it diagnose and not diagnose?
10. What are the implications of giving a patient who is on echothiophate succinylcholine? How would you treat the results?
11. What is the most reliable test of depth of paralysis? Of return of airway reflexes?

References

1. Nickalls R, Nickalls E. The first reversal of curare. *Anaesthesia.* 2007;40:572–573.
2. Stoelting RK, Hillier SC, eds. Anticholinesterase drugs and cholinergic agonists. In: *Pharmacology & Physiology in Anesthetic Practice,* 4th ed. Philadelphia: Lippincott Williams & Wilkins; 2006: 251–265.
3. Triggle D, Mitchell J, Filler R. The pharmacology of physostigmine. *CNS Drug Rev.* 1998;4:87–136.
4. Sung J-J, Kim S, Lee H, et al. Anticholinesterase induces nicotinic receptor modulation. *Muscle Nerve.* 1998;21:1135–1144.
5. Ramirez J, Sprung J, Keegan M, Hall B, Bourke D. Neostigmine-induced prolonged neuromuscular blockade in a patient with atypical pseudocholinesterase. *J Clin Anesth.* 2004;17:221–224.
6. Craig R, Hunter J. Neuromuscular blocking drugs and their antagonists in patients with organ disease. *Anaesthesia.* 2009;64 (suppl 4):55–65.

7. Juel V, Massey J. Review: myasthenia gravis. *Orph J Rare Dis.* 2007;2:44.

8. Jaretzki A, Barohn R, Ernstoff RM, et al. Myasthenia gravis: Recommendations for clinical research standards. *Neurology.* 2000;55:16–23.

9. Woodruff-Pak D. Preclinical experiments on cognition enhancement in Alzheimer's disease: drugs affecting nicotinic acetylcholine receptors. *Drug Dev Res.* 2002;56:335–346.

10. Zwart R, van Kleef R, Gotti C, Smulders C, Vijverberg H. Competitive potentiation of acetylcholine effects on neuronal nicotinic receptors by acetylcholinesterase-inhibiting drugs. *J Neurochem.* 2000;75:2492–2500.

11. Schultz U, Idelberger R, Rossaint R, Buhre W. Central anticholinergic syndrome in a child undergoing circumcision. *Acta Anaesth Scand.* 2002;46:224–226.

12. Röhm K, Riechmann J, Boldt J, Schuler S, Suttner S, Piper S. Physostigmine for the prevention of postanaesthestic shivering following general anaesthesia—a placebo-controlled comparison with nefopam. *Anaesthesia.* 2005;60:433–438.

13. Deer T, Krames E, Hassenbusch S, et al. Future directions for intrathecal pain management: a review and update from the Interdisciplinary Polyanalgesic Consensus Conference 2007. *Neuromodulation: Technology at the Neural Interface.* 2007;11(2):92–97.

14. Manelli L, Bartolini A, Ghelardini C. Neuropathy-induced apoptosis: protective effect of physostigmine. *J Neurosci Res.* 2009;87:1871–1876.

15. Zeinali F, Stulberg J, Delaney C. Pharmacological management of postoperative ileus. *Can J Surg.* 2009;52:153–157.

16. Rosman A, Chaparala G, Monga A, Spungen A, Bauman W, Korsten M. Intramuscular neostigmine and glycopyrrolate safely accelerated bowel evacuation in patients with spinal cord injury and defecatory disorders. *Dig Dis Sci.* 2008;53:2710–2713.

17. Cheng C-R, Sessler D, Apfel C. Does neostigmine administration produce a clinically important increase in postoperative nausea and vomiting? *Anesth Analg.* 2005;101:1349–1355.

18. Tramer M, Fuchs-Buder T. Omitting antagonism of neuromuscular block: effect on postoperative nausea and vomiting and risk of residual paralysis: a systematic review. *Br J Anaesth.* 1999;82:379–386.

19. Gan T. Risk factors for postoperative nausea and vomiting. *Anesth Analg.* 2006;102:1884–1898.

20. Bjerke R, Mangione M. Asystole after intravenous neostigmine in a heart transplant recipient. *Can J Anesth.* 2001;48:305–307.

21. Sawasdiwipachai P, Laussen P, McGowan F, Smoot L, Casta A. Cardiac arrest after neuromuscular blockade reversal in a heart transplant infant. *Anesthesiology.* 2007;107:663–665.

22. Shields J. Heart block and prolonged Q-Tc interval following muscle relaxant reversal: a case report. *AANA J.* 2008;76:41–45.

23. Lonsdale M, Stuart J. Complete heart block following glycopyrronium/neostigmine mixture. *Anaesthesia.* 1989;44:448–449.

24. Habib A, Gan T. Use of neostigmine in the management of acute postoperative pain and labour pain: a review. *CNS Drugs.* 2006;20:821–839.

25. Hatjia H. Bronchospasm caused by neostigmine [Letter]. *Eur J Anaesth.* 2006;23:80–87.

26. Centers for Disease Control and Prevention. Case definition: nerve agents or organophosphates. Available at: http://www.bt.cdc.gov/agent/nerve/casedef.asp. Accessed June 15, 2009.

27. Petroianu G, Hasan M, Nurulain S, Arafat M, Shafiullah M, Naseer O. Protective agents in acute high-dose organophosphate exposure: comparison of ranitidine with pralidoxime in rats. *J Appl Toxicol.* 2005;25:68–73.

28. Petroianu G, Hasan M, Nurulain S, Arafat K, Sheen R, Nagalkerke N. Comparison of two pre-exposure treatment regimens in acute organophosphate (paraoxon) poisoning in rats: tiapride vs. pyridostigmine. *Toxicol Appl Pharmacol.* 2007;219:235–240.

29. Agency for Toxic Substances and Disease Registry. Medical management guidelines for nerve agents: tabun (GA); sarin (GB); soman (GD); and VX. Available at: http://www.atsdr.cdc.gov/MHMI/mmg166.html. Accessed June 20, 2009.

30. Pascuzzi R. The edrophonium test. *Semin Neurol.* 2003;23:83–87.

31. Hofer S, Eisenbach C, Lokic IK, et al. Pharmacologic cholinesterase inhibition improves survival in experimental sepsis. *Crit Care Med.* 2008;36:404–408.

32. Murphy G, Szokol J, Marymont J, Franklin M, Avram M, Vender J. Residual paralysis at the time of tracheal extubation. *Anesth Analg.* 2005;100:1840–1845.

33. Capron F, Fortier L, Racine S, Donati F. Tactile fade detection with hand or wrist stimulation using train-of-four, double-burst stimulation, 50-hertz tetanus, 100-hertz tetanus, and acceleromyography. *Anesth Analg.* 2006;102:1578–1584.

34. Samet A, Capron F, All F, Meistelman C, Fuchs-Buder T. Single acceleromyographic train-of-four, 100-hertz tetanus or double-burst stimulation: which test performs better to detect residual paralysis? *Anesthesiology.* 2005;102:51–56.

Inhalation Anesthesia

John M. O'Donnell, DrPH, MSN, RN, CRNA

Objectives

After completing this chapter, the reader should be able to

- Recognize the historic impact of the development of inhalation anesthesia on care delivery and in relief of human suffering.
- Review the possible mechanisms of action of inhaled anesthetics.
- Review the pharmacodynamic principles related to inhaled anesthetics, including potency, minimal alveolar concentration, and system-by-system effects.
- Review the pharmacokinetic principles related to inhaled anesthetics, including solubility, equilibration, uptake, distribution, concentration effect, second gas effect, metabolism, and elimination.
- Identify other issues related to use of inhaled anesthetics, including differences by system, rare toxicity events, and environmental concerns.

Introduction

Inhalation anesthetics are the most commonly used drugs in administration of general anesthesia and have unique characteristics relative to handling and administration. Their use requires anesthesia providers to develop a unique body of knowledge and skill. Anesthetists must understand the intricacies of inhalation delivery systems (anesthesia gas machine, vaporizers, circuit) as well as the complexities of the uptake and distribution of inhaled anesthetics. Despite more than 150 years of use and recent intense investigation in attempting to identify a specific mechanism of action, inhaled anesthetics remain a conundrum. An appreciation of the target system effects (brain) and the consequent impact on other systems (side effects and toxicities) relative to the various agents are necessary for the process of drug selection, administration, and estimation of the recovery profile. Finally, an understanding of the historic context of inhalation anesthetic discovery and the evolution of the development of modern inhaled anesthetics provides perspective on how far this core component of anesthesia practice has advanced and yet in some ways has remained the same since the 1840s.

Historic Context of Inhalation Anesthetics

The evolution and use of inhaled anesthetics parallel advances in medicine and demonstrate that scientific advances are sometimes happenstance and often require advances in other fields (Table 12-1). Many experts consider the discovery of the anesthetic properties of ether and other inhaled anesthetics to be the single most important advance in medicine to reduce human suffering in the last two centuries. Before 1846 the prospect of entering the hospital and undergoing a surgical procedure was rightfully dreaded because it promised pain and suffering of a nature so extreme as to be nearly unthinkable. In *Ether Day: The Strange Tale of America's Greatest Medical Discovery and the Haunted Men Who Made It,* Fenster provides a window on this suffering and quotes a letter to the famous Scottish surgeon James Simpson to illustrate this perspective: "Suffering so great as I underwent cannot be expressed in words. The blank whirlwind of emotion, the horror of great darkness, and the sense of desertion by god and man, bordering close upon despair, which swept through my mind and overwhelmed my heart, I can never forget."[1]

Discovery of Nitrous Oxide, Ether, and Chloroform

Before the first demonstration of the surgical use of ether, the alternatives were bleak for patients undergoing surgical procedures. The quality of a surgeon was often determined by the speed of his procedures, and surgical training was,

Table 12-1 Timeline for the Synthesis or Introduction of Inhaled Anesthetic Agents

Year	Historic Figure	Comment
1540	Valerius Cordus	Synthesizes "sulfuric" ether
1540	Paracelsus	Writes of the pain-relieving qualities of ether Distills laudanum
1774	Joseph Priestly	Synthesizes nitrous oxide
1800	Humphrey Davy	Nitrous oxide manuscript in which he suggests a possible use in relief of surgical pain
1831–1832	Samuel Guthrie (U.S.) Jean Baptiste-Andre Dumas (France) Eugene Soubeiran (France)	Synthesis of chloroform occurs independently and concurrently in three locations
1800–1845	Multiple scientists, students, and the public	Widespread use of nitrous oxide and ether for frolics and exhibitions
1842	Crawford W. Long	Uses ether successfully for surgical procedures Does not publish until 1848
1845	Horace Wells	Unsuccessful demonstration of the use of nitrous oxide for surgical anesthesia
1846	William T. G. Morton	Successfully demonstrates the use of "letheon" (sulfuric ether with orange oil) as a surgical anesthetic Surgeon is John Collins Warren
1847	James Young Simpson	Uses chloroform for relief of the pain of childbirth
1920–1940	Multiple investigators	Divinyl ether, ethylene, ethyl chloride, cyclopropane are synthesized and brought to market Flammability and toxicity limit use
1951	Ross Terrell	Fluroxene
1953		Halothane
1955		Methoxyflurane
1963		Enflurane
1981		Isoflurane
1988		Desflurane
1990		Sevoflurane (first approved for use in Japan)

at best, inconsistent.[2] The use of restraints, strong men who would hold a patient down, mesmerism, stimulants, and draughts including herbs, opioids, and/or alcohol were reported to reduce the horror and pain of the experience.[3,4]

Ether was first synthesized by Valerius Cordus in 1540. Phillip von Hohenheim, who later took up the names Theophrastus Philippus Aureolus Bombastus von Hohenheim and finally Paracelsus, was a 16th century Swiss-German alchemist and contemporary of Cordus.[5] Paracelsus was experimenting with substances that relieved pain, including various opioid tinctures. He discovered that alkaloids in opium were more soluble in alcohol than water and synthesized a tincture that he termed laudanum (from the Latin *laudare*, "to praise") that included opium, alcohol, musk, amber, and other substances. Laudanum (tincture of opium in alcohol) later became widely accepted as a "cure-all" and was used to relieve pain, allow sleep, reduce irritation, and treat other nonspecific ailments.[5] Paracelsus also became aware of the properties of ether and in his writings documented its pain-relieving qualities.[5]

Nitrous oxide was first synthesized and reported on by Joseph Priestly in 1774. Priestly also isolated and described carbon dioxide, carbon monoxide, sulfur dioxide, and "dephlogisticated air," which later became known as oxygen.[6] Priestly, however, did not experiment on himself with the gas or report on its intoxicating or pain-relieving capabilities. These observations were first made by Sir Humphrey Davy in 1800 in his treatise, *Researches, Chemical and Philosophical, Chiefly Concerning Nitrous Oxide, or Dephlogisticated Nitrous Air*.[7] Davy reported that he took the drug and had relief from a toothache. Near the end of his text Davy made the following observation: "As nitrous oxide in its extensive operation appears capable of destroying physical pain, it may probably be used with advantage during surgical operations in which no great effusion of blood takes place."[7] This comment preceded the actual use of nitrous oxide for procedures by almost half of a century and represents one of the great missed opportunities of history. Davy himself was an influential figure in the scientific community but was not primarily interested in surgery or surgical care.[3]

Chloroform was first discovered almost simultaneously by three separate scientists: first by the American inventor/physician Samuel Guthrie (1831) and rapidly followed by the German chemist Justus von Liebig (1832) and the French pharmacologist Eugene Soubeiran (1832). They discovered chloroform separately and almost simultaneously and described their synthesis methods. There was some controversy over the "first" to synthesize chloroform, but it is now accepted that Guthrie preceded the other two by a few months.[8] The French chemist Jean Baptiste-Andre Dumas later named the substance and more fully described its makeup as C_2HCl_3 in 1834.[9,10] Preceding the first obstetric use of chloroform by more than a decade, it was used for treatment of asthma, pain relief during the setting of bones, and for other medically related purposes.

Early Use of Nitrous Oxide, Ether, and Chloroform

Surgical Use of Nitrous Oxide

Horace Wells is both a pivotal and tragic figure in the history of anesthesia and the evolution of the use of inhalation anesthetics. Wells, a deeply religious dentist from Hartford, Connecticut, had an interest in dental advancements and a deep revulsion for the pain he necessarily inflicted in his work. In 1844 Wells attended a demonstration of the use of nitrous oxide by the showman Gardner Quincy Colton. A young clerk named Sam Cooley breathed in the intoxicant, became excited, and rushed after an imagined enemy in the audience. Sitting near to Wells, he rolled up his trouser leg, displaying a gashed leg that he regarded with puzzlement; apparently he had not noticed the pain of the injury. Recognizing the possibility that the gas might be used in dentistry, Wells underwent removal of a wisdom tooth by his partner, Dr. Benjamin Riggs, in consultation with Colton. The operation was a success and Wells convinced Colton to teach him how to manufacture and administer the drug to his patients. After several successful procedures, his former student, mentee, and ex-business partner, William T. G. Morton, convinced him that he should conduct a "public demonstra-tion." One of the leading surgeons of the day, Dr. John Collins Warren, agreed to act as the surgeon, and the demonstration was held on December 9, 1845, before students and physicians in a surgical amphitheater at the Massachusetts General Hospital. The patient was inadequately anesthetized and by some accounts cried out during the extraction of a tooth. Many in the audience expressed their opinion that the demonstration was a "humbug" affair.

Wells' reputation was greatly damaged, but he continued his efforts to promote nitrous oxide anesthesia both at home and abroad. Unfortunately, he was unsuccessful and eventually began self-experimentation with chloroform, which after ether rapidly grew in popularity as an anesthetic. He became addicted and mentally unstable, finally attacking prostitutes with sulfuric acid on the streets of Boston in 1848. Jailed for the assault, he came to his senses in prison and in despair of his actions took his own life by opening an artery in his leg.[1]

Surgical Use of Ether

Wells is a tragic yet sympathetic figure, whereas William T. G. Morton, who is credited with the first public demonstration of the surgical properties of ether, is a renowned yet scandalous figure. Like Wells, Morton was a dentist and a student of Wells, considering Wells a mentor. Unlike Wells, Morton was reported to be avaricious and without scruples and by some was considered to be a scoundrel. Wells and Morton became partners in a dental practice, but the partnership was brief and unsuccessful. Afterward, Morton is thought to have attempted to enroll in medical school at Harvard. Whether he actually became a full-fledged medical student is debatable but it is clear that he never graduated. In 1844, Morton learned of the properties of "sulfuric ether" from a chemistry professor, Charles T. Jackson, who demonstrated that the inhalation of ether resulted in loss of consciousness. (The term "sulfuric ether" refers to products used in the distillation process: ethanol and sulfuric acid. Today we would refer to the substance as "diethyl ether.") Jackson later claimed to be the inventor of the concept of "etherization" but did not apply the concept beyond the classroom and thus was not credited with the discovery of surgical anesthesia.[4]

Morton continued his dental practice as a way to finance his education while continuing his medical studies. He had experimented with a variety of methods to reduce the pain and horror of dentistry with little success. Present at the unsuccessful demonstration of nitrous oxide by Wells, Morton consulted Jackson about the possibility of using a stronger substance. It is unclear whether Jackson advised ether, but after reportedly learning how to use ether by trying it on animals and taking it himself, he successfully used the drug to perform a dental extraction in his office. The event was published in a local paper (the *Boston Daily Journal*), and Dr. Henry Bigelow, a junior surgeon at the Massachusetts General Hospital, arranged a meeting with Dr. John Collins Warren, the chief of surgery. The intent of the meeting was to establish a time and date for a public demonstration of the new approach, and it was agreed that the demonstration would take place on October 16, 1846.[11]

On October 16, 1846 (known now as "ether day"), an audience again assembled in the surgical amphitheater at Massachusetts General Hospital, yet Morton was not present at the agreed time. Morton had been delayed by a last-minute alteration of his delivery device, which consisted of a glass ball with a wooden connecting tube equipped with a valve. The patient was Edward Gilbert Abbott, who had a "wen," or vascular mass, under his mandible. After a considerable wait, Morton finally arrived, and it is reported that

Dr. Warren stated, "Sir, your patient is ready."[3] Indeed, this is reported to be the first surgical delay as a result of the anesthesia provider! Morton then proceeded to have Abbott inhale the ether until unconscious, and the surgical procedure commenced. Much to the astonishment of the observers, the patient remained still throughout the excision, and it was reported that upon the conclusion of the procedure, Warren turned to the audience with tears in his eyes and stated, "Gentlemen, *this* is no humbug."[1,3,12] Bigelow went on to document the events in his paper "Insensibility during surgical operations produced by inhalation."[13]

Morton referred to the drug he used as "Letheon," and there are several theories as to why he might have withheld the true name and nature of the substance. The first explanation is that ether had a reputation due to several decades of use as a "social" or "party" drug and was widely used at ether frolics. It is speculated that perhaps Morton believed he would not be permitted to use it for a serious purpose because of this reputation. The second and more plausible explanation based on his known reputation and character is that Morton wished to hide the true identity of the substance to retain exclusive rights in patenting the discovery for his own profit.[1,11] Approximately 3 weeks later Warren gave his approval for the use of the substance for a "capital" or more significant procedure. Warren found Morton's subterfuge to be unscrupulous and publicly confronted him as to the true nature of the substance. When Morton admitted that it was pure "sulfuric ether" combined with oil of orange to conceal the characteristic odor, Warren gave permission, and ether was then used for the more extensive surgery.[11]

Although Morton has been given the leading position in the history of the surgical use of ether, he was, in reality, not the first to demonstrate its use. Dr. Crawford W. Long in Jefferson, Georgia first used ether for a surgical procedure on March 30, 1842. Long also demonstrated use of ether publicly and eventually published his account in 1848 in *The Southern Medical and Surgical Journal*. Despite the fact that Long used ether almost 4 years before Morton, he still does not receive full credit for the discovery. There are several reasons for this, including the delay between use and eventual publication, the more rural setting, his lack of national prominence, and the patent that Morton obtained for the discovery. Long now receives recognition for his early use but not to the same degree of notoriety or credit that have accrued to Morton and his confederates.[14–16]

Chloroform Use in Obstetrics and Surgery

Dr. James Young Simpson was a young Scottish obstetrician practicing in Edinburgh, Scotland. He, like his contemporaries across the Atlantic, was struck by the utter despair and suffering associated with surgery, dentistry, and childbirth. He also sought (unsuccessfully) for methods to alleviate the suffering. Upon hearing of the successful use of ether in Boston, Simpson first used ether to relieve the pain of childbirth in early 1847. He concluded that it was not satisfactory for labor and began experimenting with chloroform, giving the first widely publicized public demonstration of chloroform (on himself) in November 1847.[10] Interestingly, the use of chloroform for labor analgesia met with widespread resistance from religious leaders on the grounds that the pain of childbirth was "natural" and that changing the experience constituted a thwarting of God's will. Through support from important religious leaders of the day and after Queen Victoria requested the use of chloroform during her delivery, the practice became more widely accepted.[10,17]

Chloroform Versus Ether

Until the 1920s and 1930s, chloroform and ether were the principal anesthetizing agents. The debate raged as to which agent was superior. Alice Magaw, the famed nurse anesthetist, was reported in 1900 to have administered more than 10,000 consecutive ether anesthetics without a fatality, whereas a growing sense of suspicion about the safety profile of chloroform was rising.[18,19] The first documented chloroform death occurred in 1848, but its popularity continued to grow until it became the most commonly used anesthetic. It was not until 1911 that its pro-arrhythmia properties, resulting in ventricular fibrillation, were identified.[20] Despite this, chloroform continued to be used and remained the dominant anesthetic in the United Kingdom and Europe until the mid 1930s.

In 1934 Killian reviewed all previous statistical reports and calculated that risk of death in this era for an ether anesthetic was between 1:14,000 and 1:28,000 compared with risk of death with chloroform between 1:3000 and 1:6000.[20] Use of chloroform declined but was not eliminated entirely until as late as the 1970s.[10]

Development of Additional Anesthetics

Between the surgical use of nitrous oxide, ether, and chloroform and the revolution in fluorine chemistry in the 1940s was the development of several other anesthetics from the 1920s to 1940s: ethyl chloride, ethylene, cyclopropane, and divinyl ether.[21] The development of these agents was based on a conception of the structure-activity relationships of these molecules. Cyclopropane was very popular because it allowed rapid induction and clear-headed emergence.[22] However, because of their toxicity and flammability profiles, these drugs were eventually withdrawn from the market.

Ross Terrell and Fluorine Chemistry

Ross Terrell was a research chemist working for Baxter pharmaceuticals after World War II. His laboratory became known as the birthplace of modern inhaled anesthetics. Their work was based on the evolution of fluorine chemistry, which had at its roots the development of the atomic bomb (Manhattan project). The application of these scientific developments led to an acceleration in formulation of new agents in the 1940s and 1950s. The agents introduced during this time included fluroxene ($CF_3CH_2OCH = CH_2$) (1951), halothane ($CF_3CHClBr$) (1953), and methoxyflurane ($CH_3OCF_2CHCl_2$) (1955).[23]

Halothane was tremendously successful and rapidly displaced all other agents as the primary inhaled anesthetic.[24] Until recently halothane was still widely used with most applications in the pediatric setting because it was especially useful for mask inductions in children. Although the market leader for many years, halothane has associated problems that contributed to it falling into disuse, including a relatively high level of hepatic metabolism, cardiovascular problems (bradycardia, myocardial depression, arrhythmogenicity, and hypotension), and drug-induced hepatitis. The other two agents synthesized during this era enjoyed little success—fluroxene because of flammability and methoxyflurane because of liberation of fluoride ions with potential for renal damage.[23]

Terrell and his team continued to synthesize a large number of halogenated compounds from the 1950s to the 1970s. These included enflurane (CHF_2OCF_2CHFCl), isoflurane ($CF_3CHClOCHF_2$), sevoflurane ($[CF_3]_2CHOCH_2F$), and desflurane ($CF_3CHFOCHF_2$). The last three agents remain the primary agents used in modern anesthesia.[21, 23, 25]

Table 12-2 displays the pharmacologic properties of these anesthetics.[21, 25, 26]

Ideal Inhalation Anesthetics

The ideal inhalation anesthetic would be potent, have a low solubility in blood as well as in tissue beds, be nonflammable, be nonpungent, provide protection to organ systems throughout the body, provide bronchodilation (or at least avoid bronchoconstriction), have stable hemodynamics, have minimal effect on cerebral blood flow (CBF), reduce cerebral metabolic need, and elicit no seizure activity. In addition, the ideal agent would be stable in solution, nonreactive with carbon dioxide absorbents, environmentally friendly with no greenhouse gas effect, and affordable (Table 12-3).[24,25]

Importance of Halogenation

The inhaled anesthetics used in modern anesthesia care include nitrous oxide, isoflurane, desflurane, and sevoflurane. Methoxyflurane and enflurane are no longer used. Methoxyflurane was a potent agent but suffered from a low vapor pressure and high-blood-gas solubility, causing prolonged induction and emergence. Further, liberation of fluoride ions from extensive metabolism presented a risk of nephrotoxicity.[22] Enflurane was potent and had minimal pungency and a favorable solubility and vapor pressure. Myocardial depression and sensitization to catecholamines (thus increasing the chance of ventricular arrhythmias), epileptiform electroencephalographic activity in the face of hypocarbia, and metabolism with significant fluoride ion liberation were significant problems with this agent.[22,27] Halothane is no longer widely used as an anesthetic in the United States but may still be available in some areas and is

Table 12-2 Selected Pharmacologic Properties of Inhaled Anesthetics

Property	N_2O	Desflurane	Sevoflurane	Isoflurane	Halothane
MAC (30–60 yo, 37°C)	105	6.6	1.8	1.17	0.75
MAC in 60–70% N_2O		2.38	0.66	0.56	0.29
Oil-to-gas solubility	1.4	19	47	91	224
Vapor pressure at 20°C (mm Hg)	38,770	669	157	238	243
Preservative required?	No	No	No	No	Yes, thymol
Stable in moist CO_2 absorber?	Yes	Yes	No	Yes	No
Extent metabolized	—	0.02	2–5	0.2	20
Metabolites		Trifluoroacetate	Fluoride hexafluoroisopropanol	Trifluoroacetate	Trifluoroacetate
Organ system at risk due to metabolite		Liver	Kidney	Liver	Liver

MAC, minimal alveolar concentration; N_2O, nitrous oxide; yo, years old.

Source: From references 21, 25, and 26.

Table 12-3 Characteristics of the "Ideal" Inhalation Anesthetic

Nonflammable	Blunt autonomic responses
Easily vaporized	Minimal effect on cerebral blood flow
Potent	Preserves ability to monitor neurophysiologic function
Low solubility	Minimal cardiovascular effects
Minimal metabolism	Absence of toxicity: renal, hepatic, etc.
Nonarrhythmogenic/ compatible with epinephrine	Nonirritating to the pulmonary system
Provides skeletal muscle relaxation	Provides bronchodilation

Source: From references 21, 25, and 26.

discussed from the standpoint of comparing and contrasting its characteristics with the current agents. Nitrous oxide is an inorganic gas, whereas all modern *volatile* inhaled agents are hydrocarbons, with isoflurane, desflurane, and sevoflurane being ethers and halothane being an alkane.

Volatility is the characteristic of being able to change states from liquid to gas, and a volatile liquid is said to be "readily vaporizable at a relatively low temperature."[8] This is an important concept with inhaled anesthetics because *vapor pressure*, or the pressure exerted by the molecules leaving the liquid phase to enter the gas phase, determines the design of the vaporizer found on the anesthesia gas machine. Addition or substitution of molecules on the inhaled anesthetic gases determines their vaporization potential as well as several other physical properties.

Modern volatile, inhaled anesthetics are considered to be halogenated, which means that halogen molecules (chlorine, bromine, and fluorine) have been substituted for hydrogen molecules on the hydrocarbon structure. Thus halogenation has a variety of effects on the characteristics of the agents, including nonflammability, decreased solubility in blood, alterations in stability, and changes in potency (increased with combinations of fluorine, chlorine, and bromine but decreased with fluorine alone).

Pharmacokinetic Issues: Uptake and Distribution

Equilibrium, Conversion of Concentration (Percent) to Partial Pressure, and Blood-to-Gas Solubility

To achieve the desired anesthetic effect, the pharmacokinetics of inhaled anesthetics must be appreciated. Instead of the more familiar intravenous (IV) model, kinetics related to the inhaled agents require understanding of the delivery systems (anesthesia machine, vaporizer, and circuit), understanding of the conversion of concentrations to partial pressures, characteristics of the surface exchange area (lung), interindividual characteristics of patients (cardiac output), and the physiochemical characteristics of the agents (solubility, vapor pressure, halogenation).

Anesthesia providers are primarily interested in how inhaled anesthetics interact with elements of the central nervous system (CNS) to create an anesthetic effect (pharmacodynamic properties) but do not as yet have a direct measure to quantify this relationship. We therefore are limited to measuring the inspired and expired anesthetic gas concentrations via gas-analyzing systems. In a given anesthetic, when the inspired and expired concentrations of agent are equal, the agent is said to have "equilibrated," and depending on the concentration administered, a pharmacodynamic outcome (anesthesia) can be anticipated.

Volatile inhaled agents are delivered from a vaporizer that is calibrated in percent (fraction delivered [FD]). The vapor is picked up by the fresh gas flow (FGF) and delivered to the breathing circuit, which has a volume of approximately 6 L. The gas then enters the inspiratory limb of the circuit to be inspired by the patient (fraction inspired [FI]). The inspired concentration is then taken into the lungs through spontaneous or controlled ventilation and transferred to the alveoli (fraction alveolar [FA]). The gas must then cross the pulmonary and vascular membranes (alveoli and capillary) to dissolve in blood. In the alveoli and also in the blood, this concentration is, by convention, referred to as a partial pressure with the pressure units in mm Hg. The concentration of agent is directly proportional to the partial pressure exerted by the gas form of the agent. The terms pressure alveolar, pressure arterial, pressure brain, and pressure venous represent the partial pressure exerted in the alveoli and then the blood and tissues accordingly (Figure 12-1).

For example, an FD of 1% is the result of turning the vaporizer dial to 1.0%. The 1.0% of vapor delivered from the vaporizer is then increasingly diluted by the volume of the circuit and then the volume of the lung in establishing the FA. The drug must then move across the pulmonary membrane to achieve a partial pressure in the blood. Typically, the concentration from vaporizer to lung to tissue and then back to the lung is represented as a descending series of concentrations and can be written as FD > FI > FA > pressure arterial > pressure brain > pressure venous. To return to the concept of the inhalation anesthetic, each 1.0% of agent at normal atmospheric pressure represents 1.0% of 760 or 7.6 mm Hg pressure, which would also

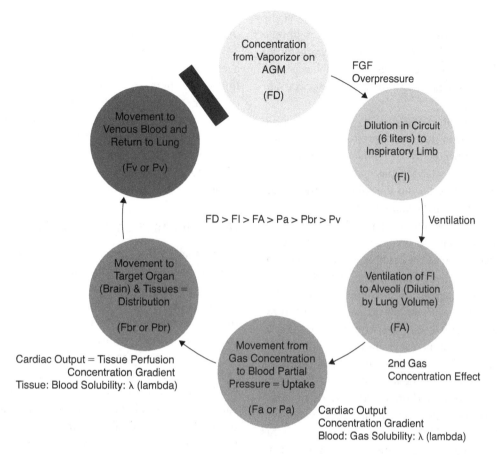

Figure 12-1 Uptake and distribution schematic with important variables.

represent a pressure in blood of 7.6 mm Hg once equilibration has occurred based on the inherent solubility of the agent. Therefore 2% would represent 15.2 mm Hg of pressure in the blood with each additional percent theoretically representing an additional 7.6 mm Hg of pressure (at 1 atmosphere) and again would depend on the blood-to-gas solubility partition coefficient.

The concept of solubility of the agent in blood and other tissues is important to the speed of movement of the agent along this series of concentration gradients toward equilibration and thus is central to the inherent titratability of the agent. The generic definition of solubility is "the concentration that a substance can achieve in a specified solvent when the solution is saturated"[28] (e.g., salt in water). When discussing solubility in the context of inhalation anesthetics, however, we speak in more specific terms and typically refer to the "relative affinity of the inhaled anesthetic for two phases (e.g. gas and blood) at equilibrium."[21,24] For example, a blood-to-gas solubility coefficient of 1.0 indicates that at equilibrium a concentration of anesthetic in arterial blood of 1.0% would mean that the concentration in the lung would be 1%. Importantly, if the blood-to-gas

partition coefficient is 2.0, the concentration in the blood must equal 2% to achieve a concentration in the lung of 1%. In other words, agents with low blood-to-gas partition coefficients equilibrate more rapidly than do agents with more robust blood-to-gas partition coefficients if the other variables are held constant.

The blood-to-gas solubility coefficient determines the rate of equilibration of the amount between the blood and gas phases. As described, direct brain site measurement of agent levels is not practical; however, the expired versus inspired concentration is measurable via mass spectrometry. The rate of equilibration of the FA toward the initial FI is therefore used to evaluate equilibration of the agents between the blood and gas phases. This parameter is termed the FA/FI ratio and is a key component to understanding uptake and distribution of inhaled anesthetics.

Overcoming Input Problems in Achieving FA

Input is the delivery of agent into the breathing circuit with resultant rise in the concentration, and, when inspired, the concentration is represented by the symbol FI, meaning fraction inspired. Because developing an alveolar concentration or fraction alveolar (FA) is necessary for uptake into blood and thus development of a concentration at the site of action (brain), understanding the variables associated with rapidly achieving FI and thus FA is important to the anesthetist.

The FD concentration is easily achieved by turning the vaporizer concentration to the desired level (percent). However, the FI is impacted by several factors: the absorption of vapor into the materials that make up the circuit, the fresh gas flow (FGF) rate, and the volume of the circuit that has potential to dilute the vapor.[22,29,30]

The absorption of vapor into the materials making up the circuit was of greater concern when circuits were composed of soluble materials, such as latex rubber. However, modern circuits are now composed primarily of polyvinyl chloride, which does not absorb significant quantities of agent.[31] The FGF can be increased to more rapidly increase the concentration of vapor inspired (FI) toward the concentration of vapor delivered (FD). Flow rate increases are limited only by the delivery parameters of the anesthesia machine. Finally, the anesthesia circuit consists of the inspiratory and expiratory connecting tubing and the carbon dioxide-absorbent canisters. The total volume of the adult circuit is approximately 6 L. Increased FGF rate and FD can be used to overcome this dilution effect in achieving the desired FI. Increasing FD to supraphysiologic levels to overcome dilution of the circuit in attempting to attain a desired FI is termed *overpressuring*. The *overpressuring* technique should be used with great caution because actual delivery of this concentration of agent as an FA could result in overdose of inhaled anesthetic and development of life-threatening side effects.

Uptake of Inhaled Anesthetics

Understanding the Uptake Equation and the Impact on FA

The variables involved in the uptake of inhaled anesthetic from the lung can be represented mathematically as follows: uptake = cardiac output (Q) × concentration gradient (alveolar to venous partial pressure difference) × blood-to-gas solubility (λ). Because uptake is a *product* of these three variables, no uptake can occur in situations that cause any of the variables to be zero. Therefore no uptake occurs if the patient has suffered cardiac arrest (Q = 0), there is no concentration gradient between the alveoli and venous blood (agent has not yet begun to cross the pulmonary exchange

membrane *or* has fully equilibrated), and if the agent is insoluble in blood (λ = 0).

Uptake therefore represents the amount or quantity of agent that crosses into the blood. Because the equation is linear, any increase in the cardiac output, concentration gradient, or solubility of agents will result in increased uptake and thus reduce the FA. A primary goal is to rapidly induce the patient (or change anesthetic level = titratability); however, increased uptake inhibits the rapid rise of the FA. To simplify this concept, we can consider the "container" analogy to describe uptake and the FA/FI ratio.

FA/FI Ratio: The "Container" Analogy

In this analogy the lungs can be viewed as a container. The level of fluid or gas in the container represents the concentration of agent in the alveoli (FA) as it rises toward the concentration of agent being delivered (FI). Assuming that the FI selected will produce general anesthesia, the rate at which the FA rises toward the FI (FA/FI ratio approaches 1.0) will determine the speed of induction of general anesthesia. The factors that will reduce the rate of rise of the FA/FI are the uptake variables in combination with the input variables (Figure 12-2). Increased uptake is associated with reduced rate of rise of the FA/FI ratio and thus a slowed induction of anesthesia. The three factors that increase uptake are increased cardiac output, increased agent solubility in blood, and increased concentration gradient.

The importance of these three variables to clinical anesthesia practice is primarily to be aware of them. Cardiac output is not manipulated for the purposes of changing induction speed. However, the practitioner should be aware that patients with high cardiac outputs may have slower induction and patients with low cardiac outputs may have sudden induction (and potentially become rapidly and deeply anesthetized). Further, differences in blood-to-gas solubility between the agents must be understood to make adjustment in technique. Finally, the alveolar to venous partial pressure gradient is most important during induction; any changes or titration of the agent during maintenance and during emergence when having the alveolar concentration as low as possible is an advantage for agent washout.

Five input variables can be altered to offset increased uptake (Table 12-4).[21,25,26] The FGF can be increased to offset the dilution offered by the anesthesia breathing circuit. A concurrent increase in alveolar ventilation offsets the dilution of the lung volume, and both methods help to increase the rate of rise of the FA. The equation for alveolar ventilation, which is respiratory rate × (tidal volume – dead space),

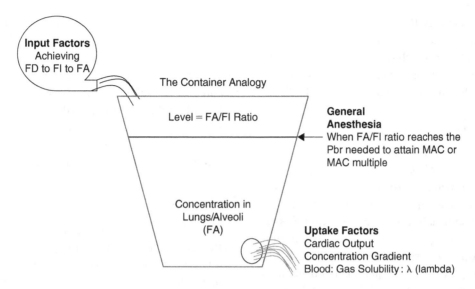

Figure 12-2 Input variable manipulation in overcoming uptake problems: The "container" analogy.

demonstrates that increasing rate and/or tidal volume helps to increase the concentration of the FA toward the FI given that the tidal volume exceeds the dead space volume.

As described, the FD can be increased to supraphysiologic levels to increase the FI, the FA, and also *the rate of rise* of the FA/FI.[25] This suraphysiologic concentration level of the inhaled anesthetic is termed *overpressuring* and has been compared with giving a bolus of an IV drug. Typically, the overpressuring phenomena are associated with use of the volatile inhalation agents. In addition, two effects

Table 12-4 Input Variables Manipulated to Offset the Impact of Uptake

Input Variable	Description
Increasing FD: overpressuring	Increasing the concentration on the vaporizer to supraphysiologic level (caution is warranted)
Increasing fresh gas flow	Increasing gas flow rates via the anesthesia gas machine
Increasing alveolar ventilation	Increasing rate and/or tidal volume (note: tidal volume must exceed dead space)
Concentration effect	The administration of a gas in high concentration will increase its own concentration and the rate of rise of its FA/FI.
Second gas effect	The administration of a gas in high concentration will increase the rate of rise of the FA/FI of a companion gas.

Source: From references 21, 25, and 26.

are unique to inhalation gases and anesthetics that can help to increase their concentration and the rate of rise of the FA/FI: the concentration effect and the second gas effect.

The *concentration effect* states that administration of a high concentration of a gas increases its own concentration in the lung and speeds the rate of rise of the FA/FI, and the *second gas effect* states that administering a high concentration of a gas increases its own concentration, the rate of rise of its own FA/FI, and the concentration and rate of rise of the FA/FI of a second (or companion) gas. The concentration effect has two components: the concentrating effect of delivery of a high concentration of a gas and the augmented gas inflow effect. The concentration effect depends on the bulk movement of a large volume of the gas from the alveoli to the blood based on the concentration gradient. If 100 total parts of gas are given and one-half of the anesthetic gas moves in bulk from blood to gas and the remaining alveolar gases do not move in bulk, the following effect occurs. If the anesthetic gas is given as 20% of the total, then 10 parts of the 20 move into the blood, leaving 10 parts remaining divided by total volume, which is 80 + 10 = 11.1%. However, should 70% concentration be given, representing 70 of the total 100 parts, 35 parts would cross into the blood, leaving 35 ÷ (30 + 35) or 54% at the end of the movement. This represents a 4.9 times increase in total concentration at the end of one bulk movement when the concentration was increased only 3.5 times (70% vs. 20%). Further, the net decrease in volume at the end of the bulk movement serves to concentrate the remaining gases in the lung. If one of the remaining gases is also an anesthetic, the resultant increase in relative concentration is termed the second gas effect. Finally, the bulk movement of a large volume of a gas from the alveoli to the blood results in an enhanced or augmented inflow that in the above case would be from the original mix of gases that further increases the concentration and also the rate of rise of the FA/FI.[22,25]

Distribution Equation

The distribution of inhaled anesthetics begins with uptake. As has been described, uptake can be defined by a linear equation. Distribution to tissue groups can also be described with a linear equation, and, importantly, the equation is nearly identical to the uptake equation. Distribution = Q (tissue group perfusion) × a-v concentration gradient (representing the tissue bed) × λ (tissue-to-blood partition coefficient). Again, the equation is linear, with increase in any variable associated with increased distribution to that tissue. The tissue group with the greatest perfusion is the vessel-rich group, which consists of the brain, liver, heart, lungs, kidneys, and other organs. An understanding of this principle helps to emphasize the importance of preferential perfusion in regard to the potential effects of inhalation anesthetics on specific tissue groups.

Time Constant

The time constant is unique to inhalation anesthetic pharmacology and is analogous to the half-time used in IV pharmacokinetics. Instead of time to a 50% change, the time constant for inhaled anesthetics is the time until a 63% change of the system toward equilibrium occurs (Table 12-5).[21]

The time constant can also be calculated for the various tissue groups through application of a second definition, which defines the time constant as the capacity of tissue/blood flow to the tissue. Capacity is defined by the equation λ (lambda or tissue-to-blood solubility for a specific

tissue bed) × k (a constant representing 100 mL of tissue). The blood flow to the tissue is also defined as flow per 100 mL of tissue per minute. For example, the time constant for the brain (which is in the vessel-rich group) can be represented in the following equation: T_cBrain = λ (~1 to 2) × 100 mL/100 mL blood per 100 mL-tissue per minute = 100–200/100 = 1 to 2 minutes. Each subsequent increment of 1 to 2 minutes therefore represents a 63% change of the remaining volume toward equilibrium (Table 12-6).[21]

FA/FI Curve

The curve representing the FA/FI for the inhalation anesthetics has a characteristic shape (Figure 12-3). The overall FA/FI curve shapes demonstrate the impact of solubility on uptake as the curves separate according to their respective blood-to-gas solubilities. The first segment of the FA/FI time curve represents the rapid rate of rise of FA toward FI before uptake begins as initially no concentration gradient exists. The curve then bends or has a first "knee" that represents rapid uptake into the blood and distribution to vessel-rich tissues. The second segment represents distribution and uptake into the muscle group tissues with the final or third segment representing distribution and uptake into fat with vessel-poor tissues receiving little or no perfusion.

Despite the muscle group having a relatively low tissue-to-blood partition coefficient, it takes significantly longer to equilibrate. This is a result of the high percentage of body composition that is muscle (as much as 75% of body mass) representing a large tissue volume combined with a relatively low perfusion of 3 mL per 100 mL of muscle tissue. The longer time constant for fat represents the effect of both a high solubility coefficient and a relatively low perfusion rate for fat (2 mL per 100 mL of tissue per minute). The movement of inhalation anesthetic into muscle and fat must be considered as a potential cause for postanesthetic

Table 12-5 Time Constants, Mathematical Computation, and Tissue Group Values

Time Constant	% Change of Volume	Unchanged Volume	63% of Unchanged Volume	Vessel-Rich Group	Muscle Group	Fat Group
1	63	37	0.63 × 37 = 23	1–2 min	33 min	2500 min
2	86 (63 + 23)	14	0.63 × 14 = 9	2–4 min	66 min	5000 min
3	95 (86 + 9)	5	0.63 × 5 = 3	3–6 min	99 min	7500 min
4	98 (95 + 3)	2	0.63 × 2 = 1	4–8 min	132 min	10,000 min

Values are rounded to whole numbers.

Source: From reference 26.

Table 12-6 Tissue Groups, Body Mass, Cardiac Output, Time Constants, and Flow per Tissue Group

Tissue Group	% Body Mass (70 kg)	% CO	Time Constant (min)	Flow per Minute— 100 mL of Tissue
Vessel rich	10	75	1–2	100
Muscle	50	19	33	3
Fat	19	6	2500	2
Vessel poor	21	0	N/A	

Source: From reference 26.

sedation. Muscle equilibration is nearly complete after 2 hours, whereas time for equilibration for fat is significantly longer and should not be considered until at least 4 hours of anesthesia have passed.[25] The exception to this understanding of fat as a potentially slow reservoir is fat surrounding organs. Some evidence suggests that this fat serves as the fourth active reservoir and due to its proximity to lean or vessel-rich tissues may serve as a significant reservoir (up to one-third of uptake) that in turn may be responsible for some cases of delayed emergence as agent exits this compartment during recovery.

Elimination of Inhaled Anesthetics

Most inhalation anesthetics are eliminated via the respiratory system. A final ratio is used to designate the washout phase. This ratio is FA/FA_0, which represents the actual expired FA divided by the FA when anesthetic was still being administered. The intent is to have this fraction approach zero—for example, the expired percent of 1%/2% (the last fraction administered) or an FA/FA_0 fraction of 0.5. A few minutes later after aggressive ventilation, the expired concentration may be 0.5%/2% and the FA/FA_0 will have

fallen to 0.25. This parameter can be used to describe the total decrement of anesthetic level and in estimating the rate of emergence after halting drug administration until the patient awakens. The same variables that govern induction of anesthesia, including solubility, perfusion or cardiac output, and concentration gradient, impact elimination of drug and thus recovery to the point of minimal alveolar concentration (MAC) awake or other specific recovery endpoints. Similarities in approach exist between inhalation anesthesia induction and elimination of drug. These include increasing the gas flows, increasing alveolar ventilation, and turning off the inspired concentration of drug to reverse the concentration gradient. Low blood and tissue solubility is valuable during emergence and contributes to a more rapid recovery profile.

Two key differences exist as well. During induction the principle of administering a high concentration of agent is used (overpressuring) to rapidly overcome dilution and establish the desired FA. During recovery there is no mechanism available to create a "negative pressure" of agent that might speed elimination of drug. Second, the anesthetist must keep in mind that solubility of the agent in blood and the various tissue groups plays a role in recovery; the longer the anesthetic, the more fully nontarget tissue groups will be equilibrated with more drug stored in these sites. Additionally, as drug levels fall in the CNS and other vessel-rich tissues, fat and muscle may actually be continuing to absorb agent until levels fall below their attained concentration. Thus solubility plays an important role during recovery as well as during initial administration. Finally, other pathways may exist for agent elimination, including via the skin, via the gut, and through "intertissue" diffusion. Losses via the skin and gut are thought to be negligible.

Pharmacodynamics and Inhaled Anesthetics

Pharmacodynamics represents the drug-receptor site interaction, whereas pharmacokinetics is the study of how drug molecules are administered, get to the receptor site, and are (eventually) eliminated. As described, when considering pharmacokinetics of inhaled anesthetics we describe their uptake and distribution. These principles are well established, and administration is predicable and measurable. Pharmacodynamics with respect to inhaled anesthetics refers to their interaction with target sites in the brain as well as interaction with other organ systems (side effects). The outcomes of the interaction are observable

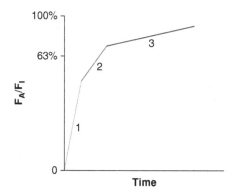

Figure 12-3 The FA/FI curve for inhalation anesthetics.

and continue to be described. The exact mechanism of the interaction between inhaled anesthetics and target sites in the brain remains an area of active investigation.

Mechanism of Action of Inhaled Anesthetics

Despite more than a decade of intense investigation, a single mechanism explaining the effects of inhaled anesthetics has not yet been discovered.[32,33] Two primary theories of inhalation anesthetic have risen to the forefront and continue to enjoy support among their proponents. In 1847, soon after the introduction of chloroform, Von Bibra and Harless hypothesized that general anesthetics act by dissolving in the fatty fraction of brain cells. This hypothesis attempts to provide a single set of physical or chemical characteristics that accurately predict anesthetic potency. The first report of anesthetic potency being related to lipid solubility was published by H. H. Meyer in 1899. Two years later a similar theory was published independently by Overton. Using the concept of lipid solubility, the Meyer-Overton hypothesis predicts that agents with higher lipid solubility have greater potency. Further, this hypothesis appears to meet the "necessary" standard (some potency is required for action), albeit not the "sufficiency" standard, because lipid solubility neither correlates perfectly with MAC nor explains all agent actions.[32–34]

The Meyer-Overton theory further suggests that the agent crosses the neuronal membrane and then dissolves in the lipid bilayer of the neuron. With as little as 0.4% increase in membrane volume, general anesthesia occurs. This very modest change in membrane characteristics is sometimes used to argue against the theory; however, it is noted that hyperbaric pressurization or "pressure reversal" results in at least partial emergence from the anesthetized state. This concept is further supported by the lipid solubility of agents (as measured by the octanol-to-water partition coefficient) relative to their respective MAC values (Table 12-2).[21,25,26] Factors that fail to support this concept include the variety of identified receptor sites for inhaled anesthetics and the optical isomer effect in which optical isomers with identical lipid solubility have very distinct pharmacologic properties, including absolute differences in potency.[32,33]

Specific Protein Theories

The second major theory relative to inhalation anesthetics is the specific receptor theory. This theory implies that a single anesthetic molecule–receptor interaction can be discovered that explains the function of all inhaled anesthetics. Multiple potential sites exist for this interaction, including inhibition of neurotransmitter release, neurotransmitter inactivation, presynaptic sites, postsynaptic sites, membrane-protein sites, voltage-gated ion channels, intracellular messenger systems, ligand-gated ion channels, and second messenger effects.[35]

GABA

γ-Aminobutyric acid (GABA) remains a viable target for inhalation agent activity. A variety of researchers have investigated the impact of inhaled anesthetics on GABA and more specifically on the interaction of inhaled agent with the receptor-based "alcohol" site.[35] Because anesthesia is produced by reduced neurotransmitter activity in the CNS, GABA would seem to be a reasonable target, with a "GABA agonist" effect likely to result in enhanced chloride conductance, neuronal hyperpolarization, and thus decreased neuronal activity.[36] However, the mechanism(s) of action underlying this depression of neuronal function relative to the $GABA_A$ interaction remains unclear.[37]

Molecule Transfer and Receptor Interaction

Two main factors—compound size and compound hydrogen bond activity—appear to primarily determine agent binding at specific yet diverse CNS receptor sites (e.g., GABA, glycine, N-methyl-D-aspartate). The two main factors that determine agent potency are compound size and compound hydrogen bond activity, with the shape of the anesthetic molecule playing only a minimal role. A two-stage mechanism of action appears to be necessary: transfer of the anesthetic to the site of action and the resultant molecule–receptor interaction. These observations appear to more accurately portray a unitary theory of the steps necessary for the anesthetic to be active but do not provide insight into a single mechanism of action.[32]

Potency and MAC

Potency represents the comparative dose of an agent required to elicit a predefined effect. This is sometimes represented graphically in the form of a quantal dose–response curve with effect on the y axis (in this case movement) and dose on the x axis. The primary clinical measure of potency is MAC, which represents the percentage of an agent required to abolish movement in response to a supramaximal stimuli (such as skin incision) at one atmosphere in 50% of subjects.[12,17,24,38–40] With respect to the inhaled anesthetics under discussion, the most potent is halothane followed by isoflurane, sevoflurane, and desflurane. The physiochemical property used to describe potency is the oil-to-gas solubility or partition coefficient. Although the exact mechanism of inhaled anesthetic action is unknown, it is known that some lipid solubility is necessary for effect. The oil-to-gas partition coefficient estimates this relationship because oil has similar properties to CNS lipid and correlates with the MAC values. The relationship is that the oil-to-gas partition coefficient is inversely related to the MAC values (oil-to-gas partition coefficient = 1/MAC).

MAC, MAC Multiples, and the Additive Effect

The most potent inhaled agent is halothane, which is no longer widely used in clinical practice. The other inhaled anesthetics, isoflurane, sevoflurane, and desflurane, are all less potent.[39] Ideally, anesthetic agents produce anesthesia while allowing the use of a high concentration of oxygen. In 30- to 60-year-old patients, MAC values for halothane, isoflurane, sevoflurane, and desflurane are 0.75%, 1.15%, 1.85%, and 6.6% at one atmosphere, respectively, which indicates they are all relatively potent and can be given with a high concentration of oxygen.[39,41] By contrast, the MAC for nitrous oxide is 105% at one atmosphere. For this reason, full anesthetic doses of nitrous oxide can only be administered in a hyperbaric chamber.[25]

Several MAC multiples are significant. A MAC multiple is the multiplication of the MAC value by a constant (k) to illustrate a different response point in the overall dose–response relationship. For example, MAC awake is a multiple that is useful during emergence from anesthesia. MAC awake ranges from 0.34 to 0.64 of MAC for modern inhaled anesthetics.[21] This means that the expired inhaled anesthetic concentration must fall to approximately one-third of the MAC value for the patient to be considered awake and able to follow commands. Further, this parameter correlates well with amnesia.[21] Other MAC multiples include MAC_{BAR} (block autonomic response), which is approximately 1.5 × MAC, and MAC_{95}, which is approximately 1.3 × MAC and represents the percentage of an agent required to abolish movement in response to a supramaximal stimuli (such as skin incision) at one atmosphere in 95% of subjects.[32,39,42,43] This corresponds to the ED_{95} parameter in IV pharmacology. Finally, a variety of factors require adjustment of dose based on the providers' understanding of their impact on MAC. These factors increase, decrease, or have no effect on MAC requirements (the dose needed) (Table 12-7).

MAC values are roughly additive. This effect is best appreciated when comparing MAC values alone versus MAC values of potent agents when combined with nitrous oxide 60% to 70%. Nitrous oxide 60% to 70% represents approximately 60% of one MAC (one full MAC of nitrous oxide requires administration of 105%). If given with a volatile inhaled anesthetic, the inhaled agent level should be reduced by approximately 60% with only 40% of the inhaled agent MAC dose required. Table 12-2 demonstrates that the dose of each inhaled agent is reduced approximately 60% when combined with 60% to 70% nitrous oxide.

Summary of Inhaled Agent Pharmacodynamics

The predominant effects of inhaled anesthetics cannot be explained by the depletion, production, or release of a single neuromodulator in the CNS. The ultimate action of inhaled anesthetics seems to occur on specific neuronal membrane proteins. These proteins allow ion movement during membrane excitement, and their inhibition results in decreased excitability.

Some combination of membrane protein and surrounding lipid membrane interaction with the inhaled agents must occur, but the mechanism is still not fully understood. What is understood is that these drugs have multiple presynaptic and postsynaptic effects in the brain and spinal cord. Of great importance is the ability of inhaled anesthetics to prevent a motor response to noxious stimulation. This effect is thought to result from agent interaction with a site(s) of action in the spinal cord and is the basis for the MAC concept. MAC represents the effective dose at 50%, or ED_{50}, for inhaled agents for absence of movement in the face of a surgical stimulus. MACs are additive, and MAC multiples can be used to evaluate outcome variables in addition to movement.

Modern Inhaled Anesthetics

Halothane (2-bromo-2-chloro-1,1,1-trifluoroethane), introduced in 1958, was the dominant anesthetic used in practice for many years. It is no longer routinely used in clinical practice but is still useful in providing context for the modern anesthetics. Advantages to halothane use are solubility (when introduced, its solubility was considered to be low; as other drugs were introduced, it was considered to be high), potency, nonpungency (has a sweet odor), and smooth muscle relaxation (including bronchial smooth muscle). Unfortunately, the disadvantages of halothane are many and include myocardial sensitization to epinephrine (ventricular arrhythmias), myocardial depression, substantial increases in CBF compared with other agents, high solubility (when compared with the newer inhaled agents such as desflurane), chemical instability (oxidative decomposition

Table 12-7 Factors With Impact on MAC

Increased MAC (Need More Agent)	No Impact on MAC	Decreased MAC (Need Less Agent)
Decreased age	Anesthetic duration	Increased age (MAC decreases 6% for every decade after age 1 year)
Acute increase in CNS neurotransmitter levels	K$^+$ levels	Metabolic acidosis
Hyperthermia	Anesthetic metabolism	Hypoxia (PaO$_2$, 38 mm Hg)
Hypernatremia	Thyroid conditions	Induced hypotension (mean arterial pressure < 50 mm Hg)
Chronic alcohol abuse	Gender	Decreased central neurotransmitter levels
Increased CNS catecholamine levels—acutely	Species	α_2-Agonist administration Hypothermia Hyponatremia Lithium Hypo-osmolality Pregnancy (progesterone) Acute ethanol intoxication Ketamine Pancuronium Physostigmine (10 times clinical doses) Neostigmine (10 times clinical doses) Lidocaine Opioids Opioid agonist-antagonist analgesics Barbiturates Chlorpromazine Diazepam Hydroxyzine Marijuana (active ingredient) Verapamil Anemia

Factors that increase MAC may require administration of additional inhalation agent, whereas factors that decrease MAC may require reduction of inhalation dose.

Source: From references 21, 25, and 26.

into HCl acid, HBr acid, chlorine, and phosgene requiring addition of thymol for chemical stabilization), relatively high percentage of metabolism (20%), trifluoroacetate metabolites (the basis of halothane hepatitis), and finally vinyl halide production through interaction with carbon dioxide absorbents. As a result of these disadvantages, halothane fell into disuse among the adult population in the 1970s and in the pediatric population by the 1990s.

Isoflurane (2-chloro-2-[difluoromethoxy]-1,1,1-trifluoroethane) is the most potent inhaled agent currently in use, with a MAC value of 1.17 (Table 12-2). Isoflurane is a halogenated methyl, ethyl ether and is known for chemical stability and clinical predictability. Introduced in the early 1980s, isoflurane represented a significant step forward because hepatic and renal toxicity was largely avoided.[44] Advantages to isoflurane use include stability and predictability, lack of toxicity,

relatively low solubility, low or absent flammability, smooth and skeletal muscle relaxation, minimal cardiac depression, and a vapor pressure that allows use of a nonheated vaporizer. Disadvantages include pungency, potential for coronary steal (although very rare), dose-dependent increase in heart rate, and reduction in vascular tone.

Desflurane (2,2,2-trifluoro-1-fluoroethyl-difluoromethyl ether) is a completely fluorinated methyl, ethyl ether. Desflurane is chemically similar and in clinical effects very similar to isoflurane. Substitution of a fluorine for the chlorine on the first ethyl carbon decreased solubility substantially (0.42). Advantages of desflurane include low blood gas solubility (titratability), skeletal muscle relaxation, low tissue-to-blood solubility (faster emergence[45]), lack of toxicity, and minimal metabolism. Disadvantages include a high vapor pressure (669, requiring a special heated vaporizer), lower potency (MAC is 6%), significant pungency, respiratory irritation, potential for coronary steal, tachycardia, hypertension, dose-dependent reduction in vascular tone, and production of carbon monoxide through interaction with desiccated carbon dioxide (CO_2) absorbent.

All agents produce some carbon monoxide when reacting with dry CO_2 absorbents; however, desflurane produces the most. Awareness of the issue, taking steps to avoid absorbent desiccation (turning off gas flows), or weekly changeover of the CO_2 absorbent can help to avoid the problem of carbon monoxide poisoning that has been reported.[46–50]

Sevoflurane(2,2,2-trifluoro-1-[trifluoromethyl]ethylfluoromethyl ether) is a methyl isopropyl ether that is completely fluorinated. Introduced in Japan in 1990, sevoflurane has replaced halothane as the anesthetic of choice in children and is the most commonly used inhalation anesthetic in clinical practice today. Advantages of sevoflurane include low solubility in blood, sweet smell, lack of bronchial irritation, smooth (bronchial) and skeletal muscle relaxation, and a vapor pressure that allows use of a nonheated vaporizer. Disadvantages include a relatively high degree of metabolism (5%) with production of inorganic fluoride, a brain-to-blood solubility coefficient higher than desflurane suggesting possible emergence delay (although multiple studies demonstrate very similar overall recovery profiles[51–54]), production of compound A, and exothermic reactions with CO_2 absorbents.

Compound A

Compound A is vinyl halide byproduct of the chemical reaction between sevoflurane and desiccated CO_2 absorbents. Compound A is clearly a nephrotoxin in the rat model, but this effect on humans has not been demonstrated.[49,55–59] In addition to CO_2-absorbent desiccation, use of low flows (below 2 L/min) during maintenance of anesthesia have been associated with accumulation of this reaction byproduct, and thus some clinicians continue to suggest maintaining flows of greater than 2 L/min during sevoflurane anesthesia as a precaution. Research in this area has demonstrated that low-flow anesthesia can be used safely even in patients with renal dysfunction[58] and that CO_2-absorbent compounds free of or with reduced amounts of strong bases such as KOH and NaOH have decreased production of compound A during the inhalation anesthetic breakdown reaction.[49,55,56,60]

Combustion and Inhalation Anesthetics

Several cases of fires, explosions, or extremely elevated temperatures within the anesthetic circuit have been reported. All severe cases occurred in 2002 and 2003 and involved sevoflurane and desiccated Baralyme CO_2-absorbent reactions.[61] In 2003 Abbot Pharmaceuticals, in combination with the FDA, issued a warning letter to all anesthesia providers in the United States, warning them of this issue. By 2005 it was clear that the strong bases in the CO_2-absorbent Baralyme reacted significantly with sevoflurane. Chemtron (the manufacturer) voluntarily pulled Baralyme from the U.S. market. Laster et al. chronicled the exothermic nature of the sevoflurane–Baralyme CO_2-absorbent reactions.[48,62] A national consensus conference was convened by the Anesthesia Patient Safety Foundation in 2005 to review this issue (as well as the carbon monoxide and compound A issues) and recommended that every provider and facility be aware of the need to avoid desiccation of CO_2-absorbent systems and also to urge CO_2-absorbent manufacturers to reduce the levels of strong bases in their products.[47]

Combustion is also a problem in use of nitrous oxide, which is an inorganic gas still used for both sedation and general anesthesia more than 150 years since the Wells exhibition. Despite the potential for combustion, a few key benefits of nitrous oxide continue to drive its use. These include a low blood gas solubility, low manufacturing cost, absence of odor, minimal metabolism, ease of use, and a second gas pharmacokinetic effect. Disadvantages in addition to combustion are many and have resulted in a sharp drop in the use of nitrous oxide for surgical anesthesia over the last decade. These disadvantages include low potency (MAC 105%), nausea and vomiting, expansion of nitrogen-filled compartments such as the endotracheal cuff or a pneumothorax (34 times more diffusible than nitrogen), diffusion hypoxia (large volume of nitrous dilutes alveolar oxygen during emergence), inhibition of B_{12}-dependent enzymes resulting in suppressed formation of methionine synthase (myelin, possible neuropathy), and thymidylate synthase (DNA, possible congenital effect) and pernicious anemia with prolonged exposure.[63–68]

Impact of Inhaled Anesthetics by System

The differences between the modern potent inhaled anesthetics (isoflurane, sevoflurane, and desflurane) on a system-by-system basis are subtle and require an in-depth understanding of the agents. This understanding is important in tailoring care to the needs of the individual. Interindividual variations in patient physiology and pathophysiology as well as variables associated with the surgical procedure and coadministered medications must all be considered in selecting agents.

Neurologic System

Flow: Metabolism Coupling, Electroencephalogram, and Autoregulation of Vasculature

In normal human physiology cerebral metabolic rate is coupled with cerebral blood flow (CBF). Because the brain has no stores of glucose or oxygen, continuous delivery of these critical substrates is necessary to maintain neuronal integrity. The inhaled anesthetics partially *uncouple* this flow metabolism relationship by increasing blood flow in a dose-dependent manner while reducing cerebral metabolic rate. Full uncoupling is not achieved because some metabolism continues and flow is available.[25]

Isoflurane, desflurane, and sevoflurane have similar effects on the cerebral metabolic rate and have the capability of producing an isoelectric electroencephalogram (EEG) reading at higher doses.[69–71] These effects occur at clinically relevant anesthetic doses such that patient hemodynamic deterioration can be managed. No further reduction in cerebral metabolic rate is attained by increasing the dose of these drugs after the EEG reading has become isoelectric.[25]

Some studies suggest sevoflurane may have proconvulsant effects as well, with case reports of seizures in pediatric patients and young adults.[72,73] These effects appear to be associated with low CO_2 levels, speed of induction, and dose of sevoflurane.[74,75] Women seem to be more susceptible than men.[24] It appears to be prudent to use sevoflurane with caution in the following situations: rapid induction in women, high doses of the drug combined with hyperventilation, and in patients with prior history of epileptic foci.[75,76]

Autoregulation of the cerebral vascular is an active response to changes in pressure. There are both myogenic components (blood vessel changes caliber in response to pressure change) and metabolic components (blood vessel changes caliber in response to metabolic mediator). Accordingly, changes in CBF are multivariate both from the standpoint of agents used and underlying brain conditions. In humans receiving inhalation anesthetics, CBF increases in a time-dependent and dose-dependent manner.[77–85] In general, as the dose of the agents increase, cerebral vasodilation occurs, although there are regional differences within the brain itself. This vasodilation is opposed by, but not overcome by, the vasoconstriction that occurs with reductions in metabolism.[77–79,82,84,85]

Preservation of autoregulation during anesthesia and surgery is a desirable outcome. Sevoflurane preserves autoregulation up to approximately 1.5 MAC, whereas isoflurane does not fully preserve autoregulation at 1.0 MAC.[86–88] This may represent a greater direct vasodilatory effect seen with isoflurane or a relatively smaller direct vasodilator effect of sevoflurane, preserving the ability of the vessel to respond to changes in blood pressure at 1.5 MAC. This concept is supported by the work of McCulloch et al.[89] In their study the authors measure both resistance and flow during isoflurane anesthesia. They suggest that changes in arteriolar tone influence CBF in two ways: controlling resistance and changing effective downstream pressure.[89] By contrast, desflurane has an even more significant effect on autoregulation that is fully abolished at 1.5 MAC.[90]

Intracranial Pressure, Cerebral Blood Flow, and Cerebrospinal Fluid

Autoregulation directly impacts the total volume within the cranium. During neuroanesthesia it is critical that the anesthesia provider understand the basic principles and variables related to intracranial dynamics. Intracranial pressure (ICP) is normally 0 to 15 mm Hg and is derived by the combination of blood, cerebrospinal fluid (CSF), and brain tissue within the rigid cranium (Monroe-Kellie physiology). CBF must be understood and is the variable that can be controlled to some extent by the anesthetist. As CBF increases, cerebral blood volume increases, and ICP then increases in a curvilinear fashion as the compliance within the cranium is reduced. Sevoflurane, desflurane, and isoflurane are all known to increase CSF pressure.[91,92] Sponheim et al. studied the effects of 0.5 and 1.0 MAC of isoflurane, sevoflurane, and desflurane on ICP and cerebral perfusion pressure in a pediatric population. All three agents increased ICP and reduced mean arterial pressure and cerebral perfusion pressure in a dose-dependent manner, with desflurane increasing ICP slightly more than the other agents.[93] Using a porcine model Holmstrom and Akeson[82] evaluated ICP change with 0.5 to 1 MAC of isoflurane, desflurane, and sevoflurane. All three drugs demonstrated dose-dependent increases in CBF and ICP, with hypocapnia blunting the vasodilatory response and thus the elevation of ICP. These authors also reported that cerebral autoregulation was preserved.[82] The concept that hypocapnia can be used to offset the CBF and ICP changes associated with inhalation anesthetics is supported by human data, which also demonstrates the value of hypocapnia.[94] It is important to note that other studies do demonstrate conflicting results, with hypocapnia being an ineffective therapy.[95]

The effects of nitrous oxide on cerebral physiology are less clear than the potent volatile agents because of broader species-related variability and the clinical reality that nitrous is rarely administered without a companion agent. However, nitrous oxide has been studied in individual human volunteers and has been demonstrated to be a significant cerebrovasodilator. The net effect is an increase in cerebral perfusion pressure and CBF.[96] In a pediatric study, nitrous oxide was added to 1.5 MAC sevoflurane, and cerebral reactivity to CO_2 was significantly reduced, reinforcing the vasodilatory effect and also the likelihood that nitrous oxide blunts autoregulation.[97]

Inhalation agents also have the potential to augment the production or decrease the absorption of CSF. Desflurane at 1 MAC causes CSF production to be unchanged or slightly increased,[98] whereas isoflurane does not appear to alter CSF production or resistance to absorption model across several dose ranges.[99] Sevoflurane at 1 MAC can depress CSF production significantly but may also slightly increase resistance to absorption with no significant net effect on overall volume.[100] The overall effect of the current inhaled anesthetics on CSF formation and absorption appears to be small.

All three of the modern inhaled anesthetics have been used successfully for neurosurgical procedures. The overall experience with isoflurane is the most robust; however, the data related to both sevoflurane and desflurane is building. Increases in CBF, cerebral blood volume (CBV), and thus ICP are possible; however, both hypocapnia and IV anesthetics such as barbiturates or propofol can be used to blunt or mediate the effects of the inhalation agents on ICP and CBF.[101,102]

Neuroprotection and Inhaled Anesthetics

Isoflurane appears to have some neuroprotective effects in both human and animal models in situations of focal ischemia. Investigators demonstrated improved outcome after carotid endarterectomy for isoflurane versus halothane and enflurane in humans and have also used animal models to demonstrate the protective effect of isoflurane.[103–109] Anesthetic preconditioning (administering an agent for a fixed period of time before an event) has been effective, with data suggesting both short- and long-term benefit. Use of other inert gases (xenon) with anesthetizing effect have also been evaluated and appear to provide some benefit,[110] especially when used in combination with other approaches such as cooling.[110,111] The value of sevoflurane and desflurane relative to neuroprotection is less understood, with preconditioning associated with some success in animal models.[103,112–117]

The full impact of inhalation anesthetic neuroprotection remains unknown, with some authors suggesting the effect of inhaled anesthetic preconditioning to be minimal or of a limited nature.[103,104] However, this area continues to be persistently investigated, and multiple cellular mechanisms have been proposed in explaining the neuroprotective mechanisms, including up-regulation of nitric oxide synthase systems, activation of ATP-dependent potassium channels, reduction or inhibition of excitatory neurotransmitter systems, augmentation of blood flow to the affected region, and up-regulation of factors preventing apoptosis.[113,116]

EEG and Evoked Potentials

Volatile anesthetics, including nitrous oxide at greater than 1 MAC levels,[118] depress neuronal activity and impulse transmission at anesthetic doses, resulting in lower EEG frequency and decreased amplitude of the signal for peripheral transmission of sensory evoked potentials (SEP) and motor evoked potentials. Increasing concentrations produce dose-dependent depression of these signals up to and including burst suppression. Using all agents within a single animal model, Murrell et al.[69] analyzed 1.25, 1.5, and 1.75 MAC doses of isoflurane, sevoflurane and desflurane, respectively. Isoflurane produced burst suppression at every dose, whereas sevoflurane and desflurane increased the amount of burst suppression to normal signal (burst suppression ratio) in a dose-dependent manner.[119] In patients with known epileptiform EEG activity, sevoflurane causes a relative acceleration of epileptiform activity synchronization,[120] although no clinical correlate of this effect has yet been identified.[121] At low doses of agents, including nitrous at less than 1 MAC, there is an excitatory effect, perhaps reflecting inhibition of inhibitory neurons. At increasing doses, the EEG and SEP signals are suppressed with decreased frequency and amplitude, respectively.[122]

Cortical somatosensory, motor, visual, auditory, and brainstem evoked potentials can be influenced by the inhalation agents. All volatile agents cause a dose-dependent increase in latency and decrease in amplitude in cortical SEP recordings. Latency is the length of time needed for the signal to travel from point A to point B. Amplitude is the height of the signal. There is a dose-dependent reduction of amplitude in these signals, with visual evoked potentials being most sensitive and brainstem evoked potentials being relatively resistant.[26,119,123] The level of sensitivity can be described in the following order: visual evoked potentials > SEP > brainstem evoked potentials. Motor evoked potentials, which evaluate the integrity of descending motor pathways, are also highly sensitive. Sudden increases in the anesthetic level (> 0.5 MAC) have more significant impact on SEPs.[26,119,123]

Autonomic Nervous System

Volatile anesthetics depress the autonomic nervous system in a dose-dependent manner, including both parasympathetic and sympathetic nervous system responses.[25,124] Baroreceptors, which are important to ensuring homeostatic vascular, respiratory, and cardiac reflexes, are inhibited with both afferent and efferent signaling systems affected.[125–129] Interestingly, although elements of the autonomic nervous system are blunted, isoflurane has the ability to increase afferent baroreceptor signals.[130,131] Desflurane and possibly isoflurane have the potential to activate the sympathetic nervous system, helping in part to explain cardiovascular changes seen with these drugs. One mechanism is believed to be through stimulation of pulmonary receptors responding to pungency, explaining also why sevoflurane (nonpungent) does not demonstrate this effect.[132,133] At low levels of inhalation anesthesia, sympathetic outflow is relatively preserved with sevoflurane, isoflurane, and desflurane. With sevoflurane, more rapid return of baroreceptor reflexes after anesthesia has been demonstrated when compared with isoflurane.[134]

Nitrous oxide stimulates the sympathetic nervous system during use and is typically administered in combination with the more potent inhaled anesthetics.[135–138] The outcome of this sympathetic activation is an improved blood pressure and a reduction in hypotension associated with use of the more potent agents. Although this effect can be partly explained by the sympathetic nervous system stimulation provided by the nitrous oxide, it may also be attributed to the lower dose of inhaled anesthetics used when nitrous is given.[25]

In summary, the overall effect of inhaled anesthetics on the limbs of the autonomic nervous system is inhibition with nitrous oxide and desflurane, demonstrating the ability to activate the sympathetic nervous system through different mechanisms. However, there are differences that are useful to understand during clinical care. Low doses of agents preserve some baroreceptor and other autonomic functions, which are useful when caring for critically ill or otherwise compromised patients. Desflurane causes some sympathetic nervous system activation, especially when the dose is rapidly increased, thus explaining the tachycardia and occasional hypertension seen during use of the agent. Finally, if rapid return of autonomic reflexes is desired, sevoflurane may be a prudent choice.

Cardiovascular System

It is important for the anesthetist to have an appreciation for and be able to accurately predict cardiovascular effects of inhalation agents relative to the drug chosen, physiology, and pathophysiology.

Blood Pressure and Myocardial Contractility

Isoflurane, sevoflurane, and desflurane administration results in a predictable, dose-related reduction in arterial blood pressure. The primary mechanism for this reduction in pressure is a decrease in systemic vascular resistance. All three agents are potent in producing these effects that are similar in their magnitude at equipotent doses.[139–147] Depression of myocardial function with reduction in contractility is a significant concern with both enflurane and halothane.[148–154] Myocardial contractility is affected at higher doses when using the modern anesthetics, but this effect is not a significant concern when using typical doses found in clinical practice.[25]

Heart Rate

Heart rate changes with inhalation anesthetics depend on multiple variables, including baseline heart rate, coexisting disease, state of the autonomic nervous system, vascular volume, and depth of anesthesia. Sevoflurane at lower doses has little effect on heart rate, whereas isoflurane and desflurane increase heart rate by 5% to 10% from baseline.[142] More dramatic changes in heart rate have been observed with rapid change of anesthetic concentration with desflurane and isoflurane.[142,155–157] As described, baroreceptor responses are at least partially blunted with the inhaled anesthetics, so the change in heart rate must be associated with a different mechanism. Muzi et al. suggested that the pungency of the agents stimulates receptors in the pulmonary system that in turn elicits reflex increases in heart rate.[133]

This effect can be moderated by blunting central sympathetic nervous system outflow with beta-blockers, α_2-agonists, or opioids.[158,159] These responses are typically seen during induction or rapid titration and during steady-state anesthesia.

Coronary Steal, Myocardial Ischemia, and Cardioprotection

The coronary steal phenomenon was first described by Buffington et al. in 1987, who went on to provide detailed characterization of this potential phenomena.[160–163] Patients with cardiac vessel occlusion, collateralization, and a fixed stenotic vascular lesion leading to the abnormal vascular bed are the variables associated with steal. Inhalation agent-induced coronary artery vasodilation was thought to be associated with diversion of blood away from vessels with inability to dilate to vessels (in healthy tissue beds) with capability to dilate (Figure 12-4). The subsequent movement of blood according to the path of least resistance was thought to represent a risk of ischemia to approximately 25% of patients with coronary artery disease having surgery.[162] This property of inhaled agents was first described with isoflurane and extended to desflurane. Subsequent and detailed investigation revealed that although these anatomic and physiologic phenomena may exist, the solution in avoidance of myocardial ischemia in the population with coronary artery disease is vigilance in maintenance of adequate coronary perfusion pressure (CPP). Steal would thus be an issue only when adequate perfusion pressure was not maintained.[164] This was demonstrated in a 1992 investigation of 200 patients who underwent coronary artery bypass grafting. Desflurane was compared with sufentanil in this population, and outcomes were similar. However, on induction, ischemia was noted in 13% of the desflurane patients, with the authors concluding that this effect was a result of inadequate adjunctive control of hemodynamic parameters, including heart rate and coronary perfusion pressure.[165] Other investigators have studied the impact of isoflurane versus sevoflurane and inhalation techniques versus opioid techniques in at-risk populations and found that inhalation anesthetic agents were not associated with increased myocardial ischemia risk in these populations.[166,167]

Not only are inhalation anesthetic agents safe to administer in these at-risk populations, there is a growing body of evidence that the inhalation anesthetics provide protection against myocardial ischemia. In coronary occlusion physiology, a brief ischemia episode initiates complex cell signaling mechanisms that attempt to reduce ischemia and last for up to 3 hours. Volatile anesthetics trigger a similar cascade of events.[25] Myocardial preconditioning is the administration of a dose of inhalation anesthetic for a fixed period of time in anticipation of possible reductions in blood flow, with myocardial ischemic preconditioning occurring after the patient has suffered a period of inadequate myocardial perfusion. Studies demonstrated that inhalation anesthetic myocardial preconditioning can reduce injury in the postinfarct period, protect against reperfusion injury, and reduce the overall size of the infarct.[168–172] Several mechanisms have been postulated for this, including the Na^+/H^+ exchange pump, the adenosine receptor, G-protein inhibition, protein kinase C, tyrosine kinase, and adenosine triphosphate-sensitive potassium channels, K_{ATP}. Drugs can be administered that mimic the ischemic preconditioning cascade, including adenosine, opioid agonists, and K_{ATP} agonists.[25]

The K_{ATP} agonists are under intense investigation, and inhalation anesthetics appear to mimic their effects.[173] A new K_{ATP} agonist, Nicorandil, now in clinical trials, is a K_{ATP} receptor agonist and must be given as a continuous IV infusion.[173] Importantly, diabetes with resultant hyperglycemia is thought to oppose the effectiveness of the K_{ATP} channel mechanism, emphasizing the importance of perioperative glucose control with insulin in this population. The K_{ATP} channel is also closed by sulfonylurea oral hyperglycemic drugs, which should be discontinued 24 to 48 hours before surgery in high-risk patients.[25,174–177] Additionally, not only does this form of preconditioning benefit the heart, there is now evidence that preconditioning with inhaled anesthetics may have benefit for other organ systems, including the brain, liver, and kidneys.[174]

Arrhythmia Generation

Inhaled anesthetics have the potential to cause arrhythmias through a variety of mechanisms that may include prolongation of the effective refractory period, increased QT interval, or even blockade of sodium currents.[21] Sevoflurane prolongs the QT interval and should be used in caution in patients with acquired prolonged QT interval conditions.[178,179]

Myocardial sensitization is a term sometimes used to describe the arrhythmogenic effects of inhaled anesthetics when combined with epinephrine. With the modern inhaled agents, the risk of arrhythmogenesis has been greatly reduced, especially when compared with drugs such as halothane, which has substantial arrhythmogenic potential.[156,180–182] However, caution should still be taken when epinephrine is administered. For healthy patients and typical MAC levels (1–1.3 MAC), the submucosal dose of epinephrine is up to 7.0 μg/kg for desflurane and up to 5.0 μg/kg for sevoflurane or isoflurane.[183]

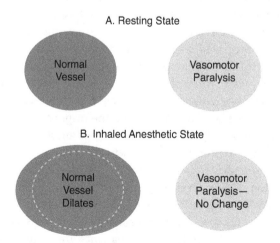

Figure 12-4 Coronary steal schematic.

Pulmonary System

Decisions in selection and use of inhaled anesthetics require an intimate understanding of these drugs. It is important that the anesthesia provider identify key differences to make informed and appropriate drug choices.

Ventilation, Intercostal Function, and Diaphragmatic Function

Inhalation anesthetics reduce both ventilatory volume and frequency. Initially, the respiratory depression seen with inhalation anesthetics demonstrates a decrease in volume with an increase in respiratory rate. During the early phases of an inhaled anesthetic induction (Guedel stage 2), ventilation may be irregular. As the patient becomes more deeply anesthetized, respiratory rate again becomes regular. Despite the increase in respiratory rate, the decrease in volume decreases overall minute ventilation, and without respiratory support, CO_2 levels begin to rise. Addition of nitrous oxide as a component of an inhalation induction is associated with an additional increase in respiratory rate, possibly due to stimulation of the sympathetic nervous system. As the patient continues to become more deeply anesthetized, intercostal muscles begin to relax as do skeletal muscles throughout the body. This loss of intercostal function during spontaneous ventilation gives rise to a diaphragmatic or "belly breathing" pattern that is sometimes observed during emergence from anesthesia as well and is an indication of significant anesthetic depth. Isoflurane, sevoflurane, and desflurane all have the ability to depress ventilation in this manner. At very deep levels of anesthesia, diaphragmatic function is also lost in a dose-dependent manner.

Functional Residual Capacity, Hypoxic Pulmonary Vasoconstriction, Carbon Dioxide, and Oxygen Responsiveness

Functional residual capacity (FRC) is defined as the sum of residual volume and expiratory reserve volume and is approximately 2400 mL in a 70-kg man. The importance of FRC during anesthesia cannot be underestimated. FRC is the volume of air remaining in the lungs after induction and when the patient has become apneic. As such it contains the oxygen upon which the patient depends until ventilation and oxygenation support begin. A healthy patient with a full FRC of oxygen (denitrogenated through breathing 100% oxygen) has as much as 8 to 10 minutes of available oxygen (FRC volume ÷ oxygen consumption per minute = 2400 mL/250 mL/min).

During inhalation anesthesia, the loss of skeletal muscle tone and spontaneous ventilatory movement allows the anterior-posterior diameter of the chest to decrease. The FRC is held open in part by this external splinting. Also, the diaphragm relaxes during deep anesthesia and ascends cephalad, thoracic blood volume increases, and the phasic activity of expiratory respiratory muscles is altered.[184–189] The net result is a reduction in the total FRC, thus decreasing the total "apneic time" available before the patient begins to desaturate without ventilatory support.

Further, other factors such as reduction in hypoxic pulmonary vasoconstriction (HPV) play a role in reducing the amount of available oxygen.[190–193] Hypoxic pulmonary vasoconstriction is the shunting of blood from alveoli with low oxygen levels to areas with higher oxygen levels. The net effect is homeostatic as the resultant movement of pulmonary arteriolar blood to oxygenated lung units improves ventilation-perfusion relationships. The shunting occurs through vasoconstriction of lung arterioles with redirection of blood flow. All inhalation anesthetics reduce hypoxic pulmonary vasoconstriction in a dose-dependent manner by vasodilation of these arterioles. The net result is an increase in ventilation-perfusion mismatch (shunt) with a resultant reduction in systemic oxygenation.

Respiratory responses to CO_2 and oxygen are mediated through both central and peripheral chemoreceptors. Central chemoreceptors are found in the medulla, whereas peripheral chemoreceptors are found in the carotid and aortic bodies. These chemoreceptors are sensitive to changes in hydrogen ion concentration (H^+). Accumulation of H^+ ion (CO_2 dissociates into hydrogen ions; therefore increased CO_2 represents increased H^+) stimulates an increase in respiratory rate and depth through a reflex mechanism. Afferent signals from the peripheral chemoreceptors ascend to the brainstem and are then distributed to medullary centers via the nucleus tractus solitarius. There they are relayed to the medullary respiratory center and integrated with input from the pontine apneustic (depth) and pneumotaxic (rate) centers, which lead to increases in ventilatory rate and depth. Additionally, peripheral chemoreceptors that sense oxygen levels send afferents in a similar manner, and the response is a similar ventilatory effort. Very low levels of anesthetic agent are needed to produce from 15% to 75% depression of the ventilatory drive from hypoxia.[25] Patients with chronic elevation of CO_2 levels (e.g., chronic obstructive pulmonary disease) desensitize their CO_2 receptors and are said to have a "hypoxic drive" or primarily oxygen-based ventilatory stimulus reflex. These patients are at increased risk after an anesthetic, including an inhalation agent, and should be carefully monitored.

The ventilatory response to elevation in CO_2 is linear and can be graphically represented (Figure 12-5). Minute ventilation increases in a linear manner to changes in $PaCO_2$ between 20 and 80.[25] The impact of inhaled anesthetic agents on CO_2 responsiveness is to reduce the overall ventilatory response in the face of an increasing H^+ concentration. This is sometimes referred to as a "shift to the right" of the curve. The inhaled anesthetics suppress both CO_2 and O_2 responsiveness in a dose-dependent fashion. All inhalation agents act in a similar manner, with even residual levels of inhaled anesthetic significantly blunting these reflex responses. This is an important consideration for postanesthetic monitoring and evaluation.

The shift to the right of the CO_2 response curve shifts the CO_2 point at which the ventilatory drive does not stimulate a breath. This point is termed the "apneic threshold" and is typically 4 to 5 mm Hg $PaCO_2$ below the $PaCO_2$ that stimulates regular respirations. For example, the normal arterial CO_2 range is 35 to 45 mm Hg. On average, regular respirations occur with $PaCO_2$ of approximately 40 mm Hg. With hyperventilation, the CO_2 falls, in this case, and when it reaches 35 mm Hg or below, the patient no longer has a stimulus to breathe as a result of his or her CO_2 level. Going back to the example of the rightward shifted CO_2 response curve, the apneic threshold will be proportionately higher as the CO_2 rises. Therefore patients who have residual inhalation agent may require a CO_2 that is significantly higher to stimulate respiratory effort. Concurrently, inhaled anesthetics also blunt the hypoxic drive. Typically, the threshold for the hypoxic drive is a PaO_2 of approximately 60 mm Hg. With residual inhalation agent, patient oxygen levels must fall below this point to respond with a normal ventilatory effort.

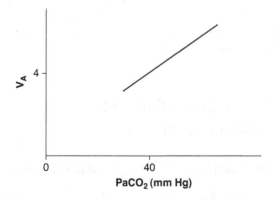

Figure 12-5 Carbon dioxide response curve schematic.

Airway Resistance, Bronchodilation, Pungency, and Mucociliary Clearance

Airway resistance is increased by inhaled anesthetics. This is a result of decreased net lung volume (see the preceding FRC description) rather than a constriction of airway smooth muscle. Inhaled anesthetics directly decrease smooth muscle tone of bronchioles in a dose-dependent manner (although the effect may be opposed in the case of the pungent agents). Volatile anesthetics relax airway smooth muscle primarily by directly depressing smooth muscle contractility and indirectly inhibiting the reflex neural pathways or by working through the nitric oxide pathway.[25,194] In the clinical setting, the most effective bronchodilator in current use is sevoflurane relative to bronchodilation and lack of pungency.[195–197] Inhaled anesthetics also have the ability to prevent bronchoconstriction in the face of an antigen challenge[194,198] and are used in management of patients with reactive airway diseases, including asthma, bronchitis, and emphysema, for this reason.[199]

Pungency is defined as a sharp or acrid taste or odor. Halothane was formerly the prototypical inhaled agent for inhalation induction because of the sweetness that characterized its vapor. Of the currently used inhalation agents, only sevoflurane is nonpungent. The pungency sequence can be denoted as D > I > S. As a result sevoflurane is typically the only agent used for inhalation anesthesia and is the dominant agent used in pediatric care.

Pungency complications include respiratory irritation with increased secretions, coughing, and even laryngospasm. In patients with preexisting reactive airway disease, these symptoms are typically those targeted to be avoided. The respiratory irritation effect of inhaled agents is thought to be a threshold phenomenon. In 81 un-premedicated, healthy volunteers at 2 MAC, 4% of sevoflurane subjects, 40% of isoflurane subjects, and 74% of desflurane subjects coughed and objected to breathing in any further agent.[200] In a second study of five un-premedicated, healthy volunteers breathing 1 MAC of desflurane, all subjects completed the test.[201] Therefore the respiratory irritation effect is absent when 1 MAC of desflurane, isoflurane, or sevoflurane is used instead of 2 MAC.[201,202] Therefore the threshold for respiratory irritation for desflurane is 1 MAC (6%). Additionally, the threshold for respiratory irritation is 1.5 MAC (1.8%) for isoflurane. Sevoflurane does not cause respiratory irritation.[24]

The corporate product monograph for desflurane acknowledges the potential for adverse airway events and warns against use in inhalation induction and during mask induction. This is prudent because the dose of inhaled anesthetics must sometimes be adjusted above 1 MAC to attain specific outcomes during induction and even through the course of a case. Use of opioids that have antitussive effects can decrease the potential for respiratory irritation responses when using desflurane or isoflurane.[24]

The trachea is a musculomembranous tube lined with ciliated columnar epithelium that extends to the terminal bronchioles. Mucociliary movement and thus secretion clearance is reduced by all inhalation anesthetics in a dose-dependent manner. This has implications for the ability to clear secretions in the postoperative period and is important in patient populations with preexisting problems clearing secretions, such as in those with chronic obstructive pulmonary disease.

In summary, the respiratory differences between the inhalation agents are subtle. Even at very low levels (0.1 MAC), responses to CO_2/O_2 can be blunted or abolished with the hypercapnic responses more resistant than the hypoxic response.[203,204] Hypoxic pulmonary vasoconstriction effects are most important in patients with significant disease. Issues related to the pungency of inhaled anesthetics play a role in induction, emergence, and (as described in the previous section) cardiovascular responses. An understanding of the bronchodilation effects is important in managing patients with reactive airway disease.

Renal and Hepatic Systems

Inhaled agents undergo little metabolism and are thus not eliminated via the kidneys. Changes in blood pressure and/or cardiac output associated with the cardiovascular effects of agents are possible. With reductions in perfusion pressure come associated, nonspecific risk to these vital organs.

Renal Issues

Only sevoflurane undergoes significant metabolism, with up to approximately 5% of an inhaled dose metabolized. Although sevoflurane is not associated with hepatotoxicity, it does undergo oxidative metabolism that results in liberation of inorganic fluoride ions as well as hexafluoroisopropanol. Clinical studies show that serum fluoride concentrations often peak above 50 µmol/L (especially in obese patients) even when sevoflurane is administered during surgery of average duration.[17,205,206] Because of sevoflurane's low blood-to-gas solubility and its rapid elimination, fluoride concentrations fall very quickly after surgery, and renal toxicities are not expected (and have not been associated) with sevoflurane administration.[58,205,207,208]

Hepatic Issues

Modern inhaled anesthetics undergo little metabolism, which represents a substantial advancement in drug-class

pharmacokinetics. Historically, metabolic byproducts (e.g., methoxyflurane metabolizing into high levels of fluorine and injuring the kidneys or chloroform breakdown, causing hepatic damage) were significant limiting factors in use of inhaled anesthetics.

All inhaled anesthetics have been associated with postoperative liver dysfunction. Two mechanisms have been identified related to inhaled anesthetic-induced hepatitis. The first and milder form is direct hepatocyte toxicity, which has a low morbidity. This direct hepatocyte injury is thought to be associated with other variables that reduce blood flow to the liver, including proximate surgery and reductions in perfusion pressure as a result of low blood pressure or low cardiac output.

The second form is more severe and is associated with both the metabolic pathway and immune modulation. Inhaled anesthetics are metabolized in the liver by cytochrome P-450 mixed-function oxidase isoenzymes, with the CP450 2E-1 subset responsible for inhaled anesthetic breakdown. Trifluoroacetate is the common breakdown product from desflurane, halothane, and isoflurane metabolism.[17] This substance is hepatotoxic and is thought to act through an immunologic mechanism involving trifluoroacetyl hapten formation and an autoimmune response.[17,209–213] The incidence of hepatic injury seems to depend on the extent of metabolism (with liver enzyme induction thought to be a variable) and subsequent formation of trifluoroacetylated compounds with initiation of immune responses. The most feared outcome is a fulminant, autoimmune-mediated hepatic failure culminating in centrilobular necrosis. This form is commonly referred to as "halothane hepatitis" because of the significantly higher incidence found with halothane. Risk factors include reexposure to the agent, and demographic variables include gender (female > male), obesity, age (> 50 years), specific genetic markers, and ethnic group (Mexican American).[17,210,211,213–216] Although very rare, this form of hepatitis is also possible with administration of isoflurane and desflurane.[217]

Other Issues Related to Inhaled Anesthetics

Genetic Effects and Effects on Fetal Development

The potential for genetic effects of the inhaled agents is not significant. Modern inhaled anesthetics have shown negative results when tested for carcinogenicity and mutagenicity, although animal models have been positive for both outcomes.[218–223]

As described earlier, nitrous oxide has direct effects on suppression of the activity of vitamin B_{12}-dependent enzymes with resultant issues with myelin formation (methionine synthetase) and DNA formation (thymidylate synthetase). The time course for initiation of these effects is short (within hours); therefore it is prudent to avoid use of nitrous oxide in women who are in their first trimester of pregnancy.

The question of impact of environmental nitrous on pregnant healthcare providers has remained a matter of interest and controversy. Specifically, epidemiologic studies done in the 1960s and 1970s seemed to indicate that the spontaneous abortion rates and congenital birth defect rates among operating room personnel were higher than comparison cohorts. Teratogenicity and mutagenicity effects were studied with congenital anomalies also reported in animal models and bench studies suggesting possible mutagenic effects.[219,220,224] No follow-up human studies have demonstrated an increased incidence,[225] and industry-wide safety measures, which include National Institute for Occupational Safety and Health regulation of agent pollution levels, high rates of room air exchange, and mandatory use of scavenging, have greatly reduced provider concern. Further, providers now have sufficient variety available in the modern anesthetic world to select total IV anesthetic techniques and/or to avoid use of nitrous oxide entirely should they so choose.

Malignant Hyperthermia

Malignant hyperthermia is an inherited and potentially fatal syndrome that susceptible patients develop when they receive inhaled anesthetics, including isoflurane, sevoflurane, desflurane, the skeletal muscle relaxant succinylcholine, and possibly nitrous oxide.[226] Inhaled anesthetics act as a trigger for this genetic "gun" and a cascade of events occurs that includes uncontrolled calcium release within skeletal muscle cells, leading to muscle rigidity and life-threatening hypermetabolism. Treatment includes dantrolene 2.5 to 10 mg/kg, cooling, and side effect management. Without treatment, mortality is as high as 90%. Diagnostic testing for malignant hyperthermia susceptibility is advancing as more is understood about its genetic nature. The caffeine-halothane contracture test remains the gold standard diagnostic test for malignant hyperthermia but has a high false-positive rate, is expensive, and is available in only eight institutions in North America.

The second test uses a blood sample to assess for a genetic mutation linked to the disease. Because the *RYR1* (malignant hyperthermia) gene is very large, testing all possible mutation sites is time-consuming and expensive. The current molecular genetic testing screens for only 17

of 60 possible mutations, yielding a positive result in only 25% to 30% of susceptible patients.[226]

Environmental Concerns

There are two primary concerns related to the environmental impact of halogenated inhalation anesthetics. The first is the impact of chlorine and bromine released into the atmosphere with potential to harm the ozone layer and thus increase ultraviolet exposure and contribute to global warming. The second and complementary fear is that the fluorinated hydrocarbons will contribute as greenhouse gases to the overall planetary warming effect.[21]

Inhalation agents are typically scavenged out of operating rooms and vented to the atmosphere without processing. Although the overall impact of these agents is minimal compared with industrial and animal sources, some authors have suggested a proactive line of attack by converting to total IV anesthetic approaches.[214] Although this may seem reasonable at first blush, the conversion from the dominant method of general anesthesia (inhalation) to the IV form would need to be analyzed from an overall carbon and greenhouse gas impact perspective because production of the additional IV tubing and other plastic parts as well as their disposal (incineration?) would need to be explored with comparison to the current system.

⬛ Key Points

- Historic developments and initial use of inhalation anesthetics lagged behind the actual scientific discoveries of the agents. First use of inhalation anesthesia represented a tremendous advance in medical care and a landmark reduction in human suffering.
- Although no "ideal" inhalation agent exists, modern agents are potent, have few side effects, and are typically chosen based on a spectrum of variables, including system effects, side effects, potential toxicity, and cost.
- Use of inhaled anesthetics requires an understanding of drug physical characteristics (solubility, pungency, vapor pressure), pharmacokinetics (uptake and distribution), and pharmacodynamics (MAC and system-by-system effects).
- Low solubility of agents in blood and tissue allows for rapid induction and emergence. The modern inhaled agents have relatively low solubilities when compared with historic predecessors.
- MAC concentration is the dose of an inhaled anesthetic required to prevent movement of 50% of patients who

experience a surgical stimulus. This parameter establishes a frame of reference when administering agents.

- Volatile anesthetics depress both ventilatory response to carbon dioxide and response to hypoxemia. Even residual amounts of inhaled agents may have this effect, requiring careful monitoring in the postanesthetic period.
- Although nitrous oxide use in clinical practice has declined significantly, providers must remain aware of the impact of nitrous oxide on enclosed air space expansion, potential for nausea and vomiting, and need for supplemental oxygen after nitrous oxide anesthesia.
- Volatile anesthetics cause dose-dependent decreases in blood pressure, neuronal function, and myocardial function.
- Volatile anesthetics cause both skeletal and smooth muscle relaxation. Important smooth muscle relaxation effects include the respiratory system (bronchial smooth muscle), vascular system (arteriolar smooth muscle), and the uterus.

Chapter Questions

1. Which inhalation anesthetic is the best choice for a patient with reactive airway disease such as asthma or chronic bronchitis?
2. The endotracheal tube cuff is typically filled with room air. Why should the cuff pressure be monitored during nitrous oxide anesthesia? In addition, why would administration of nitrous oxide be a problem during surgery for a patient having tympanoplasty?
3. Sevoflurane has a slightly higher brain-to-blood solubility coefficient than does desflurane. What is the implication for emergence, and what steps could you take to minimize the impact on your anesthetic?
4. Why must patients who receive general anesthesia with inhalation agents be carefully monitored in the postoperative period for ventilatory issues?
5. Why is it important to understand the subtle differences on organ systems between the modern inhaled anesthetics?

References

1. Fenster JM. *Ether Day: The Strange Tale of America's Greatest Medical Discovery and the Haunted Men Who Made It*, 1st ed. New York: HarperCollins; 2001.

2. Thorwald J. *The Century of the Surgeon*. New York: Pantheon Books; 1957.

3. Boston Public Library. *NOVA, Science Adventures on Television: A Series of Reading Lists*. Boston: The Library; 1974.

4. Wolfe RJ. *Tarnished Idol: William Thomas Green Morton and the Introduction of Surgical Anesthesia: A Chronicle of the Ether Controversy*. San Anselmo, CA: Norman; 2001.

5. Ball P. *The Devil's Doctor: Paracelsus and the World of Renaissance Magic and Science,* 1st American ed. New York: Farrar, Straus and Giroux; 2006.

6. Priestley J. *Experiments and Observations on Different Kinds of Air*. London: Printed for J. Johnson; 1774.

7. Davy H. *Researches, Chemical and Philosophical, Chiefly Concerning Nitrous Oxide, or Dephlogisticated Nitrous Air, and Its Respiration*. London: Smith, Elder; 1839.

8. Foy G. The discovery of chloroform. *Br Med J.* 1915;1:1103.

9. Moir JC. November 1847 and its sequel: events connected with the discovery of the anaesthetic properties of chloroform by James Y. Simpson, George S. Keith and J. Matthews Duncan. *Edinb Med J.* 1947;54:593–610.

10. Simpson D. Simpson and "the discovery of chloroform." *Scott Med J.* 1990;35:149–153.

11. Moore FD. John Collins Warren and his act of conscience: a brief narrative of the trial and triumph of a great surgeon. *Ann Surg.* 1999;229:187–196.

12. Eger EI 2nd, Sonner JM. Anaesthesia defined (gentlemen, this is no humbug). *Clin Anaesth.* 2006;20:23–29.

13. Bigelow HJ. Insensibility during surgical operations produced by inhalation. *Boston Med Surg J.* 1846;35:309–317.

14. Ehrlich TB, O'Leary JP. Crawford Williamson Long and the use of ether anesthesia. *Am Surg.* 1994;60:155–156.

15. Robinson JS Jr, Eastwood DW. Publish and perish—Crawford Long's dilemma. *South Med J.* 1972;65:600–604.

16. Keys TE. Historical vignettes. Dr. Crawford Williamson Long (1815-1878). *Anesth Analg.* 1972;51:865.

17. Bovill JG. Inhalation anaesthesia: from diethyl ether to xenon. *Handb Exp Pharmacol.* 2008;182:121–142.

18. Nelson JE, Wilstead SF. Alice Magaw (Kessel): her life in and out of the operating room. *AANA J.* 2009;77:12–16.

19. Koch E. Alice Magaw and the great secret of open drop anesthesia. *AANA J.* 1999;67:33–34.

20. Wawersik J. History of chloroform anesthesia. *Anaesth Reanim.* 1997;22:144–152.

21. Eger EI, Weiskopf RB, Eisenkraft JB. *The Pharmacology of Inhaled Anesthetics,* vol 1. San Antonio, TX: Foundation; 2002.

22. Morgan GE, Mikhail MS, Murray MJ. *Clinical Anesthesiology,* 4th ed. New York: Lange Medical Books/McGraw-Hill; 2006.

23. Terrell RC. The invention and development of enflurane, isoflurane, sevoflurane, and desflurane. *Anesthesiology.* 2008; 108:531-533.

24. Eger EI 2nd. Characteristics of anesthetic agents used for induction and maintenance of general anesthesia. *Am J Health Syst Pharm.* 2004;61(Suppl 4):S3–S10.

25. Barash PG, Ebert T. Inhalation anesthesia. In: Barash PG, ed. *Clinical Anesthesia*, 6th ed. Philadelphia: Wolters Kluwer; 2009.

26. Kossick M. Inhalational anesthetics. In: Nagelhaut J, Plaus K (Eds.) *Nurse Anesthesia*. Philadelphia: W.B. Saunders; 2009.

27. Brown BR Jr. Clinical significance of the biotransformation of inhalation anesthetics. *South Med J.* 1976;69:554–556.

28. *Merriam-Webster Unabridged Online Dictionary.* Springfield, MA; 2008. Available at: www.merriam-webster.com. Accessed August 15, 2009.

29. Smith C, Flynn C, Wardall G, Broome IJ. Leakage and absorption of isoflurane by different types of anaesthetic circuit and monitoring tubing. *Anaesthesia.* 2002;57: 686–689.

30. Coetzee JF, Stewart LJ. Fresh gas flow is not the only determinant of volatile agent consumption: a multi-centre study of low-flow anaesthesia. *Br J Anaesth.* 2002;88:46–55.

31. Dorsch JA, Dorsch SE. *Understanding Anesthesia Equipment*, 5th ed. Philadelphia: Wolters Kluwer Health; 2008.

32. Abraham MH, Acree WE Jr, Mintz C, Payne S. Effect of anesthetic structure on inhalation anesthesia: implications for the mechanism. *J Pharm Sci.* 2008;97:2373–2384.

33. Ueda I, Suzuki A. Is there a specific receptor for anesthetics? Contrary effects of alcohols and fatty acids on phase transition and bioluminescence of firefly luciferase. *Biophys J.* 1998;75:1052–1057.

34. Katz Y. Anesthesia and the Meyer-Overton rule. II. A solution theory view of anesthesia and perturbations. *J Theor Biol.* 1994;167:99–105.

35. Hemmings HC, Hopkins PM. *Foundations of Anesthesia: Basic Sciences for Clinical Practice*, 2nd ed. Philadelphia: Mosby Elsevier; 2006.

36. Mihic SJ, McQuilkin SJ, Eger EI 2nd, Ionescu P, Harris RA. Potentiation of gamma-aminobutyric acid type A receptor-mediated chloride currents by novel halogenated compounds correlates with their abilities to induce general anesthesia. *Mol Pharmacol.* 1994;46:851–857.

37. Bieda MC, Su H, Maciver MB. Anesthetics discriminate between tonic and phasic gamma-aminobutyric acid receptors on hippocampal CA1 neurons. *Anesth Analg.* 2009;108: 484–490.

38. Rehberg B, Grunewald M, Baars J, Fuegener K, Urban BW, Kox WJ. Monitoring of immobility to noxious stimulation during sevoflurane anesthesia using the spinal H-reflex. *Anesthesiology.* 2004;100:44–50.

39. Eger EI 2nd. Age, minimum alveolar anesthetic concentration, and minimum alveolar anesthetic concentration-awake [see comment]. *Anesth Analg.* 2001;93:947–953.

40. Eger EI 2nd, Raines DE, Shafer SL, Hemmings HC Jr, Sonner JM. Is a new paradigm needed to explain how inhaled anesthetics produce immobility? *Anesth Analg.* 2008;107: 832–848.

41. Mapleson WW. Effect of age on MAC in humans: a meta-analysis. *Br J Anaesth.* 1996;76:179–185.

42. Nishiyama T. Hemodynamic and catecholamine response to a rapid increase in isoflurane or sevoflurane concentration during a maintenance phase of anesthesia in humans. *J Anesth.* 2005;19:213–217.

43. Paul M, Fisher DM. Are estimates of MAC reliable? *Anesthesiology.* 2001;95:1362–1370.

44. Wade JG, Stevens WC. Isoflurane: an anesthetic for the eighties? *Anesth Analg.* 1981;60:666–682.

45. White PF, Tang J, Wender RH, et al. Desflurane versus sevoflurane for maintenance of outpatient anesthesia: the effect on early versus late recovery and perioperative coughing. *Anesth Analg.* 2009;109:387–393.

46. Ebert TJ. Renal responses to low-flow desflurane, sevoflurane, and propofol in patients. 2000;93(6):1401–1406.

47. Olympio MA. Carbon dioxide absorbent desiccation safety conference convened by APSF. *APSF Newsletter.* 2005;20:25–30.

48. Laster MJ, Eger EI. Temperatures in soda lime during degradation of desflurane, isoflurane, and sevoflurane by desiccated soda lime. *Anesth Analg.* 2005;101:753–757.

49. Struys MMRF, Bouche MPLA, Rolly G, et al. Production of compound A and carbon monoxide in circle systems: an in vitro comparison of two carbon dioxide absorbents. *Anaesthesia.* 2004;59:584–589.

50. Wissing H, Kuhn I, Warnken U, Dudziak R. Carbon monoxide production from desflurane, enflurane, halothane, isoflurane, and sevoflurane with dry soda lime. *Anesthesiology.* 2001;95:1205–1212.

51. Singh D, Rath GP, Dash HH, Bithal PK. Sevoflurane provides better recovery as compared with isoflurane in children undergoing spinal surgery. *J Neurosurg Anesthesiol.* 2009;21:202–206.

52. Magni G, Rosa IL, Melillo G, Savio A, Rosa G. A comparison between sevoflurane and desflurane anesthesia in patients undergoing craniotomy for supratentorial intracranial surgery. *Anesth Analg.* 2009;109:567–571.

53. Vallejo MC, Sah N, Phelps AL, O'Donnell J, Romeo RC. Desflurane versus sevoflurane for laparoscopic gastroplasty in morbidly obese patients. *J Clin Anesth.* 2007;19:3–8.

54. Sakata DJ, Gopalakrishnan NA, Orr JA, White JL, Westenskow DR. Rapid recovery from sevoflurane and desflurane with hypercapnia and hyperventilation. *Anesth Analg.* 2007;105:79–82.

55. Luttropp HH, Johansson A. Soda lime temperatures during low-flow sevoflurane anaesthesia and differences in deadspace. *Acta Anaesth Scand.* 2002;46:500–505.

56. Kharasch ED, Powers KM, Artru AA. Comparison of Amsorb, soda lime, and Baralyme degradation of volatile anesthetics and formation of carbon monoxide and compound A in swine in vivo. *Anesthesiology.* 2002;96:173–182.

57. Conzen PF, Kharasch ED, Czerner SFA, et al. Low-flow sevoflurane compared with low-flow isoflurane anesthesia in patients with stable renal insufficiency [see comment]. *Anesthesiology.* 2002;97:578–584.

58. Higuchi H, Adachi Y, Wada H, Kanno M, Satoh T. The effects of low-flow sevoflurane and isoflurane anesthesia on renal function in patients with stable moderate renal insufficiency. *Anesth Analg.* 2001;92:650–655.

59. Higuchi H, Adachi Y, Arimura S, Kanno M, Satoh T. Compound A concentrations during low-flow sevoflurane anesthesia correlate directly with the concentration of monovalent bases in carbon dioxide absorbents. *Anesth Analg.* 2000;91:434–439.

60. Kobayashi S, Bito H, Obata Y, Katoh T, Sato S. Compound A concentration in the circle absorber system during low-flow sevoflurane anesthesia: comparison of Dragersorb Free, Amsorb, and Sodasorb II. *J Clin Anesth.* 2003;15:33–37.

61. Fatheree RS, Leighton BL. Acute respiratory distress syndrome after an exothermic Baralyme-sevoflurane reaction. *Anesthesiology.* 2004;101:531–533.

62. Laster M, Roth P, Eger EI 2nd. Fires from the interaction of anesthetics with desiccated absorbent. *Anesth Analg.* 2004; 99:769–774.

63. O'Donnell JM. Orotracheal tube intracuff pressure initially and during anesthesia including nitrous oxide. *CRNA.* 1995; 6:79–85.

64. Singer MA, Lazaridis C, Nations SP, Wolfe GI. Reversible nitrous oxide-induced myeloneuropathy with pernicious anemia: case report and literature review. *Muscle Nerve.* 2008;37:125–129.

65. Sanders RD, Weimann J, Maze M. Biologic effects of nitrous oxide: a mechanistic and toxicologic review. *Anesthesiology.* 2008;109:707–722.

66. Lockwood AJ, Yang YF. Nitrous oxide inhalation anaesthesia in the presence of intraocular gas can cause irreversible blindness. *Br Dent J.* 2008;204:247–248.

67. Shulman RM, Geraghty TJ, Tadros M. A case of unusual substance abuse causing myeloneuropathy. *Spinal Cord.* 2007; 45:314–317.

68. Bajaj P, Nanda R, Goyal PKR. Pressure and volume changes of tracheal tube cuff following inflation with various inflating agents during nitrous oxide anesthesia. *Mid East J Anesthesiol.* 2004;17:1055–1068.

69. Murrell JC, Waters D, Johnson CB. Comparative effects of halothane, isoflurane, sevoflurane and desflurane on the electroencephalogram of the rat. *Lab Anim.* 2008;42:161–170.

70. Lukatch HS, Kiddoo CE, Maciver MB. Anesthetic-induced burst suppression EEG activity requires glutamate-mediated excitatory synaptic transmission. *Cereb Cortex.* 2005;15: 1322–1331.

71. Morimoto Y, Hagihira S, Koizumi Y, Ishida K, Matsumoto M, Sakabe T. The relationship between bispectral index and electroencephalographic parameters during isoflurane anesthesia. *Anesth Analg.* 2004;98:1336–1340.

72. Rewari V, Sethi D. Recurrence of focal seizure activity in an infant during induction of anaesthesia with sevoflurane. *Anaesth Intens Care.* 2007;35:788–791.

73. Mohanram A, Kumar V, Iqbal Z, Markan S, Pagel PS. Repetitive generalized seizure-like activity during emergence from sevoflurane anesthesia. *Can J Anaesth.* 2007;54:657–661.

74. Julliac B, Guehl D, Chopin F, et al. Risk factors for the occurrence of electroencephalogram abnormalities during induction of anesthesia with sevoflurane in nonepileptic patients. *Anesthesiology.* 2007;106:243–251.

75. Kurita N, Kawaguchi M, Hoshida T, Nakase H, Sakaki T, Furuya H. The effects of sevoflurane and hyperventilation on electrocorticogram spike activity in patients with refractory epilepsy. *Anesth Analg.* 2005;101:517–523.

76. Hisada K, Morioka T, Fukui K, et al. Effects of sevoflurane and isoflurane on electrocorticographic activities in patients with temporal lobe epilepsy. *J Neurosurg Anesthesiol.* 2001; 13:333–337.

77. Molnar C, Settakis G, Sarkany P, Kalman S, Szabo S, Fulesdi B. Effect of sevoflurane on cerebral blood flow and cerebrovascular resistance at surgical level of anaesthesia: a transcranial Doppler study. *Eur J Anaesthesiol.* 2007;24:179–184.

78. Kimme P, Ledin T, Sjoberg F. Dose effect of sevoflurane and isoflurane anesthetics on cortical blood flow during controlled hypotension in the pig. *Acta Anaesth Scand.* 2007;51:607–613.

79. Kadoi Y, Saito S, Takahashi K. The comparative effects of sevoflurane vs. isoflurane on cerebrovascular carbon dioxide reactivity in patients with hypertension. *Acta Anaesth Scand.* 2007;51:1382–1387.

80. Schlunzen L, Cold GE, Rasmussen M, Vafaee MS. Effects of dose-dependent levels of isoflurane on cerebral blood flow in healthy subjects studied using positron emission tomography. *Acta Anaesth Scand.* 2006;50:306–312.

81. Holmstrom A, Rosen I, Akeson J. Desflurane results in higher cerebral blood flow than sevoflurane or isoflurane at hypocapnia in pigs. *Acta Anaesth Scand.* 2004;48:400–404.

82. Holmstrom A, Akeson J. Desflurane increases intracranial pressure more and sevoflurane less than isoflurane in pigs subjected to intracranial hypertension. *J Neurosurg Anesthesiol.* 2004;16:136–143.

83. Oshima T, Karasawa F, Okazaki Y, Wada H, Satoh T. Effects of sevoflurane on cerebral blood flow and cerebral metabolic

rate of oxygen in human beings: a comparison with isoflurane. *Eur J Anaesthesiol.* 2003;20:543–547.

84. Luginbuehl IA, Fredrickson MJ, Karsli C, Bissonnette B. Cerebral blood flow velocity in children anaesthetized with desflurane. *Paediatr Anaesth.* 2003;13:496–500.

85. Fairgrieve R, Rowney DA, Karsli C, Bissonnette B. The effect of sevoflurane on cerebral blood flow velocity in children. *Acta Anaesth Scand.* 2003;47:1226–1230.

86. Wong GT, Luginbuehl I, Karsli C, Bissonnette B. The effect of sevoflurane on cerebral autoregulation in young children as assessed by the transient hyperemic response. *Anesth Analg.* 2006;102:1051–1055.

87. Rozet I, Vavilala MS, Lindley AM, Visco E, Treggiari M, Lam AM. Cerebral autoregulation and CO_2 reactivity in anterior and posterior cerebral circulation during sevoflurane anesthesia. *Anesth Analg.* 2006;102:560–564.

88. Endoh H, Honda T, Ohashi S, Hida S. Cerebral autoregulation during sevoflurane or isoflurane anesthesia: evaluation with transient hyperemic response. *Masui.* 2001;50:1316–1321.[Japanese]

89. McCulloch TJ, Turner MJ. The effects of hypocapnia and the cerebral autoregulatory response on cerebrovascular resistance and apparent zero flow pressure during isoflurane anesthesia. *Anesth Analg.* 2009;108:1284–1290.

90. De Deyne C, Joly LM, Ravussin P. Newer inhalation anaesthetics and neuro-anaesthesia: what is the place for sevoflurane or desflurane? *Ann Fr Anesth Reanim.* 2004;23:367–374. [French]

91. Talke P, Caldwell J, Dodsont B, Richardson CA. Desflurane and isoflurane increase lumbar cerebrospinal fluid pressure in normocapnic patients undergoing transsphenoidal hypophysectomy. *Anesthesiology.* 1996;85:999–1004.

92. Talke P, Caldwell JE, Richardson CA. Sevoflurane increases lumbar cerebrospinal fluid pressure in normocapnic patients undergoing transsphenoidal hypophysectomy. *Anesthesiology.* 1999;91:127–130.

93. Sponheim S, Skraastad O, Helseth E, Due-Tonnesen B, Aamodt G, Breivik H. Effects of 0.5 and 1.0 MAC isoflurane, sevoflurane and desflurane on intracranial and cerebral perfusion pressures in children. *Acta Anaesth Scand.* 2003;47:932–938.

94. Adams RW, Cucchiara RF, Gronert GA, Messick JM, Michenfelder JD. Isoflurane and cerebrospinal fluid pressure in neurosurgical patients. *Anesthesiology.* 1981;54:97–99.

95. Grosslight K, Foster R, Colohan AR, Bedford RF. Isoflurane for neuroanesthesia: risk factors for increases in intracranial pressure. *Anesthesiology.* 1985;63:533–536.

96. Hancock SM, Eastwood JR, Mahajan RP. Effects of inhaled nitrous oxide 50% on estimated cerebral perfusion pressure and zero flow pressure in healthy volunteers. *Anaesthesia.* 2005;60:129–132.

97. Wilson-Smith E, Karsli C, Luginbuehl I, Bissonnette B. Effect of nitrous oxide on cerebrovascular reactivity to carbon dioxide in children during sevoflurane anaesthesia. *Br J Anaesth.* 2003;91:190–195.

98. Muzzi DA, Losasso TJ, Dietz NM, Faust RJ, Cucchiara RF, Milde LN. The effect of desflurane and isoflurane on cerebrospinal fluid pressure in humans with supratentorial mass lesions. *Anesthesiology.* 1992;76:720–724.

99. Artru AA, Momota T. Rate of CSF formation and resistance to reabsorption of CSF during sevoflurane or remifentanil in rabbits. *J Neurosurg Anesthesiol.* 2000;12:37–43.

100. Sugioka S. Effects of sevoflurane on intracranial pressure and formation and absorption of cerebrospinal fluid in cats. *Masui.* 1992;41:1434–1442.[Japanese]

101. Liao R, Li J, Liu J. Volatile induction/maintenance of anaesthesia with sevoflurane increases jugular venous oxygen saturation and lumbar cerebrospinal fluid pressure in patients undergoing craniotomy. *Eur J Anaesthesiol.* 2009.

102. Bonhomme V, Demoitie J, Schaub I, Hans P. Acid-base status and hemodynamic stability during propofol and sevoflurane-based anesthesia in patients undergoing uncomplicated intracranial surgery. *J Neurosurg Anesthesiol.* 2009;21:112–119.

103. McAuliffe JJ, Loepke AW, Miles L, Joseph B, Hughes E, Vorhees CV. Desflurane, isoflurane, and sevoflurane provide limited neuroprotection against neonatal hypoxia-ischemia in a delayed preconditioning paradigm. *Anesthesiology.* 2009;111:533–546.

104. Fries M, Coburn M, Nolte KW, et al. Early administration of xenon or isoflurane may not improve functional outcome and cerebral alterations in a porcine model of cardiac arrest. *Resuscitation.* 2009;80:584–590.

105. Lee JJ, Li L, Jung HH, Zuo Z. Postconditioning with isoflurane reduced ischemia-induced brain injury in rats. *Anesthesiology.* 2008;108:1055–1062.

106. Sakai H, Sheng H, Yates RB, Ishida K, Pearlstein RD, Warner DS. Isoflurane provides long-term protection against focal cerebral ischemia in the rat. *Anesthesiology.* 2007;106:92–99; discussion 8–10.

107. Miura Y, Grocott HP, Bart RD, Pearlstein RD, Dexter F, Warner DS. Differential effects of anesthetic agents on outcome from near-complete but not incomplete global ischemia in the rat. *Anesthesiology.* 1998;89:391–400.

108. Hoffman WE, Thomas C, Albrecht RF. The effect of halothane and isoflurane on neurologic outcome following incomplete cerebral ischemia in the rat. *Anesth Analg.* 1993;76:279–283.

109. Michenfelder JD, Sundt TM, Fode N, Sharbrough FW. Isoflurane when compared to enflurane and halothane decreases the frequency of cerebral ischemia during carotid endarterectomy. *Anesthesiology.* 1987;67:336–340.

110. Thoresen M, Hobbs CE, Wood T, Chakkarapani E, Dingley J. Cooling combined with immediate or delayed xenon inhalation provides equivalent long-term neuroprotection after neonatal hypoxia-ischemia. *J Cerebr Blood Flow Metab.* 2009; 29:707–714.

111. Hobbs C, Thoresen M, Tucker A, Aquilina K, Chakkarapani E, Dingley J. Xenon and hypothermia combine additively, offering long-term functional and histopathologic neuroprotection after neonatal hypoxia/ischemia. *Stroke.* 2008;39:1307–1313.

112. Codaccioni JL, Velly LJ, Moubarik C, Bruder NJ, Pisano PS, Guillet BA. Sevoflurane preconditioning against focal cerebral ischemia: inhibition of apoptosis in the face of transient improvement of neurological outcome. *Anesthesiology.* 2009; 110:1271–1278.

113. Bantel C, Maze M, Trapp S. Neuronal preconditioning by inhalational anesthetics: evidence for the role of plasmalemmal adenosine triphosphate-sensitive potassium channels. *Anesthesiology.* 2009;110:986–995.

114. Wang C, Jin Lee J, Jung HH, Zuo Z. Pretreatment with volatile anesthetics, but not with the nonimmobilizer 1,2-dichlorohexafluorocyclobutane, reduced cell injury in rat cerebellar slices after an in vitro simulated ischemia. *Brain Res.* 2007;1152:201–208.

115. Payne RS, Akca O, Roewer N, Schurr A, Kehl F. Sevoflurane-induced preconditioning protects against cerebral ischemic neuronal damage in rats. *Brain Res.* 9 2005;1034:147–152.

116. Matchett GA, Allard MW, Martin RD, Zhang JH. Neuroprotective effect of volatile anesthetic agents: molecular mechanisms. *Neurol Res.* 2009;31:128–134.

117. Loepke AW, Priestley MA, Schultz SE, McCann J, Golden J, Kurth CD. Desflurane improves neurologic outcome after low-flow cardiopulmonary bypass in newborn pigs. *Anesthesiology.* 2002;97:1521–1527.

118. Leduc ML, Atherley R, Jinks SL, Antognini JF. Nitrous oxide depresses electroencephalographic responses to repetitive noxious stimulation in the rat. *Br J Anaesth.* 2006;96:216–221.

119. Banoub M, Tetzlaff JE, Schubert A. Pharmacologic and physiologic influences affecting sensory evoked potentials: implications for perioperative monitoring. *Anesthesiology.* 2003; 99:716–737.

120. Moshchev DA, Sazonova OB, Ogurtsova AA, Lubnin A. Effect of sevoflurane on spontaneous brain bioelectrical activity in neurosurgical patients. *Anesteziol Reanimatol.* 2008;11–16. [Russian]

121. Constant I, Seeman R, Murat I. Sevoflurane and epileptiform EEG changes. *Paediatr Anaesth.* 2005;15:266–274.

122. Sloan TB. Anesthetic effects on electrophysiologic recordings. *J Clin Neurophysiol.* 1998;15:217–226.

123. Vaugha DJ, Thornton C, Wright DR, et al. Effects of different concentrations of sevoflurane and desflurane on subcortical somatosensory evoked responses in anaesthetized, nonstimulated patients. *Br J Anaesth.* 2001;86:59–62.

124. Ogawa Y, Iwasaki K, Shibata S, Kato J, Ogawa S, Oi Y. Different effects on circulatory control during volatile induction and maintenance of anesthesia and total intravenous anesthesia: autonomic nervous activity and arterial cardiac baroreflex function evaluated by blood pressure and heart rate variability analysis. *J Clin Anesthesiol.* 2006;18:87–95.

125. Taoda M, Hashimoto K, Karasawa F, Satoh T. The effect of sevoflurane and enflurane on renal sympathetic nerve activity in sinoaortic denerved rabbits. *Masui.* 2000;49:1328–1332. [Japanese]

126. Saeki Y, Hasegawa Y, Shibamoto T, et al. The effects of sevoflurane, enflurane, and isoflurane on baroreceptor-sympathetic reflex in rabbits. *Anesth Analg.* 1996;82:342–348.

127. Huang CL, Huang HH, Chao A, Wang YP, Tsai SK. Rapid recovery of spontaneous baroreflex after sevoflurane anesthesia in ambulatory surgery. *Acta Anaesthesiol Sin.* 2001;39:23–26.

128. Ebert TJ, Perez F, Uhrich TD, Deshur MA. Desflurane-mediated sympathetic activation occurs in humans despite preventing hypotension and baroreceptor unloading. *Anesthesiology.* 1998;88:1227–1232.

129. Ebert TJ, Kotrly KJ, Vucins EJ, Pattison CZ, Kampine JP. Halothane anesthesia attenuates cardiopulmonary baroreflex control of peripheral resistance in humans. *Anesthesiology.* 1985;63:668–674.

130. Seagard JL, Elegbe EO, Hopp FA, et al. Effects of isoflurane on the baroreceptor reflex. *Anesthesiology.* 1983;59:511–520.

131. Seagard JL, Hopp FA, Bosnjak ZJ, Osborn JL, Kampine JP. Sympathetic efferent nerve activity in conscious and isoflurane-anesthetized dogs. *Anesthesiology.* 1984;61:266–270.

132. Ebert TJ. Cardiovascular and autonomic effects of sevoflurane. *Acta Anaesthesiol Belg.* 1996;47:15–21.

133. Muzi M, Ebert TJ, Hope WG, Robinson BJ, Bell LB. Site(s) mediating sympathetic activation with desflurane. *Anesthesiology.* 1996;85:737–747.

134. Tanaka M, Nishikawa T. Sevoflurane speeds recovery of baroreflex control of heart rate after minor surgical procedures compared with isoflurane. *Anesth Analg.* 1999;89:284–289.

135. Dedola E, Albertin A, Poli D, et al. Effect of nitrous oxide on desflurane MACBAR at two target-controlled concentrations of remifentanil. *Minerva Anestesiol.* 2008;74:165–172.

136. Ogawa S, Saito H, Saeki S, Suzuki H. Reflex sympathetic activities during inhalation of anaesthetics in cats: nitrous oxide. *Neurosci Lett.* 1994;168:16–18.

137. Abdulla YW, Giesecke AH, Hein HA, Cordes U. A comparison of the activity of the sympathoadrenal and adrenocortical

system under inhalation anesthesia techniques. *Acta Anaesthesiol Belg.* 1983;34:257–264.

138. Fukunaga AF, Epstein RM. Sympathetic excitation during nitrous-oxide-halothane anesthesia in the cat. *Anesthesiology.* 1973;39:23–36.

139. Zubicki A, Gostin X, Miclea D, et al. Comparison of the haemodynamic actions of desflurane/N$_2$O and isoflurane/N$_2$O anaesthesia in vascular surgical patients. *Acta Anaesth Scand.* 1998;42:1057–1062.

140. Sundeman H, Biber B, Henriksson BA, Raner C, Seeman-Lodding H, Winso O. Effects of desflurane on systemic, pre-portal and renal circulatory responses to infra-renal aortic cross-clamping in the pig. *Acta Anaesth Scand.* 1996;40(8 Pt 1):876–882.

141. McMurphy RM, Hodgson DS, Bruyette DS, Fingland RB. Cardiovascular effects of 1.0, 1.5, and 2.0 minimum alveolar concentrations of isoflurane in experimentally induced hypothyroidism in dogs. *Vet Surg.* 1996;25:171–178.

142. Ebert TJ, Harkin CP, Muzi M. Cardiovascular responses to sevoflurane: a review. *Anesth Analg.* 1995;81(6 Suppl):S11–S22.

143. Linde HW, Oh SO, Homi J, Joshi C. Cardiovascular effects of isoflurane and halothane during controlled ventilation in older patients. *Anesth Analg.* 1975;54:701–704.

144. Han RQ, Li SR, Wang BG, et al. The effect of isoflurane induced hypotension on intraoperative cerebral vasospasm in intracranial aneurysm surgery. *Zhonghua Yi Xue Za Zhi.* 2004;84:286–289.[Chinese]

145. Nathanson MH, Fredman B, Smith I, White PF. Sevoflurane versus desflurane for outpatient anesthesia: a comparison of maintenance and recovery profiles. *Anesth Analg.* 1995; 81:1186–1190.

146. Kelly RE, Hartman GS, Embree PB, Sharp G, Artusio JF Jr. Inhaled induction and emergence from desflurane anesthesia in the ambulatory surgical patient: the effect of premedication. *Anesth Analg.* 1993;77:540–543.

147. Weiskopf RB, Holmes MA, Rampil IJ, et al. Cardiovascular safety and actions of high concentrations of I-653 and isoflurane in swine. *Anesthesiology.* 1989;70:793–798.

148. Holzman RS, van der Velde ME, Kaus SJ, et al. Sevoflurane depresses myocardial contractility less than halothane during induction of anesthesia in children. *Anesthesiology.* 1996;85:1260–1267.

149. Pagel PS, Kampine JP, Schmeling WT, Warltier DC. Reversal of volatile anesthetic-induced depression of myocardial contractility by extracellular calcium also enhances left ventricular diastolic function. *Anesthesiology.* 1993;78:141–154.

150. Wolf WJ, Neal MB, Peterson MD. The hemodynamic and cardiovascular effects of isoflurane and halothane anesthesia in children. *Anesthesiology.* 1986;64:328–333.

151. Rathod R, Jacobs HK, Kramer NE, Rao LK, Salem MR, Towne WD. Echocardiographic assessment of ventricular performance following induction with two anesthetics. *Anesthesiology.* 1978;49:86–90.

152. Kaplan JA, Miller ED, Bailey DR. A comparative study of enflurane and halothane using systolic time intervals. *Anesth Analg.* 1976;55:263–268.

153. Goldberg AH. Cardiovascular function and halothane. *Clin Anesth.* 1968;1:23–60.

154. Kashimoto S, Nonaka A, Yamaguchi T, Nakamura T, Kumazawa T. Effects of inhalation anesthetics on myocardial and hepatic energy metabolism in normotensive and spontaneously hypertensive rats subjected to hemorrhage. *Acta Anaesth Scand.* 1994;38:187–191.

155. Tayefeh F, Larson MD, Sessler DI, Eger EI 2nd, Bowland T. Time-dependent changes in heart rate and pupil size during desflurane or sevoflurane anesthesia. *Anesth Analg.* 1997; 85:1362–1366.

156. Stevens WC, Cromwell TH, Halsey MJ, Eger EI 2nd, Shakespeare TF, Bahlman SH. The cardiovascular effects of a new inhalation anesthetic, Forane, in human volunteers at constant arterial carbon dioxide tension. *Anesthesiology.* 1971; 35:8–16.

157. Weiskopf RB. Cardiovascular effects of desflurane in experimental animals and volunteers. *Anaesthesia.* 1995;50(Suppl): 14–17.

158. Yonker-Sell AE, Muzi M, Hope WG, Ebert TJ. Alfentanil modifies the neurocirculatory responses to desflurane. *Anesth Analg.* 1996;82:162–166.

159. Weiskopf RB, Eger EI 2nd, Noorani M, Daniel M. Fentanyl, esmolol, and clonidine blunt the transient cardiovascular stimulation induced by desflurane in humans. *Anesthesiology.* 1994;81:1350–1355.

160. Buffington CW. Coronary steal models. *Anesthesiology.* 1992; 77:219–220.

161. Buffington CW. No coronary dilation: no coronary steal. *Anesthesiology.* 1991;75:376–377.

162. Buffington CW, Davis KB, Gillispie S, Pettinger M. The prevalence of steal-prone coronary anatomy in patients with coronary artery disease: an analysis of the Coronary Artery Surgery Study Registry. *Anesthesiology.* 1988;69:721–727.

163. Buffington CW, Romson JL, Levine A, Duttlinger NC, Huang AH. Isoflurane induces coronary steal in a canine model of chronic coronary occlusion. *Anesthesiology.* 1987;66: 280–292.

164. Agnew NM, Pennefather SH, Russell GN. Isoflurane and coronary heart disease. *Anaesthesia.* 2002;57:338–347.

165. Helman JD, Leung JM, Bellows WH, et al. The risk of myocardial ischemia in patients receiving desflurane versus

sufentanil anesthesia for coronary artery bypass graft surgery. The S.P.I. Research Group. *Anesthesiology.* 1992;77: 47–62.

166. Ebert TJ, Kharasch ED, Rooke GA, Shroff A, Muzi M. Myocardial ischemia and adverse cardiac outcomes in cardiac patients undergoing noncardiac surgery with sevoflurane and isoflurane. Sevoflurane Ischemia Study Group. *Anesth Analg.* 1997;85:993–999.

167. Searle NR, Martineau RJ, Conzen P, et al. Comparison of sevoflurane/fentanyl and isoflurane/fentanyl during elective coronary artery bypass surgery. Sevoflurane Venture Group. *Can J Anaesth.* 1996;43:890–899.

168. Lucchinetti E, Jamnicki M, Fischer G, Zaugg M. Preconditioning by isoflurane retains its protection against ischemia-reperfusion injury in postinfarct remodeled rat hearts. *Anesth Analg.* 2008;106:17–23.

169. Minguet G, Joris J, Lamy M. Preconditioning and protection against ischaemia-reperfusion in non-cardiac organs: a place for volatile anaesthetics? *Eur J Anaesthesiol.* 2007;24: 733–745.

170. Smul TM, Lange M, Redel A, Burkhard N, Roewer N, Kehl F. Desflurane-induced preconditioning against myocardial infarction is mediated by nitric oxide. *Anesthesiology.* 2006;105:719–725.

171. Ismaeil MS, Tkachenko I, Gamperl AK, Hickey RF, Cason BA. Mechanisms of isoflurane-induced myocardial preconditioning in rabbits. *Anesthesiology.* 1999;90:812–821.

172. Cason BA, Gamperl AK, Slocum RE, Hickey RF. Anesthetic-induced preconditioning: previous administration of isoflurane decreases myocardial infarct size in rabbits. *Anesthesiology.* 1997;87:1182–1190.

173. Yamanaka H, Hayashi Y. Myocardial preconditioning in anesthesia: from bench to bedside. *Masui.* 2009;58:279–287. [Japanese]

174. De Hert SG, Preckel B, Schlack WS. Update on inhalational anaesthetics. *Curr Opin Anaesthesiol.* 2009;22:491–495.

175. De Hert SG, Turani F, Mathur S, Stowe DF. Cardioprotection with volatile anesthetics: mechanisms and clinical implications. *Anesth Analg.* 2005;100:1584–1593.

176. Yu CH, Beattie WS. The effects of volatile anesthetics on cardiac ischemic complications and mortality in CABG: a meta-analysis. *Can J Anaesth.* 2006;53:906–918.

177. Gu W, Pagel PS, Warltier DC, Kersten JR. Modifying cardiovascular risk in diabetes mellitus. *Anesthesiology.* 2003;98: 774–779.

178. Carlock FJ, Brown M, Brown EM. Isoflurane anaesthesia for a patient with long Q-T syndrome. *Can Anaesth Soc J.* 1984;31:83–85.

179. Kleinsasser A, Kuenszberg E, Loeckinger A, et al. Sevoflurane, but not propofol, significantly prolongs the Q-T interval. *Anesth Analg.* 2000;90:25–27.

180. Forrest JB, Cahalan MK, Rehder K, et al. Multicenter study of general anesthesia. II. Results. *Anesthesiology.* 1990;72:262–268.

181. Golembiewski J. Considerations in selecting an inhaled anesthetic agent: case studies. *Am J Health Syst Pharm.* 2004; 61(Suppl 4):S10–S17.

182. Stachnik J. Inhaled anesthetic agents. *Am J Health Syst Pharm.* 2006;63:623–634.

183. Johnston RR, Eger EI, II, Wilson C. A comparative interaction of epinephrine with enflurane, isoflurane, and halothane in man. *Anesth Analg.* 1976;55:709–712.

184. Hedenstierna G, Strandberg A, Brismar B, Lundquist H, Tokics L. What causes the lowered FRC during anaesthesia? *Clin Physiol.* 1985;5(Suppl 3):133–141.

185. Laws AK. Effects of induction of anaesthesia and muscle paralysis on functional residual capacity of the lungs. *Can Anaesth Soc J.* 1968;15:325–331.

186. Lin CY. Uptake of desflurane. *Anaesthesia.* 1997;52:502–503.

187. Norris MC, Kirkland MR, Torjman MC, Goldberg ME. Denitrogenation in pregnancy. *Can J Anaesth.* 1989;36:523–525.

188. Villars PS, Kanusky JT, Levitzky MG. Functional residual capacity: the human windbag. *AANA J.* 2002;70:399–407.

189. Warner DO, Warner MA, Ritman EL. Human chest wall function while awake and during halothane anesthesia. I. Quiet breathing. *Anesthesiology.* 1995;82:6–19.

190. Benumof JL. AANA journal course: update for nurse anesthetists—anesthesia for thoracic surgery: lung separation. *AANA J.* 1998;66:253–261.

191. Benumof JL. Isoflurane anesthesia and arterial oxygenation during one-lung ventilation. *Anesthesiology.* 1986;64:419–422.

192. Benumof JL. One-lung ventilation and hypoxic pulmonary vasoconstriction: implications for anesthetic management. *Anesth Analg.* 1985;64:821–833.

193. Benumof JL. One-lung ventilation: which lung should be PEEPed? *Anesthesiology.* 1982;56:161–163.

194. Hirshman CA, Edelstein G, Peetz S, Wayne R, Downes H. Mechanism of action of inhalational anesthesia on airways. *Anesthesiology.* 1982;56:107–111.

195. Rooke GA, Choi JH, Bishop MJ. The effect of isoflurane, halothane, sevoflurane, and thiopental/nitrous oxide on respiratory system resistance after tracheal intubation. *Anesthesiology.* 1997;86:1294–1299.

196. Mitsuhata H, Saitoh J, Shimizu R, Takeuchi H, Hasome N, Horiguchi Y. Sevoflurane and isoflurane protect against bronchospasm in dogs. *Anesthesiology.* 1994;81:1230–1234.

197. Katoh T, Ikeda K. A comparison of sevoflurane with halothane, enflurane, and isoflurane on bronchoconstriction caused by histamine. *Can J Anaesth.* 1994;41:1214–1219.

198. Lele E, Petak F, Fontao F, Morel DR, Habre W. Protective effects of volatile agents against acetylcholine-induced bronchoconstriction in isolated perfused rat lungs. *Acta Anaesth Scand.* 2006;50:1145–1151.

199. Mutlu GM, Factor P, Schwartz DE, Sznajder JI. Severe status asthmaticus: management with permissive hypercapnia and inhalation anesthesia. *Crit Care Med.* 2002;30:477–480.

200. TerRiet MF, DeSouza GJ, Jacobs JS, et al. Which is most pungent: isoflurane, sevoflurane or desflurane? *Br J Anaesth.* 2000;85:305–307.

201. Jones RM, Cashman JN, Eger EI 2nd, Damask MC, Johnson BH. Kinetics and potency of desflurance (I-653) in volunteers. *Anesth Analg.* 1990;70:3–7.

202. Jones RM, Cashman JN, Mant TG. Clinical impressions and cardiorespiratory effects of a new fluorinated inhalation anaesthetic, desflurane (I-653), in volunteers. *Br J Anaesth.* 1990;64:11–15.

203. Pandit JJ. The variable effect of low-dose volatile anaesthetics on the acute ventilatory response to hypoxia in humans: a quantitative review. *Anaesthesia.* 2002;57:632–643.

204. Pandit JJ. Effect of low dose inhaled anaesthetic agents on the ventilatory response to carbon dioxide in humans: a quantitative review. *Anaesthesia.* 2005;60:461–469.

205. Kanbak M, Karagoz AH, Erdem N, et al. Renal safety and extrahepatic defluorination of sevoflurane in hepatic transplantations. *Transplant Proc.* 2007;39:1544–1548.

206. Takenami T, Arai M, Matsuzaki S, Anzai K, Ueno T, Hoka S. Serum and urinary inorganic fluoride concentrations with renal and hepatic functions after repeated sevoflurane anesthesia. *Masui.* 2002;51:1086–1093. [Japanese]

207. Isik Y, Goksu S, Kocoglu H, Oner U. Low flow desflurane and sevoflurane anaesthesia in children. *Eur J Anaesthesiol.* 2006;23:60–64.

208. Conzen PF, Kharasch ED, Czerner SFA, et al. Low-flow sevoflurane compared with low-flow isoflurane anesthesia in patients with stable renal insufficiency. *Anesthesiology.* 2002;97:578–584.

209. Njoku D, Laster MJ, Gong DH, Eger EI 2nd, Reed GF, Martin JL. Biotransformation of halothane, enflurane, isoflurane, and desflurane to trifluoroacetylated liver proteins: association between protein acylation and hepatic injury. *Anesth Analg.* 1997;84:173–178.

210. Qureshi MA, Saeed F, Hussain T. Halothane induced fulminant hepatic failure. *J Coll Physicians Surg Pak.* 2007;17:103–104.

211. Anderson JS, Rose NR, Martin JL, Eger EI, Njoku DB. Desflurane hepatitis associated with hapten and autoantigen-specific IgG4 antibodies. *Anesth Analg.* 2007;104:1452–1453.

212. Ihtiyar E, Algin C, Haciolu A, Isiksoy S. Fatal isoflurane hepatotoxicity without re-exposure. *Ind J Gastroenterol.* 2006; 25:41–42.

213. Spracklin DK, Emery ME, Thummel KE, Kharasch ED. Concordance between trifluoroacetic acid and hepatic protein trifluoroacetylation after disulfiram inhibition of halothane metabolism in rats. *Acta Anaesth Scand.* 2003;47:765–770.

214. Irwin MG, Trinh T, Yao CL. Occupational exposure to anaesthetic gases: a role for TIVA. *Expert Opin Drug Saf.* 2009; 8:473–483.

215. Eghtesadi-Araghi P, Sohrabpour A, Vahedi H, Saberi-Firoozi M. Halothane hepatitis in Iran: a review of 59 cases. *World J Gastroenterol.* 2008;14:5322–5326.

216. Kumar GP, Bhat VJ, Sowdi V. Fulminant hepatic failure following halothane anaesthesia. *J Clin Forensic Med.* 2005;12: 271–273.

217. Sakabe T, Tsutsui T, Maekawa T, Ishikawa T, Takeshita H. Local cerebral glucose utilization during nitrous oxide and pentobarbital anesthesia in rats. *Anesthesiology.* 1985;63: 262–266.

218. Eger EI 2nd, White AE, Brown CL, Biava CG, Corbett TH, Stevens WC. A test of the carcinogenicity of enflurane, isoflurane, halothane, methoxyflurane, and nitrous oxide in mice. *Anesth Analg.* 1978;57:678–694.

219. Marx T. Pollution of the work environment by volatile anesthetics and nitrous oxide. *Anasth Intens Notfallmed Schmerzther.* 1997;32:532–540.[German]

220. Husum B. Mutagenicity of inhalation anaesthetics studied by the sister chromatid exchange test in lymphocytes of patients and operating room personnel. *Dan Med Bull.* 1987;34:159–170.

221. Kundomal YR, Baden JM. Mutagenicity of inhaled anesthetics in *Drosophila melanogaster. Anesthesiology.* 1985;62: 305–309.

222. Baden JM, Kelley M, Mazze RI, Simmon VF. Mutagenicity of inhalation anaesthetics: trichloroethylene, divinyl ether, nitrous oxide and cyclopropane. *Br J Anaesth.* 1979; 51:417–421.

223. Baden JM, Kelley M, Wharton RS, Hitt BA, Simmon VF, Mazze RI. Mutagenicity of halogenated ether anesthetics. *Anesthesiology.* 1977;46:346–350.

224. Lane GA, Nahrwold ML, Tait AR, Taylor-Busch M, Cohen PJ, Beaudoin AR. Anesthetics as teratogens: nitrous oxide is fetotoxic, xenon is not. *Science.* 1980;210:899–901.

225. McGregor DG. Occupational exposure to trace concentrations of waste anesthetic gases. *Mayo Clin Proc.* 2000;75: 273–277.

226. Dixon BA, O'Donnell JM. Is your patient susceptible to malignant hyperthermia? *Nursing.* 2006;36(12 Pt.1):26–27.

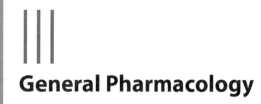

General Pharmacology

After completing this chapter, the reader should be able to

- Discuss the concepts minimum inhibitory concentration, time-dependent and dose-dependent killing, postantibiotic effect, synergism, and resistance and explain how these concepts relate to antibiotic dosing.
- Consider pharmacokinetic and pharmacodynamic principles that relate to antibiotic administration.
- Identify the classification of antibiotic compounds as defined by their chemical structure and/or mechanism of action.
- Understand the indications and clinical uses for the antibiotic classes, including β-lactam, aminoglycoside, macrolide, tetracycline, clindamycin, vancomycin, fluoroquinolones, and metronidazole.
- Review the practical aspects of antibiotic therapy as it relates to the anesthesia provider, including surgical prophylaxis, dosage and administration in the perioperative period, infective endocarditis, and the effects of antibiotics on neuromuscular blockade.

13
Antibiotics

Erica J. McCall, MSN, CRNA

is to provide nurse anesthetists with general principles related to antibiotic therapy, review the classes of agents most commonly encountered in the perioperative period, and highlight some of the most important anesthetic implications for antibiotic use.

Introduction

Antibiotics are some of the most widely used drugs, not just in the operating room but also in communities at large. Although infections are rarely the primary indication for a surgical procedure, anesthesia providers need to be knowledgeable in the use of antibiotic agents for the treatment and management of ongoing infections (i.e., the therapeutic use of antibiotics) as well as prophylactic use for the prevention of nosocomial infections.

As anesthesia providers, we are responsible for administering these drugs with awareness of possible adverse reactions, such as allergic reactions, direct organ toxicity, and altered neuromuscular function. Further, we are responsible for treating the adverse reactions if they occur, even though a surgical colleague or other healthcare provider chooses the specific agent used. Antibiotic-resistant organisms in intensive care units, hospital wards, and outpatient settings are another major concern with antimicrobial therapy.

There is an inordinate number of antibiotic, antifungal, and antiviral agents today, with newer agents being developed, tested, and released to market. The objective of this chapter is not to provide an in-depth analysis of each of these agents, because the scope is far too large for one chapter, or an entire textbook for that matter. The objective

General Principles

Minimum Inhibitory Concentration

Successful therapy of an infection depends on host defenses and the concentration of the agent at the site of the infection. Bacteriostatic agents interfere with the growth or replication of organisms but do not kill the offending organism. Bacteriostatic agents provide a minimum inhibitory concentration, which is defined as the lowest concentration of a given antimicrobial at which an organism's growth is inhibited. Bactericidal agents, or those that kill bacteria, may be needed if a host has impaired defenses (Table 13-1). If either of these concentrations is above a level that can be safely achieved in a patient, that organism is considered resistant to that drug.

In vitro susceptibility testing can be used to guide clinical therapy. However, laboratory testing does not recognize variations in tissue concentrations, and in some cases the concentration at the site of infection is lower than the serum concentration. Additional local factors such as the pH and protein concentration may also limit the drug's activity. In these cases the drug may not be effective even though the in vitro tests would assume the organism is sensitive to that drug.

Table 13-1 Bactericidal and Bacteriostatic Antibacterial Agents

Bactericidal Agents	Bacteriostatic Agents
Aminoglycosides	Clindamycin
β-Lactam antibiotics	Macrolides
Daptomycin	Tetracyclines
Ketolides	
Metronidazole	
Quinolones	
Tigecycline	
Vancomycin	

Dose-Dependent or Time-Dependent Killing

With some antibiotics, as the concentration of the drug increases, so does the rate and extent of bacterial death. This concentration-dependent killing occurs with the aminoglycosides. With other agents clinical efficacy is related to the duration of time that the minimum inhibitory concentration is maintained. For these, a greater concentration does not increase the extent of bacterial death. This time-dependent killing is seen with the β-lactam antibiotics. These distinctions are important when determining a dosing strategy for antimicrobial agents.

Postantibiotic Effect

Some antibiotic agents exhibit a phenomenon called the postantibiotic effect (PAE). When these agents are administered, bacterial growth is suppressed even after an antibiotic level is no longer detected. This effect occurs with most antibiotics; however, the type of bacteria affected and the duration of the PAE are highly variable. For example, most antibiotics have significant in vitro PAEs against gram-positive cocci, but only carbapenems, aminoglycosides, and other agents inhibiting protein or DNA synthesis have PAEs against gram-negative bacilli.

Synergism

Synergism of two antibiotic agents occurs when the bacteriostatic or bactericidal effects of two or more agents used together is greater than their effects when administered alone. This includes the dosing of two antibiotics to treat a severe infection, such as ampicillin and gentamicin in the treatment of enterococcal endocarditis, or the use of an antibiotic with an agent that inhibits its enzymatic inactivation, such as sulbactam and ampicillin.

Resistance

Antibiotic resistance is a growing problem in both community-acquired and nosocomial infections. The World Health Organization estimates that around 14,000 people are infected and die each year from nosocomial "superinfections" due to drug-resistant organisms.[1]

Microorganisms develop resistance in different forms. First, a drug may be unable to reach its target if the offending organism develops efflux pumps in its cell membranes to remove antibiotics from the cell. This type of resistance is seen with the β-lactams, tetracyclines, fluoroquinolones, and macrolides. The second includes bacterial production of enzymes that alter or inactivate the drug compound—for example, resistance to the β-lactam antibiotics when an organism is able to produce β-lactamase. Finally, an alteration in the drug's target creates resistance—for example, the mutation of bacterial topoisomerases to prevent fluoroquinolone binding.

Multiple factors have contributed to the increase in drug resistant strains of bacteria. Before selecting an antimicrobial agent, one must consider if its use is even indicated. Overuse of broad-spectrum antibiotics is a potentially dangerous practice that can lead to further pathogen resistance.

Pharmacokinetic and Pharmacodynamic Principles

The aim of antibiotic therapy should be to achieve a drug-concentration at the site of infection equal to or greater than the minimum inhibitory concentration for the infecting organism. The concentration must also be one that is tolerated by the host. Therefore the location of the infection and host factors determine the choice of drug and the route it is administered. For example, the ability of an antimicrobial to cross the blood–brain barrier varies widely among individual agents. The ability of a drug to penetrate into a site of infection also depends on its protein binding because most agents depend on passive diffusion. Drugs that are highly protein bound may not penetrate as well and will have reduced effectiveness because only the unbound portion is free to enter the site of infection.

Host Factors

The clinical efficacy of antimicrobials is also related to the host's defense mechanisms. Both cellular and humoral immunity are important. If a host has an inadequate quality or quantity of immunoglobulin, an altered cellular immune system, or a lack of phagocytic cells, treatment of an infection with a drug that has a known sensitivity may be inadequate. In an immunocompetent host, a bacteriostatic agent may be sufficient to cure an infection. However, if the host is immunocompromised, this same agent may not be adequate and a bactericidal agent may be required.

Local Factors

Local factors also influence the antimicrobial activity of a drug. The presence of pus, which contains phagocytes and proteins that may bind to or inhibit the drug, makes treatment less effective. Additionally, areas of infection such as abscess cavities have reduced blood supply so penetration of the drug is reduced. If an infected area contains a foreign body (e.g., prosthesis), successful treatment may require removal of the material.

Age

The pharmacokinetics of most drugs change as a person ages. Newborns, especially premature infants, have poorly developed renal excretion and hepatic biotransformation mechanisms. Elderly patients also have delayed drug elimination due to a reduction in creatinine clearance and may clear drugs less readily. Elderly patients also may metabolize drugs less rapidly, so dosage adjustments must be made to prevent toxic drug levels.

Pregnancy

The use of antibiotics in pregnancy may increase the risk of adverse reactions to both mother and fetus. Pharmacokinetic principles vary in pregnant females as a result of an increased blood volume, and therefore volume of distribution, as well as an increased glomerular filtration rate. Some agents, including penicillins (except ticarcillin), cephalosporins, and erythromycin, are relatively safe (Table 13-2). However, some antibiotic agents are known to cross the placental barrier and harm the growing fetus. Examples include aminoglycoside-associated hearing loss and tetracycline-associated teeth and bone problems. Tetracycline can also cause fatty necrosis of the liver, pancreatitis, and renal injury in the pregnant patient.

Antibiotic Selection and Specific Antibiotic Classes

Antimicrobial agents are classified by their chemical structure and their proposed mechanism of action (Table 13-3).

Table 13-2 Antibiotics in Pregnancy and Lactation

Antibiotic Class	Pregnancy Category
Penicillins	B
Cephalosporins	B
Tetracyclines	D
Fluoroquinolones	C
Linosinamides	B
Macrolides	B/C

Table 13-3 Classification of Antimicrobials

ß-Lactam
Penicillins
Penicillinase-susceptible
Penicillin G
Penicillin V
Penicillinase-resistant
Nafcillin, oxacillin, dicloxacillin, methicillin, ticarcillin (plus clavulanic acid), piperacillin (plus tazobactam)
Extended spectrum
Ampicillin, amoxicillin
Cephalosporins
First generation
Cephalothin, cephalexin, cefazolin, cephadrine, cephapirin
Second generation
Cefaclor, cefamandole, cefonicid, cefuroxime, cephamycins (cefoxitin, cefotetan)
Third generation
Cefotaxime, ceftazidime, ceftriaxone
Fourth generation
Cefepime
Carbapenems
Imipenem, meropenem, ertapenem
Monobactams
Aztreonam
ß-Lactamase inhibitors
Clavulanic acid, sulbactam, tazobactam
Aminoglycosides
Gentamicin, tobramycin, kanamycin, amikacin, netilmicin, neomycin, streptomycin
Macrolides
Erythromycin, clarithromycin, azithromycin
Tetracyclines
Tetracycline, doxycycline, minocycline, oxytetracycline, tigecycline
Lincosamides
Clindamycin
Vancomycin
Fluoroquinolones
Ciprofloxacin, norfloxacin, levofloxacin, gemifloxacin, moxifloxacin, ofloxacin
Miscellaneous
Metronidazole

Agents such as the β-lactams (penicillins, cephalosporins, and carbapenems) and vancomycin inhibit cell wall synthesis. Other agents bind either to the 50S or 30S ribosomal subunits and inhibit protein synthesis. In some cases this binding is reversible (tetracyclines, macrolides, lincosamides, and linezolid); in others it is irreversible (aminoglycosides). There are agents that interfere with bacterial nucleic wall synthesis such as RNA polymerase (rifampin) and topoisomerase (quinolones).

β-Lactam Compounds

The β-lactam antibiotics are a group of frequently used agents that have a common chemical structure, mechanism of action, and pharmacology. These include penicillins, cephalosporins, carbapenems, monobactams, and β-lactamase inhibitors.

Mechanism of Action

Bacterial cell walls are rigid and completely surround the cytoplasmic membrane, maintaining the cell's shape and integrity. This cell wall is made of a complex lattice of glycopeptide polymers linked between amino acid side chains. The synthesis of this glycopeptide is a three-step process involving about 30 bacterial enzymes. The cross-linking is catalyzed by a transpeptidase, an enzyme that is inhibited by penicillins and cephalosporins. Other sites of action for these compounds are the penicillin-binding proteins. Each bacterium has several such proteins, each with varying affinity for each of the β-lactam compounds. These proteins play a role in bacterial resistance.

Resistance

β-Lactamases are enzymes produced by bacteria that hydrolyze the β-lactam ring of a compound, rendering the molecule inactive. This is the most common form of resistance. Hundreds of different β-lactamases have been identified, but most bacteria produce only one form of the enzyme. The actions of these enzymes are relatively narrow and may be classified as penicillinases or cephalosporinases. There is not a distinct correlation between the susceptibility of a β-lactam compound to the lactamases and that compound's ability to kill the bacterium.

Several other forms of bacterial resistance to β-lactam compounds exist. First includes the modification of the penicillin-binding proteins. Previously susceptible strains may develop higher molecular weight penicillin-binding proteins that have a decreased affinity for β-lactam compound binding. This is the mechanism of methicillin resistance in

staphylococci. Second, a β-lactam drug may be unable to penetrate an organism penicillin-binding protein to its site of activity. This type of resistance occurs with gram-negative organisms whose inner cell membrane, similar to the cytoplasmic membrane of gram-positive organisms, is covered by a second impenetrable outer membrane. Third, active efflux pumps on gram-negative bacteria transport some of the β-lactam agents away from their site of action before they can take effect. Finally, biofilms produced by microorganisms that adhere to prosthetic devices (i.e., joints, heart valves, and catheters) are less susceptible to antibiotic therapy.

Penicillins

The basic structure of the penicillins contains a thiazolidine ring attached to a β-lactam ring (Figure 13-1). This nucleus forms the structural integrity of the compound, the alteration of which results in a loss of antimicrobial activity. An example is the hydrolysis of the β-lactam ring by bacterial β-lactamase, which renders the penicillin inactive. Side chains attach to the β-lactam ring, thereby determining the antibacterial characteristics of each agent. There are three general classifications of the penicillins based on their spectrum of activity. First, penicillin G and penicillin V are active against gram-positive organisms and gram-negative cocci but are susceptible to β-lactamases and are ineffective against most *Staphylococcus aureus* strains. The next class, penicillinase-resistant penicillins, includes nafcillin, oxacillin, dicloxacillin, and methicillin (which is discontinued in the United States). This group is resistant to β-lactamase-producing staphylococci, such as *S. aureus* and *Staphylococcus epidermidis*, which are not methicillin resistant. They are also active against streptococci but not enterococci, anaerobic bacteria, or gram-negative cocci and rods. The last class, extended-spectrum penicillins, includes ampicillin and amoxicillin. These have activity including gram-negative organisms such as *Haemophilus*

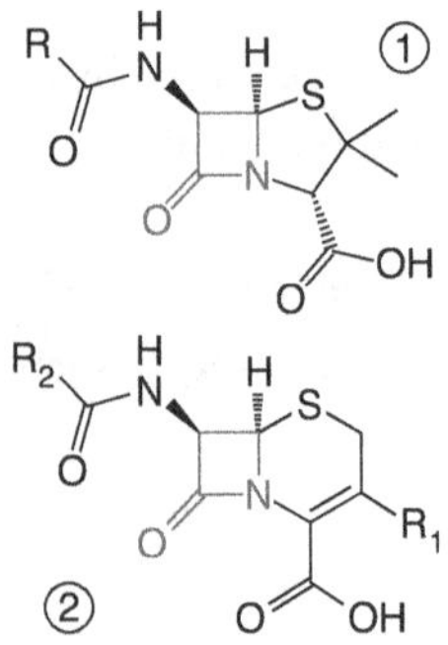

Figure 13-1 β-Lactam antibiotics basic chemical structure. (1) Penicillin. (2) Cephalosporin with β-lactam ring (shaded area).

influenzae and *Escherichia coli*. However, they are susceptible to hydrolysis by β-lactamases and thus are often administered with a β-lactamase inhibitor.

Pharmacokinetics

Several penicillins may be administered orally, but absorption varies depending on their protein binding and acid stability. Those considered acid-stable (dicloxacillin, ampicillin, and amoxicillin) may all be given orally. Penicillins, except amoxicillin, should be administered 1 to 2 hours before or after a meal to minimize acid inactivation and binding to food proteins. After absorption, these penicillins are widely distributed throughout the body. Probenecid, a uricosuric agent, may be administered simultaneously with oral penicillins. This agent competitively inhibits the renal tubular secretion of penicillins, thereby raising the serum blood levels.

Intravenous administration of penicillins results in rapid and complete absorption. Protein binding determines the concentration of free drug in serum. Nafcillin, which is highly protein bound, achieves a lower concentration than a less protein bound drug, such as penicillin G or ampicillin. Therapeutic concentrations of the penicillins are easily achieved in bodily tissue and fluids, such as pleural fluid, pericardial fluid, joint fluid, and bile. However, only low concentrations are found in intraocular fluid, prostatic secretions, and cerebrospinal fluid (CSF). In normal conditions, concentrations of penicillins in the CSF are less than 1% of plasma concentrations. In disease states, such as bacterial meningitis, where there is active inflammation of the meninges, concentrations may increase to as much as 5% of plasma concentrations. At these concentrations susceptible strains of pneumococci and meningococci may be killed.

Elimination of penicillins is mainly by the kidneys, although other routes excrete small amounts. Glomerular filtration accounts for 90% of excretion, and 10% is via tubular secretion. Concentrations of the penicillins in urine are high. Penicillin G has a half-life of approximately 30 minutes, whereas the extended-spectrum penicillins have a half-life of 1 hour. In patients with renal failure, dose adjustments must be made to one-fourth or one-third the normal dose if creatinine clearance is less than 10 mL/min (Table 13-4).

Clinical Uses and Indications

Penicillin G is an effective agent against infections caused by streptococci, meningococci, enterococci, penicillin-susceptible pneumococci, and staphylococci not producing β-lactamases. It is also useful against *Treponema pallidum* and other spirochetes, clostridium species, actinomyces, other gram-negative rods, and gram-negative anaerobic organisms not producing β-lactamases. No penicillin is effective against amoebae, plasmodia, rickettsiae, fungi, or viruses. Clinical indications include pneumococcal pneumonia, pneumococcal meningitis, streptococcal pharyngitis, streptococcal pneumonia, streptococcal necrotizing fascitis, streptococcal endocarditis, streptococcal meningitis, meningococcal infections, gonococcal infections, syphilis, actinomycosis, and prophylactic use.

Many organisms previously susceptible to penicillin G are now resistant. This includes penicillin-resistant *Streptococcus viridans* and *Streptococcus pneumoniae*. When penicillin G was first introduced, most strains of *S. aureus* were susceptible. Now, over 90% of staphylococci stains isolated from patients are resistant to penicillin G. Additionally, most *S. epidermidis* strains are resistant, and strains of gonococci-producing penicillinase are becoming more common.

Penicillinase-resistant penicillins are resistant to hydrolysis by staphylococci penicillinase, and their use should be limited to infections that are known to be caused by organisms that produce the enzyme. They are less active than penicillin G against other organisms susceptible to penicillin, including staphylococci that do not produce penicillinase. These drugs have a greater ability to penetrate the outer membrane of gram-negative bacteria than penicillins and are thus more effective against gram-negative bacteria. Within this class there are three subtypes. The aminopenicillins, including ampicillin and amoxicillin, are the most active of all the β-lactam compounds against penicillin-resistant pneumococci and are the drug of choice for infections of this type. They are also useful in treating infections caused by anaerobes, enterococci, and non-β-lactamase

Table 13-4 Antibiotic Dosing Adjustments in Patients With Renal or Hepatic Impairment

Dosage Adjustment Needed in Renal Impairment	Contraindicated in Renal Impairment	Dosage Adjustment Needed in Hepatic Impairment
Aminoglycosides, cephalosporins (except cefoperazone and ceftriaxone), clarithromycin, daptomycin, ertapenem, imipenem, meropenem, penicillins (except antistaphylococcal penicillins, e.g., nafcillin and dicloxacillin), quinolones, vancomycin	Tetracyclines	Clindamycin, erythromycin, metronidazole, tigecycline

producing strains of gram-negative cocci and bacilli. The aminopenicillins are frequently used to treat urinary tract infections, sinusitis, otitis, lower respiratory tract infections, and salmonella infections.

Carboxypenicillins, another subtype of the penicillinase-resistant penicillins, include the drugs carbenicillin and ticarcillin. Carbenicillin, the first penicillin effective against *Pseudomonas aeruginosa*, is now obsolete. Ticarcillin is very similar to carbenicillin but is two to four times more active against *P. aeruginosa*.

Finally, the ureidopenicillins, including piperacillin, mezlocillin, and azlocillin, have added activity against certain gram-negative bacilli like *Klebsiella pneumoniae*. These agents are useful in the treatment of other infections caused by gram-negative bacteria, including those acquired in hospitals.

Adverse Reactions

Hypersensitivity reactions are the most common adverse reactions seen with the penicillins. They include development of a maculopapular rash, urticarial rash, fever, bronchospasm, vasculitis, serum sickness, exfoliative dermatitis, Stevens-Johnson syndrome, and anaphylaxis (Table 13-5). All the penicillins are cross-sensitizing and cross-reacting, and allergy to one form results in a greater risk of infection if another is given. In some instances, the reaction may be mild and can disappear even if the drug is continued. In other cases, immediate cessation of the drug and supportive therapy are needed. Elimination of the drug usually results in rapid clearing of the clinical manifestations; however, some symptoms may persist weeks after therapy was stopped.

Angioedema and anaphylaxis are the most serious reactions due to penicillin usage. Angioedema, marked swelling of the tongue, lips, face, periorbital tissue, accompanied by wheezing and development of hives have been seen after topical, oral, or parenteral administration of penicillins. An acute anaphylactic reaction to penicillins is most likely to occur after injection of the drug; however, it has been observed after oral administration or after intradermal injection during skin testing. Penicillins are the most common drugs among all other classes that result in an anaphylactic or anaphylactoid reaction. The best way to prevent an adverse reaction is to avoid the use of penicillin in patients who have a history of allergy to penicillin; a drug from a different class should be administered.

Patients with renal failure should have the dose of penicillin adjusted, because high doses may cause seizures. Other adverse reactions include neutropenia (nafcillin),

Table 13-5 Antibiotic-Induced Allergic Reactions

Penicillins	Urticaria, angioedema, anaphylaxis, maculopapular skin eruptions, exfoliative dermatitis, vesicular eruptions, erythema multiforme, Stevens-Johnson syndrome, toxic epidermal necrolysis, serum sickness-like reaction, vasculitis, cytopenias
Cephalosporins	Urticaria, angioedema, anaphylaxis, maculopapular skin eruptions, erythema multiforme, Stevens-Johnson syndrome, toxic epidermal necrolysis, renal dysfunction, toxic nephropathy, hepatic dysfunction, aplastic anemia, hemolytic anemia
Macrolides	Urticaria, angioedema, anaphylaxis, mild skin eruptions, photosensitivity, Stevens-Johnson syndrome, toxic epidermal necrolysis
Fluoroquinolones	Urticaria, angioedema, pruritus, photosensitivity, flushing, fever, chills, angioedema, erythema nodosum, anaphylaxis, hyperpigmentation
Tetracyclines	Urticaria, angioedema, anaphylaxis, pericarditis, polyarthralgia, exacerbation of systemic lupus erythematosus, pulmonary infiltrates with eosinophilia
Vancomycin	Anaphylaxis, drug fever, eosinophilia, skin eruptions (including exfoliative dermatitis), Stevens-Johnson syndrome, toxic epidermal necrolysis, vasculitis

hepatitis (oxacillin), and interstitial nephritis (methicillin). Large oral dosages of penicillin may cause nausea, vomiting, and diarrhea. Secondary infections resulting from the elimination of sensitive microflora, such as vaginal candidiasis, may result.

Cephalosporins

Cephalosporins are similar to penicillins but have a broader spectrum of activity because they are stable against many bacterial β-lactamases. The chemical structure of the cephalosporins includes a 7-aminocephalosporanic acid nucleus that closely resembles the 6-aminopenicillanic acid found in penicillins. The spectrum of each individual drug's activity is due to the addition of various side chains. These compounds are highly resistant to penicillinase regardless of the nature of their side chain or their affinity for the enzyme. Cephamycins are structurally similar to cephalosporins but contain a methoxy group in the β-lactam ring of the 7-aminocephalosporanic acid nucleus.

There are four major generations of cephalosporins based on the general spectrum of antimicrobial activity. First-generation cephalosporins, including cephalothin, cephalexin, cefazolin, cephradine, and cephapirin, are active against gram-positive bacteria with some activity against gram-negative organisms. Gram-positive cocci, except enterococci, methicillin-resistant *S. aureus*, and *S. epidermidis*, are also susceptible. The first-generation cephalosporins are also active against *E. coli, K. pneumoniae*, and *P. mirabilis*. Second-generation cephalosporins, including cefaclor, cefamandole, cefonicid, and cefuroxime, along with the structurally similar cephamycins, including cefoxitin and cefotetan, are active against organisms inhibited by the first-generation drugs but have increased activity against gram-negative organisms. Third-generation cephalosporins, including cefotaxime, ceftazidime, and ceftriaxone, are less active against gram-positive cocci than first-generation agents and are more active against Enterobacteriaceae, including strains producing β-lactamase. Ceftazidime and cefoperazone are also active against *P. aeruginosa* but are not as active as other third-generation agents against gram-positive cocci. The fourth-generation cephalosporin cefepime has extended coverage when compared with the third-generation cephalosporins and is more resistant to hydrolysis by plasmid and chromosomal β-lactamases, such as those produced by *Enterobacter*.

Pharmacokinetics

Of the first-generation cephalosporins, cephalexin and cephradine may be given orally. These agents are absorbed, and tissue levels are variable, generally lower than serum levels. These agents are not metabolized, and excretion occurs via glomerular filtration and tubular secretion. As with the penicillins, probenecid may be administered simultaneously to increase the serum level of the cephalosporin. Dose adjustments should be made for patients with impaired renal function.

The only parenteral first-generation cephalosporin still in use is cefazolin. Cefazolin penetrates well into most tissues, with the exception of the central nervous system, and is relatively nontoxic. For an adult a dose of 0.5 to 2 g every 8 hours is administered. Cefazolin is highly bound to plasma proteins, about 85%, and excreted by glomerular filtration in the kidneys.

The second-generation cephalosporins, cefaclor, cefuroxime, and loracarbef, may be administered orally. They are absorbed to a varying extent and are excreted in the urine. Second-generation cephamycins, cefoxitin and cefotetan, are administered intravenously, and both are highly protein bound. Cefoxitin is widely distributed but poorly penetrates the central nervous system, even in inflammatory states. It has a half-life of 40 minutes and is excreted primarily unchanged in the urine. Cefotetan is similar to cefoxitin with a longer half-life of 3 to 5 hours and is excreted primarily in the urine and to a small extent in feces.

Cefixime, ceftibuten, and cefpodoxime are third-generation cephalosporins that may be administered orally. Parenteral third-generation agents include ceftriaxone, cefotaxime, and ceftazidime. Ceftriaxone is highly protein bound, 85% to 95%, and widely distributes throughout the body, including the CSF (and to a greater extent with inflammation). The elimination half-life is 8 hours: About half is excreted unchanged in the urine and the remainder undergoes biliary excretion. Cefotaxime has a half-time elimination of 1 to 1.5 hours and thus must be administered every 4 to 8 hours in serious infections. This drug is metabolized in the liver to an active metabolite, desacetyl cefotaxime, which acts synergistically with its parent compound. Both the unchanged drug and its metabolite are excreted in the urine. Ceftazidime is unique among the third-generation cephalosporins because of its antimicrobial activity against *Pseudomonas* and other gram-negative microorganisms. It has minimal protein binding, about 17%, and distributes throughout the body, including the CSF (at higher concentrations with inflammation). Ceftazidime has a half-life elimination of 1 to 2 hours and is excreted unchanged in the urine.

Cefepime is the only fourth-generation cephalosporin available for use in the United States. It is widely distributed and penetrates well into the CSF. The plasma half-life of cefepime is 2 hours, and it is excreted unchanged in the urine.

Clinical Uses and Indications

The cephalosporins are widely used, broad-spectrum antibiotics used therapeutically and prophylactically. They are more stable to many β-lactamases than penicillins, although a variety of bacteria is resistant to their activity.

The first-generation cephalosporins are effective in treating skin and soft tissue infections caused by *S. aureus* and *Staphylococcus pyogenes*. For this reason cefazolin is often used for surgical prophylaxis, which is covered extensively later in this chapter (see Practical Aspects of Antibiotic Use, Surgical Prophylaxis). The oral first-generation cephalosporins may be used to treat urinary tract infections, cellulitis, or soft tissue abscesses caused by staphylococci or streptococci.

The second-generation cephalosporins cefoxitin and cefotetan have been used to treat mixed anaerobic infections and for prophylaxis in colorectal surgery when intestinal anaerobic protection is desired. The oral second-generation agents may be used to treat sinusitis, otitis, or respiratory tract infection when the suspected organism is β-lactamase-producing *H. influenzae.*

Third-generation cephalosporins are often used to treat serious infections caused by *Klebsiella, Enterobacter, Proteus, Providencia, Serratia,* and *Haemophilus* species. Empirical therapy with these agents may be used in an immunocompromised or immunocompetent patient with sepsis. Cefotaxime and ceftriaxone are also used to treat nosocomial pneumonia caused by *S. aureus* or *H. influenzae.*

Fourth-generation cephalosporins are also used for empirical treatment of nosocomial infections where resistant strains are anticipated. Cefepime is also useful in treatment regimens of *Enterobacter,* methicillin-susceptible staphylococci, and many gram-negative bacilli.

Adverse Reactions

Cephalosporins exhibit many of the same hypersensitivity reactions of penicillins. Most commonly a maculopapular rash develops, although urticaria, bronchospasm, and anaphylaxis may occur. However, clinical studies indicate a frequency of skin reactions between 1% and 3% and anaphylactic reactions between 0.0001% and 0.1%.[2]

Some patients receiving cefotetan may have hypoprothrombinemia, vitamin K inhibition, and bleeding diathesis. This is preventable if vitamin K is administered. Cefotetan, cefoperazone, and other cephalosporins containing a methylthiotetrazole group may cause disulfiram-like reactions, so alcohol should be avoided.

Cephalosporin Use in Patients With Penicillin Allergy

As a result of their shared chemical structure, cross-reactivity may occur between penicillins and cephalosporins. This topic has been examined in multiple laboratory and clinical studies, and varying degrees of cross-reactivity have been documented. However, it is generally believed that the rate of cross-reactivity between penicillin and second- and third-generation cephalosporins is 5% or less. The degree of cross-reactivity between penicillins and first-generation cephalosporins is slightly greater.[3]

A review article by Kelkar and Li[2] offers several therapeutic approaches. First, avoid using any antibiotic containing a β-lactam ring in patients with penicillin allergy. This option avoids the risk of cross-sensitivity but may result in increased cost, decreased antimicrobial effectiveness, or potential for increased antimicrobial resistance.

However, it may be an attractive therapeutic approach in patients reporting a serious (or undefined) reaction to penicillin. A second option is to administer the cephalosporin to a patient with a stated penicillin allergy. Many clinicians follow this approach when the patient's previous reaction to penicillin was mild, non-life threatening or not anaphylactic, and when the risk of anaphylaxis from, or reaction to, cephalosporin is not considered high enough to warrant selection of another agent. The drawback to this approach is the increased risk of drug reaction or anaphylaxis. The third strategy is to evaluate the patient with a stated allergy to penicillin with tests for that allergy to penicillin. Although this may be an attractive option for patients in whom cephalosporin therapy is strongly indicated for their medical condition, these tests are costly and not readily available in the immediate perioperative setting. For all three approaches, a thorough clinical evaluation and patient history is of utmost importance.

Other β-Lactam Agents

Carbapenems, monobactams, and β-lactamase inhibitors have a structure similar to that of penicillins and cephalosporins but are of a distinct class. These agents have therapeutic usefulness beyond or different from the other β-lactam compounds.

Carbapenems

Carbapenems contain a fused β-lactam ring and a five-member ring system. This class, including imipenem, meropenem, and ertapenem, has a broader spectrum of activity than the penicillins and cephalosporins. Imipenem has antimicrobial activity similar to other β-lactam antibiotics, but it is resistant to hydrolysis by most β-lactamases. It is active against a variety of microorganisms, including streptococci, enterococci, staphylococci, and *Listeria.* This includes penicillin-resistant strains of *S. pneumoniae* and some strains of methicillin-resistant staphylococci. Anaerobes are also susceptible. Meropenem has an antimicrobial spectrum similar to imipenem, with greater activity against gram-negative but less activity with gram-positive aerobes. Ertapenem differs by having a longer half-life of 4 hours and has antimicrobial action against gram-positive organisms, Enterobacteriaceae, and anaerobes.

Imipenem is administered intravenously with cilastatin, a renal dehydropeptidase inhibitor that prevents its inactivation in renal tubules. When given together, the half-life is about 1 hour. About 70% of imipenem is excreted unchanged in the urine. Meropenem and ertapenem are not sensitive to renal degradation, so concomitant administration with cilastatin is not required. All the carbapenems penetrate body tissues and fluids, including the CSF.

Carbapenems are indicated for mixed aerobic and anaerobic infections resistant to treatment with other antibiotics. Carbapenems are the antibiotic of choice for cephalosporin-resistant *Enterobacter* infections because they are not susceptible to β-lactamases produced by these organisms. Hospitalized patients with serious infections may be treated with carbapenems if the suspected organism is a cephalosporin-resistant or penicillin-resistant bacterium.

Adverse reactions of carbapenems include gastrointestinal symptoms (i.e., nausea, vomiting, diarrhea, and skin rashes). In patients with renal impairment, high levels of imipenem may lead to seizures, so dosage adjustments should be made.

Monobactams

Monobactams also are similar antibiotics and contain a monocyclic β-lactam ring. Aztreonam, the only monobactam available in the United States, is relatively resistant to β-lactamases. Its spectrum of activity includes gram-negative rods, but it has no activity against gram-positive bacteria or anaerobic organisms. Aztreonam is administered intravenously, has a half-life of 1 to 2 hours, and is excreted unchanged in the urine. Aztreonam is well tolerated with little adverse reaction. Aztreonam does not have cross-reactivity in patients allergic to penicillin or cephalosporin.[4]

β-Lactamase Inhibitors

The β-lactamase inhibitors, clavulanic acid, sulbactam, and tazobactam, are structurally related to β-lactam molecules but have very weak antimicrobial action. Instead, these agents can inactivate β-lactamases, thereby protecting antibiotics from inactivation by these enzymes. The three agents have slightly different pharmacology, stability, and potency, but the paired penicillin determines their antimicrobial spectrum.

Amoxicillin paired with potassium clavulanate is effective against staphylococci, *H. influenzae*, gonococci, and *E. coli* that produce β-lactamase. Sulbactam is a β-lactamase inhibitor that may be administered intravenously with ampicillin. Together, they are active against gram-positive cocci, including *S. aureus*, gram-negative anaerobes, except *Pseudomonas*, and anaerobes. Tazobactam when combined with piperacillin extends activity to include *S. aureus, H. influenzae, Bacteroides*, and other gram-negative bacteria. Given intravenously, this pair is used to treat moderate-to-severe infections, including nosocomial pneumonia, bone and joint infections, intra-abdominal infections such as appendicitis and peritonitis, and septicemia.

Aminoglycosides

The aminoglycoside class of antimicrobials is primarily used to treat infections caused by aerobic gram-negative organisms. This class includes the agents gentamicin, tobramycin, kanamycin, amikacin, netilmicin, neomycin, and streptomycin. These agents interfere with ribosomal function and inhibit protein synthesis and thus are bactericidal. All aminoglycosides have a hexose ring nucleus to which amino sugars are attached by glycosidic linkages. The hexose ring is either streptidine, in the case of streptomycin, or 2-deoxystreptamine in all other aminoglycosides (Figure 13-2). The various amino sugars determine the individual characteristics of each drug in the class.

Mechanism of Action

The mechanism of action of aminoglycosides is an irreversible inhibition of protein synthesis. First there is passive diffusion of the agent through porin channels on the outer membrane of the target organism. Then active transport via an oxygen-dependent process occurs across the cell membrane and into the cytoplasm of the organism. Anaerobic and low extracellular pH conditions inhibit the transport of these agents because a transmembrane electrochemical gradient is necessary for this process with transport coupled to a proton pump.

Once inside the cell membrane, the 30S ribosomal subunit is the site of action for the aminoglycoside agent. There are three mechanisms of protein synthesis inhibition that occur concurrently, resulting in cell death. First, the agent may interfere with the initiation of protein synthesis. Second, they cause a misreading of mRNA that leads to incorrect amino acids being integrated into the peptide chains, resulting in a nonfunctional protein. Finally, these agents reduce polysomes into nonfunctional monosomes.

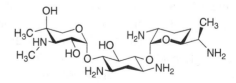

Figure 13-2 Basic chemical structure of gentamicin.

As a result of these mechanisms, the aminoglycosides are bactericidal and exhibit concentration-dependent killing. They also have a PAE, the duration of which is also concentration dependent.

Resistance

Resistance of a microorganism to an aminoglycoside mirrors its mechanism of action. The agent may be unable to penetrate the cell wall and move intracellularly, it may have a low affinity for the ribosomal subunit, or enzymes may inactivate the drug. This last mechanism, the enzymatic inactivation of aminoglycosides by adenylylation, acetylation, or phosphorylation, is the most common form of resistance. Additionally, as mentioned, the transport of the aminoglycosides into the cytoplasm of the organism is an oxygen-dependent, active process. Thus anaerobic bacteria are resistant to these agents because they lack the necessary transport system required for the agent to gain access through the cell's inner membrane.

Pharmacokinetics

Aminoglycosides are highly polar cations, which are not readily absorbed from the gastrointestinal tract, limiting oral administration. Intestinal conditions such as ulcers or inflammatory bowel may increase absorption by this route. Aminoglycosides are well absorbed after intramuscular injection and reach peak plasma concentrations within 30 to 90 minutes. The intravenous route is most common for the aminoglycosides, usually as an infusion lasting 30 to 60 minutes.

Aminoglycosides may be administered in two to three divided daily doses. However, because of their concentration-dependent and PAE characteristics, a given total dosage of an aminoglycoside may be more effective when administered in a larger, once-daily dose.

Aminoglycosides, because they are highly polar compounds, do not penetrate into most cells, including the central nervous system and the eye. With the exception of streptomycin, aminoglycosides are not highly protein bound, with the volume of distribution approximating the volume of extracellular fluid. The aminoglycosides do not occur in high concentrations in secretions of body tissues, except for the renal cortex and endolymph and perilymph of the inner ear, which likely contributes to the toxicity caused by them.

The aminoglycosides are excreted almost entirely by glomerular filtration. The half-life of aminoglycosides in serum is 2 to 3 hours but may be as long as 24 to 48 hours in patients with impaired renal function. The dose of aminoglycosides must be adjusted for these patients, and plasma concentrations should be monitored. Determination of the aminoglycosides' plasma concentration is essential for guiding dosing. These concentrations should be monitored several times per week and within 24 to 48 hours of a dose change.

Adverse Reactions

The aminoglycoside class of antibiotics are both ototoxic and nephrotoxic. These adverse reactions are more likely to occur when they are administered for more than 5 days, at higher doses, in the elderly, and in patients with impaired renal function.

Ototoxicity, in the form of vestibular and auditory dysfunction, can occur with any drug of this class. Damage to vestibular and cochlear sensory cells is largely irreversible. Once the sensory cells are lost, retrograde degeneration of the auditory nerve may follow, leading to irreversible hearing loss.

The first clinical symptom of cochlear toxicity is tinnitus, and if the aminoglycoside is not discontinued, auditory impairment may occur within days. If therapy is stopped, the tinnitus may persist for up to 2 weeks. Symptoms of vestibular dysfunction are more vague and include headache, nausea, vomiting, and difficulty with equilibrium. Again, early recognition and cessation of the drug is paramount. Of the drugs in this class, neomycin, kanamycin, and amikacin are the most ototoxic, and streptomycin and gentamicin are the most vestibulotoxic.

Nephrotoxicity occurs in approximately 8% to 26% of patients who receive an aminoglycoside for more than several days. Toxicity occurs when the aminoglycosides accumulate and are retained in the proximal tubular cells of the kidney and correlates with the total amount of the drug that is administered. Thus nephrotoxicity is more likely to occur in long courses of therapy with the drugs of this class. However, because the proximal tubular cells can regenerate, impairment due to toxicity is largely reversible after the drug is discontinued. Clinical symptoms include an increase in serum creatinine, reduced creatinine clearance, or an increase in the aminoglycoside trough level on examination. Of the drugs in this class, neomycin, tobramycin, and gentamicin are the most nephrotoxic.

Another adverse reaction of the aminoglycoside antibiotics is acute neuromuscular blockade with resulting respiratory muscle paralysis and apnea. The likely mechanism of this reaction is aminoglycosides' inhibition of prejunctional acetylcholine release and reduced postsynaptic sensitivity to acetylcholine. This phenomenon, as well as options for treatment, is addressed later (see Practical Aspects of Antibiotic

Use, Antibiotics and Neuromuscular Blockade). Other adverse reactions to aminoglycosides, including hypersensitivity, rash, and anaphylaxis, are unusual.

Clinical Uses and Indications

Gentamicin

Gentamicin is a widely used aminoglycoside due to its spectrum of activity against gram-negative and gram-positive organisms, low cost, and availability for intravenous, topical, and ophthalmic use. Gentamicin inhibits many strains of staphylococci, coliforms, and other gram-negative bacteria. When given in combination with a β-lactam antibiotic, it acts synergistically against gram-negative infections such as those due to *Pseudomonas, Proteus, Enterobacter, Klebsiella, Serratia*, and *Stenotrophomonas*, including urinary tract infections, bacteremia, infected burns, osteomyelitis, pneumonia, peritonitis, and otitis. However, due to the risk of toxicity with prolonged use, it should not be used for more than a few days unless the benefit of such use outweighs the risk of toxicity. Nephrotoxicity is usually reversible and mild with gentamicin, occurring in 5% to 25% of patients who receive the drug for longer than 3 to 5 days, so serum measurement of the drug levels is important. Ototoxicity, in the form of vestibular dysfunction, is less likely, occurring in 1% to 5% of patients receiving the drug. Other hypersensitivity reactions are unlikely.

Tobramycin

Tobramycin has an antimicrobial spectrum of activity and toxicity profile similar to that of gentamicin, and its clinical indications for use are the same. However, tobramycin is superior to other aminoglycosides in its activity against *P. aeruginosa*, and it is formulated in a solution for inhalation in respiratory infections caused by that organism. Tobramycin is also used in ophthalmic ointments and solutions.

Kanamycin and Amikacin

Kanamycin is no longer widely used, due to its limited spectrum of activity when compared with other aminoglycosides. However, amikacin, a semisynthetic derivative of kanamycin, has the largest spectrum of activity in this class because of its resistance to many aminoglycoside-inactivating enzymes. Because of this, amikacin is the drug of choice for treatment of hospital-acquired, gram-negative, bacillary infections resistant to gentamicin and tobramycin. Multidrug-resistant strains of *Mycobacterium tuberculosis* are susceptible to amikacin, including those resistant to streptomycin. Like all the other drugs of this class, amikacin is ototoxic and nephrotoxic, with auditory deficits being the most common adverse effect.

Netilmicin

The newest of the aminoglycosides to be marketed, netilmicin, has similar pharmacokinetic and dosing properties to that of gentamicin. However, like amikacin, it is not susceptible to the aminoglycoside-inactivating enzymes and may be used to treat infections caused by organisms resistant to gentamicin and tobramycin. Netilmicin has a similar toxic profile to that of gentamicin and tobramycin.

Neomycin

Neomycin is a broad-spectrum agent active against many gram-negative and gram-positive bacteria and some mycobacterium. Neomycin, in combination with erythromycin, is often used as a preparation before bowel surgery to reduce aerobic bowel flora. Other neomycin-containing solutions may be used intraoperatively for bladder irrigation and for injection into joints, the pleural cavity, tissue spaces, or abscess cavities where an infection may be present. Neomycin is often used in combination with other agents, such as polymyxin, bacitracin, or a corticosteroid, for use as a topical cream or ointment. Adverse effects include intestinal superinfection with oral use and hypersensitivity reactions associated with topical use.

Streptomycin

Streptomycin has an antimicrobial spectrum similar to the other aminoglycosides, but resistance to streptomycin by many species has limited its clinical usefulness. Streptomycin is still used as a second-line agent for treating tuberculosis, in combination with penicillin for treating bacterial endocarditis, and in combination with tetracycline for plague and tularemia.

Hypersensitivity reactions, such as fever and skin rash, may occur with prolonged contact with streptomycin. However, vestibular dysfunction is the most serious toxic result of streptomycin and is found in proportion to the blood levels of the drug and the duration of its administration.

Macrolides

Macrolides are another class of antibiotics that inhibit protein synthesis for susceptible organisms. A macrocyclic lactone ring, 14-membered for erythromycin and clarithromycin and 15-membered for azithromycin, to which one or more deoxy sugars are attached, characterizes them (Figure 13-3). Erythromycin was the first discovered drug in this class; clarithromycin and azithromycin are semi-synthetic derivatives, which have structural differences that improve acid stability, and tissue penetration, and that broaden their spectrum of activity.

Mechanism of Action

Macrolide antibiotics are bacteriostatic. They reversibly bind to 50S ribosomal subunits of susceptible organisms, thereby inhibiting protein synthesis. This binding blocks the aminoacyl translocation reaction and formation of initiation complexes. At higher concentrations erythromycin may be bactericidal against susceptible organisms.

Resistance

Resistance to macrolides is usually plasmid encoded, and several mechanisms have been identified. These include active drug efflux, chromosomal mutations that alter the 50S ribosomal protein, production of esterases by Enterobacteriaceae that hydrolyze the drug, and macrolide-inducible or constitutive production of methylase enzymes that modify the ribosomal target and decrease drug binding. Cross-resistance between drugs in this class is complete. Constitutive methylase production also leads to cross-resistance to compounds that have the same ribosomal binding site (e.g., clindamycin and type B streptogramins).

Pharmacokinetics

Erythromycin must be administered as an enteric-coated tablet, because gastric acids inactivate it. Higher plasma levels of the drug may be achieved with the intravenous

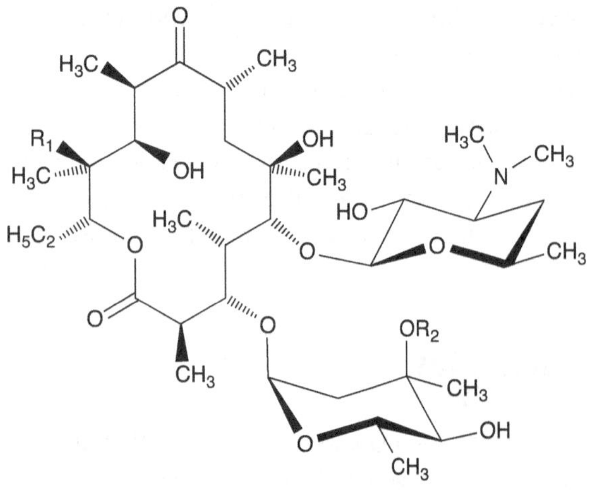

Figure 13-3 Basic chemical structure of erythromycin.

form, erythromycin lactobionate. Erythromycin is widely distributed, except to the brain and CSF, and does cross the placenta. Erythromycin is highly protein bound, around 70% to 80%, and has a plasma half-life of 1.5 hours. It is excreted in the bile and feces, with only 5% excreted in the urine, so dose adjustment in renal patients is not necessary.

Clarithromycin has improved acid stability over erythromycin and has better absorption with oral dosing. It also has a longer half-life of 6 hours and may be administered in an extended-release formulation. Clarithromycin is 40% to 70% protein bound and is widely distributed throughout the body tissues. Clarithromycin is metabolized in the liver, with an active metabolite displaying some antibacterial activity. It is partially excreted in the urine, about 10%, but dose adjustments are not necessary for patients with a creatinine clearance greater than 30 mL/min.

Azithromycin is also administered orally, but it has unique pharmacokinetic properties that set it apart from the other macrolide antibiotics. This includes extensive tissue distribution, with concentrations at the tissue level 10 to 100 times that of the plasma. It is then slowly released, such that its elimination half-life is close to 3 days. Azithromycin is excreted in the bile, with only a small fraction excreted unchanged in the urine.

Clinical Uses and Indications

Erythromycin, clarithromycin, and azithromycin are effective against most gram-positive bacteria, *S. pneumoniae*, *S. aureus*, *H. influenzae*, *Mycoplasma*, *Chlamydia pneumoniae*, and *Corynebacterium diphtheriae*. An erythromycin is the drug of choice for community-acquired pneumonia because of its broad spectrum of activity, including pneumococcus, mycoplasma, and legionella. It is also useful against infections caused by staphylococci, streptococci, or pneumococci in patients who are allergic to penicillin. An erythromycin is also useful in the treatment of chlamydial infections, pertussis disease or exposure prophylaxis, *Campylobacter* infections, and for treatment of *Helicobacter pylori* infections (in combination with amoxicillin and omeprazole).

Adverse Reactions

Serious adverse reactions with macrolides are uncommon. Gastrointestinal effects, such as anorexia, nausea, vomiting, and diarrhea, may occur with oral administration. Specifically, erythromycin acts on receptors in the gut, stimulating gastrointestinal motility, and may be used postoperatively to promote peristalsis or in patients with gastroparesis to speed gastric emptying.

Acute cholestatic hepatitis, with accompanying fever, jaundice, and impaired liver function, may occur after treatment with erythromycin. This finding usually occurs after the use of erythromycin estolate and may reflect a hypersensitivity to the estolate ester. These symptoms usually resolve a few days after the drug is stopped. Other hypersensitivity reactions such as fever, rash, and eosinophilia may also occur.

Erythromycin and clarithromycin metabolites can inhibit cytochrome P-450 enzymes, thereby increasing the serum concentrations of many other drugs. These include carbamazepine, corticosteroids, cyclosporine, digoxin, theophylline, triazolam, valproate, and warfarin. Azithromycin has a differing lactone ring structure, and thus these drug interactions do not occur.

Tetracyclines

The tetracycline class of antibiotics is bacteriostatic, protein-synthesis inhibitors with a broad-spectrum of organisms. They are active against *Rickettsia*, gram-positive and gram-negative bacteria, aerobes, and anaerobes. The tetracyclines, so named for their four hydrocarbon rings, are collectively close congeners of polycyclic napthacenecarboxamide (Figure 13-4). The first marketed agent, chlortetracycline, is no longer available in the United States, but tetracycline is a semisynthetic derivative. Other agents in this class include demeclocycline, doxycycline, minocycline, oxytetracycline, and tigecycline. The antibacterial activity of the various drugs within the class is similar, although some organisms resistant to tetracycline may be susceptible to doxycycline, minocycline, or tigecycline.

Mechanism of Action

Tetracyclines reversibly bind to 30S bacterial ribosomes and prevent access of the aminoacyl tRNA to the acceptor site on the mRNA-ribosome complex, thereby inhibiting bacterial protein synthesis. The tetracyclines gain intracellular access of the bacteria both by passive diffusion and by

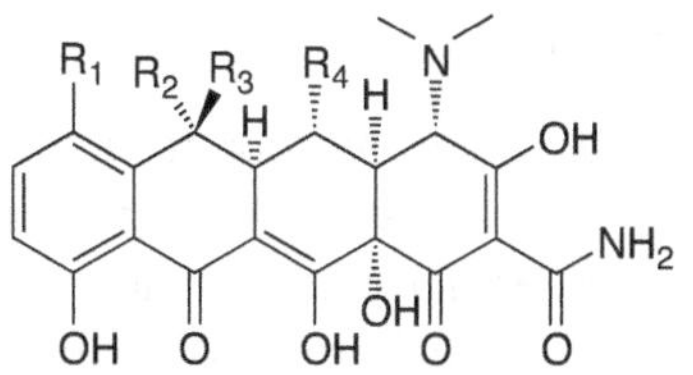

Figure 13-4 Basic chemical structure of tetracycline.

an energy-dependent process of active transport across the cytoplasmic membrane.

Resistance

Resistance to tetracyclines mirrors their mechanism of action, three of which have been defined: (1) decreased intracellular concentrations resulting from a decreased influx or the acquisition of an energy-dependent efflux pathway, (2) production of a protein that interferes with tetracycline binding to the ribosome, and (3) enzymatic inactivation of the tetracycline. The amount of cross-resistance among drugs in this class depends on which mechanism is at work.

Pharmacokinetics

Differences in clinical efficacy and use vary among the tetracyclines, mainly due to the differences in absorption, distribution, and excretion. Of the drugs in this class, absorption after oral administration is 60% to 70% for tetracycline, oxytetracycline, and demeclocycline and 95% to 100% for doxycycline and minocycline. Tigecycline is not well absorbed and is thus given intravenously. Absorption occurs in the stomach and upper small intestines and is impaired by food, calcium, magnesium, iron or zinc salts, and an alkaline pH.

Tetracyclines are 40% to 80% bound to plasma proteins and are distributed widely throughout the body tissue and fluids. Tetracyclines accumulate in the reticuloendothelial cells of the liver, spleen, and bone marrow and in bone, dentine, and enamel of unerupted teeth, which can lead to the adverse reactions listed below.

Tetracyclines are excreted both in urine, mainly by glomerular filtration, and in bile. However, doxycycline and tigecycline are eliminated by nonrenal mechanisms and do not require dosage adjustments for patients with impaired renal function.

Clinical Uses and Indications

A tetracycline is the drug of choice for rickettsial infections, including Rocky Mountain spotted fever, *Mycoplasma pneumoniae*, chlamydia, including *C. pneumoniae*, anthrax, acne, and some gastric and duodenal ulcers caused by *H. pylori*. In the past tetracyclines were used to treat bacterial gastroenteritis, gonococcal infections, and urinary tract infections, but now many strains of bacteria causing these infections are resistant to the tetracyclines.

The glycylcycline tigecycline, a derivative of minocycline, has a spectrum of activity similar to the older tetracyclines but also has activity against many tetracycline-resistant strains as well as a number of multidrug-resistant noso-comial pathogens. Among those are *S. aureus*, includ-ing methicillin-resistant, vancomycin-intermediate, and vancomycin-resistant strains; penicillin-susceptible and penicillin-resistant streptococci; enterococci, including vancomycin-resistant strains, gram-positive rods, Entero-bacteriaceae, multidrug-resistant strains of *Acinetobacter*, gram-positive and gram-negative anaerobes; rickettsiae; chla-mydia; legionella; and rapidly growing mycobacteria. Tigecy-cline is approved by the U.S. Food and Drug Administration for intra-abdominal, skin, and skin-structure infections.

Adverse Reactions

The most common adverse reaction reported with tetra-cyclines is gastrointestinal distress, including abdominal discomfort, nausea, vomiting, and diarrhea. This is likely due to direct local irritation and can be limited by adminis-tering the drug with food while avoiding dairy products or antacids. Normal flora is also suppressed with tetracycline use, which can cause intestinal functional disturbance, vag-inal or oral candidiasis, or enterocolitis.

Tetracycline may deposit in the teeth and bone as a result of its chelation with calcium. Children, especially those under 8 years of age, receiving tetracycline may have tooth discoloration, enamel dysplasia, bone deformity, or bone growth inhibition. Pregnant patients who receive tetracycline may have children born with the same result because tetracyclines cross the placenta. Other adverse reactions, such as photosensitivity, hepatic or renal toxic-ity, and hypersensitivity reactions, occur less commonly.

Clindamycin

Clindamycin is a congener of lincomycin (Figure 13-5). It has a spectrum of activity that includes streptococci, staph-ylococci, and pneumococci. Clindamycin shares many sim-ilarities with erythromycin, but it is not effective against enterococci and gram-negative aerobic organisms.

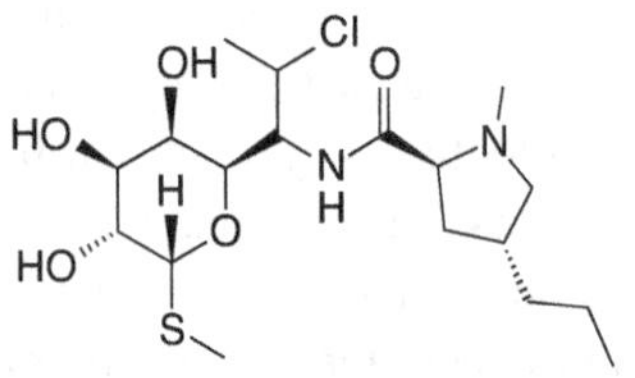

Figure 13-5 Basic chemical structure of clindamycin.

Mechanism of Action

Clindamycin is another antibiotic that inhibits protein syn-thesis. It binds to the 50S subunit of a bacterial ribosome and interferes with the formation of initiation complexes and with aminoacyl translocation reactions. Resistance to clindamycin occurs with mutation of the ribosomal recep-tor site, modification of the receptor by a constitutively produced methylase, and enzymatic inactivation. Organ-isms that are resistant to macrolide antibiotics may display cross-resistance to clindamycin (see Macrolides, Resis-tance, above).

Pharmacokinetics

Clindamycin is well absorbed after oral administration but is also frequently used in its intravenous form. Clindamy-cin is highly protein bound, about 90%, and widely distrib-utes to many body tissues, fluids, and bone and crosses the placental barrier. It does not penetrate the brain and CSF, even in meningitis. Clindamycin is actively taken up by phagocytic cells and accumulates in polymorphonuclear leukocytes, alveolar macrophages, and abscesses. The liver metabolizes clindamycin, with only about 10% excreted unchanged in the urine. Inactive metabolites are excreted in the bile and urine. No dosage adjustment is needed for patients in renal failure; however, clindamycin may accu-mulate in patients with severe hepatic disease, so dosage adjustments in these patients may be required.

Clinical Uses and Indications

Clindamycin is used to treat anaerobic infections, espe-cially those due to *Bacteroides fragilis*. It is also used to treat penetrating wounds of the abdomen and gut, infec-tions originating in the female genital tract, and aspiration pneumonia, alone or in combination with an aminoglyco-side or cephalosporin. Clindamycin is recommended for endocarditis prophylaxis in patients undergoing certain dental or surgical procedures (see Practical Aspects of Antibiotic Use, Infective Endocarditis, below). Topical for-mulations of clindamycin may be used for acne and bacte-rial vaginosis.

Adverse Reactions

The most common adverse reaction to clindamycin is diar-rhea. The incidence of severe pseudomembranous colitis, characterized by abdominal pain, diarrhea, fever, and mucus and blood in the stool, ranges from 0.01% to 10% of patients. Because this is a potentially lethal side effect, clindamycin should only be used to treat infections that are resistant to less toxic agents. Other adverse effects such as skin rashes, elevated liver enzymes, and neutropenia occur less frequently.

Clindamycin produces prejunctional and postjunctional effects at the neuromuscular junction. Large doses of clindamycin can induce profound and long-lasting neuromuscular blockade that is not readily antagonized by calcium or anticholinesterase agents. Concurrent administration of clindamycin with a neuromuscular blocking agent may potentiate the neuromuscular block (see Practical Aspects of Antibiotic Use, Antibiotics and Neuromuscular Blockade, below).

Vancomycin

Vancomycin is a glycopeptide antibiotic that is bactericidal against gram-positive bacteria. It is bactericidal against most staphylococci, including strains resistant to nafcillin, methicillin, and those producing β-lactamase. Vancomycin is only bactericidal against cells that are actively dividing; thus its action is relatively slow.

Mechanism of Action

Vancomycin is a complex tricyclic glycopeptide that inhibits cell wall synthesis in susceptible microorganisms (Figure 13-6). It binds to the cell wall precursor unit and inhibits transglycosylase, preventing elongation of peptidoglycan and cross-linking, which renders the cell susceptible to lysis. Vancomycin also conveys an antibacterial effect as the cell membrane is damaged.

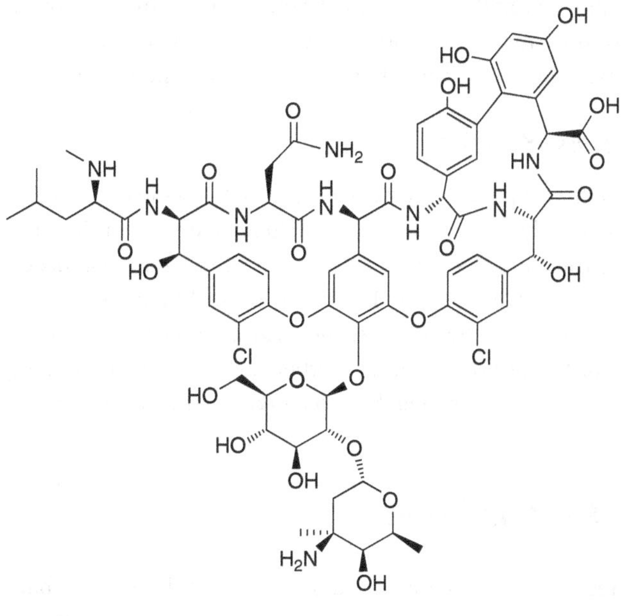

Figure 13-6 Basic chemical structure of vancomycin.

Resistance

Resistance of enterococci to vancomycin has become a major problem for hospitals in the United States, particularly *E. faecium* and *E. faecalis*. This resistance is due to a modification of the binding site on the peptidoglycan building block and a loss of affinity for vancomycin at the binding site, and thereby a loss of activity. Some strains of *S. aureus* also have these resistance determinants.

Pharmacokinetics

Vancomycin is poorly absorbed after oral administration and is only given this way for the treatment of staphylococcal enterocolitis and antibiotic-associated enterocolitis caused by *Clostridium difficile*. Vancomycin hydrochloride is a sterile powder that is diluted and administered intravenously over at least 1 hour. After intravenous administration, vancomycin widely distributes throughout the body and body fluids, including the CSF when the meninges are inflamed, bile, pleural, pericardial, synovial, and ascitic fluids. About 30% of vancomycin is plasma protein bound, and its serum half-life is about 6 hours. The total daily dose is divided two to three times to maintain therapeutic levels, and serum concentration monitoring is often used. Vancomycin is excreted by glomerular filtration, and clearance is proportional to creatinine clearance, so dosage adjustments must be made for patients with renal impairment.

Clinical Uses and Indications

Vancomycin is used clinically for the treatment of severe infections, specifically staphylococcal infections resistant to methicillin, including pneumonia, empyema, endocarditis, osteomyelitis, and soft-tissue abscesses in patients who are allergic to penicillin and cephalosporins. Vancomycin is also used in combination with cefotaxime, ceftriaxone, or rifampin for the treatment of penicillin-resistant pneumococcal meningitis. Vancomycin may also be a useful prophylactic agent in patients undergoing cardiac or orthopedic implantation of prosthetic materials. Treatment of enterocolitis with oral vancomycin is reserved for infections refractory to metronidazole.

Adverse Reactions

Vancomycin may cause hypersensitivity reactions, including macular skin rash, chills, fever, and anaphylaxis. If vancomycin is administered rapidly, extreme flushing, erythematous or urticarial reactions, tachycardia, and hypotension may occur. This phenomenon, called "red man" syndrome, is not an allergic reaction but a drug-induced histamine release due to a direct toxic effect of vancomycin on mast cells. Approximately 5% to 14% of adults who receive vancomycin report this reaction.[5] It may be prevented by prolonging the infusion time of vancomycin to 1 to 2 hours or by increasing the dosing interval.

Ototoxicity may also occur when excessive plasma levels of vancomycin are reached. Nephrotoxicity is also unlikely with appropriate dosing and monitoring of plasma drug levels. However, greater attention must be paid when other ototoxic or nephrotoxic drugs such as an aminoglycoside are administered at the same time as vancomycin.

Fluoroquinolones

Fluoroquinolones are synthetic fluorinated analogs of nalidixic acid (Figure 13-7). They are broad-spectrum antibiotics active against many gram-positive and gram-negative bacteria. These agents have very few side effects, and resistance to them does not develop rapidly. Some of the agents in this class include ciprofloxacin, norfloxacin, levofloxacin, gemifloxacin, moxifloxacin, and ofloxacin.

Mechanism of Action

The fluoroquinolones are bactericidal by two mechanisms. First, they inhibit bacterial DNA gyrase, thereby preventing normal DNA transcription and replication. This seems to be the target of fluoroquinolones on gram-negative bacteria. Second, they inhibit bacterial topoisomerase IV, which interferes with separation of replicated chromosomal DNA to daughter cells during cell division. This is the primary activity of fluoroquinolones for many gram-positive bacteria. Bactericidal activity of fluoroquinolones is concentration dependent and does not exhibit significant PAE.

Resistance

Resistance to fluoroquinolones is related to the specific agent's mechanism of action. Mutations in the bacterial chromosomal genes encoding DNA gyrase or topoisomerase IV may occur, or the drug may be actively transported out of the bacteria.

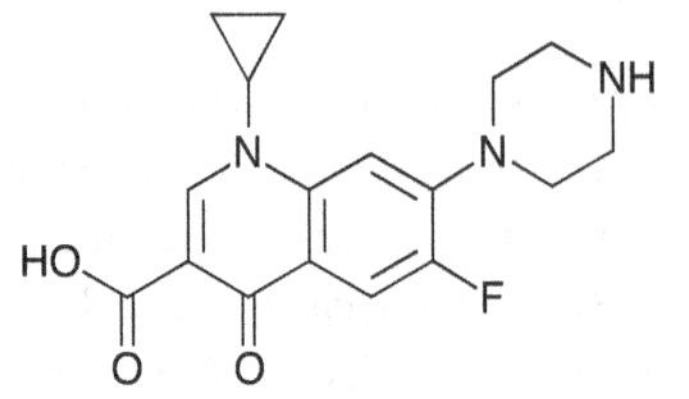

Figure 13-7 Basic chemical structure of ciprofloxacin.

Pharmacokinetics

Fluoroquinolones are readily absorbed after oral administration, and some agents are useful when administered intravenously. They are widely distributed throughout the body, with concentrations in the urine, kidney, lung, prostate tissue, bile, and macrophages and neutrophils higher than the serum levels. CSF, bone, and prostatic fluid levels are lower. The serum half-lives of the various fluoroquinolones range from 3 to 10 hours. Most are eliminated by tubular secretion or glomerular filtration, so dose adjustments in renal impairment are important. However, moxifloxacin is metabolized by the liver and should not be used in patients with hepatic dysfunction.

Clinical Uses and Indications

Fluoroquinolones are potent agents against *E. coli, Salmonella, Shigella, Enterobacter, Campylobacter,* and *Neisseria.* Fluoroquinolones also display activity against some staphylococci, but not methicillin-resistant strains. Levofloxacin and moxifloxacin are effective against streptococci, and gemifloxacin is effective against anaerobic bacteria.

Fluoroquinolones are the drug of choice in treating urinary tract infections. Fluoroquinolones, except norfloxacin, may also be used to treat infections of soft tissue, bone, and joints, and in intra-abdominal and respiratory infections. Some agents, including norfloxacin, ciprofloxacin, and ofloxacin, are effective in the treatment of prostatitis and some sexually transmitted diseases. Levofloxacin, gemifloxacin, and moxifloxacin have better activity against gram-positive organisms and atypical pneumonia caused by chlamydia, mycoplasma, and legionella and therefore are used frequently in the treatment of respiratory tract infections.

Adverse Reactions

The fluoroquinolones are generally well tolerated. The most commonly reported reactions include nausea, vomiting, and diarrhea; however, headache and dizziness may also occur. Rare occurrences of QT interval prolongation have been reported with fluoroquinolones. Concurrent use with class IA or III antiarrhythmics, or other agents known to prolong the QT interval, should be avoided or used with caution.

Metronidazole

Metronidazole, a nitroimidazole (Figure 13-8), is a bactericidal agent active against most anaerobic protozoal parasites and anaerobic bacteria. Metronidazole has antibacterial activity against all anaerobic cocci, anaerobic gram-negative bacilli, and anaerobic spore-forming gram-positive bacilli.

Mechanism of Action

Metronidazole is a prodrug: The nitro group is chemically reduced in anaerobic bacteria and sensitive protozoans. The products of this reduction are responsible for the antimicrobial activity of metronidazole. It has selective toxicity for anaerobic microorganisms: Increasing levels of oxygen inhibit metronidazole activity.

Resistance

Resistance to metronidazole, as seen in *Trichomonas vaginalis* and *Giardia lamblia*, is likely due to impaired oxygen scavenging, leading to higher oxygen concentration and decreased activation of the drug.

Pharmacokinetics

Metronidazole is available for oral, intravenous, intravaginal, and topical use. It is well absorbed after oral administration, but for serious anaerobic infections it is administered intravenously. Metronidazole is widely distributed in all body tissues and fluids, including vaginal secretions, seminal fluid, saliva, breast milk, and CSF. Protein binding is low, about 20%, and its volume of distribution approximates that of total body water. The half-life of metronidazole is about 7.5 hours. Metronidazole metabolism occurs in the liver: 75% of the drug is eliminated as metabolites in the urine, and only 10% is eliminated unchanged. Dosage adjustments should be made in patients with severe liver or kidney disease. Metabolism of metronidazole is induced by phenobarbital, prednisone, and rifampin, whereas cimetidine inhibits its metabolism.

Clinical Uses and Indications

Metronidazole is used for the treatment of anaerobic or mixed intra-abdominal infections, vaginitis, *C. difficile* colitis, and brain abscess. It is often used in the operative setting for prophylaxis in elective colorectal surgery. Metronidazole is also used to treat amebiasis, including amebic colitis and amebic liver abscess, giardiasis, and trichomoniasis.

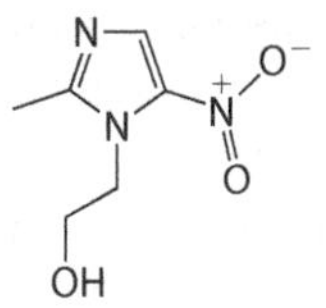

Figure 13-8 Basic chemical structure of metronidazole.

Adverse Reactions

The most common adverse effects of metronidazole include nausea, headache, metallic taste, and dry mouth. Less frequently, vomiting, diarrhea, stomatitis, insomnia, weakness, thrush, rash, neutropenia, and peripheral neuropathy can occur. Alcohol should be avoided with metronidazole to avoid a disulfiram-like effect. Metronidazole is mutagenic in bacteria. Although data on teratogenicity are inconsistent, metronidazole should be avoided in pregnant and nursing women.

Practical Aspects of Antibiotic Use

Surgical Prophylaxis

In surgical patients, antimicrobials may be used therapeutically to treat an ongoing infection or may be administered prophylactically before an event to prevent the formation of an infection. Postoperative surgical site infections are a major category of nosocomial infections, at an estimated annual cost in the United States of $1.5 billion.[6] These include incisional infections, either superficial or deep, or infections of an organ or other organs or spaces manipulated during an operation.

Seminal work by the National Research Council[7] determined wound classification, which has been the basis for the recommendation for surgical antimicrobial prophylaxis (Table 13-6). The most common pathogens causing postoperative, surgical site infections vary according to the type of surgery (Table 13-7). In general, *S. aureus* from the environment or the patient's skin flora is the most likely pathogen in clean procedures where the gastrointestinal, gynecologic, and respiratory tracts have not been entered. In other procedures, such as clean-contaminated, contaminated, and dirty, the "polymicrobial aerobic and anaerobic flora closely resembling the normal endogenous microflora of the surgically resected organ are the most frequently isolated pathogens."[8(p220)]

As early as 1974, the Centers for Disease Control and Prevention began their Study of the Efficacy of Nosocomial Infection Control. They later identified four risk factors for patients developing postoperative infections: operations on the abdomen, operations lasting more than 2 hours, contaminated or dirty wound classification, and a diagnosis of at least three medical conditions.[9] Antimicrobial prophylaxis is needed in contaminated and clean-contaminated operations, clean procedures placing prosthetic materials, procedures in an immunocompromised host, and in any other procedure in which a postoperative infection would

Table 13-6 Wound Classification

Clean

No inflammation
No break in technique
Neither GI nor respiratory tract entered, but transection of appendix or cystic duct considered clean in absence of acute inflammation
Entrance of genitourinary or biliary tract considered clean in absence of infected urine or bile
Subdivided into refined-clean (elective, not drained, and primarily close) and other clean (clean cases other than refined-clean)

Clean-Contaminated

GI or respiratory tract entered without significance
Minor break in technique
Entrance of genitourinary or biliary tract in presence of infected urine or bile

Contaminated

Major break in technique (e.g., emergency cardiac massage)
Acute bacterial inflammation without puss
Spillage from GI tract
Traumatic wound, fresh from relatively clean source

Dirty

Presence of pus
Perforated viscus
Traumatic wound, old or from dirty source

GI, gastrointestinal.

be devastating.[6] Table 13-8 lists the general principles of antimicrobial surgical prophylaxis.

Dosage and Administration

In 2002 the Centers for Medicare and Medicaid Services and the Centers for Disease Control and Prevention implemented the National Surgical Infection Prevention Project. Their goal was "to decrease the morbidity and mortality associated with postoperative surgical site infections by promoting appropriate selection and timing of administration of prophylactic antimicrobial agents."[10(p1706)] This work group endorsed the practice that the infusion of the first dose of an antimicrobial agent should begin within 60 minutes of surgical incision. The infusion should begin within 120 minutes when vancomycin or a fluoroquinolone is indicated. Additional recommendations included initial dose and time to redose (Table 13-9), antibiotic selection (Table 13-10), and discontinuation of prophylactic antimicrobials within 24 hours of the end of surgery.

Table 13-7 Common Pathogens Causing Postoperative Infections

Operative Site	Aerobes	Anaerobes
Mouth and esophagus	Streptococci	Bacteroides (not *B. fragilis*), peptostreptococci, fusobacteria
Stomach	Enteric gram-negative bacilli Streptococci	Bacteroides (not *B. fragilis*), peptostreptococci, fusobacteria
Biliary	Enteric gram-negative bacilli Streptococci *S. aureus*	
Intestinal	Enteric gram-negative bacilli	*B. fragilis, Clostridia*
Gynecologic	Enteric gram-negative bacilli Streptococci	Gram-positive bacilli *B. fragilis*, Enterobacteriaceae Fusobacteria, peptostreptococci
Urologic	Enteric gram-negative bacilli Streptococci	
Prostate	Gram-negative bacilli, enterococci	
Cardiac	*S. aureus, Staphylococcus epidermis,*	
Thoracic	*S. aureus, S. epidermis,* streptococci	Bacteroides (not *B. fragilis*) peptostreptococci
Peripheral vascular	*S. aureus, S. epidermis*	
Head and neck	Gram-positive cocci	
Neurosurgical	*S. aureus, S. epidermis* Gram-negative bacilli	
Orthopedic	*S. aureus, S. epidermis* Streptococci	

Table 13-8 General Principles of Antimicrobial Surgical Prophylaxis

1. Antibiotic should be active against common surgical wound pathogens.
2. Antibiotic should have proven efficacy in clinical trials.
3. Antibiotic must achieve concentrations greater than the minimum inhibitory concentration of the suspected pathogens by the time incision is made.
4. The shortest possible course and most effective/least toxic antibiotic should be used.
5. The newer broad-spectrum antibiotics should be reserved for therapy of resistant infections.
6. If all else is equal, the least expensive antibiotic should be chosen.

Table 13-9 Suggested Initial Dose and Time to Redosing for Antimicrobial Drugs Commonly Utilized for Surgical Prophylaxis.

Antimicrobial	Renal half-life, h Patients With Normal Renal Function	Renal half-life, h Patients With End-Stage Renal Disease	Recommended Infusion Duration	Standard Dose	Weight-Based Dose Recommendation[a]	Recommended Redosing Interval,[b] h
Aztreonam	1.5–2	6	3–5 min,[c] 20–60 min[d]	1–2 g IV	2-g maximum (adults)	3–5
Ciprofloxacin	3.5–5	5–9	60 min	400 mg IV	400 mg	4–10
Cefazolin	1.2–2.5	40–70	3–5 min,[c] 15–60 min[d]	1–2 g IV	20–30 mg/kg (if < 80 kg, use 1 g; if > 80 kg, use 2 g)	2–5
Cefuroxime	1–2	15–22	3–5 min,[c] 15–60 min[d]	1.5 g IV	50 mg/kg	3–4
Cefamandole	0.5–2.1	12.3–18[e]	3–5 min,[c] 15–60 min[d]	1 g IV		3–4
Cefoxitin	0.5–1.1	6.5–23	3–5 min,[c] 15–60 min[d]	1–2 g IV	20–40 mg/kg	2–3
Cefotetan	2.8–4.6	13–25	3–5 min,[c] 20–60 min[d]	1–2 g IV	20–40 mg/kg	3–6
Clindamycin	2–5.1	3.5–5.0[f]	10–60 min (do not exceed 30 mg/min)	600–900 mg IV	If <10 kg, use at least 37.5 mg; if > 10 kg, use 3–6 mg/kg	3–6
Erythromycin base	0.8–3	5–6	NA	1 g PO 19, 18, and 9 h before surgery	9–13 mg/kg	NA
Gentamicin	2–3	50–70	30–60 min	1.5 mg/kg IV[g]	...[g]	3–6
Neomycin	2–3 (3% absorbed under normal gastrointestinal conditions)	12–24 or longer	NA	1 g PO 19, 18, and 9 h before surgery	20 mg/kg	NA
Metronidazole	6–14	7–21; no change	30–60 min	0.5–1 g IV	15 mg/kg initial dose (adult); 7.5 mg/kg on subsequent doses	6–8
Vancomycin	4–6	44.1–406.4 (CCR < 10 mL/min)	1 g over 60 min (use longer infusion time if dose > 1 g)	1 g IV	10–15 mg/kg (adult)	6–12

CCR, creatinine clearance rate.

[a] Data are primarily from published pediatric recommendations. [b] For procedures of long duration, antimicrobials should be readministered at intervals of 1–2 times the half-life of the drug. The intervals in the table were calculated for patients with normal renal function. [c] Dose injected directly into vein or via running intravenous infusion. [d] Intermittent intravenous infusion. [e] In patients with a serum creatinine level of 5–9 mg/dL. [f] The half-life of clindamycin is the same or slightly increased in patients with end-stage renal disease, compared with patients with normal renal function. [g] If the patient's body weight is 130% higher than the ideal body weight (IBW), the dosing weight (DW) can be determined as follows: DW = IBW + [0.4 × (total body weight − IBW)].

Source: From reference 10.

Table 13-10 Guidelines for Antimicrobial Use in Surgical Prophylaxis

Antibiotic Dosing

Infusion of the first antibiotic dose should begin 1 hour before skin incision (120 minutes for fluoroquinolone or vancomycin).
Prophylactic antimicrobials should be discontinued 24 hours after surgery.
Initial antimicrobial dose should be adequate based on the patient's body weight, or body mass index.
Additional antimicrobial dose should be provided intraoperatively if the operation continues 2 half-lives after the initial dose.

Antibiotic Selection	Procedure
Abdominal or vaginal hysterectomy	Cefotetan preferred; cefazolin or cefoxitin alternative Metronidazole monotherapy also used In ß-lactam allergy; clindamycin combined with gentamicin or ciprofloxacin or azetronam; metronidazole with gentamicin or ciprofloxacin; or clindamycin monotherapy
Hip or knee arthroplasty	Use cefazolin or cefuroxime. In ß-lactam allergy, vancomycin or clindamycin
Cardiothoracic and vascular surgery	Use cefazolin or cefuroxime. In ß-lactam allergy, vancomycin or clindamycin
Colon surgery	For oral antimicrobial prophylaxis; neomycin plus erythromycin base or neomycin plus metronidazole. For parenteral, use cefotetan, cefoxitin, or cefazolin plus metronidazole. In ß-lactam allergy, use clindamycin combined with gentamicin, ciprofloxacin, or azetronam, or use metronidazole combined with gentamicin or ciprofloxacin.

Infective Endocarditis

As early as 1955 the American Heart Association began publishing recommendations in an attempt to guide patients and healthcare providers in the prevention of infective endocarditis (IE). The fundamental principles behind these recommendations were as follows:

(1) IE is an uncommon but life-threatening disease, and prevention is preferable to treatment of an established infection; (2) certain underlying cardiac conditions predispose to IE; (3) bacteremia with organisms known to cause IE occurs commonly in association with invasive dental, GI, or GU tract procedures; (4) antimicrobial prophylaxis was proven to be effective for prevention of experimental IE in animals; and (5) antimicrobial prophylaxis was thought to be effective in humans for prevention of IE associated with dental, GI, or GU tract procedures.[11(p1738)]

More recently numerous publications have questioned the validity of the last principle. Therefore in 2007 the American Heart Association revised its guidelines for prophylactic antimicrobial use. The complete listing of guidelines may be found elsewhere, but several key points relevant to anesthesia providers are listed here.[11]

Certain cardiac conditions are associated with the highest risk of adverse outcomes from IE in which antimicrobial prophylaxis is reasonable. These include patients with prosthetic cardiac valves or prosthetic material used for cardiac valve repair, patients with prior history of IE, cardiac transplantation patients who have developed valvuloplasty, and some congenital heart disease (CHD) patients. The specific forms of CHD included are unrepaired cyanotic CHD, including palliative shunts and conduits; CHD that has been completely repaired with prosthetic material or device placed by catheter intervention or surgery; during the first 6 months after the procedure; and repaired CHD with residual defects at the site of or adjacent to a prosthetic patch or device that limits endothelialization. Only in patients with those conditions listed is antibiotic prophylaxis considered reasonable for dental procedures that involve manipulation of gingival tissues or the periapical region of teeth or perforation of oral mucosa, invasive procedures on the respiratory tract involving an incision or biopsy of respiratory mucosa (including tonsillectomy and adenoidectomy), or procedures on infected skin, skin structures, or musculoskeletal tissues. If a patient with the listed cardiac conditions is scheduled to undergo a procedure and an infection is already established, antimicrobial therapy should be directed at the most likely causative microorganism. Antibiotic prophylaxis is not recommended solely to prevent IE for gastrointestinal or genitourinary tract procedures such as diagnostic esophagogastroduodenoscopy or colonoscopy.

Antibiotics and Neuromuscular Blockade

One of the most relevant adverse effects related to antimicrobial therapy for the anesthesia provider is the interaction these agents have on the neuromuscular system, especially when they are administered in the perioperative period along with other agents affecting the neuromuscular junction. The antibiotic classes aminoglycosides, tetracyclines, clindamycin, and the polymyxins have the ability to produce neuromuscular blockade. Of the β-lactams, penicillin G and V only produce neuromuscular block in concentrations not usually seen clinically, and cephalosporins do not have any neuromuscular blocking activity. The extent of blockade of all the antibiotic agents is further potentiated when used in combination with nondepolarizing neuromuscular blocking agents, such as vecuronium, anesthetics, and other drugs used during anesthesia, such as lidocaine. In addition, patients with underlying disease states, such as myasthenia gravis, are at increased risk for displaying these effects.[12] Table 13-11 summarizes the different proposed mechanisms of action at the neuromuscular junction for each antibiotic class and degree of reversibility.

Site of Neuromuscular Blocking Action Between Antibiotic Classes

In an early review by Sokoll and Gergis, the effect of the individual antibiotic drug classes on neuromuscular function was explored.[13] The aminoglycoside agents, probably the most recognized classes of antibiotics for causing neuromuscular blockade, display discrete differences between the individual agents. The effect of streptomycin is thought to be caused by postsynaptic receptor blockade, inhibition

of acetylcholine release from the nerve terminal, and an additional nonspecific local anesthetic-type action. This block is at least partially reversed by neostigmine and to a greater extent by the administration of calcium. Neomycin has depressant activity on the nerve terminal by inhibiting acetylcholine release and also has some weak postsynaptic blocking action. This block is reversed by both neostigmine and calcium, although calcium is reported to be more effective. Gentamicin has a presynaptic site of action and produces neuromuscular blockade by depressing the release of acetylcholine. Calcium antagonizes a gentamicin-induced neuromuscular block.

The mode of neuromuscular block seen with clindamycin is multifactorial. It has a local anesthetic effect on myelinated nerves and stimulates the nerve terminal and blocks the postsynaptic cholinergic receptor. The clindamycin-induced block is difficult to reverse, either with calcium or neostigmine. The neuromuscular block associated with tetracyclines is weak and may be related to calcium chelation and a resulting inhibition of acetylcholine release. Thus the block is usually reversed with calcium but not with neostigmine.

According to Sokoll and Gergis,[13] antibiotic-induced or potentiated neuromuscular blockade should be suspected if there is delayed recovery from a nondepolarizing neuromuscular blocking agent and increased depth of neuromuscular blockade after the administration of an antibiotic, difficulty reversing a nondepolarizing neuromuscular agent when antibiotics have been used, or a recurarization occurs in the postoperative setting when an antibiotic is administered. The anesthesia provider should evaluate the patient's response to train-of-four and titanic stimulation and evaluate the patient for clinical signs of adequate neuromuscular function such as maximum inspiratory force and head lift.

Table 13-11 Antibiotics and Neuromuscular Blockade

Antibiotic	Site of Action	Reversal Regimen
Gentamicin	Presynaptic, possibly postsynaptic	Calcium; neostigmine (partially)
Amikacin	Presynaptic	Calcium; neostigmine (partially)
Kanamycin	Presynaptic, possibly postsynaptic	Calcium or 4-aminopyridine
Neomycin	Presynaptic, also weak postsynaptic	Calcium (partially); neostigmine (poorly)
Streptomycin	Presynaptic and postsynaptic	Calcium (partially); neostigmine (poorly)
Clindamycin	Postsynaptic	Difficult with any method
Lincomycin	Postsynaptic, also slightly presynaptic	Neostigmine (poorly); calcium (poorly)
Piperacillin	Postsynaptic	Neostigmine
Penicillin G	Presynaptic, possibly nerve terminal	Calcium
Tetracycline	Presynaptic	Calcium
Polymyxins A or B	Postsynaptic	4-Aminopyridine
Polymyxin E	Postsynaptic	Calcium (poorly)

Key Points

- Anesthesia providers should be knowledgeable about various antibiotic agents, as they are widely used in the perioperative period.
- An agent's minimum inhibitory concentration, dose- or time-dependent killing, postantibiotic effect, and synergism will guide antibiotic therapy. Additional local and host factors should also be considered.
- Successful antibiotic therapy requires attention to specific agents' mechanism of action, resistance, pharmacokinetics, and potential for adverse reaction.
- Choice for surgical antibiotic prophylaxis should include the type of surgery and a patient's risk factors.

Timing and discontinuation of the agent should follow established guidelines.

■ Special caution should be used when an anesthesia provider administers an aminoglycoside, tetracycline, clindamycin, or a polymyxin due to potential neuromuscular effects.

Chapter Questions

1. Define the minimum inhibitory concentration, and describe how it relates to antibiotic therapy.
2. Explain the concepts dose-dependent killing, time-dependent killing, and postantibiotic effect. Identify how these guide antibiotic dosing regimens.
3. Define antibiotic resistance and strategies to limit its emergence.
4. Discuss the mechanism of action, clinical use, and possible adverse reactions with each of the following drugs/drug classes: β-lactam, aminoglycoside, macrolide, tetracycline, clindamycin, vancomycin, fluoroquinolones, and metronidazole.
5. Describe the indications for surgical prophylaxis and the recommended dosage and administration guidelines.
6. Characterize infective endocarditis and distinguish the types of patients and surgical procedures that require prophylactic antibiotic coverage.
7. Review the neuromuscular blocking effects of antibiotics, the proposed mechanism of action, and treatment options.

References

1. World Health Organization. World Health Organization report on infectious diseases 2000. Overcoming antimicrobial resistance. Available at: http://www.who.int/infectious-disease-report/2000/index.html. Accessed April 15, 2009.
2. Kelkar PS, Li JT-C. Cephalosporin allergy. *N Engl J Med.* 2001; 354:804–809.
3. Riedl MA, Casillas AM. Adverse drug reactions: types and treatment options. *Am Fam Physician.* 2003;68:1781–1790.
4. Solensky R. Hypersensitivity to beta-lactam antibiotics. *Clin Rev Allerg Immunol.* 2003;24:201–219.
5. Hepner DL, Castells MC. Anaphylaxis during the perioperative period. *Anesth Analg.* 2003;97:1381–1395.
6. Lampiris HW, Maddix D. Clinical use of antimicrobial agents. In: Katzung BG, ed. *Basic & Clinical Pharmacology*, 10th ed. Available at: http://www.accessmedicine.com/content.aspx?aID=2510929. Accessed October 30, 2008.
7. Howard JM. Report of an ad hoc committee of the Committee on Trauma, Division of Medical Sciences, National Academy of Sciences-National Research Council, postoperative wound infections: the influence of ultraviolet irradiation of the OR and various other factors. *Ann Surg.* 1964; 160:9–192.
8. Nichols RL. Preventing surgical site infections: a surgeon's perspective. *Emerg Infect Dis.* 2001;7:220–224.
9. Haley RW, Culver DH, Morgan WM, White JW, Emori TG, Hooton TM. Identifying patients at high risk of surgical wound infection: a simple multivariate index of patient susceptibility and wound contamination. *Am J Epidemiol.* 1985;121:206–215.
10. Bratzler DW, Houck PM. Antimicrobial prophylaxis for surgery: an advisory statement from the National Surgical Infection Prevention Project. *Clin Infect Dis.* 2004;38:1706–1715.
11. Wilson W, Taubert KA, Gewits M, et al. Prevention of infective endocarditis: guidelines from the American Heart Association. *Circulation.* 2007;116:1736–1754.
12. Cheng EY, Nimphius N, Hennen CR. Antibiotic therapy and the anesthesiologist. *J Clin Anesth.* 1995;7:425–439.
13. Sokoll MD, Gergis SG. Antibiotics and neuromuscular function. *Anesthesiology.* 1981;55:148–159.

Objectives

After completing this chapter, the reader should be able to

- Describe the physiology of vomiting.
- Describe the various receptors within the chemoreceptor trigger zone that may be blocked to prevent or treat postoperative nausea and vomiting.
- Identify patients at high risk of postoperative nausea and vomiting.
- Discuss various classes of medications that may be efficacious in preventing or treating postoperative nausea and vomiting.
- Discuss alternatives to pharmacologic interventions for prevention of postoperative nausea and vomiting.

14

Antiemetic Drugs and Therapies

Nancy L. Tierney, DMP, CRNA
Priscilla P. Walkup, DMP, CRNA
William A. White, Jr., DMP, CRNA

Introduction

Nausea, retching, and vomiting are universally recognized as unpleasant experiences that are often associated with surgery and anesthesia. Chemotherapy-induced nausea and vomiting (CINV) is a common adverse consequence of anticancer therapy.[1]

Twenty percent to 30% of all surgical patients experience postoperative nausea and vomiting (PONV).[2] Among high-risk populations the incidence may reach 70%.[3] Nausea and vomiting are the most common adverse effects in the postanesthesia care unit (PACU) and are the most common reasons that adults and children have protracted stays in the PACU or unexpected hospital admissions due to anesthesia.[4] Patients often rate nausea and vomiting as more distressing than postoperative pain. Nausea and vomiting can delay hospital discharge, increase costs, and cause serious comorbidities such as wound dehiscence, pulmonary aspiration, tachycardia, hypertension, and postoperative pain.[5]

Prevention and treatment of nausea and vomiting continue to present challenges for healthcare providers. This is especially true in areas such as anesthesia and chemotherapeutics where nausea and vomiting are all too common and where no single therapy has proven completely effective.[6]

Risk factor assessment for PONV is necessary for formulating effective individualized prevention and treatment plans for each patient. Risk factors may be categorized as patient related (Table 14-1),[7–9] anesthesia related (Table 14-2),[7,10] or surgery related (Table 14-3).[7,10]

Nausea and vomiting may be manifestations of a wide variety of conditions, including adverse effects from medications, systemic disorders or infections, pregnancy, vestibular dysfunction, central nervous system infection or increased pressure, peritonitis, hepatobiliary disorders, radiation, and

Table 14-1 Patient-Related Risk Factors for PONV

Young age
Female gender
Obesity
Pain
Anxiety
History of motion sickness
Presence of food in stomach
Gastroparesis
Diabetes mellitus
Nonsmoker
Pregnancy

Table 14-2 Anesthesia-Related Risk Factors for PONV

Opioid analgesics
Potent inhalation anesthetics
Nitrous oxide
Barbiturates
Etomidate
Ketamine
Anticholinesterase drugs

Table 14-3 Surgical Procedures Associated With Increased Incidence of PONV

Adults	Children
Laparoscopy	Adenotonsillectomy
Mastectomy	Orchiopexy
Dilatation and curettage	Middle ear surgery
Tooth extraction	Otoplasty
Head and neck surgery	Strabismus repair
Gastrointestinal surgery	

gastrointestinal disorders.[11] It is beyond the scope of this chapter to discuss the management of nausea and vomiting related to all these etiologies. Instead, this chapter focuses on prevention and treatment of PONV.

Physiology of Emesis

Vomiting is one of the ways that the body eliminates noxious, toxic substances. Actually, vomiting is thought to be an evolutionary protective mechanism for ejecting toxic substances from the stomach. Nausea and vomiting educate and remind animals about which foods are safe to eat, because the unpleasant effects of nausea and vomiting caused by toxins are so well remembered.[7,10]

The stimuli that cause vomiting can originate in any part of the gastrointestinal tract, although distention or irritation of the duodenum provides the strongest stimulus.[12] The act of vomiting involves coordination of the gastrointestinal, abdominal, and respiratory musculature and is controlled by the emetic center, a group of neurons located in the reticular formation of medulla oblongata (Figure 14-1).[7,10,13]

The emetic center consists of various scattered groups of neurons that control the components of the vomiting act.[13] Sensory input from many areas of the body can activate the emetic center. Afferent impulses from the pharynx, gastrointestinal tract, and mediastinum and direct stimulation from the cerebral cortex (anticipation, fear, memories), signals from the sensory organs (disturbing sights, smells, pain), input from the chemoreceptor trigger zone (CTZ) in the fourth ventricle, or signals from the vestibular apparatus of the inner ear can all stimulate the emetic center to initiate vomiting.[7,10,11,14,15]

The CTZ is an area of importance to anesthesia providers because it is not protected by the blood–brain barrier and is an anatomic site at which multiple pharmacologic interventions may be directed to prevent or treat PONV.[9] The CTZ can be activated by the agonist molecules serotonin, dopamine, histamine, acetylcholine, and neurokinin-1 (substance P) to stimulate the emetic center. Specific receptors exist for each of these agonists. Blockade of these receptors is believed to be an important mechanism of action of antiemetic drugs.[7,16] Specific pharmacologic agents have been developed that successfully block the transmission of these neurotransmitters at the level of the CTZ; however, no single agent will block all pathways.[2]

Selective Serotonin Receptor Antagonists

In the past, dopamine antagonists, corticosteroids, anticholinergics, and antihistamines were commonly used in the prevention and treatment of PONV; however, many of these demonstrated undesirable side effects such as dry mouth, excessive sedation, dysphoria, restlessness, and extrapyramidal symptoms. Serotonin (5-hydroxytryptamine [5-HT]) is a widely distributed endogenous vasoactive substance (autacoid) that evokes complex changes in the cardiovascular system (cerebral, coronary, and pulmonary vascular vasoconstriction) and functions as an important neurotransmitter in emesis and pain transmission.[17] Serotonin is released from the enterochromaffin cells of the small intestine, stimulates the vagal afferents through 5-hydroxytryptamine type 3 (5-HT$_3$) receptors, and can initiate the vomiting reflex.

A newer class of antiemetic agents, the 5-HT$_3$ receptor antagonists, initially used for the treatment of CINV, is now widely used for the prevention and treatment of PONV, with few undesirable side effects. The two most commonly reported side effects of 5-HT$_3$ antagonists are mild, transient headache and dizziness. Some patients have shown transient, clinically insignificant electrocardiographic changes after the administration of 5-HT$_3$ antagonists.[7]

Serotonin receptors are located in the enterochromaffin cells of the gastrointestinal tract, the CTZ, and the area postrema. These receptors play an important role in the activation of the CTZ, especially with drug-induced emesis. Therefore by blocking the 5-HT$_3$ receptors in the area postrema, the CTZ is less sensitive to the effects that anesthetic drugs can have in inducing PONV. Although other drugs are more effective in treating nausea, 5-HT$_3$ antagonists are more effective in treating vomiting.[3] Serotonin antagonists produce antiemetic activity by selectively inhibiting 5-HT$_3$ receptors in the central and peripheral nervous systems, the CTZ, and the vagus nerve within the gastrointestinal tract, respectively.[18]

Currently, there are six different 5-HT$_3$ antagonists identified as having therapeutic efficacy in managing nausea and vomiting: ondansetron, dolasetron, granisetron, tropisetron, palonosetron, and ramosetron. Only four of these have been approved in the United States for PONV: ondansetron, dolasetron, granisetron, and palosetron.[19] Tropisetron (Navoban) is used for treating PONV and CINV in some other countries.[20,21] Ramosetron (Nasea, Yamanouchi, Tokyo, Japan) is used elsewhere to treat CINV and is under investigation for the treatment of PONV.[22,23] Table 14-4[8,24] lists doses and timing of a variety of antiemetic medications used by anesthesia providers. Table 14-5 [25,26] lists doses of antiemetic medications for children.

Ondansetron

Ondansetron (Zofran), the prototype and first drug of this class, was also the first serotonin receptor antagonist

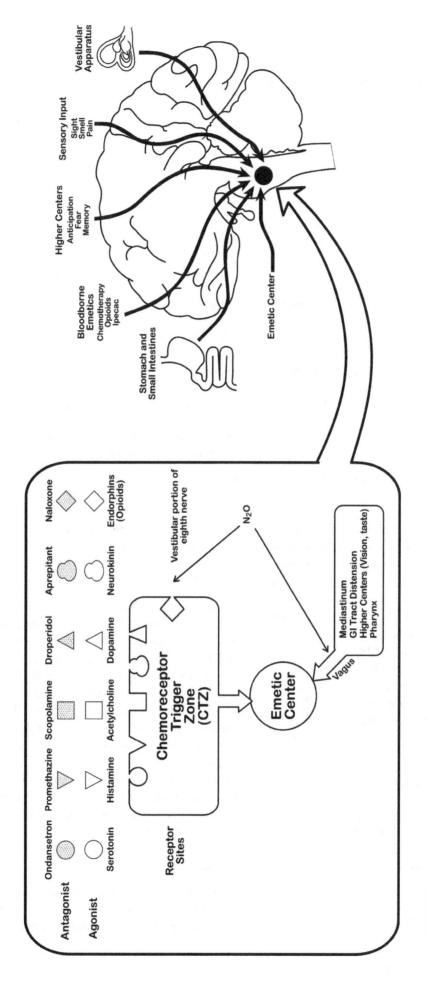

Figure 14-1 The chemoreceptor trigger zone and the emetic center.

Source: From references 7 and 10.

Table 14-4 Antiemetic Doses and Timing for Administration in Adults

Drug	Receptor Site of Action	Dose	Timing	Onset Time (min)	Duration ($T_{\beta_{1/2}}$) (h)
Ondansetron (Zofran)	5-HT$_3$	4–8 mg IV	At end of surgery	~30	3–6
Dolasetron (Anzemet)	5-HT$_3$	12.5 mg IV	At end of surgery	~15	6–8
Granisetron (Kytril)	5-HT$_3$	0.35–1 mg IV	At end of surgery	~30	5–9
Palonosetron (Aloxi)	5-HT$_3$	0.25 mg IV	Before start of chemotherapy	~30	40
Dexamethasone (Decadron)		4–10 mg IV	Before induction	15–30	36–54
Droperidol (Inapsine)	D$_2$	0.625–1.25 mg IV	At end of surgery	~30	2.3
Prochlorperazine (Compazine)	D$_2$	5–10 mg IV	At end of surgery	~5–10	7
Promethazine (Phenergan)	H$_1$, D$_2$, M$_1$	12.5–25 mg IV	At end of surgery	3–5	9–16
Metoclopramide (Reglan)	D$_2$	10 mg IV	Before induction	1–3	4–6
Scopolamine (Transderm-Scop)	M$_1$	Transdermal patch	Applied evening before or 4 h before end of surgery	120–240	Releases 1 mg over 72 h

D$_2$, dopamine type 2; H$_1$, histamine type 1; IV, intravenously; M$_1$, muscarinic cholinergic type 1.

approved for the prevention and treatment of PONV in oral and intravenous forms and has been designated as a first-line treatment regimen for nausea and vomiting.[27,28] A single 4-mg dose is very efficacious in preventing PONV but is less efficacious in the prevention of PONV beyond an interval of 2 hours after surgery.[28] Sadhasivam et al. found that ondansetron used as a single agent decreased PONV from 81% to 33% compared with placebo.[29]

Ondansetron is structurally similar to serotonin and has specific 5-HT$_3$ receptor antagonist properties. The usual adult dosage is 4 to 8 mg intravenously (IV) given over 2 to 5 minutes. The onset of action is approximately 30 minutes, and the elimination half-time is approximately

Table 14-5 Antiemetic Doses for Children

Drug	Dose
Ondansetron	50-100 µg/kg up to 4 mg
Dolasetron	350 µg/kg up to 12.5 mg
Dexamethasone	150 µg/kg up to 8 mg
Droperidol	50-75 µg/kg up to 1.25 mg
Dimenhydrinate	0.5 mg/kg
Perphenazine	70 µg/kg

4 hours.[24] The most efficacious dose in children older than 2 years is 50 to 100 µg/kg (maximum, 4 mg).

Dolasetron

Dolasetron (Anzemet) is a potent, highly selective 5-HT$_3$ receptor antagonist. Dolasetron is rapidly metabolized to hydrodolasetron, which is responsible for the antiemetic effects. Hydrodolasetron has an elimination half-time of 8 hours and is approximately 100 times more potent than dolasetron. Hydrodolasetron appears in the urine within 30 minutes after administration. The recommended adult dosage of dolasetron is 12.5 mg by injection given approximately 15 minutes before the end of anesthesia.[24] Dolasetron oral tablets 50 to 100 mg given 2 hours before induction of anesthesia has been found to be comparable with ondansetron 4 mg IV for PONV prophylaxis. Dizziness, headache, and increased appetite are among the more prevalent side effects.[30]

Granisetron

Granisetron (Kytril) is a more selective 5-HT$_3$ receptor antagonist than ondansetron and has been widely used in the prevention and treatment of nausea and vomiting in patients receiving chemotherapy. The elimination half-time of granisetron is approximately 9 hours. A single dose may be effective for 24 hours. Although granisetron is approved for use in the United States, its relatively high cost may limit its clinical application.[31] Granisetron 1 mg is the optimal dose when administered immediately before induction. Some researchers have found this dose to be effective in PONV prevention; others have determined granisetron 20 to 40 μg/kg to be the optimal dose for adults and children.[32,33] Side effects are mild and include diarrhea, sedation, and headache.

Palonosetron

Palonosetron (Aloxi) is the newest 5-HT$_3$ receptor antagonist introduced for the prevention of acute and delayed CINV and approved by the U.S. Food and Drug Administration (FDA). Palonosetron has not been shown to be effective in terminating nausea or vomiting once it occurs and should not be used for this purpose. Palonosetron differs from the other 5-HT$_3$ receptor antagonists in that it has a much longer half-life. The half-lives of the 5-HT$_3$ receptor antagonists are as follows: palonosetron, 40 hours; ondansetron, 3 to 6 hours; dolasetron, 6 to 8 hours; and granisetron, 5 to 9 hours.[24] Common side effects of palonosetron are headache, constipation, diarrhea, and dizziness. Less common side effects may be bradycardia, hypotension, and tachycardia. The adult dose of palonosetron is 0.25 mg IV 30 minutes before the start of chemotherapy administration. Currently, palonosetron is not recommended for use in PONV.

Although many studies have recommended that 5-HT$_3$ receptor antagonists be administered at the beginning of anesthesia, more recent consensus guidelines for managing PONV have determined that all three 5-HT$_3$ receptor antagonists used for PONV (ondansetron, dolasetron, and granisetron) are most effective when administered at the end of surgery.[34] Furthermore, consensus guidelines have determined no difference in efficacy and safety among these serotonin receptor antagonists.

Corticosteroids

Glucocorticoids (analogs of cortisol, which is synthesized in the adrenal cortex) play a useful role in the prevention and treatment of PONV.[35] These drugs are also useful antiemetics when administered before chemotherapy. Unlike other antiemetic medications administered by anesthesia providers, corticosteroids do not appear to exert their effects

through activation or inhibition of receptors for serotonin, histamine, acetylcholine, or dopamine. Corticosteroids manifest their effects by interacting with intracellular receptors that regulate expression of corticosteroid-responsive genes. The prolonged amount of time required for gene expression and protein synthesis results in an onset time of several hours.[36,37] The exact mechanism of antiemetic action of corticosteroids is not completely understood.

Dexamethasone

The corticosteroid used most frequently to prevent PONV is dexamethasone. Onset time for dexamethasone is longer than for other classes of antiemetics; therefore it should be given approximately 1 hour before surgery and anesthesia. Slower onset makes dexamethasone less useful for treating PONV than for preventing it. Of importance, a single dose of dexamethasone has a biologic half-life of 36 to 56 hours—longer than that of any other antiemetic medication.[37,38] Corticosteroids work best as part of a multimodal approach for prophylaxis of PONV.

Corticosteroids exert powerful effects on every organ system of the body. Hyperglycemia, fluid retention, and hypertension occur. Wound infection and wound dehiscence may occur more frequently after corticosteroid administration. Corticosteroids are metabolized via hepatic reduction.[36,37] The effective antiemetic dose of dexamethasone for adults is 4 to 10 mg IV.

Butyrophenones

Butyrophenones have proven to be very effective antiemetics in the postoperative settting.[39] These drugs are older, standard, neuroleptic-type antipsychotics that possess significant sedative and antiemetic properties. Important side effects include extrapyramidal symptoms, motor restlessness, and severe anxiety.[40]

Most neuroleptics protect against the nausea- and emesis-inducing effects of a variety of endogenous and exogenous agonists that stimulate the CTZ in the medulla. The main routes of metabolism of butyrophenones are oxidative and conjugative processes in the liver.[40]

Droperidol

Since the 1970s droperidol has been a useful first-line antiemetic for patients undergoing surgery. In 2001 the FDA changed the labeling requirements for droperidol injection because of reports of QT interval prolongation and torsade de pointes. Twenty reported cases of torsades and five deaths were reported; most of those patients received doses in excess of 50 mg in a 24-hour period. It appears that QT prolongation is a dose-related phenomenon. Nevertheless, cases of QT prolongation and/or torsade de pointes have been reported in patients receiving droperidol at doses at or below recommended antiemetic doses. Some cases have occurred in patients with no known risk factors for QT prolongation, and some of these cases were fatal.[41]

Before administering droperidol, it is now recommended that a 12-lead electrocardiogram should be recorded. If the QT interval measures greater than 440 ms for men or greater than 450 ms for women, then droperidol should not be given. If the QT interval is normal and droperidol is given, the electrocardiogram should be monitored for 2 to 3 hours.[2]

Droperidol is contraindicated in patients with known or suspected QT prolongation, including patients with congenital long QT syndrome. Droperidol should be administered with extreme caution to patients who may be at risk for development of prolonged QT syndrome (e.g., congestive heart failure, bradycardia, use of a diuretic, cardiac hypertrophy, hypokalemia, hypomagnesemia, or administration of other drugs known to increase the QT interval).[41]

Because of its potential for serious proarrhythmic effects and death, droperidol is best reserved for use in the treatment of patients who fail to show an acceptable response to other treatments, because of either insufficient effectiveness or the inability to achieve an effective dose due to intolerable adverse effects from those drugs.[41]

One frequently administered adult dose for PONV prophylaxis is 0.625 mg IV. Doses as low as 1.25 mg can produce untoward effects (restlessness) in the postoperative period.[42] In children the recommended antiemetic dose is 50 to 75 $\mu g/kg^{-1}$.[43]

Interestingly, the mean elimination half-life of droperidol is approximately 120 minutes, which does not correlate with the well-known, relatively prolonged duration of its pharmacologic action.[44] Because of these rare but catastrophic side effects, the use of droperidol has fallen out of favor among most of the anesthesia community.

Haloperidol

Haloperidol is a butyrophenone antipsychotic that blocks postsynaptic mesolimbic dopaminergic D_1 and D_2 receptors in the brain. It is believed to depress the reticular activating system, thus affecting basal metabolism, body temperature, wakefulness, vasomotor tone, and emesis.[24]

Haloperidol is antiemetic at doses that are considerably lower than those used for treatment of psychosis or to control agitation.[45] Doses less than 5 mg are associated with minimal risk. Antiemetic dose ranges are as low as 0.5 to 1 mg IV or intramuscularly (IM) given immediately before emergence. Antiemetic effects occur within 30 minutes and last for 4 hours.[39] Haloperidol 2 mg IM has been demonstrated to successfully treat PONV.[45] The half-life of haloperidol is 24 hours.[40]

Benzamides

Metoclopramide

Metoclopramide is a gastrointestinal prokinetic drug of the benzamide class of dopamine antagonists. Metoclopramide blocks dopaminergic receptors in the CTZ, increases lower esophageal sphincter tone, relaxes the pylorus and duodenum, and enhances gastric and small bowel motility.[7,14] Metoclopramide does not alter gastric pH but does speed gastric emptying. Within the gastrointestinal tract, dopamine antagonism may potentiate cholinergic smooth muscle stimulation.[11] This prokinetic effect is the most valuable pharmacologic property of metoclopramide. Metoclopramide blocks D_2 receptors in the CTZ, resulting in antinausea and antiemetic action.[11]

In addition to being a potent dopamine antagonist, metoclopramide has cholinomimetic properties that contribute to the stimulant effects on the gastrointestinal tract. Patients with gastric motor failure, particularly those with diabetic gastroparesis, can receive significant benefit.

The antiemetic efficacy of metoclopramide is not firmly established. Some researchers demonstrated benefit verses placebo, whereas others showed no significant difference.[46–48] Metoclopramide is not routinely used as a first-line intervention for treating or preventing PONV.

Common side effects include somnolence, nervousness, agitation, and dystonic reactions. If the drug is given preoperatively, the clinician may wish to administer an amnesic drug first to protect the patient from unpleasant recollections.

The usual dose of metoclopramide is 10 mg IV over several minutes. Its elimination half-life is 2 to 4 hours. The drug is excreted mainly by the kidneys.[49]

Phenothiazines

Chlorpromazine and promethazine have been used for many years in the prevention and treatment of postoperative emesis, particularly if opioids have been administered.[7]

Similar to the butyrophenones, the phenothiazines are believed to exert their antiemetic effects primarily by antagonism of central dopaminergic receptors in the CTZ.[7,23] These drugs also antagonize histamine 1 and cholinergic receptors.[14] All phenothiazines are capable of producing extrapyramidal symptoms and sedation.[23] The degrees of extrapyramidal reactions and sedation vary between phenothiazines. Phenothiazines used as antipsychotics produce little sedation, whereas those that are used as antiemetics are potent sedatives.[14,23] Extrapyramidal reactions may consist of dystonic reactions, feelings of motor restlessness (akathisia), and parkinsonian signs and symptoms. Dystonic reactions occur more frequently in pediatric patients, and parkinsonian symptoms are more common in geriatric patients.[50] Extrapyramidal symptoms may be treated with anticholinergic agents such as diphenhydramine or benztropine.[24,50] Avoid using phenothiazines in patients with Reye's syndrome. There is an FDA black box warning that promethazine should not be used in pediatric patients less than 2 years of age because of the potential for fatal respiratory depression. In pediatric patients 2 years of age and older, it is recommended that the lowest effective dose of promethazine be used and concomitant administration of other respiratory depressants be avoided.

The phenothiazines cause a reversal of the vasopressor effects of epinephrine with a further decrease in blood pressure. Treat phenothiazine-induced hypotension with phenylephrine or norepinephrine.[50] The phenothiazines undergo hepatic metabolism and are not dialyzable.[24]

Prochlorperazine (Compazine)

Prochlorperazine is the prototype for the phenothiazine class. It is a piperazine phenothiazine that blocks postsynaptic mesolimbic dopaminergic (D$_1$ and D$_2$) receptors in the brain, including the CTZ; exhibits a strong α-adrenergic and anticholinergic blocking effect; and depresses the release of hypothalamic and hypophyseal hormones. Prochlorperazine is believed to depress the reticular activating system, thus affecting basal metabolism, body temperature, wakefulness, vasomotor tone, and emesis.[24] Its antiemetic action may be exerted more at dopamine receptors than at histamine receptors.

Prochlorperazine has a more rapid onset of action than does promethazine.[24] In comparison with ondansetron, prochlorperazine effectively reduced PONV and the need for rescue antiemetics in patients undergoing total hip or knee replacement.[24] Prochlorperazine has a marked sedating effect but produces less sedation than promethazine.[24] Prochlorperazine can produce adverse side effects such as central nervous system depression, hypotension, and extrapyramidal symptoms. The usual adult dose is 5 to 10 mg IV. A buccal form has been developed.

Promethazine (Phenergan)

Promethazine is a piperazine phenothiazine that has long been used to treat PONV, breakthrough nausea and vomiting in CINV, and opioid-induced nausea and vomiting.[7,14,51] Promethazine blocks D$_1$ and D$_2$ receptors in the brain, exhibits a strong α-adrenergic blocking effect, and depresses the release of hypothalamic and hypophyseal hormones. Promethazine competes with histamine for the H$_1$ receptor and reduces stimuli to the brainstem reticular system.[24] The antiemetic action is mediated via the CTZ.[50]

Promethazine is also used for the treatment of allergic blood reactions and anaphylaxis. Promethazine produces marked sedation. Extrapyramidal symptoms may occur, especially with large doses and with concomitant administration of monoamine oxidase inhibitors.[50] Hypotension is more common if the patient is hypovolemic. The usual adult dose is 10 to 25 mg IV, IM, or rectally. Promethazine should not be given subcutaneously or intra-arterially. Promethazine is a venous irritant and should be diluted in 10 to 20 mL of saline and administered through a rapidly infusing intravenous catheter to prevent tissue damage. Promethazine undergoes hepatic metabolism, primarily oxidation.[24]

Antihistamines (H$_1$ Receptor Antagonists)

All of the available H$_1$ receptor antagonists are reversible competitive inhibitors of the interaction of histamine with H$_1$ receptors. Histamine's myriad effects are mediated by histamine receptors that are distributed widely throughout the body. Histamine plays a central role in hypersensitivity and allergic responses. The actions of histamine on bronchial smooth muscles and blood vessels account for many of the symptoms of such responses. In addition to histamine, mast cells secrete a variety of other inflammatory mediators, such as kinins and prostaglandins that contribute to hypersensitivity reactions. Histamine has a major role in gastric acid secretion and also modulates neurotransmitter release.[52] At least four histamine receptor subtypes have been classified: H$_1$, H$_2$, H$_3$, and H$_4$.

The H$_1$ receptor antagonists (promethazine, hydroxyzine, cyclizine, and dimenhydrinate) are effective antiemetics used in the treatment of various conditions, including motion sickness, pruritus, and PONV. The H$_1$

receptor antagonists may be classified as first-generation or second-generation agents. Second-generation H_1 receptor antagonists (cetirizine, loratadine, and fexofenadine) have little sedating activity and are used to treat allergic rhinitis. They exert little or no antiemetic effect and are not discussed further. First-generation H_1 receptor antagonists are effective antiemetics. They are readily distinguished by their strong sedative effects and are more likely to block autonomic receptors that are involved in the initiation of nausea and vomiting.[31,53] Many of the first generation H_1 receptor antagonists are extensively metabolized by microsomal systems in the liver; little is excreted unchanged.[52,53]

The H_1 receptor antagonists that are primarily used to treat nausea and vomiting are cyclizine and dimenhydrinate. Prochlorperazine, which has antidopaminergic as well as antihistamine actions, is used to treat severe nausea and vomiting. Because it has a second site of action, prochlorperazine is valuable for treating nausea and vomiting despite its marked sedation and numerous side effects.

The H_2 receptor antagonists cimetidine, ranitidine, and famotidine are used in the treatment of peptic ulcers and gastroesophageal reflux disease but are of limited use as antiemetic agents; therefore they are not discussed here. Ondansetron, dolasetron, and granisetron are H_3 receptor antagonists. All three are of great value in the prevention and treatment of nausea and vomiting and are discussed more thoroughly in the section on selective serotonin receptor antagonists.

The H_4 receptor is similar to and binds with many H_3 agonists. H_4 receptor antagonists offer promise for treating inflammatory conditions involving mast cells and eosinophils, such as allergic rhinitis, asthma, and rheumatoid arthritis.[52]

Diphenhydramine (Benadryl)

Diphenhydramine is the prototype for the first generation H_1 receptor antagonists. Much like dimenhydrinate, diphenhydramine can be used for antiemetic prophylaxis in patients with a history of PONV. It has been used to control the symptoms of Parkinson's disease and to treat symptoms for drug-induced extrapyramidal reactions.[24,50] Diphenhydramine is useful for treating histamine-mediated effects from blood transfusion reactions and from radiocontrast dyes.[31] The sedating and drying properties of diphenhydramine make it a useful preoperative medication. Additional pharmacologic effects include dry mouth, blurred vision, and urinary retention. Less common side effects include dizziness, fatigue, blurred vision, euphoria, nervousness, insomnia, and tremors. The usual adult dose is 25 to 50 mg orally (PO), IM, or IV. Its duration of action is 4 to 6 hours.

Cyclizine (Marezine)

Cyclizine is used as prophylaxis and therapy for nausea and vomiting associated with vertigo, motion sickness, and after middle ear surgery.[7,23,52,53] Several drugs inhibit the action of histamine at H_1 sympathetic pathways, which are predominantly involved in signaling from the vestibular center, but only cyclizine is used to treat PONV. Cyclizine, which has both antimuscarinic and antihistamine actions, has gained some favor, probably due to its multiple routes of administration (intravenous, subcutaneous, intramuscular, and oral) and low incidence of side effects. Cyclizine 50 mg IV immediately after elective cesarean birth has been shown to decrease the incidence and severity of nausea and vomiting and the need for rescue antiemetic therapy compared with dexamethasone.[54] Common mild side effects are a consequence of its antimuscarinic actions and include sedation and dry mouth. The usual adult dose is 50 mg IV.

Dimenhydrinate (Dramamine)

Dimenhydrinate possesses antihistaminic and weak anticholinergic properties. It is used primarily as an antiemetic to prevent and treat nausea and vomiting associated with vertigo (Ménière's disease), motion sickness, radiation sickness, and less frequently PONV.[10,53] Dimenhydrinate produces marked sedation, drowsiness, and dry mouth.[23,52] The usual adult dose is 50 mg IV.

Hydroxyzine (Atarax, Vistaril)

Hydroxyzine may be used as a preoperative medication to potentiate a lesser dosage of opioid.[7,53] Intravenous hydroxyzine is not recommended because it can cause thrombosis. Side effects are drowsiness, involuntary motor activity, dry mouth, and electrocardiographic changes (T-wave abnormalities). Hydroxyzine produces considerable central nervous system depression, which may contribute to its prominent antipruritic action.[52] Sedation limits the applicability of hydroxyzine to PONV.[53] Doses are 50 to 100 mg PO and 25 to 100 mg IM.

Meclizine (Antivert)

Meclizine is used primarily as an antiemetic to treat nausea and vomiting associated with vertigo and motion sickness.[51,53] It produces slight sedation. Meclizine, when used in combination with other antiemetic drugs such as ondansetron, has been studied for the prevention of PONV.[51] This long-acting drug (12 to 24 hours[52]) has few side effects and may be beneficial as a prophylactic component of multi-modal therapy for patients at risk for PONV.[51] The usual adult dose is one 50-mg chewable tablet before surgery.

Anticholinergics

Scopolamine

Anticholinergic drugs are known to be effective antiemetics, especially in regard to motion sickness. It is well known that motion sickness is caused by stimulation of the vestibular apparatus, a structure rich in muscarinic cholinergic type 1 receptors (M_1).[7,31,52] Atropine and scopolamine are nonselective competitive muscarinic receptor antagonists that are believed to act on the vestibular component.[7,24] Both are tertiary amines, but scopolamine more readily crosses the blood–brain barrier, allowing greater access to the emetic center.[31,55] Thus scopolamine, a centrally acting anticholinergic, is a pure anticholinergic agent that has its effect at M_1 receptors where it acts as a muscarinic antagonist. It is the only suitable anticholinergic in clinical use for PONV. Scopolamine is one of the oldest remedies for motion sickness and continues to be used for this purpose because it has no superior.[53,56]

Scopolamine has been shown to significantly reduce the risk of suffering from emetic symptoms in the postoperative period.[57] Scopolamine also is highly effective in preventing and treating motion sickness.[58] Since the introduction of the transdermal scopolamine patch (TDS), scopolamine is being used singularly or as part of a multimodal preventive approach to prevent PONV.[24,31,53,56]

Transdermal scopolamine is safe and effective for the treatment and prevention of PONV; however, the transdermal route is a poor choice for the acute treatment of PONV due to its delayed onset of action.[59] TDS is considered a first-line drug in the prophylaxis of nausea and vomiting associated with PONV, motion sickness, and CINV, and in palliative care where it is used to sedate, dry upper airway secretions, and ease breathing at the end of life.

Scopolamine may be of use in patients for whom the main emetic stimulus is vestibular (nausea and vomiting associated with movement or ear, nose, and throat surgery). TDS is commonly used in conjunction with other antiemetics as a part of the multisystem approach of reducing nausea and vomiting. TDS is a delivery system that allows gradual, sustained drug release, providing for longer therapeutic efficacy. Because scopolamine is absorbed in low antiemetic doses, TDS produces few side effects. The most common side effects of scopolamine are sedation and dry mouth.[56] Other possible side effects are visual disturbances, dizziness, drowsiness, blurred vision, confusion, hallucinations, and difficulty with urination (use cautiously with patients who have benign prostatic hypertrophy).[2,24,35]

TDS is contraindicated with closed-angle glaucoma; gastrointestinal or urinary tract obstruction; or hepatic, renal, or metabolic dysfunction.[2,24,58] Each TDS contains 1.5 mg and delivers ~1 mg over 72 hours. Transdermally, scopolamine's time of onset is approximately 2 hours; IV onset is approximately 10 minutes. The intravenous effects last about 2 hours, and TDS effects last for up to 72 hours. For good effect, the TDS should be applied to a hairless area at least 2 to 4 hours before the end of surgery. TDS should be applied 1 hour before cesarean birth. If applied sooner, the newborn risks exposure. TDS may contain metal, so remove the patch before magnetic resonance imaging to prevent the possibility of burns. Remove TDS after 24 hours. The pharmacologic effects may last up to 72 hours due to continued absorption from the skin. Scopolamine is metabolized by the hepatic route; excretion is via the urine. Scopolamine has an elimination half-life of almost 5 hours.

Neurokinin-1 Receptor Antagonists

Aprepitant

Aprepitant (Emend) is a highly selective, brain-penetrating, neurokinin-1 receptor antagonist with a long half-life of 9 to 12 hours. Substance P, the primary endogenous ligand at the neurokinin-1 receptor, is a regulatory peptide that is found in the gastrointestinal tract (vagal afferents) and areas of the central nervous system thought to be involved with the vomiting reflex.[60] Aprepitant has little or no affinity for serotonin (5-HT$_3$), dopamine, and corticosteroid receptors.

When aprepitant is used for prevention of PONV, the recommended adult dose is 40 mg PO, taken within 3 hours of induction. Safety and effectiveness have not been established in children. Common adverse effects are constipation, diarrhea, headache, hiccoughs, and fatigue. Serious adverse effects of aprepitant administration are sinus tachycardia, febrile neutropenia, sepsis, Stevens-Johnson syndrome, and hypersensitivity reactions. Aprepitant decreases the effectiveness of oral contraceptives.

Metabolism of aprepitant is primarily hepatic, via the CYP3A4 enzyme. Aprepitant is not excreted renally. This is the only neurokinin-1 receptor antagonist approved by the FDA. Aprepitant is indicated alone or in combination with other antiemetics for the prevention of PONV and CINV. Aprepitant is not intended for treatment of existing nausea and vomiting or for chronic continuous therapy.[24]

Miscellaneous Drugs and Therapies

Numerous drugs and treatments have been purported to possess antiemetic qualities. Benzodiazepines, especially lorazepam, are recommended as adjunct therapy in treating CINV.[10] Preoperative replacement of fluid deficit can reduce the incidence of PONV in physical status 1 patients undergoing laparoscopic cholecystectomy.[61] Aromatherapy, such as sniffing isopropyl alcohol from an alcohol wipe, is sometimes useful for quickly treating PONV. Of these varied drugs and treatments, few have enough merit to be included in the treatment of nausea and vomiting. This discussion is limited to those drugs that are supported by controlled clinical trials.

Propofol

Regardless of anesthetic technique or anesthetic drugs chosen, the incidence of PONV is decreased when propofol is included.[31,62,63] A total intravenous technique with propofol greatly reduces the incidence of PONV compared with a pure inhalation technique.[64] Subhypnotic doses of propofol have been used as rescue therapy for emesis in acute care settings. Although the mechanism of antiemetic action remains obscure, propofol is popular in the outpatient setting, in part because of its antiemetic effects.[2,65] Propofol has also proven effective in preventing CINV.[7,31,65]

The antiemetic properties of propofol make it particularly useful for anesthesia in patients at high risk for PONV and perhaps for all patients for whom it is not contraindicated.[64] However, propofol alone is not a satisfactory antiemetic for most patients.[2,62,64]

Ephedrine

Ephedrine, an indirectly acting sympathomimetic drug, may be of value as an antiemetic for inpatient and outpatient surgery.[34] Ephedrine has a similar antiemetic action to that of droperidol but with less sedation.[66] Ephedrine IM appears to be best suited for treating nausea and vomiting resulting from postural changes or hypotension.[7] The usual adult dose is 5 to 10 mg intravenous push repeated every

5 to 10 minutes as needed, then every 3 to 4 hours not to exceed 150 mg in 24 hours. Pediatric patients should not receive more than 3 mg/kg in 24 hours.[24]

Cannabinoids

Cannabinoids (marijuana-related compounds) are effective oral antiemetics used to treat CINV that has failed to respond adequately to conventional antiemetic therapy.[7,67] Although not common in nurse anesthesia practice, sublingual dronabinol (Marinol) is effective in treating intractable PONV.[7] Nabilone (Cesamet), a Schedule II synthetic drug, is a longer acting cannabinoid.[67] (Oral nabilone duration is 8 to 12 hours vs. oral dronabinol, 4 to 6 hours.)

Drugs of this class are not commonly used for PONV because they are associated with a high incidence of side effects (confusion, postural hypotension, vision disturbances, dizziness, ataxia, euphoria, sedation, depression, and hallucinations).[7,68,70] Although side effects may contraindicate cannabinoids for use in the treatment of PONV, some of these same side effects may be viewed as beneficial in patients being treated for CINV (euphoria, sedation, drowsiness, somnolence).[69] The oral dose of dronabinol is 2.5 mg twice daily, and the oral dose of nabilone is 1 to 2 mg twice daily.

Acupuncture and Acupressure

Acupuncture is a technique that can be traced back at least 2500 years and is one of the main forms of treatment in traditional Chinese medicine. Acupuncture is based on the premise that throughout the body patterns of energy can be identified and that stimulation of specific areas can result in diagnosis and treatment of various physiologic disorders.[70] Acupuncture is based on the principle of qi or chi, the energy present in living organisms. When the flow of qi is stagnant, the physical condition is affected. The application of pressure to specific points on the body unblocks abnormal energy flow and relieves signs and symptoms of illness. Scattered across the surface of the body are more than 400 acupuncture points and 20 meridians connecting these points (which are areas of high electrical conductance).[71] The two Chinese meridian points that are effective in lessening nausea and vomiting are Nei-Guan P6 and Zu-San-Li ST36.[72]

Acupuncture responses can occur locally or may be mediated by sensory neurons to many structures within the central nervous system. Placing needles into these specific areas results in several identifiable physiologic events, including stimulation of the myelinated afferent nerve fibers, release of endogenous opioids, release of neurotransmitters (substance P and serotonin), and activation of the nuclei of the dorsal horn, the brainstem, and the hypothalamic-pituitary axis.[73] PONV, headache, fibromyalgia, osteoarthritis, and asthma are other areas showing promising results from acupuncture.[70]

Stimulation of the P6 acupoint decreases the incidence of PONV.[74] The P6 acupuncture site is located between the palmaris longus tendon and flexor carpi radialis tendon of the forearm, one-sixth of the distance between the distal wrist crease and the cubital crease (Figure 14-2).[74] Stimulation of this acupoint can be accomplished through acupuncture, electroacupuncture, transcutaneous acupoint electrical stimulation, or acupressure. Acupressure is based on the same principles as acupuncture. Firm and steady pressure applied to P6 point with the fingers or a wristband causes a significant reduction in the incidence of PONV and the requirement for rescue medication in the first 6 hours after laparoscopic cholecystectomy, similar to that of ondansetron 4 mg IV.[75] Acupressure has no side effects or drug interactions and is simple to use. Acupressure bands are very inexpensive.

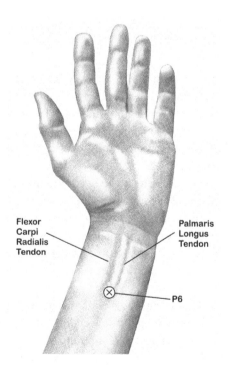

Figure 14-2 The P6 acupoint.

Source: From reference 74.

Anesthetic Techniques for Preventing PONV

Despite considerable efforts by many researchers, PONV continues to be an important cause of patient discomfort and dissatisfaction. Unfortunately, no single intervention is completely efficacious and free of side effects (Table 14-6).[34]

Considerations for PONV prophylaxis and treatment should include the following: the patient's level of PONV risk, potential adverse events associated with the various antiemetics, efficacy of antiemetics, costs of antiemetics, and increased healthcare costs associated with caring for the patient who experiences PONV.[34]

Not all patients need PONV prophylaxis. Those at low risk for PONV are unlikely to benefit from prophylaxis and would be put at unreasonable risk from the potential side effects of antiemetics, such as prolonged somnolence. Thus prophylaxis should be reserved for those patients who are at moderate to high risk of PONV or who could be harmed by the act of vomiting.[34] Patients at moderate risk may benefit from a single intervention. Multiple interventions should be reserved for patients at high risk of PONV.[76]

Ondansetron, dexamethasone, and droperidol are equally efficacious antiemetic agents. Because they are similarly effective and act independently, the safest or least expensive should be used first. The combination of low cost and apparent safety make dexamethasone an attractive first-line agent.[77] A treatment algorithm for prevention of PONV for moderate- to high-risk adult patients is presented in Figure 14-3.[14,15,77]

All children at high risk for postoperative vomiting should receive combination therapy using a 5-HT$_3$ antagonist and a second drug. Rescue antiemetic therapy should be administered to children who vomit after surgery.[25,26,34]

The Society of Ambulatory Anesthesia consensus statement on PONV recommends that if vomiting occurs

Table 14-6 Strategies to Reduce Baseline Risk for PONV

Use regional anesthesia.
Use propofol for induction and maintenance of general anesthesia.
Use intraoperative supplemental oxygen.
Maintain hydration.
Avoid nitrous oxide.
Minimize the use of intraoperative and postoperative opioids.
Minimize the use of neostigmine.

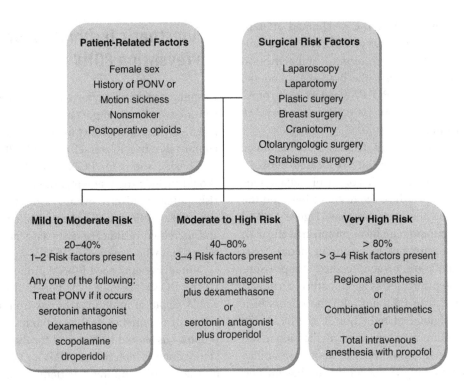

Figure 14-3 Risk factors for PONV and guidelines for prophylactic antiemetic therapy. PONV = Postoperative nausea and vomiting. Percentages denote risk of developing PONV.

Source: Modified from 14, 15, 77.

within 6 hours postoperatively, patients should not receive a repeat dose of the same prophylactic antiemetic because of lack of evidence for effectiveness in this time frame. The guidelines recommend using a drug that is of a different class from those used for prophylaxis, such as promethazine.[4,18,34] When assessing the patient who experiences PONV, the anesthesia provider must remain vigilant for other causes of nausea and vomiting, such as pain, hypotension, hypoxia, hypoglycemia, increased intracranial pressure, or gastric bleeding.[64]

Conclusion

PONV has been a bothersome problem since the days of the first anesthetics. Although PONV can be notoriously difficult to prevent, many advances have been made in understanding its etiology and in formulating effective interventions. Judicious patient assessment for risk factors, plus the utilization of pharmacologic interventions and anesthetic techniques with proven efficacy (such as hydration, oxygenation, normothermia, and freedom from pain), may one day relegate this complication of surgery and anesthesia to a place of little importance.

Key Points

- Twenty percent to 30% of all surgical patients experience PONV.
- Nausea and vomiting are the most common reasons that adults and children have protracted stays in the PACU or unexpected hospital admissions due to anesthesia.
- The act of vomiting involves coordination of the gastrointestinal, abdominal, and respiratory musculature and is controlled by the emetic center, a group of cells located in the medulla oblongata.
- The CTZ is located in the fourth ventricle in the area postrema and is not protected by the blood–brain barrier.
- The CTZ contains numerous receptors for serotonin, dopamine, histamine, acetylcholine, and opioids.
- Some patients demonstrate transient, clinically insignificant electrocardiographic changes after the administration of 5-HT$_3$ antagonists.
- The half-lives of the 5-HT$_3$ receptor antagonists are as follows: ondansetron, 3 to 6 hours; dolasetron, 6 to 8 hours; granisetron, 5 to 9 hours; and palonosetron, 40 hours.

- Consensus guidelines for managing PONV have determined that all three 5-HT$_3$ receptor antagonists used for PONV (ondansetron, dolasetron, and granisetron) are most effective when administered at the end of surgery.
- Dexamethasone has a biologic half-life of 36 to 56 hours—longer than that of any other antiemetic.
- Because of its potential for serious proarrhythmic effects and death, droperidol is best reserved for use in the treatment of patients who fail to show an acceptable response to other treatments, because of either insufficient effectiveness or the inability to achieve an effective dose due to intolerable adverse effects from those drugs.
- Phenothiazines such as chlorpromazine and promethazine are potent sedatives.
- First-generation H$_1$ receptor antagonists such as diphenhydramine and dimenhydrinate are effective antiemetics that possess strong sedative effects and are more likely to block autonomic receptors that are involved in the initiation of nausea and vomiting.
- Regardless of anesthetic technique or anesthetic drugs chosen, the incidence of PONV is decreased when propofol is included.
- PONV prophylaxis should be reserved for those patients who are at moderate to high risk or who could be harmed by the act of vomiting. Patients at moderate risk may benefit from a single intervention. Multiple interventions should be reserved for patients at high risk of PONV.
- All children at high risk for postoperative vomiting should receive combination therapy using a 5-HT$_3$ antagonist and a second drug.

Chapter Questions

1. Are there known risk factors that increase the incidence of PONV? If so, what are they?
2. Which premedications have the ability to alter the incidence of PONV?
3. Would an 18-year-old man with attention deficit hyperactivity disorder who smokes two packages of cigarettes a day and is scheduled for a cystoscopic procedure be at increased risk for PONV?
4. How will you attempt to minimize the risk of PONV for an anxious 32-year-old woman who is scheduled for the surgical removal of an astrocytoma? How will you treat her if nausea still occurs after surgery?
5. Should all surgical patients be treated prophylactically for PONV?

References

1. Seigel LJ, Longo DL. The control of chemotherapy-induced emesis. *Ann Intern Med.* 1981;95:352–359.
2. Morgan GE, Mikhail MS, Murray MJ. *Clinical Anesthesiology,* 4th ed. New York: Lang Medical Books/McGraw-Hill; 2006:179-204, 237-241, 1005–1008.
3. Gan TJ. Postoperative nausea and vomiting—can it be eliminated? *JAMA.* 2002;287:1233–1236.
4. Lichtor JL. Ambulatory anesthesia. In: Barash PG, Cullen BF, Stoelting RK, Cahalan MK, Stock MC, eds. *Clinical Anesthesia,* 6th ed. Philadelphia: Lippincott Williams & Wilkins; 2009:833–846.
5. Macario A, Weinger M, Carney S, Kim A. Which clinical anesthesia outcomes are important to avoid? *Anesth Analg.* 1999;89:652–658.
6. Bryson WO, Frost EA, Rosenblatt M. Management of the patient at high risk for postoperative nausea and vomiting. *Middle East J Anesthesiol.* 2007;9:15–35.
7. Watcha MF, White PF. Postoperative nausea and vomiting: its etiology, treatment, and prevention. *Anesthesiology.* 1992;77:162–184.
8. Nicholau D. Postanesthesia recovery. In: Stoelting RK, Miller RD, eds. *Basics of Anesthesia,* 5th ed. Philadelphia: Churchill Livingstone; 2007:563–579.
9. Cotton JW, Rowell LR, Hood RR, et al. A comparative analysis of isopropyl alcohol and ondansetron in the treatment of postoperative nausea and vomiting from the hospital setting to the home. *AANA J.* 2007;75:21–26.
10. Garrett K, Tsuruta K, Walker S, Jackson S, Sweat M. Managing nausea and vomiting. *Crit Care Nurse.* 2003;23:31–50.
11. McQuaid KR. Drugs used in the treatment of gastrointestinal diseases. In: Katzung BG, ed. *Basic & Clinical Pharmacology* 9th ed. New York: Lange Medical Books/McGraw-Hill; 2004:1034–1063.
12. Gutton AC, Hall JE. *Human Physiology and Mechanisms of Disease,* 6th ed. Philadelphia: W.B. Saunders Company; 1997: 545–546.
13. Ganong WF. *Review of Medical Physiology,* 22nd ed. New York: Lange Medical Books/McGraw-Hill; 2005:232–265.
14. Norred CL. Antiemetic prophylaxis: pharmacology and therapeutics. *AANA J.* 2003;71:133–140.
15. Gan TJ. Postoperative nausea and vomiting: can it be eliminated? *JAMA.* 2002;287:1233–1236.
16. Peroutka SJ, Snyder SH. Antiemetics: neurotransmitter receptor binding predicts therapeutic action. *Lancet.* 1982:1; 658–659.
17. Hindle AT. Recent developments in the physiology and pharmacology of 5-hydroxytryptamine. *Br J Anaesth.* 1994;73: 395–407.

18. Habib AS, Reuveni J, Taguchi A, et al. A comparison of ondansetron with promethazine for treating postoperative nausea and vomiting in patients who received prophylaxis with ondansetron: a retrospective database analysis. *Anesth Analg.* 2007;104:548.

19. Scuderi, PE. Management of postoperative nausea and vomiting. *Curr Rev Clin Anesth.* 2003;23:297–308.

20. Chan MTV, Chui PT, Ho WS. Single-dose tropisetron for preventing postoperative nausea and vomiting after breast surgery. *Anesth Analg.* 1998;87:931–935.

21. Capouet V, DePauw C, Vernet B, et al. Single dose i.v. tropisetron in the prevention of postoperative nausea and vomiting after gynaecological surgery. *Br J Anaesth.* 1996;76:54–60.

22. Fujii Y, Saitoh Y, Tanaka H, et al. Ramosetron for preventing postoperative nausea and vomiting in women undergoing gynecological surgery. *Anesth Analg.* 2009;90:472–475.

23. Rose JB, Watcha MF. Postoperative nausea and vomiting in paediatric patients. *Br J Anaesth.* 1999;83:104–117.

24. Donnelly AJ, Baughman VL, Gonzalez JP, et al. *Anesthesiology & Critical Care Drug Handbook,* 8th ed. Hudson, OH: Lexi-Comp; 2008:118–119, 408–411, 452–453, 611–612, 973–976, 992–993, 1077–1084.

25. Rowley MP, Brown TCK. Postoperative vomiting in children. *Anaesth Intens Care.* 1982;10:309–313.

26. Sinclair DR, Chung F, Mezei G. Can postoperative nausea and vomiting be predicted? *Anesthesiology.* 1999;91:109–118.

27. Tramèr MR, Reynolds DJM, Moore RA, McQuay HJ. Efficacy, dose-response, and safety of ondansetron in prevention of postoperative nausea and vomiting. *Anesthesiology.* 1997;87:1277–1289.

28. Leeser J, Lip H. Prevention of postoperative nausea and vomiting using ondansetron, a new, selective, 5-HT$_3$ receptor antagonist. *Anesth Analg.* 1991;72:751–755.

29. Sadhasivam S, Saxena A, Kathirvel S, et al. The safety and efficacy of prophylactic ondansetron in patients undergoing modified radical mastectomy. *Anesth Analg.* 1999;89:1340–1345.

30. Wolf H. Preclinical and clinical pharmacology of the 5-HT$_3$ receptor antagonists. *Scand J Rheumatol.* 2000;29:37–45.

31. Stoelting RK, Hillier SC. *Pharmacology & Physiology in Anesthetic Practice,* 2nd ed. Philadelphia: Lippincott Williams & Wilkins; 2006:151–178, 266–275, 429–443, 444–455.

32. Fujii Y, Hidenori T. Current prevention and treatment of postoperative nausea and vomiting with 5-hydroxytryptamine type 3 receptor antagonists: a review. *J Anesth.* 2001;5:223–232.

33. Kovac AL. Prevention and treatment of postoperative nausea and vomiting. *Drugs.* 2000;59:212–243.

34. Gan TJ, Meyer T, Apfel CC, et al. Consensus guidelines for managing postoperative nausea and vomiting. *Anesth Analg.* 2003;97:62–71.

35. Rose JB, Watcha MF. Postoperative nausea and vomiting. In: Benumof JL, Saidman LJ, eds. *Anesthesia and Perioperative Complications,* 2nd ed. St. Louis, MO: Mosby; 1999:425–440.

36. Haynes R. Adrenocorticotropic hormone: adrenocortical steroids and their synthetic analogues—inhibitors of the synthesis and actions of adrenocortical hormones. In: Gilman AG, Rall TW, Nies AS, Taylor P, eds. *Goodman & Gilman's the Pharmacological Basis of Therapeutics,* 8th ed. New York: Pergamon Press; 1990:1431–1462.

37. Schimmer BP, Parker KL. Adrenocorticotropic hormone: adrenocortical steroids and their synthetic analogues: inhibitors of the synthesis and actions of adrenocortical hormones. In: Brunton LL, Lazo JS, Parker KL, eds. *Goodman & Gilman's the Pharmacological Basis of Therapeutics,* 11th ed. New York: McGraw-Hill; 2006:1587–1612.

38. Henzi I, Walder B, Tramer MR. Dexamethasone for the prevention of postoperative nausea and vomiting: a quantitative systemic review. *Anesth Analg.* 2000;90:186–194.

39. Smith JC II, Wright EL. Haloperidol: an alternative butyrophenone for nausea and vomiting prophylaxis in anesthesia. *AANA J.* 2005;73:273–275.

40. Baldessarini RJ, Tarazi FI. Drugs and the treatment of psychiatric disorders: psychosis and mania. In: Hardman JG, Limbird LE, eds. *Goodman and Gilman's the Pharmacological Basis of Therapeutics,* 10th ed. New York: McGraw-Hill; 2001:485–520.

41. FDA strengthens warnings for droperidol. Available at: http://www.fda.gov/bbs/topics/ANSWERS/2001/ANS01123.html. Accessed July 1, 2009.

42. Lichtor JL, Wetchler BV. Anesthesia for ambulatory surgery. In: Barash PG, Cullen BF, Stoelting RK, eds. *Clinical Anesthesia.* Philadelphia: Lippincott-Raven; 1997:1137–1158.

43. Watcha MF, Simeon RM, White PF, Stevens JL. Effect of propofol on the incidence of postoperative vomiting after strabismus surgery in pediatric outpatients. *Anesthesiology.* 1991;75:204.

44. Fischler M, Bonnet F, Trang H, et al. The pharmacokinetics of droperidol in anesthetized patients. *Anesthesiology.* 1986;64:486–489.

45. Buttner MB, Walder B, von Elm E, Tramer MR. Is low-dose haloperidol a useful antiemetic? A meta-analysis of published and unpublished randomized trials. *Anesthesiology.* 2004;1:1454–1463.

46. Cooke RD, Comyn DJ, Ball RW. Prevention of postoperative nausea and vomiting by domperidone: a double blind randomized study using domperidone, metoclopramide and a placebo. *S Afr Med J.* 1979;56:827–829.

47. Cohen SE, Woods WA, Wyner J. Antiemetic efficacy of droperidol and metoclopramide. *Anesthesiology.* 1984;60:67–69.

48. Henzi I, Walder B, Tramer MR. Metoclopramide in the prevention of postoperative nausea and vomiting: a quantitative

systematic review of randomized, placebo-controlled studies. *Br J Anaesth*. 1999;83:761–771.

49. Altman DF. Drugs used in gastrointestinal diseases. In: Katzung BG, ed. *Basic and Clinical Pharmacology*, 4th ed. Norwalk, CT: Appleton & Lange; 1989:793–799.

50. Omoigui S. *The Anesthesia Drug Handbook*. St. Louis, MO: Mosby Year Book; 1992:166–170.

51. Forrester, CM, Benfield, DA, Matern CE, et al. Meclizine in combination with ondansetron for prevention of postoperative nausea and vomiting in a high-risk population. *AANA J*. 2007;75:27–33.

52. Skidgel RA, Erdos EG. Histamine, bradykinin, and their antagonists. In: Brunton LL, Lazo JS, Parker KL, eds. *Goodman & Gilman's the Pharmacological Basis of Therapeutics*, 11th ed. New York: McGraw-Hill; 2006:628–651.

53. Katzung BG. Drugs with important actions on smooth muscle: histamine, serotonin, & the ergot alkaloids. In: Katzung BG, ed. *Basic & Clinical Pharmacology*, 9th ed. New York: Lang Medical Books/McGraw-Hill; 2004:259–280.

54. Nortcliffe SA, Shah J, Buggy DJ. Prevention of postoperative nausea and vomiting after spinal morphine for caesarean section: comparison of cyclizine, dexamethasone and placebo. *Br J Anaesth*. 2003;90:665–670.

55. Rédai I, Mets B. Sympathomimetic, sympatholytic drugs, parasympathomimetic, and parasympatholytic drugs. In: Evers AS, Maze M, eds. *Anesthetic Pharmacology: Principles and Clinical Practice*. Philadelphia: Churchill Livingstone; 2004:599–620.

56. Pappano AJ, Katzung BG. Cholinoceptor-blocking drugs. In: Katzung BG, ed. *Basic & Clinical Pharmacology*, 9th ed. New York: Lang Medical Books/McGraw-Hill; 2004:109–121.

57. Kranke P, Morin AM, Roewer N, et al. The efficacy and safety of transdermal scopolamine for the prevention of postoperative nausea and vomiting: quantitative systemic review. *Anesth Analg*. 2002;95:33–43.

58. Scholz J, Steinfath M, Tonnre PH. Antiemetics. In: Evers AS, Maze M, eds. *Anesthetic Pharmacology: Principles and Clinical Practice*. Philadelphia: Churchill Livingstone; 2004: 777–791.

59. Jones S, Strobl R, Crosby D, et al. The effect of transdermal scopolamine on the incidence and severity of postoperative nausea and vomiting in a group of high-risk patients given prophylactic intravenous ondansetron. *AANA J*. 2006; 74:127–132.

60. Gan TJ, Apfel CC, Kovac A, et al. A randomized, double-blind comparison of the NK$_1$ antagonist, aprepitant, versus ondansetron for the prevention of postoperative nausea and vomiting. *Anesth Analg*. 2007;104:1082–1089.

61. Adanir T, Aksun M, Özgürbüz U, et al. Does preoperative hydration affect postoperative nausea and vomiting? A randomized, controlled trial. *J Laparoendosc Adv Surg Techn*. 2008;8:1–4.

62. Tramèr M, Moore A, McQuay H. Propofol anesthesia and postoperative nausea and vomiting: quantitative systematic review of randomized controlled studies. *Br J Anesth*. 1997;78:247–255.

63. Borgeat A. Subhypnotic doses of propofol do not possess antidopaminergic properties. *Anesth Analg*. 1997;84: 196–198.

64. Fowler MA, Spiess BD. Postanesthesia recovery. In: Barash PG, Cullen BF, Stoelting RK, Cahalan MK, Stock MC, eds. *Clinical Anesthesia*, 6th ed. Philadelphia: Lippincott Williams & Wilkins; 2009:1421–1443.

65. Tomioka S, Kurio T, Takaishi K, et al. Propofol is effective in chemotherapy-induced nausea and vomiting: a case report with quantitative analysis. *Anesth Analg*. 1999;89: 798–799.

66. Rothenberg DM, Parnass SM, Litwack K, et al. Efficacy of epinephrine in the prevention of postoperative nausea and vomiting. *Anesth Analg*. 1991;72:58–61.

67. Sutton IR, Daeninck P. Cannabinoids in the management of intractable chemotherapy-induced nausea and vomiting and cancer-related pain. *J Support Oncol*. 2006;4:531–535.

68. McCaffrey R. Make PONV a priority. *OR Nurse*. 2007;1: 39–45.

69. Tramèr MR, Carrol D, Campbell FA, et al. Cannabinoids for control of chemotherapy induced nausea and vomiting: quantitative systematic review. *BMJ*. 2001;323:1–8.

70. NIH Consensus Conference. Acupuncture. *JAMA*. 1998;280: 1518–1524.

71. Shang C. The mechanism of acupuncture. Available at: http:// www.acupuncture.org/Acup/Mech. 2002.htm. Accessed June 29, 2009.

72. Garrett K, Tsuruta K, Walker S, Jackson S, Sweat M. Managing nausea and vomiting: current strategies. *Crit Care Nurse*. 2003;23:31–50.

73. Tony V. Western views of acupuncture. *Family Practice News*. 2001;31:1–39.

74. Wang S, Kain Z. P6 acupoint injections are as effective as droperidol in controlling early postoperative nausea and vomiting in children. *Anesthesiology*. 2002;97:359–360.

75. Agarwal A, Bose N, Gaur A, Singh U, Gupta MK, Singh D. Acupressure and ondansetron for postoperative nausea and vomiting. *Can J Anesth*. 2002;49:554–560.

76. White PF. Prevention of postoperative nausea and vomiting—a multimodal solution to a persistent problem. *N Engl J Med*. 2004;350:2511–2512.

77. Apfel CC, Korttila K, Abdala M, et al. A factorial trial of six interventions for the prevention of postoperative nausea and vomiting. *N Engl J Med*. 2004;350:2441–2451.

Prophylaxis for Aspiration Pneumonitis

Allan Schwartz, DDS, CRNA

Allan Schwartz, DDS, CRNA

Objectives

After completing this chapter, the reader will be able to

- Define terms associated with aspiration and the gastrointestinal system.
- Review the anatomy and physiology of the gastrointestinal system.
- Learn the body's natural protective mechanisms against aspiration.
- List factors that affect our natural protective mechanisms against aspiration.
- Discuss the pathophysiologic process of aspiration pneumonitis.
- Discuss treatments for aspiration pneumonitis.
- Learn physical and pharmaceutical means of preventing aspiration pneumonitis.
- Discuss the legal implications of patients developing aspiration pneumonitis.

Introduction

The *American Journal of Obstetrics and Gynecology* published a landmark article in the July–December 1946 issue entitled, "The aspiration of stomach contents into the lungs during obstetric anesthesia," by Curtis L. Mendelson, MD.[1] Dr. Mendelson meticulously observed the causes for the morbidity and mortality experienced by some of his obstetric patients who aspirated gastric contents. He performed careful animal studies, whose outcomes formed the basis for our present-day anesthesia theory and practice for the prophylaxis used to prevent aspiration pneumonitis (AP).

Definitions

- Aspirate is derived from the Latin words, *a spirare*, meaning to breathe upon. Aspiration is the inhalation of a bolus of a solid and/or a liquid bolus into the airway.[2,3]
- Aspiration pneumonia is an infectious process caused by the aspiration of secretions containing pathogenic oropharyngeal bacteria into the lungs.[4,5]
- Aspiration pneumonitis is a direct chemical injury to lung tissues caused by the aspiration of highly acidic gastric contents into the lungs.[4,5] Pulmonary aspiration of gastric contents is believed to occur in 1 in 3216 anesthetics.[6]

- Mendelson's syndrome describes AP: a severe respiratory condition caused by the inhalation of acidic gastric contents into the lungs.[2]
- Reflux is from the Latin *refluere*, which means to flow back.[2] Oral and gastric contents normally progress in a one-way direction from the mouth into the stomach, which then empties into the duodenum. Patients with depressed protective reflexes or who have abnormal anatomic structures can reflux solids or liquids into the esophagus, which can then possibly be aspirated into the lungs.
- Stomach is from the Greek word *stomakhos*, meaning gullet. It is the organ that serves as a food reservoir and is the first major site for the beginning of the digestion of food. Figure 15-1a shows the anatomy of the stomach and Figure 15-1b, the histology of the stomach.[7,8] Gastric secretions begin the process of digestion, which is the breakdown of foods and liquids into their basic components for absorption into the bloodstream to support the organs and tissues of the body.

Box 15-1 provides a complete list of the contents and functions of gastric secretions.[2,8,9]

Physiology of Swallowing, Coughing, Gagging, and Laryngospasm as Normal Protective Mechanisms

Swallowing

Swallowing (deglutition) is the complex coordinated effort of the mouth, tongue, pharynx, and esophagus. The pharynx must function in a dual role, first as a passageway for

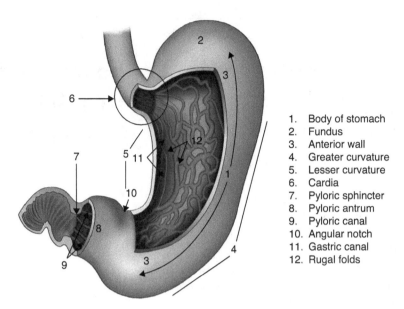

1. Body of stomach
2. Fundus
3. Anterior wall
4. Greater curvature
5. Lesser curvature
6. Cardia
7. Pyloric sphincter
8. Pyloric antrum
9. Pyloric canal
10. Angular notch
11. Gastric canal
12. Rugal folds

Figure 15-1a The anatomy of the stomach.

Source: Obtained from public domain Cancer.gov website: http://training.seer.cancer.gov/ugi/Anatomy/stomach.html.

inspiratory and expiratory gases (respiration) of the lungs and, second, as a passageway for the delivery of solids and liquids down the esophagus into the stomach (swallowing). Conduction of respiratory gases is the dominant function of the nose, mouth, and pharynx each day. Swallowing requires only a few seconds of oropharyngeal time. Swallowing involves both voluntary and involuntary stages, with built-in protective mechanisms to prevent compromise or interference to respiration (Box 15-2).[8]

Stomach contents are swept through the stomach from the cardia to the pylorus by peristaltic waves, at a rate of three to four waves per minute. These powerful peristaltic waves serve to stir and mix the gastric contents. One percent to 3% of the gastric content (chyme) enters the duodenum

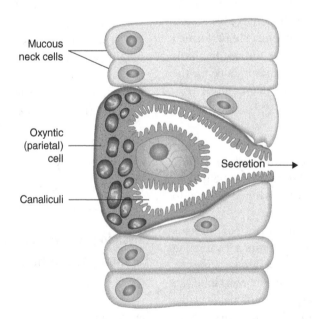

Mucous neck cells

Oxyntic (parietal) cell

Secretion

Canaliculi

Figure 15-1b The histology of the stomach.

Source: Medical Physiology, 11th edition. Guyton AC, Hall JE. Secretory Functions of the Alimentary Tract, Page 796, Copyright Elsevier 2006.

Box 15-1 Contents and Functions of Gastric Secretions

Hydrochloric acid: a potent acid with a pH of 1–2, used for the digestion of food. The parietal cells of the stomach secrete hydrochloric acid when stimulated by cranial nerve X, the vagus nerve.

Gastrin: a hormone whose secretion is triggered by protein-rich foods, which stimulates the release of histamine

Histamine: an endogenous substance that is synthesized by the degradation of the amino acid histidine, which stimulates gastric hydrochloric acid secretion

Intrinsic factor: a substance used to absorb vitamin B_{12} in the ileum

Mucus: a substance that lubricates the bolus of food and protects the stomach wall

Pepsin: a proteolytic enzyme used for the digestion of proteins

Pepsinogen: a substance that converts to pepsin upon contact with hydrochloric acid

Source: From references 2, 8, and 9.

Box 15-2 Voluntary and Involuntary Stages of Swallowing, Stomach Physiology, and Normal Protective Mechanisms

Voluntary initiation of swallowing.

Involuntary upward pull of the soft palate to close the posterior nares from the reflux of swallowed oral contents.

Involuntary funneling of oral contents into the trachea by the palatopharyngeal folds.

Involuntary closure of the trachea by the tight approximation of the vocal cords and the rigidity of the epiglottis caused by muscular contraction.

Involuntary peristaltic propulsion of the oral contents from the posterior pharynx past the relaxed upper esophageal sphincter (the upper 3–4 cm of the esophagus).

Involuntary closure of the upper esophageal sphincter for protection against reflux.

Involuntary peristaltic contracture of the esophagus, propelling the oral contents past the relaxed gastroesophageal sphincter into a receptive and relaxed stomach. The gastroesophageal sphincter is normally held tightly closed and requires 30 torr of pressure to open.

Source: From reference 8.

per minute. The higher the gastric content, the higher the volume of chyme entry into the duodenum.[8,10]

The duodenum possesses a powerful inhibitory reflex to delay gastric emptying, called the enterogastric inhibitory nervous reflex.[8,10] This reflex can be strongly activated within 30 seconds and can thus increase the probability of stomach contents being regurgitated and then aspirated. Box 15-3 lists some factors that can trigger the enterogastric inhibitory reflex.

Digestion and metabolism of most of the medications administered in anesthesia and those used for the treatment of AP are performed by the cytochrome P-450 system of enzymes. There are 20 known pharmacogenetic cytochrome enzyme subtypes found in the liver and intestines.[11,12] Nearly half of the medications used in anesthesia are metabolized by one specific pharmacogenetic enzyme variant: CPY3A4. Interestingly, components of grapefruit juice and grapefruit pulp can interfere with CYP3A4 and other CYP enzyme variants, resulting in delay or prevention of metabolism of drugs metabolized by these enzymes. Thus higher blood

Box 15-3 Some Factors That Can Trigger the Enterogastric Inhibitory Reflex

The degree of distension of the duodenum

Irritation of the duodenal mucosa: can be due to low pH chyme, hypo-osmolar or hyperosmolar chyme, the breakdown products of proteins, and to a lesser extent fats

Source: From references 8 and 10.

levels of these medications occur, causing potential negative effects due to high levels of bioavailability.[13,14]

Protective Mechanism of Coughing

Coughing begins with stimulation of the very sensitive trachea and bronchi by foreign matter. The larynx and the carina are also very sensitive to stimulation. Corrosive chemicals can stimulate the cough reflex as far as the terminal bronchi and the alveoli. Stimulation by foreign matter is conducted along the vagus nerve to the medulla of the brain.[8] The process of coughing is outlined in Box 15-4.

Pharyngeal Protective Reflex of Gagging

The pharyngeal reflex (gagging) begins with a noxious stimulus to the soft palate or the posterior pharynx through the afferent conduction of the glossopharyngeal nerve (cranial nerve IX). The noxious stimulus is conducted to the nucleus solitarius of the medulla and part of the lower pons. Efferent stimulation then occurs through the nucleus ambiguus of the medulla to the vagus nerve (cranial nerve X). A noxious thought can also stimulate the pharyngeal reflex. The reflex elicits abdominal walls tightening, closure of the glottis, symmetric lifting of the soft palate, and tongue protrusion, which causes the noxious substance

---

Box 15-4 The Process of Coughing

1. Up to 2.5 liters of air is rapidly inspired.

2. The vocal cords tightly close and the epiglottis tightens, trapping the rapidly inspired air.

3. The abdominal muscles and the internal intercostals muscles (which cause voluntary expiration) contract forcefully.

4. Pressures in the lungs can rise ≥ 100 torr.

5. The vocal cords and epiglottis open quickly so that air explodes outward.

6. The resulting negative pressure created in the lungs causes the noncartilaginous portions of the trachea and bronchi to form slits, propelling the foreign substance out of the lungs.

(The expiration reflex is forceful expiration through the open glottis without the initial inspiration found with the coughing reflex.[15])

Source: From reference 8.

---

to be repelled.[2,8] The pharyngeal reflex can proceed to the process of vomiting. Interestingly, stimulation of 5-HT$_3$ serotonin receptors in the brainstem can trigger both the pharyngeal reflex and vomiting.[16]

Protective Mechanism of Laryngospasm

Laryngospasm is a forceful closure of the glottis due to contraction of the laryngeal muscles caused by stimulation from a foreign substance (e.g., saliva, excised tissue, foreign body, excessive positive pressure, certain potent inhaled anesthetics).[11,15] This powerful reflex is used to prevent entry of the foreign substance into the airway but can quickly prevent airway exchange through the glottis, demanding prompt assessment of the laryngospasm along with appropriate treatment.[12]

Mechanisms of AP

Many factors can compromise the body's protection against the aspiration of gastric contents into the lungs. Three broad categories of disorder can lead to airway protective mechanism failure and increase the possibility of AP:

1. Depression of protective reflexes
2. Alteration or deviation of normal anatomic structures and functions
3. Iatrogenic disorders

Box 15-5 presents a comprehensive list of factors that can affect our natural protective mechanisms of gastric contents.[5,6,10–12,17–28]

Pathophysiology of AP

Aspiration of highly acidic liquid gastric contents with a volume greater than 0.3 mL/kg (usually > 25 mL of gastric volume) and an aspirate pH ≤ 2.5 triggers an instant severe inflammatory reaction with acutely damaging histologic effects to surfactant-producing cells and the pulmonary capillary endothelium. (Note: A pH > 2.5 elicits a similar response as if distilled water was administered; a pH ≤ 1.5 produces maximal pulmonary damage.[5]) Hydrochloric acid from the stomach stimulates bronchiolar spasm and tachypnea. Hydrochloric acid causes a first-phase severe chemical burn of the tracheobronchial tree and the capillary endothelium. Gastric solids may also be aspirated, causing tracheal or bronchial occlusion.[11,23,25,28,30,31] Liquid and solid aspirate immediately obstruct the airways, impairing gas exchange and the ability to institute immediate direct treatments to the airway tissues.[25]

Four to 6 hours after exposure, a second-phase inflammatory response occurs with the infiltration of neutrophils,

Box 15-5 Factors That Can Affect Normal Protective Mechanisms Against Aspiration of Gastric Contents

Depression of protective reflexes

Alcohol

Antipsychotics

Cardiac arrest

Cerebrovascular accident

Depression of consciousness

Depression of gag, coughing, swallowing reflexes

Drug overdose

Extremes of age

Head injury

Neurologic diseases

Neuromuscularly impaired reflexes

Opioids

Sedatives

Seizures

Severe hypotension

Stress

Trauma

Alteration or deviation of normal anatomic structures and functions

Achalasia (spasm of the lower portion of the esophagus)

Ascites

Cardiac arrest

Delayed gastric emptying

Diabetes mellitus

Difficult airway

Esophageal motility disorders

Foreign body aspiration

Full stomach (gastrodistension)

Dysphagia

Esophageal strictures

Gastroesophageal reflux disease (GERD)

Gastrointestinal obstruction

Gastroparesis (diabetes, medications, infection, uremia)

High gastric pressure

Hiatal hernia

Hyperchlorhydria

Hypotension

Laryngeal incompetency

Reduced lower esophageal sphincter tone

Nausea

Obesity (can be associated with hiatal hernia and GERD)

Obstetrics*

Peptic ulcer disease

Scleroderma

Vomiting

Presence of a Zenker's diverticulum

Iatrogenic disorders

Anesthetic medications

After-hours surgery

Difficult airway management

Improperly applied cricoid pressure

Inadequate anesthesia

Emergency surgery

Outpatient surgery

Patient positioning (especially lithotomy position)

Poorly compliant patient

Presence of a nasogastric tube

Placement of artificial oral airways

Residual neuromuscular relaxation

Trauma surgery

*Obstetric patients are always considered to be a full stomach condition, regardless of their nothing-by-mouth status, and should be treated as such before any anesthetic therapy. During pregnancy, the pylorus is displaced cephalad by the gravid uterus, which decreases gastric emptying, and progesterone decreases gastric motility. Also, gastrin is secreted by the placenta.[11,29]

Source: From references 5, 6, 10–12, and 17–28.

inflammatory mediators, other inflammatory cells, adhesion molecules, and enzymes. Because of the low pH of the aspirate, bacteria are not present, and bacterial infection does not have a role in early AP.[23]

Severely damaged tissues produce a peribronchiolar exudate, which causes severe congestion. The patient develops wheezes, a cough, becomes short of breath, and develops both cyanosis and pulmonary edema. Later, hypotension and hypoxemia present with rapid progression to adult respiratory distress syndrome, as well as tracheal and bronchial infarction, followed by severe hypotension and death.[2,5,11,23,30,31] Animal studies show that gastric volumes that are buffered and are twice the critical volume of aspirate (> 0.3 mL/kg; usually > 25 mL of gastric volume) present less damage to the tracheobronchial tree and capillary endothelium.

Treatments for AP

Immediate lavage of the tracheobronchial tree can be performed if an endotracheal tube is immediately placed. Inject a small volume (5–10 mL) of sterile normal saline endotracheally. Large volumes of saline only serve to push the aspirate further into the lungs. Box 15-6 lists other early interventions to be considered for AP in an intubated patient.

Interventions for the Prevention of AP

The nurse anesthetist has many choices to preemptively assuage the morbid effects produced by the aspiration of acidic gastric contents. Box 15-7 outlines both physical methods used to prevent entry of acidic gastric contents into the respiratory tract and current pharmaceutical methods used to mobilize gastric contents into the intestinal tract, neutralize gastric contents, or prevent emesis.[5,6,11,24,32–35] These methods reduce chances for accidental entry of noxious substances into the respiratory tract. We discuss the most current aspiration prophylaxis protocols in the following sections.

Careful attention must be paid to the diabetic patient. Diabetic patients experience microvascular blockage, tissue damage, along with autonomic neuropathy, which leads to decreased circulation and paralytic nerve damage to the stomach (gastroparesis).[2,8]

Physical Methods Used for the Prevention of AP

Predicting Risk Factors for Aspiration of Gastric Contents

Box 15-5 presents a comprehensive list of factors that should alert the anesthetist to the possibility of AP in patients presenting with certain signs and symptoms.[6,24]

Box 15-6   Early Interventions for an Intubated Patient with Aspiration Pneumonitis

- Consider tilting the operating room table to a 30-degree Trendelenburg position (head down), with a turn to right lateral decubitus position to allow for mechanical drainage out of the tracheobronchial tree and the mouth.

- Promptly and carefully suction the oropharynx followed by the airway through the endotracheal tube.

- Carefully and slowly continue to lavage the airway with 5–10 mL sterile normal saline.

- Deliver an increased fraction of inspired oxygen.

- Begin titrating positive end-expiratory pressure as necessary to maintain oxygen saturation.

- Auscultate breath sounds periodically for wheezing, rhonchi, and rales.

- Administer β_2 agonists such as albuterol to relieve bronchospasm.

- Place an orogastric or nasogastric tube (Salem sump) carefully.

- Measure the pH of any remaining gastric fluid.

- Obtain an initial chest radiograph. (The effects of AP may not be seen for 6–12 hours; early changes could be seen in the lower right lobes of the lung.)

- Perform a fiberoptic bronchoscopy if aspiration of liquid substance is suspected. Rigid bronchoscopy may be necessary for the removal of solid substances.

- Provide comfort and emotional support when needed.

- The use of initial antibiotic therapy has not improved outcomes of AP.

- Intravenous corticosteroid use remains controversial, although some may consider the empirical use of methylprednisolone 30 mg/kg intravenously or dexamethasone 1 mg/kg intravenously.

- Transfer to the intensive care unit with mechanical ventilator support as necessary.

Source: From references 5, 10, 11, 25, 26, 30, and 31.

Box 15-7 Physical and Pharmaceutical Methods Used for the Prevention of Aspiration Pneumonitis

Physical methods

Predicting risk factors for the aspiration of gastric contents

Avoidance of general anesthesia

Proper fasting

Cricoid pressure (Sellick's maneuver)

Preoperative placement of an orogastric or naso-gastric tube

Use of a cuffed endotracheal tube

Use of an LMA Proseal or LMA Supreme

Preoperative prediction of the potential for nausea and vomiting

Extubation of patients only when they are fully awake and fully able to protect their airway

Pharmaceutical methods

Alkalizers (systemic): citric acid, sodium citrate (Bicitra, Oracit)

Antiemetics

Anticholinergics: scopolamine (Transderm Scop)

Butyrophenones: droperidol (Inapsine)

Nonbarbiturate anesthetic induction drugs: propofol, fospropofol disodium (Lusedra)

P/neurokinin 1 (NK_1) receptor antagonists: aprepitant (Emend)

Serotonin 5-HT_3 receptor blockers: ondansetron (Zofran), alosetron (Lotronex), palonosetron (Aloxi), dolasetron (Anzemet), granisetron (Kytril)

Synthetic corticosteroids: dexamethasone

Gastric motility prokinetic agents

Metoclopramide (Reglan), cisapride (Propulsid), trimethobenzamide (Tigan), prochlorperazine (Compazine)

Histamine (H_2) receptor antagonists

Cimetidine (Tagamet), famotidine (Pepcid), nizatidine (Axid), ranitidine (Zantac)

Proton pump (hydrogen ion) inhibitors

Omeprazole (Prilosec), esomeprazole (Nexium), lansoprazole (Prevacid), pantoprazole (Protonix), rabeprazole (AcipHex)

Source: From references 5, 6, 11, 24, and 33–35.

Avoidance of General Anesthesia

The morbid effects of inhaled general anesthetic agents, especially light planes of general anesthesia combined with the use of potent opioids, can precipitate nausea and vomiting in patients.[10] The anesthetist can consider using no anesthesia whatsoever; delaying anesthesia as long as safely possible; performing monitored anesthesia care; using local anesthesia, regional anesthesia, or combinations of these techniques when feasible.[6,28]

Fasting

General practice guidelines for fasting allow time for normal gastric emptying and normal transit time of chyme through the intestines. Guidelines do not guarantee gastric emptying or a positive outcome and do not serve as an absolute standard of care for the nurse anesthetist. Water administered 2 hours preoperatively promotes gastric emptying in patients with normal gastrointestinal function. It is found that gastric pH did not differ in groups that were administered water preoperatively from those that only fasted using available guidelines.[36]

The use of portable, two-dimensional ultrasound imaging is undergoing study to assess gastric volume. This non-invasive tool (which has found its way into other aspects of anesthetic care, such as regional anesthesia) could provide preoperative visual evidence of gastric contents, thus adding another dimension to the prevention of AP.[37]

Consideration of both fasting guidelines and pharmaceuticals for the prevention of AP provide optimum patient safety.[6,38] Table 15-1 describes current fasting guidelines to reduce the risk of pulmonary aspiration in healthy children and adults undergoing elective procedures and excludes women in labor.

Table 15-1 A Summary of Current Fasting Recommendations to Reduce Risk of Pulmonary Aspiration for Healthy Children and Adults

Ingested Material	Minimum Fasting Period (h)
Clear liquids*	2
Breast milk	4
Infant formula	6
Nonhuman milk†	6
Light meal‡	6

*Clear liquids are those that allow the clear passage of light through them. Examples are water, carbonated beverages, clear tea, and black coffee.

†Nonhuman milk is considered the same as solid food in regard to gastric clearance.

‡A light meal compares with toast and clear liquids. A full meal should not be considered because this meal can require increased time until gastric emptying.

Source: From references 11, 37, and 38.

Children fasting for long periods can experience morbidity before nonemergent surgery. Fasting leads to intravascular volume depletion, resulting in a reflex tachycardia and low blood pressure.

Insertion of intravenous catheters can be more difficult. The use of intraosseous venous access serves as an equivalent to intravenous access in urgent/emergent situations. Potent inhaled anesthetic induction can cause a precipitous drop in blood pressure, decreasing perfusion pressures to the brain, and can precipitate vomiting.[20]

Cricoid Pressure (Sellick's Maneuver)

In August 1961 the *Lancet* published a landmark article by Dr. Brian Sellick.[39] The simple maneuver he described consisted of temporarily occluding the upper end of the esophagus with backward pressure applied to the cricoid cartilage of the trachea against the bodies of the cervical vertebrae. Cricoid pressure serves two purposes: to control the regurgitation of gastric or esophageal contents and to prevent inflation of the stomach before endotracheal intubation with a cuffed endotracheal tube.[11,39] Cricoid pressure is exerted by a second person applying pressure to the cricoid cartilage with the thumb and index finger. Initially, apply the necessary pressure that an awake person can comfortably tolerate. A greater amount of force is applied after induction of general anesthesia (specifically, a force of 30–40 Newtons after loss of consciousness [1 Newton of acceleration = 1 kg m/s^2] or about 3–4 kg [6.7–9 pounds] of force).[12,15]

Vigorous application of cricoid pressure to an awake patient or to a patient not deeply induced before intubation can precipitate pain, retching, and vomiting.[6,15] Cricoid pressure can precipitate tachycardia and hypertension during induction.[15] Manual ventilation can still occur during the application of cricoid pressure. Cricoid pressure is held until purchase of the airway has been accomplished, and the laryngoscopist designates release of the pressure.

Preoperative Placement of a Nasogastric Tube

The preoperative placement of a nasogastric tube allows the evacuation of gastric contents, provides an alternate conduit for the flow of gastric contents or regurgitation away from the airway, and does not interfere with the application of cricoid pressure. Certain conditions such as closed head injury, trauma, esophageal disease such as esophageal erosion or esophageal varices, and life-threatening emergency can preclude the safe placement of a nasogastric tube.[6,11,24]

Use of a Cuffed Endotracheal Tube

A properly positioned and well-secured, high-volume/low-pressure cuffed endotracheal tube is the gold standard for protection of the trachea from both liquid and solid debris. Small amounts of regurgitated material could still potentially leak around the longitudinal folds of the endotracheal cuff and can be prevented by using water-soluble lubrication around the cuff before insertion.[15]

Use of an LMA Proseal or LMA Supreme

Two models of laryngeal mask airways possess a drain tube that allows passage of a small-bore Salem sump and allows suctioning of gastric contents with the laryngeal mask airways inserted. This greatly reduces the chances of aspiration.[40]

Preoperative Prediction of the Potential for Nausea and Vomiting

In 1999 Rhodes and McDaniel introduced an index to assess the likelihood of patients who could develop nausea, vomiting, and retching. Although this index is intended for use by oncology nurses and physicians, knowledge and awareness of its use by anesthesia providers, along with the other techniques and methods used in clinical anesthesia practice, are discussed. This index helps to make anesthetic care more safe and effective for patients.[41] Box 15-8 presents the Rhodes index of nausea, vomiting, and retching (attempting to vomit without bringing anything up), which can be used as a preoperative assessment tool for patients undergoing anesthetic care.[41,42]

Pharmaceutical Methods Used for the Prevention of AP

It is essential to review the anatomy and physiology of the vomiting center within the brain and spinal cord to better understand the variable receptors involved in sensing and transmitting the signal for the vomiting reflex. The vomiting reflex forcefully propels gastric solids and liquids that can be potentially aspirated.

The vomiting center is a complex area of sensory and motor nuclei, located mainly within the medullary and pontile reticular formation, with possible extension into the spinal cord (Figure 15-2). The vomiting center contains different receptors that can trigger sensory and motor receptors responsible for the sensation and the act of vomiting.[6,8] This area contains receptors for histamine (H$_1$ receptors), serotonin (5-hydroxytryptamine [5-HT],

Box 15-8 Rhodes Index of Nausea, Vomiting, and Retching

Patient Initials _____

Date _____

Day of Week _____

Time of Day _____

Directions: Please mark the box in each row that most clearly corresponds to your experience. Please make **one** mark on **each line**.

1. In the last 12 hours I threw up _____ times.

   ❑ 7 or more   ❑ 5–6   ❑ 3–4   ❑ 1–2   ❑ I did not throw up

2. In the last 12 hours, from retching and dry heaves, I have felt _____ distress.

   ❑ no   ❑ mild   ❑ moderate   ❑ great   ❑ severe

3. In the last 12 hours, from vomiting or throwing up, I have felt _____ distress.

   ❑ severe   ❑ great   ❑ moderate   ❑ mild   ❑ no

4. In the last 12 hours, I have felt nauseated or sick to my stomach.

   ❑ not at all   ❑ 1 hour or less   ❑ 2–3 hours   ❑ 4–6 hours   ❑ more than 6 hours

5. In the last 12 hours, from nausea/sickness to my stomach, I have felt _____ distress.

   ❑ no   ❑ mild   ❑ moderate   ❑ great   ❑ severe

6. In the last 12 hours, each time I threw up, I produced a _____ amount.

   ❑ very large   ❑ large   ❑ moderate   ❑ small   ❑ I did not throw up
     (3 cups or more)   (2–3 cups)   ($\frac{1}{2}$–2 cups)   (up to $\frac{1}{2}$ cup)

7. In the last 12 hours, I have felt nauseated or sick to my stomach _____ times.

   ❑ 7 or more   ❑ 5–6   ❑ 3–4   ❑ 1–2   ❑ no

8. In the last 12 hours, I have had periods of retching or dry heaves without bringing anything up _____ times.

   ❑ no   ❑ 1–2   ❑ 3–4   ❑ 5–6   ❑ 7 or more

Source: From reference 41.

specifically 5-HT$_3$ receptors), dopamine (D$_2$), acetylcholine (M$_1$), and substance P (NK$_1$). Figure 15-3 shows a schematic representation of the receptors within the chemoreceptor trigger zone (CTZ).[43] The vomiting center receives stimulus via the circulation from multiple stimuli: the nucleus vestibularis, the nucleus tractus solitarius, the CTZ found in the area postrema of the medulla, the labyrinth of the inner ear, and the gastrointestinal tract.

Other receptors within these areas are yet to be discovered. Many of the medications we discuss in this section block specific receptors within the vomiting center itself.[8,35,44]

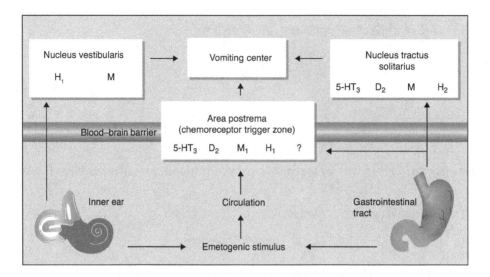

Figure 15-2 Anatomy of the vomiting center.

Source: Anesthetic Pharmacology: Physiologic Principles and Clinical Practice. Evers AS, Maze M. Page 778. Copyright Elsevier, 2004; *Gray's Anatomy for Students.* Drake RL, Vogl W, Mitchell AWM. Page 283. Copyright Elsevier 2005.

Alkalizers (Systemic): Citric Acid and Sodium Citrate (Bicitra, Oracit)

- Mechanism of action: The combination of sodium citrate and citric acid, [34,35,45,46] along with flavoring agents is a tolerably palatable liquid that mixes quickly with gastric fluid, rapidly buffers gastric fluid, and raises gastric pH.
- Clinical pharmacology
  - Pharmacokinetics: 0.34 Molar sodium citrate with pH 8.4 is administered along with pH 0.32 molar citric acid; the combination has a pH of approximately 3.15 in the stomach.
    - ◆ Absorption: Sodium citrate/citric acid passes through the stomach into the small intestine, where it is absorbed into the bloodstream and is metabolized to sodium bicarbonate and rapidly raises the systemic pH.
    - ◆ Distribution: Sodium citrate/citric acid is rapidly soluble in gastric fluid. Sodium bicarbonate circulates systemically.
    - ◆ Metabolism: Sodium citrate is rapidly and efficiently metabolized to sodium bicarbonate.
    - ◆ Elimination: Sodium bicarbonate is excreted in the urine, and sodium citrate/citric acid can be used to alkalinize urine to prevent the formation of renal calculi. Less than 5% of sodium citrate is excreted unchanged in the urine.

- Pharmacodynamics: For anesthesia use, sodium citrate dissociates to sodium ions and citrate ions. Citrate anions and chloride ions are free to combine with gastric hydrogen cations. The presence of sodium citrate with citric acid (Bicitra) also provides a continuous buffering environment in the stomach.
- Clinical uses/indications: Sodium citrate/citric acid (30 mL) is administered by mouth in a preanesthesia preparation or holding area 10 to 20 minutes before induction of anesthesia. Sodium citrate makes the solution slightly more palatable. This medication is especially useful in obstetric patients who are about to undergo certain surgical procedures.[11] Sodium citrate/citric acid is usually combined with other therapies to be discussed later for the prevention of AP.

  Sodium citrate/citric acid is also used for the alleviation of chronic metabolic acidosis. It is valuable as an alternative systemic alkalizer in patients where potassium salts are undesirable and contraindicated such as in chronic renal failure or renal tubular acidosis.[45]
- Comparative pharmacology to other drugs in class: The combination sodium citrate/citric acid and potassium citrate (Tricitra) is used as a urine alkalizer for treatment of renal calculi.
- Side effects/contraindications: Sodium citrate/citric acid is considered unpalatable by some patients

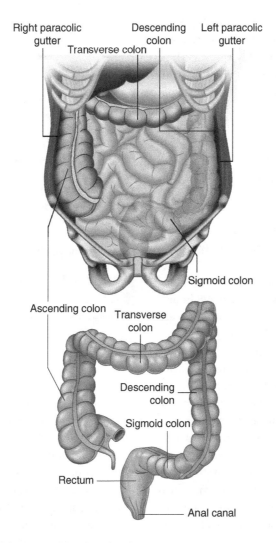

Figure 15-3 Schematic representation of the receptors within the chemoreceptor trigger zone.

Source: Anesthetic Pharmacology: Physiologic Principles and Clinical Practice. Evers AS, Maze M. Page 778. Copyright Elsevier, 2004.

and may induce a feeling of nausea or vomiting. It is contraindicated for patients on sodium-restricted diets. The medication may cause a saline laxative effect in patients.

- Drug interactions: Sodium citrate/citric acid should not be administered to patients concurrently taking aluminum-based antacids because aluminum-based antacids slow gastric emptying.[34,35]
- Guidelines/precautions: Sodium citrate/citric acid should be used with caution by patients with low urinary output or in patients with cardiac failure, hypertension, impaired renal function, peripheral edema, pulmonary edema, and toxemia of pregnancy.
- Dosage and administration: Fifteen to 30 mL sodium citrate/citric acid is administered by mouth

10 to 20 minutes before the induction of general anesthesia. Cricoid pressure must be used at induction, because gastric volume is increased by the ingestion of sodium citrate/citric acid liquid. Onset is immediately with contact of gastric acids. Duration is based on the gastric emptying time into the duodenum.

Antiemetics

Anticholinergics: Scopolamine (Transderm Scop)

- Mechanism of action: Scopolamine is an anticholinergic agent that blocks the action of acetylcholine on gastrointestinal tract peristalsis.[2,3,8,33–35] Peristalsis is the movement of digested nutrients along the intestines to expose intestinal nutrients for absorption. Acetylcholine release also facilitates the secretion of gastric acids, and medullary stimulation from the inner ear vestibular apparatus, which can signal motion sickness and nausea.

- Clinical pharmacology
  - Pharmacokinetics
    - Absorption: The transdermal scopolamine patch time releases scopolamine into the bloodstream. The transdermal patch is the commonly used form for anesthesia.
    - Distribution: Scopolamine circulates systemically. It is highly lipid soluble, and easily crosses the blood–brain barrier.
    - Metabolism: Scopolamine is efficiently metabolized in the liver, with a half-life of 4.8 hours.
    - Elimination: Scopolamine metabolites are excreted in the urine, with < 1% appearing as the unchanged parent molecule.
  - Pharmacodynamics: Scopolamine competes with acetylcholine receptor sites and reversibly combines with each of the five cholinergic muscarinic subtypes (Box 15-9). The neurotransmitter acetylcholine is responsible for mediating the action between nerves and smooth muscle, skeletal muscle, or cardiac muscle. Acetylcholine also stimulates the vestibular apparatus of the inner ear, which is responsible for balance along with the sense of position and is involved in the sensation of motion sickness (Figure 15-2).

    Motion stimulates the cilia in the labyrinth of the vestibular apparatus within the inner ear. This stimulus is then sent to the vestibular apparatus of the cerebellum, which relays its signal to the CTZ and finally on to the vomiting center. The vomiting center is a complex area of sensory and motor nuclei mainly located in the medullary and pontile reticular formation and can extend into the spinal cord (Figure 15-3).[5]
- Clinical uses/indications: Transdermal scopolamine is used as an effective and relatively inexpensive means to prevent nausea preoperatively. It can be used safely before general anesthetic induction for women having gynecologic surgery or obstetric cesarean section. It is also used as an antiemetic adjunct in patients receiving postoperative epidural morphine. High doses of scopolamine are required to block gastric acid secretion. Other medications,

---

> ### Box 15-9 The Five Cholinergic Muscarinic Receptor Subtypes
>
> **M₁:** Found at neurons and nerve endings in the central nervous system (CNS) and stomach
>
> **M₂:** Found on the heart, neurons and nerve endings, and airway smooth muscle
>
> **M₃:** Found on exocrine glands (such as the salivary glands), smooth muscle, and neurons and nerve endings
>
> **M₄:** Found on the heart and in the CNS; function unknown
>
> **M₅:** Found in the CNS; function unknown
>
> *Source:* From reference 35.

to be discussed later, are efficaciously used due to the numerous side effects of scopolamine at increased dosage.

- Comparative pharmacology to other drugs in class: Scopolamine and atropine are naturally occurring belladonna alkaloids. The molecules of scopolamine and atropine are highly lipid soluble tertiary amines, possessing a cationic portion that fits into muscarinic cholinergic receptors.

  Glycopyrrolate is a quaternary ammonium compound, is poorly lipid soluble, and also possesses an affinity for the muscarinic cholinergic receptor. Ipratropium is a synthetic quaternary ammonium analog of atropine, which is inhaled and used primarily for treating bronchospasm.
- Side effects/contraindications: Side effects of scopolamine are dizziness, drowsiness, confusion, blurred vision, dilated pupils causing photophobia, and difficult urination. Scopolamine in low doses (0.1 mg) can produce vagal mimetic effects causing paradoxical bradycardia. High doses of scopolamine can cause tachycardia and should therefore not be used in patients with coronary insufficiency, myocardial infarction, or coronary artery disease. Scopolamine is contraindicated in patients with narrow-angle glaucoma due to the production of mydriasis (dilation of the eye pupil, which inhibits the passage of

intraocular fluid into the venous circulation) and cycloplegia (relaxation of the ciliary muscle of the eye, occluding the angular space), causing a hazardous raise in intraocular pressure. Scopolamine is contraindicated in patients where conditions of inhibited peristalsis of the ureters would be detrimental, such as in prostatic hypertrophy or urinary retention. Transdermal scopolamine is slowly released into the bloodstream and can be safely administered without these side effects in most patients.

- Drug interactions: Scopolamine effects increase with patients consuming alcohol, opioids, antihistamines, tricyclic antidepressants, or phenothiazine antipsychotics.

- Guidelines/precautions: Place the transdermal scopolamine patch on a hairless area behind the ear. Avoid contact of the medication with the eye, because this can cause anisocoria (an unequal size of the pupils). The transdermal patch may contain metal and should be removed from patients before receiving magnetic resonance imaging.

- Dosage and administration: Transdermal scopolamine is available as 0.5- or 1-mg doses and is delivered within 72 hours. In anesthesia a 1-mg patch is applied to a hairless area behind the ear at least 4 hours before the induction of general anesthesia and is used for the duration of the anesthetic and up to 72 hours postoperatively.
  - Onset: 4 hours before surgery
  - Duration: up to 7 hours

Butyrophenones: Droperidol (Inapsine)

- Mechanism of action: Droperidol and haloperidol are each a butyrophenone-type molecule, which are dopaminergic antagonists binding to dopamine receptor sites in the central nervous system (CNS). Droperidol binds and blocks D_2 receptors in the CTZ of the medulla.[33–35,44]

- Clinical pharmacology
  - Pharmacokinetics
    - Absorption: Droperidol is usually administered intravenously and can be rapidly absorbed if administered intramuscularly.
    - Distribution: Droperidol is extensively protein bound and can cross the blood–brain barrier and the placenta. Its volume of distribution in children is approximately 0.25 to 0.9 L/kg and approximately 2 L/kg in adults.

- Metabolism: Droperidol is metabolized in the liver. It has a half-life of 2.3 hours in adults.
- Elimination: Droperidol metabolites are excreted 75% in urine and 22% in feces. Less than 1% of the unchanged parent drug is found in the urine, and 11% to 50% of the unchanged parent drug is found in feces.

- Pharmacodynamics: Droperidol blocks the action of the neurotransmitter dopamine on the D_2 receptors within the CTZ. Droperidol has prolonged CNS effects, which is not believed to be due to its rapid hepatic metabolism but to retention for prolonged periods on D_2 receptors. Droperidol does not affect vomiting originating from vestibular apparatus-induced motion sickness.

- Clinical uses/indications: Droperidol is a powerful antiemetic used as a treatment to prevent postoperative nausea and vomiting (PONV) caused by anesthetic medications. Present-day use of droperidol has greatly diminished due to potentially lethal alterations of cardiac electrical conduction.

- Comparative pharmacology to other drugs in class: Haloperidol is not routinely used as an anesthetic antiemetic but is an antipsychotic agent used for the management of schizophrenia, the vocal utterances caused by Tourette's disorder, and severe behavioral problems in children. Haloperidol has also found use in treating nonschizophrenic psychosis, in emergency sedation in patients with severe agitation or delirium, as an adjunct in the treatment of alcohol dependence, and as an antiemetic.

- Guidelines/precautions: Droperidol may prolong the QT_c interval of the electrocardiogram, which can precipitate torsades de pointes (polymorphic ventricular tachycardia). Prolonged QT_c is defined as greater than 440 ms in males and greater than 450 ms in females. Prolongation has occurred with droperidol doses ranging from 0.625 to 1.25 mg and up to 2.5 mg. The U.S. Food and Drug Administration (FDA) issued a black box warning in December 2001 (the most serious warning for an FDA-approved drug) requiring extreme caution before using droperidol. Patients to receive droperidol should undergo a 12-lead electrocardiogram before surgery. Patients must be monitored with a continuous electrocardiogram for 2 to 3 hours after receiving droperidol. Prolonged QT_c can develop in patients with congestive heart failure, ischemia, myocarditis, bradycardia, cerebrovascular disease, hypokalemia, hyperthyroidism/hypothyroidism, the elderly, and the concomitant use of other QT_c prolonging medications (Box 15-10).[35,47]

- Dosage and administration: Give 0.625 to 1.25 mg intravenously at the end of the surgical procedure, upon emergence from anesthesia.
  - Onset: rapid
  - Duration: up to 12 hours

Nonbarbiturate Anesthetic Induction Drugs: Propofol (Diprivan) and Fospropofol (Lusedra)

- Mechanism of action: Propofol reacts with γ-aminobutyric acid receptors subtype A ($GABA_A$) in subcortical centers of the CNS. Propofol has a postulated function as an antiemetic by either modulation of subcortical neuropathways or as a direct inhibitor within the vomiting center.[33–35,48,49]
- Clinical pharmacology (prototype)
  - Pharmacokinetics
    - Absorption: Propofol is administered intravenously and is highly protein bound in the plasma.
    - Distribution: Propofol is highly lipophilic, is rapidly distributed throughout the body to fat stores, and crosses the blood–brain barrier to react with brain $GABA_A$ receptors. Its volume of distribution is 2 to 10 L/kg.
    - Metabolism: Propofol's desirable rapid action is due to uptake by lipophilic tissues, which also accounts for 50% of its rapid decrement effects when used to produce induction of general anesthesia or sedation effect. Propofol is metabolized in the liver to water-soluble sulfate and glucuronide conjugates.
    - Elimination: Propofol has a biphasic pattern of elimination. Initial elimination occurs within 40 minutes, primarily in the urine (88%) and the feces (< 2%). Terminal elimination is 4 to 7 hours. If propofol is administered for a prolonged period of time, such as in an intensive care unit, elimination is 1 to 3 days.
  - Pharmacodynamics: Propofol interacts with the $GABA_A$ receptor of the CNS. GABA is the principal inhibitory neurotransmitter of the CNS. Propofol is postulated to act by modulation of several subcortical pathways in the CNS, inhibiting nausea and vomiting, or by direct effects on the vomiting center.

Box 15-10 Some Medications Associated With the Prolonging of the QTc Interval

Antibiotics: azithromycin, clarithromycin, erythromycin, metronidazole

Antifungals: fluconazole, ketoconazole

Antivirals: nelfinavir

Antimalarials: chloroquine

Antidysrhythmics: disopyramide, procainamide, quinidine amiodarone, sotalol

Antidepressants: amitriptyline, clomipramine, imipramine, doxepin

Antipsychotics: riperidone, haloperidol, clozapine

Inhaled anesthetics: halothane

Source: From reference 47.

- Clinical uses/indications: Propofol is a highly favored and useful medication for the induction and maintenance of anesthesia. It is also used off-label as a postoperative antiemetic. Propofol administered in subhypnotic doses is effective in chemotherapy-induced nausea and vomiting and is a rapidly effective rescue medication for PONV. It has been found to be as effective as ondansetron in the prevention of PONV. Propofol should be used in conjunction with other medications for the prevention of PONV. When used as an induction and maintenance agent for general anesthesia, it is found more effective than ondansetron for the prevention of PONV.
- Comparative pharmacology to other drugs in class: The FDA recently approved a water-soluble prodrug of propofol, called fospropofol disodium (Lusedra), which is undergoing U.S. Drug Enforcement Agency classification before its release. Fospropofol disodium is hydrolyzed to propofol by alkaline phosphatase found on the surface of endothelial cells and does not cause discomfort when injected intravenously. It can also be administered as an induction agent or used as bolus doses for anesthetic sedation.[50]
- Side effects/contraindications: Side effects of propofol are pain on injection, especially into small peripheral veins; sedation; diminished respiration;

tachycardia; decreased blood pressure; and bradycardia. Propofol is contraindicated in patients with hypersensitivity to eggs, egg products, soybeans, and soy products.

- Drug interactions: Propofol is additive to the effects of other classes of CNS depressants; hypnotic anesthetic medications such as the benzodiazepines (e.g., midazolam, lorazepam); barbiturates such as thiopental; opiates such as fentanyl, sufentanil, alfentanil, remifentanil; and alcohol.
- Guidelines/precautions: Propofol produces sedation and general anesthesia in high doses. It is contraindicated for use by anyone without advanced training in general anesthesia and advanced airway maintenance. It should not be administered by the person conducting the therapeutic or diagnostic procedure for the patient. Use strict aseptic technique
- Dosage and administration: The antiemetic effects of propofol can be achieved with a single intravenous dose of 10 mg, and effects can be maintained with an infusion of 10 μg/kg/min.

Substance P/Neurokinin 1 (NK$_1$) Receptor Antagonists: Aprepitant (Emend)

- Mechanism of action: Aprepitant is an antagonist to human substance P/neurokinin 1 (NK$_1$) receptors in the brain.[8,32–35] This receptor is found in the vomiting center of the brain. Substance P is a neurotransmitter of noxious and adverse pain information into the CNS. Pain sensation is enhanced or aggravated by substance P. Substance P/NK$_1$ regulates vomiting and is present in the final common pathway in the metabolism of substance P.
- Clinical pharmacology (prototype)
  - Pharmacokinetics
    - Absorption: Aprepitant is administered orally with absorption from the gastrointestinal tract. Aprepitant is able to cross the blood–brain barrier.
    - Distribution: Aprepitant has a volume of distribution of 70 L. It is more than 95% protein bound. Peak plasma levels are achieved in about 3 to 4 hours.
    - Metabolism: Aprepitant is metabolized in the liver.
    - Elimination: Metabolites of aprepitant are found primarily in the feces. Terminal elimination is within 9 to 13 hours.
  - Pharmacodynamics: Aprepitant crosses the blood–brain barrier and blocks the neurotransmitter

substance P/NK$_1$ from binding to receptors in the vomiting center.

- Clinical uses/indications: Aprepitant is primarily used for chemotherapy-induced nausea and vomiting. It can be used to prevent PONV if administered 3 to 4 hours before induction. Aprepitant can be used in conjunction with 5-HT$_3$ receptor antagonists (e.g., ondansetron) or corticosteroid receptor (e.g., dexamethasone) antagonists.
- Comparative pharmacology to other drugs in class: Other substance P antagonists are in development and are being tested in clinical trials.
- Side effects/contraindications: Aprepitant is contraindicated in patients sensitive to the parent drug or to its components of formulation. It is contraindicated in patients receiving pimozide (Orap), which is an atypical antipsychotic drug used to treat serious motor and verbal tics associated with Tourette's syndrome.
- Drug interactions: Aprepitant is extensively metabolized in the liver and competes with common medication metabolic pathways such as the benzodiazepines, corticosteroids, diltiazem, hormone-containing contraceptives (estrogen), rifampin, warfarin, and azole antifungal agents. Patients taking any of these medications could see prolonged effects due to a decrease in the rate of their metabolism.
- Guidelines/precautions: Aprepitant requires no dosage modification for patients with renal impairment or mild to moderate hepatic impairment due to its predominant hepatic metabolism.
- Dosage and administration: Administer 40 mg orally. Time to peak plasma levels is in approximately 3 to 4 hours.

Serotonin 5-HT$_3$ Receptor Blockers: Ondansetron (Zofran), Alosetron (Lotronex), Dolasetron (Anzemet), Granisetron (Kytril), Palonosetron (Aloxi)

- Mechanisms of action: The serotonin 5-HT$_3$ receptor blockers are highly specific competitive antagonists of the 5-HT$_3$ receptors in the vomiting center and readily cross the blood–brain barrier.[6,32–35,44,46,51–53] The 5-HT$_3$ receptor blockers also inhibit vagal nerve terminals (cranial nerve X) by distributing to peripheral vagal receptors, which play a role in the process of nausea. Serotonin is released from the enterochromaffin cells located within the mucosa of the duodenum and stimulates efferent vagal nerves with pathways to the vomiting center.

- Clinical pharmacology: Ondansetron
  - Pharmacokinetics
    - Absorption: Ondansetron is administered intravenously and has an onset of approximately 30 minutes. It can also be administered orally and intramuscularly.
    - Distribution: Ondansetron has a volume of distribution of 1.7 to 3.7 L/kg in children and 2.2 to 2.5 L/kg in adults. It is 70% to 76% protein bound in the plasma.
    - Metabolism: Ondansetron is extensively metabolized in the liver. It is also metabolized in the plasma by the platelets and the endothelial lining of blood vessels. Its half-life is 2 to 7 hours in healthy children younger than 15 years and 3 to 6 hours in healthy adults.
    - Elimination: Ondansetron is 44% to 60% excreted as metabolites. Five percent to 10% of ondansetron is excreted unchanged in the urine and approximately 25% unchanged in the feces.
  - Pharmacodynamics: Fourteen 5-HT receptor subtypes have been discovered thus far. The 5-HT receptor is part of the nicotinic GABA family of receptors. Ondansetron has negligible attraction to any of the other 5-HT receptors but is highly attracted to the 5-HT$_3$ receptors.
- Clinical uses/indications: Ondansetron is used for patients with moderate to severe cancer chemotherapy-induced nausea, in patients receiving total body or abdominal cancer radiotherapy, and as a preventive or as a rescue for PONV. Ondansetron has not been found useful for treatment of motion-induced nausea and vomiting. Ondansetron is found to block the symptoms of opioid withdrawal and is being investigated as part of the treatments needed for patients with opioid addiction.[52]
- Comparative pharmacology to other drugs in class: The 5-HT$_3$ receptor antagonists differ only in their therapeutic half-life. Dolasetron differs in that it is rapidly metabolized by the liver to hydrodolasetron, which is also a highly potent antiemetic. Table 15-2 lists the half-life of the serotonin 5-HT$_3$ receptor antagonists.
- Side effects/contraindications: The serotonin 5-HT$_3$ receptor antagonists should not be administered to patients with a hypersensitivity to the medication or any of its components of formulation.
- Drug interactions: Ondansetron is metabolized in the hepatic cytochrome P-450 (CYP3A4) enzyme

Table 15-2 Half-Life of the Serotonin 5-HT$_3$ Receptor Antagonists in Adults

Name	$t_{1/2}$
Ondansetron (Zofran)	3–6 h (2–7 h)*
Alosetron (Lotronex)	1.5 h
Dolasetron (Anzemet)	Dolasetron 10 m; Hydrodolasetron 6–8 h (4–6 h)*
Granisetron (Kytril)	5–9 h
Palonosetron (Aloxi)	40 h

*Values in parentheses are the half-lives in children.
Source: From references 34 and 43.

pathway in the liver. Therefore other medications metabolized by this pathway increase the clearance of ondansetron and shorten its therapeutic half-life, although the manufacturer recommends no dosage adjustments.

- Guidelines/precautions: There are few reported reactions to ondansetron. Ondansetron can precipitate cardiac dysrhythmias, prolonged QT$_c$ interval, and atrioventricular conduction disturbances when administered rapidly.[53] It can precipitate headaches, especially in patients prone to migraine headaches. It also can cause malaise, fatigue, or dizziness and either constipation or diarrhea in some patients.
- Dosage and administration: Administer 4 to 8 mg ondansetron intravenously in adults and 0.05 to 0.15 mg/kg in children over 2 to 5 minutes immediately before the induction of general anesthesia[18,19] or 30 minutes before the end of surgery.[34] Administration of ondansetron with other serotonin 5-HT$_3$ receptor antagonists has not been found to be useful. Ondansetron can be administered concomitantly with dexamethasone in patients more prone to PONV. (Droperidol was used concomitantly with ondansetron before to its FDA black box warning.)
  - Onset: within 30 to 60 minutes after intravenous administration
  - Duration: 3 to 6 hours in healthy patients

Synthetic Corticosteroids: Dexamethasone Sodium Phosphate (Decadron)

- Mechanism of action: The antiemetic action of dexamethasone is currently unknown but is postulated to inhibit prostaglandin synthesis caused from surgery-induced inflammation.[6,32–35] As a steroid dexamethasone may also stabilize the cell membranes of structures involved with producing PONV or penetrate to receptors in the CNS. Dexamethasone also releases endorphins, which elevate patient mood and stimulate the appetite.

- Clinical pharmacology
  - Pharmacokinetics
    - Absorption: Dexamethasone is administered intravenously for treatment of PONV but may also be administered orally or intramuscularly.
    - Distribution: Dexamethasone sodium phosphate is water soluble and is rapidly distributed throughout the circulation.
    - Metabolism: Dexamethasone is metabolized in the liver.
    - Elimination: Dexamethasone is excreted in the urine and feces.
  - Pharmacodynamics: Dexamethasone is a fluorinated derivative of the glucocorticoids prednisolone and is the isomer of betamethasone. Dexamethasone is six times more potent than prednisolone. The elimination half-life is 1.8 to 3.5 hours in a patient with normal renal function. The antiemetic effects of dexamethasone can persist for 24 hours. The use of dexamethasone is discussed in Box 15-6 as an adjunct for treatment of AP.
- Clinical uses/indications: Dexamethasone can be used in conjunction with other single-use antiemetics such as ondansetron or palonosetron for the prevention of PONV and can be used alone for chemotherapy-induced nausea and vomiting.
- Comparative pharmacology to other drugs in class: Betamethasone is used for the treatment of dermatitis, pruritus, psoriasis, and the inflammatory phase of xerosis, which is abnormal skin dryness. Betamethasone is ineffective for use for the prevention of PONV. None of the other synthetic glucocorticoids possesses the antiemetic property of dexamethasone.
- Side effects/contraindications: Dexamethasone can exhibit intense perineal discomfort such as burning or itching when administered to patients. Consider administering dexamethasone to a sedated patient due to this discomfort. Dexamethasone is contraindicated in patients with an active fungal infection, an ophthalmic herpes simplex viral infection, or tuberculosis infection. Dexamethasone reduces the humoral inflammatory response, which can inhibit both the time and quality of wound healing. It is contraindicated in patients who are sensitive to the preservative sodium bisulfite.

- Drug interactions: There are no drug interactions.
- Guidelines/precautions: Administer the smallest dose possible to prevent PONV due to impairment of the inflammatory response and wound healing. PONV dosages of Decadron are considered relatively small and are also usually a one-time event. Precaution should be considered for repeated dexamethasone administration to patients requiring multiple surgeries. Dexamethasone has been implicated as increasing the risk of postoperative bleeding in children undergoing tonsillectomy, probably due to its impairment of wound healing, and should be avoided in these patients.[54]
- Dosage and administration: Administer 0.5 mg/kg (up to 8 mg) in pediatric patients. Adult dosage is typically 4 mg intravenously. Administer dexamethasone at the time of induction of anesthesia.
  - Onset: immediate
  - Duration: ≥ 24 hours

Gastric Motility Prokinetic Medication: Metoclopramide (Reglan), Cisapride (Propulsid, no longer available), Trimethobenzamide (Tigan), Prochlorperazine (Compazine)

Metoclopramide (Reglan)

- Mechanism of action: Metoclopramide is a dopamine antagonist that blocks dopaminergic receptors in the CTZ and in high doses blocks serotonin receptors in the CTZ.[6,11,33–35,44,46] Metoclopramide is a gastrointestinal prokinetic agent: It promotes peristaltic propulsion of gastrointestinal contents through the stomach and intestines by sensitizing gastrointestinal smooth muscle to the effects of acetylcholine.
- Clinical pharmacology
  - Pharmacokinetics
    - Absorption: Metoclopramide is administered intravenously or intramuscularly but can also be administered orally, where it is absorbed directly in the gastrointestinal tract.
    - Distribution: Metoclopramide is 30% protein bound, has a volume of distribution of 2 to 4 L/kg, and readily crosses the blood–brain barrier and placenta.
    - Metabolism: Approximately 70% of intravenously administered metoclopramide is conjugated in the liver with sulfate or glucuronic acid for elimination. Orally administered metoclopramide undergoes rapid first-pass hepatic metabolism, which limits its bioavailability to 75%.

- ◆ Elimination: Intravenously administered metoclopramide is excreted 30% unchanged in the
  urine and 70% as conjugated forms, which are
  excreted in the urine and in the bile.
- ● Pharmacodynamics: Metoclopramide, which produces strengthening of the lower esophageal
  sphincter and the fundus of the stomach, sensitizes
  gastrointestinal tissue to acetylcholine and then
  motility increases in the stomach and small intestine. The pylorus and the duodenum then become
  relaxed in order to accept the gastric contents.
- ■ Clinical uses/indications: Metoclopramide is used
  preoperatively to stimulate gastric emptying as an aid
  for the prevention of AP and can even be used preoperatively for the obstetric patient.[9] It is also used
  clinically as a treatment for diabetic gastroparesis,
  as an antiemetic postoperatively or from the effects
  of chemotherapy, for symptomatic treatment of gastroesophageal reflux, for postpyloric placement of
  enteral feeding tubes, and for promoting transit of
  radiopaque dyes in radiologic examinations.
- ■ Comparative pharmacology to other drugs in class:
  Metoclopramide is structurally similar to procaine
  (Novocain), an ester local anesthetic that is no longer used, and procainamide, a benzamide antiarrhythmic without any local anesthetic effect.

  Cisapride (Propulsid) is a gastrointestinal prokinetic agent that is no longer available since 2000 in the
  United States, due to reports of severe cardiac dysrhythmias associated with its use.[55] Trimethobenzamide (Tigan) is an antiemetic agent that acts centrally
  as a dopaminergic antagonist in the CTZ. Trimethobenzamide can produce seizures and extrapyramidal
  symptoms, which is an old term referring to dysfunc-
  tions of motor control.[8]

  Prochlorperazine (Compazine) is a piperazine phenothiazine antipsychotic and is chemically unrelated
  to metoclopramide and the other gastrointestinal
  prokinetic agents already discussed. Prochlorperazine blocks dopamine receptors in the CTZ. It has the
  advantage of rectal administration as a suppository for
  patients who are experiencing active nausea and vomiting, are unable to take oral medications, or are unable
  to receive intravenous dosing for nausea and vomiting.

  The antibiotic erythromycin stimulates cholinergic activity, which increases lower esophageal
  sphincter tone and promotes gastric emptying. It
  can be used as an effective gastric prokinetic agent
  and can be administered to any patient not allergic
  to the medication.

- ■ Side effects/contraindications: Metoclopramide is
  contraindicated in patients experiencing extrapyramidal symptoms, Parkinson's disease, and seizures.
  It is contraindicated in patients with gastric obstruction and/or bowel obstruction and in patients who
  have had gastrointestinal surgery.
- ■ Drug interactions: Metoclopramide inhibits the
  effects of plasma cholinesterase and can produce
  prolongation of the anesthetic muscle relaxants succinylcholine and mivacurium (which was discontinued in 2006).
- ■ Guidelines/precautions: Metoclopramide should
  be administered slowly over 1 to 2 minutes intravenously to avoid side effects of abdominal cramping,
  hypotension, tachycardia, bradycardia, and cardiac
  dysrhythmias.
- ■ Dosage and administration: Metoclopramide 10 mg
  is administered intravenously.
  - ● Onset: 1–3 minutes
  - ● Duration: 1–2 hours

Histamine (H_2) Receptor Antagonists: Cimetidine (Tagamet), Famotidine (Pepcid), Nizatidine (Axid), Ranitidine (Zantac)

Ranitidine (Zantac)

- ■ Mechanisms of action: Ranitidine (Zantac) competitively inhibits histamine H_2 receptors in the gastric
  parietal cells, stopping the secretion of gastric acid and
  hydrogen ions, which reduces gastric volume.[6,8,33–35,46]
- ■ Clinical pharmacology
  - ● Pharmacokinetics
    - ◆ Absorption: Ranitidine is administered intra-
      venously for the preoperative treatment of AP.
    - ◆ Distribution: Ranitidine has a volume of dis-
      tribution of 1.7 L/kg and minimally penetrates
      the blood–brain barrier.
    - ◆ Metabolism: Ranitidine undergoes hepatic
      metabolism to N-oxide, S-oxide, and N-
      desmethyl metabolites.
    - ◆ Elimination: Ranitidine is excreted 70% un-
      changed in the urine when administered intra-
      venously, whereas metabolites are excreted in
      the feces.
  - ● Pharmacodynamics: Histamine (Figure 15-4) is
    an endogenous substance that is synthesized by
    the degradation of the amino acid histidine (Fig-
    ure 15-5). Mast cells, found in human connective
    tissue, store large basophilic granules containing

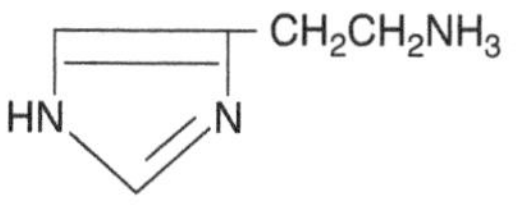

Figure 15-4 The molecular structure of histamine.

Source: From reference 35.

histamine, serotonin, bradykinin, and heparin. These substances are released from the mast cells in response to infection, inflammation, immunologic stimulation, and mechanical injury or by certain medications or chemicals.[2,3,35,46] There are three histamine receptor subtypes: H_1, H_2, and H_3. Box 15-11 describes the effects of the histamine receptor subtypes. All three histamine receptor subtypes are found on the heart. Ranitidine is a specific histamine H_2 subtype receptor antagonist that competes with histamine for attachment to the basolateral membranes of the hydrogen ion-secreting gastric parietal cells.

- Clinical uses/indications: Ranitidine is administered preoperatively for the prevention of AP and can be used in obstetric patients.[11]
- Comparative pharmacology to other drugs in class: Cimetidine was the first commercially successful H_2 receptor antagonist introduced in the 1970s. Pharmacologist Sir James W. Black was awarded the 1988 Nobel Prize in medicine for the development of cimetidine and for the development of the cardiac β receptor antagonist propanolol.[56] Cimetidine retains the imidazole ring structure similar to histamine and is assigned a relative H_2 antagonist potency of 1.

  Ranitidine uses a furan ring structure that increases its potency 4 to 10 times that of cimetidine. Nizatidine and famotidine each use a thiazole ring structure, giving nizatidine a potency 4 to 10 times that of cimetidine and famotidine, which is 20 to 50 times more potent than cimetidine.
- Side effects/contraindications: Ranitidine is contraindicated in patients sensitive to its chemical structure

and components of its formulation. Adverse reactions to ranitidine are low and are characterized as dysrhythmias, dizziness, mental confusion, and somnolence.

- Drug interactions: Ranitidine is metabolized in the hepatic cytochrome P-450 system and can reduce the absorption of atazanavir (an antiretroviral protease inhibitor for the treatment of HIV-1), some cephalosporin antibiotics (cefuroxime, cefpodoxime), antifungals (itraconazole, ketoconazole), and warfarin (Coumadin), which has produced either an increase or decrease in prothrombin time.
- Guidelines/precautions: Ranitidine must be diluted to avoid adverse reactions. Some H_2 receptor antagonists may also block H_3 receptors. H_3 receptors inhibit the synthesis and release of histamine when occupied by an agonist. Therefore histamine release may be enhanced when medications are given that evoke the release of histamine, such as atracurium, morphine, or succinylcholine (slight release), and should be used cautiously or avoided if possible.[12,35]

  There is evidence of rapid tolerance (within 2–7 days) to the antisecretory effects of H_2 antagonists in patients who ingest high doses by mouth (ranitidine 150 mg qid) or who take frequent or rapid intravenous doses (ranitidine 100 mg q6h or 50-mg bolus and 0.25 mg/kg/h). It is therefore suggested that other medications such as proton pump inhibitors be used instead of H_2 receptor antagonists.[56]

  New information was published that all patients, and especially those with osteoporosis, who use histamine receptor antagonists or proton pump antagonists (discussed in the following section) are subject to an increased risk of hip fractures. The risk of hip fracture was found to decrease with the use of lower doses. Therefore the lowest effective dose of these medications should be used.[57]
- Dosage and administration: Ranitidine 50 mg diluted in 20 mL of normal saline or D_5W administered intravenously over 5 minutes or by intravenous piggyback over 15 to 20 minutes. The dose of ranitidine does not need to be adjusted in patients with hepatic impairment but must be adjusted in patients with renal insufficiency.
  - Onset: within minutes when administered intravenously
  - Duration: elimination half lives—cimetidine 1.5 to 2.3 hours, famotidine 2.5 to 4 hours, nizatidine 1.1 to 1.6 hours, ranitidine 1.6 to 2.4 hours

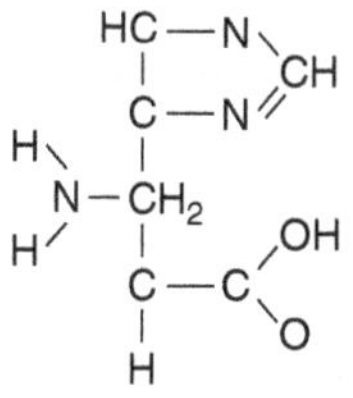

Figure 15-5 The molecular structure of the amino acid histidine.

Proton Pump (Hydrogen Ion) Inhibitors: Omeprazole (Prilosec), Esomeprazole (Nexium), Lansoprazole (Prevacid), Pantoprazole (Protonix), Rabeprazole (AcipHex)

Omeprazole

- Mechanisms of action: As discussed previously,
  hydrochloric acid (with pH 0.8, which is 3 million
  times more acidic than arterial blood) is secreted by
  the parietal cells of the gastric lining (Figures 15-1a
  and 15-1b). [2,6,33–35,44,46] Hydrogen ions are produced in

the parietal cells by a postulated mechanism involving
the following steps:

1. Active transport of chloride ions from the parietal cytoplasm into the parietal canaliculi
2. Sodium ions actively transported out of the canaliculi into the parietal cytoplasm.
3. Dissociation of water into hydrogen ions (H^+) and
   hydroxyl ions (OH^-)
4. Active *pumping* of potassium ions (K^+) into the
   parietal cytoplasm for hydrogen ions (H^+)

This results in hydrogen ion secretion into the
canaliculi of the parietal cells. This pump is called H^+/
K^+ ATPase (adenosine triphosphate) proton pump,
whose mechanism is inhibited (Figure 15-6). [8]

- Clinical pharmacology: omeprazole
  - Pharmacokinetics
    - Absorption: Omeprazole can be administered
      orally, where it passes through the stomach
      into the small bowel (experiencing the first-
      pass effect by the liver). It is also available for
      intravenous administration.
    - Distribution: Omeprazole is 95% protein
      bound and is distributed via the bloodstream
      to reach the gastric parietal cells. Omeprazole
      (a benzimidazole) diffuses into the parietal
      cell and accumulates in the canaliculi, where
      it is converted to its active component: a sul-
      phenamide. Its bioavailability is approximately
      30% to 60% with peak serum concentration
      reached in 0.5 to 4 hours.

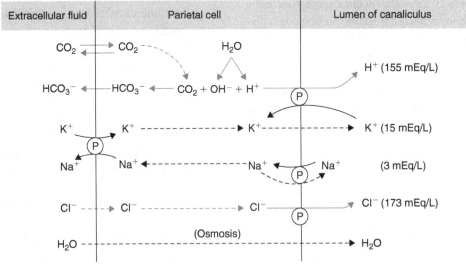

Figure 15-6 The postulated mechanism for the secretion of hydrochloric acid H^+/K^+ ATPase proton pump.

Source: Medical Physiology, 11th ed. Guyton AC, Hall JE. Secretory Functions of the Alimentary Tract, Page 796, © Elsevier 2006.

- Metabolism: Omeprazole undergoes extensive hepatic metabolism to inactive metabolites.
- Elimination: Omeprazole has a half-life of 0.5 to 1 hour and is eliminated in the urine: 77% as inactive metabolites and a negligible amount as the active drug. Metabolites also appear in breast milk and feces.
- Pharmacodynamics: The active sulphenamide form of omeprazole covalently binds to the H^+/K^+ ATPase proton pump and ceases the function of the pump. As a result, omeprazole increases gastric pH and decreases gastric fluid volume.

- Clinical uses/indications: Proton pump inhibitors are used in the treatment of gastroesophageal reflux disease (GERD), treatment of active duodenal ulcers or active benign gastric ulcers (peptic ulcers), erosive esophagitis, hypersecretory disorders such as Zollinger-Ellison syndrome, and as a multidrug regimen for the eradication of *Helicobacter pylori*. It is also used off-label for the prevention or healing of nonsteroidal anti-inflammatory drug (NSAID)-induced ulcers. Although proton pump inhibitors are not currently commonly administered as a first-line therapy for the prevention of AP, patients should continue this medication as ordered by their physician to aid in the prevention of AP, along with additional therapies previously discussed.

- Comparative pharmacology to other drugs in class
  - Esomeprazole (Nexium) is the S-enantiomer of omeprazole and is therefore structurally and pharmacologically similar to omeprazole. It has a bioavailability of 85% and a serum half-life of 1.5 hours.
    - Oral dosage for GERD
      Children < 20 kg: 10 mg once daily
      Children ≥ 20 kg: 10 to 20 mg once daily
      Adults: 20 mg once daily
  - Lansoprazole (Prevacid): capsule and oral disintegrating tablets available in 15 mg or 30 mg; intravenous 30 mg to be reconstituted in 60 mg liquid mannitol: has the same indications for usage as omeprazole.
    - Oral dosage for GERD
      Children ≤ 30 kg: 15 mg once daily
      Children > 30 kg: 30 mg once daily
      Adults: 30 mg once daily
  - Pantoprazole (Protonix): oral tablets available in 20 mg or 40 mg; intravenous 40 mg to be reconstituted in 100 mL normal saline or D_5W to be administered over 2 to 15 minutes; has the same indications for usage as omeprazole.
    - Oral dosage for GERD
      Adults: 40 mg once daily

- Rabeprazole (AcipHex): oral tablets available in 15 mg or 30 mg; has the same indications for usage as omeprazole.
  - Oral dosage for GERD
    Adults > 18 years and the elderly: 20 mg once daily

- Side effects/contraindications: Omeprazole is contraindicated in patients who are hypersensitive to the medication or components of its formulation or to any other benzamide proton pump inhibitors. Because omeprazole crosses the blood–brain barrier, rare side effects such as headache, dizziness, agitation, and confusion can occur. There are also rare instances of nausea, vomiting, diarrhea, constipation, flatulence, and abdominal pain.

  Because gastric acid levels are decreased by use of the proton pump inhibitors, serum gastrin levels increase. However, there has been no experience of significance with long-term proton pump inhibitor use, and eventually gastrin levels become maintained at normal levels.

  As mentioned in the section on histamine receptor blockers, any patients who use either histamine receptor antagonists or proton pump antagonists are subject to an increased risk of hip fractures. The risk of hip fracture was found to decrease with the use of lower doses, and the lowest effective dose of these medications should be used.[57]

- Drug interactions: Omeprazole may decrease the absorption of the protease inhibitors (atazanavir, indinavir) and should not be used concurrently. Omeprazole may increase the levels and the effects of the R-isomer of warfarin, so warfarin levels should be continuously monitored.

  Absorption of drugs dependent on low gastric pH, such as the imidazole antifungals (itraconazole, ketoconazole), ampicillin esters, and iron, may be affected by the profound acid suppression effects of omeprazole. Phenytoin elimination may be prolonged in patients taking omeprazole, and the levels and effects of omeprazole may be decreased in these same patients. Because omeprazole is metabolized by the cytochrome P-450 enzyme system, levels of benzodiazepines that are metabolized by oxidation within the cytochrome P-450 system (diazepam, midazolam, triazolam) become increased.

- Guidelines/precautions: Omeprazole should be used with caution in lactating women.

- Dosage and administration: Omeprazole is available either as a 10- or 20-mg oral capsule and in 40-mg vials. Vials must be reconstituted in 100 mL of normal saline or D_5W and infused over 30 minutes.

- For GERD

    Children < 2 years: 10 mg once daily

    Children ≥ 2 years: 20 mg once daily

    Adults: 20 mg/day for up to 4 weeks (anesthesia providers may consider a one-time dosage as part of their preoperative treatment regimen for patients with GERD)

    For patients with an indwelling patent nasogastric tube who are unable to swallow the medication, capsules may be opened and flushed with water into the stomach.

- Onset: Omeprazole 20 mg by mouth has a gastric acid antisecretory onset within 2 to 6 hours. Preoperative administration of omeprazole should occur more than 3 hours before the time of induction of anesthesia. Omeprazole administered intravenously has gastric acid antisecretory effects within 3 minutes to more than 2 hours and can be used to maintain plasma levels of the drug necessary for the treatment of bleeding gastric or duodenal ulcers.[58]

- Duration: Despite the short half-life of omeprazole, its effects may last longer than 24 hours because of its concentration within the acidic environment of the gastric parietal cells, and its acid-inhibitory effects increase with repeated dosing.

Summary and Anesthesia Implications

Respiration is the dominant function of the nose, mouth, and pharynx. The swallowing pathway shares a parallel conduit with the respiratory pathway with both voluntary and involuntary protective mechanisms to protect the respiratory pathway. Coughing and the pharyngeal reflex (gagging) are two quick and strong protective mechanisms. Coughing forcefully and explosively expels foreign matter from the respiratory pathway, whereas the pharyngeal reflex blocks the respiratory pathway and allows pharyngeal and/or gastric contents to be forcefully expelled. The body's protective mechanisms can become ineffective or fail by the depression of protective reflexes, the alteration or deviation of normal anatomic structures, and iatrogenic disorders.

AP is the inflow of a critical volume of highly acidic gastric contents, which triggers a severe inflammatory reaction and produces injurious histologic effects to the trachea, bronchioles, lung tissue, and the pulmonary capillary endothelium. The anesthetist has tools available to assess the patient's probable risks of developing AP and can use both physical and pharmaceutical methods to prevent this catastrophic event from occurring.

Conclusions

Legal Considerations

Code 1.2 of the American Association of Nurse Anesthetists Code of Ethics for the Certified Registered Nurse Anesthetist in "Responsibility to Patients" states the following: "The CRNA protects the patient from harm and is an advocate for the patient's welfare."[61] This statement states a duty for certified registered nurse anesthetist to diligently guard for the safety and well-being of the patient at all times, especially to those patients with a potential to develop AP.

A duty of care is a requirement that a person act toward others and the public with the watchfulness, attention, caution, and prudence that a reasonable person in the circumstances would use. If a person's actions do not meet this standard of care, then the acts are considered negligent, and any damages resulting may be claimed in a lawsuit for negligence.[59]

Negligence is a failure to exercise care toward others (our patients), which a reasonable or prudent person would do in similar circumstances, or by taking action, which such a reasonable person would not. Negligence is one of the greatest sources of litigation. For negligence to be a claim for damages, the injured party (plaintiff) must prove three things:

1. The party alleged to be negligent had a duty to the injured party, specifically to the one injured or to the general public.
2. The defendant's action (or failure to act) was negligent: not what a reasonably prudent person would have done.
3. The damages were caused ("proximately caused") by the negligence.

An added factor in the formula for determining negligence is whether the damages were "reasonably foreseeable" at the time of the alleged carelessness. If the injury is caused by neglect of common standards of care, negligence can be found based on the doctrine of *res ipsa loquitur* (Latin for "the thing speaks for itself").[60]

Although we have discussed physical and pharmaceutical methods used for the prevention of AP (Box 15-7), no guarantee can be afforded the certified registered nurse anesthetist that AP will be averted by the use of the materials and methods discussed. But if the certified registered nurse anesthetist acts *with the watchfulness, attention, caution, and prudence that a reasonable person in the circumstances would use,* the plaintiff could have a difficult time claiming damages.[61]

Closed-Claim Studies for AP

With the advent of physical methods, pharmaceutical methods, and well-taught protocols commonly used for the prevention of AP, it is helpful to put AP into perspective by studying malpractice claims pertaining to the occurrence of aspiration and for respiratory events from the most recent malpractice closed-claim data. The American Society of Anesthesiologists studies closed anesthesia malpractice claims data from 35 insurance companies, representing 14,500 anesthesiologists. Most malpractice claims arise from death (22%), nerve injury (21%), and brain damage (7%).[62]

Aspiration-related malpractice claims have remained a constant 3% to 3.5% of all respiratory malpractice claims from the 1970s to the 1990s. The highest incidence of aspiration malpractice claims was during the induction of a general anesthetic. Damaging respiratory-related events have decreased from 30% to 15% from the 1970s to the 1990s. This led the author to conclude, and for us to realize, that the current practice of treating AP is effective and that the hazard of gastric aspiration is not a major liability hazard.[62,63]

Other conclusions reached from the American Society of Anesthesiologists closed anesthesia malpractice claims were as follows:

1. Forty nine percent of all obstetric anesthesia malpractice claims were due to maternal death (19% of claims), headache/pain during anesthesia, and back pain/emotional distress. It is important to note that 30% of respiratory complications in obstetrics (5% is attributed to AP) that lead to maternal injury (difficult intubation, pulmonary aspiration, esophageal intubation, inadequate ventilation/oxygenation, bronchospasm, etc.) were low in leading to malpractice claims.[64]
2. Pediatric anesthesia malpractice claims were led by cardiovascular events (27%), respiratory events (25%), equipment events (17%: intravenous line placement, airway equipment, warming device burns, electrocautery), and medication-related events (14%: adverse drug reactions, malignant hyperthermia, wrong dose). Pediatric anesthesia malpractice claim trends are decreasing due to the vast improvements in techniques, medications, monitors, and other adjunctive equipment.[65]
3. Trauma anesthesia malpractice claims show aspiration to be a rare event (2.6% of claims) and that anesthetic care during trauma appears to be adequate.[66]

Key Points

- Define terms associated with aspiration and the gastrointestinal system.
- Review the anatomy and physiology of the gastrointestinal system.
- Learn the body's natural protective mechanisms against aspiration.
- List factors that affect our natural protective mechanisms against aspiration.
- Discuss the pathophysiologic process of aspiration pneumonitis.
- Discuss treatments for aspiration pneumonitis.
- Learn physical and pharmaceutical means of preventing aspiration pneumonitis.
- Discuss the legal implications of patients developing aspiration pneumonitis.

Chapter Questions

1. Aspiration pneumonitis is a chronically developed infection of lung tissues. True or False?

2. Aspiration pneumonitis can develop because of all but one of the following:
   a. A diminished cough reflex
   b. Reduced lower esophageal sphincter tone
   c. Inadequate reversal of neuromuscular blockade
   d. Gastric pH ≥ 2.5

3. The certified nurse anesthetist may anticipate the likelihood of aspiration pneumonitis by the preoperative assessment of all but one of the following physical findings:
   a. Fasting for > 6 hours
   b. An obtunded motorcycle injury patient
   c. Awake patient with reflexes intact
   d. An obstetric patient

4. Which of the following pharmaceutical types is not currently recommended as a first-line medication for the prevention of aspiration pneumonitis?
   a. Proton pump (hydrogen ion) inhibitors
   b. Histamine (H_2) receptor antagonists
   c. Antiemetics
   d. Alkalizers (systemic)

5. Aspiration pneumonitis and respiratory claims are the major cause for anesthesia-related malpractice claims. True or False?

Answers and Discussion

1. False. Aspiration pneumonitis is an acute direct chemical injury to lung tissues caused by the aspiration of highly acidic gastric contents, whereas aspiration pneumonia is an infectious process caused by the continual aspiration of secretions containing pathogenic oropharyngeal bacteria.

2. d. The pH of gastric contents is typically 1 to 2. Aspiration pneumonitis is most damaging with aspirated gastric contents of a pH $\leq$ 2.5 with a critical gastric fluid volume of 0.3 mL/kg or greater.

3. c. An awake patient with reflexes intact on assessment has the least chance of developing aspiration pneumonitis. Consideration should be made for alternatives to general anesthesia, because many different factors could increase chances for aspiration. Also, fasting for more than 6 hours does not guarantee empty stomach contents.

4. a. Proton pump inhibitors are not currently routinely used as a first-line pharmaceutical for the preoperative treatment of aspiration pneumonitis. The proton pump inhibitors are used in the treatment of gastroesophageal reflux disease, duodenal and peptic ulcers, and other ulcerative diseases. These medications should be used concurrently with other pharmaceuticals used for the preoperative prevention of aspiration pneumonitis.

5. False. Current practices for the treatment and prevention of aspiration pneumonitis are effective, and the hazard of gastric aspiration is not a major liability hazard. Aspiration-related malpractice claims have remained constant at 3% to 3.5% of all respiratory malpractice claims from the 1970s to the 1990s as practitioners are acutely aware of both the dire consequences to the patient who aspirates and aspiration pneumonitis prevention protocols.

Acknowledgments

For their devoted assistance in the preparation of this chapter, I acknowledge and thank Anita Schwartz; David Brodsky; Leonard and Lita Schwartz; Judy Feintuch, MA, MLS; Boone Hospital Center of Columbia, Missouri; The Bernard Becker Medical Library of Washington University of St. Louis, Missouri; St. Elizabeth's Hospital of Belleville, Illinois; Anesthesia Care of Effingham, Illinois; and AMSOL of Highpoint, North Carolina.

References

1. Mendelson CL. The aspiration of stomach contents into the lungs during obstetric anesthesia. *Am J Obstet Gynecol.* 1946;52:191–204.

2. Myers T, ed. *Mosby's Dictionary of Medicine, Nursing & Health Professions.* St. Louis, MO: Mosby Elsevier; 2009.

3. Friel JP, ed. *Dorland's Illustrated Medical Dictionary,* 25th ed. Philadelphia: W.B. Saunders; 1974.

4. Drake RL, Vogl W, Mitchell AWM. *Gray's Anatomy for Students.* Philadelphia: Churchill Livingstone; 2005:272.

5. Yao FSF, Artusio F. *Yao & Artusio's Anesthesiology Problem-Oriented Patient Management.* Philadelphia: Lippincott Williams & Wilkins; 2003:52-56, 464–468, 1144.

6. Fleisher LA, ed. *Evidence-Based Practice of Anesthesiology.* Philadelphia: W.B. Saunders; 2004:118–129.

7. Bloom W, Fawcett DW. *A Textbook of Histology.* Philadelphia: W.B. Saunders; 1975:645, 656.

8. Guyton AC, Hall JE. *Textbook of Medical Physiology.* Philadelphia: W.B. Saunders; 2005:480, 600–601, 688–689, 776–777, 782–790, 796–799, 823–824, 972–974.

9. Hollinshead WH. *Textbook of Anatomy.* Hagerstown, MD: Harper & Row; 1974:604–609.

10. Aitkenhead AR, Smith G, Rowbotham DJ. *Textbook of Anaesthesia.* Edinburgh, UK: Churchill Livingstone; 2007:376–377, 459–460, 542–550.

11. Nagelhout JJ, Plaus KL. *Nurse Anesthesia.* St. Louis: Saunders 2010: 122–126, 462–463, 605–610, 818–819, 878–880, 899–900, 1036, 1106, 1121–1122, 1191–1192, 1307.

12. Miller RD. *Miller's Anesthesia.* Philadelphia: Churchill Livingstone; 2005:99, 395, 511–512, 1028–1030, 1619–1620, 1635, 2290, 2384–2385, 2539, 2598–2601.

13. U.S. Food and Drug Administration. Avoiding drug interactions. Available at: http://www.fda.gov/consumer/updates/interactions112808.html. Accessed May 14, 2009.

14. Mayo Clinic. Grapefruit juice: can it cause drug interactions? Available at: http://www.mayoclinic.com/print/food-and-nutrition/AN00413/METHOD=print. Accessed May 14, 2009.

15. Barash PG, Cullen BF, Stoelting RK. *Clinical Anesthesia.* Philadelphia: Lippincott Williams & Wilkins; 2006:494–495, 1054–1056, 1154, 1163, 1393–1395.

16. Yoshioka M, Goda Y, Ikeda T. Involvement of 5-HT3 receptors in the initiation of pharyngeal reflex. *Am J Physiol Regul Integr Comp Physiol.* 1994;266:R1652–R1658.

17. Aouad MT, Berzina CE, Baraka AS. Aspiration pneumonia after anesthesia in a patient with Zenker diverticulum. *Anesthesiology.* 2000;92:1837–1839.

18. Sieber FE. *Geriatric Anesthesia.* New York: McGraw-Hill; 2007:233.

19. Taussig LM, Landau LI. *Pediatric Respiratory Medicine.* Philadelphia: Mosby; 2008:337–344.

20. Bissonnette B, Dalens BJ. *Pediatric Anesthesia Principles and Practice.* New York: McGraw-Hill; 2002:410–411, 492–494.

21. Chernick V, Boat TF, Wilmott RW. *Kendig's Disorders of the Respiratory Tract in Children.* Philadelphia: W.B. Saunders; 2006:328, 478–483.

22. Albert RK, Spiro SG, Jett JR. *Clinical Respiratory Medicine.* Philadelphia: Mosby; 2008:334–336, 348–350.

23. Marik PE. Aspiration pneumonitis and aspiration pneumonia. *N Engl J Med.* 2001;344:665–671.

24. Benington S, Severn A. Preventing aspiration and regurgitation. *Anesth Intens Care Med.* 2007;8:368–372.

25. Boysen PG, Modell J. Pulmonary aspiration. In: Shoemaker WC, ed. *Textbook of Critical Care.* Philadelphia: W.B. Saunders; 2000:1432–1439.

26. Urden LD, Stacy KM, Lough ME. *Thelan's Critical Care Nursing Diagnosis and Management.* St. Louis, MO: Mosby; 2006:632–635.

27. Hutton P, Cooper GM, James FM. *Fundamental Principles and Practice of Anaesthesia.* London: Martin Dunitz Ltd.; 2002:86–88.

28. Koda-Kimble MA, Young LY, Kradjan WA. *Applied Therapeutics: The Clinical Use of Drugs.* Philadelphia: Lippincott Williams & Wilkins; 2001:8-5–8-6, 58-15–58-17.

29. Stoelting RK, Miller RD. *Basics of Anesthesia.* Philadelphia: Churchill Livingstone; 2007:173–175, 479–480.

30. Magalini SI, Magalini SC. *Dictionary of Medical Syndromes.* Philadelphia: Lippincott-Raven; 1997:532–533.

31. Stoelting RK, Dierdorf SF. *Anesthesia and Co-existing Disease.* Philadelphia: Churchill Livingstone; 2002:208, 447–448, 580–581.

32. Engel K. *Physicians' Desk Reference 2008.* Montvale, NJ: Thomson Healthcare; 2007:1644–1652.

33. Skidmore-Roth L. *Mosby's Nursing Drug Reference 2008.* St. Louis, MO: Mosby 2008:146–147, 344–346, 383–384, 396–398, 435, 519–520, 597–598, 673–674, 760–763, 780–781, 786–787, 860–861, 880–881, 919–921.

34. Donnelly AJ, Baughman VL, Gonzales JP. *Anesthesiology & Critical Care Drug Handbook.* Hudson, OH: Lexi-Comp; 2008.

35. Stoelting RK, Hillier SC. *Pharmacology & Physiology in Anesthetic Practice.* Philadelphia: Lippincott Williams & Wilkins; 2006:158–159, 266–275, 413, 429–443, 461–467, 496–504, 708–709.

36. McGrady EM, MacDonald AG. Effect of the preoperative administration of water on gastric volume and pH. *Br J Anaesth.* 1988;60:803–805.

37. Brull SJ. Gastric ultrasonography: a non-invasive tool to determine gastric volume. Development of a quantitative model. *APSF Newsletter.* 2008;23:54–55.

38. Warner MA, Caplan RA, Epstein BS. Practice guidelines for preoperative fasting and the use of pharmacologic agents to reduce the risk of pulmonary aspiration: application to healthy patients undergoing elective procedures. *Anesthesiology.* 1999;90:896–905.

39. Sellick BA. Cricoid pressure to control regurgitation of stomach contents during induction of anaesthesia. *Lancet.* 1961; 2:404–406.

40. LMA North America. LMA proseal; LMA supreme. Available at: http://www.lmana.com/proseal.php and http://www.lmana.com/supreme.php. Accessed May 6, 2009.

41. Rhodes VA, McDaniel RW. The index of nausea, vomiting, and retching: a new format of the index of nausea and vomiting. *Oncol Nurs Forum* 1999;26:889–894.

42. Rhodes VA, McDaniel RW. Nausea, vomiting, and retching: complex problems in palliative care. *CA: Cancer J Clin* 2001;51:232–248. Available at: http://caonline.amcancersoc.org/cgi/reprint/51/4/232. Accessed April 22, 2009.

43. Leslie JB. Lecture presented at the Arizona Association of Nurse Anesthetists semiannual meeting, March 27, 2009.

44. Evers AS, Maze M. *Anesthetic Pharmacology: Physiologic Principles and Clinical Practice.* Philadelphia: Churchill Livingstone; 2004:763–792.

45. Pharmaceutical Associates Inc., Greenville, SC. Package insert sodium citrate and citric acid USP. NDC 0121–0595.

46. Morgan GE, Mikhail MS, Murray MJ. *Clinical Anesthesiology.* New York: Lange Medical Books/McGraw-Hill; 2006:276–281, 286–289, 833–834, 868–869.

47. Jayasinghe R, Kovoor P. Drugs and the QT_c interval. *Austral Prescrib.* 2002;25:63–65.

48. Teva Parenteral Medicines, Inc., Irvine, CA. Package insert propofol injectable emulsion. NDC 0703-2856-04.

49. Lusedra® Highlights of Prescribing Information. Available at: http://www.eisai.com/pdf_files/FDA%20Approved%20%20Labeling%20Text%2012.12.08.pdf. Accessed March 23, 2009.

50. Personal conversation. Munoz K, Adewale AS. Eisai Inc. May 26, 2009.

51. Rupniak NM. Elucidating the antidepressant actions of substance P (NK1 receptor) antagonists. *Curr Opin Invest Drugs.* 2002;3:257–261.

52. Lacey L. Ondansetron can be useful in treating opioid addiction. *AANA Newsbulletin.* 2009;63:8–9.

53. Aloxi® Highlights of Prescribing Information. Eisai, Inc. 2008.

54. Lacey L. Medication used to reduce nausea following tonsillectomies linked with increasing risk of bleeding. *AANA Newsbulletin.* 2009;63:11.

55. U.S. Food and Drug Administration. Janssen pharmaceutica stops marketing cisapride in the U.S. *FDA Talk Paper.* Available at: http://www.fda.gov/bbs/topics/ANSWERS/ANS01007.html. Accessed April 7, 2009.

56. Hirota K, Kushikata T. Preanaesthetic H_2 antagonists for acid aspiration pneumonia prophylaxis. Is there evidence of tolerance? *Br J Anaesth*. 2003;90:576–579.

57. Reuters. Heartburn drugs may raise risk of hip fractures: study. Available at: http://www.reuters.com/articlePrint?articleId=USTRE5505OU20090601. Accessed June 1, 2009.

58. Wilder-Smith CH, Bettschen HU, Merki HS. Individual and group dose-responses to intravenous omeprazole in the first 24h: pH-feedback-controlled and fixed-dose infusions. *Br J Clin Pharmacol*. 1995;39:15–23.

59. Law.com law dictionary. Duty of care. Available at: http://dictionary.law.com/default2.asp?selected=599&bold. Accessed April 28, 2009.

60. Law.com law dictionary. Negligence. Available at: http://dictionary.law.com/default2.asp?selected=1314&bold. Accessed April 28, 2009.

61. American Association of Nurse Anesthetists. Code of ethics for the certified registered nurse anesthetist. Available at: http://www.aana.com/resources.aspx?ucNavMenu_TSMenu TargetID=51&ucNavMenu_TSMenuTargetType=4&ucNavMenu_TSMenuID=6&id=665. Accessed April 28, 2009.

62. Cheney FW. Aspiration: a liability hazard for the anesthesiologist? *ASA Newsletter*. 2000;64:5–6, 26.

63. Posner KL. Closed claim project shows safety evolution. Available at: http://www.apsf.org/resource_center/newsletter/2001/fall/02closedclaims.htm. Accessed April 28, 2009.

64. Chadwick HS. Obstetric anesthesia closed claims update II. *ASA Newsletter*. 2000;63:12–15. Available at: http://www.asahq.org/Newsletters/1999/06_99/Obstetric_0699.html. Accessed April 29, 2009.

65. Jimenez N. Trends in pediatric anesthesia malpractice claims over the last three decades. *ASA Newsletter*. 2005;69:8–9, 12.

66. Tsai YK, Sharar SR, Posner KL. Does anesthetic care for trauma present increased risk for patient injury and professional liability? Abstract presented at the 14th Annual Trauma Anesthesia and Critical Care Symposium 2001. Available at: http://depts.washington.edu/asaccp/ASA/Newsletters/itaccs2000tsai.shtml. Accessed April 28, 2009.

Objectives

After completing this chapter, the reader should be able to

- Explain the anatomy and physiology associated with urine formation.
- Explain how diuretics alter the physiology of urine formation.
- Explain how diuretics affect the fluid and electrolyte balances.
- Identify factors that affect the delivery of anesthetic management associated with the use of diuretics.

16

Diuretics

Clifford Gonzales, MSN, CRNA

Introduction

The kidneys maintain the water and electrolyte balance of our body. Certain conditions in our body demand the kidneys to alter the physiology by excreting greater amounts of water and electrolytes than usual through pharmacologic interventions. Diuretic comes from the Greek word *diourétos*, which means to urinate.[1] In the healthcare setting and in this chapter, diuretics are pharmacologic interventions that increase urine output. Urine implies not only water but also solutes such as electrolytes (e.g., sodium), waste products (e.g., creatinine), and pharmacologic metabolites. In this chapter we review the basic anatomy and physiology associated with the processes of urine formation and flow and discuss the pharmacologic interventions that increase urine output.

Anatomy and Physiology Associated With Urine Formation

The Kidney

The urinary system consists of two kidneys, two ureters, a urinary bladder, and a urethra. The kidneys are posteriorly located at the abdomen outside the peritoneal cavity (retroperitoneal space). Each kidney has a medially indented area called the hilum, which faces the vertebral column. The kidneys can be palpated using the reference of costovertebral angle, which is the angle formed on either side of the vertebral column where the last rib and the lumbar vertebrae meet. Each kidney weighs about 150 grams.

The kidneys have three regions: the cortical, medullary, and renal pelvic regions. The cortical region is the outer region of the kidneys. The medullary region is the inner region of the kidneys that contains the pyramids. The pyramids are composed of long loops of Henle, medullary collecting ducts, and collecting tubules. The terminal openings of the pyramids, called papilla, drain the urine from the collecting ducts to the minor calices. Urine then drains to the major calices where it leads to a large collecting area called the renal pelvis.

The blood vessels, nerves, and lymphatic drains enter the hilum. The blood supply to the kidneys comes from the aorta through the renal arteries. The renal arteries progressively divide into interlobar, arcuate, and radial (interlobular) arteries.[2] The arcuate arteries terminally end at the afferent arteriole. The afferent arterioles progressively divide into glomerular capillaries (glomeruli) that connect to the efferent arterioles and then branch to the peritubular capillaries. For the deeper juxtamedullary nephrons, these peritubular capillaries are the vasa recta. The blood from the peritubular capillaries drains to the interlobular vein and then proceeds to the arcuate, interlobar, and renal veins.[2] The arteries and veins run parallel to each other.

The innervations of the kidneys come from the renal plexus. The renal plexus branches to lesser splanchnic nerves, which provide the sympathetic stimulation to the kidneys.

The kidneys are known to excrete body wastes, pharmacologic metabolites, and excess water and electrolytes. Several other functions of the kidneys are maintenance of acid–base balance; production of erythropoietin, renin, and calcitriol, which is the active form of vitamin D; regulation of arterial blood pressure; and maintenance of the blood glucose through gluconeogenesis.

The Nephron

The nephron is the functional unit of the kidneys. It is composed of the renal corpuscle and tubules. The renal corpuscle is composed of the glomerulus and Bowman's capsule. The tubules connect the Bowman's capsule to the collecting duct. The tubules include the proximal convoluted tubule (PCT), loop of Henle, distal convoluted tubule (DCT), and collecting tubules. The nephron performs three main processes to produce urine: filtration, reabsorption, and secretion.

There are about 1 million nephrons in each kidney.[2] There are two types of nephrons: cortical nephrons and juxtamedullary nephrons. The renal corpuscle of the juxtamedullary nephron is located near the border of the cortical and medullary region, whereas the cortical nephrons are located at the higher region of the cortex. In contrast to the cortical nephron having a short loop of Henle, the juxtamedullary nephron's loop of Henle descends deep in the inner medulla.

Process of Urine Formation

Urine is obtained by subtracting the sum of the processes of reabsorption and secretion from the amount of filtration. The reabsorption of solutes requires passive and active transport from the nephron's tubules to the kidneys' interstitial space, which is then reabsorbed to the peritubular capillaries. Passive transport includes diffusion and osmosis. The sodium-potassium pump and cotransport are examples of active transport. An example of cotransport, also called symporter, is 1-sodium, 2-chloride, 1-potassium symporter.[3]

The kidneys receive about 22% of cardiac output.[2] Nearly all components of plasma are filtered through glomeruli. Large substances such as blood and protein are not normally filtered through the glomeruli. The difference between the hydrostatic pressure and oncotic pressure in the glomerulus and the capsular hydrostatic pressure at the Bowman's capsule pushes the filtrate to reach the Bowman's capsule. The filtrate then moves to the PCT. Nearly three-fourths of the filtrate is absorbed from the PCT. The filtrate includes but is not limited to bicarbonates (HCO_3), sodium, chloride, potassium, and water. HCO_3 does not readily cross the cellular membrane of the epithelial cells of the tubules. HCO_3 and hydrogen ion combine to form carbonic acid (H_2CO_3). H_2CO_3 dissociates to water and carbon dioxide in the presence of carbonic anhydrase. Carbon dioxide passes easily to the epithelial membrane of the tubule. Once inside the epithelial cell, it combines with water in the presence of carbonic

anhydrase to form H_2CO_3, which dissociates into hydrogen ion and bicarbonate. Carbonic anhydrase is an enzyme that catalyzes the dehydration of carbonic acid and hydration of CO_2. The hydrogen ions inside the epithelial cells are secreted to the lumen of tubules through the sodium-hydrogen countertransport mechanism. HCO_3 exits the epithelial cell via the sodium-bicarbonate symporter to the interstitial and then reabsorbs to the peritubular capillaries.

The descending loop of Henle continuously reabsorbs water. The solutes, such as sodium, stay inside the lumen. The filtrate then becomes too concentrated as it reaches the turn of the loop. When the filtrate reaches the thick ascending loop of Henle, sodium, potassium, and chloride are reabsorbed through the 1-sodium, 2-chloride, 1-potassium symporter. In contrast to the descending and thin ascending loop of Henle, the thick ascending loop of Henle is impermeable to water. The terminal end of the thick ascending loop of Henle marks the beginning of DCT. This point also serves as a location for macula densa. The macula densa is important in sensing sodium concentration in the tubule to initiate compensatory mechanism such as secretion of renin.

The DCT reabsorbs minimal sodium and water. Most of the sodium reabsorptions are facilitated by aldosterone, which stimulates the sodium-potassium pump to reabsorb sodium from the lumen and secrete potassium to the lumen.

The rest of the filtrate reaches the collecting duct system. Antidiuretic hormone stimulates the reabsorption of water at the collecting ducts. About 180 L of filtrate pass the nephron. Ninety-nine percent are reabsorbed. The rest of the filtrate, about 1 to 2 L/day, continues down the ureters to the bladder and finally to the urethra for excretion.

■ Diuretic Agents

Carbonic Anhydrase Inhibitor (Acetazolamide)

Carbonic anhydrase is present in high concentrations in the eyes, pancreas, intestines, red blood cells,[4] and PCT of kidneys. Carbonic anhydrase is an enzyme that catalyzes the reversible reaction of CO_2 and HCO_3, resulting in H_2CO_3. The carbonic anhydrase inhibitor blocks this reaction. Acetazolamide is a prototype of the carbonic anhydrase inhibitor.

Mechanism of Action

Acetazolamide inhibits the carbonic anhydrase present in high concentration at the PCT. As discussed above, carbonic anhydrase catalyzes the dehydration of carbonic acid at the lumen of tubules to form CO_2 and water. When CO_2

and water are in the epithelial cells, carbonic anhydrase catalyzes the hydration of CO_2 to form H_2CO_3. The H_2CO_3 in the cell dissociates to form hydrogen ion and HCO_3. The hydrogen ion is secreted to the lumen of the tubule through the sodium-hydrogen countertransport mechanism. HCO_3 is transported out of epithelial cells to the interstitium and is then reabsorbed in blood through the sodium bicarbonate symporter mechanism.

Because acetazolamide inhibits carbonic anhydrase, hydrogen ion stays in the epithelial cells of the tubules. The reabsorption of sodium is inhibited. HCO_3 reabsorption is also blocked. As a result the presence of sodium and HCO_3 in the lumen of the tubules prevents reabsorption of water, leading to diuresis.

Clinical Pharmacology

Pharmacokinetics

Acetazolamide is commonly administered orally and absorbed in the gastrointestinal (GI) tract. Its onset is between 30 minutes and 1 hour, and peak time is 2 hours. It is insoluble to lipid, and protein binding is more than 93%.[5] The kidneys are the main organs of excretion.

Pharmacodynamics

Acetazolamide causes excretion of sodium and HCO_3. The diuresis and alkalinization of urine are the result for excretion of these substances. However, the kidneys compensate by reabsorbing sodium chloride. With the depletion of HCO_3, there is an increased reabsorption of sodium chloride and retention of hydrogen ion; these lead to hyperchloremic acidosis. The HCO_3 depletion leads to significant decrease in the efficacy of acetazolamide after several days.

Clinical Uses and Indications

The major indication of acetazolamide is for treatment of open-angle glaucoma. Other indications include relief of edema through diuresis, treatment and prevention of mountain sickness, and epilepsy.

Comparative Pharmacology

Methazolamide, another carbonic anhydrase inhibitor, is more lipophilic than acetazolamide.[6] The onset of methazolamide is 1 to 2 hours longer than acetazolamide.[7]

Side Effects and Contraindications

The side effects of acetazolamide include metabolic hyperchloremic acidosis due to the reabsorption of sodium chloride and excretion of HCO_3; drowsiness and paresthesias that could be due to the metabolic acidosis; renal stones due to the formation of calcium salts in an alkaline urine; hypokalemia; hyperammonemia due to the decrease in secretion of hydrogen ion in the kidneys; and hypersensitivity to sulfa drugs.

Drug Interactions

Patients taking digoxin and droperidol may have increased risk of digitalis toxicity and QT prolongation, respectively, due to hypokalemia. There may be an increased concentration of phenytoin level in the blood. The alkaline urine produced by acetazolamide increases the reabsorption of un-ionized quinidine. Salicylates decrease the excretion of acetazolamide.

Guidelines and Precautions

Preoperative assessments include evaluation of electrolytes and acid–base balance, level of consciousness, and any paresthesias. The presence of hyperchloremic metabolic acidosis may limit the intraoperative use of normal saline solution and cisatracurium. Monitor the electrocardiogram for evidence of any QT prolongation.

Dosages

Adult

- Glaucoma: oral or intravenous, 250 to 1000 mg divided one to four times daily.[8]
- Edema: oral or intravenous, 250 to 375 mg once daily in morning for 1 or 2 days, alternating with day of rest.[8]
- Acute mountain sickness: oral, 500 to 1000 mg orally daily, divided two to four times a day.
  - During rapid ascent, 1000 mg/day is recommended.
  - Initiate 24 to 48 hours before ascent and continue for 48 hours or longer while at high altitude.[8]
- Epilepsy: oral or intravenous, 8 to 30 mg/kg daily, divided every 8 to 12 hours.[8]

Pediatric

- Glaucoma: oral, 8 to 30 mg/kg daily, divided every 6 to 8 hours.[9]
  - Intravenous, 5 to 10 mg/kg intravenously every 6 hours.[10]
- Epilepsy: oral, initial, 4 mg/kg daily; maintenance, 8 to 30 mg/kg daily, divided every 8 to 12 hours.[9]
- Acute mountain sickness: oral (12 years and older), 500 to 1000 mg once a day.
  - During rapid ascent, 1000 mg/day is recommended.
  - Initiate 24 to 48 hours before ascent and continue for 48 hours or longer while at high altitude.[9]

Loop Diuretics (Furosemide)

Mechanism of Action

Furosemide inhibits the sodium, potassium, and chloride symporter, resulting in decreased reabsorption of sodium, potassium, and chloride ions from the ascending thick loop of Henle. Furosemide also inhibits the feedback mechanism from macula densa, thereby increasing the glomerular filtration rate (GFR).[11] In addition, the GFR increases due to the increased production of the prostaglandins.[12]

Clinical Pharmacology

Pharmacokinetics

Furosemide taken by mouth is absorbed in the GI tract. Intravenous administration has a peak time of 5 to 20 minutes, whereas oral administration peaks at 1 to 1.5 hours.[8] It has a 93% protein binding.[13] Ten to 30% of furosemide is metabolized in the liver. The kidneys account for 60% to 90% of furosemide excretion. The bile and fecal route are the other avenues of excretion. Hemodialysis does not affect the excretion of furosemide.

Pharmacodynamics

As the sodium-potassium-chloride symporter is inhibited, sodium, potassium, and chloride ions are not reabsorbed from the thick ascending loop of Henle. An increased volume of water stays in the renal tubules, causing large amount of diuresis and excretion of potassium and sodium. Furosemide increases the synthesis of prostaglandins, which results in venous dilation from the peripheral circulation, thereby decreasing pulmonary and left ventricular congestion, and increased renal blood flow that increases GFR. In addition, the inhibition of the feedback mechanism of macula densa by furosemide[11] promotes increased GFR. Blood pressure is reduced because of a decreased extracellular volume. However, in the presence of normal fluid volume in the body, the reduction in blood pressure could be compensated by the response of the baroreceptors.

The chronic use of furosemide may lead to resistance. The resistance may be due to the compensatory actions of the distal tubule through the secretion of aldosterone or chronic reduction in extracellular volume.[7] The maintenance of adequate fluid volume or through the combination of thiazide and furosemide may prevent the resistance to furosemide.

Clinical Uses and Indications

Furosemide's effective diuresis and increased synthesis of the prostaglandins make it a commonly used drug for the treatment of pulmonary edema related to congestive heart failure. Hypercalcemia as a result of illnesses such as squamous cell carcinoma can be treated by furosemide. It is also used as an adjunct therapy for the treatment of hypertension. Intracranial pressure is reduced through the reduction of extracellular volume. Furosemide is used to treat hyperkalemia. Although it causes natriuresis, the treatment of hyponatremia includes a combination of fluid restriction and administration of normal saline and furosemide.

Comparative Pharmacology

Ethacrynic acid, torsemide, and bumetanide are the other three loop diuretics. Furosemide, torsemide, and bumetanide are sulfa derivatives. Ethacrynic acid is a phenoxyacetic acid derivative.[14] Bumetanide is the most potent loop diuretic. Bumetanide has a shorter half-life (60–90 minutes) than furosemide.[8] Torsemide is absorbed more rapidly in the GI tract than furosemide when given through the oral route. The duration of torsemide (6–8 hours) is longer than furosemide (2 hours) when administered intravenously.[8] Ethacrynic acid produces hypoglycemia with convulsions when given to uremic patients at a higher than recommended dose.[12]

Side Effects and Contraindications

A common side effect of furosemide is alteration in the fluid and electrolyte balance. The electrolyte imbalances include hypomagnesemia, hypokalemia, and hypochloremia. The excretion of hydrogen ion may result in metabolic alkalosis. Hypotension can result when a fluid deficit is present. Uric acid may increase, leading to the exacerbation of gout. A rapid or large administration of furosemide or concomitant use of drugs such as aminoglycoside antibiotics may produce ototoxicity.[15] Precaution is advised for patients with allergy to sulfonamide drugs. Furosemide is a Pregnancy Category C drug.

Drug Interactions

The administration of probenecid and indomethacin can reduce the effect of furosemide. Hypokalemia can increase digitalis toxicity for patients on digoxin. Increased risk of lithium toxicity may result with the administration of furosemide.[16]

Guidelines and Precautions

Furosemide is commonly administered perioperatively. Rapid administration should be avoided. The bolus intravenous administration is 4 mg/min. Review the electrolytes and electrocardiogram before surgery for patients on loop diuretics. The maintenance of fluid volume is necessary to avoid hypotension. Monitor for urine output, heart rhythm, and blood pressure when administering furosemide. Cranial surgeries most often necessitate a $PaCO_2$ of 25 to 30 mm Hg that promotes hypokalemia, and the administration of furosemide might further contribute to hypokalemia.

Dosages

Adult

- Edema: intravenous, initial dose of 20 to 40 mg may be repeated after 1 to 2 hours. Addition of 20 mg intravenously no sooner than 2 hours from the previous dose may increase effectiveness of the drug. Do not exceed more than 1000 mg/day.[10]
  - Maintenance dose: the minimum effective dose administered once or may be divided to be given twice a day.[10]
- Hypertension: oral, 80 mg/day, may be divided into 40 mg twice a day.[8]
- Hypercalcemia: intravenous, initial dose of 80 to 100 mg administered at 1- to 2-hour intervals. Administer the dose with normal saline solution.[10]
- Acute pulmonary edema: intravenous, initial dose of 40 mg, may increase to 80 mg if not effective.[10]
- Acute renal failure: intravenous, initial dose of 100 mg; do not exceed 1-g intravenous bolus dose. Larger doses require infusion. Highest total intravenous dose is 6 g.[10]

Pediatric

- Edema: intravenous, initial dose of 1 mg/kg, may be repeated after 2 hours. Adding 1 to 2 mg/kg from the previous dosage may increase effectiveness of the drug. Do not exceed more than 6 mg/kg per day.[8]

Thiazide Diuretics (Chlorothiazide)

Chlorothiazide was produced to prevent the excessive loss of sodium bicarbonate seen in carbonic anhydrase inhibitor use. It is a drug used to excrete sodium and chloride to promote extracellular volume loss without causing or minimally causing acid–base imbalances.

Mechanism of Action

Chlorothiazide is a sulfonamide derivative that inhibits the sodium-chloride symporter at the DCT. As a result, increased undiluted urine is excreted. The DCT normally prevents water reabsorption. Natriuresis is not as pronounced as in loop diuretics because most of the sodium is reabsorbed from the filtrate in the PCT and loop of Henle before reaching the DCT. Upon reaching the collecting duct, the secretion of aldosterone reabsorbs some of the sodium in exchange for potassium.

Clinical Pharmacology

Pharmacokinetics

Chlorothiazide is absorbed from the GI tract. When taken orally, diuresis starts in 2 hours.[8] Intravenous chlorothiazide produces diuresis promptly (15 minutes).[8] The oral form of chlorothiazide lasts 6 to 12 hours,[8] whereas the intravenous form lasts 2 hours. Oral administration has longer benefit from the drug. It is primarily excreted through the urine.

Pharmacodynamics

Chlorothiazide can be a primary drug or an adjunct drug for the treatment of hypertension through two mechanisms. First, it inhibits the sodium-chloride symporter at the DCT. As a result extracellular volume excretion is achieved. The same mechanism is behind the relief of edema. It is a weak inhibitor of carbonic anhydrase, which does not cause metabolic acidosis such as seen in carbonic anhydrase inhibitor. Second, by an unknown mechanism chlorothiazide relaxes peripheral vascular smooth muscle.[17]

Along with sodium excretion, magnesium is also excreted by an unknown mechanism. Chlorothiazide competes with the uric acid secretion at the PCT, thereby increasing the uric acid in the body. Because of the increased presence of sodium in the collecting duct, some sodium reabsorption takes place along with potassium secretion through the influence of aldosterone.

Clinical Uses and Indications

Chlorothiazide is used for the treatment of hypertension as well as mobilization of the excess extracellular fluid such as seen in congestive heart failure and nephrogenic diseases. The effectiveness of chlorothiazide depends on its presence in the lumen of tubules. Therefore its therapeutic action is decreased in patients with renal problems.

Comparative Pharmacology

Chlorothiazide is very similar to hydrochlorothiazide. Both are sulfonamides derivatives. All thiazide diuretics have a better absorption in the GI tract other than chlorothiazide. Hydrochlorothiazide is more potent than chlorothiazide,[8] and their duration of action is similar.[8] Chlorothiazide is a weak carbonic anhydrase inhibitor compared with acetazolamide.

Chlorthalidone, metolazone, and indapamide are pharmacologically similar to thiazides and thus are called thiazide-like or thiazide-related diuretics. Chlorthalidone, metolazone, and indapamide have a longer duration of action[8] than chlorothiazide. Thiazide-like derivatives do not inhibit carbonic anhydrase enzyme. All thiazides and thiazide-like derivatives produce similar benefits and side effects.

Side Effects and Contraindications

Electrolyte imbalances, which include hypokalemia, hypomagnesemia, hyponatremia, hypophosphatemia, and hypercalcemia, may result from the administration of chlorothiazide. Hypercalcemia may produce calcium nephrolithiasis. Hyperlipidemia,[18] hyperglycemia, and hyperuricemia occur with chronic administration of the drug.

Photosensitivity[19] and skin rash may develop. As a sulfonamide drug, side effects related to sulfonamides need to be addressed.

Drug Interactions

Increased risk of digitalis toxicity may develop due to hypokalemia. Lithium toxicity has been shown to develop due to decreased excretion of lithium in patients treated with thiazide and lithium. Decreased therapeutic effects of pressors such as amines are noticeable.[17] Hypotension may be observed during the administration of inhalational anesthetics, barbiturates, or narcotics. Hypokalemia might produce synergistic effects with the drugs promoting muscle paralysis.[20]

Guidelines and Precautions

Check electrolyte levels preoperatively, particularly when patients verbalize weakness. The optimal potassium level prevents dysrhythmias from patients on digitalis or with ischemic heart disease. Adequate fluid administration is necessary to prevent hypotension, especially during the administration of inhalational anesthetics, barbiturates, or narcotics. Caution in the administration of muscle paralytics is advised, particularly when the potassium level is unknown.

Dosages

Adult

- Edema: oral/intravenous, 0.5 to 1 g once or twice a day administered on alternate days.[8]
- Hypertension: oral, 0.5 to 1 g/day, may be given in four divided doses.[8]

Pediatric

- Edema/hypertension: oral, 10 to 20 mg/kg per day, may be given in two divided doses.
  - Maximum dosage of 375 mg/day for infants and 1 g/day for children older than 2 years old is recommended.[8]

Osmotic Diuretics (Mannitol)

Osmotic diuretics produce diuresis through the osmotic property of the drug, which makes it different from other diuretics. Mannitol is used widely as an osmotic diuretic due to its availability and efficiency.

Mechanism of Action

Mannitol is freely filtered through the glomerulus. The osmotic pressure that the drug exerts prevents the reabsorption of water mainly from the PCT and descending loop of Henle. The reabsorption of mannitol from the tubules is very minimal. A large volume of water is then excreted. By mechanisms not clearly understood, mannitol reduces oxygen free radicals.[21]

Clinical Pharmacology

Pharmacokinetics

Mannitol is poorly absorbed in the GI system, so it is only administered intravenously. The metabolism of mannitol is very minimal; hence 80%[8] can be recovered from the urine. Mannitol is excreted within 30 to 60 minutes.

Pharmacodynamics

Upon intravenous administration of mannitol, it immediately exerts osmotic pressure intravascularly, causing an increase in the extracellular volume. The increase in extracellular volume causes hyponatremia initially. Its osmotic property increases the amount of filtrate in the tubules, particularly at the PCT and descending loop of Henle. The larger amount of filtrate in the tubules means lesser contact of electrolytes such as sodium to the lumen of the tubules, causing minimal natriuresis but larger diuresis. However, the large diuresis can later cause hypovolemia, which can lead to hypernatremia.

Clinical Uses and Indications

Mannitol is used to treat increased intracranial pressure by decreasing the formation rate of cerebrospinal fluid and decreasing the intracranial volume through reduction of the brain tissue water content.[22] It is used to reduce intraocular pressure through its hypotensive effect or contraction of vitreous.[23] It is used to prevent or treat oliguria during acute renal failure through diuresis.[24] Furthermore, the diuresis produced by mannitol excretes the toxins from overdose of drugs or pigments from hemolysis that can cause renal damage. Mannitol is also used in surgical procedures such as cardiovascular surgery to prevent renal failure or to reduce excess extracellular volume. Mannitol is also used in transurethral surgeries as irrigation.

Comparative Pharmacology

Other osmotic diuretics include sterile urea, glycerin, and isosorbide. Glycerin and isosorbide are taken orally and have a faster onset (10–30 minutes).[8] The peak times of all four drugs are almost similar (60–90 minutes).[8] Glycerin is metabolized the most (80%) and has the shortest half-life (30–45 minutes).[8]

Side Effects and Contraindications

The increased extracellular volume causes the exacerbation of pulmonary edema or congestive heart failure. Mannitol is contraindicated in patients with advanced renal failure with anuria, dehydration, and presence of intracranial hemorrhage without surgical intervention. Hyponatremia is produced initially and then later hypernatremia that results from hypovolemia. Skin irritation and thrombophlebitis may occur when the intravenous site is infiltrated. The intravenous infiltration of 50 g mannitol can pull 1 L of fluid from intracellular to extracellular compartment.[25] Treatment of extravasation of mannitol includes the subcutaneous infiltration along the affected site's edges with hyaluronidase (diluted with normal saline or 1% lidocaine to a concentration of 10–15 units/mL) for a total dose of 150 to 900 units.[25] A fasciotomy may be indicated for the higher severity of extravasation. A larger vein and smaller gauge needle can prevent venous irritation.

Drug Interactions

Increased risk of digitalis toxicity may develop due to hypokalemia. A decreased therapeutic effect of lithium is due to its increased excretion.

Guidelines and Precautions

The administration of mannitol, with equal or greater than 20% concentration, needs a filter set to prevent infusion of crystallized mannitol. Mannitol should be stored at room temperature because cold temperature crystallizes the drug. A white precipitate during infusion is a sign to stop the infusion and use a different intravenous line. Blood and mannitol combined may form clumps or agglomerates.

A test dose is necessary when mannitol is used in patients with renal problems. A test dose is initiated using 0.2 g/kg over 3 to 5 minutes. A urine flow of 30 to 50 mL/h is assessed within 2 to 3 hours. If this is not attained, a second dose may be administered. Do not attempt to administer more than two test doses. The rate of administration depends on the production of 30 to 50 mL of urine per 1 hour.

Dosages

- Reduction of cerebral edema, intracranial pressure, and intraocular pressure: intravenous, 1.5 to 2 g/kg in 30 to 60 minutes.[8]
- Oliguria: intravenous, 50 to 100 g as 5% to 25% solution.[8]
- Hemolytic transfusion reaction: intravenous, 20 g over 5 minutes, may repeat same dose if no diuresis resulted from the initial dose.[8]

Potassium-Sparing Diuretics (Spironolactone)

Spironolactone, eplerenone, amiloride, and triamterene are the most commonly used potassium-sparing diuretics. Two classes of potassium-sparing diuretics exist. Spironolactone and eplerenone are aldosterone antagonists, whereas amiloride and triamterene block the sodium transportation channels. All these diuretics act on the DCT and collecting ducts.

Mechanism of Action

Spironolactone is a synthetic steroid that competes with aldosterone at the receptor sites, resulting in sodium retention in the tubules and decreased secretion of potassium to the tubules. Most of the sodium reabsorption takes place at the PCT and loop of Henle. Therefore, the diuretic effect of spironolactone is less than other previously discussed diuretics. However, spironolactone is an effective diuretic in patients with primary or secondary hyperaldosteronism. The examples of secondary hyperaldosteronism are nephrotic syndrome, congestive heart failure, and liver cirrhosis. The mechanism of action differs from amiloride and triamterene because their actions are not affected by the presence of aldosterone. In contrast to spironolactone, they block the sodium transportation channels such as the sodium-hydrogen or sodium-potassium channels.

Clinical Pharmacology

Pharmacokinetics

Spironolactone is very well absorbed from the GI tract. Food intake facilitates the absorption in the GI tract. It is extensively metabolized in the liver, producing an active metabolite, canrenone. The onset of spironolactone takes days, and its half-life is 20 hours.[8]

Pharmacology

Spironolactone inhibits the actions of aldosterone at the DCT that results in the reabsorption of sodium and inhibition of potassium secretion. Hyperaldosteronism produces edema, which is the rationale for using this drug. The diuretic effect, though weak, may treat mild to moderate hypertension with or without hyperaldosteronism. The inhibition of potassium secretion prevents potassium loss but may produce hyperkalemia.

Clinical Uses and Indications

Spironolactone is used to diagnose and treat primary hyperaldosteronism. Presumptive diagnosis of primary hyperaldosteronism is confirmed when the discontinuation of spironolactone produces an increase in potassium and/or increase in blood pressure. The short-term therapy in primary hyperaldosteronism is indicated when a patient is a good candidate for surgical intervention. Spironolactone also is used as an adjunct treatment for mild to moderate essential hypertension and in the treatment of hypokalemia. Because of its weak diuretic effect and potassium-sparing properties, it is commonly combined with thiazide or loop diuretics to enhance diuresis and prevent hypokalemia.

Comparative Pharmacology

Spironolactone is the slowest in onset among the potassium-sparing diuretics (1–2 days).[8] It has the longest duration (up to 3 days) compared with amiloride and triamterene (≤ 24 hours).[8] Amiloride is not metabolized in the liver; therefore no metabolite exists. The active metabolite of triamterene is hydroxytriamterene. Triamterene may produce blue-colored urine.

Side Effects and Contraindications

Hyperkalemia may be observed due to the inhibition of secretion of potassium at the DCT. Spironolactone is not recommended in conditions associated with hyperkalemia,

such as significant impairment of kidney functions. The deficit in hydration that results from the use of spironolactone may produce central nervous system effects such as confusion and lethargy. Spironolactone has been associated with carcinogenesis in animals.[26] Gynecomastia is associated with use of spironolactone by altering the peripheral metabolism of testosterone, resulting in changes in the ratio of testosterone to estradiol.[27] The discontinuation of spironolactone resolves gynecomastia. Agranulocytosis, although rare, may develop with the use of spironolactone.[28]

Drug Interactions

Hyperkalemia may result with concomitant use of potassium supplements, angiotensin-converting enzyme inhibitors, angiotensin receptor antagonists, and indomethacin. Narcotic analgesic and barbiturates may increase the hypotensive effect of spironolactone. Nonsteroidal anti-inflammatory drugs, such as indomethacin and salicylates, and digoxin may reduce the therapeutic effect of spironolactone. Lithium toxicity can result with the use of any diuretic such as spironolactone due to decreased lithium excretion.

Guidelines and Precautions

Patients are instructed to protect the medicine from sunlight. Just like with any other diuretic, check the electrolytes and electrocardiogram preoperatively. The administration of packed red blood cells and succinylcholine may increase the potassium level, which makes it imperative to preoperatively check the potassium level. The regional and general anesthetics can exacerbate the hypotensive effects of spironolactone.

Dosages

- Edema: oral, initial dose 25 to 200 mg/day in single or divided doses. It should be continued for 5 days when administered as a sole agent for diuresis. Adjust dose for maintenance according to therapeutic effect.[8]
- Hypertension: oral, initial dose 50 to 100 mg/day in single or divided doses. It should be continued for 2 weeks to achieve therapeutic effect and then adjusted for maintenance dose depending on therapeutic effect.[8]
- Hirsutism in women: oral, 50 to 200 mg/day in one to two divided doses.[8]

- Primary aldosteronism test: oral.
  - Short test: 400 mg for 4 days. Primary hyperaldosteronism is presumptively diagnosed when the blood potassium level increases during therapy and then decreases upon discontinuation.[8]
  - Long test: 400 mg for 3 to 4 weeks. Presumptive diagnosis of primary aldosteronism is given when normal blood pressure and blood potassium level are achieved.[8]

Anesthetic Implications

Diuretics are mainly used to excrete water from the body. The balance of electrolytes such as sodium, magnesium, calcium, and potassium are affected. Common side effects from the diuretics are hypotension and electrolyte imbalances. It is imperative to perioperatively maintain optimal electrolyte levels and blood pressure. Electrolyte imbalances such as hyperkalemia may promote metabolic acidosis that might affect the duration of neuromuscular-blocking agents such as cisatracurium. Hypokalemia as a result of chronic diuretic use except the potassium-sparing diuretics may decrease the dose of neuromuscular drugs such as pancuronium and increase the dose of neostigmine.[20] However, acute hypokalemia does not affect dose requirement for nondepolarizing neuromuscular-blocking drugs.[29] The furosemide dose either antagonizes or potentiates the nondepolarizing neuromuscular-blocking drugs.[29] A furosemide dose of greater than 100 μm/kg inhibits phosphodiesterase, which results in an increase in cAMP, which increases muscle contraction thereby antagonizing the nondepolarizing neuromuscular-blocking dugs.[29] In contrast to a higher dose of furosemide, a lower dose (less than 100 μm/kg) potentiates nondepolarizing neuromuscular-blocking drugs by blocking a protein kinase that results in decreased influx of calcium at the motor nerve ending.[29] Vigilance in the rate of intravenous bolus administration of furosemide and mannitol will avoid further complications such as ototoxicity for furosemide. A summary of diuretics discussed in this chapter is presented in Table 16-1.

Table 16-1 Summary of Diuretics

Diuretic Drug	Mechanism of Action	Major Site of Action	Indications	Anesthetic Implications
Carbonic anhydrase inhibitor (acetazolamide)	Inhibits the carbonic anhydrase, which is an enzyme that catalyzes the reversible reaction of CO_2 and HCO_3 resulting in H_2CO_3	PCT	Open-angle glaucoma, edema, treatment and prevention of mountain sickness, and epilepsy	Evaluation of electrolytes and acid–base balance. May interfere with neuromuscular drugs.
Thiazide diuretics (chlorothiazide)	Inhibits the sodium-chloride symporter	DCT	Hypertension and edema	Check electrolyte levels, particularly potassium. May interfere with neuromuscular drugs.
Loop diuretics (furosemide)	Inhibits the sodium, potassium, and chloride symporter	Thick ascending loop of Henle	Pulmonary edema, hypertension, hypercalcemia, and reduction of intracranial pressure	Check for electrolyte imbalances, blood pressure, and urine output. Bolus intravenous dose is 4 mg/min.
Osmotic diuretics (mannitol)	Exerts osmotic pressure that prevents the reabsorption of water	PCT and descending loop of Henle	Reduction of cerebral edema, intracranial pressure, and intraocular pressure; oliguria; and hemolytic transfusion reaction	Check for electrolyte imbalances, blood pressure, and intravenous infiltration; use filter with administration.
Potassium-sparing diuretics (spironolactone)	Competes with aldosterone at the receptor sites	DCT	Edema, hypertension, hirsutism, and diagnosis of primary aldosteronism	Check electrolytes, particularly potassium.

Key Points

- The urinary system consists of two kidneys, two ureters, a urinary bladder, and a urethra. The kidneys have three regions: the cortical, medullary, and renal pelvic regions. The cortical region is the outer region of the kidneys. The medullary region is the inner region of the kidneys that contains the pyramids. The pyramids are composed of long loops of Henle, medullary collecting ducts, and collecting tubules.
- The kidneys are known to excrete body wastes, pharmacologic metabolites, and excess water and electrolytes. Several other functions of the kidneys are maintenance of acid–base balance; production of erythropoietin, renin, and calcitriol, which is the active form of vitamin D; regulation of arterial blood pressure; and maintenance of the blood glucose through gluconeogenesis.
- The kidneys receive about 22% of cardiac output. Their blood supply comes from the aorta through the renal arteries.
- The difference between the hydrostatic pressure and oncotic pressure in the glomerulus and the capsular hydrostatic pressure at the Bowman's capsule pushes the filtrate to reach the Bowman's capsule. Reabsorption and secretion are continuous throughout the different tubules. The rest of the filtrate, about 1 to 2 L/day, continues down the ureters to the bladder and finally to the urethra for excretion.
- The carbonic anhydrase inhibitor blocks the carbonic anhydrase from catalyzing the dehydration of carbonic acid at the lumen of tubules to form CO_2 and water. The side effects of acetazolamide include metabolic hyperchloremic acidosis due to the reabsorption of sodium chloride and excretion of HCO_3.
- Furosemide inhibits the sodium, potassium, and chloride symporter, resulting in decreased reabsorption of sodium, potassium, and chloride ions from the ascending thick loop of Henle. The bolus intravenous administration is 4 mg/min.
- Osmotic diuretics produce diuresis through the osmotic property of the drug, which makes it different from other diuretics.
- Mannitol is contraindicated in patients with advanced renal failure with anuria, dehydration, and presence of intracranial hemorrhage without surgical intervention.
- The administration of mannitol, with equal or greater than 20% concentration, needs a filter set to prevent infusion of crystallized mannitol. Mannitol should be stored at room temperature because cold temperature crystallizes the drug.
- The intravenous infiltration of 50 g mannitol can pull 1 L of fluid from intracellular to extracellular compartment.
- Spironolactone is not recommended in conditions associated with hyperkalemia, such as significant impairment of kidney functions.
- It is imperative to perioperatively maintain optimal electrolyte levels and blood pressure.
- Hypokalemia as a result of chronic diuretic use, except the potassium-sparing diuretics, may decrease the dose of neuromuscular drugs such as pancuronium and increase the dose of neostigmine.[20] However, acute hypokalemia does not affect dose requirement for nondepolarizing neuromuscular-blocking drugs.

Chapter Questions

1. Why is diuresis lesser for diuretics acting on anatomic structures past the ascending loop of Henle?
2. How does hypokalemia affect the management of anesthesia?
3. The surgeon asked an anesthesia provider to administer 1 g/kg mannitol to the patient. How fast can the anesthesia provider administer the mannitol?

References

1. *Webster's Third New International Dictionary of English Unabridged.* Springfield, MA: Merriam Webster; 1981:682.
2. Guyton AC, Hall JE. *Textbook of Medical Physiology,* 10th ed. Philadelphia: W.B. Saunders; 2000:279–294.
3. Copstead LC, Banasik JL. *Pathophysiology: Biological and Behavioral Perspectives,* 2nd ed. Philadelphia: W.B. Saunders; 2000:625–648.
4. Sly WS, Hu PY. Human carbonic anhydrases and carbonic anhydrases deficiencies. *Annu Rev Biochem.* 1995;64:375–401.
5. Ellis PP, Price PK, Kelmenson R, Rendi MA. Effectiveness of generic acetazolamide. *Arch Ophthalmol.* 1982; 100:1920–1922.
6. Teppema LJ, Bijl H, Gourabi BM, Dahan A. The carbonic anhydrase inhibitors methazolamide and acetazolamide have different effects on the hypoxic ventilatory response in the anaesthetized cat. *J Physiol.* 2006;574:565–572.

7. Wecker L, Crespor LM, Dunaway G, Faingold C, Watts S. *Brody's Human Pharmacology: Molecular to Clinical,* 5th ed. Philadelphia: Mosby Elsevier; 2010:226–241.

8. *Drug Facts and Comparisons.* St. Louis, MO: Wolters Kluwer Health; 2009:921–948.

9. Lacy CF, Armstrong LL, Goldmann MP, Lance LL. *Drug Information Handbook: A Comprehensive Resource for All Clinicians and Healthcare Professionals,* 17th ed. Hudson: Lexi-Comp; 2008.

10. Gahatt BL, Nazareno AR. *Intravenous Medications: A Handbook for Nurses and Health Professionals,* 25th ed. St. Louis, MO: Mosby Elsevier; 2009.

11. Schattler E. The tubuloglomerular feedback mechanism is inhibited by diuretics such as furosemide. Effect of various diuretics on membrane voltage of macula densa cells. *Pflügers Arch Eur J Physiol.* 1993;423:74–77.

12. Johnston GD, Hiatt WR, Nies AS, et al. Factors modifying the early nondiuretic vascular effects of furosemide in man: the possible role of renal prostaglandins. *Circ Res.* 1983;53:630–635.

13. Forrey AW, Kimpel B, Blair AD, Cutler RE. Furosemide concentrations in serum and urine, and its binding by serum proteins as measured fluorometrically. *Clin Chem.* 1974;20:152–158.

14. Ives HE. Diuretics. In: Katzung B, ed. *Pharmacology,* 10th ed. New York: McGraw-Hill; 2007:236–253.

15. Ho KM, Sheridan DJ. Meta-analysis of furosemide to prevent or treat acute renal failure. *BMJ.* 2006;333:420.

16. Reyes JL, Aldana I, Barbier O, Parralles AA, Melendez E. Indomethacin decreases furosemide-induced natriuresis and diuresis on the neonatal kidney. *Pediatr Nephrol.* 2006; 21:1690–1697.

17. Stier CT Jr. Diuretics. In: DiPalma JR, DiGregorio GJ, Barbieri EJ, Ferko AP, eds. *Basic Pharmacology in Medicine,* 4th ed. West Chester, PA: Medical Surveillance; 1994:455–467.

18. Chrysant SG, Neller GK, Dillard B, Frohlich ED. Effects of diuretics on lipid metabolism in patients with essential hypertension. *Angiology.* 1976;27:707–711.

19. Johnston GA. Thiazide-induced lichenoid photosensitivity. *Clin Exp Dermatol.* 2002;27:670–672.

20. Miller RD, Roderick LL. Diuretic-induced hypokalemia, pancuronium neuromuscular blockade and its antagonism by neostigmine. *BMJ.* 1978;50:541–544.

21. Scott JA, Khaw BA, Locke E, Haber E, Homey C. The role of free radical-mediated processes in oxygen-related damage in cultured murine myocardial cells. *Circ Res.* 1985; 56:72–77.

22. Donato T, Shapira Y, Artru A, Powers K. Effect of mannitol on cerebrospinal fluid dynamics and brain tissue edema. *Anesth Analg.* 1994;78:58–66.

23. Mauger TF, Nye CN, Boyle KA. Intraocular pressure, anterior chamber depth and axial length following intravenous mannitol. *J Ocular Pharmacol Therap.* 2000;16:591–594.

24. Eneas JF, Schoenfeld PY, Humphreys MH. The effect of infusion of mannitol-sodium bicarbonate on the clinical course of myoglobinuria. *Arch Intern Med.* 1979;139:801–805.

25. Kumar MM, Sprung J. The use of hyaluronidase to treat mannitol extravasation. *Anesth Analg.* 2003;97:1199–1200.

26. Marselos M, Vainio H. Carcinogenic properties of pharmaceutical agents evaluated in the IARC monographs programme. *Carcinogenesis.* 1991;12:1751–1766.

27. Rose LI, Underwood R, Newmark SR, Kisch ES, Williams GH. Pathophysiology of spironolactone-induced gynecomastia. *Ann Intern Med.* 1977;87:398–403.

28. Ibañez L, Vidal X, Ballarín E, Laporte JR. Population-based drug-induced agranulocytosis. *Arch Intern Med.* 2005;165:869–874.

29. Azar I, Cotrell J, Gupta B, Turndorf H. Furosemide facilitates recovery of evoked twitch response after pancuronium. *Anesth Analg.* 1980;59:55–57.

Antihypertensive Drugs

Sandra M. Ouellette, MEd, CRNA, FAAN

Objectives

After completing this chapter, the reader should be able to

- Classify antihypertensive drugs by primary site or mechanism of action.
- List and discuss practical uses for α₂ agonists used in anesthesia.
- Identify drugs classified as adrenergic neuronal blockers, and describe contraindications to their use.
- List and discuss major contraindications to β-adrenergic receptor antagonists.
- Describe mechanisms associated with adverse effects in acute withdrawal from β-adrenergic receptor antagonists.
- Compare mechanism of action of labetalol with other α- and β-adrenergic antagonists used in the perioperative period.
- Identify the first approved intravenous dihydropyridine calcium channel blocker, and discuss its perioperative use.
- Describe the physiologic effects of the renin angiotensin system, and discuss its role in hypertension.
- Describe adverse effects of angiotensin II receptor inhibition.
- Identify three drugs classified as arterial vasodilators; list major advantages and disadvantages of these drugs.
- Compare nitroglycerin with nitroprusside in mechanisms of action, indications, and adverse effects.
- Describe mechanism of action of fenoldopam; list and discuss advantages and disadvantages associated with its use.
- Identify signs and symptoms associated with cyanide toxicity associated with the use of nitroprusside; develop a treatment plan for this adverse drug effect.
- Describe the etiology of perioperative hypertension, and identify common drugs used for treatment perioperatively.
- Discuss advantages, disadvantages, and overall effectiveness of drugs commonly used to manage perioperative hypertension.

Introduction

The prevalence of high blood pressure in the Unites States continues to increase, and it is now estimated that 73 million individuals have chronic hypertension.[1] It is estimated that 16% of these patients are undiagnosed, 27% are untreated, and 45% are uncontrolled.[2] Chronic hypertension is the most common cardiovascular disease encountered in the United States, and these patients present a challenge to the anesthetist.

Many of these patients receive one or more antihypertensive drugs preoperatively, and side effects associated with these drugs should be appreciated. In addition, perioperative hypertensive emergencies may be encountered in this patient population, and complications associated with acute hypertension and treatment options must be appreciated by anesthetists.

This chapter discusses six classes of antihypertensive drugs: sympatholytics, calcium channel blockers, angiotensin-converting enzyme inhibitors, angiotensin II receptor antagonists, adrenergic antagonists, and vasodilators. Mechanisms of action of each drug class and common drugs found in each class are discussed. The class prototype drug is fully discussed, and others in the class are then compared in regard to pharmacokinetic and pharmacodynamic profiles as well as advantages, disadvantages, side effects, and anesthetic implications. This chapter ends with a discussion of acute perioperative hypertension and its management.

Mechanisms of Action of Antihypertensive Drugs

Hypertension is defined in adults as a systemic blood pressure persistently elevated above 140 mm Hg, 90 mm Hg diastolic, or both.[3] Hypertension is divided into two types: primary and secondary. Primary hypertension accounts for approximately 95% of all cases. Although the etiology is poorly understood, a number of mechanisms alone or in combination seem to play a role in its development. The renin-angiotensin-aldosterone system and mechanisms controlling sodium excretion are implicated. The renin-angiotensin-aldosterone system is generally activated in response to low renal perfusion states, decreased sodium delivery to the distal nephron, or sympathetic stimulation.

Activation of this system results in renal retention of sodium and water and excretion of potassium, which is exchanged for sodium in the distal tubule. Hypertension that can be explained by a specific disease entity is termed secondary hypertension. Some typical causes of secondary hypertension include renovascular disease, aldosteronism, pheochromocytoma, coarctation of the aorta, renal artery stenosis, and renal failure. Pheochromocytoma, coarctation of the aorta, and renal artery stenosis are considered surgically correctable forms of hypertension.

Table 17-1 classifies antihypertensive drugs by their primary site of action. Examples of major drugs found in each class are listed in tables throughout the chapter and their pharmacologic properties explored. Common side effects as well as pertinent issues related to their use in the surgical patient are highlighted.

Table 17-1 Classification of Antihypertensives by Primary Site or by Mechanism of Action

Sympatholytics	Mechanism of Action
Centrally acting	Centrally acting α_2-adrenergic receptor agonist
Adrenergic neuron	Peripheral-acting adrenergic blocker
Blockers	
α-Adrenergic	α-Adrenergic receptor antagonist
Antagonists	
β-Adrenergic	β-Adrenergic receptor antagonist
Mixed adrenergic	α- and β-adrenergic antagonist
Calcium channel blockers	Modulates the influx of calcium in arterial smooth muscle and/or myocardial cells
ACE inhibitors	Competitive inhibitor of ACE, decreasing formation of angiotensin II
Angiotensin II receptor	Angiotensin II receptor antagonist and reduces aldosterone
Vasodilators	Peripheral vasodilators affecting the arterial, venous, or both arterial and venous circulation

ACE, angiotensin-converting enzyme.

Sympatholytics

Sympatholytics represent a class of antihypertensives that depress the sympathetic nervous system by several different mechanisms. This broad class of antihypertensives is divided into five subtypes according to their mechanism of action: centrally acting sympatholytics, adrenergic neuron blockers, α-adrenergic receptor antagonists, β-adrenergic receptor antagonists, and mixed adrenergic receptor antagonists.

Centrally Acting Sympatholytics

Methyldopa (Aldomet) stimulates central α-adrenergic receptors by formation of a false neurotransmitter that results in decreased sympathetic outflow to the heart, kidneys, and peripheral vasculature. It is used for the treatment of essential hypertension, especially pregnancy-induced hypertension. Although it crosses the placenta, it appears to be safe in pregnancy and lactation.

Central nervous system (CNS) effects of methyldopa include sedation, headache, dizziness, and decreased mental acuity. It lowers heart rate, blood pressure, and systemic vascular resistance. Patients may have dry mouth, diarrhea, nausea, and vomiting. Miscellaneous side effects include positive Coombs test, hemolytic anemia, bone marrow depression, impotence, rash, and increased liver function tests and renal function tests.

Guanabenz Acetate (Wytensin)

Guanabenz acetate is also a centrally acting α_2-adrenergic agonist. It lowers blood pressure primarily by stimulating central α receptors, which leads to inhibition of sympathetic outflow from the brain. It has no effect on potassium levels and does not cause sodium to be excreted or retained.

Like methyldopa, guanabenz may cause headache, dizziness, and drowsiness. Like other centrally acting sympatholytics, it may cause dry mouth and lower heart rate, blood pressure, and systemic vascular resistance. In addition to serving as an antihypertensive, it has been used for opioid withdrawal syndrome. Its central effect causes it to possess both anesthetic and analgesic-sparing effects.

Guanfacine Hydrochloride (Tenex)

Guanfacine acts in a similar fashion to other central sympatholytics. In the cerebral cortex, stimulation of α_2-adrenergic receptors triggers inhibitory neurons to reduce sympathetic outflow to the heart and blood vessels. This results in decreased peripheral vascular resistance and a slight reduction in heart rate. Cardiac output is not altered by the drug.

Major side effects associated with use of guanfacine include dry mouth, sedation, dizziness, somnolence, fatigue, and confusion. It reduces heart rate, blood pressure, and systemic vascular resistance. Acute withdrawal of the drug may result in rebound hypertension. Pharmacologic effectiveness is antagonized in patients who receive naloxone. The antihypertensive effects are also reduced in patients receiving estrogens, nonsteroidal anti-inflammatory drugs, and tricyclic antidepressants.

Clonidine (Catapres, Dixarit, Duraclon)

Clonidine is a centrally acting antiadrenergic agent that also stimulates α_2-adrenergic receptors in the CNS. This inhibits sympathetic vasomotor centers and lowers systolic and diastolic blood pressure and heart rate. The central action also reduces plasma concentrations of norepinephrine and inhibits renin release from the kidneys. Practical uses for α_2 agonists in anesthesia are listed in Box 17-1.

The ratio of α_2-to-α_1 effect with clonidine is 220:1. It is rapidly and almost completely absorbed after oral administration and reaches a peak plasma level within 60 to 90 minutes. Clonidine can also be delivered through a time-release transdermal patch. By this route a minimum of 2 days is required to reach therapeutic plasma concentrations. The elimination half-life of clonidine is 9 to 12 hours. Approximately one-half of the drug is metabolized in the liver to inactive metabolites, and the rest is excreted unchanged in the urine.

Clonidine has been used as an antihypertensive agent for over two decades. It is useful for hypertension of various

---

- Premedication
- Sedation
- Anesthetic sparing effect
- Regional anesthesia
- Intrathecal administration
- Epidural administration
- Caudal administration
- Peripheral nerve block
- Postoperative analgesia
- Analgesia for labor
- Treatment of chronic pain
- Prevention or treatment of drug withdrawal
- Prevention or treatment of postoperative shivering

---

etiologies (renal, renovascular), and the incidence of serious side effects is low. Dry mouth and sedation occur, but these side effects diminish with continued use. A modest reduction in heart rate is noted, but symptomatic bradycardia or orthostatic hypotension is not generally seen. A withdrawal syndrome may be seen with sudden discontinuation of therapy after a prolonged period. Withdrawal results in dangerous hypertension secondary to increased sympathetic nervous system activity.

Other manifestations of withdrawal include tachycardia, restlessness, insomnia, headache, and nausea. It takes 6 days of therapy to produce the adaptive changes necessary to elicit clonidine withdrawal. It is the most serious side effect associated with use of α_2 agonists.[4]

Clonidine has also been used in the treatment of patients with chronic stable angina pectoris and in those with acute myocardial infarction complicated by systemic hypertension. It has been shown to decrease myocardial ischemia, infarction, and mortality after cardiovascular surgery. The decrease in overall mortality associated with clonidine is superior to that observed with beta-blockers, and clonidine has been found to reduce the incidence of postoperative mortality for the first 2 years after surgery.[5]

Central effects of clonidine make it a useful agent in the pharmacologic management of a number of psychiatric disorders. It reduces the physiologic signs of opiate withdrawal and has been a mainstay in the management of acute detoxification from opiate addiction. It is useful in reducing the hyperadrenergic response associated with drug withdrawal from benzodiazepines and alcohol. Other disorders managed with clonidine include anxiety syndromes, memory disorders, spasticity, and chronic pain states. It has been useful in management of anxiety and panic attacks, manic symptoms, and hyperactivity in children. Memory impairment and memory disorders associated with Korsakoff's psychosis are effectively treated with low-dose clonidine. Spasticity of the lower extremities associated with multiple sclerosis and hyperactive reflexes associated with spinal cord injury respond to treatment with α_2 agonists such as clonidine.

In addition to a positive effect on blood pressure, premedication with 3 μg/kg clonidine reduced propofol and thiopental requirements by 30% to 35%.[6] Watanabe et al.[7] evaluated whether oral clonidine (150–300 μg) premedication is an alternative to N_2O in terms of shortening induction time and attenuating the adrenergic response to tracheal intubation during inhalation induction with sevoflurane. The premedication was given 90 minutes before induction, and patients were anesthetized with a triple deep breath with either 5% sevoflurane or 60% N_2O and 5% sevoflurane. Induction times were shorter and increases in mean arterial pressure and heart rate after tracheal intubation were less in those who received either dose of clonidine. Anesthesia was smoother in those who received clonidine versus N_2O with sevoflurane without clonidine.[7]

α_2 Agonists have been used to supplement regional blocks. Dannelli et al.[8] evaluated the effects of adding 50 μg clonidine to 150 mg ropivacaine for superficial cervical plexus block in patients undergoing elective carotid endarterectomy. They found adding clonidine to ropivacaine shortened the onset time and improved the quality of anesthesia. The first postoperative analgesia requirement occurred after 17 hours in the group receiving ropivacaine alone and 20 hours in the ropivacaine–clonidine group.[8] Dexmedetomidine (Precedex) is a selective α_2-receptor agonist with sedative properties. With an affinity for α_2 to α_1 blockade of 1620:1, it has eight times greater affinity for α_2 receptors than clonidine. After intravenous (IV) administration, there is a rapid distribution phase with a distribution half-life of 6 minutes. The terminal elimination half-life is approximately 2 hours. Dexmedetomidine undergoes complete biotransformation with very little unchanged drug excreted in the urine. It is possible that metabolites may accumulate after long-term infusion in patients with impaired renal function. Dexmedetomidine may impair the metabolism of alfentanil. Table 17-2 compares the pharmacologic characteristics of clonidine and dexmedetomidine, a newer α_2 agonist.

Although not typically used solely as an antihypertensive, dexmedetomidine does have multiple uses in the perioperative period, and its potent central effect and sedation may prevent hypertension in the surgical patient. The drug has been used effectively in both pediatric and adult patients. Box 17-2 lists safety precautions in the use of dexmedetomidine. Tables 17-3a and 17-3b compare pharmacologic characteristics of major α-adrenergic agonists, including clonidine.

Table 17-2 Pharmacologic Comparisons of α_2 Agonists

Clonidine	Dexmedetomidine
Half-life 8 h	Half-life 2 h
Administered epidurally, by patch or by epidural route	Administered intravenously
An antihypertensive	A sedative-analgesic
An analgesic adjunct	Primary action is sedation
IV formulation not available	Only IV α_2 agonist available in United States

IV, intravenous.

Adrenergic Neuronal Blockers

Adrenergic neuronal blockers inhibit the function of peripheral postganglionic adrenergic neurons. Guanadrel, reserpine, and metyrosine are antihypertensive agents found in this class of sympatholytics. The pharmacokinetic profile of adrenergic neuronal blockers is found in Tables 17-4a and 17-4b.

Guanadrel (Hylorel) is a peripheral-acting adrenergic blocker. It is an adrenergic ganglionic blocking agent pharmacologically related to guanethidine. It blocks the release of norepinephrine from the adrenal medulla and adrenergic nerve endings that normally occurs with stimulation of the sympathetic nervous system. It acts as an exogenous false neurotransmitter that is accumulated, stored, and released like norepinephrine but is inactive at adrenergic receptors. When given intravenously it causes increased

---

Box 17-2 Safety Precautions for Use of Dexmedetomidine (Precedex)

- Exercise caution when administering to patients with advanced heart block or severe ventricular dysfunction.
- Significant episodes of bradycardia and sinus arrest are possible in patients with high vagal tone or after rapid bolus administration of the drug.
- Less than 1% of patients experience respiratory adverse events with continuous IV infusion in the ICU.
- Administration by continuous infusion should not exceed 24 hours.
- There is reduced need for morphine in patients treated with Precedex.
- The most frequent adverse effects include:
  - Hypotension
  - Hypertension
  - Bradycardia
  - Nausea, vomiting
  - Fever
  - Hypoxia
  - Tachycardia

ICU, intensive care unit; IV, intravenous.

Table 17-3a Centrally Acting α_2-Adrenergic Agonists

Drug	Onset	Peak	Duration	Half-life	Metabolism	Elimination
Methyldopa	1–2 h	2–6 h	24 h	1.7 h	Liver	Kidneys
Guanabenz	1 h	2–5 h	6–12 h	4–14 h	Liver	Kidneys
Guanfacine	2 h	6 h	24 h	17 h	Liver	Kidneys
Clonidine PO	0.5–1 h	2–4 h	8 h	6–20 h	Liver	Kidneys 80% GI 20%
Transdermal	1–3 days	2–3 days	7 days			

PO, oral.

blood pressure by initially releasing norepinephrine from the nerve terminal. With oral administration, the small amount of norepinephrine released is metabolized by monoamine oxidase, and hypertension is generally not an issue. It does have a potential to release norepinephrine, however, and its use is contraindicated in patients with pheochromocytoma.

Blocking the release of norepinephrine leads to catecholamine depletion and a reduction in peripheral vascular resistance that follows α receptor vasoconstrictor inhibition. There is lowering of systolic and diastolic blood pressure and an increase in parasympathetic tone. Standing blood pressure is reduced more than supine blood pressure, and it is more effective in lowering systolic than diastolic blood pressure. During adrenergic neuronal blockade with guanadrel, effector cells become supersensitive to norepinephrine, and this supersensitivity is similar to that noted with postganglionic sympathetic denervation.

Guanadrel is administered orally twice a day, generally starting at 5 mg. This dose may be increased up to 20 to 75 mg/day in two to four divided doses. The drug is rapidly absorbed from the gastrointestinal tract and has an onset of 0.5 to 2 hours. Drug effect peaks at 4 to 6 hours and has a duration of 4 to 14 hours. The half-life is 10 to 12 hours, and it is cleared by renal and nonrenal mechanisms. Its elimination is impaired in patients with renal insufficiency, and total body clearance is reduced four- to fivefold in patients with severe renal dysfunction.

Contraindications to the use of guanadrel include pheochromocytoma, congestive heart failure, and patients taking monoamine oxidase inhibitors. Side effects include orthostatic hypotension, which may be intensified by ingestion of alcohol or use of reserpine. There is increased sensitivity to catecholamines in patients receiving this drug. Adequate hydration before induction of anesthesia decreases the risk of acute intraoperative hypotension.

Table 17-3b Common Adverse Effects Associated With Centrally Acting α_2-Adrenergic Agonists

System	Methyldopa	Guanabenz	Guanfacine	Clonidine
CNS	Sedation, headache, dizziness, fatigue, paresthesias, parkinsonism, < mental acuity	Drowsiness, headache, dizziness, sedation, ataxia, fatigue, weakness	Dizziness, somnolence, confusion, fatigue, insomnia	Drowsiness, dizziness, depression
CV	< HR, BP, SVR	< BP, HR, SVR	< HR, BP, SVR	< BP, HR, SVR
	Orthostatic hypotension, angina	Chest pain, edema, arrhythmia		< Renin activity, rebound > BP
GI	Dry mouth, nausea, vomiting, > liver FTs	Dry mouth, nausea, vomiting	Dry mouth, nausea	Dry mouth, nausea, vomiting, > liver FTs
Other + Coombs test	Hemolytic anemia, bone marrow, depression, arthralgias, gynecomastia, galactorrhea, rash, > BUN pedal edema	Blurred vision, muscle aches	Impotence, > growth hormone levels, pruritis	Fluid retention, pruritis, diaphoresis

BP, blood pressure; BUN, blood urea nitrogen; CV, cardiovascular; FTs, functions tests; GI, gastrointestinal; HR, heart rate; SVR, systemic vascular resistance.

Table 17-4a Pharmacokinetics of Adrenergic Neuronal Blockers

Drug	Onset	Peak	Duration	Half-life	Metabolism	Elimination
Guandrel	0.5–2 h	4–6 h	4–14 h	10–12 h		Kidney
Reserpine	3–6 days	2–6 wk	50–100 h		Hepatic	GI, Kidney
Metyrosine	< 2 h	2–3 days	3–4 days	3–8 h		Kidney

Reserpine (Serpalan) is an alkaloid of rauwolfia serpentina that interferes with the binding of serotonin at receptor sites. It also decreases synthesis of norepinephrine by depleting dopamine, its precursor, and competitively inhibits reuptake of norepinephrine in storage granules. The result is depletion of norepinephrine and serotonin in the CNS, peripheral nervous system, heart, and other organs and tissues. Because reserpine depletes amines in both the central and peripheral nervous systems, antihypertensive effects are probably related to combined peripheral and central effects.

Sympathetic inhibition results in decreased blood pressure, bradycardia, and reduced cardiac output. Most adverse effects are related to effects on the CNS. Sedation and inability to concentrate or perform complex tasks are the most common adverse effects. Psychotic depression, which may lead to suicide, may occur, and the drug should never be given to a patient with a history of suicidality. The use of reserpine has diminished because of these serious side effects.

In the treatment of hypertension, the initial adult dose is 0.5 mg/day, which is reduced to 0.1 to 0.25 mg/day. It is often administered with a diuretic, and in this case a usual daily dose of 0.25 mg can often be reduced to 0.05 mg/day. Reserpine is widely distributed, especially to adipose tissue.

It crosses the blood–brain barrier and placenta and is distributed in breast milk. Peak drug effect is 2 hours, and the half-life is 4.5 to 11.3 hours. Reserpine is totally metabolized and is excreted in the feces and urine. Metyrosine (Demser) blocks the enzyme tyrosine hydroxylase to inhibit the conversion of tyrosine to dihydroxyphenylalanine, which is the initial and rate-setting step in the synthesis of catecholamines. Its major use has been in the short-term management of pheochromocytoma or long-term control when surgery cannot be performed. In patients with pheochromocytoma, catecholamine synthesis is reduced by 35% to 80%, and this reduces hypertension and other symptoms.

For management of patients with pheochromocytoma, metyrosine is started orally at 250 mg in four divided doses daily. It can be increased to 2 to 3 g/day in divided doses to a maximum of 4 g/day. Its peak effect is 2 to 3 days, duration 3 to 4 days, and half-life 3.4 to 7.2 hours. It is excreted in the urine.

Because metyrosine may cause crystalluria, daily urine volume should be greater than 2 L. Other adverse effects include orthostatic hypotension, sedation, extrapyramidal signs, diarrhea, anxiety, and psychic disturbances. Alcohol and other CNS depressants add to sedation and CNS depression. Administration of droperidol, haloperidol, and phenothiazines in patients receiving metyrosine potentiate

Table 17-4b Adverse Effects Associated With Adrenergic Neuronal Blockers

System	Guanadrel	Reserpine	Metyrosine
CNS	Fatigue, headache, drowsiness, tremors, paresthesias, depression, confusion	Drowsiness, sedation, lethargy, depression > dreaming, dizziness	Sedation, fatigue extrapyramidal signs, trismus, psychic disturbances
CV	Orthostatic hypotension, palpitations, chest pain, > heart rate	< Heart rate, edema, orthostatic hypotension, > A-V conduction	
RS	Respiratory cough, shortness of breath, > wheezing		Pulmonary fibrosis
Other	Other visual disturbances, nasal stuffiness, nocturia, urine retention, urinary urgency, hematuria, impotence	Nasal congestion, blurred vision, miosis, ptosis thrombocytopenic purpura, anemia, > bleeding time	Eosinophilia, nasal stuffiness, shortness of breath

A-V, atrioventricular; CV, cardiovascular.

extrapyramidal effects. The cardiovascular effects of phenothiazines and vasodilators are increased in patients receiving this drug. Adequate hydration is critical during surgery to avoid hypotension. Patients receiving metyrosine may have arrhythmias during volatile anesthesia.

α-Adrenergic Blockers

α-Adrenergic receptor blockers generally selectively block α_1 receptors (postsynaptic) without affecting α_2 receptors (presynaptic). Older drugs of this class that used to manage patients with pheochromocytoma include phentolamine and phenoxybenzamine. Both drugs are nonselective compounds available for IV use. α-Adrenergic receptor blockers used in the management of hypertension include prazosin, terazosin, and doxazosin.

Phentolamine mesylate (Regitine) competitively blocks α-adrenergic receptors, but the action is transient and incomplete. By blocking α-adrenergic receptors, it causes vasodilation and decreases general vascular resistance and pulmonary artery pressure. Adrenergic receptor antagonists reduce arteriolar resistance and increase venous capacitance, and this causes a sympathetically mediated reflex increase in heart rate and plasma renin activity.

Phentolamine has been used in the diagnosis of pheochromocytoma and to prevent or control hypertensive episodes during surgical resection of pheochromocytoma. The adult dose used to prevent hypertensive episodes during surgery is 1 to 5 mg intramuscularly or intravenously as needed. The effective dose is variable, but it is rare to need more than 1 mg at a time to adequately treat hypertension. In children the dose is 1 mg or 0.1 mg/kg to a maximum of 5 mg. Unlabeled uses for phentolamine are to prevent necrosis and sloughing after extravasation of norepinephrine. Treatment of extravasation of catecholamines in adults and children consists of 5 to 10 mg phentolamine diluted in 10 mL normal saline injected into the affected area within 12 hours of extravasation.

The peak pharmacologic effect of phentolamine is reached within 2 minutes after IV administration and 15 to 20 minutes after intramuscular administration. Duration of action is 10 to 15 minutes intravenously and 3 to 4 hours intramuscularly. Half-life is 19 minutes, and it is excreted in the urine. Adverse effects may include flushing, orthostatic hypotension, tachycardia, cardiac arrhythmias, abdominal pain, nausea, vomiting, and exacerbation of peptic ulcer disease.

Phenoxybenzamine hydrochloride (Dibenzyline) is a long-acting α-adrenergic blocking agent that produces noncompetitive blockade at α receptor sites. This antagonism prevents α receptors from reacting to endogenous or exogenous catecholamines. Its major use is in the preoperative preparation of patients with pheochromocytoma.

The adult dose for management of pheochromocytoma is 5 to 10 mg twice daily, and the dose is increased by 10 mg/day at 4-day intervals until the desired response is obtained. The usual dose range is 20 to 60 mg/day in two to three divided doses. The usual range in a child is 0.4 to 1.2 mg/kg/day. Onset of action is 2 hours, peak 4 to 6 hours, and duration 3 to 4 days. The half-life is 24 hours. Elimination is by urine (80%) and bile.

Adverse effects include dizziness, fainting, sedation, postural hypotension, tachycardia, and palpitation. Nasal congestion, miosis, and drooping of eyelids have also been reported. The drug is contraindicated in instances when a fall in blood pressure is dangerous. Both phentolamine and phenoxybenzamine are rarely used clinically today, but they are prototypes of α-adrenergic antagonists and are useful when comparing newer drugs in this class.

Prazosin (Minipress) produces a selective, reversible inhibition of α_1-adrenoceptors resulting in vasodilation in both resistance (arterioles) and capacitance (veins). Both peripheral resistance and blood pressure are reduced. It lowers blood pressure in the supine and standing position, and the most pronounced effect is on diastolic pressure. It has minor effects on heart rate and blood pressure in the supine position and does not cause renin release. Although its primary use is in the treatment of hypertension, it is rarely used alone because it supports retention of sodium and water. It is effective when used with β-adrenergic blockers and diuretics.

The oral dose in adults is generally 1 mg twice or three times a day to a dose of 20 mg daily. Approximately 60% of an oral dose reaches the systemic circulation. It has an onset of action of 2 hours, peak of 2 to 4 hours, and duration of less than 24 hours. Its half-life is 2 to 4 hours. It is extensively metabolized in the liver. Approximately 6% to 10% is excreted in the urine with the remainder lost in the bile or feces.

Side effects noted with treatment with prazosin may include dizziness, drowsiness, nervousness, and weakness. Postural hypotension, syncope, edema, palpitations, and abdominal cramps have been reported. Other side effects associated with drug use may include nausea, vomiting, elevated liver function tests, myalgia, pruritus, and diaphoresis. Its use in patients having general anesthesia with volatile agents or spinal block accentuates hypotensive effects. Administration of diuretics with prazosin also increases hypotensive effects.

Terazosin (Hytrin) is a quinazoline antihypertensive and vasodilating agent chemically similar to prazosin. It selectively blocks α_1-adrenergic receptors in vascular smooth muscle, resulting in relaxation that lowers peripheral vascular resistance and blood pressure. Vasodilation results in a mild reflex increase in heart rate.

The usual adult dose is 1 to 5 mg daily with a maximum dose of 20 mg/day. After rapid absorption from the gastrointestinal tract, the drug effects peak in 1 to 2 hours. It has a half-life of 9 to 12 hours. It is metabolized in the liver, and 60% is excreted in the feces and 40% in the urine. Side effects may include somnolence, headache, nervousness, nausea, and nasal congestion. Other reported side effects associated with use of terazosin may include orthostatic hypotension, arrhythmias, palpitations, pedal edema, dyspnea, thrombocytopenia, blurred vision, and muscle pain. Use of volatile anesthetics or spinal anesthesia may result in hypotension. Because nasal congestion is a side effect of drug administration, nasal intubation should be avoided in patients receiving terazosin.

Doxazosin (Cardura) is a selective α_1-adrenergic blocker that is 50% as potent as prazosin.[9] By selective competitive inhibition of α_1 receptors, it produces vasodilation in both resistance and capacitance vessels. Vasodilatation in arterioles and venules results in reduced peripheral vascular resistance and reduction in blood pressure.

The starting adult dose is generally 1 mg daily in the adult titrated up to 16 mg/day in divided doses. The average dose is 1 to 8 mg/day. In geriatric patients the starting dose is reduced to 0.5 mg initially. Doxazosin is readily absorbed from the gastrointestinal tract, and 62% to 69% of the dose reaches the systemic circulation. Peak drug effect after oral administration is 2 to 6 hours, and the duration is up to 24 hours. The half-life of the drug is 9 to 12 hours. Approximately 35% of the dose is metabolized in the liver and is eliminated in the urine and feces.

Pharmacodynamic effects associated with the use of doxazosin include somnolence, fatigue, and vertigo. It may also cause orthostatic hypotension, angina, edema, increased heart rate, and arrhythmia. Other side effects noted may include nausea, vomiting, dyspnea, and fluid retention. When used with β-adrenergic blockers, hypotension is increased. Use of doxazosin with volatile anesthetics and central neuronal blocking drugs accentuate hypotensive responses.

β-Adrenergic Antagonists

β-Adrenergic antagonists inhibit the interaction of epinephrine, norepinephrine, and sympathetic drugs with β receptors and are excellent drugs for chronic and acute management of hypertension. These drugs block β_1 and β_2 or may be effective at only β_1 receptors. Those drugs that block both postsynaptic receptors are known as nonselective β-adrenergic blockers, whereas those that are antagonistic only at β_1 receptors are selective beta-blockers.

Predicting the effect of β-adrenergic blockade depends on a good understanding of adrenergic receptor location and physiology. Major therapeutic effect from this class of drugs is on the cardiovascular system. Because catecholamines have positive chronotropic and inotropic effects on the heart, β receptor blockade results in reduced contractility and reduced heart rate. These drugs decrease spontaneous rate of depolarization of ectopic pacemakers, slow conduction in the atria and atrioventricular (A-V) node, and increase the functional refractory period of the A-V node. With some of these drugs, peripheral vascular resistance may be increased initially due to blockade of the β_2 dilating effects. With continued use peripheral vascular resistance returns to normal or decreases.

Antagonism of β_2 receptors in bronchial smooth muscle by nonselective drugs may increase airway resistance in patients with hyperactive airway. This may lead to life-threatening bronchospasm. Although β_1 selective agents are less likely to cause bronchoconstriction, they have a preferential selectivity for β_1 receptors. In large doses they block β_2 receptors as well.

Catecholamines promote glycogenolysis and mobilize glucose in response to hypoglycemia. Nonselective β antagonists blunt these responses and may delay recovery from hypoglycemia. These drugs can also block clinical signs of hypoglycemia such as nervousness, tremor, and tachycardia. These drugs should thus be used with caution in labile diabetics and those with frequent episodes of hypoglycemia. If a β antagonist must be used in a diabetic, a β_1 selective is preferred.

Beta-blockers reduce β_1-stimulated release from the kidney of renin, and this lowers blood pressure. Although the mechanism is unclear, prolonged administration of beta-blockers reduces peripheral vascular resistance. The fall in peripheral vascular resistance and cardiac output plays a major role in the antihypertensive effect of this class of drugs. Some beta-blockers produce peripheral vasodilation through production of nitric oxide, β_2 receptor agonism, α_1 receptor antagonism, calcium channel blockade, and opening of the potassium channel. Contraindications to use of β antagonists are noted in Box 17-3.

Nonselective β Receptor Antagonists

Propranolol (Inderal) is a nonselective beta-blocker of both cardiac and bronchial adrenergic receptors and

Box 17-3 Contraindications to Use of β-Adrenergic Blockers

1. Severe bradycardia
2. Greater than first-degree heart block
3. Cardiogenic shock
4. Most, but not all, contraindicated in congestive heart failure

competes with epinephrine and norepinephrine for available β receptor sites. At higher doses it depresses cardiac function, reducing contractility and arrhythmias. It lowers both supine and standing blood pressure in hypertensive patients. It is a Class II antiarrhythmic, and it depresses automaticity at the sinus node and ectopic pacemaker and decreases A-V and intraventricular conduction velocity.

Hypotensive effects are the result of decreased cardiac output, suppressed renin activity, and β blockade. Propranolol also decreases platelet aggregation. Propranolol has been used in the management of migraine headache. Although its mechanism of action in this situation is not clearly known, the positive effect in this situation is thought to be due to inhibition of cerebral vasodilation and arteriolar spasm. Other unlabeled uses for propranolol include acute panic symptoms or stage fright, anxiety states, tremors, schizophrenia, tardive dyskinesia, recurrent gastrointestinal bleeding in patients with cirrhosis, and treatment of aggression and rage. Its primary use is in the management of hypertension, angina, and arrhythmias. It is also used in the medical management of idiopathic hypertrophic subaortic stenosis, thyrotoxicosis, and pheochromocytoma. In the case of pheochromocytoma, beta-blockers should not be administered unless the patient has been alpha blocked. Without alpha-blockade, high levels of catecholamines can stimulate alpha receptors and cause hypertensive crisis.

Primary contraindications to the use of propranolol include greater than first-degree heart block, congestive heart failure, and bronchial asthma or bronchospasm. Other contraindications include cardiogenic shock, significant aortic or mitral valvular disease, severe chronic obstructive pulmonary disease (COPD), allergic rhinitis, or concurrent use with adrenergic-augmenting psychotropic drugs or within 2 weeks of monoamine oxidase inhibition therapy. Caution is advised for the use of propranolol in patients with peripheral arterial insufficiency, bronchitis or emphysema, renal or hepatic impairment, diabetes prone to hypoglycemia, and Wolf-Parkinson-White syndrome.

The drug is typically given orally, although IV administration is preferred in the acute treatment of arrhythmias. The dose given depends on its indication for use and age of the patient. The IV dose is 0.5 to 3 mg, which can be repeated every 2 minutes. The oral dose is 60 to 480 mg/day in two divided doses. Absorption after oral administration is complete, but it undergoes extensive first-pass metabolism, and only 25% of an oral dose reaches the systemic circulation. Onset is less than 2 minutes after IV administration and 30 minutes with oral administration. Peak action is under 5 minutes intravenously and 1 to 1.5 hours orally. The duration is less than 10 minutes intravenously and 12 hours orally.

Propranolol is almost completely metabolized in the liver to an active metabolite called 4-hydroxypropranolol and is 90% to 95% eliminated by the kidneys. Propranolol is highly lipophilic and readily enters the CNS, causing fatigue or depression. When propranolol is administered with other antihypertensives, hypotensive effects are greater. The bronchodilating effects of β agonists and sympathomimetic drugs are reduced when patients are receiving propranolol. In the diabetic there is a reduction in hypoglycemic effects of insulin and glyburide. Gastrointestinal absorption of antacids and alcohol is reduced in patients receiving propranolol. Higher doses of propranolol may increase the effect of neuromuscular blocking drugs, and volatile anesthetics given to patients receiving this drug may increase the incidence of arrhythmias. Severe bradycardia has been reported in patients receiving neostigmine for reversal of neuromuscular-blocking drugs. Chronic blockade of β-adrenergic receptors results in up-regulation of receptors, which increase receptor density. Abrupt withdrawal of the drug can then lead to severe hypertension and tachycardia followed by myocardial ischemia, myocardial infarction, or serious arrhythmias. The drug should be gradually reduced over a period of 1 to 2 weeks, and the patient should be monitored closely during this time.

Although propranolol is considered the prototype drug in this class, it is rarely used today. In a study only 1% of patients received propranolol compared with 60% who received metoprolol and 39% who received atenolol.[10] β_1 Selective agents are safer in most patients, especially those with hyperactive airway.

Nadolol (Corgard) is a nonselective β-adrenergic blocking drug pharmacologically and chemically similar to propranolol. It is a long-acting adrenergic blocker with equal affinity for β_1 and β_2 receptors. Its actions are similar to those seen with propranolol on major organ systems. Nadolol is water soluble, and only 30% to 40% is absorbed from the gut. Its onset is 0.5 to 1 hour, and it has a peak action at

2 to 4 hours and a duration of 12 to 24 hours. Its elimination half-life is 20 hours. Nadolol is not metabolized and is excreted in the urine. It is used for pretension either alone or in combination with a diuretic. The usual adult dose is 20 to 40 mg orally, increased to 40 to 80 mg/day.

There is decreasing bronchodilatation by β agonists and sympathomimetics in patients receiving nadolol. It may mask the signs of hypoglycemia or hyperthyroidism as well as inadequate anesthesia. Airway stimulation in an inadequately anesthetized patient receiving nadolol may trigger bronchospasm.

Timolol (Blocadren, Betimol, Timoptic, Timoptic XE) is a nonselective beta-blocker used as an antihypertensive, antiarrhythmic, and antianginal agent. It can also be used topically to lower normal and elevated intraocular pressure. It appears to lower intraocular pressure by reducing formation of aqueous humor and by increasing outflow of aqueous humor. The ophthalmic formulation of Timoptic is used for the treatment of glaucoma. It may be extensively absorbed from the eye into the systemic circulation, resulting in asthma or congestive heart failure in some patients.

Timolol is well absorbed from the gastrointestinal tract when given orally. The usual oral dose is 10 to 40 mg daily. Onset of action is less than 30 minutes, peak action is 1 to 2 hours, and duration is 6 to 12 hours. Its half-life is 4 hours. The drug undergoes first-pass hepatic metabolism and is excreted by the kidneys.

Like most β-adrenergic blockers, the use of timolol is contraindicated in patients with asthma, severe COPD, advanced heart block, profound bradycardia, or congestive heart failure. It increases muscle weakness in patients with myasthenia gravis and bradycardia, and myocardial depression is increased when patients receiving digoxin, verapamil, or diltiazem receive timolol. Anesthetics and opioids increase hypotension and bradycardia in patients receiving the drug. Arrhythmias may be increased in patients receiving volatile anesthetic.

Pindolol (Visken) is a nonselective beta-blocking agent that possesses slight intrinsic sympathomimetic activity or partial β agonist effect in therapeutic dose ranges. Its primary use is in the management of chronic hypertension. Through competitive blockade at β receptors on the heart, it leads to negative chronotropic, inotropic, and dromotropic effect on the heart, and this along with a decrease in peripheral resistance reduces blood pressure. Blockade of β_2 receptors in bronchial smooth muscle leads to wheezing in patients with active bronchospastic disease.

The average daily oral dose of pindolol is 10 to 40 mg. It has an onset of 30 minutes, peak action of 1 to 2 hours, and a duration of 24 hours. Its elimination half-life is 3 to 7 hours.

Pindolol is rapidly absorbed from the gastrointestinal tract with 50% to 95% reaching the systemic circulation. Forty percent to 60% is metabolized in the liver. Penbutolol (Levatol) is a nonselective β_1 and β_2 blocking agent with many pharmacologic characteristics similar to propranolol. It is used to treat mild to moderate hypertension, and the oral dose in adults is generally 10 to 40 mg daily. Its onset is less than 1 hour, peak action 1 to 3 hours, and duration 12 to 24 hours. The elimination half-life is 5 hours. It is metabolized in the liver and excreted in the urine. Carteolol (Cartrol, Ocupress) is a nonselective β_1 and β_2 blocking drug used for hypertension and lowering of intraocular pressure when used as an ophthalmic solution. It is a long-acting beta-blocker with intrinsic sympathomimetic effect. The initial dose is 2.5 mg initially, increased to 10 mg daily. Onset of action is less than 1 hour, peak action 1 to 3 hours, and duration 24 hours. The half-life is 6 hours. It is metabolized in the liver to an active metabolite and excreted primarily in the urine. A summary of adverse effects of nonselective beta-blockers is found in Table 17-5a.

Selective β Receptor Antagonists

Metoprolol (Lopressor, Toprol XL) is a β-adrenergic blocker agent with preferential selectivity for β_1 receptors located primarily on cardiac muscle. At higher doses, metoprolol also inhibits β_2 receptors located on bronchial and vascular musculature. Antihypertensive action may be due to antagonism of catecholamines at cardiac adrenergic neuron sites, reduced sympathetic outflow to the periphery, and suppression of renin levels.

Metoprolol may be given intravenously or orally. Its onset of action is 5 minutes intravenously with a peak less than 1 hour and duration of 5 to 8 hours. The elimination half-life is 3 to 7 hours. It is extensively metabolized in the liver and eliminated by the kidney. For hypertension, the usual oral dose is 100 mg daily, increasing at weekly intervals until blood pressure is controlled. It is also used in the management of angina, myocardial infarction, and congestion heart failure.

Because the β_1 selectively makes it less likely to aggravate bronchospastic disease, metoprolol is a popular agent to manage hemodynamic problems perioperatively. When used in this setting, the IV dose is 1 to 5 mg every 2 or 3 minutes for three doses or until the problem is resolved. An effect is usually seen within 2 to 3 minutes and may last up to 4 hours.[11] If metoprolol is given to patients receiving amiodarone or other antihypertensives, hypotensive effects are enhanced. Its use enhances the CNS depressant effects of benzodiazepines, and when neostigmine is used in the presence of this drug to reverse neuromuscular blocking agents, marked bradycardia may occur. Like other beta-blockers, it masks signs of hypoglycemia and hyperthyroidism, and acute withdrawal may result in rebound tachycardia and hypertension, which is dangerous in patients with cardiac disease.

Atenolol (Tenormin) selectively blocks β_1 receptors located in cardiac muscle. With large doses preferential selectivity is lost, and blockade of β_2 receptors may lead to wheezing and bronchospasm. Mechanisms for antihypertensive action include central action, suppression of the renin-angiotensin-aldosterone system, and competitive inhibition of catecholamine binding at β- adrenergic receptors. Atenolol is given orally, and 50% of the oral dose is absorbed. It peaks in 2 to 4 hours after oral administration and in 5 minutes after IV administration. The half-life is 6 to 7 hours and duration of action 24 hours. The adult oral dose is 25 to 100 mg and the IV dose is 5 mg every 5 minutes for two doses. The drug does not undergo hepatic metabolism and is excreted by the kidneys and gastrointestinal system.

In addition to treating hypertension, atenolol is also used to manage angina, acute myocardial infarction, and tachyarrhythmias. Like other beta-blockers, it should not be discontinued abruptly because of the risk of hypertension, tachyarrhythmias, and myocardial ischemia. Although its slow onset makes it less suitable for perioperative use than other drugs, data in noncardiac surgery suggest a valuable effect in reducing cardiovascular risk.[12] It may be more suitable than metoprolol in managing perioperative cardiovascular risk due to its prolonged duration of action.[13] It is often the drug selected for prophylactic β-adrenergic blockade in at-risk cardiac patients

Acebutolol (Monitan, Sectral) is a selective β_1-adrenergic blocking agent with mild intrinsic sympathomimetic activity. It produces negative chronotropic and inotropic effects and decreases both systolic and diastolic blood pressure. It decreases exercise-induced heart rate, inhibits reflex orthostatic tachycardia, and decreases cardiac output at rest and during exercise. It is used in the management of moderate hypertension and recurrent stable ventricular arrhythmias. Unlabeled uses include management of stable ventricular arrhythmias.

The adult dose for management of hypertension is 400 to 800 mg daily orally in one or two divided doses. In geriatric patients the dose should be reduced to 200 to 400 mg/day orally. The maximum dose in the adult is 1200 mg and in geriatric patients 800 mg daily. Acebutolol is well absorbed after oral administration and undergoes extensive first-pass metabolism in the liver. The average bioavailability is 40%, but in the geriatric patient bioavailability increases twofold. The peak effect is seen in 3 hours, and the half-life is 3 to 4 hours. Acebutolol is metabolized in the liver to diacetolol with activity equipotent to the parent compound. The metabolite is excreted in 8 to 13 hours by the kidney and gastrointestinal tract.

Betaxolol (Betoptic, Betoptic S, Kerlone) is a selective β_1-adrenergic blocker used to treat hypertension and intraocular hypertension in open-angle glaucoma. Its antihypertensive effects are thought to be due to decreased cardiac output, reduced sympathetic nervous system outflow to the periphery resulting in vasodilation, and suppression of renin activity in the kidney.

The usual adult dose for treatment of hypertension is 5 to 10 mg/day orally. The maximum dose is 20 mg/day in divided doses. It is well absorbed, and 90% of the oral dose reaches the systemic circulation. Its onset is 0.5 to 1 hour, peak effect is 2 hours, and duration of action is over 12 hours. Its half-life is 3 to 4 hours, and it is metabolized in the liver to at least five metabolites. It is eliminated through the urine, feces, and bile. Bisoprolol fumarate (Zebeta) is a long-acting, cardioselective, adrenergic blocking agent used in the treatment of hypertension. It does not possess membrane-stabilizing properties or have intrinsic sympathomimetic activity. To maintain cardioselectivity, the lowest possible dose should be used. Bisoprolol decreases heart rate, blood pressure, contractile force, and cardiac workload; reduces myocardial oxygen consumption; and increases blood flow to the myocardium.

The adult dose for management of chronic hypertension is 2.5 to 5 mg once daily. The maximum dose is 20 mg daily. Bisoprolol is readily absorbed from the gastrointestinal tract, with 82% to 94% reaching the systemic circulation. Peak therapeutic effect is seen in 2 to 4 weeks, and duration is 24 hours. The half-life is 10 to 12 hours, and it is metabolized in the liver to inactive metabolites. It is excreted in the urine.

Esmolol (Brevibloc) is a competitive β_1-adrenergic blocker with little to no effect at β_2 receptors except at high dose. It has no intrinsic sympathomimetic activity and no membrane-stabilizing activity. Esmolol is used to treat hypertension, especially perioperative hypertension. It is also used to treat supraventricular tachycardia and to control the ventricular response to atrial fibrillation or atrial flutter. Esmolol is a short-acting β_1 antagonist and must be infused for optimum effect. When used to treat intraoperative hypertension or tachycardia, a bolus of 1 mg/kg is followed by an infusion of 150 µg/kg/min. The infusion is adjusted as necessary up to a maximum of 300 µg/kg/min. For control of postoperative hypertension, one-third of patients may require the maximum dose to control blood pressure.

The onset of action of esmolol is 1 to 10 minutes after IV administration. Onset is quicker with a loading dose of 0.5 to 1 mg/kg. The duration of hemodynamic effects is 10 to 30 minutes with longer action noted after administration of higher cumulative doses for extended periods of time. The half-life is 9 minutes, and it is metabolized in the blood by red blood cell esterases. Patients with end-stage renal disease have decreased elimination of metabolites of esmolol. Infusions must be administered with an infusion pump. The concentrate (250-mg/mL ampule) is not for direct IV administration. The 250-mg/mL ampule must be diluted to a final concentration of 10 mg/mL by placing 2.5 g in 250-mL solutions.

Esmolol is commonly used to manage perioperative hypertension. Because the total duration of effect is short, a return to baseline blood pressure levels occurs in approximately 20 to 30 minutes. It is truly a "titratable" beta-blocker and has been used to prevent or treat acute hypertension associated with induction of anesthesia and laryngoscopy and intubation.[14,15] It is frequently used during surgery, during emergency, and at the time of endotracheal extubation to prevent or treat emergence hypertension of tachycardia.[16,17]

Kindler et al.[18] evaluated the efficacy of IV lidocaine 1.5 mg/kg and two doses of esmolol (1 mg/kg and 2 mg/kg) for attenuating the cardiovascular response to laryngoscopy and intubation and assessed whether a combination of both drugs is more effective than either drug alone. Esmolol 1 and 2 mg/kg was reliably effective in attenuating the heart rate response to tracheal intubation. Neither the two doses tested nor lidocaine affected the blood pressure response.[18] Atlee et al.[19] evaluated the effect of esmolol 1 mg/kg and nicardipine 30 μg/kg in combination to blunt hemodynamic changes after laryngoscopy and tracheal intubation. They found the peak increase in blood pressure is best blunted with the combination, but no single drug or combination of the doses tested opposed the increase in heart rate.[19] Small doses of esmolol (0.2–0.4 mg/kg) before laryngoscopy and intubation may blunt the increase in heart rate and blood pressure.[20]

Esmolol is very useful in the management of severe postoperative hypertension and in situations where cardiac output, heart rate, and blood pressure are increased.[21] Caution must be used with administration of esmolol in patients with COPD, but it can be used safely. Gold et al.[22] studied the impact of esmolol on ventilatory function in patients with COPD. Despite marked hemodynamic response, there was no adverse effect on pulmonary function. It was concluded that beta-blockade with esmolol could be achieved in patients with COPD and cardiac disorders with little risk of bronchospasm.[22] A summary of adverse effects of all selective beta-blockers is found in Table 17-5b.

Mixed Adrenergic Antagonists

Labetalol hydrochloride (Normodyne, Trandate) is an adrenergic receptor blocking agent that combines selective α activity (α$_1$ antagonist only) with nonselective β-adrenergic blocking actions. Both actions contribute to blood pressure reductions. Alpha blockade results in vasodilation, decreased peripheral resistance, and orthostatic hypotension while only slightly affecting cardiac output and coronary artery blood flow. Beta-blocking effects at the sinus node, A-V node, and ventricular muscle result in bradycardia and depression of myocardial contractility.[23]

Labetalol is used to treat mild to moderate hypertension and can be given intravenously to manage hypertension in the perioperative period. It is one-fifth to one-tenth as potent as phentolamine at α receptors and one-third to one-fourth as potent as propranolol at β receptors. The ratio of alpha-to-beta blockade is 1:3 after oral administration and 1:7 after IV administration. Labetalol is readily absorbed from the gastrointestinal tract, but only 25% reaches the systemic circulation due to first-pass hepatic metabolism. Table 17-5c presents the pharmacokinetic profile for labetalol. The adult oral dose to treat hypertension is 100 mg twice daily; it may be gradually increased to a maximum dose of 1200 to 2400 mg daily. The dose may be reduced to 100 mg twice daily in the elderly.

Clinical uses for labetalol include attenuation of hypertension and tachycardia after surgery. It attenuates the hypertensive response associated with pheochromocytoma and clonidine withdrawal. The general IV dose in the adult is 20 mg slowly over 2 minutes with 20 to 80 mg every 10 minutes up to a total dose of 300 mg. It may be given by continuous infusion at a rate of 2 mg/min. The hypotensive effect of labetalol begins within 2 to 5 minutes after IV administration and lasts 2 to 4 hours.[24] Its major side effect is orthostatic hypotension. Its use is associated with less tachycardia than other vasodilators. Its side effect profile is the same as other beta-blockers. It is useful in controlling transient hyperdynamic responses during surgery in patients with adequate anesthesia and analgesia. Adequate fluid replacement minimizes risk of postural hypotension.

Labetalol has been evaluated for treatment of acute perioperative hypertension after cardiac, vascular, intracranial, and general surgery and has been found to be a safe and effective agent.[25–27] It has been shown to be more effective than esmolol for management of perioperative hypertension and is effective in a variety of clinical settings.[28,29]

Carvedilol (Coreg, Kredex) is an adrenergic receptor antagonist that combines selective α activity and nonselective blocking actions. Both activities contribute to

Table 17-5a Adverse Effects of Nonselective Beta-Blockers

System	Propranolol	Nadolol	Timolol	Pindolol	Penbutolol	Carteolol
CNS	Psychosis, sleep disturbances, depression, confusion, agitation, light headedness, fatigue, syncope, drowsiness, insomnia, vivid dreams		Fatigue, lethargy, weakness, somnolence, confusion, psychic disturbances	Fatigue, confusion, dizziness, insomnia, drowsiness	Dizziness, fatigue, headache, insomnia	Headache, dizziness, drowsiness, insomnia, tremor, paresthesias
CV	Palpitations, profound bradycardia, A-V block, hypotension, acute CHF, angina	Bradycardia, CHF hypotension, conduction disturbance	Palpitation, A-V conduction disturbance, bradycardia, CHF	Bradycardia, hypotension	Bradycardia, A-V block	Hypotension, bradycardia, CHF
RS	Respiratory distress, dyspnea, laryngospasm, bronchospasm	Respiratory distress, laryngospasm	Difficulty breathing, bronchospasm	Bronchospasm, pulmonary edema, dyspnea	Cough, dyspnea	Bronchospasm
GI	Dry mouth, nausea, vomiting, diarrhea, abdominal cramps	Dry mouth	Anorexia, dyspepsia	Nausea, diarrhea	Nausea, vomiting, dyspepsia	Nausea, abdominal pain, diarrhea
Other	Dry eyes, visual disturbances, tinnitus, hearing loss, nasal stuffiness, eosinophilia, thrombocytopenia, agranulocytosis (rare), hyperglycemia, hypocalcemia	Blurred vision, dry eyes	Hypokalemia, hypoglycemia	Agranulocytosis (rare), hypoglycemia		Hyperglycemia

CHF, congestive heart failure; CV, cardiovascular; GI, gastrointestinal; RS, respiratory.

Table 17-5b Adverse Effects of Selective Beta-Blockers

System	Metoprolol	Atenolol	Acebutolol	Betaxolol	Bisoprolol	Esmolol
CNS	Dizziness, fatigue, insomnia, depression, dreaming	Dizziness, vertigo, light-headedness, syncope, fatigue, lethargy, insomnia, drowsiness	Fatigue, confusion, dizziness, insomnia, syncope	Depression	Dizziness, fatigue, tiredness, sleep disturbance	Headache, dizziness, somnolence, confusion, agitation
CV	Bradycardia, palpitation, CHF, A-V block, complete heart block, cardiac arrest, Raynaud's phenomenon	Bradycardia, CHF, hypotension, leg pain, dysrhythmias	Hypotension, bradycardia, CHF	Bradycardia, hypotension	Bradycardia, hypotension, angina	Dose-related hypotension, bradycardia, myocardial depression
RS	Laryngospasm, respiratory distress, bronchospasm, shortness of breath	Dyspnea, pulmonary edema, bronchospasm	Bronchospasm, pulmonary edema, dyspnea	> Airway resistance	Asthma, bronchospasm, cough, dyspnea	Dyspnea, chest pain, bronchospasm

(continues)

Table 17-5b Adverse Effects of Selective Beta-Blockers *(continued)*

System	Metoprolol	Atenolol	Acebutolol	Betaxolol	Bisoprolol	Esmolol
GI	Nausea, gastric pain, heartburn, diarrhea	Nausea, vomiting	Nausea, diarrhea	Nausea, vomiting	Abdominal pain, nausea, vomiting, diarrhea	Nausea, vomiting
Other	Eosinophilia, thrombocytopenia, agranulocytosis, dry mouth, dry mucous membrane, hypoglycemia	Masks signs of hypoglycemia		Athralgia, hyperglycemia	Arthralgia, hyperkalemia	

CHF, congestive heart failure; CV, cardiovascular; GI, gastrointestinal; RS, respiratory.

Table 17-5c Pharmacokinetics of β-Adrenergic Blockers

Drug	Onset	Peak	Duration	Half-life	Metabolism	Elimination
Nonselective						
Propranolol						
PO	0.5 h	1.5 h	12 h	3–5 h	First pass	Kidney
IV	< 2 min	5 min	< 10 min		Hepatic	
Nadolol	0.5–1 h	2–4 h	12–24 h	20 h	Hepatic	Kidney
Timolol	< 30 min	1–2 h	6–12 h	4 h	Hepatic	Kidney
Pindolol	< 30 min	1–2 h	24 h	3–7 h	Hepatic	Kidney
Penbutolol	< 1 h					
	1–3 h	12–24 h	5 h		Kidney	
Carteolol	< 1 h	1–3 h	24	6 h		Kidney
Selective						
Metoprolol						
PO	15 min	< 1 h	6–12 h	3–7	Hepatic	Kidney
IV	< 5 min	5–8 min				
Atenolol	1 h	2 h	12–24 h	6–7 h		Kidney
Acebutolol	1.5 h	2–3 h	24 h	3–4 h	Hepatic	GI
Betaxolol	< 1 h	4 h	12–24 h	14–22 h	Hepatic	Kidney, GI
Bisopropol	< 1 h	1–4 h	24 h	9–12 h	Hepatic	Kidney
Esmolol						
IV	< 5 min	< 30 min	30 min	8–12 min	Red blood cell esterases	Kidney
Mixed Adrenergic Antagonists						
Labetalol						
PO	20 min	2 h	1–4 h	3–8 h	Hepatic	Kidney, bile
IV	2–5 min	5–15 min	2–4 h			
Carvedilol	< 1 h	1–2 h	7–10 h	7–10 h	Hepatic	Bile, GI

GI, gastrointestinal; PO, oral.

Table 17-5d Adverse Effects of Mixed Adrenergic Antagonists

System	Labetalol	Carvedilol
CNS	Dizziness, fatigue, headache, tremors, transient paresthesias, mental depression, nightmares, drowsiness	Dizziness, headache, paresthesias
CV	Postural hypotension, palpitation, bradycardia, syncope, pedal and peripheral edema, pulmonary edema, CHF	Bradycardia, hypotension, syncope, A-V block, angina
RS	Dyspnea, bronchospasm	Sinusitis, bronchitis
GI	Nausea, vomiting, diarrhea, taste disturbances, dry mouth, cholestasis	Nausea, vomiting, diarrhea, abdominal pain
Other	Myalgia, cramps	Thrombocytopenia, hyperglycemia, arthralgia

CHF, congestive heart failure; CV, cardiovascular; GI, gastrointestinal; RS, respiratory.

Box 17-4 Anesthetic Considerations in Patients Receiving Beta-Blockers

- Drug should not be abruptly stopped due to rebound hypertension and tachycardia.
- Drug should not be discontinued before surgery because of risk of postoperative myocardial ischemia, hypertension, and tachyarrhythmia.
- Cardiovascular depressant effects of anesthetics increased in beta-blocked patient.
- May mask signs of hyperthyroidism and hypoglycemia under anesthesia.
- May mask signs of inadequate anesthesia.
- Reversal of neuromuscular blocking drugs with anticholinesterases may result in marked bradycardia.
- Reflex tachycardia due to intraoperative blood loss may be blunted.
- Anesthetics and opioids analgesics are associated with increased hypotension and bradycardia in the beta-blocked patient.
- Adequate fluid administration minimizes the risk of orthostatic hypotension.

---

blood pressure–reducing properties. Decreased peripheral vascular resistance and vasodilation result from α_1 blocking effects. It is three to five times more potent than labetalol in reducing blood pressure. It is also used to treat angina, dysrhythmias, and congestive heart failure because it lowers myocardial oxygen demand and cardiac work. The starting dose to treat hypertension is 6.25 mg twice daily increased to a maximum dose of 25 mg. The drug is rapidly absorbed from the gastrointestinal tract, and 25% to 35% reaches the systemic circulation. Peak antihypertensive effect is seen in 7 to 14 days. The half-life is 7 to 10 hours. It is metabolized in the liver and partially excreted in the bile. Adequate perioperative hydration before ambulation minimizes postural hypotension and postoperative nausea and vomiting after surgery. A summary of adverse effects of mixed adrenergic antagonists is found in Table 17-5d. Anesthetic considerations in patients receiving beta-blockers is found in Box 17-4.

Calcium Channel Blocking Agents

Voltage-sensitive calcium channels (L-type or slow channels) mediate the entry of extracellular calcium into smooth muscle and cardiac myocytes as well as the conduction system of the heart. Calcium is a trigger for contraction in both smooth muscle and cardiac muscle. Calcium antagonists or calcium entry blockers inhibit calcium function, leading to relaxation in vascular smooth muscle, and may produce negative inotropic and chronotropic effects on the heart.

Calcium channel blockers can be grouped according to their diverse chemical structure: phenylalkylamines, dihydropyridines, benzothiazepines, diphenylpiperazines, and diarylaminopropylamine. All drugs within this chemical class bind to a calcium channel and reduce calcium flux through the channel. The drugs differ, however, in regard to pharmacologic characteristics, drug interactions, and toxicity.

Nifedipine (Adalat, Procardia) is from the dihydropyridine class and is the prototype drug for calcium channel blockers. It selectively blocks calcium flux across calcium channels in cardiac and vascular smooth muscle without changing serum calcium concentration. Although it has minimal to no effect on cardiac conduction or contractility, it decreases peripheral vascular resistance and increases cardiac output. Vasodilation of peripheral and coronary vessels is greater than that produced by other calcium blockers, and reflex tachycardia follows. Nifedipine is used in the treatment of hypertension as well as angina, especially that caused by coronary spasm. Unlabeled uses include treatment for esophageal disorders, vascular headache, asthma, cardiomyopathy, and primary pulmonary hypertension.

The usual oral dose of nifedipine to treat hypertension in the adult is 10 to 20 mg three times a day up to 180 mg/day or 30 to 90 mg sustained release once daily. It is readily absorbed from the gastrointestinal tract but undergoes first-pass hepatic metabolism, and only 45% to 75% reaches the systemic circulation. It has an onset of 10 to 30 minutes, peaks in 30 minutes, and has a half-life of 2 to 5 hours. It is metabolized in the liver and excreted in the urine and feces.

Although intranasal nifedipine has been used to treat poorly controlled hypertension preoperatively, the practice has been condemned.[30] Varon and Marik condemned the use of sublingual nifedipine for hypertensive emergencies.[31] Others have called for a moratorium on its use intranasally for safety reasons.[32] There have been cases of neurologic and cardiac effects reported with sublingual nifedipine. Neurologic effects include dizziness, aphasia, hemiparesis, loss of consciousness, and stupor. Cardiac effects include electrocardiographic changes, syncope, heart block, palpitations, myocardial infarction, and sinus arrest. Intranasal use today is considered unacceptable because of the inability to control heart rate and degree of blood pressure reduction.[33]

Felodipine (Plendil), a dihydropyridine, is a calcium antagonist with high vascular selectivity that reduces both systolic and diastolic blood pressure. Blood pressure reduction is due to a reduction in peripheral vascular resistance or afterload against which the heart has to work. By reducing afterload, myocardial oxygen demand is also reduced. Therefore in addition to being useful to treat hypertension, felodipine is also useful in management of stable angina.

The oral dose of felodipine to treat hypertension is 5 to 10 mg daily for a maximum dose of 20 mg/day. It is completely absorbed from the gastrointestinal tract but undergoes first-pass hepatic metabolism, and only 15% reaches the systemic circulation. Its onset is less than 1 hour, peak 2 to 4 hours, and duration 20 to 24 hours. The half-life of felodipine is 10 hours. It is metabolized by the hepatic cytochrome P-450 system and is excreted in the urine within 72 hours. The starting dose should be reduced by 50% in older patients or in those with liver dysfunction.

Nicardipine (Cardene, Cardene IV) is a dihydropyridine calcium antagonist that inhibits transmembrane influx of calcium ions into cardiac muscle and smooth muscle. It more selectively alters vascular smooth muscle but may reduce myocardial contractility. It significantly decreases systemic vascular resistance and thus lowers blood pressure. It is used to manage essential hypertension and has also been used to manage chronic stable hypertension.

Nicardipine is 100 times more water soluble than nifedipine and can be administered orally or intravenously. It was the first dihydropyridine calcium channel blocker approved for IV administration in the United States. The oral dose is 20 to 60 mg twice daily, and the IV dose is 0.625 to 2.5 mg IV bolus followed by 0.5 to 5 mg/h. Its pharmacokinetic profile is listed in Table 17-6a and its adverse effects in Table 17-6b. It may prolong the QT segment on the electrocardiogram and is contraindicated in patients with hepatorenal impairment or congestive heart failure.

Table 17-6a Pharmacokinetic Profile of Calcium Channel Blockers

Drug	Onset	Peak	Duration	Half-life	Metabolism	Elimination
Dihydropyridines						
Nifedipine	0.5 h	5 h	8–24 h	2–5 h	Hepatic	Kidney, GI
Felodipine	< 1 h	2–4 h	20–24 h	10 h	Hepatic	Kidney
Nicardipine						
PO	20 min	1–2 h	12 h	2–4 h	Hepatic	Kidney, GI
IV	< 2 min	< 5 min				
Isradipine	1 h	2–3 h	12 h	8 h	Hepatic	Kidney, GI
Amlodipine	Gradual	6–9 h	24 h	28–120 h	Hepatic	Kidney, GI
Clevidipin	< 5 min	< 10 min	10–20 min	20 min	Nonspecific esterases	Kidney, GI
Phenylalkylamines						
Verapamil	< 30 min	1–2 h	2–10 h	6–12 h	Hepatic	Kidney
Benzothiazepines						
Diltiazem						
PO	30–60 min	2–3 h	6–24 h	3.5–6 h	Hepatic	Kidney
IV	3 min					

GI, gastrointestinal; PO, oral.

Nicardipine has been successful in the management of perioperative hypertension, control of hypertension associated with pheochromocytoma, controlled hypertension, prevention of cerebral vasospasm, and myocardial preservation during cardiopulmonary bypass.[34] Its efficacy for control of intraoperative and postoperative blood pressure has been demonstrated in both cardiac and noncardiac surgical patients. Goto et al.[35] evaluated nicardipine for control of intraoperative hypertension during gastrectomy. Patients received either enflurane, nicardipine 0.5 to 2 μg/kg/min, or atrial natriuretic factor 0.5 to 0.2 μg/kg/min to control hypertension. Although all three drugs controlled blood pressure, an increase in urine output was seen with nicardipine and atrial natriuretic factor, suggesting a direct effect of nicardipine on the proximal tubule.[35] It compared favorably with nitroprusside in the treatment of hypertension during coronary artery bypass graft.[36] Nicardipine is very effective in the management of postoperative hypertension.[37–39] It was given by an infusion or bolus followed by infusion and titrated until a therapeutic level was achieved. It does not cause "coronary steal syndrome," a problem associated with use of nitroprusside, and results in favorable myocardial oxygen supply and demand balance.[40]

Isradipine (DynaCirc) is another dihydropyridine used in the management of chronic hypertension. It inhibits calcium ion influx into cardiac muscle and smooth muscle without changing calcium concentrations. It significantly decreases systemic vascular resistance and reduces blood pressure. It may also be used to treat angina. The usual dose to treat chronic hypertension is 1.25 to 10 mg orally twice daily for a maximum dose of 20 mg/day. It undergoes first-pass hepatic metabolism and is excreted in the urine and feces.

Amlodipine (Norvasc) is also a dihydropyridine calcium channel antagonists that predominantly acts on the peripheral circulation, decreasing peripheral vascular resistance and increasing cardiac output. It reduces systolic, diastolic, and mean arterial blood pressure and is used to treat mild to moderate hypertension chronically. The oral dose is 5 to 10 mg daily but should be reduced by half in the elderly or in those with hepatic impairment. It is absorbed readily and has a gradual onset with peak effect of 6 to 9 hours and a duration of 24 hour. It has a half-life of 28 to 69 hours in those under age 45, and 40 to 120 hours in those over age 60. The administration of adenosine in patients receiving amlodipine may increase the risk of bradycardia. Herbal preparations such as ephedra and ma huang and melatonin may antagonize antihypertensive effects.

Clevidipine (Clevelox) is used to treat perioperative hypertension. It is an ultra–short-acting calcium channel blocker that is metabolized in blood (hydrolysis) and tissues by nonspecific esterases. It has an onset of less than 5 minutes, peak of less than 10 minutes, and duration of 10 to 20 minutes. It is excreted in the urine and feces.

Table 17-6b Adverse Effects of Calcium Channel Blockers

System	Nifedipine	Felodipine	Nicardipine	Verapamil	Diltiazem
CNS	Dizziness, light-headedness, nervousness, weakness, blurred vision, headache	Dizziness, fatigue, headache	Dizziness, headache, fatigue, depression, paresthesias, insomnia, somnolence, nervousness	Dizziness, vertigo, headache, fatigue, sleep disturbances, depression, syncope	Headache, fatigue, dizziness, drowsiness, nervousness, insomnia, tremor
CV	Facial flushing, hypotension, palpitations, peripheral edema	Flushing, palpitations, peripheral edema, tachycardia	Flushing, pedal edema, hypotension, tachycardia	Hypotension, CHF, bradycardia, A-V block, peripheral edema, pulmonary edema	Edema, arrhythmias, second- and third-degree heart block, bradycardia, CHF, hypotension
RS	Nasal congestion, dyspnea, cough, wheezing				
GI	Nausea, diarrhea, cramps, gingival hyperplasia	Nausea, diarrhea, dyspepsia	Anorexia, nausea, vomiting, dry mouth, dyspepsia	Nausea, abdominal discomfort, > hepatic enzymes	Nausea, anorexia, vomiting, diarrhea, impaired taste
Other	Joint stiffness, muscle cramps, pruritus, urticaria	Small < hemoglobin, hematocrit, red blood cell count	Arthritis, arthralgia	Flushing, muscle fatigue, diaphoresis, pruritus	Rash

CHF, congestive heart failure; CV, cardiovascular; GI, gastrointestinal; RS, respiratory.

Clevidipine lowers blood pressure by reducing peripheral vascular resistance. It may cause flushing and reduces gastric emptying. The dose is 0.3 to 3 μg/kg/min to a maximum of 16 μg/kg/min. In patients with a pseudocholinesterase deficiency, clearance is reduced and recovery is prolonged.

Verapamil (Calan, Isoptin, Verelan) is a phenylalkamine that inhibits calcium ion influx through slow calcium channels into myocardial and arterial smooth muscle. It dilates coronary arterioles and inhibits coronary artery spasm. It slows conduction through the sinoatrial and A-V node without altering intraventricular conduction. Vasodilation of arterioles lowers peripheral vascular resistance and reduces blood pressure. In addition to management of hypertension, verapamil may be used to treat angina, arrhythmias, supraventricular tachycardia, hypertropic cardiomyopathy, and migraine headache. It can be administered orally or intravenously. The initial oral dose is 40 to 80 mg initially followed by 120 to 480 mg every 6 to 8 hours. The IV dose is 0.075 to 0.15 mg/kg or 5 to 10 mg IV bolus that can be repeated in 15 to 30 minutes. After oral administration, 90% is absorbed, but only 25% to 30% reaches the systemic circulation due to first-pass metabolism. Table 17-6a shows the pharmacokinetic profile of verapamil.

Diltiazem (Cardizem) is a benzothiazepine calcium channel blocker used in the treatment of hypertension, angina, and atrial tachyarrhythmias. It is a slow calcium channel blocker with pharmacologic actions similar to verapamil. It inhibits calcium ion influx through slow calcium channels in the myocardium and arterial smooth muscle of peripheral and coronary vessels. It slows conduction at the sinoatrial and A-V node without affecting intraventricular conduction.

The usual adult dose for treatment of hypertension is 60 to 120 mg sustained release twice daily with a range of 240 to 360 mg/day. Approximately 80% is absorbed from an oral dose, but only 40% reaches the systemic circulation. Its onset is 30 to 60 minutes after an oral dose, peak effect is 2 to 3 hours, and duration is 6 to 24 hours. Its half-life is 3.5 to 6 hours. It can be given intravenously at a dose of 0.25 mg/kg followed by 15-mg/h infusion. Onset time with IV administration is 3 minutes and half-life is 2 hours. It is metabolized in the liver and primarily excreted by the kidneys, with some elimination in the feces. A list of anesthetic considerations in patients receiving calcium channel blockers is found in Box 17-5.

Angiotensin-Converting Enzyme Inhibitors

The renin-angiotensin-aldosterone system is an important physiologic mechanism and one that may contribute to hypertension.[41] Renin is stored in the afferent and

---

Box 17-5 Anesthetic Considerations in Patients Receiving Calcium Channel Blockers

1. Calcium channel blockers increase hypotensive effect of anesthetic and analgesic drugs.

2. Adequate hydration reduces risk of hypotension in the perioperative period.

3. Calcium channel blockers increase vasodilating properties of anesthetic and analgesic drugs.

4. Calcium channel blockers increase volume of fluids required during perioperative period.

5. Calcium channel blockers possess anesthetic and opioid-sparing properties during surgery.

6. Calcium channel blockers increase cardiovascular depressant effects of general anesthetics.

7. Patients with pseudocholinesterase deficiency have reduced clearance and prolonged recovery of clevidipine.

8. Clevidipine reduces gastric emptying.

9. Diltiazem increases the sedative effect of midazolam.

10. Patients receiving diltiazem with β-adrenergic blockers are more prone to hypotension and bradyarrhythmias.

---

efferent vessels of the nephron and is normally released with reduced renal perfusion or β_1-adrenergic stimulation. Once released, renin combines with angiotensinogen from the liver to form angiotensin I. Angiotensin I goes to the lung and under the influence of angiotensin-converting enzyme (ACE) in the lung becomes angiotensin II. Angiotensin II causes vasoconstriction and increased blood pressure. It also stimulates the release of aldosterone from the zona glomerulosa of the adrenal cortex. Aldosterone in turn results in sodium reabsorption in the distal convoluted tube and collecting duct of the nephron. In this segment of the nephron, potassium or hydrogen ion is secreted for every sodium ion saved. Table 17-7a provides the pharmacokinetic profile of ACE inhibitors, and Table 17-7b the adverse effects.

A number of drugs are available to alter the renin-angiotensin-aldosterone system. Important pharmacologic agents for the control of hypertension are ACE inhibitors and angiotensin II receptor antagonists. Captopril (Capoten)

Table 17-7a Pharmacokinetic Profile of ACE Inhibitors

Drug	Onset	Peak	Duration	Half-life	Metabolism	Elimination
Captopril	15 min	1–2 h	6–12 h	2 h	Hepatic	Kidney
Lisinopril	1 h	6–8 h	24 h	12 h		Kidney only
Enapril						
PO	1 h	4–8 h	12–24 h	2 h	Hepatic	Kidney, GI
IV	15 min	4 h	6 h	2 h		
Ramipril	2 h	6–8 h	24 h	2 h	Hepatic	Kidney
Benazepril	1 h	2–6 h	20–24 h	22 h	Hepatic	Kidney
Fosinopril	1 h	3 h	24 h	3–4 h	Hepatic	Kidney
Moexipril	0.5 h	1–2 h	6–12 h	2 h	Hepatic	Kidney
Perindopril	1 h	1 h	24 h	0.8–1 h	Hepatic	Kidney
Trandolapril	1–4 h	4–10 h	24 h	6 h	Hepatic	Kidney
Quinapril	1 h	2–4 h	24 h	2 h	Hepatic	Kidney

GI, gastrointestinal.

lowers blood pressure by specific inhibition of the ACE. This blocks formation of angiotensin II from renin. Angiotensin II is a powerful vasoconstrictor. Peripheral vascular resistance is lowered without reflex tachycardia or changes in cardiac output that often accompanies vasodilation. Inhibition of ACE also lowers aldosterone levels, which reduces reabsorption of sodium by the kidney, thus saving potassium. Captopril is the prototype in this class of drugs.

ACE inhibitors such as captopril are used to manage hypertension and have a positive effect in some patients with a history of congestive heart failure.[42] Patients in heart failure have a reduction in central venous pressure andiapulmonary wedge pressure when administered captopril. A decrease in dyspnea and improved exercise tolerance is also noted.

Captopril is well tolerated across the life span or from the premature infant to the adult. The usual oral adult dose to manage hypertension is 6.25 to 25 mg three times a day, which may be increased to 50 mg three times a day for a maximum dose of 450 mg daily. Absorption is 60% to 75%, and onset is 15 minutes. Peak effect is 1 to 2 hours, and duration is 6 to 12 hours. It is distributed to all tissues except the CNS. It is metabolized in the liver and excreted primarily by the kidneys.

Table 17-7b Adverse Effects of ACE Inhibitors

System	Captopril	Lisinopril	Enapril	Ramipril
CNS	Dizziness, fainting	Headache, fatigue, dizziness	Headache, fatigue, dizziness, insomnia, paresthesias, somnolence, nervousness	Dizziness, fatigue, headache
CV	First-dose hypotension, tachycardia, angioedema	Hypotension, chest pain	Postural hypotension, syncope, chest pain, palpitations, angioedema	Angiodema
RS	Cough	Cough, dyspnea	Cough	Cough
GI	Altered taste, weight loss	Nausea, vomiting, anorexia	Nausea, diarrhea, abdominal pain, dyspepsia	Nausea, vomiting, diarrhea
Other	Hyperkalemia, neutropenia, agranulocytosis, impaired renal function, nephritic syndrome	Neutropenia, azotemia, > BUN, > creatine levels, rash	< Hemoglobin, hematocrit, hyperkalemia	Hyperkalemia, hyponatremia, pruritus

BUN, blood urea nitrogen; CV, cardiovascular; GI, gastrointestinal; RS, respiratory.

Lisinopril (Zestril, Prinivil) acts by the same mechanism as captopril. It is used to treat hypertension and congestive heart failure, and improved survival after myocardial infarction is observed when patients receive lisinopril. The usual adult oral dose to treat hypertension begins with 10 mg daily and is increased to 20 to 40 mg one or two times daily. The maximum dose is 80 mg/day. Initial and maintenance are reduced by 50% in the elderly. Its onset of action is 1 hour, peak effect is 6 to 8 hours, and duration is 24 hours. The half-life is 12 hours. It is not metabolized and is excreted primarily by the kidneys. It is contraindicated in patients with renovascular disease and must be used cautiously in the hyperkalemic patient.

Enalapril (Vasotec) is similar to the prototype drug captopril in suppressing the renin-angiotensin-aldosterone system. Its antihypertensive effect is due to vasodilation secondary to suppression of the renin-angiotensin-aldosterone system. It is useful in mild to moderate hypertension as well as in malignant and accelerated hypertension. It is also used to manage renovascular hypertension except in bilateral renal artery stenosis. A 10% decrease in arterial blood pressure may occur after a single dose of enalapril in normotensive subjects. This is due to additional effects of ACE inhibition such as interference with degradation of bradykinin or accumulation of prostaglandins.[43] Enalapril can be administered orally or intravenously. The usual oral dose in the adult for hypertension is 5 mg/day, which can be increased to 10 to 40 mg/day in one or two divided doses. The IV dose is 1.25 mg every 6 hours, and as much as 5 mg every 6 hours is given in hypertensive emergencies. The IV dose should be given slowly over a 5-minute period. After oral administration 70% is absorbed from the gastrointestinal tract. Onset is within 1 hour, peak effect is in 4 to 8 hours, and duration is 12 to 24 hours. The half-life is 2 hours. The oral dose undergoes first-pass metabolism in the liver to an active form, enalaprilat. It is excreted in the urine and feces within 24 hours.

Ramipril (Altace), like other drugs of this class, lowers blood pressure by reducing peripheral vascular resistance secondary to inhibition of formation of angiotensin II. The adult dose to manage hypertension or congestive heart failure is 2.5 to 5 mg daily. This dose may be increased to 20 mg/day in two divided doses. After 60% absorption from the gastrointestinal tract, it has an onset of 2 hours, peak effect of 6 to 8 hours, duration of 24 hours, and half-life of 2 to 3 hours. It is actively metabolized in the liver to an active metabolite, ramiprilat, and is excreted by the kidney and gastrointestinal system. Benazepril (Lotensin) lowers blood pressure by suppression of the renin-angiotensin-aldosterone system. It should be used cautiously in patients with renal impairment, renal artery stenosis, hypovolemia, and in those receiving diuretics. The usual adult oral dose is 10 to 40 mg daily. It is readily absorbed from the gastrointestinal tract with 37% reaching the systemic circulation. Onset is within 1 hour, peak effect 2 to 6 hours, duration 20 to 24 hours, and half-life 22 hours. It is metabolized in the liver to an active metabolite, benazeprilat, and the metabolite is excreted primarily in the urine.

Fosinopril (Monopril) lowers blood pressure by altering the renin-angiotensin-aldosterone system and lowering angiotensin II. The oral adult dose to treat hypertension is 5 to 40 mg daily with a maximum dose of 80 mg. It is readily absorbed from the gastrointestinal tract and converted in the liver to its active form, fosinoprilat. Its onset is in 1 hour, peak effect 3 hours, duration 24 hours, and half-life 3 to 4 hours. It is hydrolyzed by intestinal and hepatic esterases to the active form, fosinoprilat, and is eliminated by the kidneys and gastrointestinal tract.

Moexipril (Univasc) is also a competitive inhibitor of ACE and results in reduced angiotensin II. It is used to treat hypertension, congestive heart failure, and diabetic nephropathy. The oral dose is 7.5 mg/day, which can be increased to 30 mg/day for a maximum of 60 mg. Its onset of action is 30 minutes, peak effect 1 to 2 hours, duration 6 to 12 hours and half-life 2 hours.

Perindopril (Aceon) lowers blood pressure by ACE inhibition and reduction of the vasoconstrictor angiotensin II. The adult oral dose to treat hypertension is 4 mg daily up to 8 mg daily in divided doses for a maximum of 16 mg/day. The drug is readily absorbed from the gastrointestinal tract and is metabolized in the liver to its active metabolite, perindoprilat. Onset is 1 hour, peak 3 to 7 hours, duration 24 hours, and half-life 30 to 120 hours. It is excreted primarily in the urine and should be used with caution in patients with renal insufficiency, volume depletion, or hyperkalemia, or with potassium-sparing drugs.

Trandolapril (Mavik) also lowers blood pressure by inhibition of ACE and lowering of angiotensin II levels. The usual adult dose is 1 to 2 mg/day, which may be increased to a maximum of 8 mg daily. It is readily absorbed from the gastrointestinal tract and converted in the liver to the active form, trandolaprilat. It is eliminated by the kidneys.

Quinapril (Accupril) is a potent, long-acting, second-generation ACE inhibitor that lowers angiotensin II and aldosterone levels. It lowers blood pressure through vasodilation and lowers pulmonary capillary wedge pressure, vascular resistance, and mean arterial pressure. Cardiac output and stroke volume are increased, which is useful in patients with congestive heart failure as well as hypertension. The usual starting adult oral dose is 10 to 20 mg daily to a maximum of 80 mg in two divided doses. It is rapidly absorbed from the gastrointestinal tract and has an onset of 1 hour, peak effect of 2 to 4 hours, duration of 24 hours, and half-life of 2 hours. It is extensively metabolized in the liver to its active metabolite, quinaprilat, and is mostly eliminated through the kidneys with a smaller elimination pathway in the feces.

When ACE inhibitors are maintained until the day of surgery, the incidence of hypotension after induction of anesthesia in hypertensive patients is 75% to 100%.[44,45] The main reason for this complication is decreased left ventricular preload and cardiac output. The risk of hypotension is increased with use of combined antihypertensive drugs or complete renin-angiotensin system blockade or with severe hypertension and left ventricular dysfunction. Some believe the risk of hypotension after anesthetic induction is reduced by drawing ACE inhibitors the day before surgery. It should be noted, however, that data on safe use of ACE inhibitors when combined with general anesthesia are conflicting.[46,47] Although some recommend discontinuation of ACE inhibitors preoperatively, others report safe use during anesthesia.[48] When hypotension does occur, IV fluids and vasopressors such as ephedrine or phenylephedrine are effective treatments in most cases. In severe cases of hypotension, the vasopressin analogue terlipressin has been used successfully.[49] A list of anesthetic considerations for patients receiving ACE inhibitors is found in Box 17-6.

Angiotensin II Receptor Antagonists

Angiotensin receptors are designated as AT_1 and AT_2. The AT_1 receptors are located in vascular and myocardial tissue as well as in the brain, kidney, and adrenal glomerulosa cells that produce aldosterone. Adverse effects of inhibition of angiotensin II include hypotension, hyperkalemia, and reduced renal function. Hypotension is more severe in patients who depend on angiotensin II function to maintain it. This includes those with volume depletion, renovascular hypertension, cardiac failure, and cirrhosis. As with ACE inhibitors, reports of refractory hypotension have been reported with angiotensin II receptor blockade.[50,51] Cough is much less of a problem with angiotensin II antagonists, and angioedema rarely occur. Table 17-8a lists the pharmacokinetics of angiotensin II receptor antagonists and Table 17-8b the adverse effects.

Losartan potassium (Cozaar) selectively blocks the binding of angiotensin II to the AT_1 receptor, and antihypertensive

---

Box 17-6 Anesthetic Considerations for Patients Receiving ACE Inhibitors

1. Hypotensive effects of ACE inhibitors are increased when patient also receives diuretic.

2. Antacids decrease absorption of captopril.

3. NSAIDs and ASA may decrease hypertensive effects of ACE inhibitors.

4. Intraoperative hypotension should first be treated with fluids.

5. Hypotensive risk is increased with vasodilators and anesthetic drugs.

6. Hypotension in patients under general anesthesia receiving ACE inhibitors may need to be treated with vasopressin agonists.

7. Lisinopril increases the muscle relaxant effects of curare-like neuromuscular-blocking drugs.

8. There is a risk of hyperkalemia with potassium-containing solutions.

ASA, acetylsalicylic acid; NSAIDs, nonsteroidal anti-inflammatory drugs.

---

effects result from blocking the vasoconstriction effects of angiotensin and lowering aldosterone secretion from the adrenal cortex. It is primarily used for the treatment of chronic hypertension. The adult oral dose for treatment of hypertension is 25 to 50 mg in one or two divided doses. The maximum daily dose is 100 mg. It is rapidly absorbed from the gastrointestinal tract, and 25% to 33% reaches the systemic circulation. Onset is less than 30 minutes, peak effect is 6 hours, duration is 24 hours, and half-life is 1.5 hours. The half-life of the active metabolite is 6 to 9 hours. It is extensively metabolized by the hepatic cytochrome P-450 enzyme system and is eliminated through the kidneys and gastrointestinal tract.

Candesartan (Atacand) selectively blocks binding of angiotensin II to angiotensin I receptors in vascular smooth muscle and the adrenal gland. This results in blocking the vasoconstriction and the aldosterone-secreting effects of angiotensin II, resulting in antihypertensive effects. The starting adult dose is 16 mg daily, and the dose range is 8 to 32 mg in divided doses. Candesartan is rapidly absorbed from the gastrointestinal tract and activated by ester

Table 17-8a Pharmacokinetics of Angiotensin II Receptor Antagonists

Drug	Onset	Peak	Duration	Half-life	Metabolism	Elimination
Losartan	6 h	24 h	1.5–2 h	6–9 h	Hepatic metabolite	Kidney, GI
Candesartan	< 1 h	3–4 h	24 h	9 h	Unchanged	Kidney, bile
Irbesartan				11–15 h	Hepatic	GI
Valsartan	< 2 h	2–4 h	24 h	6 h	Hepatic	GI
Telmisartan	1–2 h	0.5–3 h	24 h	5–24 h	Minimal hepatic metabolism	Kidney, GI
Eprosartan	1–2 h	1–2 h	24 h	5–9 h	Minimal hepatic metabolism	Kidney, GI

GI, gastrointestinal.

hydrolysis during absorption. Fifteen percent reaches the systemic circulation. Its onset is in less than 1 hour, peak effect 3 to 4 hours, and duration 24 hours. The half-life is 9 hours, and therapeutic effect is reached in 2 to 4 weeks. It is minimally metabolized in the liver and excreted unchanged in the bile and urine.

Irbesartan (Avapro) also blocks the effect of angiotensin II at the AT_1 receptor, lowering blood pressure by vasodilation and reduction in aldosterone levels. The beginning dose is 150 mg daily, which can be increased to 300 mg daily. It is rapidly absorbed from the gastrointestinal system, and 60% to 80% is bioavailable. It has a half-life of 11 to 15 hours and is metabolized in the liver and excreted in the feces.

Valsartan (Diovan) is an angiotensin antagonist used to treat hypertension and congestive heart failure. The oral adult dose to treat hypertension is 80 mg/day, and the maximum dose is 320 mg/day. It is rapidly absorbed from the gastrointestinal system and has 25% bioavailability. Peak plasma levels are reached in 2 to 4 hours, and blood pressure effects are seen in 4 weeks. Its half-life is 6 hours, and it is metabolized in the liver and eliminated in feces.

Telmisartan (Micardis) is also an angiotensin receptor antagonist used to treat chronic hypertension. The oral adult dose is 40 to 80 mg daily, and absorption is dose dependent. It is minimally metabolized and is primarily excreted in the feces as unchanged drug. Eprosartan mesylate (Teveten) is also an angiotensin antagonist used to treat hypertension. The usual daily dose is 600 mg daily with a maximum dose of 800 mg daily recommended. Only 13% of an oral dose reaches the systemic circulation. Its peak effect is seen in 1 to 2 hours, and the half-life is 5 to 9 hours. It is minimally metabolized and eliminated in the feces and urine. Anesthetic considerations for patients receiving angiotensin receptor antagonists are listed in Box 17-7.

Arterial Vasodilators

Hydralazine (Apresoline) reduces blood pressure mainly by direct effects on vascular smooth muscle of arterial resistance vessels. It has little effect on venous capacitance vessels. Hydralazine vasodilation is associated with powerful sympathetic responses caused by baroreceptor reflexes

Table 17-8b Adverse Effects of Angiotensin II Receptor Antagonists

System	Losartan	Candesartan	Valsartan	Telmisartan
CNS	Dizziness, headache, insomnia	Fatigue	Headache, dizziness	Headache, fatigue, dizziness
CV		Chest pain, peripheral edema		Hypotension, hypertension, chest pain, peripheral edema
RS	Nasal congestion, cough, upper respiratory tract infection, sinusitis	Cough, sinusitis, upper respiratory tract infection	Cough, sinusitis	Sinusitis, pharyngitis
GI	Dyspepsia, nausea	Nausea, vomiting, diarrhea	Nausea, diarrhea	Dyspepsia, abdominal pain
Other	Muscle cramps, back pain	Back pain, arthralgia, albuminuria	Arthralgia, hyperkalemia	

CV, cardiovascular; GI, gastrointestinal; RS, respiratory.

Box 17-7 Anesthetic Considerations for Patients Receiving Angiotensin Receptor Antagonists

1. Marked hypotension can occur during anesthesia in volume-depleted patients.

2. Increased neuromuscular block can occur with curare-like muscle relaxants.

3. Increased hypotensive effects of anesthetic and analgesia drugs can occur.

and has been shown to increase circulating catecholamine levels.[52] The result is increased heart rate and contractility, increased renin activity, and fluid retention. The response on diastolic blood pressure is often better than on systolic pressure. Vasodilation reduces peripheral resistance and substantially improves cardiac output and renal and cerebral blood flow.

Hydralazine can be administered orally, intramuscularly, or intravenously. The usual adult oral dose is 10 to 50 mg four times a day. It can be given intramuscularly at a dose of 10 to 50 mg every 4 to 6 hours or intravenously 10 to 20 mg every 4 to 6 hours. It is well absorbed from the gastrointestinal tract and has an onset of 20 to 30 minutes. Peak effect is 2 hours, and duration is 2 to 6 hours. Its half-life is 2 to 8 hours. It can be difficult to titrate blood pressure response and may be associated with an unpredictable decrease in blood pressure lasting for up to 12 hours.[53] It is metabolized in the intestinal wall and liver and eliminated in the urine and feces.

Sympathetic stimulation associated with administration of hydralazine increases myocardial oxygen demand and may result in myocardial ischemia. It does not dilate epicardial coronaries and may steal blood from ischemic myocardium, further contributing to ischemia. Its use is not advised in patients with coronary artery disease or hypertensive patients with risk factors for coronary disease. It increases intracranial pressure and should be avoided in patients at risk for intracranial hypertension. Hydralazine has been the drug of choice for hypertension associated with preeclampsia,[54] but more recent studies suggest that compared with other drugs, hydralazine is associated with increased maternal and fetal complications.[55]

Minoxidil (Loniten, Rogaine) is a direct-acting vasodilator with pronounced hypotensive effects. It acts by blocking calcium uptake through cell membranes and reduces systolic and diastolic blood pressure by decreasing peripheral vascular resistance. Hypotensive effects are accompanied

by activation of the sympathetic nervous system and renin-angiotensin-aldosterone system. The net result is increased heart rate and cardiac output and sodium retention and edema. Salt and water retention results from increased proximal tubular reabsorption due to reduced renal perfusion pressure. The oral dose to treat hypertension is 5 mg/day increased every 3 to 5 days to a dose of 40 mg/day. The maximum dose is 100 mg/day. It is readily absorbed from the gastrointestinal tract and has an onset of 30 minutes, peak action of 2 to 8 hours, duration of 3 to 5 days, and half-life of 4.2 hours. It is metabolized in the liver and eliminated in the urine and feces.

Diazoxide (Hyperstat, Proglycem) directly relaxes arteriolar smooth muscle and decreases pancreatic secretion of insulin. It reduces blood pressure by direct vasodilatory on vascular smooth muscle by direct competition for calcium receptor sites. It causes sodium and water retention and decreases urine output because of increased proximal tubular absorption secondary to reduced glomerular filtration rate. Hypotensive effects may be accompanied by marked reflex tachycardia and increased cardiac output and stroke volume. Cerebral and coronary blood flows are usually maintained. The dose of diazoxide to treat severe hypertension in the adult or child is 1 to 3 mg/kg up to 150 mg intravenously. It can be repeated every 5 to 15 minutes as needed. The onset is 30 to 60 seconds after IV administration, peak effect is 5 minutes, and duration is 2 to 12 hours. The half-life is 21 to 45 hours. It is partially metabolized in the liver and eliminated in the urine. Vasoactive drugs, general anesthetics, and acute intraoperative blood loss increase the hypotensive effects of diazoxide. It lowers blood glucose, and careful monitoring of perioperative glucose levels is recommended.

Fenoldopam mesylate (Corlopam) is a rapid-acting vasodilator that is a dopamine 1 receptor agonist. It binds selectively to dopamine 1 receptors without interaction with dopamine 2 or α- or β-adrenergic receptors. It exerts hypotensive effects by decreasing peripheral vascular resistance while increasing renal blood flow, diuresis, and natriuresis. It is used to treat severe, malignant hypertension and is administered intravenously. The IV dose is 0.025 to 0.3 μg/kg/min by continuous infusion.[56] The dose range is 0.01 to 1.6 μg/kg/min. The onset of action is 5 minutes, peak effect is 15 minutes, and duration is 15 to 30 minutes. The half-life of fenoldopam is 5 minutes. It is recommended that it be titrated no more than every 15 minutes. It is conjugated in the liver and excreted predominantly in the urine.

There is a low incidence of hypotension associated with the use of fenoldopam. Its longer half-life, lack of dependence on venodilation for blood pressure effect, and receptor-mediated mechanisms of action allow for slower reduction in blood pressure compared with nitroprusside.[57] This allows for standard blood pressure monitoring during administration of the drug.

Adverse effects associated with high-dose fenoldopam include headache, restless legs, diaphoresis, and nausea. ST-T wave changes on the electrocardiogram have been reported. Nonspecific ST-T wave changes are known consequences of vasodilator therapy and appear to be benign. They appear to be related to myocardial repolarization rather than myocardial ischemia.[58]

Fenoldopam maintains or improves renal hemodynamics despite decreased systemic blood pressure. It predictably increases renal blood flow and causes natriuresis and diuresis. Intraocular pressure rises slightly during fenoldopam infusion, and it is recommended that the drug be avoided or used cautiously in patients with glaucoma.[59] Safety and effectiveness of this drug in children have not been established. Electrocardiographic changes consisting of nonspecific T wave changes or inversion and ventricular arrhythmias have been reported with this drug. Unlike nitroprusside or nitroglycerin at high doses, no activating or inhibitory effects on hemostasis in either plasma coagulation or platelet function has occurred. Adverse effects include flushing, dizziness, headache, and hypotension. The incidence and severity of hypotension is worse with concomitant administration of other antihypertensives. The use of these agents seems to have an additive effect when used with fenoldopam. Caution should definitely be exercised with the use of beta-blockers in conjunction with fenoldopam. The reflex response of increased heart rate in response to hypotension may be attenuated with beta-blockade, and severe hypotension can occur. Hypokalemia has been reported, and the mechanism by which this happens is unknown. It is uncertain whether the hypokalemia occurs as a result of diuresis and natriuresis associated with the drug or as a direct effect.

A major advantage of the use of fenoldopam rests in its positive renal effects. α Receptor stimulation causes renal vasoconstriction; renal DA_1 receptor stimulation causes renal vasodilation, natriuresis, and diuresis. Because of DA_1 stimulation, it has the potential to be renal protective. Its selection as an antihypertensive takes high priority when maintenance of renal function is desired. It may be especially beneficial in patients at high risk for renal ischemia, patients with preexisting hepatic or renal impairment, and when increased urine flow is desired.

Unlike nitroprusside, it is not light labile, and there are no toxic metabolites. It offers significant advantages as an IV agent for management of blood pressure in both hypertensive emergencies and in the perioperative setting.

Arterial and Venous Vasodilators

Nitroglycerin (Tridil) is an organic nitrate and potent vasodilator that relaxes vascular smooth muscle, resulting in dose-related dilation of both venous and arterial blood vessels. It is a venous vasodilator producing predominantly venodilation at usual doses but arterial dilator at higher doses. It owes its vascular effects to the production of nitric oxide and subsequent increase in cyclic guanosine monophosphate (GMP) and smooth muscle relaxation. It promotes peripheral pooling of blood, reduction in peripheral resistance, and decreased venous return to the heart. Cardiac preload and afterload are reduced, and myocardial oxygen consumption is reduced. Table 17-9a provides the pharmacokinetic profile of vasodilators, Table 17-9b the adverse effects of arterial vasodilators, and Table 17-9c the adverse effects of mixed vasodilators.

Nitroglycerin is used to treat perioperative hypertension and is used for prophylaxis or treatment of angina. It may be used for controlled hypotension during some surgical procedures. The IV dose is 0.5 to 10 μg/kg/min titrated to effect. Its onset is within 1 minute, and its duration is 3 to 5 minutes. It has a half-life of 1 to 4 minutes. It is extensively metabolized in the liver, and the inactive metabolite is excreted through the kidney.

Nitroprusside sodium (Nipride, Nitropress) acts directly on vascular smooth muscle to produce peripheral vasodilation with marked lowering of blood pressure and a slight increase in heart rate. It is an arterial and venous vasodilator and thus decreases both cardiac preload and afterload. Its major use is in hypertensive emergencies, acute congestive heart failure, and controlled hypotension, and it has been considered the drug of choice for acute perioperative hypertension, especially after cardiac surgery.[59] The dose is 0.5 to 10 μg/kg/min with an average dose of 3 μg/kg/min. The infusion must be wrapped to protect it from sunlight. It has an onset of action after IV administration of 0.5 to 1 minutes, peak effect of 2 to 3 minutes, and duration of 5 to 10 minutes. Because of its potent and labile effects, its use requires invasive blood pressure monitoring. It is rapidly converted to cyanogens in erythrocytes and other tissue, which is metabolized to thiocyanate in the liver. It is excreted in the urine primarily as thiocyanate.

Nitroprusside increases cerebral blood flow and intracranial pressure. Its use is associated with reflex tachycardia and rebound hypertension when the drug is discontinued. It lowers pulmonary vascular resistance and increases pulmonary perfusion ventilation mismatch due to inhibition of hypoxic pulmonary vasoconstriction. It lowers renal blood flow and decreases renal function when compared with other

Table 17-9a Pharmacokinetic Profile of Vasodilators

Drug	Onset	Peak	Duration	Half-life	Metabolism	Elimination
Hydralazine						
PO	0.5 h	0.5–1 h	4–6 h	3–7 h	Intestinal wall;	Kidney
IV	0.5 h		2–6 h		liver	
Minoxidil	0.5 h	2–8 h	2–5 days	4.2 h	Liver	Kidney, GI
Diazoxide						
PO	1 h		8 h	21–45 h	Liver	Kidney
IV	< 1 min	5 min	2–12 h			
Fenoldopam IV	5 min	15 min	15–30 min	5 min	Liver	Kidney
Nitroglycerin IV	1 min		3–5 min	1–4 min	Liver	Kidney
Nitroprusside IV	< 1 min	2–3 min	5–10 min	2.7–7 days	Liver	Kidney

GI, gastrointestinal; PO, oral.

antihypertensives.[60] Its use is contraindicated in congenital Leber's optic atrophy and severe hypovolemia. Its use with spinal or general anesthesia increases intraoperative hypotension.

A major adverse effect associated with large doses of nitroprusside is cyanide toxicity. Data suggest that nitroprusside infusion rates in excess of 4 μg/kg/min for 2 to 3 hours may lead to cyanide levels in the toxic range.[61] Hemolysis associated with cardiopulmonary bypass increases the release of free cyanide.[62] Nitroprusside also causes cytotoxicity through the release of nitric oxide, which generates hydroxyl radicals and peroxynitrite, leading to lipid peroxidation.[63]

Signs and symptoms of toxicity associated with nitroprusside toxicity are related to metabolic changes as well as changes in the CNS and cardiovascular systems. Changes associated with CNS dysfunction include alterations in mental status, seizures, and coma. Signs of cardiovascular instability include tachyphylaxis to the drug with hypertension, arrhythmias, and ST segment changes. There is a close association between cyanide toxicity and metabolic acidosis.[64] Treatment of cyanide toxicity is found in Box 17-8. Sodium nitrite converts hemoglobin to methemoglobin, which competes with cytochrome oxidase for cyanide radicals. Sodium thiosulfate provides a continuous source of sulfur donors and prevents accumulation of cyanide radicals. Vitamin B_{12} binds cyanide and acts as a reservoir that can be excreted in the urine.

Table 17-9b Adverse Effects of Arterial Vasodilators

System	Hydralazine	Minoxidil	Diazoxide	Fenoldopam
CNS	Headache, dizziness, tremors	Fatigue	Headache, weakness, dizziness, insomnia, extrapyramidal symptoms	Headache, anxiety, dizziness, insomnia
CV	Palpitations, angina, tachycardia, flushing	Tachycardia, angina, ECG changes, tamponade, rebound hypertension, pulmonary edema	Palpitations, atrial, ventricular dysrhythmias, orthostatic hypotension	Hypotension, tachycardia, T wave inversion, flushing, postural hypotension
GI	Anorexia, nausea, vomiting, abdominal pain, paralytic ileus		Nausea, vomiting, ileus, impaired hepatic function	Nausea, vomiting, abdominal pain
Other	< Hemoglobin, hematocrit, anemia, agranulocytosis, nasal congestion, muscle cramps, edema	Hypertrichosis, pruritus, skin darkening, Stevens-Johnson syndrome	Blurred vision, papilledema, neutropenia, eosinophilia	Nasal congestion, dyspnea

CV, cardiovascular; ECG, electrocardiographic; GI, gastrointestinal.

Table 17-9c Adverse Effects of Mixed Vasodilators

System	Nitroglycerin	Nitroprusside
CNS	Headache, apprehension, blurred vision, vertigo, dizziness, faintness	Restlessness, apprehension, muscle twitching, headache, dizziness
CV	Postural hypotension, palpitations, > heart rate, syncope, circulatory collapse	Profound hypotension, palpitations, > heart rate, < heart rate, retrosternal discomfort
GI	Nausea, vomiting, abdominal pain, dry mouth	Nausea, vomiting, abdominal pain
Other	Methemoglobinemia (high dose), flushing, rash, anaphylactoid reaction, oral and conjunctival edema	Nasal stuffiness, > serum creatinine, thiocyanate toxicity (hypotension, blurred vision, fatigue, metabolic acidosis, pink skin, absence of reflexes, faint heart sounds)

CV, cardiovascular; GI, gastrointestinal.

Anesthetic Management of Acute Perioperative Hypertension

Perioperative hypertension and arterial blood pressure lability affect up to 80% of patients undergoing cardiac surgery and up to 25% of patients undergoing noncardiac surgery.[65–67] There are many reasons for perioperative hypertension (Box 17-9). Patients with poor blood pressure controlled preoperatively or recent development of moderate to severe hypertension have a higher incidence of perioperative hypertension. Perioperative hypertension is also seen in patients with high spinal cord injury (mass reflex) and

Box 17-8 Treatment of Sodium Nitroprusside Cyanide Toxicity

1. Stop the infusion of nitroprusside.

2. Administer 100% oxygen.

3. Correct metabolic acidosis.

4. Administer 3% sodium nitrite 4–6 mg/kg slowly intravenously.

5. Administer sodium thiosulfate 150–200 mg/kg intravenously over 15 minutes.

6. Consider hydroxocobalamin (vitamin B_{12}) 25 mg/h.

in certain surgical procedures such as intracranial procedures, carotid endarterectomy, heart and neck surgery, and major cardiovascular procedures. Treatment modalities for hypertension in patients with intracranial pathology require special consideration. It requires an understanding of the pathophysiology of intracranial hypertension and determinants of cerebral perfusion pressure. Treatment modalities in this circumstance should control blood pressure while considering the impact of treatment on cerebral blood flow and intracranial pressure.[68] Perioperative hypertension is primarily caused by increased sympathetic discharge with sympathetic systemic vasoconstriction and is often treated with an IV vasodilator.

The incidence of perioperative hypertension is rising as a result of an aging population, increase in cardiovascular procedures, decrease in deep opioid anesthesia, and prolonged sedation after surgery. Hypertension can be a serious complication in the surgical patient. Complications associated with hypertension may include cerebral vascular accident, myocardial ischemia, myocardial infarction,

Box 17-9 Etiology of Perioperative Hypertension

- Inadequate anesthesia
- Airway manipulation
- Hypercarbia
- Hypoxia
- Pharmacologic adjuncts
- Distention of urinary bladder
- Aortic cross-clamp
- Hypervolemia
- Hypothermia
- Tourniquet pain
- Medication noncompliance; poorly controlled preoperative blood pressure
- Disease-related factors
  - Pheochromocytoma
  - Hyperthyroid storm
  - Autonomic hyperreflexia
  - Malignant hyperthermia
  - Intracranial hypertension
  - Renovascular hypertension
- Accelerated hypertension in a patient with preexisting hypertension.

left ventricular dysfunction, cardiac arrhythmias, tension on suture lines, hemorrhage, pulmonary edema, and cognitive dysfunction.[69-71] Once recognized, the etiology of hypertension must be aggressively pursued. When general measures such as correcting physiologic parameters and deepening anesthesia fail to correct the problem, pharmacologic therapy is indicated.

Blood pressure management in hypertensive emergencies requires the use of parenteral agents because rapid control is critical. In the perioperative period the oral route is generally unavailable, and speed and ability to titrate the drug to the desired response is desirable. The profile of an ideal perioperative antihypertensive drug is found in Box 17-10.

Traditional pharmacologic agents used for acute hypertension are IV preparations of adrenergic antagonists, calcium channel blockers, direct-acting vasodilators, angiotensin enzyme (ACE) inhibitors, and dopamine 1 agonists. The dopamine 1 agonist fenoldopam and calcium channel blocker clevidipine are newer drugs that are well suited for management of perioperative hypertension. The choice of antihypertensive in critical care and perioperative settings varies widely. One study found that labetalol is the initial IV antihypertensive selected, accounting for 32% of patients with severe hypertension, followed by metoprolol,

nitroglycerin, and hydralazine at 16%, 15%, and 15%, respectively. Nicardipine and sodium nitroprusside were administered at rates of 8% and 6%, respectively.[72] Intermittent IV labetalol is most often administered initially for patients without stroke (21%) followed by nicardipine (20%) and sodium nitroprusside (19%). Nicardipine is most often administered initially for patients with acute hemorrhagic stroke (35%) followed by IV labetalol (21%) and sodium nitroprusside (16%).[73]

Comparison studies of clevidipine, nitroglycerin, sodium nitroprusside, and nicardipine for acute hypertension treatment in cardiac surgical patients have been done. There were no differences in the incidence of myocardial infarction, stroke, or renal dysfunction for clevidipine-treated patients compared with other treatment groups. There was no difference in mortality between the clevidipine, nitroglycerin, or nicardipine groups. Mortality was significantly higher in the sodium nitroprusside group compared with the clevidipine group. Clevidipine was more effective than nitroglycerin or sodium nitroprusside and equivalent with nicardipine in maintaining blood pressure within the prescribed blood pressure range.[74]

Commonly used adrenergic antagonists for management of perioperative hypertension include esmolol and labetalol. Advantages and disadvantages of both drugs are listed in Table 17-10. Esmolol is a cardioselective beta-blocker with a rapid onset and short duration of action. It is primarily used to treat tachycardia but lowers blood pressure primarily by inhibiting renin release and decreasing cardiac output. Major drawbacks to the use of esmolol include the possibility of worsening cardiac conduction defects, ventricular function, and bronchospastic problems. Esmolol is particularly useful in severe postoperative hypertension in tachycardiac patients.[75] It is given as a 0.5- to 1-mg/kg loading dose followed by an infusion at 50 μg/kg/min increased up to 300 μg/kg/min.

Labetalol, a combined α_1, β_1, and β_2 antagonist, which slightly reduces heart rate, reduces systemic vascular resistance and maintains cardiac output. Cerebral, renal, and coronary blood flow are maintained. It is a first line for prophylaxis for surgical hypertension. Labetalol can be given as a loading dose of 20 mg followed by doses of 20 to 80 mg. It can be infused at a rate of 1 to 2 mg/min and increased until the desired blood pressure is achieved. Bolus injections of 1 to 2 mg/kg can cause a serious drop in blood pressure and should be avoided.[76]

Nicardipine and clevidipine are calcium channel blockers with a pharmacokinetic profile that is well suited for perioperative control of hypertension. Advantages and disadvantages of these drugs are listed in Table 17-11. Nicardipine is more potent in vascular smooth muscle than

Box 17-10 Profile of Ideal Perioperative Antihypertensive Drug

- Parenteral administration
- Rapid onset and offset (seconds or minutes)
- Easy titratability
- Reliable efficacy
- Ease of use
- Minimal need for continuous blood pressure monitoring
- Few to no drug interactions
- Minimal hypotension
- Little to no potential for exacerbation of comorbidity
- No acute tolerance or tachyphylaxis
- Safe: no toxic metabolites
- Minimal sympathetic activation
- Preservation of renal blood flow and glomerular filtration
- Cost effectiveness

Table 17-10 α- and β-Adrenergic Blocking Drugs

Drug	Advantages	Disadvantages
Esmolol (Brevibloc)	Easy to titrate Short $t_{1/2}$ 8 min β$_1$ selective antagonist Quick onset, rapid offset Metabolized by red blood cell esterases Myocardial depression Preserves myocardial oxygen supply Bolus dosing or IV infusion possible	Depresses myocardial contractility May cause conduction defects Contraindicated in heart failure, A-V block, severe bradycardia Hypotension at high doses Caution advised with poor ventricular function and hyperactive airway Potential for exaggerated effect when used with volatile agents
Labetalol (Trandate Normodyne)	Half-life 4–6 h Alpha-, beta-blocker: no reflex tachycardia Less potential for bradycardia and hypotension than esmolol Minimal effect on renal function Bolus dosing or IV infusion	Caution in patients with COPD Can depress myocardial contractility Potential excess response with volatiles Can depress myocardial contractility Same contraindications as for other beta-blockers

in cardiac muscle and has strong cerebral and coronary vasodilating properties. The degree of vascular selectivity exceeds that of nifedipine. Its major drawback is its very long half-life. Nicardipine is indicated for short-term IV management of hypertension, reduction of postoperative myocardial ischemia, prevention of perioperative myocardial infarction, and prophylaxis for postsurgical coronary artery spasm. The initial infusion rate is 5 mg/h and is increased by 2.5 mg/h every 5 minutes to a maximum of 15 mg/h or until the desired blood pressure is achieved.

Clevidipine, the first, third-generation IV dihydropyridine calcium channel blocker, exerts arterial-specific vasodilating effects and is characterized by an ultrafast onset and offset of decreasing blood pressure.[77] After IV administration clevidipine is quickly cleared from the blood by nonspecific blood and tissue esterases, resulting in rapid elimination with a half-life of approximately 1 minute. In healthy volunteers, arterial blood pressure and heart rate returned to normal in 10 to 15 minutes after discontinuation of a short infusion.[78] Rapid elimination of clevidipine is maintained after stopping either a 24-hour or short infusion.[79]

The initial dose of clevidipine for blood pressure control is 1 to 2 mg/h. The dose can be doubled at 90-second

Table 17-11 Calcium Channel Antagonists Available in Parenteral Form

Drug	Advantages	Disadvantages
Nicardipine (Cardene)	Dose-dependent arterial vasodilation Arterial catheter not mandatory No coronary steal Cerebral, coronary vasodilation Minimal effects on cardiac contractility, conduct Mild natriuretic effect	Slow onset, offset May accumulate Variable duration of action Hypotension possible Venous irritation May cause sympathetic activity, tachycardia Marked fluctuations in blood pressure possible
Clevidipine (Cleviprex)	Ultrashort $t_{1/2}$ Rapid onset, offset Targeted arterial vasodilation Metabolized by blood esterases Reduced need for other antihypertensives Reliable control Reliable transition to other antihypertensives Non–weight-based dosing No dose adjustment needed in patients with renal and hepatic disease Ready to use vial; no mixing No significant myocardial depression No effect on venous return (preload) Potential for drug interactions is low	Lipid emulsion Because of lipid restrictions, no more than 1000 mL or average of 21 mg/h recommended In geriatrics, start at low dose and titrate Photosensitivity during storage, not during administration Continuous monitoring required during administration

intervals initially. The desired therapeutic response for most patients occurs at a dose of 4 to 6 mg/h. Patients with severe hypertension may need up to 16 mg/h. Patients not transitional to other medications should be closely monitored for rebound hypertension for 8 hours after discontinuation of the infusion. Clevidipine contains 0.2 g lipid/mL (2 kcal). Because of lipid load restrictions, no more than 1000 mL or an average of 21 mg/h of clevidipine is recommended over a 24-hour period. It is contraindicated in patients with allergies to soy beans, eggs, or egg products. It is also contraindicated in patients with defective lipid metabolism such as pathologic hyperlipidemia or acute pancreatitis. This class of calcium channel blockers can produce negative inotropic effects and exacerbate heart failure.

Clevidipine gives no protection against abrupt beta-blocker withdrawal. Pollack et al.[80] evaluated the use of clevidipine for the treatment of acute severe hypertension. Within 30 minutes of starting clevidipine, 88.9% had achieved target blood pressure range. Median time to target range was 10.9 minutes. No concurrent IV antihypertensives were needed, and clevidipine was well tolerated with successful transition to oral antihypertensive therapy after infusion.[80] It has also been evaluated for treatment of preoperative hypertension in cardiac surgical patients. Patients treated with clevidipine demonstrated a 92.5% rate of treatment success at a median of 6 minutes. A modest increase in heart rate occurred during administration, but the drug was well tolerated in patients having cardiac surgery.[81] Finally, Singla et al.[82] examined the efficacy and safety of clevidipine in treating postoperative hypertension in cardiac surgical patients. Treatment success was achieved in 91.8% of patients, and median time to target blood pressure was 5.3 minutes. In this study no significant increase in heart rate from baseline was observed.[82] It appears, therefore, that clevidipine is effective and safe for management of acute severe hypertension as well as preoperative and postoperative hypertension in cardiac surgical patients. Advantages and disadvantages of calcium channel antagonists for management of hypertension are listed in Table 17-11.

Direct-acting vasodilators often used in the perioperative period to manage hypertension are nitroglycerin, sodium nitroprusside, and hydralazine. Advantages and disadvantages of each are listed in Table 17-12. Nitroglycerin is a nitric oxide compound that produces vasodilation by principally affecting venous capacitance vessels and preload. At higher doses, arteriolar relaxation occurs and thus afterload is altered.

Nitroglycerin must be prepared in glass bottles and administered through special infusion sets intended for nitroglycerin. The initial IV dose is 5 μg/min followed by a 5-μg/min increase every 3 to 5 minutes to 20 μg/min. If no response is noted at 20 μg/min, the infusion can be increased at increments of 10 μg/min up to 200 μg/min. Its onset and peak effects are immediate, and duration when the infusion is discontinued is 3 to 5 minutes.

Table 17-12 Direct-Acting Vasodilators

Drug	Advantages	Disadvantages
Nitroglycerin (Tridil)	Rapid onset Short duration of action Coronary vasodilator Reduced myocardial oxygen consumption No major toxicities No coronary steal Reduced pulmonary vascular resistance	Decreased diastolic blood pressure Reflex tachycardia Potential for hypotension Variable efficacy Tachyphylaxis Methemoglobinemia Intrapulmonary shunting Prolonged bleeding time
Sodium nitroprusside (Nipride)	Immediate onset Short duration of action Reduced myocardial oxygen demand	Reflex tachycardia Cyanide toxicity Intrapulmonary shunting Precipitous drop in blood pressure possible Photodegradation Methemoglobinemia Coronary steal Enhanced bleeding Cerebral vasodilator
Hydralazine (Apresoline)	Maintains or increases cerebral blood flow Duration of action 2–4 h Increased cardiac output Stroke volume	Reflex tachycardia Reduced pressor response to ephedrine Drug interactions Sodium, water retention

Sodium nitroprusside is a nitric oxide compound with equal arteriolar and venous dilating effects. Its onset and offset are rapid, but hypotensive effects can be unpredictable. Like nitroglycerin it may cause intrapulmonary shunting, which may lead to hypoxia. Unlike nitroglycerin it may reduce coronary perfusion pressure and cause coronary steal. Cyanide toxicity is a concern with large doses for a prolonged period of time, and invasive monitoring of blood pressure is required.

The initial dose of Nipride for acute hypertension is 0.3 to 0.5 μg/kg/min increased in increments of 0.5 μg/kg/min to the desired hemodynamic effect. The usual dose is 0.3 μg/kg/min, and a dose higher than 0.4 μg/kg/min is rarely needed. The maximum dose is 10 μg/kg/min. When administered by prolonged infusion faster than 2 μg/kg/min, cyanide is generated fasted than an unaided patient can handle. Onset of action is under 2 minutes, and duration is 1 to 10 minutes.

Hydralazine lowers blood pressure almost exclusively by a direct relaxant effect on arteriolar smooth muscle. The vasodilator probably reflects interference with calcium transport in vascular smooth muscle. Reduction in blood pressure may result in reflex tachycardia that is poorly tolerated in some patients, such as those with coronary artery disease. Onset is slower, 5 to 10 minutes, and duration longer, 2 to 4 hours, than with nitroglycerin or nitroprusside. Enhanced hypotensive effects may be seen in patients taking diuretics, monoamine oxidase inhibitors, diazoxide, and other antihypertensive drugs.

Fenoldopam, approved by the U.S. Food and Drug Administration in 1997, is a selective dopamine receptor (DA$_1$) agonist that can lower blood pressure while maintaining or improving renal blood flow. It causes systemic vasodilation and regional vasodilation, especially renal. It does not bind to DA$_2$, α$_1$, or renal blood flow (Table 17-13). It does not cross the blood–brain barrier and therefore does not interact with receptors in the CNS. Selectivity for the dopamine

Table 17-13 Fenoldopam: Dopamine Receptor Agonist Compared With Dopamine

	Actions of DA$_1$ Agonists	
	Dopamine	Fenoldopam
DA$_1$ (vasodilation)	+++	+++
DA$_2$ (vasodilation, emesis)	+++	—
α$_1$ (vasoconstriction)	++	—
β$_1$ (inotropic, chronotropic effect)	+++	—
β$_2$ (vasodilation)	+	—

+++, major action; ++, moderate action; +, mild action; —, no action.

1 receptor is the most unique property of fenoldopam. The blood pressure–lowering effects are predictable and stable with constant dose infusion. For severe hypertension in the adult, the initial infusion is 0.1 to 0.3 μg/kg/min. It may be increased in increments of 0.05 to 0.1 μg/kg/min every 15 minutes until target blood pressure is reached. Boluses should never be given. The maximal infusion rate reported in clinical studies was 1.6 μg/kg/min. Because blood pressure lowering with fenoldopam is predictable, invasive monitoring of blood pressure may not be necessary. The use of an arterial line is at the discretion of the anesthetist, but frequent monitoring of blood pressure is recommended.

The half-life is short, 4 to 5 minutes, and the drug is rapidly eliminated after the infusion is discontinued. The drug is metabolized by the cytochrome P-450 system. No dose adjustments are necessary for patients with renal or hepatic impairment. It increases renal blood flow and glomerular filtration rate. Advantages and disadvantages of its use are noted in Table 17-14. It should be noted that fenoldopam contains sodium bisulfite, and this may result in allergic-type reactions, including anaphylactic symptoms or life-threatening or less severe asthmatic episodes in some patients. The overall prevalence of sulfite sensitivity is unknown but probably low.

Table 17-14 Dopamine 1 Agonists

Drug	Advantages	Disadvantages
Fenoldopam (Corlopam)	Rapid onset Short duration of action No precipitous fall in blood pressure Easily titrated Preserves renal function No coronary steal No negative inotropic, chronotropic effect No invasive arterial monitoring needed No known drug interactions	Reflex tachycardia ECG changes Mild tolerance after long-term infusion May reduce serum potassium Contains sodium bisulfite Mild increase in intraocular pressure Potentially high cost

ECG, electrocardiographic.

Key Points

- There are five classes of antihypertensives: sympatholytics, calcium channel blockers, ACE inhibitors, angiotensin receptor antagonists, and vasodilators.
- There are five subtypes of sympatholytics.
- For clonidine, the ratio of α_2-to-α_1 effect is 220:1; for dexmedetomidine the ratio is 1620:1.
- β-Adrenergic antagonists used to treat hypertension have a nonselective or selective action at the β receptor.
- There are three primary contraindications to the use of the prototypical drug propranolol: greater than first-degree heart block, congestive heart failure, and bronchial asthma or bronchospasm.
- The ratio of alpha-to-beta blockade with oral and IV labetalol is 1:3 and 1:7, respectively.
- Calcium channel antagonists inhibit calcium entry into cardiac and smooth muscle, resulting in vascular relaxation and negative inotropic and chronotropic effects.
- Clevidipine is an ultra–short-acting calcium channel antagonist metabolized in blood and tissues by nonspecific esterases.
- The renin-angiotensin-aldosterone system contributes to hypertension by vasoconstriction (angiotensin II) and sodium and water retention (aldosterone).
- ACE inhibitors inhibit formation of angiotensin II and bradykinin; refractory hypotension has been reported when patients taking these drugs receive anesthesia.
- Fenoldopam is a selective dopamine 1 agonist used in the management of acute perioperative hypertension.
- Acute treatment of hypertension in patients with intracranial pathology should consider the pathophysiology of intracranial hypertension and determinants of cerebral perfusion pressure.
- Perioperative hypertension is primarily caused by increased sympathetic discharge with vasoconstriction; it is often treated with vasodilators.

Chapter Questions

1. List five classes of antihypertensives, and describe their primary mechanism of action.
2. Describe the mechanism of action of five types of sympatholytics.
3. List and discuss the use of α_2 agonists in anesthesia.
4. Compare the pharmacokinetic and pharmacodynamic profiles of clonidine and dexmedetomidine.
5. List and discuss safety precautions in the use of dexmedetomidine.
6. Why should beta-blockers not be given to patients with pheochromocytoma if alpha blockade is not present?
7. What is the major advantage(s) of selective versus nonselective beta-blockers?
8. Why is esmolol generally more useful perioperatively than other selective or nonselective β antagonists?
9. How does labetalol compare with other α- and β-adrenergic blockers?
10. List and discuss major anesthetic considerations for patients receiving β-adrenergic blocking drugs.
11. What are common anesthetic considerations for patients receiving calcium channel blockers?
12. What are major anesthetic considerations for patients chronically receiving ACE inhibitors?
13. What are three adverse effects of inhibition of the angiotensin II receptors?
14. Dopamine and fenoldopam are both dopamine receptor agonists. Why is dopamine a positive inotrope and fenoldopam an antihypertensive?
15. What is the major effect of fenoldopam over other vasodilators?
16. Compare nitroglycerin with nitroprusside in mechanism of action, advantages, and disadvantages.
17. Identify factors responsible for perioperative hypertension.
18. List and discuss pharmacologic characteristics of an ideal IV antihypertensive.
19. Why is clevidipine more useful for acute hypertension than nifedipine or nicardipine?
20. What are the advantages and disadvantages of perioperative alpha- and beta-blockers in the management of hypertension? Calcium channel blockers? Direct-acting vasodilators? Dopamine 1 agonists?

References

1. Hajjar I, Kotchen TA. Trends in prevalence, awareness, treatment, and control of hypertension in the United States, 1988–2000. *JAMA*. 2003;290:199–206.
2. Steinberg JS. Angiotensin II receptor antagonists: mechanisms and therapeutic utility. *Hosp Pharm*. 1998;33(1): 53–65.
3. Walker JR. Antihypertensive agents. *J Periop Nurs*. 1999;14: 278–283.

4. Maze M, Tranquilli W. Alpha-2 adrenoreceptor agonists: defining the role in clinical anesthesia. *Anesthesiology.* 1991; 74:581–605.

5. Wallace AW, Galindez D, Salahieh A, et al. Effect of clonidine on cardiovascular morbidity and mortality after noncardiac surgery. *Anesthesiology.* 2004;101:284–293.

6. Marinangel F, Cocco C, Ciccozzi A, et al. Hemodynamic effects of intravenous clonidine on propofol and thiopental reduction. *Acta Anaesth Scand.* 2000;44:150–156.

7. Watanabe T, Inagaki Y, Ishibe Y. Clonidine premedication effects on inhaled induction with sevoflurane in adults: a prospective, double-blind, randomized study. *Acta Anaesth Scand.* 2006;50:180–181.

8. Dannelli G, Cabertih L, Buti M, et al. Does clonidine 50 ug improve cervical plexus block obtained with ropivacaine 150 mg for carotid endarterectomy? A randomized, double-blind study. *J Clin Anesth.* 2006;18:585–588.

9. Militello MA, Mauro V. *Drug Information Handbook for Cardiology.* Hudson, OH: LexiCorp; 2006:317.

10. Armanious S, Wong DT, Etchells E, et al. Successful implementation of perioperative beta-blockade utilizing a multidisciplinary approach. *Can J Anaesth.* 2003;50:131–136.

11. Kirshenbaum JM, Kloner RA, Antman EM, et al. Use of an ultra-short acting beta-blocker in patients with acute myocardial ischemia. *Circulation.* 1985;72:873–880.

12. Wallace A, Layug B, Tateo I, et al. Prophylactic atenolol reduces postoperative myocardial ischemia. *Anesthesiology.* 1998;88:7–17.

13. Redelmeier D, Scales D, Kopp A, et al. Beta blockers for elective surgery in elderly patients: population based, retrospective cohort study. *BMJ.* 2005;331:932.

14. Singh H, Vichitvejpaisal P, Gaines GY, et al. Comparative effects of lidocaine, esmolol, and nitroglycerin in modifying hemodynamic response to laryngoscopy and intubation. *J Clin Anesth.* 1995;7:5–8.

15. Sharma S, Mitra S, Grover VK, et al. Esmolol blunts the haemodynamic response to tracheal intubation in treated hypertensive patients. *Can J Anaesth.* 1996;43:778–782.

16. Lim SH, Chin NM, Tai HY, et al. Prophylactic esmolol infusion for the control of cardiovascular responses to extubation after cranial surgery. *Ann Acad Med Singapore.* 2000;29:447–451.

17. Fuhrman TM, Ewell CL, Pippin WD, et al. Comparison of esmolol and alfentanil to attenuate hemodynamic responses to emergence and extubation. *J Clin Anesth.* 1992;4:444–447.

18. Kindler CH, Schumaker PG, Schneider MC. Effects of intravenous lidocaine and/or esmolol on hemodynamic responses to laryngoscopy and intubation: a double-blind controlled clinical trial. *J Clin Anesth.* 1996;8:491–496.

19. Atlee JL, Dhamee SM, Olund TL, et al. The use of esmolol, nicardipine, or their combination to blunt hemodynamic changes after laryngoscopy and tracheal intubation. *Anesth Analg.* 2000;90:280–285.

20. Bensky KP, Donahue-Spencer L, Hertz E, et al. The dose related effects of bolus esmolol on heart rate and blood pressure following laryngoscopy and intubation. *AANAJ.* 2000;68:437–441.

21. Smerling A, Gersong WM. Esmolol for severe hypertension following repair of aortic coarctation. *Crit Care Med.* 1990;18:1288–1290.

22. Gold MR, Dee WG, Corea-Spofford D, et al. Esmolol and ventilatory function in cardiac patients with COPD. *Chest.* 1991;100:1215–1218.

23. Lund-Johasen P. Pharmacology of combined alpha-beta blockers II. Hemodynamic effects of labetalol. *Drugs.* 1984; 28:35–50.

24. Kanto J, Allonen H, Kleimola T, et al. Pharmacokinetics of labetalol in healthy volunteers. *Int J Pharmacol Ther Toxicol.* 1981;19:41–44.

25. Cruise CJ, Skeobik Y, Webster RE, et al. Intravenous labetalol versus sodium nitroprusside for treatment of hypertension post coronary bypass surgery. *Anesthesiology.* 1989; 71:835–839.

26. Geniton DJ. A comparison of the hemodynamic effects of labetalol and sodium nitroprusside in patients undergoing endarterectomy. *AANAJ.* 1990;58:281–287.

27. Leslie JB, Kalayjian RW, Sirgo MA, et al. Intravenous labetalol for treatment of postoperative hypertension. *Anesthesiology.* 1987;67:413–416.

28. Sladen RN, Klamerus KJ, Swafford MW, et al. Labetalol for the control of elevated blood pressure following coronary artery bypass grafting. *J Cardiothorac Anesth.* 1990;4:210–221.

29. Singh PP, Dimich I, Sampson I, et al. A comparison of esmolol and labetalol for treatment of perioperative hypertension in geriatric ambulatory surgical patients. *Can J Anaesth.* 1992;39:559–562.

30. Wetsler N, Klein M, Szendro G, et al. The dilemma of immediate preoperative hypertension: to treat and operate or to postpone surgery. *J Clin Anesth.* 2003;15:179–183.

31. Varon J, Marik PE. The diagnosis and management of hypertensive crisis. *Chest.* 2000;118:214–227.

32. Grossman E, Messert FH, Grodzicki T, et al. Should a moratorium be placed on sublingual nifedipine capsules given for hypertensive emergencies and pseudoemergencies? *JAMA.* 1996;276:1328–1331.

33. Chobanian AV, Bakeis GI, Black HR, et al. The seventh report of the Joint National Committee on Prevention, Detection,

Evaluation and Treatment of High Blood Pressure. The JNC 7 Report. *JAMA.* 2003;289:2560–2571.

34. Tobias JD. Nicardipine: applications in anesthetic practice. *J Clin Anesth.* 1995;7:525–533.

35. Goto F, Kato S, Sudo I. Treatment of intraoperative hypertension with enflurane, nicardipine, or human atrial natriuretic peptide: hemodynamic and renal effects. *Can J Anaesth.* 1992;39:932–937.

36. Van Wezel HB, Koolen JJ, Visser CA, et al. Antihypertensive and anti-ischemic effects of nicardipine and nitroprusside in patients undergoing coronary bypass grafting. *Am J Cardiol.* 1989;84:22H–27H.

37. Kross RA, Ferri E, Leung D, et al. A comparison study between calcium channel blockers (nicardipine) and a combined alpha-beta blocker (labetalol) for control of emergence hypertension during craniotomy for tumor surgery. *Anesth Analg.* 2000;91:904–909.

38. Dorman T, Thompson DA, Bueslou MJ, et al. Nicardipine versus nitroprusside for breakthrough hypertension following carotid endarterectomy. *J Clin Anesth.* 2001;13:16–19.

39. Vincent JL, Berlot G, Presiser JC, et al. Intravenous nicardipine in the treatment of postoperative arterial hypertension. *J Cardiothorac Vasc Anesth.* 1997;11:160–164.

40. Cohn JN, Franciosa JA, Francis GS. Effect of short term infusion of sodium nitroprusside on mortality in acute myocardial infarction complicated by left ventricular failure: results of the Veterans Administration cooperative study. *N Engl J Med.* 1982;306:1129–1135.

41. Colson P, Rychwaert F, Coriat P. Renin angiotensin system antagonists and anesthesia. *Anesth Analg.* 1999;89:1143–1155.

42. Powers ER, Chiaramida A, Demaria AN, et al. A double-blind comparison of lisinopril and captopril in patients with symptomatic congestive heart failure. *J Cardiovasc Pharmacol.* 1987;9:82–88.

43. Kiowski W, Linder L, Kleinbloes C, et al. Blood pressure control by the renin-angiotensin system in normal subjects. *Circulation.* 1992;85:1–8.

44. Corait P, Richer C, Douraki T, et al. Influence of chronic angiotensin-converting enzyme inhibitor on anesthetic induction. *Anesthesiology.* 1994;81:299–307.

45. Colson P, Saussine M, Sequin JR, et al. Hemodynamic effects of anesthesia in patients chronically treated with angiotensin converting enzyme inhibitors. *Anesth Analg.* 1992;74:805–808.

46. Hohne C, Meier L, Boemke W, et al. ACE inhibition does not exaggerate the blood pressure decrease in the early phase of spinal anesthesia. *Acta Anaesth Scand.* 2003;47:891–896.

47. Ryckwaert F, Colson O. Hemodynamic effects of anesthesia in patients with ischemic heart failure chronically treated with angiotensin-converting enzyme inhibitors. *Anesth Analg.* 1997;84:945–949.

48. Comfere T, Sprung J, Kumar MM, et al. Angiotensin system inhibitors in a general surgical population. *Anesth Analg.* 2005;100:636–644.

49. Moreilli A, Tritapepe L, Rocco M, et al. Terlipressin versus norepinephrine to counteract anesthesia-induced hypotension in patients with renin-angiotensin system inhibitors: effects on systemic and regional hemodynamics. *Anesthesiology.* 2005;102:12–19.

50. Betrand M, Godet G, Meersschaert K, et al. Should the angiotensin II antagonists be discontinued before surgery? *Anesthesia Analg.* 2001;92:26–30.

51. Brabant S M, Bertrand M, Eyrand D, et al. The hemodynamic effects of anesthetic induction in vascular surgical patients chronically treated with angiotensin II receptor antagonists. *Anesth Analg.* 1999;89:1388–1392.

52. Shepherd AM, Irvine NA. Differential hemodynamic and sympathoadrenal effects of sodium nitroprusside and hydralazine in hypertensive subjects. *J Cardiovasc Pharmacol.* 1986;8:527–533.

53. Shepherd AM, Ludden TM, Mcnay JL, et al. Hydralazine kinetics after single repeated oral dose. *Clin Pharmacol Ther.* 1980;28:804–811.

54. Powers DR, Papadakos PJ, Wallin JD. Parenteral hydralazine revisited. *J Emerg Med.* 1998;16:191–196.

55. Magee LA, Cham C, Waterman E J, et al. Hydralazine in treatment of severe hypertension in pregnancy: metanalysis. *BMJ.* 2003;327:955–960.

56. Tumlin JA, Dunbar LM, Oparil S, et al. Fenoldopam, a dopamine agonist for hypertensive emergency: a multicenter randomized trial. Fenoldopam Study Group. *Acad Emerg Med.* 2000;7:655–662.

57. Oparil S, Aronson S, Deeb MG, et al. Fenoldopam: a new parenteral antihypertensive. *Am J Hypertens.* 1999;12:635–664.

58. Grether DD, Elliott WJ, Moscucci M, et al. Electrocardiographic changes during the treatment of hypertensive emergencies with sodium nitroprusside or fenoldopam. *Arch Intern Med.* 1992;152:2445–2448.

59. Estafonous FG. Hypertension in the surgical patient: management of blood pressure and anesthesia. *Cleve Clin J Med.* 1998;56:385–393.

60. Elliott WJ, Weber RR, Nelson KS, et al. Renal and hemodynamic effects of intravenous fenoldopam versus nitroprusside in severe hypertension. *Circulation.* 1990;81:970–977.

61. Pasch T, Schutlz V, Hoppelshauser G. Nitroprusside induced formation of cyanide and its detoxification with thiosulphate during deliberate hypotension. *J Cardiovasc Pharmacol.* 1983;5:77–85.

62. Cheung AT, Cruz-Shiavone GE, Meng QC, et al. Cardiopulmonary bypass, hemolysis, and nitroprusside induced cyanide production. *Anesth Analg.* 2007;105:29–33.

63. Niknahad H, O'Brien PJ. Involvement of nitric oxide in nitroprusside-induced hepatocyte cytotoxicity. *Biochem Pharmacol.* 1996;51:1031–1039.

64. Friederich JA, Butterworth F. Sodium nitroprusside: Twenty years and counting. *Anesth Analg.* 1995;81:152–162.

65. Haas CE, LeBlanc JM. Acute postoperative hypertension: a review of therapeutic options. *Am J Health Syst Pharm.* 2004;61:1661–1675.

66. Cheung AT. Exploring an optimum intra/postoperative management strategy for acute hypertension in the cardiac surgery patient. *J Cardiol Surg.* 2006;21(suppl 1):S8–S14.

67. Dix P, Howell S. Survey of cancellation rate of hypertensive patients undergoing anesthesia and elective surgery. *Br J Anaesth.* 2001;86:789–793.

68. Tietjen CS, Hurn PD, Ulatowski JA, et al. Treatment modalities for hypertensive patients with intracranial pathology: options and risks. *Crit Care Med.* 1996;24:311–322.

69. Aronson S, Boisvert D, Lapp W, et al. Isolated systolic hypertension is associated with adverse outcomes from coronary bypass grafting surgery. *Anesth Analg.* 2002;94:1079–1084.

70. Reich DL, Bennett-Guerrero E, Bodian CA, et al. Intraoperative tachycardia and hypertension are independently associated with adverse outcome in noncardiac surgery of long duration. *Anesth Analg.* 2002;95:273–277.

71. Charlson ME, McKenzie CR, Gold JP, et al. Intraoperative blood pressure: what patterns identify patients at risk for postoperative complications? *Ann Surg.* 1990;212:567–580.

72. Granger C, Katz J, Kleinschmidt K, et al. Acute severe hypertension is associated with high morbidity and mortality: interim results of STAT registry. Poster presented at the 37th Annual Critical Care Congress, Honolulu, Hawaii, February 2–6, 2008.

73. Dasta JF, Bollinger JE, Gerlach AT, et al. National survey of acute hypertension management. *Crit Care Med.* 2007; 12(suppl):A89.

74. Aronson S, Dyke CM, Stierer KA, et al. The ECLIPSE Trials: comparative studies of clevidipine to nitroglycerin, sodium nitroprusside, and nicardipine for acute hypertension treatment in cardiac surgery patients. *Anesth Analg.* 2008;107:1110–1121.

75. Baiser JR, Martinez EA, Winters BD, et al. Beta-adrenergic blockade accelerates conversion of postoperative supraventricular tachyarrhythmias. *Anesthesiology.* 1998;89:1052–1059.

76. Rosei EA, Trust PM, Brown JJ, et al. Letter: Intravenous labetalol in severe hypertension. *Lancet.* 1975;2:1093–1094.

77. Kieler-Jensen N, Jolin-mellgard A, Norlander M, et al. Coronary and systemic hemodynamic effects of clevidipine, an ultra short acting calcium antagonist, for treatment of hypertension after coronary artery surgery. *Acta Anaesth Scand.* 2000;44:186–193.

78. Ericsson H, Fakt C, Hohlund L, et al. Pharmacokinetics and pharmacodynamics of clevidipine in healthy volunteers after intravenous infusion. *Eur J Clin Pharmacol.* 1999;55:61–67.

79. Ericsson H, Bredberg U, Eriksson U, et al. Pharmacokinetics and arteriovenous differences in clevidipine concentration following a short-term and long-term intravenous infusion in healthy volunteers. *Anesthesiology.* 2000;92:993–1001.

80. Pollack CV, Varon J, Garrison NA, et al. Clevidipine, an intravenous dihydropyridine calcium channel blocker, is safe and effective for treatment of patients with acute severe hypertension. *Ann Emerg Med.* 2009:53:329–338.

81. Levy JH, Mancao MY, Gitter R, et al. Clevidipine effectively and rapidly controls blood pressure preoperatively in cardiac surgery patients: the results of the randomized, placebo-controlled efficacy study of clevidipine assessing its preoperative antihypertensive effect in cardiac surgery. *Anesth Analg.* 2007;105:918–925.

82. Singla N, Warltier DC, Gandhi SD, et al. treatment of acute postoperative hypertension in cardiac surgical patients: an efficacy study of clevidipine assessing its postoperative antihypertensive effect in cardiac surgery-2 (ESCAPE-2), a randomized, double-blind, placebo-controlled trial. *Anesth Analg.* 2008;107:59–67.

18
Steroids

Sass Elisha, EdD, CRNA
Mark Gabot, MSN, CRNA
Sarah Giron, MS, CRNA

Objectives

After completing this chapter, the reader should be able to

- Describe the physiologic components of the hypothalamic-pituitary-adrenal axis.
- Discuss the anesthetic considerations related to hypothalamic-pituitary-adrenal axis suppression.
- Identify the recommended dose of steroid needed for supplementation based on the degree of surgical stress produced.
- Discuss the pharmacokinetic and pharmacodynamic profiles of a variety of steroid compounds.
- Implement a treatment strategy for acute adrenal crisis.

Introduction

Neurophysiology Associated With Glucocorticoid Production

Corticosteroids, primarily cortisol, are necessary to maintain homeostasis of many physiologic functions. Glucocorticoids play an essential role in maintaining (1) carbohydrate, protein, and lipid metabolism; (2) fluid and electrolyte regulation; (3) cardiovascular, central nervous, immune, endocrine, and renal system stability; and (4) inhibition of the inflammatory response. Approximately 95% of all glucocorticoid activity is mediated via cortisol.[1] The process of corticosteroidogenesis begins as the hypothalamus secretes corticotropin-releasing hormone (CRH), also known as corticotropin-releasing factor, into a venous capillary network of the hypophysial portal system called the median eminence. Once CRH interacts with the cells within the anterior pituitary gland, adrenocorticotropic hormone (ACTH) is synthesized. ACTH is released from the anterior pituitary gland and has the effect of increasing cortisol production with the adrenal cortex. The primary mechanism of action of ACTH to stimulate corticosteroidogenesis is by enhancing the enzymatic activity that catalyzes the conversion of cholesterol to pregnenolone, primarily from the zona fasciculata and secondarily by the zona reticularis of the adrenal cortex. Because this process involves the hypothalamus, pituitary, and adrenal glands, it is referred to as the hypothalamic-pituitary-adrenal (HPA) axis (Figure 18-1).

Three layers comprise the adrenal cortex:

1. Outermost layer, zona glomerulosa: primarily produces mineralocorticoids (aldosterone)
2. Middle layer, zona fasciculata: primarily produces glucocorticoids (cortisol) and androgens
3. Innermost layer, zona reticularis: primarily produces glucocorticoids (cortisol) and androgens

It is theorized that most cortisol is produced within the zona fasciculata.

A negative feedback process either stimulates or inhibits the continued production of steroids. It is well known that steroid plasma concentrations fluctuate throughout the day with the peak quantities released at approximately 8:00 AM. Decreased plasma concentrations of steroids are sensed within the hypothalamus, which initiates the release

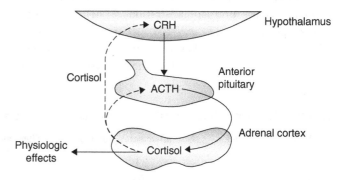

Figure 18-1 Neurophysiology associated with glucocorticoid production.

of CRH, and corticosteroidogenesis ensues. Conversely, increased glucocorticoids within the blood have an inhibitory effect primarily on the hypothalamus and secondarily on the anterior pituitary gland to decrease CRH and ACTH production and release, respectively. Exogenous steroids ingested over a period of time mimic endogenous cortisol and have an inhibitory effect on corticosteroidogenesis. Adrenocortical atrophy occurs, and during a period of physiologic stress output of cortisol from the adrenal gland may be limited. Therefore HPA axis suppression may result in acute adrenal crises. Recovery of normal HPA axis and adrenocortical function can take up to 1 year.

Clinical Pharmacology

Pharmacokinetics

Synthetic glucocorticoids have been created for therapeutic use in a variety of clinical situations. Although all endogenous and synthetic glucocorticoids have a common 21-carbon steroid nucleus (e.g., gonane), specific alterations in the chemical structure alter its pharmacokinetic and pharmacodynamic profile. These alterations include potency, rate of metabolism, degree of protein binding, and glucocorticoid and mineralocorticoid activity.

Hydrocortisone is synthetically produced cortisol, the primary glucocorticoid in humans. Therefore hydrocortisone is often used as the gold standard of comparison for glucocorticoid potency. Table 18-1 compares the properties of various synthetic glucocorticoids.[2]

Glucocorticoids can be administered via the oral, intramuscular, and intravenous routes. Parenteral administration results in a rapid increase in plasma concentration compared with oral administration. Systemic absorption of glucocorticoids may also occur from local sites of administration (i.e., skin, conjunctiva, epidural space, synovial spaces, and respiratory tract). Systemic effects of glucocorticoids depend on the glucocorticoid potency, route of administration, and duration of therapy.

After systemic absorption, 90% or more of cortisol is bound to plasma proteins. Albumin and transcortin (e.g., corticosteroid-binding globulin) are the principal proteins responsible for steroid binding. Most synthetic glucocorticoids predominately bind to albumin, having a relatively lower affinity to transcortin.[3] Clinical situations that decrease (i.e., malnutrition and liver disease) or increase (i.e., pregnancy and estrogen therapy) the amount of extracellular albumin and transcortin alter the level of bound cortisol. Only the free fraction of unbound corticosteroid ($\leq 10\%$) is able to enter cells, exert physiologic effects, and undergo metabolic degradation.

Pharmacodynamics

Hydrocortisone and other synthetic glucocorticoids exert their pharmacologic effects in a similar fashion to endogenous cortisol. After administration and subsequent distribution, only the free fraction of unbound glucocorticoid is able to exert physiologic effects. These physiologic effects are initiated by the active transport of the glucocorticoid into the intracellular cytoplasm. Subsequent binding between the glucocorticoid and cytoplasmic receptors (e.g., glucocorticoid receptors or mineralocorticoid receptors) occurs. For many synthetic glucocorticoids, the binding specificity to glucocorticoid receptors or mineralocorticoid receptors occurs in a dose-dependent manner. As an example, hydrocortisone given at supraphysiologic doses (i.e., > 30 mg/day) causes activation of the mineralocorticoid receptors.[4] Mineralocorticoid receptor activation contributes to fluid and electrolyte regulation through subsequent increased sodium reabsorption, increased water reabsorption, and increased renal excretion of potassium. Table 18-1 compares the properties of various synthetic glucocorticoids.

The glucocorticoid receptor is expressed in most cell types, resides predominantly within the cytoplasm, and is a ligand-activated transcription factor. Upon binding

Table 18-1 Comparative Properties of Various Synthetic Glucocorticoids

Synthetic Glucocorticoid	Anti-inflammatory Potency	Sodium-retaining Potency	Duration of Action (h)	Equivalent Dose (mg)
Cortisol	1	1	8–12	20
Cortisone	0.8	0.8	8–36	25
Dexamethasone	25	0	36–54	0.75
Prednisone	4	0.8	18–36	5
Methylprednisolone	5	0.5	12–36	4
Betamethasone	25	0	36–54	0.75

with glucocorticoids, the inactive glucocorticoid receptor becomes activated, separates from its associated proteins, and translocates to the cellular nucleus. The glucocorticoid receptor then interacts with specific regulatory regions of affected genes; also known as glucocorticoid responsive elements.[5] These glucocorticoid responsive elements provide specificity to gene modulation by glucocorticoids. The effects of glucocorticoids are mediated by (1) repression or activation of specific genes, (2) interaction with other transcription factors, (3) messenger RNA modulation, and (4) altered protein production that mediates the tissue-specific effects of hormones.[6] In addition to these genomic effects, there is increasing evidence that the actions of corticosteroids are also mediated by glucocorticoid interaction with membrane-associated receptors and second messengers.[6]

Steroids are stress hormones, and there is a biphasic response to steroid secretion with increased physiologic stress, immediate and delayed. However, the primary homeostatic action of steroids when prolonged sympathetic nervous system stimulation occurs is to modulate the delayed stress response. The time that is ultimately required for gene expression modulation and protein synthesis reflects this delayed response. Box 18-1 describes the physiologic effects of glucocorticoids.

Metabolism

The serum half-life of synthetic glucocorticoids varies from 80 minutes (hydrocortisone) to 270 minutes (dexamethasone).[5] The biotransformation of glucocorticoids occurs primarily in the liver, where endogenous glucocorticoids (e.g., cortisol) and synthetic glucocorticoids undergo oxidation-reduction reactions to form the metabolites dihydrocortisol and tetrahydrocortisol. These metabolites undergo further hepatic conjugation with sulfate or glucuronide and are further degraded to inactive water-soluble metabolites.

Elimination

Water-soluble inactive metabolites are excreted in the urine by the kidneys. Urinary cortisol level (e.g., unbound, active cortisol filtered by the kidney) is the most accurate measure of cortisol activity. Although the elimination half-time of cortisol is 1.5 to 3 hours, the physiologic effects of cortisol occur for several hours, due to the gene modulation by glucocorticoids.[7] The kidneys excrete approximately 95% of the conjugated, water-soluble, inactive metabolites, whereas the remainder is excreted in the intestinal tract.[5]

Side Effects and Contraindications

Side Effects

The pharmacologic actions and tissue-specific physiologic effects of glucocorticoids are mediated by activation of the same corticosteroid receptor. As a result, synthetic glucocorticoids have side effects that parallel their therapeutic effectiveness.[5] High-dose or prolonged glucocorticoid therapy has multiple side effects. Systemic effects of glucocorticoids depend on the glucocorticoid potency, route of administration, and duration of therapy. For example, recent evidence has determined that at least 5 mg/day of prednisone can cause HPA axis suppression for up to a year after the cessation of therapy.[2] As the duration of glucocorticoid therapy increases beyond 1 week, the adverse side effects increase in a time- and dose-dependent manner. Table 18-2 describes side effects of glucocorticoid therapy.

A risk and benefit analysis for each patient must be undertaken before instituting therapy. After therapy is initiated, the lowest dose required to control the condition and produce the desired effect should be used. When a reduction in dosing is deemed possible, it should be completed in a gradual manner. Abrupt reduction or cessation of therapy may be life threatening due to HPA axis suppression. Box 18-2 describes the signs and symptoms associated with acute adrenal crisis.

Contraindications

Relative contraindications to glucocorticoid therapy include those clinical situations that augment the inherent side effects of these physiologically potent agents. These clinical situations include active systemic infection (i.e.,

---

Box 18-1 Physiologic Effects Associated with Glucocorticoids

- Increased cardiac output
- Increased respiratory rate
- Increased gluconeogenesis
- Decreased inflammation
- Decreased immune response
- Inhibition of digestion
- Enhanced analgesia
- Redistribution of central nervous system blood flow

Table 18-2 Side Effects Associated With Glucocorticoid Therapy

Organ System	Side Effect
Endocrine	Adrenal atrophy
	HPA axis suppression, secondary adrenal insufficiency
	Cushing's syndrome
	Diabetes mellitus, glucose intolerance
Cardiovascular	Dyslipidemia
	Hypertension
	Thrombosis
	Vasculitis
Central nervous	Cataracts, glaucoma
	Changes in mood, behavior, cognition, and/or memory
	Headache
	Glucocorticoid-induced psychosis, steroid dependence
	Cerebral atrophy
Immune	Immunosuppression
	Increased susceptibility to infection (i.e., *Candida* infection)
	Latent virus activation (i.e., cytomegalovirus, latent tuberculosis)
Renal	Increased sodium and water retention
	Increased potassium and hydrogen ion excretion, hypokalemic alkalosis
	Edema
Gastrointestinal	Peptic ulcer disease
	Gastrointestinal bleeding
	Pancreatitis
Musculoskeletal	Osteoporosis, osteonecrosis, osteopenia
	Skeletal muscle atrophy, myopathy, proximal muscle weakness
	Retardation of normal longitudinal bone growth
Integumentary	Atrophy, striae rubrae distensae
	Acne, dermatitis
	Delayed wound healing
	Erythema, petechia, ecchymosis, hirsutism, telangiectasia, hyperpigmentation
Reproductive	Delayed puberty, hypogonadism
	Fetal growth inhibition
	Menstrual disorder

Box 18-2 Signs and Symptoms Associated With Acute Adrenal Crisis

- Hypotension unresponsive to vasopressor therapy
- Hyperdynamic circulation
- Hypoglycemia
- Hyperkalemia
- Hyponatremia
- Hypovolemia
- Metabolic alkalosis
- Decreased level of consciousness

viral, bacterial, fungal, helminthic, or protozoan), immunosuppression (i.e., chemotherapy), acute psychosis, primary glaucoma, hypokalemia, congestive heart failure, Cushing's syndrome, diabetes, hypertension, osteoporosis, and hyperthyroidism.[3] A risk and benefit analysis for each patient must be undertaken before instituting therapy. Hypersensitivity, anaphylactoid, or anaphylactic reactions to synthetic glucocorticoids or their preparation (i.e., preservatives) are absolute contraindications.

Drug Interactions

Pharmacologic interactions of glucocorticoids can pose significant risks to the patient. Many pharmacologic agents used in anesthesia interact with glucocorticoids. Drug interaction does not preclude the use of these medications during anesthetic management. However, the effects on the patient and the clinical pharmacology profile of glucocorticoids should always be considered. Table 18-3 describes possible drug interactions of glucocorticoids.

Practical Aspects of Drug Administration

Glucocorticoids are indicated for treatment of a variety of conditions, including anaphylactoid/anaphylactic reactions, asthma, chronic obstructive pulmonary disease, autoimmune diseases (i.e., rheumatoid arthritis), and sepsis. With the exception of replacement therapy for primary or secondary adrenal insufficiency, the therapeutic effects

Table 18-3 Drug Interactions Associated With Glucocorticoids

Type of Drug Interaction	Class of Drug	Specific Interaction
Accentuate glucocorticoid side effects	Loop diuretics Nonsteroidal anti-inflammatory agents	Increased risk of hypokalemia Increased risk of gastrointestinal side effects (i.e., peptic ulcer disease)
Glucocorticoid metabolism	Estrogens, oral contraceptives, and macrolide antibiotics Barbiturates and phenytoin	Decreased hepatic metabolism due to cytochrome P-450 inhibition Increased glucocorticoid metabolism due to cytochrome P-450 induction
Accentuate secondary drug effects	Digitalis glycosides Depolarizing muscle relaxants (e.g., succinylcholine) Ester local anesthetics Etomidate	Increased risk of arrhythmia due to hypokalemia Increased duration of action due to inhibition of hepatic pseudocholinesterase synthesis Increased duration of action due to inhibition of hepatic pseudocholinesterase synthesis Increased adrenocortical suppression
Altered secondary drug response	Oral anticoagulants Anticholinesterase Antidiabetic	Decreased response to warfarin therapy Increased risk of the development of severe weakness in patients with myasthenia gravis Increased blood glucose concentrations

of glucocorticoids (e.g., inflammation modulation and immunosuppression) are palliative and not curative.[3]

Parenteral administration results in a rapid increase in plasma concentration as compared with oral administration. Inhalation administration, preferably via metered-dose inhaler, allows administration in the awake or anesthetized patient. Glucocorticoid administration in the epidural space has been widely used in the pain management of chronic back pain. Many dosing regimens for anesthetic perioperative administration of corticosteroids have been proposed. Invariably, the dosing of corticosteroids and their gradual discontinuation depend on the type of surgery and associated stress response.

Clinical Uses and Indications

Although there is a broad spectrum for the indications and the clinical use of corticosteroids, prophylactic replacement for patients who are at risk for adrenal deficiency such as in Addison's disease or to treat chronic inflammatory conditions such as asthma or rheumatoid arthritis is indicated. Intraoperatively, the administration of intraoperative corticosteroids is used to prevent postoperative nausea and vomiting (PONV), inhibit the delayed inflammatory response (anaphylaxis), and avoid HPA axis suppression, which can lead to acute adrenal crises.

Corticosteroids are composed of two specific groups of steroids, glucocorticoids and mineralocorticoids, and are differentiated based on their difference in action, metabolism, and structure. Glucocorticoids control fat, protein, and carbohydrate metabolism and also possess anti-inflammatory properties. The anti-inflammatory actions of glucocorticoids make these drugs attractive for the treatment of cerebral edema, dermatitis, allergic reactions, inflammatory bowel diseases such as Crohn's disease and ulcerative colitis, lumbar disc disease, asthma, arthritis, ocular inflammation, sepsis, and laryngeal edema. Mineralocorticoids function to regulate sodium retention and to monitor electrolyte and water balance in the body.

Approximately 1% to 3% of adults worldwide take corticosteroids on a long-term basis to help manage a chronic condition or disease. It has been shown that as many as 20% of patients have taken oral glucocorticoids for more than 6 months, and almost 5% of patients remain on oral therapy longer than 5 years.[8] In the United States 14% of patients take glucocorticoids for skin and musculoskeletal conditions.[9] Steroids are an integral part of the medication regimen because it is estimated that 38% of patients who have rheumatoid arthritis take steroids.[10] Between 1998 and 1999, over 1 million epidural steroid injections were performed to relieve back pain and improve functional mobility for patients.[11] Because of the high volume of patients who use corticosteroids, this population represents a significant group of patients who will undergo surgical procedures and are at risk for HPA axis suppression and acute adrenal crises.

There are advantages to administering steroids during the perioperative period. Dexamethasone is commonly administered to help and prevent PONV during anesthetic management; dexamethasone acts synergistically when added to a protocol that uses a multiple anti-PONV pharmacologic modality. In a 1999 study by Wang and colleagues, patients undergoing laproscopic cholecystectomies were given intravenous dexamethasone or saline before induction of anesthesia. Overall, the addition of dexamethasone to the anesthetic reduced the rate of PONV from 63% (saline group) to 23% (8 mg dexamethasone).[12] In a 2001 study by Mitsuta et al. the perioperative administration of corticosteroid was shown to decrease the inflammatory process in pulmonary parenchyma caused by decreased cytokine production. The administration of a preoperative corticosteroid was also effective in preventing "asthmatic attacks during the perioperative period."[13]

Corticosteroid administration to surgical patient with suspected HPA axis suppression is necessary. The first reported case of patient death attributed to acute adrenal insufficiency caused by preoperative withdrawal of glucocorticoid therapy was reported in 1952.[14] Another case study emerged a year later describing another patient who died after acute discontinuation of corticosteroid therapy 6 hours after surgery.[15] Since the 1950s multiple recommendations have been published specifying which patients might be at risk for HPA axis inhibition and thus quantifying how much corticosteroid to give pre-, intra-, and postoperatively to treat HPA axis suppression. Assessing for the potential for HPA axis suppression during the preoperative period is essential to avoid the potential for acute adrenal crises.

Comparative Pharmacology of Other Drugs in Class

All corticosteroids have a basic three hexane and one pentane ring structure. With modifications to this basic cholesterol structure, agents have varying degrees of potency, metabolism, mineralocorticoid effect, and duration of action as illustrated in Figure 18-2.

Because of the similarity of the chemical structure common to all steroids, patients who have allergies to a specific agent have the potential to be allergic to other synthetic steroids. Allergic reactions caused by steroids are rare; however, steroid use should be avoided if a true allergic reaction has occurred.[16] The subclasses of corticosteroids are shown in Table 18-4.

The plasma half-lives of glucocorticoids range from 1 to 5 hours, but the duration of clinical action can be measured

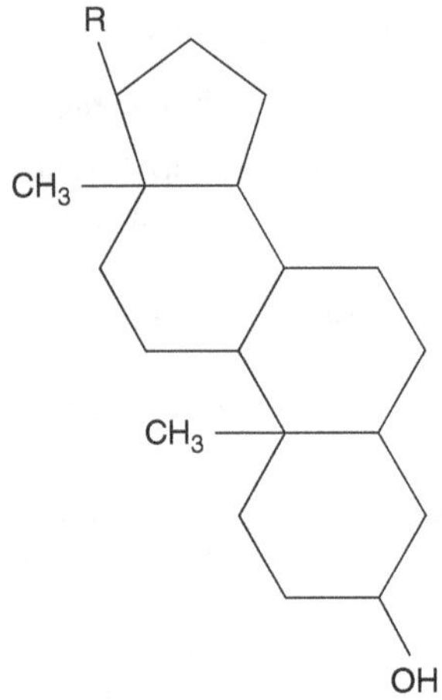

Figure 18-2 Cholesterol structure common to all glucocorticoids.

by monitoring the length of ACTH suppression. Therefore based on the time of ACTH suppression, glucocorticoids are classified as short- (8- to 12-hour effect), intermediate- (24- to 36-hour effect), or long-acting agents (> 48-hour effect). Corticosteroid treatment for patients outside the operating room who will not need chronic therapy (< 3–4 weeks) usually aims to use short- to intermediate-acting agents dosed early in the morning on alternate days to facilitate HPA axis recovery on the second day.[17]

In addition to the glucocorticoid effects that occur, all steroids have various degrees of mineralocorticoid effects due to their structural similarity with aldosterone. Clinically significant mineralocorticoid actions target the kidneys and promote active reabsorption of sodium and passive reabsorption of water. This can be of concern in cases where kidney function is impaired or when retention of sodium and water can lead to fluid overload or other undesirable effects.

Table 18-4 Classification of Commonly Used Steroids

Subclass	Steroid
Subclass 1	Hydrocortisone, hydrocortisone acetate, cortisone acetate, prednisolone, methylprednisolone, and prednisone
Subclass 2	Triamcinolone acetonide, triamcinolone alcohol
Subclass 3	Betamethasone, betamethasone sodium phosphate, dexamethasone, dexamethasone sodium phosphate
Subclass 4	Hydrocortisone-17-butyrate, hydrocortisone-17-valerate, betamethasone valerate, betamethasone dipropionate

The anti-inflammatory action of the specific steroids depends on their ability to support lysosomal membranes and to prevent leukocyte migration into inflamed vascular tissue. Glucocorticoids also decrease the ability of macrophages to respond to microorganisms and are known inhibitors of inflammatory substances. Thus the anti-inflammatory effects provided by steroids occur by stabilization of membranes and blockage of innate immune responses that would cause further cellular destruction.[18,19] A comparison of the pharmacokinetic and pharmacodynamic effects of various steroids is presented in Table 18-5.

Dosage and Administration

Cortisol is secreted at a rate of 20 mg/day from the adrenal cortex. Glucocorticoids function to maintain cardiac function, blood pressure, hemodynamic responsiveness to catecholamines, metabolism, growth, and immunity. During periods of stress the levels of cortisol can increase to 150 to 300 mg/dL per day.[18] By initiating systemic corticosteroid therapy for the treatment of a disease, HPA axis suppression can occur due to the dose that is administered and the duration of treatment primarily caused by adrenocortical atrophy. Adrenal suppression can occur at doses of 5.0 to 7.5 mg/day prednisone in as little as 4 weeks. Therefore short- or intermediate-acting steroids are taken once a day early in the morning to mimic the natural cycle of cortisol. Other methods to decrease HPA axis suppression include dosing on alternate mornings and tapering the agent to the lowest possible dose to avoid adrenocortical atrophy.[17]

If acute adrenal insufficiency occurs, a loading dose of cortisol 100-mg bolus is administered followed by 100 mg intravenously every 6 hours for 24 hours. Chronic adrenal insufficiency requires an oral dosage regimen of typically 25 mg cortisone every morning followed by a 12.5-mg dose in the afternoon. It is critical that these patients who present to the operating room receive a stress dose of steroids to help prevent hemodynamic instability secondary to HPA axis suppression. The use of etomidate has been implicated in causing adrenocortical suppression after a single dose for as long as 24 hours after administration. The proposed mechanism of the suppression is by inhibition of the enzyme 11β-hydroxylase, which is necessary for the chemical conversion of cholesterol to cortisol. Figure 18-3 illustrates one algorithm that can be used for patients who have suspected HPA axis suppression.

Inhaled glucocorticoids are part of the medication regimen indicated for patients who have asthma. Glucocorticoids directly and indirectly stabilize membranes, decrease proteolytic enzymes released by inflammatory mediators, and modulate cytokines released through the inflammatory process.[18,19] One to four daily metered inhaled doses of glucocorticoid may be required for relief depending on the severity of the asthma. To decrease intubation-related bronchoconstriction in patients with known bronchial hyperactivity, a thorough preoperative management includes 40 mg of an oral corticosteroid combined with inhaled salbutamol 0.2 mg per puff for 5 days preoperatively.[17]

It has been determined that dexamethasone decreases the risk of PONV in both adult and pediatric surgical patients. In a study done in 2003 by Elhakim and colleagues,[20]

Table 18-5 Comparison of Pharmacokinetics and Pharmacodynamics of Commonly Used Steroids

Steroid	Anti-inflammatory Potency	Equivalent Dose (mg)	Elimination Half-time (h)	Duration of Action (h)	Sodium Retaining Potency	Route of Administration
Cortisol	1	20	1.5–3.0	8–12	1	O, T, IV, IM, IA
Cortisone	0.8	25	0.5	8–36	0.8	O, T, IV, IM, IA
Prednisolone	4	5	2–4	12–36	0.8	O, T, IV, IM, IA
Prednisone	4	5	2–4	12–36	0.8	O
Methylprednisolone	5	4	2–4	12–36	0.5	O, T, IV, IM, IA, E
Betamethasone	25	0.75	5	36–54	0	O, T, IV, IM, IA
Dexamethasone	25	0.75	3.5–5.0	36–54	0	O, T, IV, IM, IA
Triamcinolone	5	4	3.5	12–36	0	O, T, IV, IM, E
Fludrocortisone	10	2		24	250	O, T, IV, IM
Aldosterone	0				3000	

E, epidural; IA, intra-articular; IM, intramuscular; IV, intravenous; O, oral; T, topical.

pediatric patients aged 4 to 11 were given a dexamethasone dose of 0.5 mg/kg as soon as intravenous access was established. Overall, only 4% of these patients required a rescue antiemetic, whereas the placebo control group required a rescue antiemetic at a rate of 22%. Lee and colleagues[21] demonstrated that with an 8-mg dose of dexamethasone, PONV was decreased from 56.1% in the control group to 23.8% in the dexamethasone group. The antiemetic effects frequently last longer than 24 hours in duration.[11] To decrease cost, avoid postsurgical complications, decrease recovery stay, and improve patient outcome

and satisfaction, corticosteroids should be used to prevent PONV. Decadron administration should be used cautiously in patients who have diabetes because a substantial increase in blood sugar can occur.

Although there have been several case reports of death attributed to acute adrenal insufficiency related to abrupt discontinuation of corticosteroids, many reviews advocate a lower stress dose than previously used in protection against HPA axis suppression. The estimated risk of hypotensive crisis secondary to adrenal suppression in chronic corticosteroid therapy patients was 1% to 2% in

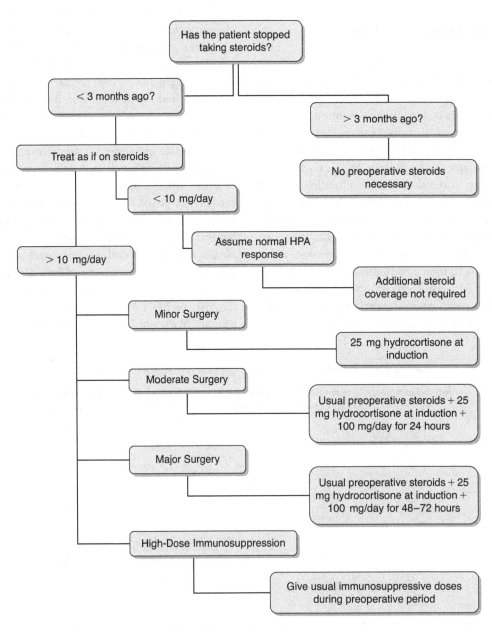

Figure 18-3 Decision algorithm for preoperative steroid supplementation.

a study by Brown and Buie.[22] The authors also found that in patients who were allowed to take their usual maintenance doses of corticosteroids preoperatively, there were no complications related to adrenal insufficiency even during major surgery.[22] Bhansali and colleagues stated that not all patients require stress doses of corticosteroids. Through preoperative assessment of patients with pituitary macroadenomas, it was determined that 65% of those patients did not have significant HPA axis depression despite exogenous steroid use.[23]

Anesthetists commonly administer a stress dose of corticosteroids to prevent hemodynamic instability secondary to adrenal insufficiency for patients who are taking steroids. The dosage and redosage routine vary dramatically when comparing studies, but most recommendations take into account the type of surgery, amount of surgical stress encountered, the dosage and duration of current corticosteroid therapy, and a tapering schedule postoperatively. Regardless of institution policy or personal preference, all these variables should be considered by anesthetists and incorporated into their practice if possible for the safety of their patients.

Nicholson and colleagues[24] suggested that minimal doses of corticosteroids are effective to avoid adrenal insufficiency. Disadvantages to administering large doses of steroids include delayed wound healing, immunosuppression, decreased glucose tolerance, and fluid and electrolyte imbalances. These authors advocated that patients are grouped into those that currently take greater than or less than a prednisone dosage of 10 mg/day (or equivalent); whether the surgery is considered minor, moderate or major; or if the patient has stopped corticosteroid therapy within the past 3 months.[24] A detailed schematic of their postoperative corticosteroid replacement schedule is shown in Table 18-6.

Table 18-6 Postoperative Steroid Replacement Schedule

Postoperative Day	Steroid Tapering Dosage
1	Hydrocortisone 100 mg intravenously q 8 h, starting with induction of anesthesia
2	If patient is stable and major postoperative stress has resolved, lower dose of hydrocortisone to 50 mg q 8 h
3	Hydrocortisone 25 mg q 8 h
4	Hydrocortisone 25 mg twice a day
5	Maintenance dose resumed (i.e., 15–20 mg in AM and 5–10 mg in PM)

In a study by Jabbour,[25] in patients receiving more than 20 mg/day prednisone (or equivalent) for greater than 3 weeks within the previous year, a stress dose of corticosteroids was administered preoperatively and possibly every 8 hours thereafter. The study designates the degree of surgical stress as either minor or major, and a tapering dose of hydrocortisone is recommended through postoperative day 5.[25]

Key Points

- Hypothalamic pituitary adrenal (HPA) axis suppression can result during anesthesia for patients who are taking steroids on a chronic basis.
- Glucocorticoids (primarily cortisol) exert a powerful physiologic effect on every body system.
- Acute adrenal crises can occur perioperatively in patients who have developed adrenocortical atrophy.
- The amount of steroid administered preoperatively to patients with presumed HPA axis suppression should be dependent on the degree of surgical stress that will be encountered.
- The pharmacokinetic and pharmacodynamic profile of the individual steroid preparation vary.

Chapter Questions

1. Which hormone secreted by the anterior pituitary stimulates corticosteroidogenesis?
   a. ACTH
   b. CRH
   c. Cortisol
   d. Aldosterone

2. Which layer of the adrenal gland secretes the majority of cortisol?
   a. Zona glomerulosa
   b. Zona fasciculata
   c. Zona reticularis
   d. Adrenal medulla

3. The degree of HPA axis suppression depends on which of the following?
   a. Amount of cortisol produced
   b. Dose and duration of glucocorticoid therapy
   c. Concentration of aldosterone secreted by the zona glomerulosa
   d. Amount of surgical stress that is encountered as determined by the surgical procedure

4. Which physiologic effect is associated with cortisol?
   a. Decreased cardiac contractility
   b. Inhibition of gluconeogenesis
   c. Increased peristalsis
   d. Inhibition of inflammation

5. Which is not a sign that is associated with acute adrenal crises?
   a. Hypoglycemia
   b. Hypokalemia
   c. Hyponatremia
   d. Hypotension

Answers and Discussion

1. a. Adrenocorticotropic hormone increases the rate of steroid production in the adrenal gland.

2. b. The majority of cortisol is secreted by the zona fasciculata.

3. b. The degree of HPA axis suppression is dependent on the dose and duration of glucocorticoid therapy.

4. d. Inhibition of the inflammatory response is a physiologic effect that is associated with cortisol.

5. b. Acute adrenal crises are associated with hyperkalemia, not hypokalemia.

References

1. Guyton AC, Hall JE. *Textbook of Medical Physiology*, 11th ed. Philadelphia: Elsevier Saunders; 2006:945–957.

2. Nagelhout J, Elisha S, Waters E. Should I continue or discontinue that medication? *AANA J*. 2009;77:59–73.

3. Shimmer BP, Parker KL. Adrenocorticotropic hormone; adrenocortical steroids and their synthetic analogs; inhibitors of the synthesis and actions of adrenocortical hormones. In: Brunton LL, Lazo JS, Parker KL, eds. *Goodman & Gilman's The Pharmacological Basis of Therapeutics*, 11th ed. Columbus, OH: McGraw-Hill; 2006:1587–1612.

4. Roizen MF, Fleisher LA. Anesthetic implications of concurrent diseases. In: Miller RD, ed. *Miller's Anesthesia*, 6th ed. Philadelphia: Elsevier; 2005:1017–1150.

5. Schacke H, Docke WD, Asadullah K. Mechanisms involved in the side effects of glucocorticoids. *Pharmacol Therap*. 2002;96:23–43.

6. Rhen T, Cidlowski JA. Antiinflammatory action of glucocorticoids—new mechanisms for old drugs. *N Engl J Med*. 2005;353:1711–1723.

7. Stoelting RK, Hillier SC. Hormones as drugs. In: Stoelting RK, Hillier SC, eds. *Pharmacology & Physiology in Anesthetic Practice*, 4th ed. Philadelphia: Lippincott Williams & Wilkins; 2006:456–476.

8. van Staa TP, Leufkens HG, Abenhaim L, Begaud B, Zhang B, Cooper C. Use of oral corticosteroids in the United Kingdom. *Q J Med*. 2000;93:105–111.

9. Steinbuch M, Youket TE, Cohen S. Oral glucocorticoids use is associated with an increased risk of fracture. *Osteo Int*. 2004;15:323–328.

10. Wolfe F, Caplan L, Michaud K. Treatment for rheumatoid arthritis and the risk of hospitalization for pneumonia: associations with prednisone, disease-modifying antirheumatic drugs, and antitumor necrosis factor therapy. *Arthritis Rheum*. 2006;54:628–634.

11. Carrino JA, Morrison WB, Parker L, Schweitzer ME, Levin DC, Sunshine JH. Spinal injection procedures: volume provider distribution, and reimbursement in the US Medicare population from 1993 to 1999. *Radiology*. 2002;225:723–729.

12. Wang JJ, Ho ST, Liu YH, et al. Dexamethasone reduces nausea and vomiting after laproscopic cholecystectomy. *Br J Anaesth*. 1999;85:772–775.

13. Mitsuta K, Shimoda T, Fukushima C, et al. Preoperative steroid therapy inhibits cytokine production in the lung parenchyma in asthmatic patients. *Chest*. 2001;120:1175–1183.

14. Fraser CG, Preuss FS, Bigford WD. Adrenal atrophy and irreversible shock associated with cortisone therapy. *JAMA*. 1952;149:1542–1543.

15. Lewis L, Robinson RF, Yee J, Hacker LA, Eisen G. Fatal adrenal cortical insufficiency precipitated by surgery during prolonged continuous cortisone treatment. *Ann Intern Med*. 1953;39:116–126.

16. Wolverton SE. *Comprehensive Dermatologic Drug Therapy*. Philadelphia: W.B. Saunders; 2001.

17. Jackson S, Gilchrist H, Nesbitt LT Jr. Update on the dermatologic use of systemic glucocorticosteroids. *Dermatol Ther*. 2007;20:187–205.

18. Stoelting RK, Hillier SC. *Pharmacology and Physiology in Anesthetic Practice*. Philadelphia: Lippincott Williams and Wilkins; 2005.

19. Nagelhout JJ, Zaglaniczny KL. *Nurse Anesthesia*. St. Louis, MO: Elsevier Saunders; 2005.

20. Elhakim M, Ali NM, Rashed I, Riad MK, Refat M. Dexamethasone reduces postoperative vomiting and pain after pediatric tonsillectomy. Can J Anaesth. 2003;50:392–397.

21. Lee Y, Lai H, Lin P, Huang S, Lin Y. Dexamethasone prevents postoperative nausea and vomiting more effectively in women with motion sickness. Can J Anaesth. 2003;50:232–237.

22. Brown CJ, Buie WD. Perioperative stress dose steroids: do they make a difference? *J Am Coll Surg.* 2001;193:678–686.

23. Bhansali A, Dutta P, Bhat MH, Mukherjee KK, Rajput R, Bhadada S. Rational use of glucocorticoid during pituitary surgery—a pilot study. *Indian J Med Res.* 2008;128:294–299.

24. Nicholson G, Burrin JM, Hall GM. Peri-operative steroid supplementation. *Anaesthesia.* 1998;53:1091–1104.

25. Jabbour SA. Steroids and the surgical patient. *Med Clin North Am.* 2001;85:1311–1317.

Herbal and Dietary Supplements

Anthony Chipas, PhD, CRNA

Objectives

After completing this chapter, the reader should be able to

- Discuss the implications of the 11 herbal supplements that most impact anesthesia and surgery.
- Describe why herbal supplements are not considered drugs.
- Identify with which pharmacologic effects herbal supplements may interfere.
- Identify some of the alkaloids that are the active ingredients in herbal supplements.

Introduction

The use of complementary and alternative medicine (CAM) predates the advent of modern organized health care. CAM includes herbal medications and dietary supplements, meditation, massage therapy, aromatherapy, acupuncture, reflexology, and relaxation therapy, including the use of music and soothing imagery. Although many patients we serve use and believe in CAM, many anesthesia providers are wary of this type of "voodoo" medicine and the "health nuts" who use them. Despite our skepticism, the widespread use of these medications and supplements impacts the care we deliver. Their use demands that we become aware of their pharmacologic effects and the potential for adverse reactions during surgery and anesthetic care.

Historic Perspective

Though alternative medicines are not mainstream health care in the United States, they are so in many other countries. These ancient compounds, originally preparations used by native healers and shamans, are the primary ingredients of some of today's front-line medicines. These preparations include plants such as foxglove (digitalis), Madagascar periwinkle (vincristine), and ma huang (ephedrine). The ancient Chinese and Egyptian writings and lore handed down by native American Indian tribes describe many of these plants and their medicinal uses. Indeed, most indigenous cultures used herbs in their healing rituals or traditional medicines.[1] Before the discovery of antibiotics, the herb echinacea was widely prescribed for infections. Today, research confirms that this herb does stimulate the immune system by increasing the production of white blood cells.[2]

In the early 19th century methods of chemical analysis became available, and scientists began extracting and modifying active ingredients from plants.[3] Later, chemists began isolating the active alkaloid ingredients and producing their own version of plant compounds, transitioning from raw herbs to modern pharmaceuticals.

It is estimated that as many as 80% of the world's population, 4 billion people, use some form of herbal medication or supplements. According to the World Health Organization, herbal medicine is a large part of naturopathy, homeopathic, Native American, and traditional Asian medicine.[4] In the United States it is estimated that in 2002 as many as 35% of the adult populations used CAM, and that number is growing by approximately 20% per year.[4,5] The complementary and alternative market is growing in the United States at approximately $3 billion per year.[2]

Legislative Intervention

In 1991 Congress established the Office of Alternative Medicine, which in 1998 became the National Center for Complementary and Alternative Medicine within the National Institutes of Health. In 2006 more than twice as many CAM-related English language research articles were published as in 1996.[6]

Vitamins, herbs, and other supplements are not tested by any governmental organization. Herbal medications are not regulated by the U.S. Food and Drug Administration (FDA), as are other drugs. In 1994 herbal medications were classified as dietary supplements by the U.S. Dietary Supplement Health and Education Act (DSHEA) and as such do not undergo the same rigorous animal and human trials as other medications. In addition, these preparations do not need a physician's prescription. They can be sold over the counter at any health food or grocery store as long as they are marketed as supplements and not as medicines. The DSHEA does require that herbal supplements be manufactured according to good manufacturing practices, but because of regional variation in growing practices, there is no guarantee that each bottle has the same bioequivalence or is in fact safe. Herbal supplements may be contaminated with pesticides, organic and inorganic fertilizers, or any number of other contaminants. To have a product removed from the market, the manufacturer does not have to demonstrate equivalence in bioavailability or purity; rather, it is up to the FDA to prove that a supplement is not safe for human consumption. Despite the widespread use of herbal preparations by our patients, there is not a great deal of evidence-based practice regarding their efficacy, and many anesthesia providers remain under-educated about the consequences of patients taking herbal preparations.[7]

Anesthesia Implications

With as many as 35% of our patients using one or more herbal or dietary supplements, along with prescription medications, it is prudent to have an understanding of the implications of these therapies. Herbal medications are pharmacologically active agents that have various effects on our patients, including intrinsic pharmacologic effects; pharmacodynamic interactions, including the alteration of drug receptors; and pharmacokinetic interactions, including altering absorption, metabolism, and elimination of anesthetic medications.

The more medications a patient takes, the more potential there is for drug interactions. If a patient is taking seven prescribed medications, there is a potential for 42 possible drug interactions ($n \times (n - 1)$). If you add two additional herbal supplements to those that are prescribed, the chance for an interaction jumps to 72 possible interactions. With the administration of five anesthetic medications, the provider now has the potential for 182 drug interactions.

Preoperative Assessment

The provider needs to ask specifically about the use of alternative medicines and dietary supplements during the preanesthetic evaluation. When asked what medications they take, many patients will not include dietary supplements or herbal remedies. Studies indicate that the general use of herbal supplements in elective surgical patients is between 7% and 39%. Yet less than 30% of patients tell their healthcare providers about them.[8,9] Patients assume that "natural" equates to safe and harmless, whereas anesthesia providers understand that without scientific evidence these dietary supplements may be either harmless, therapeutic, or, in some cases, dangerous when combined with prescription medications. Popular herbal medications and dietary supplements are frequently used to self-medicate for headaches, digestive disorders, depression, sleep disorders, menopausal symptoms, weight loss, muscular enhancement, weight loss, joint health, and fatigue (energy-boosting compounds).

Interactions vary with the supplement used. Supplements such as ginseng and garlic may interfere with coagulation and potentiate bleeding, which are important considerations when doing neuraxial anesthesia, whereas kava could cause increased somnolence from general anesthesia. The health risks posed by these supplements include coagulopathies, hypertension, alterations in the pharmacokinetics and pharmacodynamics of anesthetic medications, and increased somnolence.

Of the many dietary supplements currently on the market, 11 are particularly troubling for anesthesia and surgery (Table 19-1). Those patients presenting to a preoperative assessment clinic need to be encouraged to discontinue their medications at least 2 weeks before the scheduled surgery. Many herbal supplements, such as valerian, need to be tapered over a 1-week period to prevent acute withdrawal.

If a patient is not seen in advance, the anesthesia provider needs to weigh the risks versus the benefits. If the patient has an increased risk of intraoperative bleeding or if the plan calls for neuraxial anesthesia, then a platelet transfusion might be considered.

Commonly Used Dietary Supplements

Table 19-2 outlines some commonly used herbal supplements. Some of these dietary supplements may interfere with surgery and anesthesia.

Table 19-1 Herbal Supplements With Anesthetic Implications

Dietary Supplement	Uses	Implications	Discontinue
Echinacea	Anti-infective agent Antagonizes immunosuppressants	Allergic reactions	No data
Ephedra	Weight loss, bronchospasm, and congestion	No longer available in United States Cardiac dysrhythmias, hypertension, depletes catecholamine stores	24 h
Feverfew	Headache, fever, menstrual irregularities	Inhibits platelet activity	No data
Garlic	Hyperlipidemia, atherosclerosis	Increased bleeding times Increases fibrinolysis	7 days
Ginger	Nausea, vomiting, and motion sickness	Increased bleeding times	No data
Ginkgo biloba	Memory impairment, dementia, peripheral vascular disease	Increased bleeding times by inhibiting platelet-activating factor	36 h
Ginseng	Improves concentration Hypoglycemia	Increased bleeding times	7 days
Kava	Anxiety, stress, and insomnia Increases anesthetic dose with long-term use	Potentiates barbiturates	24 h
Saw palmetto	Benign prostatic hypertrophy Inhibits cyclooxygenase	Potentiates barbiturates?	No data
St. John's wort	Moderate depression Anesthetic drugs Delayed emergence	Affects CYP4503A4, which metabolizes 50% of herb	5 days
Valerian	Insomnia Increases anesthetic dose with long-term use	Potentiates barbiturates To be tapered over 7 days	No data but need

Table 19-2 Herbal Supplements

Herbal Supplement	Aloe Vera [2,4,5,7,9,12]
Scientific Name	*Aloe vera, aloe barbadensis*
Indication	Topically: Heals wounds and skin conditions, sunburns, burns
Orally	Diabetes, osteoarthritis, asthma, epilepsy, and laxative
How Used	Green leaf contains strong laxatives and may lower blood glucose.
Implications	May inhibit the healing of deep surgical wounds when applied topically.

Herbal Supplement	Bitter Orange [2,4,5,7,9,12]
Scientific Name	*Citrus aurantium*
Indication	Heartburn, loss of appetite, nasal congestion, and weight loss. May be antifungal.
How Used	Eating dried fruit or topically
Implications	May cause tachycardia or hypertension. Avoid with heart conditions or on antihypertensive medications or monoamine oxidase inhibitors. May increase risk of sunburn.

(continues)

Table 19-2 Herbal Supplements *(continued)*

Herbal Supplement	Black Cohosh [2,4,5,7,9,12,14]
Scientific Name	*Actaea racemosa, Cimicifuga racemosa*
Indication	Menstrual disorders, general malaise, sore throat, coughs, backaches
How Used	Dried herbs or capsules
Implications	No evidence that it helps menstrual disorders. Mild sedative, anti-inflammatory and antispasmodic properties. May decrease blood pressure with continued use.

Herbal Supplement	Chamomile [2,4,5,7,9,12]
Scientific Name	*Matricaria recutita, Chamomilla recutita*
Indication	Upset stomach, gas, diarrhea, anxiety, sleeplessness
How Used	Flowers used in tea or used as cream or ointments.
Implications	No evidence of efficacy. Contains coumarins, which are naturally occurring alkaloids that are appetite depressants. May cause rash or anaphylaxis.

Herbal Supplement	Echinacea [2,4,5,7,9,10,12,14] (anesthetic or surgical implication)
Scientific Name	*Echinacea purpurea, Echinacea angustifolia*
Indication	Treats and prevents upper respiratory infections, stimulates immune system
How Used	Member of daisy family. Flowers dried for teas; juices used for external use.
Implications	Evidence does not prove the prevention of colds or flu. Some immunostimulatory effects; should be avoided before or after transplants. May stimulate asthma or allergic rhinitis.

Herbal Supplement	Ephedra [2,4,5,7,9–14] (anesthetic or surgical implication)
Scientific Name	*Ephedra sinica*
Indication	Ancient Chinese medicine to prevent colds, flu, asthma, wheezing, and nasal congestion. Contains alkaloids, including ephedrine, pseudoephedrine, and norephedrine. Elimination half-life is 5.2 hours and mostly eliminated by kidneys.
How Used	Dried plants used in teas or extracts.
Implications	Hypertension, stroke, worsening heart conditions, restlessness; avoid if pregnant or breast-feeding. Little evidence of effectiveness in weight loss. Long-term use can lead to catecholamine depletion and profound hypotension upon induction. FDA banned sale in United States in 2004 but available in other countries.

Herbal Supplement	Feverfew [2,4,5,7,9–12] (anesthetic or surgical implication)
Scientific Name	*Tanacetum parthenium, Chrysanthemum parthenium*
Indication	Migraine headaches, rheumatoid arthritis, psoriasis, asthma, tinnitus
How Used	Dried leaves ground or eaten fresh.
Implications	May inhibit platelet function. Rebound aches if discontinuation not tapered.

Herbal Supplement	Garlic [2,4,5,7,9,10,12,14] (anesthetic or surgical implication)
Scientific Name	*Allium sativum*
Indication	Lowers cholesterol, heart disease, hypertension, stomach and colon cancer. May slow atherosclerosis.
How Used	Dried and powdered or cloves eaten raw or cooked. One of most extensively researched plants.
Implications	Decreased coagulation similar to aspirin and may decrease blood pressure. Should be discontinued 1 week before surgery. May interfere with saquinavir, drug used for HIV. Safe in most adults.

Table 19-2 Herbal Supplements *(continued)*

Herbal Supplement	Ginger [2,4,5,7,9–12] (anesthetic or surgical implication)
Scientific Name	*Zingiber officinale*
Indication	Stomachaches, diarrhea, nausea from motion sickness, chemotherapy, pregnancy or surgery, rheumatoid arthritis, osteoarthritis
How Used	Root is cooked fresh or dried. Ground root used in capsules or teas.
Implications	Evidence of effectiveness is questionable. Decreased coagulation similar to aspirin. Should be discontinued 1 week before surgery.

Herbal Supplement	Ginkgo [1–4,6,9–12] (anesthetic or surgical implication)
Scientific Name	*Ginkgo biloba*
Indication	Many pharmacologic ingredients including flavonoid glycosides (antioxidants) and terpene lactones (platelet antagonists). Impaired memory, dementia, peripheral vascular disease, tinnitus and scavenging free radicals. May stabilize or improve cognitive dysfunction in Alzheimer's disease and dementia.
How Used	Leaves dried and ground.
Implications	Tolerated by most adults. Some concern with bleeding because of increased risk of bleeding for platelet inactivation.

Herbal Supplement	Ginseng [2,4,5,7,9–12,14] (anesthetic or surgical implication)
Scientific Name	*Panax ginseng*
Indication	Boosts immune system; improves mental and physical performance, erectile dysfunction, hepatitis C, menopause, lowering blood glucose and blood pressure. Protects body against stress and restores homeostasis.
How Used	Dried root made into capsules, ointments, or teas.
Implications	Evidence for lowering blood glucose and possibly beneficial for immune system. Use with caution in patient on insulin, as it lowers postprandial blood glucose. Decreased coagulation similar to aspirin. Should be discontinued 1 week before surgery.

Herbal Supplement	Hawthorn [2,4,5,7,9,12,14]
Scientific Name	*Crataegus laevigata, Crataegus monogyna*
Indication	Heart disease, digestive and kidney problems, angina
How Used	Dried and used in capsules
Implications	May lower blood pressure but limited research.

Herbal Supplement	Horse Chestnut [2,4,5,7,9,12]
Scientific Name	*Aesculus hippocastanum*
Indication	Chronic venous insufficiency, ankle swelling, leg cramps
How Used	Topical preparations. Active ingredient aescin.
Implications	Raw horse chestnut is poisonous.

Herbal Supplement	Kava [2,4,5,7,9–12] (anesthetic or surgical implication)
Scientific Name	*Piper methysticum*
Indication	Insomnia, asthma, urinary tract infections, anxiety, menopausal symptoms
How Used	Root used to prepare beverages, capsules, and topical solutions.
Implications	May cause liver damage, hepatitis or liver failure, dystonia (muscle spasms), scaly yellow skin eruptions, drowsiness that may potentiate benzodiazepines. May inhibit platelet function.

(continues)

Table 19-2 Herbal Supplements *(continued)*

Herbal Supplement	Lavender [2,4,5,7,9,12]
Scientific Name	*Lavandula angustifolia*
Indication	Antiseptic, anxiety, restlessness, insomnia, depression, headache, hair loss
How Used	Essential oils
Implications	Oil on skin may cause irritation. Generally considered safe.

Herbal Supplement	Licorice Root [2,4,5,7,9,12,14]
Scientific Name	*Glycyrrhiza glabra, Glycyrrhiza uralensis*
Indication	Stomach ulcers, bronchitis, sore throat, viral infection like hepatitis
How Used	Dried powder
Implications	High amounts can cause hypertension and arrhythmias due to hypokalemia. Caution in use with diuretics, lower cortisol levels. May cause preterm labor.

Herbal Supplement	Peppermint Oil [2,4,5,7,9,12]
Scientific Name	*Mentha x piperita*
Indication	Indigestion, nausea, cold symptoms, headaches, muscle pain, irritable bowel
How Used	Essential oil
Implications	Some evidence of effectiveness for irritable bowel. Generally safe in small amounts.

Herbal Supplement	Saw Palmetto [2,4,5,7,9–12] (anesthetic or surgical implication)
Scientific Name	*Serenoa repens, Sabal serrulata*
Indication	Urinary symptoms from enlarged prostate, pelvic pain, bladder disorders, decreased libido, hair loss, hormone imbalances
How Used	Ground fresh or dried fruit for capsules or teas
Implications	Potentiates barbiturates? May increase bleeding because of anti-inflammatory effects that inhibit cyclooxygenase.

Herbal Supplement	St. John's Wort [2,4,5,7,9–12] (anesthetic or surgical implication)
Scientific Name	*Hypericum perforatum*
Indication	Mild depression, anxiety, sleep disorders, sedative, malaria. Inhibits reuptake of serotonin, dopamine, and norepinephrine.
How Used	Teas and concentrated extracts for capsules
Implications	Increased sensitivity to sunlight, fatigue, sexual dysfunction. Interaction with pharmacokinetics and dynamics of many drugs: antidepressants, birth control pills, cyclosporine (transplant rejection), digoxin, indinavir (HIV), irinotecan (cancer), anticoagulants (Coumadin). Should not be used by patients on monoamine oxidase inhibitors. Interferes with other drugs metabolized by CYP4503A4 pathway.

Herbal Supplement	Soy [2,4,5,7,9,12]
Scientific Name	*Glycine max*
Indication	Lowers cholesterol, menopausal symptoms, osteoporosis, improves memory, hypertension, breast and prostate cancer
How Used	Tablets and capsules. Active ingredient isoflavones.
Implications	Daily use may lower low-density-lipoprotein cholesterol, inconsistent reduction of hot flashes. May lower estrogen so women with breast cancer or risk for other cancers should use only after discussion with physician.

Table 19-2 Herbal Supplements *(continued)*

Herbal Supplement	Valerian [2,4,5,7,9–12] (anesthetic or surgical implication)
Scientific Name	*Valerian officinalis*
Indication	Anxiety, sleep disorders, depression, irregular heartbeat. Mediates through GABA pathways.
How Used	Root used in capsules or teas.
Implications	May potentiate benzodiazepines.

Herbal Supplement	Yohimbe [2,4,5,7,9,12]
Scientific Name	*Pausinystalia yohimbe*
Indication	Low libido and erectile dysfunction.
How Used	Bark used in capsules and teas.
Implications	Hypertension, tachycardia, anxiety, sleeplessness. Used with caution if taking monoamine oxidase inhibitors (MAOIs) and should not be used with tricyclic antidepressants or phenothiazines.

Summary

Patients are bombarded with information about the benefits of herbal supplements by mail, television, and radio and see these products displayed in health food stores and pharmacies. Many of these consumers are aware of the positive benefits of taking these products, but few know the side effects. These side effects could cause interactions with prescription medications, making these patients susceptible to hypertension, bleeding, pregnancy, and even the rejection of transplanted organs.

Seventy percent of individuals who use alternative medicines do not discuss it with their healthcare providers but self-diagnose and self-treat their illnesses.[15] The prudent anesthesia provider should include questions about the patient's use of CAM during their interview. When asked what medications they take, most people do not include herbal supplements because they believe the supplements are not "medicines" but safe, nutritional supplements. Other patients do not talk about these non-mainstream health alternatives because they fear being ridiculed. The consequences of not specifically asking about herbal supplements may be dangerous for our patients by adding to the morbidity of their care.

Although neither the American Association of Nurse Anesthetists nor the American Society of Anesthesiologists have a standard or guidelines concerning discontinuation of herbal supplements, it is a general recommendation that they be discontinued 1 or 2 weeks before any surgery. Patients need to be instructed to taper these supplements because rapid discontinuation may lead to dangerous rebound phenomena.

The Internet has increased access to information about medical diagnosis and treatment. Much of the information available to consumers on the web can be linked directly or indirectly to commercial sites and manufacturers of dietary supplements. Many of these sites list the benefits but provide little discussion about the implications and possible drug interactions. This leaves the consumer as uninformed as many of the anesthesia providers concerning the downside of taking these supplements. There are, however, many governmental and private sources of information concerning herbal and food supplements, and some of these are listed in Table 19-3.

Key Points

- Not all dietary and complementary supplements have the same bioequivalence.
- When we do a preoperative history, we need to specifically ask whether patients are taking dietary supplements.
- Dietary supplements may interfere with prescribed medications by either enhancing the other drugs' activity or competing for binding sites.
- Many dietary and complementary supplements are effective in the treatment of certain diseases.
- The federal government does not regulate dietary supplements unless there is a problem.

Table 19-3 Available Information for Practitioners and Consumers

Site	Web Address	Information
Center for Food Safety and Applied Nutrition, U.S. Food and Drug Administration	http://www.fda.gov/Food/default.htm	This site contains safety, industry, and regulatory information about supplements. All adverse events should be reported on this site.
National Center for Complementary and Alternative Medicine, National Institutes of Health	http://nccam.nih.gov	Database of facts concerning alternative therapies, including herbal supplements.
Quackwatch	http:// www.quackwatch.com	Quackwatch is an international network about health-related frauds, myths, fads, fallacies, and misconduct. Its primary focus is on *quackery*-related information that is difficult or impossible to get elsewhere.
ConsumerLab	http:// www.consumerlab.com	Independent testing laboratory that compares the efficacy and bioavailability of all dietary supplements.
HerbMed	http://www.herbmed.org	Information on many herbal medications, including warnings.
Physicians' Desk Reference for Herbal Medicines		Addendum to Physicians' Desk Reference.

Chapter Questions

1. Why was ephedra removed from the market in the United States?
2. How does valerian root cause sedation, and what effect does that have on the anesthetic care plan?
3. What questions do anesthesia providers need to add to their preanesthetic assessment and why?
4. Why should patients awaiting organ transplant be warned to stop taking echinacea or St. John's wort?
5. Which supplements cause coagulopathies?
6. Which supplements cause increased sedation?
7. Why are herbal supplements not regulated by the FDA?

References

1. Brinks J, Grimley Evans J. Ginkgo biloba for cognitive impairment and dementia. *Cochran Database Syst Rev.* 2007;2:CD003120.
2. Yang XX, Hu ZP, Duan W, Zhu YZ, Zhou SF. Drug-herb interactions: eliminating toxicity with hard drug design. *Curr Pharm Des.* 2006;12:2629–2664.
3. Knox J, Gaster B. Dietary supplements for the preventions and treatment of coronary artery disease. *J Altern Complement Med.* 2007;13:83–95.
4. Tindle HA, Davis RB, Phillips RS, Eisenberg DM. Trends in use of complementary and alternative medicine by US adults: 1997–2002. *Altern Ther Health Med.* 2005;11:42.
5. Messina B. Herbal supplements: facts and myth—talking to your patients about herbal supplements. *J Perianesth Nurs.* 2006;21:268–278.
6. Ang-Lee M, Yuan CS, Moss J. *Complementary and Alternative Therapy in Miller's Anesthesia*, 7th Ed.. New York: Churchill-Livingston; 2008.
7. Ashar BH, Rice TN, Sisson SD. Physicians' understanding of the regulation of dietary supplements. *Arch Intern Med.* 2007;167:966.
8. American Society of Anesthesiologists. What you should know about your patients' use of herbal medicines and other dietary supplements [brochure]. Philadelphia: American Society of Anesthesiologists; 2003:1–2.
9. Ruda A, Chatterjee S, Sengupta S, et al. Herbal medications and their anesthetic implications. *Internet J Anesthesiol.* 2009;19(1).
10. Kaye AD, Clarke RC, Sabar R. Herbal medications: current trends in anesthesiology practice—a hospital survey. *J Clin Anesth.* 2000;12:468.
11. Council for Public Interest in Anesthesia. Herbal products and your anesthetic, AANA Publications [brochure].
12. Moss J. Herbal medicines and perioperative care [Editorial]. *Anesthesiology.* 2006;105:441–445.
13. Murphy J. Perioperative considerations with herbal medicines. *J Am Operat Room Nurses Assoc.* 2000;69;173–183.
14. Using Dietary Supplements Wisely. National Center for Complementary and Alternative Medicine. Available at: http://nccam.nih.gov/health. Accessed June 1, 2009.
15. Norred C, Zamudio S, Palmer S. Use of complementary and alternative medicines by surgical patients. *J Am Assoc Nurse Anesth.* 2000;68:13–19.

Objectives

α- and β-Adrenergic Receptor Agonists and Antagonists

John P. McDonough, EdD, CRNA
Kiran Macha, MBBS, MPH
Lillia Loriz, PhD, ARNP

After completing this chapter, the reader should be able to

- Describe the synthesis, storage, effects, and metabolism of endogenous catecholamines in the human body.
- List the different types of α- and β-adrenergic receptors.
- Compare and contrast agonist and antagonist drugs that act on α and β receptors.
- Use appropriate caution regarding these drugs in the geriatric population.

Introduction

Both the sympathetic and parasympathetic divisions of the autonomic nervous system are controlled by neurotransmitters that are specifically found in a "lock and key" arrangement with certain types of receptors. Each of these receptors, when either stimulated or blocked, produces a specific physiologic result. Frequently during the course of anesthesia management we are called on to create, or correct, changes in physiologic parameters such as heart rate, blood pressure, and/or the lumen size of various tubular structures such as bronchi or blood vessels. Although when dealing with adrenergic receptors the sympathetic division is the one most commonly affected, one must also be aware that potential parasympathetic changes may result from our actions.

Catecholamines

Catecholamines are made up of a basic structure called a catechol (Figure 20-1). Catecholamines have an aromatic ring attached to the amine group. Catecholamines include epinephrine, norepinephrine, and dopamine and are produced in the adrenal medulla. Sympathetic nerve fibers also produce norepinephrine, and dopamine is synthesized in the brain.

Catecholamine Synthesis

Catecholamines are derivatives of phenylalanine amino acids. Tyrosine hydroxylase, which is the rate-limiting enzyme, converts phenylalanine to tyrosine and then tyrosine to 3,4-dihydroxy-L-phenylalanine, or DOPA. Dopa decarboxylase converts DOPA to dopamine. Norepinephrine is produced from dopamine by the action of dopamine β-hydroxylase. Norepinephrine and epinephrine differ in the number of methyl groups they possess. Methylation of norepinephrine takes place in the adrenal medulla through the action of phenylethanolamine N-methyltransferase enzyme.[126] Synthesis of epinephrine occurs only in the adrenal medulla due to the concentration of the methylation enzyme in the adrenal medulla (Figure 20-2).

Catecholamines are stored in the chromaffin vesicles found in chromaffin cells that are located in the adrenal medulla. Norepinephrine forms a complex with ATP and is bonded to a protein called chromogranin in these chromaffin cells. The catecholamine is released by exocytosis due to localized depolarization of the membranes. Calcium is essential for the exocytosis of catecholamines. The release of amines can be modulated by the activation of the presynaptic α_2-adrenergic receptor, which exerts inhibitory control. An active amine pump exists on the neuronal membrane that recaptures excess or unused catecholamines.

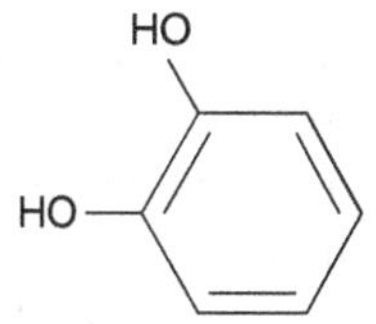

Figure 20-1 Catechol.

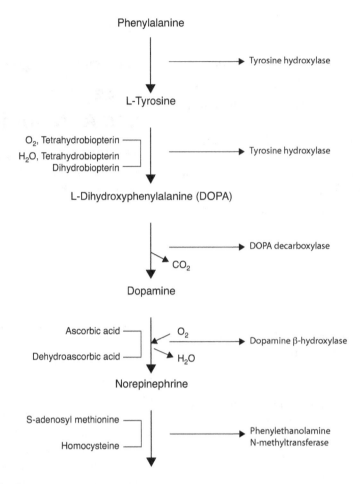

Figure 20-2 Catecholamine synthesis.

Metabolism of Catecholamines

Catecholamines are metabolized by enzymatic action of the following pathways[52] (Figure 20-3):

- Monoamine oxidase (MAO) deaminates amino neurotransmitters in the cells. This enzyme is found in the sympathetic nerve fibers on the outside of the mitochondrial membrane. Two types of MAO exist:
  - Monoamine oxidase A: deaminates epinephrine, norepinephrine, and dopamine
  - Monoamine oxidase B: deaminates only dopamine

  The deamination of the catecholamines with MAO produces catechol-aldehydes, which are further reduced to alcohols. The end product of epinephrine and norepinephrine metabolism is vanillylmandelic acid.[15] Dopamine is metabolized to homovanillic acid.
- Catechol-*O*-methyl transferase (COMT) causes methylation of catecholamines in the extraneuronal tissues. Epinephrine and norepinephrine are reduced to metanephrine and normetanephrine, respectively. Vanillylmandelic acid is the eventual

end product of this degradation process. COMT also metabolizes dopamine to homovanillic acid.[16]

The end products of the catecholamine metabolism are conjugated with glucuronic acid in the liver and are excreted in urine.

Types of Adrenergic Receptors

Ahlquist[5] was the first to demonstrate the existence of α- and β-adrenergic receptors through his pharmacologic studies. Later, the subtypes of α- and β-adrenergic receptors, α_1, α_2 and β_1, β_2, β_3, respectively, were identified.[28,72] α and β receptors belong to the G-protein coupled receptor (GPCR) family. GPCR has seven membrane domains, which are arranged in the form of a pocket, analogous to a lock mechanism, so that the agonists and antagonists are able to, as would a key, fit into this space (Figure 20-4).

α_1 Receptors are GPCRs, specifically subtype G_q-protein coupled receptors. The agonist binding with the receptor

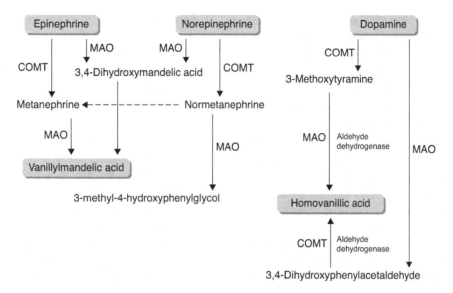

Figure 20-3 Metabolism of catecholamines.

causes the activation of phospholipase C to yield second messengers. In this case these messengers are inositol-1,4,5-triphosphate and diacylglycerol. These cause phosphorylation of the calcium channel ions. The calcium ions mediate the effects in the end organ. α_2 Receptors are GPCRs, specifically subtype G_i-protein coupled receptors. Activation of these receptors decreases the activity of the enzyme adenylyl cyclase, which in turn decreases the cAMP levels in the neuronal cells. The release of neurotransmitters from the presynaptic neurons is blocked. This inhibition causes decrease in sympathetic or adrenergic outflow.[37]

β_1, β_2, and β_3 receptors belong to GPCR subtype G_s-protein coupled receptor group. The receptor stimulation increases the second messenger, cAMP, levels in the cells. Both β_1 and β_2 receptors are located in the cardiac muscle. However, there are greater numbers of β_1 than β_2 receptors in cardiac muscle. There are three extracellular and intracellular loops in the GPCRs. The first and second extracellular loops, connected by a disulfide bridge, play an important role in the development of receptor conformation. The phosphorylation site in the GPCR is responsible for the β receptor desensitization and down-regulation processes.[23,99]

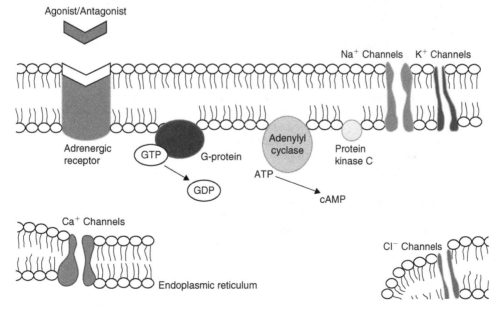

Figure 20-4 Adrenergic components at the cellular level.

The β receptor desensitization process involves (1) binding of the agonist to the G-protein receptor, (2) activation of the protein kinases, (3) phosphorylation of the receptor, and (4) the uncoupling of the receptor. Such uncoupled receptors are removed from the sarcolemma membranes through a process known as internalization or sequestration. The down-regulation, or decrease in number of the receptors, is due to prolonged exposure of the receptors to the agonists. Prolonged exposure to agonist results in cAMP-dependent destabilization of the messenger RNA. This decreases the synthesis of the β-adrenergic receptors. Desensitization and down-regulation processes regulate the number of β receptor on the cell membranes. The increase of second messenger, cAMP, causes the release of calcium ions from the sarcoplasmic reticulum. Calcium ions mediate the end responses such as the increase in force of contraction in cardiac muscle due to the stimulation of β_1 receptors. β_3 receptors are present on the adipocytes. They are involved in the process of lipolysis (Table 20-1).

A few terms used in the chapter are defined here:

- **Agonist:** Any molecule that couples with a receptor on a cell membrane and brings effective changes.
- **Antagonist:** Any molecule that occupies the receptor site and does not activate the receptor. The presence of an antagonist at the receptor site prevents an agonist from occupying and activating the receptor.
- **Sympathomimetic drugs:** Drugs that produce the same effects as catecholamines on various organs of the body. They are classified as follows:
  - Direct-acting drugs produce effects in different organ systems of the body by acting directly on α- and β-adrenergic receptors. Examples of this classification of drugs are phenylephrine and albuterol.
  - Indirect-acting drugs produce effects by:
    - Releasing endogenous catecholamines from the sympathetic nerve endings. Examples of this classification of drugs are amphetamines.

Table 20-1 Effects of α and β Receptor Stimulation

α Receptors		β Receptors		
α_1 (α_{1A}, α_{1B}, α_{1D})	α_2 (α_{2A}, α_{2B}, α_{2C})	β_1	β_2	β_3
GPCR family	GPCR family	GPCR family	GPCR family	GPCR family
G_q, ↑ phospholipase C, ↑ phospholipase D, ↑ phospholipase A_2	G_i, ↓ adenylyl cyclase	G_s, ↑ adenylyl cyclase	G_s, ↑ adenylyl cyclase	G_s, ↑ adenylyl cyclase
Location: heart, blood vessels, glands, and gut	Location: brain (thermo-regulatory center, cerebellar cortex and prefrontal cortex), pancreatic cells, platelets, and blood vessels	Location: heart and kidneys	Location: blood vessels, bronchi, uterus, urinary tract, and eyes	Location: adipose tissue
a) Contraction of smooth muscles of peripheral blood vessels, bladder neck, prostrate capsule, and prostrate fibro-muscular stroma b) Relaxes intestinal smooth muscles c) Pupil dilatation d) Platelet aggregation e) Decreases insulin release	a) Presynaptic inhibition—adrenergic transmission b) Decreases insulin release c) Arterial vasoconstriction d) Venous constriction e) Platelet aggregation and thrombus stabilization	a) Increase in heart rate, contractility, excitability, and conduction b) Increases renin and angiotensin secretion c) Increases blood pressure d) Enhances lipolysis e) Relaxation of intestinal muscles	a) Relaxation of vascular, bronchial, gastro-intestinal, and genitourinary smooth muscles b) Increases insulin release	a) Lipolysis

- Inhibiting the reuptake of the catecholamines into the neurons. An example of this classification of drugs is cocaine.[7]
- Inhibiting enzymes such as MAO and COMT that metabolize catecholamines increases the presence of catecholamines in the synaptic cleft. Examples of this classification of drugs are pargyline, phenelzine, selegiline, tolcapone, and entacapone.

- Mixed-acting sympathomimetic drugs that act on both α- and β-adrenergic receptors and also release catecholamines from the vesicles. An example of this classification of drugs is ephedrine.

Adrenergic Receptor Agonists

Epinephrine (adrenaline) is an agonist of α_1, α_2, β_1, and β_2 receptors (Figure 20-5).[91] It is secreted in the adrenal medulla and may have a transmitter role in the brain.

Mechanisms of Action

Cardiovascular Effects

The stimulation of β_1 receptors in the cardiac muscle increases chronotropism, inotropism, stroke volume, and cardiac output. The conduction velocity is increased in cardiac tissue. Peripherally, it acts on α_1 receptors and increases systemic vascular resistance. These combined effects lead to the increase in blood pressure. Myocardial oxygen demand increases due to the cardiac and vascular effects of epinephrine. The contraction of the smooth muscle in the blood vessels at the level of arterioles causes the increase in the vascular tone. Because of this, local blood flow decreases in the periphery. This may result in tissue hypoxia. Epinephrine has little or no effect on the cerebral vasculature. Cerebral autoregulation mitigates the effects of increases in blood pressure. Along with the peripheral vasoconstriction, renal blood flow is decreased.

Central Nervous System (CNS) Effects

Although theoretically the action of epinephrine on α_2 receptors in the brain should decrease heart rate and blood

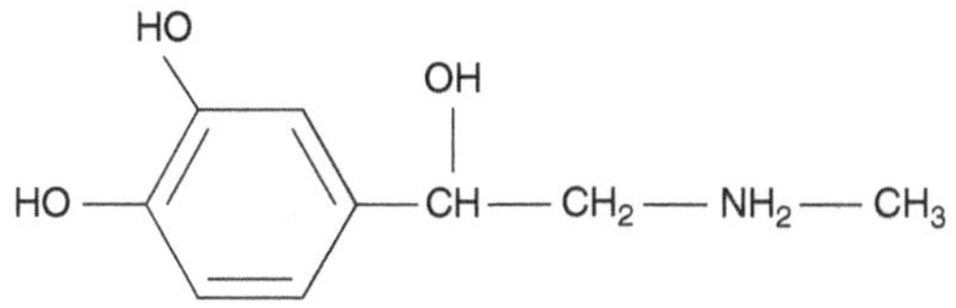

Figure 20-5 Epinephrine.

pressure, these reactions are not seen due to the effects of epinephrine on the heart.

Pulmonary Effects

Epinephrine stimulates β_2 receptors on the smooth muscles of bronchioles. This results in bronchodilatation. Bronchiole decongestion may result from the stimulation of α_1 receptors that cause vasoconstriction in the bronchial mucosa.

Gastrointestinal Effects

Epinephrine stimulation of α and β receptors on the smooth muscles cells in the gut results in slowing of peristaltic movements and constriction of sphincters.

Genitourinary Effects

The predominant α receptor presence on the smooth muscle cells in the trigone area of urinary bladder, bladder neck, and prostatic capsule stimulation causes urinary retention.[30]

Metabolic Effects

Epinephrine stimulation of α_2 receptors on the beta cell of the pancreas inhibits insulin secretion.[48] β Receptor stimulation on alpha cell of the pancreas increases glucagon release. Glucose clearance from blood is also decreased. These effects increase the blood glucose levels.[39] The inhibition of insulin release and triglyceride lipase enzyme and stimulation of β_2 receptors on adipocytes result in an increase in free fatty acid concentrations. Glycogenolysis and lipolysis cause a rise in glucose and free fatty acids, respectively.[110]

Ophthalmic Effects

Epinephrine stimulation of β-adrenergic receptors on the ciliary body and trabecular cells increase both the rate of formation of aqueous humor and rate of outflow in the eye, respectively. Mydriasis occurs due to the contraction of iris muscle.[82]

Platelets

Epinephrine stimulation of adrenergic receptors on the platelet membrane causes platelet aggregation and inhibition of synthesis of eicosanoids (prostaglandins, prostacyclins, thromboxanes, and leukotrienes) and prostaglandin I_2. The endothelial eicosanoid synthesis is also suppressed. These actions, in combination with the increased levels of free fatty acids, blood viscosity, and elevated blood pressure, increase the risk of vascular endothelial dysfunction.[10]

Pharmacokinetics

Oral administration of catecholamines is not effective. Catecholamines are absorbed through the intestines and are immediately metabolized by MAO and COMT in the liver.

Clinical Uses

- Epinephrine is used in the treatment of anaphylaxis. Epinephrine stabilizes mast cell membrane, increases blood pressure, and dilates bronchioles.
- Epinephrine is used in the treatment of acute exacerbation of asthma due to its bronchodilator effects.[118]
- Epinephrine is used in combination with local anesthetic agents to increase the duration of local anesthetic drugs and decrease local anesthetic drug toxicity and blood loss.[25]

Side Effects

Epinephrine is known to cause sweating, headache, tremors, nausea, dizziness, and arrhythmias.

Route of Administration

Epinephrine is administered parenterally or by injection or prefilled disposable devices, ophthalmic route, or aerosol.

Norepinephrine (noradrenaline) is an agonist of α_1, α_2, β_1 receptors (Figure 20-6). It is the major hormone produced in sympathetic postganglionic fibers except hair follicles and sweat glands.

Mechanisms of Action

Cardiovascular Effects

Norepinephrine effects on the heart include an increase in chronotropism, stroke volume, and cardiac output. These effects increase blood pressure.

CNS Effects

A decrease in norepinephrine levels in the brain leads to depression, anxiety, and attention disorders.

Genitourinary Effects

Norepinephrine causes urinary retention due to smooth muscle contraction in the urinary bladder.

Metabolic Effects

Metabolic effects include glycogenolysis.

Ophthalmic Effects

Norepinephrine causes mydriasis.

Clinical Uses

Norepinephrine is used as a vasopressor.[94]

Side Effects

Norepinephrine is known to produce headache, sweating, and arrhythmias.

Route of Administration

Norepinephrine is administered by intravenous infusion.

Dopamine is an agonist of α, β_1, D_1, D_2, D_3, D_4, and D_5 receptors (Figure 20-7). It is a major hormone in the extrapyramidal system and the anterior pituitary gland in the brain.

Mechanisms of Action

Cardiovascular Effects

At higher doses, β_1 receptor and α_1 receptor stimulation causes an increase in cardiac contractility and peripheral vasoconstriction, respectively.

Pulmonary Effects

Dopamine has no inhibitory action on the bronchial smooth muscles.[29]

CNS Effects

Dopamine acts centrally and is one of the important neurotransmitters in the brain. It is involved in memory,

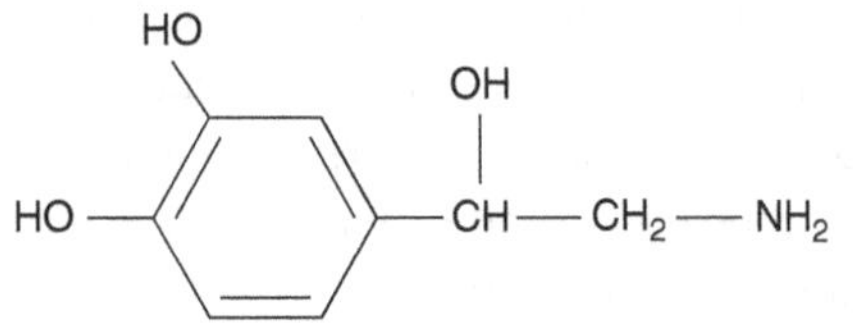

Figure 20-6 Norepinephrine.

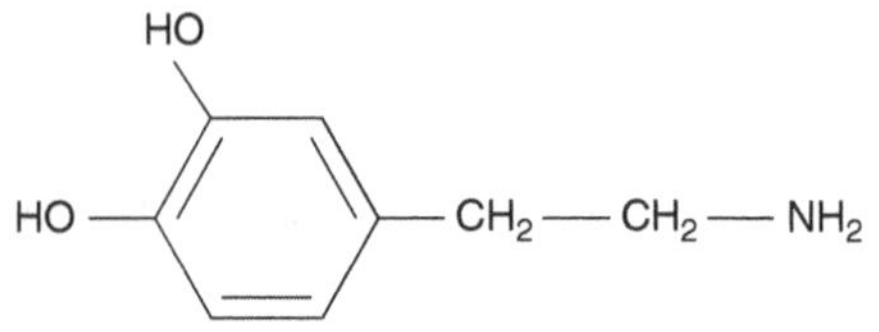

Figure 20-7 Dopamine.

attention, and neurocognitive functions. It regulates motor and limbic functions. Dopamine depletion in the brain causes schizophrenia, attention deficit hyperactivity disorder, and Parkinson's disease. Increased levels in the brain can cause mania.[53,96,105]

Dopamine produced in the hypothalamus inhibits D_2 receptors in the anterior pituitary gland. This inhibition decreases the secretion of prolactin in the brain. Prolactin is an important hormone that regulates lactation.[22]

Renal Effects

Dopamine stimulation of the D_1 receptors leads to the vasodilation of the renal and mesenteric vascular beds and coronary arteries.[38] Natriuretic effect is due to the inhibition of sodium potassium ATPase activity in the proximal tubule and medullary thick ascending limb of loop of Henle.[107]

Clinical Uses

- Dopamine is used to induce a positive inotropic effect.
- Dopamine is used in low cardiac output and oliguric conditions such as shock.[131]

Side Effects

Dopamine is known to cause tachycardia and arrhythmias.

Route of Administration

Dopamine is administered by intravenous infusion. Dopamine administered intravenously does not cross the blood–brain barrier.

Dobutamine is an α and β agonist (Figure 20-8). It is a derivative of dopamine and has no action on dopamine receptors. It is a synthetic catecholamine. Dobutamine

Figure 20-8 Dobutamine.

stereoisomers dextro(-) isomer acts on α receptors, and levo(+) isomer acts on β receptors.

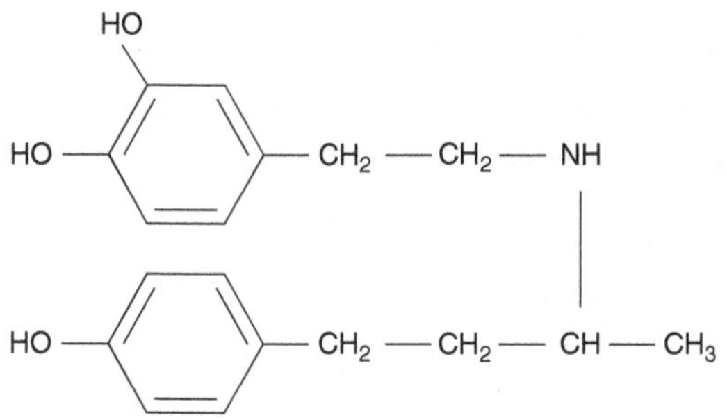

Mechanisms of Action

Cardiovascular Effects

Dobutamine improves systolic function, increases inotropism, stroke volume, cardiac output, and cardiac index.[112] It lowers the left ventricular end diastolic pressure, but mean aortic pressure is unchanged. It decreases peripheral vascular resistance due to α_1 antagonism and has minimal vascular effects compared with cardiac effects.[92] When compared with equipotent doses of dopamine, dobutamine is less arrhythmogenic. It causes pulmonary arterial vasodilatation.

Renal Effects

Dobutamine increases renal perfusion by increasing cardiac output. It does not stimulate dopamine receptors in the kidneys.[80]

Pharmacokinetics

Elimination half-life is 2 minutes. COMT and MAO enzymes metabolize the drug. Major end metabolite excreted in urine is 3-*O*-methyldobutamine.[133]

Clinical Uses

It is used in the short-term management of low perfusion states that would benefit from increased inotropism.

Side Effects

Dobutamine causes tachycardia and is less arrhythmogenic compared to dopamine.

Route of Administration

Dobutamine is administered by intravenous infusion.

Ephedrine is an agonist of α and β receptors and also releases catecholamines from vesicles (Figure 20-9). It is a

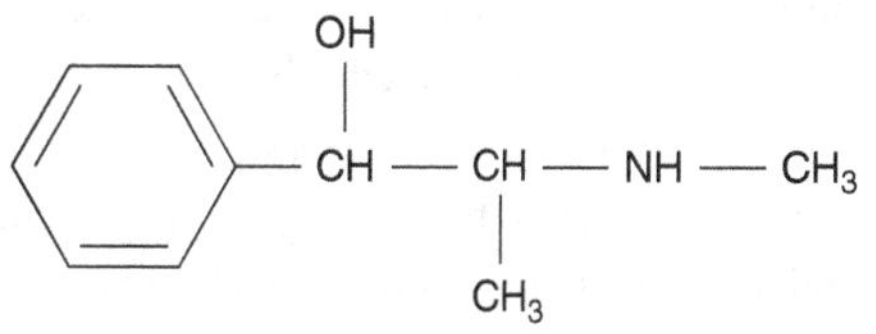

Figure 20-9 Ephedrine.

mixed-acting sympathomimetic drug. It was originally isolated from the plant *Ephedra vulgaris*.

Mechanisms of Action

Cardiovascular Effects

Ephedrine increases blood pressure by increasing heart rate (β receptor), cardiac output, and peripheral vascular tone (α receptors). It is used to manage hypotension in obstetric anesthesia because it is thought to preserve uteroplacental blood flow due to predominant β receptor stimulation (i.e., increase in cardiac output and arterial pressure) compared with α effect (i.e., vasoconstriction). It can cause coronary vascular spasm.[130]

CNS Effects

Ephedrine crosses the blood–brain barrier and acts as a CNS stimulant.

Pulmonary Effects

Ephedrine dilates bronchioles due to its agonist action on β_2 receptors on bronchial smooth muscles.

Genitourinary Effects

Urinary retention may occur due to the urinary bladder sphincter constriction.

Adipose Tissue Effects

Ephedrine, through its action on β_3 receptors on brown adipose tissue, induces thermogenesis. It causes weight loss.[69]

Pharmacokinetics

Elimination half-life is 6 hours. The metabolites benzoic acid and 1,2-dihydroxy-1-phenylpropane are excreted in the urine.

Clinical Uses

- Ephedrine is used in the treatment of asthma due to its bronchodilator effects.
- Ephedrine is used as a nasal decongestant due to its action on α receptors, which causes vasoconstriction of the mucosal blood vessels.
- Ephedrine is used to manage hypotension during spinal anesthesia in obstetric patients because it preserves uteroplacental blood flow.
- Ephedrine is used in patients suffering from narcolepsy due to its stimulant actions in the brain.

Side Effects

Ephedrine is known to produce hypertension, insomnia, urinary retention, headache, weakness, tremor, palpitations, psychosis, and tachyphylaxis.

Route of Administration

Ephedrine is administered by intravenous infusion and orally (MAO enzyme has little or no effect on the ephedrine).

Phenylephrine is a α_1 agonist (Figure 20-10).

Mechanisms of Action

Cardiovascular Effects

Phenylephrine increases blood pressure by peripheral vasoconstriction.

Pulmonary Effects

Phenylephrine acts as a bronchial decongestant. This is due to constriction of bronchial mucosa blood vessels.[66]

Ophthalmic Effects

Phenylephrine causes mydriasis and does not paralyze ciliary muscles.[75] It decreases intraocular pressure by the constriction of the smooth muscle cells in the blood vessels of the ciliary body. Phenylephrine should not be used in narrow-angle glaucoma patients due to rebound congestion. It is also contraindicated in those who are taking MAO inhibitors.

Male Genital Organs

Phenylephrine may be used to treat drug-induced priapism. The intracavernous injection of phenylephrine causes detumescence. It is not associated with the cardiac β effects such as tachycardia. Detumescence relieves pressure on veins and improves blood flow.

Obstetric Anesthesia

Phenylephrine use in obstetric anesthesia is considered to be controversial. Studies have shown that it can be

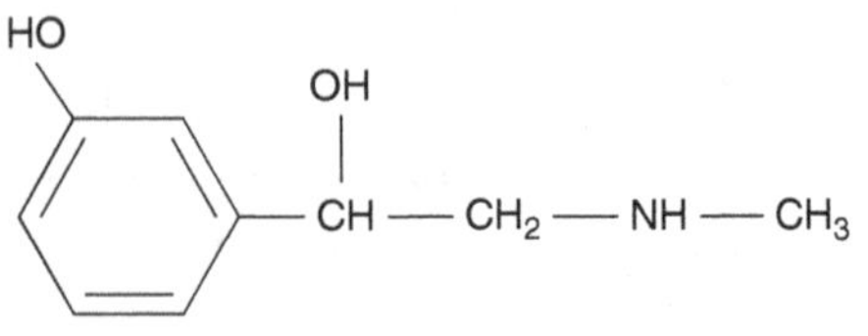

Figure 20-10 Phenylephrine.

used to manage hypotension during obstetric anesthesia because it is found to cause less fetal acidosis compared with ephedrine.[88]

Pharmacokinetics

Phenylephrine is metabolized by MAO and sulfotransferase enzymes in the enterocytes and liver. The metabolites 3-hydroxymandelic acid and phenylephrine sulfate are excreted in the urine. They have no affinity to the adrenergic receptors.

Clinical Uses

- Phenylephrine is used in the management of hypotension.
- Phenylephrine is used as a nasal decongestant.
- Phenylephrine is used as a mydriatic agent.
- Phenylephrine is used to relieve drug-induced priapism.[102]

Side Effects

Phenylephrine is known to cause reflex bradycardia and hypertension.[98]

Route of Administration

Phenylephrine is administered by oral, nasal, ophthalmic, and parenteral routes.

Amphetamines are agonists of α and β receptors and release catecholamines (norepinephrine and dopamine) from vesicles (Figure 20-11). They are mixed-acting sympathomimetic drugs. Modafinil, levoamphetamine, dextroamphetamine, and meta-amphetamine drugs belong to the amphetamine group.

Mechanisms of Action

Cardiovascular Effects

Amphetamine effects on the cardiovascular system are not marked. The changes in blood pressure and heart rate are not clinically significant.

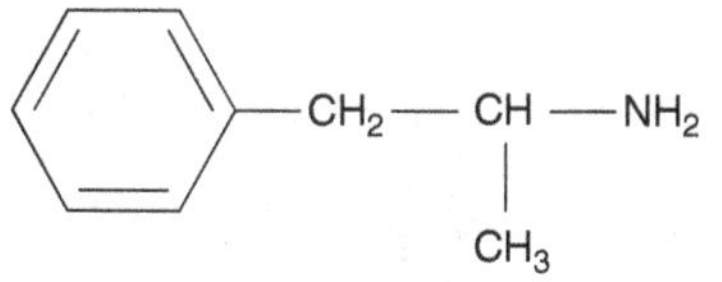

CNS Effects

Amphetamine crosses the blood–brain barrier and acts as a CNS stimulant. It increases alertness, concentration, and motor and speech activity as well as improves skeletal muscle performance. The stimulation of the reticular activating system causes wakefulness. Amphetamines also suppress physical fatigue due to sleep deprivation, stimulate the respiratory center, and increase the rate and depth of respiration.[45]

Genitourinary Effects

Amphetamines increase urinary bladder sphincter tone and may cause urinary retention.

Pharmacokinetics

The amphetamines are metabolized in the liver and kidneys. Elimination half-life is 6 to 12 hours. They are weak bases, and amphetamine toxicity/overdose can be treated by acidification of urine.

Clinical Uses

Amphetamines are known to treat narcolepsy and attention deficit hyperactivity disorder.

Side Effects

Amphetamines are known to cause restlessness, dizziness, tremor, hyperactivity reflexes, hyperpyrexia, decreased libido, insomnia, fatigue, depression, palpitations, hypertension, arrhythmias, hepatic failure, renal failure, dependence, and tolerance.

Route of Administration

Amphetamines are administered orally.

Table 20-2 provides a synopsis of other adrenergic receptor agonists not covered extensively here.

Adrenergic Receptor Antagonists

Phenoxybenzamine is an α_1 and α_2 receptor antagonist (Figure 20-12).[7]

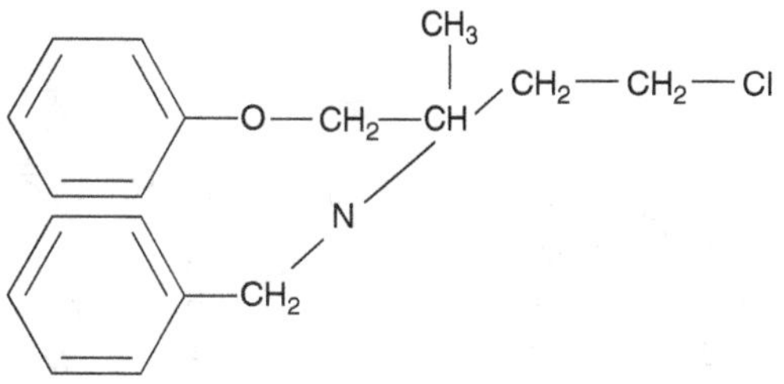

Figure 20-11 Amphetamine.

Figure 20-12 Phenoxybenzamine.

Table 20-2 Other α- and β-Adrenergic Receptor Agonists

Drug	Receptor	Actions	Pharmacokinetics	Clinical Uses	Side Effects
Clonidine[11,25,26,43,108,128]	α₂ Receptors in the vasomotor center in central nervous system	Vasodilatation Lowers blood pressure Decreases cardiac output Antirenin effect	Clonidine is metabolized in the gut and liver. Hydroxy-clonidine, an inactive predominant metabolite, is excreted in the urine. Renal clearance, protein binding, and metabolism in the liver influence clonidine clearance.	Antihypertensive Route of administration: oral	Hypotension Dryness of mouth Sedation Sexual dysfunction Contact dermatitis
Methyldopa[100,103,117]	α₂ Receptors in the vasomotor center in central nervous system	Vasodilatation Lowers blood pressure Decreases cardiac output Decreases renin secretion	Elimination half-life is 2 h. Methyldopa sulfate is the metabolite excreted in urine.	Antihypertensive used in pregnancy-induced hypertension Route of administration: oral and parenteral	Bradycardia Transient sedation Parkinsonian signs Gynecomastia Galactorrhea
Salbutamol/albuterol[6,27,31,63]	β₂ receptors	Relaxation of smooth muscles in bronchioles	Salbutamol mean half-life is 3.8 h.	Asthma COPD Route of administration: aerosol	Tremor Tachycardia Electrolyte imbalance
Terbutaline Salmeterol					
Ritodrine[32,62,86]	β₂ receptors	Relaxes uterine smooth muscle	Both the fetus and mother excrete ritodrine in a free and conjugated form.	To arrest premature labor Route of administration: oral and parenteral	Tachycardia Cardiac arrhythmias Pulmonary edema Hyperglycemia

Table 20-2 Other α- and β-Adrenergic Receptor Agonists *(continued)*

Drug	Receptor	Actions	Pharmacokinetics	Clinical Uses	Side Effects
Isoproterenol/isoprenaline[40]	β > α receptors nonselective	Increases cardiac muscle contractility Increases cardiac output Decreases vascular resistance	It is excreted as 3-O-methyl isoprenaline in the urine.	Shock Route of administration: parenteral	Palpitations Tachycardia Headache Arrhythmias
Pseudophedrine[54,111]	α and β receptors nonselective	Vasoconstrictor, especially mucosa and skin Mild CNS effects	Elimination half-life is 5–6 h. Mostly it is excreted in unchanged form.	Nasal decongestant Route of administration: oral	Avoid in hypertension
Methylphenidate[8,32,83,89]	α and β receptors nonselective. Blocks reuptake of dopamine and norepinephrine into presynaptic neurons	CNS stimulant	Duration of action is 1–4 h. Elimination half-life is 2–3 h.	Attention deficit hyperactivity disorder Narcolepsy Route of administration: oral	Nervousness Insomnia Palpitations Weight loss Dependence Addiction

CNS, central nervous system; COPD, chronic obstructive pulmonary disease.

Mechanisms of Action

Phenoxybenzamine is metabolized to an intermediate metabolic product, called ethyleneimine ions, that react with α receptors. These ions cause irreversible receptor blockade by forming covalent bonds with the α receptors.

Cardiovascular Effects

Phenoxybenzamine blocks α_1 receptors, leading to decreased peripheral vascular tone and thus lowering blood pressure. An increase in norepinephrine levels due to α_2 blockade can cause increased heart rate and cardiac output.

CNS Effects

Phenoxybenzamine crosses the blood–brain barrier and acts as a CNS stimulant. As a result it can cause nausea, vomiting, sedation, depression, tiredness, and lethargy.

Other Receptors

Phenoxybenzamine also partially blocks serotonin, histaminergic, and cholinergic receptors. It has no effect on β-adrenergic receptors.

Pharmacokinetics

Elimination half-life is 24 hours. It is excreted in urine and feces.

Clinical Uses

- Phenoxybenzamine is used to manage hypertension in pheochromocytoma.[42]
- Phenoxybenzamine is used to relieve ischemic effects in peripheral vascular diseases.
- Phenoxybenzamine is used to treat patients with benign prostatic hypertrophy to improve urinary flow.[61]

Side Effects

Phenoxybenzamine is known to cause postural hypotension, tachycardia, arrhythmias, headache, nausea, and vomiting.

Route of Administration

Phenoxybenzamine is administered orally and by intravenous infusion.

Phentolamine is an α_1 and α_2 receptor antagonist (Figure 20-13).

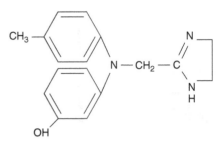

Figure 20-13 Phentolamine.

Mechanisms of Action

Cardiovascular Effects

Phentolamine causes peripheral vasodilatation and lowers blood pressure by blocking α_1 receptors. The release of norepinephrine from the vesicles occurs due to α_2 receptor antagonism. The excess accumulation of norepinephrine in the synaptic cleft can cause reflex tachycardia.

Pulmonary Effects

Phentolamine has been shown to decrease airway resistance and improve symptoms in asthmatic patients.[71]

Male Genital Organs

In the male genitalia, phentolamine causes relaxation of corporal smooth muscles. Because of this, blood flow into the cavernosal spaces increases and causes penile erection.

Pharmacokinetics

Elimination half-life is 19 minutes. It is excreted in both free and conjugated forms.

Clinical Uses

- Phentolamine is used in the management of hypertension in pheochromocytoma.
- Phentolamine is used in the management of hypertension due to clonidine withdrawal.
- The drug has shown to improve male erectile dysfunction.[64]

Side Effects

Phentolamine is known to cause tachycardia, arrhythmias, nausea, and abdominal pain. Intrapenile injections can cause priapism.

Route of Administration

Phentolamine is administered by intravenous infusion.

Prazosin is an α_1 receptor antagonist (Figure 20-14). It does not increase norepinephrine levels in the synaptic cleft because it has little effect on presynaptic α_2 receptors.

Mechanisms of Action

Cardiovascular Effects

Prazosin causes peripheral vasodilatation due to α_1 receptor antagonism. It lowers blood pressure and increases heart rate. The effect of prazosin is greater on arterioles than veins.[79]

Pulmonary Effects

Prazosin is not shown to produce any effect on bronchioles.[19]

Genitourinary Effects

Prazosin blocks α_1 receptors on smooth muscle cells of the urinary bladder trigone and prostate. These effects improve urinary flow.[9]

Metabolic Effects

The effects of prazosin on fat metabolism include decrease in cholesterol, low-density lipoprotein, and triglyceride levels in the plasma. These effects are due to α_1 receptor blockade.[90]

Pharmacokinetics

Prazosin is absorbed through the gut and is metabolized in the liver. The peak concentration in the plasma is reached after 1 to 3 hours after oral intake in normal subjects. The mean elimination half-life is 2.5 hours. The metabolites are excreted in the urine. In patients with congestive heart failure, liver diseases, and renal diseases, the drug elimination is not normal and dose should be adjusted accordingly.[81]

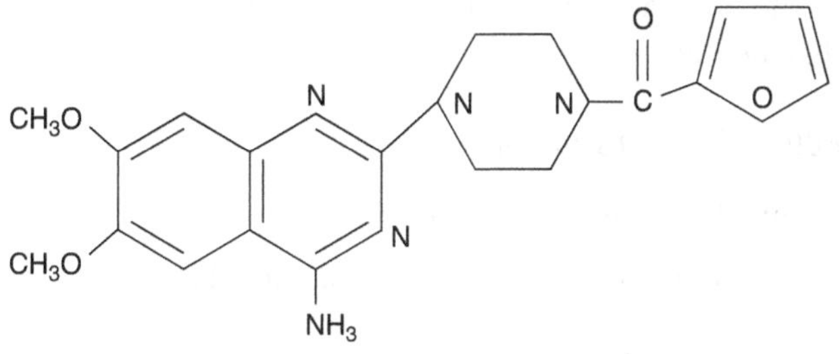

Clinical Uses

- Prazosin is a preferred drug in hypertensive patients with prostate enlargement that causes problems with the urinary flow. An additional advantage is prazosin may cause reduction of lipids and consequently decreases vascular risk.[120]
- Prazosin is used to improve urinary flow in patients with benign prostatic hypertrophy.[84]

Side Effects

Prazosin is known to produce a generalized decrease in blood pressure,[65] known as postural hypotension, occasionally resulting in syncope.

Route of Administration

Prazosin is administered orally.

Yohimbine is an α_2 receptor antagonist (Figure 20-15). It is an alkaloid obtained from the African plant *Pausinystalia yohimbe*.

Mechanisms of Action

Cardiovascular Effects

Yohimbine increases heart rate and blood pressure by releasing norepinephrine from the presynaptic vesicles due to α_2 receptor antagonism.

CNS Effects

Yohimbine crosses the blood–brain barrier and acts as a CNS stimulant. The adrenergic activation leads to increased motor activity and anxiety and can cause tremors.

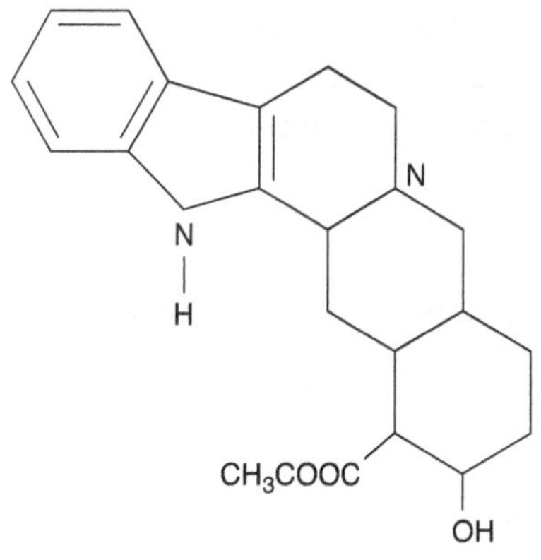

Figure 20-14 Prazosin.

Figure 20-15 Yohimbine.

Genitourinary Effects

Yohimbine improves male erectile function by improving the blood flow into the cavernosal spaces. It enhances the release of nitric oxide and cGMP levels in the corporal smooth muscle cells.[47,121]

Pharmacokinetics

Yohimbine is rapidly absorbed orally and is metabolized in the liver. The mean elimination half-life is 0.6 hours. The metabolites are eliminated in the urine.[74]

Clinical Uses

Yohimbine is available by prescription and is marketed as a dietary supplement "over the counter" to individuals seeking relief from erectile dysfunction.[101]

Side Effects

Yohimbine is known to produce dizziness, tremors, tachycardia, and abnormal behavior.

Route of Administration

Yohimbine is administered orally.

Atenolol is a β_1 antagonist (Figure 20-16).

Mechanisms of Action

Atenolol lacks what has been described as "intrinsic sympathomimetic activity" and anesthetic-like membrane-stabilizing activity.

Cardiovascular Effects

Atenolol causes peripheral vasodilatation and lowers blood pressure. It has also been shown to improve blood pressure control in the elderly and in pregnant women.[127] In peripheral vascular disease patients, it increases local blood flow and decreases ischemic effects.

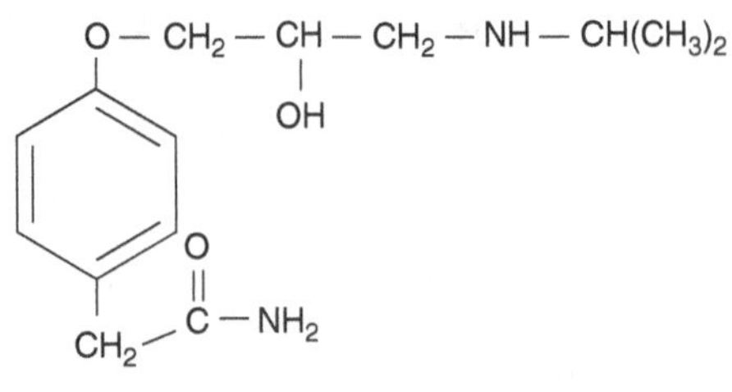

Figure 20-16 Atenolol.

CNS Effects

Atenolol has low lipid solubility. Atenolol penetration into the brain is not significant and therefore has mild CNS effects.

Metabolic Effects

Atenolol increases the plasma levels of total triglycerides and decreases high-density lipoprotein levels. This is due to the unopposed stimulation of the α receptors that inhibits lipoprotein lipase. Long-term use of atenolol may increase the vascular risk.[44,45]

Anesthetic Effect

Atenolol has no anesthetic action.

Drug Safety

The drug can be safely used in diabetics and asthmatic patients. It does not block β_2 receptors in the liver and lungs that are important in the recovery from hypoglycemia and bronchodilatation, respectively.

Pharmacokinetics

The drug is rapidly absorbed orally, and peak blood levels are observed after 2 to 4 hours.[60] The drug effect starts after 4 hours (both oral and intravenous administration), and effects persist for up to 24 hours. It is usually administered once daily. It is eliminated in the urine unchanged.[76] The dosage should be adjusted based on renal function.

Clinical Uses

Atenolol is used in the management of hypertension and may be recommended as a treatment in angina pectoris because the drug decreases heart rate and myocardial oxygen demand.

Side Effects

Atenolol is known to produce hypotension, fatigue, nausea, diarrhea, and dizziness.

Route of Administration

Atenolol is administered orally.

Timolol is a nonselective β antagonist (Figure 20-17).

Mechanisms of Action

Timolol lacks intrinsic sympathomimetic activity and membrane-stabilizing activity.

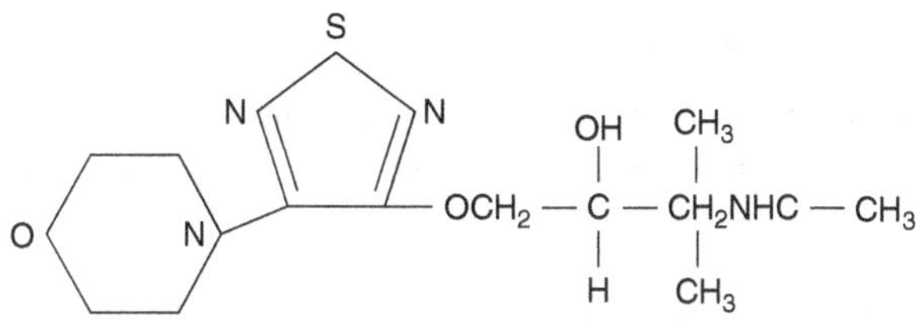

Figure 20-17 Timolol.

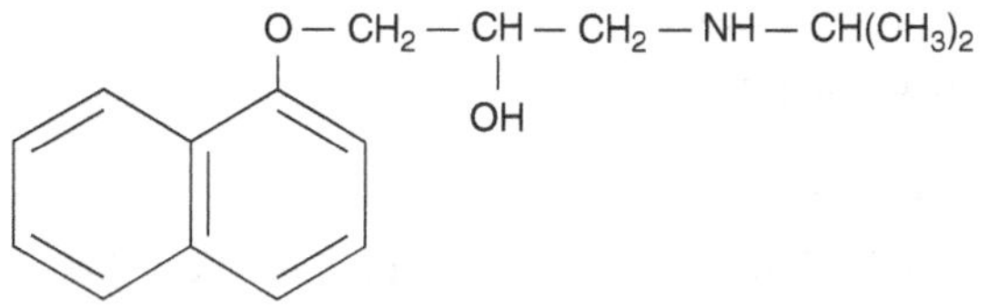

Figure 20-18 Propranolol.

Cardiovascular Effects

Blood pressure is lowered by the reduction of peripheral vascular tone.

Pulmonary Effects

Timolol is known to increase airway resistance.[119]

Ophthalmic Effects

Timolol blocks β receptors on smooth muscle cells in the ciliary body blood vessels. As a result aqueous humor production is reduced, and this results in a decrease of intraocular pressure. It has no effect on the trabeculae, and therefore no change is noted in the outflow of aqueous humor.[104]

Anesthetic Effect

Timolol has no local anesthetic action.

Pharmacokinetics

After oral administration of timolol, peak plasma levels are attained within 1 to 2 hours. Average elimination half-life from plasma is 2.5 hours. It is partially metabolized in the liver and eliminated in the urine.

Clinical Uses

Timolol is used in the treatment of glaucoma and hypertension.[135]

Side Effects

Timolol is known to cause blurred vision, confusion, depression, bradycardia, arrhythmias, and bronchospasm.[124]

Routes of administration

Timolol is administered orally, and ophthalmic preparations are also available.

Propranolol is a β_1 and β_2 antagonist (Figure 20-18).

Mechanisms of Action

Propranolol lacks intrinsic sympathomimetic activity but has anesthetic-like membrane-stabilizing activity.

Cardiovascular Effects

Propranolol causes decreased inotropism, chronotropism, and cardiac output. It depresses the automaticity in the sinoatrial node and conduction velocity in the atrioventricular junction. It decreases myocardial oxygen demand and may increase peripheral vascular resistance due to β_2 receptor antagonism.[14,106,122]

Pulmonary Effects

Propranolol blocks β_2 receptors on the bronchial smooth muscle cells, causing bronchoconstriction and increased resistance to airflow.[56]

CNS Effects

Propranolol crosses the blood–brain barrier. It acts as a short-term anxiety reliever. The somatic symptoms arising from increased adrenergic tone associated with conditions such as anxiety and social phobia may be ameliorated.[67,87] Other CNS effects include dreaming, nightmares, and forgetfulness.

Metabolic Effects

Propranolol decreases insulin release by blocking β_2 receptors on the beta cells of the pancreas that produce and store insulin. The adrenergic-mediated effects on lipid and carbohydrate metabolism such as lipolysis and glycogenolysis are inhibited. It depresses sympathetic warning signs such as tachycardia and tremors in hypoglycemic patients.[46] Sweating is not suppressed.[34]

Musculoskeletal Effects

Propranolol decreases the energy supply to the skeletal muscles due to its inhibitory effects on the carbohydrate and lipid metabolism (glycogenolysis and lipolysis). Tremors are also suppressed.[51]

Ophthalmic Effects

Propranolol blocks β_2 receptors in the ciliary body and decreases the production of aqueous humor, lowering intraocular pressure.

Renal Effects

Propranolol decreases renin release in the kidneys by blocking β_1 receptors.

Anesthetic Actions

Propranolol has anesthetic properties, but because of its irritant effects it is not in clinical use as an anesthetic.

Pharmacokinetics

Propranolol is metabolized in the liver, and metabolites such as 4-hydroxypropranolol are excreted in the urine. The metabolism depends on the hepatic blood flow. Elimination half-life is 4 hours. Conditions such as hepatic, renal, and thyroid diseases as well as malnutrition, hypertension, and hypothermia can alter propranolol elimination. Drugs such as cimetidine may interfere in the process of propranolol elimination.[57]

Clinical Uses

Propranolol may be used in the management of hypertension, angina, supraventricular arrhythmias, ventricular arrhythmias, migraine prophylaxis, tremors, social phobia, and generalized anxiety disorder.

Side Effects

Propranolol is known to cause myocardial depression, bradycardia, bronchoconstriction, hypoglycemia, angina, depression, and sexual dysfunction.[109] Furthermore, it may exacerbate peripheral vascular disease symptoms due to vasoconstriction.

Routes of Administration

Propranolol is administered orally and parenterally.

Esmolol is a selective β_1-adrenergic antagonist (Figure 20-19).

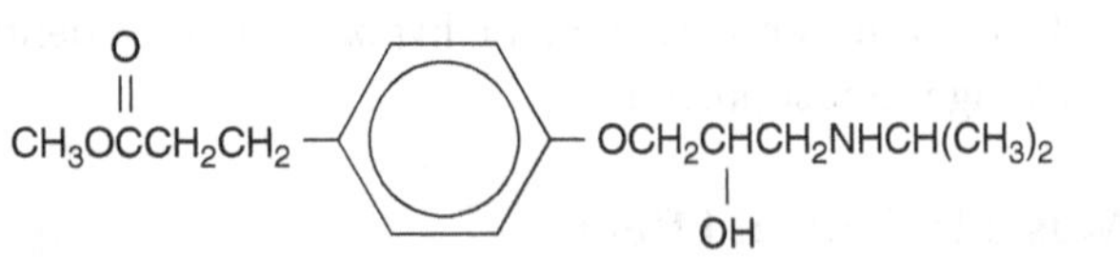

Figure 20-19 Esmolol.

Mechanisms of Action

Esmolol is an ultra–short-acting drug. Esmolol lacks intrinsic sympathomimetic activity, membrane-stabilizing activity and alpha blocking activity.

Cardiovascular Effects

Esmolol decreases heart rate, myocardial oxygen demand, and blood pressure. It lacks direct vascular effects. Esmolol acts as an antiarrhythmic by decreasing the conduction velocity and increasing the refractoriness of atrioventricular junction cells. It does not block the peripheral vascular sympathomimetic effects of the adrenergics.[35]

CNS Effects

Esmolol is not known to have a direct effect on cerebral circulation. It does not interfere with cognitive functions.[78]

Pulmonary Effects

Esmolol does not cause increased airway resistance.[115]

Pharmacokinetics

The average elimination half-life of esmolol is 9 minutes. The drug is metabolized rapidly by the red cell esterases to an acid metabolite and methanol. The elimination of esmolol is independent of renal and hepatic function because it is metabolized by the red blood cell esterases.[129]

Clinical Uses

- Esmolol is used to manage heart rate and blood pressure in situations where the dosage of the drug can be easily titrated to response and adverse effects can be rapidly managed by the termination of infusion. It is most useful in surgeries and in critically ill patients.[11,18,68]
- It is also used in the management of supraventricular arrhythmias and in the early treatment of myocardial ischemia.[2,4]

Side Effects

Esmolol is known to produce bradycardia, hypotension, dizziness, confusion, headache, and nausea.

Route of Administration

Esmolol is administered parenterally.

Table 20-3 provides a synopsis of other adrenergic receptor antagonist drugs not covered extensively here.

Table 20-3 Other α- and β-Adrenergic Receptor Antagonists

Drug	Receptor	Actions	Pharmacokinetics	Clinical Uses	Side Effects
Terazosin[3,17,20,36,123] Doxazosin[41] Tamsulosin	α₁ Antagonists	Decreased peripheral vascular resistance Peripheral vasodilatation Causes hypotension Reduces smooth muscle tone in the urinary bladder neck and prostate Reduction in LDL and total cholesterol, increase in HDL	Terazosin mean elimination half-life is 12 h. It is metabolized in liver and excreted in bile. Doxazosin elimination half-life is 9 h. Tamsulosin elimination half-life is 9–13 h.	Antihypertensive Benign prostatic hypertrophy Route of administration: oral	Reflex tachycardia Marked postural hypotension Syncope
Labetalol[24,93,95]	α, β Nonselective antagonists	Decreases in heart rate Reduces peripheral vascular resistance Has less effect on cardiac output Lowers blood pressure	Elimination half-life is 5.5 h. Metabolized in liver and eliminated in urine and bile as conjugates of glucuronides.	Antihypertensive Used in the treatment of essential hypertension, renal hypertension, pheochromocytoma, pregnancy hypertension, and hypertensive emergencies Routes of administration: oral and parenteral	Posture-related dizziness Tiredness Headache Skin rash Urinary retention Impotence
Nadolol[50,97,113]	β Nonselective antagonists	Lacks intrinsic sympatho-mimetic or anesthetic-like membrane-stabilizing activity Lowers heart rate and contractility Lowers blood pressure	Elimination half-life is 7.3–15.7 h. Single dose per day. It is eliminated as unmetabolized in urine. It is excreted in breast milk.	Antihypertensive Angina pectoris Migraine Route of administration: oral	Fatigue Hypotension Abdominal cramps Impotence
Sotalol[12,59,85,116]	β Nonselective antagonists	Lacks intrinsic sympatho-mimetic, anesthetic-like membrane-stabilizing activity and cardioselectivity Lengthens repolarization and effective refractory period in all cardiac tissues Antiarrhythmic (class III) Lowers blood pressure	Elimination half-life is 7–15 h. Excreted through kidneys, and liver has no role.	Paroxysmal supraven-tricular tachycardias Ventricular tachycardia Ventricular fibrillation Antihypertensive Route of administration: oral	Bradycardia Dyspnea Dizziness Fatigue Hypotension Bronchospasm Congestive heart failure
Metoprolol[1,21,114]	β₁ Antagonists	Decrease in heart rate Decrease in blood pressure No effect on the systemic vascular resistance	Elimination half-life 3–4 h. It is metabolized in liver to hydroxymetoprolol and o-demethylmetoprolol. It is safe to be used in patients suffering with asthma and diabetes.	Angina pectoris Essential hypertension Postmyocardial infarction Routes of administration: oral and parenteral	Fatigue Dizziness Headache

HDL, high-density lipoprotein; LDL, low-density lipoprotein.

Caution in α- and β-Adrenergic Drug Usage in the Geriatric Population

It is important to take caution when using medications in elderly patients because physiologic changes related to aging can affect the patient's response to medications. Drug absorption is not noted to change significantly in the elderly; however, changes in gastrointestinal motility and rate of gastric emptying can be appreciated. Drug distribution can demonstrate a significant change, particularly because the elderly are known to experience a decrease in total body water composition and lean body mass. In addition, the elderly also have increases in body fat and slight decreases in plasma albumin. These changes in body composition can affect the distribution of both lipid-soluble and water-soluble drugs. Drug excretion is another factor that can be significantly affected by changes in the renal system. It is important to be aware of the potential for hepatic and renal failure.

α-Adrenergic receptor blockers can cause clinical conditions that are of particular concern with the elderly. Some of these conditions include orthostatic hypotension and sodium and water retention. On the other hand, β-adrenergic receptor blockers can be responsible for heart failure in patients with cardiac disease or increase the incidence of hypoglycemic episodes. In addition, β-adrenergic antagonist drugs can also increase airway resistance, creating additional problems for individuals with obstructive pulmonary disease. Increased fatigue, sedation, sleep disturbances, and depression are other side effects of these drugs that present additional problems for the elderly. Many elderly struggle with balance and stability, and side effects such as orthostatic hypotension, fatigue, and sedation can lead to patient falls and the cascade of complications that accompany falls in the acute postoperative period. Sodium and water retention can be of particular concern to individuals with heart failure and renal disease.

Zaugg and colleagues[134] suggested many benefits from perioperative use of β-adrenergic antagonists in the elderly. Some of these benefits include decreased analgesic requirements, faster recovery from anesthesia, and improved hemodynamic stability.

It is sometimes necessary to administer or prescribe these types of drugs to the elderly. Caution is essential. The main caveat when administering drugs to the elderly is to start low and go slow. Take into account other medications and those side effects to avoid potentiating negative effects.

Current advances in drug development have led to a newer generation of selective α and β agonists and antagonists that results in fewer side effects than the previous nonselective drugs. When prescribing for the elderly, these selective drugs are the drugs of choice because the side effects are fewer and often less severe. These new selective drugs make them better options for the elderly population.

Key Points

- Catecholamines play important roles in balancing the parasympathetic influence on different organ systems, influencing energy metabolic pathways, modulating the immune system, and may act as a neurotransmitter.
- Even though the α- and β-adrenergic receptors belong to the GPCRs, the difference in internal organization of proteins, the receptor location (pre- or postsynaptic), and second messengers associated with them produce either excitatory or inhibitory effects.
- The drugs that are nonselective may cause a wide range of actions that may not be desirable. Their use should be limited to reduce the number of adverse reactions. For example, propranolol should not be used in asthmatics and diabetics because it inhibits bronchodilatation and prolongs hypoglycemia. Receptor-specific drugs should be administered to those patients suffering from multiple clinical conditions to produce specific desirable effects and to minimize drug interactions.
- Pregnancy (first trimester) and breast-feeding should limit the use of drugs because some of them can act as a teratogen or may damage immature liver in infants.
- Even though a drug acts specifically on a receptor, it may not produce the same degree of effects as the other drug on the same organ system. For example, ritodrine is a β_2-adrenergic receptor agonist used as a uterine relaxant and not as a bronchodilator even though it has effects on the smooth muscle cells in bronchioles.
- Some drugs may interfere in the metabolism of other drugs by enabling or suppressing the enzyme systems in the liver. For example, cimetidine interferes with the metabolism of propranolol.
- In those who suffer from liver diseases, drugs metabolized in the kidneys or other organ systems should be preferred and vice versa. For example, esmolol is metabolized by red cell esterases and is safe to be used in patients diagnosed with liver and kidney diseases.
- Chronic usage of drugs can cause tolerance and dependence (e.g., amphetamines). Long-term use of β-adrenergic receptor agonists may not produce desirable effects even with the increase in dosage due to cellular mechanisms such as receptor desensitization and down-regulation processes.
- In patients suffering from multiple clinical conditions, clinicians should limit the number of drugs used. Teamwork is encouraged.
- Table 20-4 provides an overview of the drugs discussed in this chapter.

Table 20-4 Drug, Route of Administration, and Dosage

Drug	Route of Administration and Availability
Epinephrine	Intravenous therapy: 0.01 mg/mL, 0.1 mg/mL, 0.5 mg/mL, 1 mg/mL Aerosol: 160 μg, 200 μg, 220 μg, 250 μg EpiPen autoinjectors: 0.3 mg, 0.15 mg Nebulizer: 1%. 1.25%, 2.25% Ophthalmic: 0.5%, 1%, 2%
Norepinephrine	Intravenous: 1 mg/mL
Dopamine	Intravenous: 40 mg/mL, 80 mg/mL, 160 mg/mL Dopamine hydrochloride in dextrose 5%: 80 mg/mL, 160 mg/mL, 320 mg/100 mL
Dobutamine	Intravenous: 12.5 mg/mL
Ephedrine	Oral: 8 mg, 12.5 mg, 25 mg Injection: 50 mg/mL Intranasal spray: 0.25%
Clonidine	Oral: 0.1 mg, 0.2 mg, 0.3 mg Transdermal: 2.5 mg, 5 mg, 7.5 mg Intravenous for epidural: 100 μg/mL, 500 μg/mL
Methyldopa	Oral: 250 mg, 500 mg Intravenous: 50 mg/mL
Salbutamol/albuterol	Aerosol: 90 μg Oral: 2 mg, 4 mg Oral extended release: 4 mg, 8 mg Oral solution: 2 mg/5 mL
Terbutaline	Intravenous: 1 mg/mL
Salmeterol	Inhalation: 50 μg per inhalation
Isoproterenol	Intravenous: 0.2 mg/mL, 0.02 mg/mL Aerosol: 80 μg per inhalation
Pseudoephedrine	Oral tablets: 30 mg, 60 mg Capsules: 60 mg Capsules extended release: 120 mg, 240 mg Syrup: 30 mg/5 mL Oral solutions: 15 mg/mL, 30 mg/5 mL
Methylphenidate	Oral: 5 mg, 10 mg, 20 mg; sustained release: 20 mg
Phenoxybenzamine	Oral : 10 mg
Phentolamine	Intravenous: 5 mg per vial
Prazosin	Oral: 1 mg, 2 mg, 5 mg
Yohimbine	Oral: 5.4 mg
Atenolol	Oral: 25 mg, 50 mg, 100 mg
Timolol	Ophthalmic: 0.25%, 0.5% Oral: 5 mg, 10 mg, 20 mg
Propranolol	Oral: 10 mg, 20 mg, 40 mg, 60 mg Intravenous: 1 mg/mL Extended release: 60 mg, 80 mg, 120 mg
Esmolol	Intravenous: 10 mg/mL
Terazosin	Oral: 1 mg, 2 mg, 5 mg, 10 mg
Doxazosin	Oral: 1 mg, 2mg, 4 mg, 8 mg
Tamsulosin	Oral: 0.4 mg
Labetalol	Oral: 100 mg, 200 mg, 300 mg Intravenous: 5 mg/mL
Nadolol	Oral: 20 mg, 40 mg, 80 mg, 120 mg, 160 mg
Sotalol	Oral: 80 mg, 120 mg, 160 mg, 240 mg
Metoprolol	Oral: 50 mg, 100 mg Extended release: 50 mg, 100 mg, 200 mg

Chapter Questions

1. Describe the metabolic pathway of catecholamines.
2. List drugs that are safe to be used in those diagnosed with both liver and kidney disorders.
3. Discuss the safety of alpha- and beta-blockers in pregnancy.
4. Why should nonselective drugs not be administered to patients diagnosed with asthma or diabetes?
5. Describe the effects of different adrenergic agonist and antagonist drugs on the central nervous system.
6. List the short-acting drugs and the clinical situations where they can be useful.
7. Describe the mechanisms of the adrenergic drugs that influence glucose metabolism.
8. List and discuss the adrenergic drugs that increase vascular risk.
9. Describe the drugs that can produce multiple beneficial effects when used in patients with more than two clinical conditions.
10. Discuss the drugs that may potentiate the effects of other adrenergic drugs.
11. List reasons why we should limit the number of drugs in geriatric patients.
12. Describe the adrenergic drugs that can be used in the treatment of central nervous system disorders.

References

1. Ablad B, Borg KO, Carlsson E, et al. A survey of the pharmacological properties of metoprolol in animals and man. *Acta Pharmacol Toxicol (Copenh)*. 1975;36(Suppl 5):7–23.
2. Abrams J, Allen J, Allin D, et al. Efficacy and safety of esmolol vs propranolol in the treatment of supraventricular tachyarrhythmias: a multicenter double-blind clinical trial. *Am Heart J*. 1985;110:913–922.
3. Achari R, Laddu A. Terazosin: a new alpha adrenoceptor blocking drug. *J Clin Pharmacol*. 1992;32:520–523.
4. Adamson PC, Rhodes LA, Saul JP, et al. The pharmacokinetics of esmolol in pediatric subjects with supraventricular arrhythmias. *Pediatr Cardiol*. 2006;27:420–427.
5. Ahlquist RP. A study of the adrenotropic receptors. *Am J Physiol*. 1948;153:586–600.
6. Ahrens RC, Smith GD. Albuterol: an adrenergic agent for use in the treatment of asthma pharmacology, pharmacokinetics and clinical use. *Pharmacotherapy*. 1984;4:105–121.
7. Alousi A. The regulation of norepinephrine synthesis in sympathetic nerves: effect of nerve stimulation, cocaine, and catecholamine-releasing agents. *Proc Natl Acad Sci USA*. 1966;56:1491.
8. Anderson VR, Scott LJ. Methylphenidate transdermal system: in attention-deficit hyperactivity disorder in children. *Drugs*. 2006;66:1117–1126.
9. Andersson KE, Lepor H, Wyllie MG. Prostatic alpha 1-adrenoceptors and uroselectivity. *Prostate*. 1997;30:202–215.
10. Anfossi G. Role of catecholamines in platelet function: pathophysiological and clinical significance. *Eur J Clin Invest*. 1996;26:353.
11. Angaran DM, Schultz NJ, Tschida VH. Esmolol hydrochloride: an ultrashort-acting, beta-adrenergic blocking agent. *Clin Pharm*. 1986;5:288–303.
12. Antonaccio MJ, Gomoll A. Pharmacology, pharmacodynamics and pharmacokinetics of sotalol. *Am J Cardiol*. 1990;65:12A–21A; discussion 35A–36A.
13. Ashton H, Rawlins MD. Central nervous system depressant actions of clonidine and UK-14,304: partial dissociation of EEG and behavioural effects. *Br J Clin Pharmacol*. 1978;5:135–140.
14. Astrom H. Haemodynamic effects of beta-adrenergic blockade. *Br Med J*. 1968;30:44.
15. Axelrod J. Studies on the metabolism of catecholamines. *Circ Res*. 1961;9:715.
16. Axelrod J. Enzymatic O-methylation of epinephrine and other catechols. *J Biol Chem*. 1958;233:702.
17. Babamoto KS, Hirokawa WT. Doxazosin: a new alpha 1-adrenergic antagonist. *Clin Pharm*. 1992;11:415–427.
18. Barbier GH, Shettigar UR, Appunn DO. Clinical rationale for the use of an ultra-short acting beta-blocker: esmolol. *Int J Clin Pharmacol Ther*. 1995;33:212–218.
19. Barnes PJ, Ind PW, Dollery CT. Inhaled prazosin in asthma. *Thorax*. 1981;36:378–381.
20. Basar MM, Yilmaz E, Ferhat M, Basar H, Batislam E. Terazosin in the treatment of premature ejaculation: a short-term follow-up. *Int Urol Nephrol*. 2005;37:773–777.
21. Benfield P, Clissold SP, Brogden RN. Metoprolol. An updated review of its pharmacodynamic and pharmacokinetic properties, and therapeutic efficacy, in hypertension, ischaemic heart disease and related cardiovascular disorders. *Drugs*. 1986;31:376–429.
22. Ben-Jonathan N. Dopamine as a prolactin (PRL) inhibitor. *Endocrinol Rev*. 2001;22:724.
23. Bouvier M, Collins S, O'Dowd BF, et al. Two distinct pathways for cAMP-mediated down-regulation of the beta 2-adrenergic receptor. Phosphorylation of the receptor and regulation of its mRNA level. *J Biol Chem*. 1989;264:16786–16792.
24. Brogden RN, Heel RC, Speight TM, Avery GS. Labetalol: a review of its pharmacology and therapeutic use in hypertension. *Drugs*. 1978;15:251–270.

25. Brown RRS. Epinephrine and local anesthesia revisited. *Oral Surg Oral Med Oral Pathol Oral Radiol Endodont.* 2005;100:401–408.

26. Buchanan ML, Easterling TR, Carr DB, et al. Clonidine pharmacokinetics in pregnancy. *Drug Metab Dispos.* 2009; 37:702–705.

27. Buchwald A, Hochhaus G. Pharmacokinetic and pharmaco-dynamic aspects of salmeterol therapy. *Int J Clin Pharmacol Ther.* 1998;36:652–660.

28. Bylund DB. Subtypes of alpha 1- and alpha 2-adrenergic receptors. *FASEB J.* 1992;6:832.

29. Cabezas GA, Lezama Y, Velasco M. Dopaminergic modulation of human bronchial tone. *Arch Med Res.* 2001;32:143–147.

30. Caine M, Raz S, Zeigler M. Adrenergic and cholinergic receptors in the human prostate, prostatic capsule and blad-der neck. *Br J Urol.* 1975;47:193–202.

31. Cazzola M, Testi R, Matera MG. Clinical pharmacokinetics of salmeterol. *Clin Pharmacokinet.* 2002;41:19–30.

32. Challman TD, Lipsky JJ. Methylphenidate: its pharmacology and uses. *Mayo Clin Proc.* 2000;75:711–721.

33. Chalon S, Berlin I, Sachon C, Bosquet F, Grimaldi A. Pro-pranolol in hypoglycaemia unawareness. *Diabetes Metab.* 1999;25:23–26.

34. Chang KKC. Interactions of esmolol and adenosine in atrio-ventricular nodal-dependent supraventricular tachycardia: implication for the cellular mechanisms of adenosine. *Car-diology.* 2002;97:138–146.

35. Chapple CR, Wyndaele JJ, Nordling J, Boeminghaus F, Ypma AF, Abrams P. Tamsulosin, the first prostate-selective alpha 1A-adrenoceptor antagonist. A meta-analysis of two ran-domized, placebo-controlled, multicentre studies in patients with benign prostatic obstruction (symptomatic BPH). Euro-pean Tamsulosin Study Group. *Eur Urol.* 1996;29:155–167.

36. Civantos Calzada BB. Alpha-adrenoceptor subtypes. *Phar-macol Res.* 2001;44:195–208.

37. Clark BJ. Dopamine receptors and the cardiovascular sys-tem. *Postgrad Med J.* 1981;57(Suppl 1):45–54.

38. Clutter WE. Epinephrine plasma metabolic clearance rates and physiologic thresholds for metabolic and hemodynamic actions in man. *J Clin Invest.* 1980;66:94.

39. Conolly ME, Davies DS, Dollery CT, Morgan CD, Paterson JW, Sandler M. Metabolism of isoprenaline in dog and man. *Br J Pharmacol.* 1972;46:458–472.

40. Cox DA. The antihypertensive effects of doxazosin: a clinical overview. *Br J Clin Pharmacol.* 1986;21(Suppl 1):83S.

41. Crout JR. Anesthetic management of pheochromocytoma: the value of phenoxybenzamine and methoxyflurane. *Anes-thesiology.* 1969;30:29.

42. Davies DS, Wing AM, Reid JL, Neill DM, Tippett P, Dollery CT. Pharmacokinetics and concentration-effect relationships of intervenous and oral clonidine. *Clin Pharmacol Ther.* 1977;21:593–601.

43. Day JJL. Adrenergic mechanisms in control of plasma lipid concentrations. *BMJ.* 1982;284:1145–1148.

44. de la Torre R, Farre M, Navarro M, Pacifici R, Zuccaro P, Pichini S. Clinical pharmacokinetics of amphetamine and related substances: monitoring in conventional and non-conventional matrices. *Clin Pharmacokinet.* 2004;43:157–185.

45. Deacon SP, Barnett D. Comparison of atenolol and pro-pranolol during insulin-induced hypoglycaemia. *Br Med J.* 1976;2:272–273.

46. Dean RC, Lue TF. Physiology of penile erection and patho-physiology of erectile dysfunction. *Urol Clin North Am.* 2005;32:379–395.

47. Deibert DC, DeFronzo RA. Epinephrine-induced insulin resistance in man. *J Clin Invest.* 1980;65:717–721.

48. Devlin RG, Duchin KL, Fleiss PM. Nadolol in human serum and breast milk. *Br J Clin Pharmacol.* 1981;12:393–396.

49. Dupont E. Treatment of benign essential tremor with pro-pranolol: a controlled clinical trial. *Acta Neurol Scand.* 1973;49:75.

50. Eisenhofer G, Kopin IJ, Goldstein DS. Catecholamine metabolism: a contemporary view with implications for physiology and medicine. *Pharmacol Rev.* 2004;56:331–349.

51. Emilien G, Maloteaux JM, Geurts M, Hoogenberg K, Cragg S. Dopamine receptors—physiological understand-ing to therapeutic intervention potential. *Pharmacol Ther.* 1999;84:133–156.

52. Empey DW. Cardiovascular effects of pseudoephedrine. *Br J Clin Pharmacol.* 1980;9:351.

53. England JDF. The effect of metoprolol and atenolol on plasma high density lipoprotein levels in man. *Clin Exp Pharmacol Physiol.* 1980;7:329–333.

54. Fallowfield JM. Propranolol is contraindicated in asthma. *BMJ.* 1996;313:1486.

55. Feely J, Wilkinson GR, Wood AJ. Reduction of liver blood flow and propranolol metabolism by cimetidine. *N Engl J Med.* 1981;304:692–695.

56. Firth BG, Ratner AV, Grassman ED, Winniford MD, Nicod P, Hillis LD. Assessment of the inotropic and vasodilator effects of amrinone versus isoproterenol. *Am J Cardiol.* 1984;54:1331–1336.

57. Fitton A, Sorkin EM. Sotalol. An updated review of its pharmacological properties and therapeutic use in cardiac arrhythmias. *Drugs.* 1993;46:678–719.

58. Fitzgerald JD, Ruffin R, Smedstad KG, Roberts R, McAinsh J. Studies on the pharmacokinetics and pharmacodynamics of atenolol in man. *Eur J Clin Pharmacol.* 1978;13:81–89.

59. Gerstenberg T, Blaabjerg J, Nielsen ML, Clausen S. Phenoxy-benzamine reduces bladder outlet obstruction in benign

prostatic hyperplasia. A urodynamic investigation. *Invest Urol.* 1980;18:29–31.

60. Gezginc K, Gul M, Karatayli R, Cander B, Kanat F. Noncardiogenic pulmonary edema due to ritodrine usage in preterm labor. *Taiwan J Obstet Gynecol.* 2008;47:101–102.

61. Goldstein DA, Tan YK, Soldin SJ. Pharmacokinetics and absolute bioavailability of salbutamol in healthy adult volunteers. *Eur J Clin Pharmacol.* 1987;32:631–634.

62. Goldstein I, Carson C, Rosen R, Islam A. Vasomax for the treatment of male erectile dysfunction. *World J Urol.* 2001;19:51–56.

63. Graham RM, Thornell IR, Gain JM, Bagnoli C, Oates HF, Stokes GS. Prazosin: the first-dose phenomenon. *Br Med J.* 1976;2:1293–1294.

64. Grandordy BM, Paiva de Carvalho J, Regnard J, et al. The effect of intravenous phenylephrine on airway calibre in asthma. *Eur Respir J.* 1995;8:624–631.

65. Granville-Grossman K. Propranolol, anxiety and the central nervous system. *Br J Clin Pharmacol.* 1974;1:361.

66. Gray RJ. Managing critically ill patients with esmolol. An ultra short-acting beta-adrenergic blocker. *Chest.* 1988;93:398.

67. Greenway FL. The safety and efficacy of pharmaceutical and herbal caffeine and ephedrine use as a weight loss agent. *Obes Rev.* 2001;2:199–211.

68. Griffith RK. Adrenergics and adrenergic-blocking agents. *History (London).* 2003;26:1.

69. Gross GN, Souhrada JF, Farr RS. The longterm treatment of an asthmatic patient using phentolamine. *Chest.* 1974;66:397–401.

70. Guimaraes S, Moura D. Vascular adrenoceptors: an update. *Pharmacol Rev.* 2001;53:319–356.

71. Guthrie SK, Hariharan M, Grunhaus LJ. Yohimbine bioavailability in humans. *Eur J Clin Pharmacol.* 1990;39:409–411.

72. Haddad NJ, Moyer NJ, Riley FC Jr. Mydriatic effect of phenylephrine hydrochloride. *Am J Ophthalmol.* 1970;70:729–733.

73. Heel RC, Brogden RN, Speight TM, Avery GS. Atenolol: a review of its pharmacological properties and therapeutic efficacy in angina pectoris and hypertension. *Drugs.* 1979;17:425–460.

74. Heinke W. The effect of esmolol on cerebral blood flow, cerebral vasoreactivity, and cognitive performance: a functional magnetic resonance imaging study. *Anesthesiology.* 2005;102:41.

75. Hess HJ. Prazosin: biochemistry and structure-activity studies. *Postgrad Med.* 1975;9–17.

76. Ichai C, Soubielle J, Carles M, Giunti C, Grimaud D. Comparison of the renal effects of low to high doses of dopamine and dobutamine in critically ill patients: a single-blind randomized study. *Crit Care Med.* 2000;28:921–928.

77. Jaillon P. Clinical pharmacokinetics of prazosin. *Clin Pharmacokinet.* 1980;5:365–376.

78. Kacere RD. Intravenous epinephrine stimulates aqueous formation in the human eye. *Invest Ophthalmol Vis Sci.* 1992;33:2861.

79. Kimko HC, Cross JT, Abernethy DR. Pharmacokinetics and clinical effectiveness of methylphenidate. *Clin Pharmacokinet.* 1999;37:457–470.

80. Kirby RS, Coppinger SW, Corcoran MO, Chapple CR, Flannigan M, Milroy EJ. Prazosin in the treatment of prostatic obstruction. A placebo-controlled study. *Br J Urol.* 1987;60:136–142.

81. Kirschenbaum HL, Rosenberg JM. Clinical experience with sotalol in the treatment of cardiac arrhythmias. *Clin Ther.* 1994;16:346–364.

82. Kuhnert BR, Gross TL, Kuhnert PM, Erhard P, Brashar WT. Ritodrine pharmacokinetics. *Clin Pharmacol Ther.* 1986;40:656–664.

83. Laverdure B, Boulenger JP. Beta-blocking drugs and anxiety. A proven therapeutic value. *Encephale.* 1991;17:481–492.

84. Lee A. A quantitative, systematic review of randomized controlled trials of ephedrine versus phenylephrine for the management of hypotension during spinal anesthesia for cesarean delivery. *Anesth Analg.* 2002;94:920.

85. Leonard BE, McCartan D, White J, King DJ. Methylphenidate: a review of its neuropharmacological, neuropsychological and adverse clinical effects. *Hum Psychopharmacol.* 2004;19:151–180.

86. Leren P, Foss PO, Helgeland A, Hjermann I, Holme I, Lund-Larsen PG. Effect of propranolol and prazosin on blood lipids. The Oslo Study. *Lancet.* 1980;2:4–6.

87. Levitzki A. From epinephrine to cyclic AMP. *Science.* 1988;241:800.

88. Loeb HS. Superiority of dobutamine over dopamine for augmentation of cardiac output in patients with chronic low output cardiac failure. *Circulation.* 1977;55:375.

89. MacCarthy EP, Bloomfield SS. Labetalol: a review of its pharmacology, pharmacokinetics, clinical uses and adverse effects. *Pharmacotherapy.* 1983;3:193–219.

90. Martin C, Viviand X, Leone M, Thirion X. Effect of norepinephrine on the outcome of septic shock. *Crit Care Med.* 2000;28:2758–2765.

91. McNeil JJ, Louis WJ. Clinical pharmacokinetics of labetalol. *Clin Pharmacokinet.* 1984;9:157–167.

92. Mehler-Wex C, Riederer P, Gerlach M. Dopaminergic dysbalance in distinct basal ganglia neurocircuits: implications for the pathophysiology of Parkinson's disease, schizophrenia and attention deficit hyperactivity disorder. *Neurotox Res.* 2006;10:167–179.

93. Mehta AV, Chidambaram B, Rice PJ. Pharmacokinetics of nadolol in children with supraventricular tachycardia. *J Clin Pharmacol.* 1992;32:1023–1027.

94. Meyer SM, Fraunfelder FT. 3. Phenylephrine hydrochloride. *Ophthalmology*. 1980;87:1177–1180.

95. Molinoff PB. Alpha- and beta-adrenergic receptor subtypes properties, distribution and regulation. *Drugs*. 1984; 28(Suppl 2):1–15.

96. Montan S. Effects of methyldopa on uteroplacental and fetal hemodynamics in pregnancy-induced hypertension. *Obstet Gynecol*. 1993;168:152.

97. Morales A, Condra M, Owen JA, Surridge DH, Fenemore J, Harris C. Is yohimbine effective in the treatment of organic impotence? Results of a controlled trial. *J Urol*. 1987;137:1168–1172.

98. Muruve N, Hosking DH. Intracorporeal phenylephrine in the treatment of priapism. *J Urol*. 1996;155:141–143.

99. Myhre E, Rugstad HE, Hansen T. Clinical pharmacokinetics of methyldopa. *Clin Pharmacokinet*. 1982;7:221–233.

100. Neufeld AH. Experimental studies on the mechanism of action of timolol. *Surv Ophthalmol*. 1979;23:363–370.

101. Nieoullon A. Dopamine and the regulation of cognition and attention. *Prog Neurobiol*. 2002;67:53–83.

102. Nies AS. Clinical pharmacology of propranolol. *Circulation*. 1975;52:6.

103. Olsen NV. Effects of dopamine on renal haemodynamics tubular function and sodium excretion in normal humans. *Dan Med Bull*. 1998;45:282–297.

104. Onesti G. Antihypertensive effect of clonidine. *Circ Res*. 1971;28:53.

105. Parker WA. Propranolol-induced depression and psychosis. *Clin Pharm*. 1985;4:214–218.

106. Rizza RA. Adrenergic mechanisms for the effects of epinephrine on glucose production and clearance in man. *J Clin Invest*. 1980;65:682.

107. Roth RP, Cantekin EI, Bluestone CD, Welch RM, Cho YW. Nasal decongestant activity of pseudoephedrine. *Ann Otol Rhinol Laryngol*. 1977;86(2 pt. 1):235–242.

108. Ruffolo RR Jr. The pharmacology of dobutamine. *Am J Med Sci*. 1987;294:244–248.

109. Ryan RE. Nadolol: its use in the prophylactic treatment of migraine. *Headache*. 1983;23:26.

110. Sannerstedt R. Acute haemodynamic effects of metoprolol in hypertensive patients. *Br J Clin Pharmacol*. 1977;4:23.

111. Sheppard D, DiStefano S, Byrd RC, et al. Effects of esmolol on airway function in patients with asthma. *J Clin Pharmacol*. 1986;26:169–174.

112. Singh BN, Deedwania P, Nademanee K, Ward A, Sorkin EM. Sotalol. A review of its pharmacodynamic and pharmacokinetic properties, and therapeutic use. *Drugs*. 1987;34:311–349.

113. Skerjanec A, Campbell NR, Robertson S, Tam YK. Pharmacokinetics and presystemic gut metabolism of methyldopa in healthy human subjects. *J Clin Pharmacol*. 1995;35:275–280.

114. Smith DD. Intravenous epinephrine in life-threatening asthma. *Ann Emerg Med*. 2003;41:706–711.

115. Spiritus EM, Casciari R. Effects of topical betaxolol, timolol, and placebo on pulmonary function in asthmatic bronchitis. *Am J Ophthalmol*. 1985;100:492–494.

116. Stanaszek WF, Kellerman D, Brogden RN, Romankiewicz JA. Prazosin update. A review of its pharmacological properties and therapeutic use in hypertension and congestive heart failure. *Drugs*. 1983;25:339–384.

117. Tam SW, Worcel M, Wyllie M. Yohimbine: a clinical review. *Pharmacol Ther*. 2001;91:215–243.

118. Tarazi RC, Dustan HP, Bravo EL. Haemodynamic effects of propranolol in hypertension: a review. *Postgrad Med J*. 1976;52(Suppl 4):92–100.

119. Titmarsh S, Monk JP. Terazosin. A review of its pharmacodynamic and pharmacokinetic properties, and therapeutic efficacy in essential hypertension. *Drugs*. 1987;33:461–477.

120. Van Buskirk EM. Adverse reactions from timolol administration. *Ophthalmology*. 1980;87:447–450.

121. van Zwieten PA, Thoolen MJ, Timmermans PB. The hypotensive activity and side effects of methyldopa, clonidine, and guanfacine. *Hypertension*. 1984;6(5 pt 2):II28–II33.

122. Von Euler US. Pathophysiological aspects of catecholamine production. *Clin Chem*. 1972;18:1445.

123. Wadworth AN, Murdoch D, Brogden RN. Atenolol. A reappraisal of its pharmacological properties and therapeutic use in cardiovascular disorders. *Drugs*. 1991;42: 468–510.

124. Weber MA, Case DB, Baer L, et al. Renin and aldosterone suppression in the antihypertensive action of clonidine. *Am J Cardiol*. 1976;38:825–830.

125. Wiest D. Esmolol. A review of its therapeutic efficacy and pharmacokinetic characteristics. *Clin Pharmacokinet*. 1995;28:190–202.

126. Wooltorton E. Ephedra/ephedrine: cardiovascular and CNS effects. *Can Med Assoc J*. 2002;166:633.

127. Worthley LI, Tyler P, Moran JL. A comparison of dopamine, dobutamine and isoproterenol in the treatment of shock. *Intensive Care Med*. 1985;11:13–19.

128. Yaju Y, Nakayama T. Effectiveness and safety of ritodrine hydrochloride for the treatment of preterm labour: a systematic review. *Pharmacoepidemiol Drug Saf*. 2006;15:813–822.

129. Yan M, Webster LT, Jr, Blumer JL. 3-O-methyldobutamine, a major metabolite of dobutamine in humans. *Drug Metab Dispos*. 2002;30:519–524.

130. Zaugg M, Tagliente T, Lucchinetti E, et al. Beneficial effects from beta-adrenergic blockade in elderly patients undergoing noncardiac surgery. *Anesthesiology*. 1999;91:1674–1686.

131. Zimmerman TJ, Kaufman HE. Timolol. A beta-adrenergic blocking agent for the treatment of glaucoma. *Arch Ophthalmol*. 1977;95:601–604.

Objectives

After completing this chapter, the reader should be able to

- Discuss the role of histamine as a biologic active protein.
- Identify and describe the histamine molecule.
- Differentiate between the effects of histamine agonists and antagonists on the respiratory system.
- Discuss the clinical use of H_1 antagonists.
- List two H_2 receptor antagonists and describe their effects on the gastric mucosa.
- Discuss the side effects of cimetidine and ranitidine.
- Relate basic concepts of bradykinin and its actions.
- Summarize the synthesis and metabolism of serotonin agonists and antagonists.
- Discuss the synthesis and mechanism of action of prostaglandins.

21
Drug Therapy Associated With Autocoids

Henry C. Talley, PhD, CRNA, APRN

Introduction

In this chapter we discuss drug therapy associated with autocoids. Autocoids include an array of biologically active substances that are synthesized at the site of action and mediate the initial response to tissue injury. Autocoids neither circulate to the site of action nor are stored and released from glands. The origin of the term "autocoid" is derived from *autos* (meaning "self") and *akos* (meaning "remedy"). Receptors for autocoids are characterized by subtypes, and subtype-specific agents have been successful in treating their responses. Many different kinds of substances have been used to alter the biologic activity of substances that mediate the response to injury. Of these substances, drugs associated with the therapeutic response to autocoids should be viewed as one of the most significant pharmaceutical advancements in modern medicine.

In this chapter we reflect on the diverse pharmacologic and physiologic actions of these substances. Likewise, we discuss those drugs used in the practice of anesthesia that either antagonize or inhibit their action where possible. Although we present these biologic substances in a separate chapter, it should be noted that an important exception in this chapter is a discussion of the growing interest in cytokines and lymphokines: similar substances that mediate humoral and cellular interactions involved in the immune response. Generation of autocoids occurs during the immune response (i.e., interleukin-1) and is but one example of substances that exhibit pyrogenic actions and are mediated by the formation of prostaglandins.[1]

Histamine Agonists and Antagonists

The role of histamine (β-aminoethylimidazole) as a biologically active protein has a long history since the molecule was initially isolated as a contaminate of ergot in 1910 by the British physiologist Sir Henry Dale and his colleagues. Histamine is well known as an important inflammatory mediator and can affect the function of dendritic cells, monocytes, and lymphocytes.[2]

Storage and Release

Histamine is a naturally occurring, low-molecular-weight, hydrophilic endogenous vasoactive amine (autocoid) that produces an immediate response to tissue injury and causes an array of other physiologic and pathologic responses through G-protein coupled transmembrane receptors (Figure 21-1). Histamine is synthesized in tissues by the decarboxylation of the amino acid histidine, stored in an intricate composite with heparin, and released in response to stimulation by human basophils, mast cells, and neurons.[3-5] Histamine genetic polymorphisms are responsible for differences in histamine metabolism[6] and are associated with several diseases.

The stimulus to examine compounds able to counteract the pathologic responses to histamine began in the 1930s at the Pasteur Institute in Paris after indications

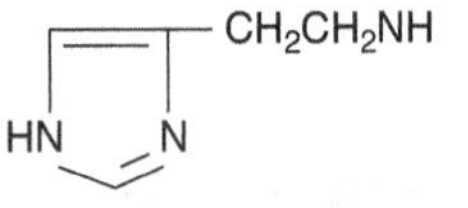

Figure 21-1 Histamine.

that histamine had an active role in allergic reactions and anaphylaxis.[7] Bouvet and Staub provided evidence that histamine played a pivotal role as a mediator of allergic reactions after demonstrating that guinea pigs were protected from anaphylaxis when exposed to a series of compounds with antihistamine activity.[5,7] Bovet was awarded the Nobel Prize for Physiology or Medicine in 1957 for his work on antihistamines and curare. The histamine molecule contains an imidazole ring and an amino group connected by two methylene groups. Pharmacologic studies on select agonists and antagonists established the existence of four types of histamine receptor and histamine receptor antagonists and led to some very important therapeutic applications for these agents. Histamine is metabolized primarily via two pathways. The pathway most important to the anesthesia provider entails methylation, which is catalyzed by histamine-*N*-methyltransferase and further degraded by monoamine oxidase.[8]

As previously stated, histamine has an array of important physiologic functions. Its release from the mast cell results in an interaction between antigens, and immunoglobin E (IgE) reaginic antibodies are thus generated and bound on the surface of the mast cell, playing a crucial role in hypersensitivity and the allergic response. Other clinically relevant conditions in which histamine release occurs in response to other stimuli include solar, cholinergic, and cold urticarias.[1] These responses are primarily mediated through mast cell and cell-fixed IgE secretory responses.[3,5,6,9,10] Although histamine release provides a wide range of effects as a result of hypersensitive responses and the allergic response (bronchoconstriction, increased capillary permeability, edema), several other mast cell mediators of inflammation are produced.

Histamine Receptors

Several agents administered during the perioperative period, because of their varied molecular structures, release histamine in a dose-dependent manner. Once released, histamine exerts extensive effects on smooth muscle, gastric acid secretion, stimulation of sensory nerve endings, and edema. It is believed that antigens interacting with antigen-specific IgE-bound receptors on the surface of nasal mast cells stimulate the release of mediators that produce the symptoms of allergic rhinitis. Additionally, the effects of all histamine subtypes fluctuate in the heart to some degree; however, these effects, in the heart and throughout the body, are mediated by four currently recognized histamine receptor subtypes, classified as H_1, H_2, H_3, and H_4.[5,7,11,12] These four histamine subtypes vary in their binding characteristics, location, and second messenger generation and appear to bind at different histamine receptor agonist and antagonist sites.[10,13] A fifth subtype has been defined within cell types that is not usually linked to histamine (H_{IC}).[10] Histamine is a neurotransmitter and mediator of several cell functions. Knowledge of the physiologic effect of histamine on organ systems helps to clarify the therapeutic agent action on these receptors. A complete discussion of the various histamine receptors agonist and antagonist is beyond the scope of this chapter; therefore, we discuss only the H_1 and H_2 histamine receptor subtypes and how these autocoids influence anesthesia drug therapy.

H_1 Agonists

Histamine-induced excitation is mediated by the H_1 receptor in primary sensory neurons. Three sources of histamine in humans, mast cells and basophils, gastric enterochromaffin-like (ECL) cells, and histaminergic nerves in the brain, are widely accepted. The first-generation antihistamines are lipophilic and readily penetrate the blood–brain barrier and also possess anticholinergic properties.[14,15] Histamine can be found in all body tissue, especially smooth muscle, glandular cells, and on nerve endings, including cardiac receptors.[15] Stimulation of the H_1 receptors at these sites provokes several systemic reactions, including skin wheals, mucous secretion, bronchial constriction, nasal congestion and irritation, and bronchospasm in asthmatics.[4,9,15,16]

H_1 receptors have been characterized by the pharmacologic actions of their respective agonists and antagonists. Although some actions are similar, there is an assortment of H_1 antihistamine receptor pharmacokinetic and pharmacodynamic differences. Prostacyclin release from vascular endothelium is mediated via H_1 receptors as a result of phospholipase enzyme activation.

H_1 Agonists and the Cardiovascular System

H_1 receptors are found in cardiac tissue and manifest as a decrease in atrioventricular node conduction. Likewise, the cardiac H_1 receptors mediate vasoconstriction in the epicardial coronary vessels. In 1988 first-generation H_1 antihistamines were found to inhibit IgE-mediated secretion of histamine from basophils.[10] Because these cells did not convey the H_1 receptor, these effects were believed to be due to alterations in signal processing in the cells. Since then, both first- and second-generation compounds have been found to have a wide variety of effects not attributable to H_1 receptor binding.[4,8–10,15,16] Research suggests that histamine reduces atrial natriuretic peptide release. Because cardiac mast cells are the primary source of histamine release in the heart, it has been theorized that cardiac mast cells are involved in the regulation of atrial natriuretic peptide release.[17] Accordingly, cardiac mast cell–cardiomyocyte communication via the histamine–atrial natriuretic peptide pathway may be associated with cardiac disorders that are related to mast cell degranulation, such as in acute coronary syndrome or cardiac hypertrophy.[2,6,7,17,18]

H_1 and H_2 histamine receptors represent successful therapeutic targets.[7] Pretreatment with antihistamines before the administration of drugs that are known to rerelease histamine during the perioperative period do not contain histamine themselves; instead, these agents compete with histamine at specific receptor sites. As a result there may be a decrease in blood pressure and other cardiovascular symptoms. Agents known to stimulate histamine release include morphine and atracurium.[19,20] The subsequent effects on vascular resistance are multifaceted and difficult to understand due to the diverse effects that these agents have on the vasculature and on myocardial function.[6,7]

Histamine causes flushing, reduced peripheral resistance, and systolic blood pressure decreases as a result of blood vessel dilation when H_1 receptors are activated. Likewise, histamine influences on capillary permeability cause edema via the apparent passage of plasma protein, lymph, and fluid into the extracellular spaces. This increase in capillary permeability is primarily a result of histamine acting on postcapillary venules, providing the basis for the free movement of plasma protein and fluid between endothelial cell gaps, which is caused by the contraction of these cells and subsequent exposure of the basement membrane.

H_1 Agonists and the Airway

H_1 receptor stimulation is responsible for the spasmogenic response seen in human bronchial muscle; however, H_2 receptor stimulation causes dilator responses. Hence, in vitro histamine-stimulated bronchospasm may be potentiated by blockage of the H_2 receptor. Although histamine stimulates several nerve endings and bronchoconstrictor response in normal patients is negligible, histamine-induced bronchospasm in the asthmatic patient causes marked increases in airway resistance and may involve afferent stimulation of the vagus nerve.[21,22]

H_2 Agonists and Gastric Secretions

Histamine is a potent gastric acid stimulus when H_2 receptors are activated. H_2 receptors are primarily found on the gastric parietal cells located in the body of the stomach. H_2 receptors on gastric parietal cells work synergistically with gastrin and acetylcholine, causing histamine to increase the secretion of HCl at a concentration of approximately 160 mmol/L or pH 0.8, with a median daily pH approximately 1.4. The mechanism of action is related primarily to parietal cell acid secretion causing intracellular increase of calcium, cyclic AMP, or both followed by a cascade that activates the translocation of the proton pump, HpKpATPase, from cytoplasmic tubulovesicles to the apical plasma membrane.[23,24] Histamine is secreted in the stomach by ECL cells, which in turn are regulated by gastrin, the main hormonal stimulant for acid secretion during meal ingestion.[23–25] Clinically significant conditions related to increased gastric acid secretion include gastroesophageal reflux disease, peptic ulcer disease, and stress-related erosion/ulcer disease; these are common and potentially serious clinical conditions. As we improve our understanding of histamine and its agonists in health and disease, we should expect this knowledge to be used to develop more effective strategies to prevent and manage these disorders.

Histamine has a direct effect on blood vessels and causes vasodilation that is mediated by H_1 and H_2 receptors that are free from autonomic nervous system innovation resulting in maximal dilation of the vasculature. Activation of H_2 receptors results in a more sustained generalized vasodilation with a slower onset than that seen after H_1 receptor activation. Furthermore, when histamine causes H_2 receptor activation in the heart, positive chronotropic effects are elicited with resultant cardiac dysrhythmias as a consequence of histamine-induced catecholamine release.

Allergic Reactions and Anaphylaxis

During allergic reactions and anaphylaxis, several potent autocoids are released; histamine and its relative importance in these reactions vary widely and depend on the species and tissues studied. Additionally, the protection provided by histamine receptor antagonists likewise varies in species and tissue. In humans, antihistamines (histamine receptor antagonists) successfully avert edema and urticaria; however, control of hypotension is managed less effectively, whereas bronchoconstriction is hardly reduced at all, highlighting the impact of other mediators to this condition.

Clinical Uses of Histamine

Histamine has been used in clinical settings as a diagnostic mediator. Histamine is used to evaluate parietal cell secretion of hydrogen ions and to determine parietal cell mass. Additionally, histamine has been used to evaluate nonspecific bronchial hyperreactivity and as a local skin test for allergy. Although hyposecretion of hydrogen ions is prevalent in pernicious anemia, gastric carcinoma, and atrophic gastritis, the fact that these entities demonstrate some degree of anacidity is a sign of the condition. Histamine is not used to diagnose the abnormal state. Zollinger-Ellison syndrome is a rare disorder characterized by one or more gastrinomas (tumors that secrete gastrin) in the pancreas, duodenum, or both. Consequently, this syndrome is often found in the presence of duodenal and peptic ulcers that are refractory to conventional medical treatment and exhibit hypersecretion of hydrogen ions in response to histamine. Histamine-induced untoward effects are often treated by the preoperative administration of H_2 receptor antagonists that do not inhibit histamine-induced gastric secretions.

Histamine Receptor Antagonists

Although histamine receptor agonist development has been expanding, due to the selective actions at specific receptor sites, this chapter is limited to the properties and clinical uses of H_1 and H_2 receptor antagonists (Tables 21-1 and 21-2) and so are discussed together.

H_1 Antagonists

H_1 receptors are classified as first- and second-generation receptor antagonists.[1,4,26] Histamine-induced responses to H_1 receptor stimulation are competitively suppressed by specific receptor antagonists (Table 21-2). With the exception of the mast cell, each cell type expresses only one type

of histamine receptor.[10] The currently available H_1 receptor antagonists exhibit reversible, competitive inhibition at the receptor site. Although many H_1 antagonists have a tertiary amino group linked by a two- or three-atom chain to two aromatic substituents, histamine contains only a primary amino group and a single aromatic ring.

The traditional histamine H_1 receptor antagonists do not exhibit H_1 receptor site selectivity; however, there is an array of dopaminergic, serotonergic, and cholinergic responses (somnolence, diminished alertness, delayed reaction time, and cognitive dysfunction) that leads to significant adverse effects involving the central nervous system (CNS). These responses are presumed to be related to both their pharmacologic nonselectivity and their ability to readily cross the blood–brain barrier.[1,9,15] CNS manifestations after overdose with the H_1 receptor antagonists include toxic psychoses accompanied by hallucinations resembling schizophrenia and other psychiatric emergencies.[18,27,28] These toxic manifestations were assumed to result from the anticholinergic properties of these drugs that are evident during poisoning with atropine and its associated compounds.

The second-generation antihistamines have contributed to some major advances in treatment regimens; they do not cross the blood–brain barrier as rapidly and are intended to exhibit greater specificity at H_1 receptor sites.[1,9] Given their superior selectivity for the H_1 receptor site, fewer undesirable CNS responses are demonstrated (unless their recommended dosages are exceeded), and their efficacy is similar to that of the classic antihistamines. Selecting among these antihistamines has focused on their pharmacokinetics and CNS profile. Because the potential for cardiotoxicity is likely when their metabolism is inhibited, caution when prescribing these agents is warranted. For the clinician, deciding among H_1 receptor antagonists necessitates a wide-ranging understanding of their diverse property.

Table 21-1 H_1 Receptor Antagonist Classifications

Agent	Sedative Effects	Anticholinergic Activity	Terminal Serum Elimination Half-life (h)	Adult Dose (mg)
Diphenhydramine*	Marked	Marked	2.4–9.3	50
Chlorpheniramine*	Mild	Mild	13.2–43	4
Promethazine*	Moderate	Marked	12–15	25–50
Hydroxyzine*	Mild	Mild	20	50–100
Loratadine†	At higher doses	Mild	8.0	10
Cetirizine†	Minimal	Indeterminable	6–9	5–10

*First-generation H_1 agonists.

†Second-generation H_1 agonists.

Pharmacokinetics and Side Effects

H_1 receptor antagonists are readily absorbed after oral administration, and a detailed understanding of the histamine–H_1 receptor interaction has resulted in clinicians being able to better predict their relative effects. First-generation H_1 antagonists are the foremost representative of the "classical antihistamines" and are widely used as sleep aids (Table 21-2). Peak plasma concentrations are reached within 2 to 3 hours after oral administration; however, plasma concentrations are relatively low due to first-pass hepatic extraction. Most of the H_1 receptor antagonists are

Table 21-2 H_1 and H_2 Antagonists

	Receptor Type	Action
Receptor–effector coupling	H_1	Stimulates phosphoinositide turnover and influx of C^{++}
	H_2	Increases cAMP by stimulating adenylate cyclase
	H_3	Presynaptic regulation of neurotransmitter release (dopamine, GABA, glutamate, ACH, norepinephrine, 5-HT)
Effect on smooth muscles		Contract (gut, bronchi) or relax (capillaries)
	H_1/H_2	Combined receptor response causing hypotension from vasodilation
		Decreased peripheral resistance; vascular effects produce flushing
	H_1	Effect is rapid and transient; receptors sensitive to lower histamine concentration
	H_2	Response is slow and sustained
Bronchi	H_1	Contracts bronchi; predominant response
	H_2	Relaxes bronchi
Heart	H_1	Slows AV conduction and increases automaticity
	H_2	Increases inotropic (promotes C^{++} flux) and chronotropic response (increased diastolic depolarization of the S-A node)

ACH; A-V, atrioventricular; GABA, γ-aminobutyric acid; 5-HT, 5-hydroxytryptamine; S-A, sinoatrial.

Source: Modified from Crawford KW. Pharmacology of autocoids. Available at: http://www.med.howard.edu/pharmacology/handouts/inflamm.htm. Accessed June 14, 2009.

metabolized via the microsomal mixed-function oxidase system in the liver. First-generation H_1 antagonists cause stimulation and depression of the CNS. First-generation H_1 antagonists are often associated with CNS toxicity in the clinical literature because of the anticholinergic and local anesthetic activity associated with class of substances. Although manifestations of CNS activity are not identical with all H_1 antagonists, most include somnolence, reduced alertness, and diminished reaction times. H_1 antagonists also blunt smooth muscle responses to histamine in the respiratory systems of some species. Most cells convey at least one histamine receptor subtype in the respiratory system; however, blockade of these receptors does not totally arrest the inflammatory response. This feature is widely publicized during in vivo and in vitro studies of animals; however, this feature is not as remarkable in humans. For instance, asphyxiation causes death in guinea pigs after small doses of histamine; however, when given an H_1 antagonists in advance, these animals can survive several lethal doses without incidence.[18] Human exposure is more complicated due to the numerous other mediators of allergic bronchoconstriction (leukotrienes and platelet activating factor) in addition to histamine.

Cortical influence of the H_1 antagonists is primarily indirect; however, they illustrate how their effect on neuromodulation can promote synchronized burst firing. H_1 antagonists with antimuscarinic activity may inhibit acetylcholine-mediated increases of thalamic interneuron neuromodulation to increase γ-aminobutyric acid release to thalamic relay neurons.[18] As a result sedation is a key feature of the first-generation H_1 antagonists but not a feature of second-generation antagonists when administered in therapeutic doses. Although sedation may be a desirable feature for select patients, activities requiring attentiveness are affected and further complicated with the concomitant ingestion of alcohol and other CNS depressants. Other side effects include impaired cognitive function, tinnitus, somnolence, tremors, and euphoria. Anticholinergic effects consist of urinary retention, impotence, blurred vision, and xerostomia (dry mouth). Finally, gastric-related effects are attenuated when not taken with meals and include decreased appetite, epigastric distress, and bowel movement irregularities.

The second-generation H_1 antagonists astemizole, loratadine, and terfenadine are unlikely to produce side effects associated with their use. Second-generation H_1 antagonists, although unlikely, exhibit CNS side effects when therapeutic doses are exceeded (Table 21-2). However, because hemodialysis does not remove second-generation H_1 antagonists, patients with impaired hepatic function, prolonged QTc intervals, and metabolic disorders may be predisposed to adverse cardiovascular effects. Although rare, QTc prolongation may occur with the use of terfenadine and astemizole, resulting in torsades de pointes (polymorphic ventricular tachycardia).[1]

Clinical Uses of H₁ Antagonists

H₁ antagonists are widely used in the acute symptomatic treatment of hypersensitivity reactions. Allergies of the respiratory system are particularly responsive to H₁ antagonist therapy. Rhinitis, conjunctivitis, and urticaria systems are suppressed due to the effect on antigen–antibody reactions. H₁ antagonism is relatively ineffective in the treatments of bronchial asthma unless used in combination with other agents. Acute urticaria responds well to H₁ antagonist therapy, whereas chronic conditions are treated less favorably. Diphenhydramine has shown some benefit in treating phenothiazine-related extrapyramidal side effects and early stages of Parkinson's disease (more effective agents are currently available). Most often, these agents are currently used as mild anxiolytics due to their sedative action.

H₂ Receptor Antagonists

Cimetidine and ranitidine are two new H₂ receptor antagonists. The newer histamine H₂ receptor antagonists (second-generation H₂ receptor antagonists) have recently been reported to promote gastric mucosal defenses.[26] Cimetidine was the first H₂ receptor antagonist to be commercialized. Cimetidine displayed competitive antagonism against histamine to produce a dose-related inhibition after oral and intravenous administration of histamine-stimulated gastric acid secretion.[26,29] Other H₂ receptor antagonists with similar properties are famotidine and nizatidine.

Mechanism of Action

H₂ receptor antagonism has led to a renewal of interest in the function of histamine in physiology and disease. Major advances have been made in the value of the role of histamine and its receptors in controlling gastric secretions. The primary stimulants of gastric parietal cell acid secretion are histamine, gastrin, and acetylcholine. Histamine binds to H₂ receptors in ECL cells, activating adenylate cyclase and generating cAMP. Gastrin activates phospholipase C and stimulates the parietal cells directly and, more significantly, indirectly by releasing histamine from ECL cells.[24,30–32] The fact that histamine H₂ receptor antagonists reduced gastric acid secretions that were stimulated by histamine, gastrin, and acetylcholine positioned histamine at the center of

secretory control. This was also supported by the capacity of H₂ receptor antagonists to inhibit secretions that resulted from vagal stimulation and from the physiologic stimulus of food ingestion.[7,10,26] The ability of H₂ receptor antagonists to inhibit virtually all forms of secretions (stimulated and basal) led to their clinical effectiveness.

The most important inhibitor of acid secretion is somatostatin. Somatostatin is synthesized by the proteolytic cleavage of prosomatostatin, a pre-prosomatostatin precursor molecule. Somatostatins are found in stomach, pancreatic islets, and enteric neurons as well as in the small intestine. In the stomach, somatostatin cells are closely coupled to their target cells (e.g., parietal, ECL, and gastrin cells) either directly via cytoplasmic processes or indirectly via local circulation.[25,30]

Pharmacokinetics and Side Effects

Oral administration of cimetidine and ranitidine causes rapid absorption of these two substances. Clinical trials established that cimetidine was useful in the treatment of acid-related diseases, such as peptic ulcer and gastroesophageal reflux disease, and further demonstrated cytoprotective and gastroprotective actions. Bioavailability is decreased by half as a result of extensive first-pass hepatic metabolism.[33,34] Protein binding also occurs because the volume of distribution of these substances exceeds total body water content.[33,34] As a result obesity exhibits less effective treatment responses with cimetidine, because greater than half of the total body content of cimetidine is found in muscle.

Although there are varied interindividual differences among patients, gastrointestinal physiology and transfer properties can significantly influence the pharmacokinetics of an orally administered drug in vivo.[35] Metabolism occurs primarily by conversion by cytochrome P-450 in the liver. Cimetidine is also known to cause drug interactions with other organic cations in the kidney in a concentration-dependent manner.[36] Therefore it has the potential to cause side effects if given concurrently with other drugs that rely on cytochrome P-450 for metabolism. Renal dysfunction prolongs the elimination half-life of these drugs (particularly with famotidine and nizatidine) and should be decreased in patients with kidney disease. Likewise, patients with acute burns should be closely monitored when receiving H₂ receptor antagonists. As with hepatic and acute burn patients, age also exhibits pharmacokinetic influences on H₂ receptor antagonists given that cimetidine clearance decreases in older adults. There is a difference of approximately 75% between ages 20 and 70 years in clearance, a 40% volume of distribution decline, and an increased elimination half-life between these groups.[8,33,34] Therefore care must be taken when administering H_2 receptor antagonists to older adults.

Clinical Uses of H_2 Receptor Antagonists

Histamine H_2 receptor antagonists were initially developed to manage peptic ulcers. Acid production was decreased by reducing the action of histamine on gastric parietal cells. The U.S. Food and Drug Administration approved the use of cimetidine in 1979, and consequently three other H_2 receptor antagonists have been marketed: ranitidine, famotidine, and nizatidine. The preoperative administration of H_2 receptor antagonists offers a suitable means of providing extensive prophylaxis in patients scheduled to undergo elective surgery. Patients with a pH greater than 2.5 (reduced risk of acid pneumonitis) were 90% after famotidine, 91% after ranitidine, and 52% after placebo when taken the evening before and morning of surgery.[37–40] Subsequent gastric acidity is unpredictable after the administration of H_2 receptor antagonists. However, in contrast to antacids, H_2 receptor antagonists exhibit no influence on gastric pH already present in the stomach.[8] Findings that antibiotics with characteristics of a base are affected by cimetidine support the presence of an acidic storage pool.[41–44] Therefore H_2 receptor antagonists may be useful adjuncts in *Helicobacter pylori* infections by increasing gastric concentrations of antibiotics that behave as weak bases.[45]

Histamine release can occur in response to certain drugs during anesthesia. Narcotics and muscle relaxants demonstrated significant in vitro and in vivo histamine release. However, H_2 receptor antagonists offer no protection against histamine release after the administration of certain drugs (morphine, atracurium, mivacurium, protamine) alone or in combination with other H_1 receptor antagonists.[46–48]

Bradykinin Agonists and Antagonists

Bradykinin is one of the most important nonapeptide inflammatory mediators involved in the development of neurogenic inflammation after tissue injury.[49,50] Bradykinin is a product of the biochemical cascade known as the kallikrein-kinin system. The kallikrein-kinin system consists of two mammalian kininogens: high-molecular-weight and low-molecular-weight kininogens that are derived from a single hepatic gene.[1,47,51,52] Kinins are the most potent endogenous vasodilators generated after allergic reactions and tissue damage and modulate several of the events accompanying inflammation (vasodilatation,

increased cell permeability, hyperalgesia, and pain).[49,51,52] Knowing that these substances act on specific receptors, therapeutic interventions may be possible.

Kallikrein-Kinin System

Bradykinin-related peptides are blood-derived vasoactive peptides that are among the most potent autocoids involved in inflammation and are believed to be stored in neuronal elements of the CNS where they may have a role as cerebral neuromodulators.[49,51,52] Kallikreins circulate in an inactive form and are activated by plasma proteases.[1] High-molecular-weight kininogens are precursors of bradykinin, whereas low-molecular-weight kininogens generate kallidin, both displaying specific biologic activities.[52] The kininogens have a plasma half-life of about 15 seconds, with a pulmonary destruction rate of 80% to 90% after a single pass.

Bradykinin Receptors

Two distinct types of receptors for kinins have been identified for bradykinin, B_1 and B_2, with both being G-protein coupled receptors.[52] Bradykinin receptor B_1 selectively binds to bradykinin and kallidin metabolites and is less prevalent than bradykinin B_2 receptors. Bradykinin receptor B_2 mediates most bradykinin- and kallidin-related effects exhibited in the absence of inflammation, and bradykinin itself is the preferred agonist for the B_2 receptor.[1,50] Kallidin can also act on the B_2 receptor after conversion to bradykinin by aminopeptidase.[50] Bradykinin is normally present in small amounts because it circulates as an inactive substance known as prekallikrein. Alteration in pH and temperature can activate prekallikrein and lead to the conversion of prekallikrein to bradykinin after tissue damage. Bradykinin is a potent algesic, causing pain and the release of neuropeptides (substance P, calcitonin gene–related peptide, and neurokinin).[1,50,53] Research also suggests that kinin-induced bronchoconstriction in guinea pig trachea may actually be a previously unanticipated function of bradykinin B_2 receptors.[1,54–56]

Bradykinin in Mammals

Bradykinin is more potent than histamine as a vasodilator (approximately ten times as powerful). Bradykinin may increase sympathetic outflow and possibly induce the sympathetic nervous system to cause hypertension. Phospholipase C activation and protein kinase C stimulation increase membrane sodium ion conductance, causing depolarization of sensory fibers.[50] Activation of bradykinin receptors has also been shown to stimulate the production of arachidonic acid and its metabolites in the brain.[57] It is also speculated that hereditary angioedema may be partially due to the formation of excess bradykinin.[1] Two other diseases that may be associated with abnormal kinin levels include carcinoid syndrome and septic shock. Kinin receptor antagonists continue to be studied. Snake venom potentiates kinins, and treatment of this ailment may shed light on the development of therapeutic treatments.

Serotonin Agonists and Antagonists

Serotonin (5-hydroxytryptamine [5-HT]) and its receptors are known to play significant roles in a variety of physiologic and pathophysiologic processes (Table 21-3). 5-HT is a CNS neurotransmitter with a long history of effector cell activity on smooth muscle and as a mediator for increased platelet aggregation. 5-HT is found throughout the gastrointestinal tract, platelets, and areas of the CNS. Due to the widespread distribution of serotonin, therapeutic drugs that target specific subtypes of serotonin receptors may support the clinical development of available treatment regimens.

Chemistry, Synthesis, and Metabolism

Neurons interact with one another through excitatory and inhibitory synaptic mediators. Excitatory synapses excite and inhibitory synapses inhibit postsynaptic neurons, causing varying degrees of responsiveness in mammals. The distribution of regulatory transmitters determines how and where theses responses occur. Likewise, specific receptors respond to certain transmitters in one way, whereas others respond differently or not at all, depending on the nature of the receptor. 5-HT belongs to one family of regulatory mediators responsible for these responses. 5-HT is one of three biogenic monoamines (dopamine, norepinephrine, and serotonin) that are responsible for several activities throughout the body that include affective states (mood, feelings, and motivation), self-awareness (sleep and wakefulness, consciousness, and personality), and the regulation of smooth muscle contraction. 5-HT receptors respond to these transmitters. Numerous pharmacologically active (naturally and synthetic) byproducts of 5-HT have hallucinogenic actions. There are 14 5-HT receptor subtypes, among which the 5-HT$_{1A}$ receptor subtype is thought to be implicated in psychiatric disorders, immunomodulation, and ischemic cerebral conditions.[58] The origin and evolution of the 5-HT$_3$ receptor subtype place it as the oldest of the 5-HT receptor subtypes, with all 14 subtypes that emerged from a single primitive 5-HT receptor that belongs to the

Table 21-3 Serotonin Agonists and Antagonists With Associated Indications

Drug	Buspirone, ipsapirone
Indication	Management of anxiety disorders or short-term relief of symptoms of anxiety and depression
Receptor	5-HT$_{1A}$
Action	Partial agonist
Drug	Cisapride
Indication	Gastrointestinal disorders. Increases esophageal sphincter muscle tone in people with gastroesophageal reflux disease. It also stimulates gastric emptying in people with diabetic gastroparesis. It has been used to treat constipation.
Receptor	5-HT$_4$
Action	Agonist
Drug	Sumatriptan
Indication	Useful in the treatment of migraine and cluster headaches
Receptor	5-HT$_{1D}$
Action	Agonist
Drug	Ondansetron
Indication	Highly effective in decreasing incidence of postoperative nausea and vomiting; also, very useful in treatment of chemotherapy-induced emesis
Receptor	5-HT$_3$
Action	Antagonist
Drug	Methysergide
Indication	Prophylaxis against development of migraine and other vascular headaches; also useful in the treatment of malabsorption and diarrhea in patients with carcinoid syndrome and for dumping syndrome with postgastrectomy.
Receptor	5-HT$_{2A/2C}$
Action	Antagonist
Drug	Ketanserin
Indication	Includes treatment of patients with carcinoid syndrome and management of systemic hypertension
Receptor	5-HT$_{2A/2C}$
Action	Antagonist
Drug	Fluoxetine, sertraline
Indication	Includes treatment of patients with depression and bipolar disorder
Receptor	5-HT$_{Transporter}$
Action	Inhibitor

G-protein coupled receptors. 5-HT is quickly removed from plasma by platelets, liver, and endothelium.

Synthesis of 5-HT occurs via a two-step pathway from the essential amino acid tryptophan. Cerebral uptake of tryptophan occurs via a carrier that also transports other amino acids; therefore tryptophan is influenced by its plasma concentration and the concentration of other amino acids competing for the uptake carrier. Serotonin is metabolized to its inactive form by oxidative deamination of the lateral amino chain by monoamine oxidase. Other pathways of metabolism have also been suggested that may lead to the formation of hallucinogenic agents. The outer membranes of serotonergic terminals are responsible for the termination of 5-HT action at the synaptic junction and in the outer membrane of platelets where it is taken up from the blood.

Serotonin and Physiologic Functions

In 1989 benzamides, such as metoclopramide, renzapride, cisapride, and zacopride, were easily accepted as potent agonists.[59,60] Studies have shown that multiple actions of 5-HT can only be explained by interactions between multiple 5-HT receptor subtypes. Recent cloning of cDNA receptors supports this assumption. 5-HT receptor subtypes are the largest and most important class of membrane proteins in mammalian cells and figure significantly in disease and drug development.[61] 5-HT_4 receptors control many important functions at the periphery, including those of the gastrointestinal and urinary tracts, human heart, and adrenal gland.[60] However, 5-HT receptors are located primarily on cerebral and CNS nerve cells. Therefore the most important physiologic functions of the 5-HT receptor are exhibited in the brain and CNS. As previously stated, serotonin receptors belong to the G-protein coupled class of transmembrane regulatory receptors. G-protein coupled receptors play a significant role in regulating pain signaling in the context of inflammation. G-protein coupled receptor kinases modulate signaling through these receptors.[62] There are several distinct yet overlapping patterns communicated by 5-HT receptor subtypes[63] joined to an array of diverse transmembrane signaling mechanisms. Of the 14 HT receptor subtypes, the most widely accepted classification system, 7 subgroups have been proposed.[64]

5-HT_1 Receptor Subtypes

There are five subgroups within the 5-HT_1 subtype; all are negatively attached to adenylyl cyclase. Of these subgroups the 5-HT_{1A} receptor activates a receptor-operated K^+ channel and inhibits a voltage-gated Ca^{++} channel. This is a common property of the pertussis toxin-sensitive G-protein coupled class of receptors.[65] Another subtype, the 5-HT_{1D} receptor, inhibits 5-HT as an autoreceptor on axon terminals and may influence the rate of firing and release of dopamine at dopamine-containing cells.[65]

The serotonin $5\text{-HT}_{1B/1D}$ agonists (triptans) are an effective class of migraine therapeutics but are contraindicated in patients with coronary artery disease. $5\text{-HT}_{1B/1D}$ agonists have been shown to narrow human coronary artery in vitro, and case reports of myocardial infarction in patients using sumatriptan have been publicized.[66] However, preclinical in vivo studies with sumatriptan failed to reveal an effect on coronary flow.[66]

5-HT_2 Receptor Subtypes

There are three subgroups within the 5-HT_2 subtype, all linked to phospholipase C with two second messengers. Several pertussis toxin-insensitive G-protein coupled classes of receptors are found within this subtype. The serotonin 5-HT_{2A} agonist has been found in abundance throughout the CNS, whereas 5-HT_{2B} was originally illustrated in the gastric fundus. 5-HT_{2C} has a high attraction to the choroid plexus, the primary site for the production of cerebrospinal fluid; however, its function is virtually unknown.

5-HT_3 Receptor Subtypes

A great deal is currently known about the structure and function of 5-HT_3 receptors. The 5-HT_3 receptor has strong structural and functional relation with the nicotinic acetylcholine receptor.[67,68] A number of studies have mapped the distribution of 5-HT_3 receptor expression in the CNS, consistently finding its highest levels within the dorsal vagal complex in the brainstem[69–71] and in the parasympathetic terminals in the gastrointestinal tract.[65] The dorsal vagal complex includes those regions responsible for the initiation and coordination of the vomiting reflex (the nucleus tractus solitarius, area postrema, and dorsal motor nucleus of the vagus nerve). Antagonism of the 5-HT_3 receptors probably contributes to the antiemetic action of 5-HT_3 receptor antagonists. Likewise, several descriptions of polymorphisms of the HT_{3A} receptor and HT_{3B} genes suggest a role for this agent in psychiatric disorders.[72,73] As evidenced by these findings, there are several components of the 5-HT_3 receptor.

5-HT_4 Receptor Subtypes

The clinical use of 5-HT_4 receptor drugs has met some resistance. Some drugs, like cisapride or maleate tegaserod, have been used to treat gastroesophageal reflux, constipation, or irritable bowel syndromes but were removed from use because of adverse cardiac problems.[59] The cautious use of 5-HT$_4$ partial agonists for cognitive deficiencies, particularly in Alzheimer's disease, is still ongoing. The use of 5-HT$_4$ ligands in bulimia or anorexia, but in addition to depression, is still an ongoing continual challenge. New methods that can attack these fundamental issues more reliably, more generally, and with greater ease of implementation will continue to build our understanding of this G-protein coupled receptor's functions.

Prostaglandins

Prostaglandins are naturally occurring, physiologically active endogenous substances that have been shown to mediate a variety of biologic functions throughout tissues and cells.[74] Prostaglandins are the cyclooxygenase metabolites of arachidonic acid containing a cyclopentane ring with two side chains. Metabolites of arachidonic acid are endogenous mediators of inflammation.

Synthesis and Mechanism of Action

Prostaglandins are synthesized and released upon cell stimulation and act on cells in the vicinity of their synthesis where they exert their actions. They are G-protein coupled receptors with seven transmembrane domains. Historically, substances were considered to be produced by the prostate gland because of the initial belief that a lipid-soluble acid present in semen that caused uterine relaxation was a secretion of the prostate.

Prostaglandins are intracellular products of arachidonate metabolism via the cyclooxygenase pathways[75] (Figure 21-2). Prostaglandin E$_2$ and other arachidonic acid metabolites are products derived from both non-neuronal and neuronal pools of two isoforms of cyclooxygenases (COX-1 and COX-2) and play an important role in the inflammatory process.[76] It is unclear if COX-1 contributes to the inflammatory process; however, COX-2 is induced at the site of inflammation and its amount in the cell rapidly increases during inflammation.[77] COX-2 also plays a significant role in the production of prostaglandin E$_2$.[76] As a rule COX-1 produces the physiologic pools of prostaglandin necessary for cellular function, whereas after adequate stimulation COX-2 has the potential to generate pathologic quantities of prostaglandins.[78]

The COX-2 isoform in neurons shows some constitutive activity; however, its functional status can be markedly altered by synaptic events.[74,78,79] Notably, neuronal synthesis of prostaglandins is hastened via increases in Ca^{++} and N-methyl-D-aspartate receptor activation.[77,78,80,81] This COX-2 isoform predominates in the spinal cord, especially in lamina I, II, and X.[78,79,81]

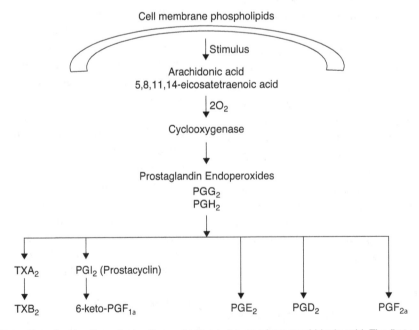

Cell membrane phospholipids

↓ Stimulus

Arachidonic acid
5,8,11,14-eicosatetraenoic acid

↓ 2O$_2$

Cyclooxygenase

↓

Prostaglandin Endoperoxides
PGG$_2$
PGH$_2$

↓

TXA$_2$ PGI$_2$ (Prostacyclin)   PGE$_2$ PGD$_2$ PGF$_{2a}$

TXB$_2$ 6-keto-PGF$_{1a}$

Formation of series 2 prostaglandins and a thromboxane from arachidonic acid. The first two pathways are catalyzed by cyclooxygenase with subsequent conversion of arachidonic acid to PGH$_2$, and all ensuing prostaglandins are catalyzed by their respective synthases.

Figure 21-2 Biosynthetic pathways of prostanoids.

Metabolism

Prostaglandin is initially metabolized very rapidly followed by a slow breakdown into inactive substances. Metabolism is catalyzed by specific enzymes found throughout the body in the gastrointestinal tract, kidneys, lung, and liver. The liver is the primary site for oxidation of existing inactive metabolites with the resultant substances excreted in urine. However, after one pass of infused prostaglandin, 95% is inactivated. Lung physiology permits the filtration of many prostaglandins and acts as a cardioprotective agent for this system and for other organs.

Effect on Body Systems

The effects of prostaglandins on the body are multifaceted (Table 21-4). For instance, the effect of the cardiovascular system often depends on the activity of the sympathetic nervous system corresponding to parasympathetic output and the metabolic status of the area affected.[8] Prostaglandins can both promote and contain atherothrombosis. Although nonsteroidal anti-inflammatory drugs selective for inhibition of COX-2 predispose to cardiovascular insult (myocardial infarction, heart failure, hypertension, and stroke), suppression of COX-1 products, such as thromboxane A_2, can trigger cardioprotection from low-dose aspirin.[82] Increased appearance of several subtypes of prostaglandin receptors has recently been demonstrated in clinical and experimental myocardial ischemia and reperfusion injury.[83] Prostaglandin E_2 has been shown to mediate anti-ischemic effects and cardiac myocyte hypertrophy, and there is support for the involvement of the prostaglandin E_{P3} receptor subtypes in this effect.[84] Mesenteric traction during cardiac surgery can produce hypotension and systemic vascular resistance, tachycardia, increased cardiac output, and cardiac index, which may be mediated by prostacyclin.[85]

The thromboxane-to-prostacyclin ratio is important in maintaining platelet activity and coagulation. Thromboxane is a strong platelet agonist involved in the pathogenesis of thrombotic diseases that stimulates platelet aggregation and vasoconstriction through the activation of adenylate cyclase and the subsequent decreased synthesis of cAMP. Prostacyclin is a powerful cytoprotective agent that exerts its action through activation of adenylate cyclase, followed by an intracellular accumulation of cAMP in various types of cells to oppose the effects of thromboxane.[86–88] High-dose aspirin prevents the effects of thromboxane and prostacyclin. Low-dose aspirin prevents thromboxane from opposing the effects of prostacyclin, preventing platelet aggregation. Therefore care must be taken so as not to disrupt this balance.

The lungs are a primary site for prostaglandin synthesis. Bronchoconstrictive disease (asthma) may be exacerbated in the presence of prostaglandins and other related substances. Circulating thromboxane and prostaglandin may result in pulmonary vasoconstriction. Drugs used to treat prostaglandin imbalance must be used with care in patients susceptible to their effects. For example, adverse hemodynamic reactions after protamine neutralization of heparin are infrequent but can pose an important clinical problem in these patients. Protamine may cause pulmonary hypertension, pulmonary vasoconstriction, and bronchospasm by stimulating the production of thromboxane.[89] Combined, these results offer valuable insight into the roles of these arachidonic metabolites in the development of atherothrombosis, emphasizing the need to reevaluate the use of selective prostacyclin- and thromboxane-based therapies in cardiovascular and pulmonary disease.[88]

Prostaglandins have displayed several roles in uterine physiology. Endometrial prostaglandin synthesis is speculated to be a cause of dysmenorrhea and may be important in the initiation of contractions and maintenance during labor. In the gravid and nongravid uterus, infusions of prostaglandins have exhibited the ability to predictably initiate and sustain contractions.

Table 21-4 Comparison of Select Prostaglandin Effects

	Systemic Vascular Resistance	Airway Resistance	Platelet Aggregation	Uterine Muscle Tone
Thromboxane	↑	↑	↑	
Prostacyclin	↓	↑	↓	
Iloprost	↓	↓	↓	
Alprostadil	↓	↑	↓	↑
Dinoprost	↑ ↓	↑		↑
Dinoprostone				↑

Table 21-5   Select Histamine Antagonists: Classification and Agents

Classification	Ethanolamine Derivatives (Aminoalkyl Ethers)
Aminoalkyl ethers exhibit substantial anticholinergic action and sedative effects.	

Agent	Dimenhydrinate
Indications	Prevention and treatment of nausea, vomiting, dizziness, or vertigo of motion sickness.
Dosage and Administration	Adults: • Oral: 50–100 mg every 4–6 h. Do not exceed 400 mg in 24 h. • IM: 50 mg, as needed • IV: 50 mg in 10 mL sodium chloride administered over 2 min Children: • Oral (6–12 yr): 25–50 mg every 6 to 8 h; not to exceed 150 mg in 24 h • Oral (2–6 yr): Up to 12.5–25 mg every 6–8 h; do not exceed 75 mg in 24 h • IM: 1.25 mg/kg or 37.5 mg/m^2 4 times/day; do not exceed 300 mg/day *Children (younger than 2 years of age): Only on advice of a physician.*
Actions	Pharmacology: Consists of equimolar proportions of diphenhydramine and chlorotheophylline. Pharmacokinetics: A depressant action on hyperstimulated labyrinthine function. The precise mode of action is not known. The antiemetic effects are believed to be caused by the diphenhydramine, an antihistamine also used as an antiemetic agent.
Contraindications	Neonates and patients that are hypersensitive to dimenhydrinate or its related components. Note: Most IV products contain benzyl alcohol, which has been associated with a fatal "gasping syndrome" in premature infants and low-birth-weight infants.
Warnings/Precautions	Use with caution in conditions that might be aggravated by anticholinergic therapy (e.g., prostatic hypertrophy, stenosing peptic ulcer, pyloroduodenal obstruction, bladder neck obstruction, narrow-angle glaucoma, bronchial asthma, cardiac arrhythmias). Children: For infants and children especially, an overdose of antihistamines may cause hallucinations, convulsions, or death. Mental alertness may be diminished. In the young child dimenhydrinate may produce excitation. Do not give to children under 2 years of age unless directed by a physician.
Adverse Reactions	Drowsiness, headache, blurred vision, tinnitus, dryness of the mouth and respiratory passages, incoordination, palpitation, dizziness, hypotension.
Agent	Clemastine
Indications	For the symptomatic treatment of allergic rhinitis.
Dosage and Administration	Adults and children 12 years of age and older: 1.34 mg every 12 h but should not exceed 8.04 mg daily.
Actions	Rapidly and almost completely absorbed from the GI tract. Peak plasma concentrations are attained within 2–5 h; maximal effect within 5–7 h and persists for 10–12 h. Appears to be extensively metabolized with renal excretion of metabolites in urine.
Contraindications	Lower dosage should be considered in adults over the age of 60 years; patients being treated with MAO inhibitors; patients with lower respiratory tract infection, narrow-angle glaucoma, bladder neck obstruction.
Warnings/Precautions	Pediatric: should not be used in premature or full-term neonates.
Adverse Reactions	Urinary retention, xerostomia (dry mouth), sedation.
Agent	Diphenhydramine
Indications	First-generation antihistamine; used as an antitussive for temporary relief of cough such as may occur with common colds or inhaled irritants; effective for the prevention and treatment of nausea, vomiting; over the counter agent used for motion sickness and sleep aid to manage short-term insomnia.
Dosage and Administration	Adult: oral and IV dosage is 25–50 mg 3 or 4 times daily at 4- to 6-h intervals, not to exceed 300 mg in 24 h (not to exceed 25 mg/min IV; IV and IM maximal dose is 400 mg in 24 h).

Table 21-5 Select Histamine Antagonists: Classification and Agents

Agent *(continued)*	Diphenhydramine
Actions	Well absorbed after oral administration, undergoes first-pass metabolism in the liver with only about 40–60% of an oral dose reaching systemic circulation unchanged with peak plasma concentrations attained within 1–4 h; rapidly and apparently almost completely metabolized (substantial first-pass metabolism in the liver) and also undergoes dealkylation with metabolites excreted in urine.
Contraindications	Contraindicated in neonates and premature infants, women who are breast-feeding, those with known hypersensitivity.
Warnings/Precautions	Glaucoma, emphysema, chronic bronchitis, or difficulty urinating due to prostatic hypertrophy.
Adverse Reactions	Marked drowsiness, blurred vision, xerostomia (dry mouth).

Classification	**Propylamine Derivatives (Alkylamines)**
Alkylamines cause less sedation; they are a common ingredient in cold and allergy preparations.	

Agent	Brompheniramine
Indications	Symptomatic relief of seasonal (e.g., hay fever) or perennial (nonseasonal) allergic rhinitis or nonallergic (vasomotor) rhinitis; used in fixed combination with other agents (e.g., phenylephrine, pseudoephedrine) for self-medication and temporary relief of itching and/or other symptoms associated with the common cold (e.g., nasal congestion).
Dosage and Administration	Administer with food, water, or milk to minimize gastric irritation. Adults: 4–6 mg every 4 h; extended release 6–12 mg every 12 h; maximum dosage of 24 mg in 24 h.
Actions	First-generation antihistamine.
Contraindications	Neonates and premature infants, women who are breast-feeding, those with peptic ulcer disease, within 2 weeks of MAO inhibitor therapy, acute asthma symptoms, known hypersensitivity.
Warnings/Precautions	Third trimester of pregnancy; neonates and premature infants; patients with prostatic hypertrophy, pyloroduodenal obstruction, or bladder neck obstruction.
Adverse Reactions	Restlessness, insomnia, anxiety, tension, nervousness, marked drowsiness, blurred vision, xerostomia (dry mouth), thickened bronchial secretions.

Agent	Chlorpheniramine
Indications	Controls the symptoms of cold or allergies (red, itchy, watery eyes; sneezing; itchy nose or throat; and runny nose).
Dosage and Administration	For self-medication of allergic rhinitis in adults and children 12 years of age and older, the usual oral dosage alone or in fixed-combination preparations is 4 mg every 4–6 h, not to exceed 24 mg in 24 h.
Actions	Rapidly and extensively metabolized with substantial metabolism in the GI mucosa during absorption and on first pass through the liver after oral administration.
Contraindications	Neonates and premature infants, women who are breastfeeding.
Warnings/Precautions	Individuals with phenylketonuria (i.e., homozygous genetic deficiency of phenylalanine hydroxylase).
Adverse Reactions	Marked drowsiness, blurred vision, xerostomia (dry mouth), nausea, vomiting, loss of appetite.

Agent	Triprolidine
Indications	Used as an antitussive for temporary relief of cough such as may occur with common colds.
Dosage and Administration	For self-medication in adults and children 12 years of age and older, the usual dosage is 2.5 mg every 4–6 h, not to exceed 10 mg in 24 h.
	Under the direction of a physician, children aged 4–6 yr may receive 0.938 mg every 4–6 h, not to exceed 3.744 mg in 24 h; children aged 2–4 yr may receive 0.625 mg every 4–6 h, not to exceed 2.5 mg in 24 h; and children aged 4 mo to 2 yr may receive 0.313 mg every 4–6 h, not to exceed 1.252 mg in 24 h.

(continues)

Table 21-5   Select Histamine Antagonists: Classification and Agents *(continued)*

Agent *(continued)*	Triprolidine
Actions	Triprolidine competes with histamine for the normal H$_1$ receptor sites on effector cells of the GI tract, blood vessels, and respiratory tract providing temporary relief of sneezing, watery and itchy eyes, and runny nose due to hay fever and other upper respiratory allergies.
Contraindications	Neonates and premature infants, women who are breast-feeding, those with angle-closure glaucoma, patients treated with MAO inhibitors, patients with lower respiratory tract infection or acute asthma.
Warnings/Precautions	Asthma, bladder neck obstruction, children, COPD, elevated intraocular pressure, older adult patients, heart disease, hypertension, hyperthyroidism, hypertrophic prostatic disease, pyloric obstruction, stenotic peptic ulcer.
Adverse Reactions	Marked drowsiness, xerostomia (dry mouth), loss of appetite, pharyngeal and bronchial secretion thickening.

Classification	**Piperazine Derivatives**
Agent	Buclizine
Indications	Prevention and treatment of nausea, vomiting, and dizziness associated with motion sickness and vertigo.
Dosage and Administration	Adults: 50-mg dose usually alleviates nausea. In severe cases 150 mg/day may be taken. Usual maintenance dose is 50 mg, 2 times/day. In prevention of motion sickness, 50 mg at least hour before beginning travel. For extended travel, a second 50-mg dose may be taken after 4–6 h.
Actions	Rapidly absorbed after oral administration and acts to block the histamine receptors in the vomiting center and thus reduce activity along these pathways. Furthermore, because buclizine possesses anticholinergic properties as well, the muscarinic receptors are similarly blocked.
Contraindications	Hypersensitivity and renal disease.
Warnings/Precautions	Bladder neck and GI obstruction, children, COPD, elevated intraocular pressure, older male adult patients with prostatic hypertrophy.
Adverse Reactions	Marked drowsiness, restlessness, insomnia, anxiety, tension, nervousness, blurred vision, xerostomia (dry mouth).

Agent	Cyclizine
Indications	Prevention and treatment of nausea, vomiting, and dizziness associated with motion sickness and vertigo.

Dosage and Administration	50 mg (as hydrochloride)
	
	• Oral
	
	   Adults: 50 mg taken a half hour before departure; repeat every 4–6 h. Do not exceed 200 mg/day.
	
	   Children (6–12 yr): 25 mg, up to 3 times/day
	
	• Parenteral: For IM use only. Not recommended for use in children.
	
	Adults: 50 mg every 4–6 h, as necessary.

Actions	Antiemetic, anticholinergic, and antihistaminic properties; onset of action of 30–60 min, depending on dosage; their duration of action is 4–6 h.
Contraindications	Hypersensitivity; cannot be combined with diclofenac (crystallization).
Warnings/Precautions	Bladder neck and GI obstruction, children, COPD, elevated intraocular pressure, older male adult patients with prostatic hypertrophy.
Adverse Reactions	Hypotension, palpitations, tachycardia, drowsiness, restlessness, nervousness, insomnia, euphoria, blurred vision, diplopia, vertigo, tinnitus, auditory and visual hallucinations (particularly when recommended dosages are exceeded), urticaria and rash, xerostomia (dry mouth), decreased appetite, nausea, vomiting, diarrhea, constipation, cholestatic jaundice, urinary dysfunction, pharyngeal dryness.

Table 21-5 Select Histamine Antagonists: Classification and Agents

Agent	Meclizine
Indications	Prevention and treatment of nausea, vomiting, and dizziness associated with motion sickness and vertigo; meclizine is "possibly effective" for the management of vertigo associated with diseases affecting the vestibular system.
Dosage and Administration	12.5, 25, and 50 mg.
Actions	Antiemetic, anticholinergic, and antihistaminic properties; onset of action of 30–60 min, depending on dosage; duration of action is 12–24 h; depresses labyrinth excitability and vestibular stimulation and may affect the medullary chemoreceptor trigger zone.
Contraindications	Hypersensitivity.
Warnings/Precautions	Bladder neck and GI obstruction, children, COPD, elevated intraocular pressure, older male adult patients with prostatic hypertrophy.
Adverse Reactions	Hypotension, palpitations, tachycardia, drowsiness, restlessness, nervousness, insomnia, euphoria, blurred vision, diplopia, vertigo, tinnitus, auditory and visual hallucinations (particularly when recommended dosages are exceeded), urticaria and rash, xerostomia (dry mouth), decreased appetite, nausea, vomiting, diarrhea, constipation, urinary dysfunction, pharyngeal dryness.

Agent	Hydroxyzine
Indications	Symptomatic relief of anxiety and tension associated with psychoneurosis and as an adjunct in organic disease states in which anxiety is manifested (alcohol withdrawal, preoperative sedation). Treatment of chronic urticaria, dermatitis, histamine-mediated pruritus, and effective as an antiemetic.
Dosage and Administration	Adults: 50–100 mg q.i.d.; children under 6 years, 50 mg daily in divided doses; children over 6 years, 50–100 mg daily in divided doses.
	Management of pruritus due to allergic conditions and in histamine-mediated pruritus: in adults, 25 mg t.i.d. or q.i.d.; children under 6 years, 50 mg daily in divided doses and over 6 years, 50–100 mg daily in divided doses.
	As a sedative when used as a premedication and after general anesthesia: 50–100 mg in adults, and 0.6 mg/kg of body weight in children.
Actions	Rapid-acting true ataraxic that is absorbed from the GI tract. Sedative properties of hydroxyzine probably occur at the subcortical level by suppressing key locations of the CNS. It also exerts bronchodilating, antispasmodic, antihistaminic, analgesic, and antiemetic effects.
Contraindications	Early pregnancy and hypersensitivity.
Warnings/Precautions	Asthma and concurrent administration of other CNS depressants.
Adverse Reactions	Xerostomia (dry mouth), headache, somnolence.

COPD, chronic obstructive pulmonary disease; GI, gastrointestinal; IM, intramuscular; IV, intravenous; MAO, monoamine oxidase.

Conclusion

The physiologic and pathophysiologic importance of the identified drug therapy associated with autocoid use remains unclear. The availability of drugs to address conditions requiring treatment with these substances and the development of therapeutics that selectively manipulate autocoid-mediated processes continue to grow. Autocoid pathways are sometimes redundant, regulatory, and even convergent. Opportunities may emerge from our studies of these substances that can open new conceptual paradigms in the study of drug therapy and further our understanding and appreciation of autocoids.

Key Points

- Autocoids include an array of biologically active substances that are synthesized at the site of action and mediate the initial response to tissue injury.
- Histamine is well known as an important inflammatory mediator and can affect the function of dendritic cells, monocytes and lymphocytes.
- Histamine has an array of important physiologic functions.
- Histamine exerts extensive effects on smooth muscle, gastric acid secretion, stimulation of sensory nerve endings, and edema.

- First-generation antihistamines are lipophilic and readily penetrate the blood–brain barrier and possess anticholinergic properties.
- First-generation H_1 antagonists cause stimulation and depression of the CNS.
- H_1 antagonists are used in the acute symptomatic treatment of hypersensitivity reactions.
- Bradykinin is an important nonapeptide inflammatory mediator involved in the development of neurogenic inflammation after tissue injury.
- Serotonin and its receptors play significant roles in a variety of physiologic and pathophysiologic processes.
- Prostaglandins are physiologically active endogenous substances that mediate a variety of biologic functions throughout tissues and cells.

Chapter Questions

1. Why must we be cautious in the use of cimetidine and ranitidine in the elderly population?
2. Why is bradykinin more potent than histamine as a vasodilator?
3. Why has the clinical use of 5-HT$_4$ receptor drugs met some resistance?

References

1. Skidgel RA, Erdos EG. Autacoids: drug therapy of inflammation. In: Brunton LL, Lazo JS, Parker KL, eds. *Goodman & Gilman's The Pharmacological Basis of Therapeutics*, 11th ed. New York: McGraw-Hill; 2005:1984.
2. Furukawa F, Yoshimasu T, Yamamoto Y, Kanazawa N, Tachibana T. Mast cells and histamine metabolism in skin lesions from MRL/MP-lpr/lpr mice. *Autoimmun Rev.* 2009; 8:495–499.
3. Frigas E, Park MA. Acute urticaria and angioedema: diagnostic and treatment considerations. *Am J Clin Dermatol.* 2009;10:239–250.
4. Stahl SM. Selective histamine H1 antagonism: novel hypnotic and pharmacologic actions challenge classical notions of antihistamines. *CNS Spectr.* 2008;13:1027–1038.
5. Marone G, Granata F, Spadaro G, Genovese A, Triggiani M. The histamine-cytokine network in allergic inflammation. *J Allerg Clin Immunol.* 2003;112(4 Suppl):S83–S88.
6. Garcia-Martin E, Ayuso P, Martinez C, Blanca M, Agundez JA. Histamine pharmacogenomics. *Pharmacogenomics.* 2009;10:867–883.
7. Parsons ME, Ganellin CR. Histamine and its receptors. *Br J Pharmacol.* 2006;147(Suppl 1):S127–S135.
8. Stoelting RK, Hillier SC. *Histamine and Histamine Receptor-Antagonists,* 4th ed. Philadelphia: Lippincott Williams & Wilkins; 2006.
9. Deml KF, Beermann S, Neumann D, Strasser A, Seifert R. Interactions of histamine H1-receptor agonists and antagonists with the human histamine H4-receptor. *Mol Pharmacol.* 2009;76:1019–1030.
10. MacGlashan D Jr. Histamine: a mediator of inflammation. *J Allerg Clin Immunol.* 2003;112(4 Suppl):S53–S59.
11. Connelly WM, Shenton FC, Lethbridge N, et al. The histamine H4 receptor is functionally expressed on neurons in the mammalian CNS. *Br J Pharmacol.* 2009;157:55–63.
12. Gemkow MJ, Davenport AJ, Harich S, Ellenbroek BA, Cesura A, Hallett D. The histamine H3 receptor as a therapeutic drug target for CNS disorders. *Drug Discov Today.* 2009;14:509–515.
13. Vonakis BM, Macglashan DW Jr, Vilarino N, Langdon JM, Scott RS, MacDonald SM. Distinct characteristics of signal transduction events by histamine-releasing factor/translationally controlled tumor protein (HRF/TCTP)-induced priming and activation of human basophils. *Blood.* 2008;111:1789–1796.
14. Alagarsamy V, Rupeshkumar M, Kavitha K, et al. Synthesis and pharmacological investigation of novel 4-(2-methylphenyl)-1-substituted-4H-[1,2,4]triazolo[4,3-a]quinazolin-5-one as a new class of H(1)-antihistaminic agents. *Eur J Med Chem.* 2008; 43:2331–2337.
15. Du Buske LM. Clinical comparison of histamine H1-receptor antagonist drugs. *J Allerg Clin Immunol.* 1996; 98(6 Pt 3):S307–S318.
16. Noubade R, Milligan G, Zachary JF, et al. Histamine receptor H1 is required for TCR-mediated p38 MAPK activation and optimal IFN-gamma production in mice. *J Clin Invest.* 2007;117:3507–3518.
17. Li D, Wen JF, Jin JY, Quan HX, Cho KW. Cardiac mast cells regulate myocyte ANP release via histamine H2 receptor in beating rabbit atria. *Regul Pept.* 2009;155:33–38.
18. Sangalli BC. Role of the central histaminergic neuronal system in the CNS toxicity of the first generation H1-antagonists. *Prog Neurobiol.* 1997;52:145–157.
19. Gong YX, Lv M, Zhu YP, et al. Endogenous histamine inhibits the development of morphine-induced conditioned place preference. *Acta Pharmacol Sin.* 2007;28:10–18.
20. Mobarakeh JI, Takahashi K, Yanai K. Enhanced morphine-induced antinociception in histamine H3 receptor gene knockout mice. *Neuropharmacology.* 2009;57:409–414.
21. Hur GY, Sheen SS, Kang YM, et al. Histamine release and inflammatory cell infiltration in airway mucosa in methylene

diphenyl diisocyanate (MDI)-induced occupational asthma. *J Clin Immunol.* 2008;28:571–580.

22. Purokivi M, Koskela HO, Koistinen T, et al. Utility of cough response during hypertonic histamine challenge in diagnosing asthma. *Respir Med.* 2008;102:1379–1384.

23. Schubert ML. Gastric secretion. *Curr Opin Gastroenterol.* 2008;24:659–664.

24. Schubert ML. Hormonal regulation of gastric acid secretion. *Curr Gastroenterol Rep.* 2008;10:523–527.

25. Larsson LI. Developmental biology of gastrin and somatostatin cells in the antropyloric mucosa of the stomach. *Microsc Res Tech.* 2000;48:272–281.

26. Ichikawa T, Hotta K, Ishihara K. Second-generation histamine H(2)-receptor antagonists with gastric mucosal defensive properties. *Mini Rev Med Chem.* 2009;9:581–589.

27. Jones J, Dougherty J, Cannon L. Diphenhydramine-induced toxic psychosis. *Am J Emerg Med.* 1986;4:369–371.

28. Roman D. Schizophrenia-like psychosis following "Mandrax" overdose. *Br J Psychiatry.* 1972;121:619–620.

29. Brimblecombe RW, Duncan WA, Durant GJ, Ganellin CR, Parsons ME, Black JW. The pharmacology of cimetidine, a new histamine H2-receptor antagonist. *Br J Pharmacol.* 1975;53:435P–436P.

30. Schubert ML, Peura DA. Control of gastric acid secretion in health and disease. *Gastroenterology.* 2008;134:1842–1860.

31. Vuyyuru L, Harrington L, Arimura A, Schubert ML. Reciprocal inhibitory paracrine pathways link histamine and somatostatin secretion in the fundus of the stomach. *Am J Physiol.* 1997;273(1 Pt 1):G106–G111.

32. Vuyyuru L, Schubert ML. Histamine, acting via H3 receptors, inhibits somatostatin and stimulates acid secretion in isolated mouse stomach. *Gastroenterology.* 1997;113:1545–1552.

33. Feldman M, Burton ME. Histamine2-receptor antagonists. Standard therapy for acid-peptic diseases. 2. *N Engl J Med.* 1990;323:1749–1755.

34. Feldman M, Burton ME. Histamine2-receptor antagonists. Standard therapy for acid-peptic diseases. 1. *N Engl J Med.* 1990;323:1672–1680.

35. Willmann S, Edginton AN, Kleine-Besten M, Jantratid E, Thelen K, Dressman JB. Whole-body physiologically based pharmacokinetic population modelling of oral drug administration: inter-individual variability of cimetidine absorption. *J Pharm Pharmacol.* 2009;61:891–899.

36. Matsushima S, Maeda K, Inoue K, et al. The inhibition of human multidrug and toxin extrusion 1 is involved in the drug-drug interaction caused by cimetidine. *Drug Metab Dispos.* 2009;37:555–559.

37. Andrews AD, Brock-Utne JG, Downing JW. Protection against pulmonary acid aspiration with ranitidine. A new histamine H2-receptor antagonist. *Anaesthesia.* 1982;37:22–25.

38. Coombs DW. Aspiration pneumonia prophylaxis. *Anesth Analg.* 1983;62:1055–1058.

39. de Souza DG, Gaughen CL. Aspiration risk after esophagectomy. *Anesth Analg.* 2009;109:1352.

40. Gallagher EG, White M, Ward S, Cottrell J, Mann SG. Prophylaxis against acid aspiration syndrome. Single oral dose of H2-antagonist on the evening before elective surgery. *Anaesthesia.* 1988;43:1011–1014.

41. Imai Y, Kawata S, Uchida K, Tarui S. Effect of a high dose of cimetidine on biliary, intestinal and fecal bile acids in rats. *Jpn J Pharmacol.* 1991;55:299–302.

42. Mok HY. Effects of cimetidine on biliary lipids in patients with reflux esophagitis. *Gastroenterology.* 1981;81:340–344.

43. Moron F, Mozsik G, Javor T. Effects of cimetidine administered in cytoprotective and antisecretory doses on the membrane-bound ATP-dependent energy systems in the gastric mucosal lesions induced by HCl in rats. *Acta Physiol Hung.* 1984;64:293–299.

44. Mozsik G, Moron F, Fiegler M, et al. Membrane-bound ATP-dependent energy systems and gastric cytoprotection by prostacyclin, atropine and cimetidine in the rat. *Int J Tissue React.* 1983;5:263–278.

45. Westblom TU, Duriex DE. Enhancement of antibiotic concentrations in gastric mucosa by H2-receptor antagonist. Implications for treatment of *Helicobacter pylori* infections. *Dig Dis Sci.* 1991;36:25–28.

46. Moss J. Histamine release in anesthesia and surgery. *N Engl Reg Allerg Proc.* 1985;6:28–36.

47. Moss J, Rosow CE. Histamine release by narcotics and muscle relaxants in humans. *Anesthesiology.* 1983;59:330–339.

48. Rosow CE, Philbin DM, Keegan CR, Moss J. Hemodynamics and histamine release during induction with sufentanil or fentanyl. *Anesthesiology.* 1984;60:489–491.

49. Calixto JB, Cabrini DA, Ferreira J, Campos MM. Kinins in pain and inflammation. *Pain.* 2000;87:1–5.

50. Walker K, Perkins M, Dray A. Kinins and kinin receptors in the nervous system. *Neurochem Int.* 1995;26:1–16; discussion 17–26.

51. Marceau F, Sabourin T, Houle S, et al. Kinin receptors: functional aspects. *Int Immunopharmacol.* 2002;2:1729–1739.

52. Regoli D, Nsa Allogho S, Rizzi A, Gobeil FJ. Bradykinin receptors and their antagonists. *Eur J Pharmacol.* 1998;348:1–10.

53. Bertrand C, Nadel JA, Yamawaki I, Geppetti P. Role of kinins in the vascular extravasation evoked by antigen and mediated by tachykinins in guinea pig trachea. *J Immunol.* 1993;151:4902–4907.

54. Gibson C, Schnatbaum K, Pfeifer JR, et al. Novel small molecule bradykinin B2 receptor antagonists. *J Med Chem.* 2009;52:4370–4379.

55. Kaman WE, Wolterink AF, Bader M, Boele LC, van der Kleij D. The bradykinin B2 receptor in the early immune response against Listeria infection. *Med Microbiol Immunol.* 2009;198:39–46.

56. Shirasaki H, Kanaizumi E, Himi T. Immunohistochemical localization of the bradykinin B1 and B2 receptors in human nasal mucosa. *Mediators Inflamm.* 2009;2009:102406. Published online 2009 Apr doi 10.1158/2009/10240.

57. Bhattacharya SK, Rao PJ, Brumleve SJ, Parmar SS. Effects of intracerebroventricular administration of bradykinin on rat brain serotonin and prostaglandins. *Res Commun Chem Pathol Pharmacol.* 1986;54:355–366.

58. Mondick JT, Oo C, Patel D, Fujitani T, Shimizu K, Barrett JS. Population pharmacokinetics of the selective serotonin 5-HT1A receptor partial agonist piclozotan. *Am J Ther.* 2009;16:106–115.

59. Bockaert J, Claeysen S, Compan V, Dumuis A. 5-HT(4) receptors: history, molecular pharmacology and brain functions. *Neuropharmacology.* 2008;55:922–931.

60. Bockaert J, Sebben M, Dumuis A. Pharmacological characterization of 5-hydroxytryptamine4(5-HT4) receptors positively coupled to adenylate cyclase in adult guinea pig hippocampal membranes: effect of substituted benzamide derivatives. *Mol Pharmacol.* 1990;37:408–411.

61. Blois TM, Bowie JU. G-protein-coupled receptor structures were not built in a day. *Protein Sci.* 2009;18:1335–1342.

62. Eijkelkamp N, Heijnen CJ, Elsenbruch S, Holtmann G, Schedlowski M, Kavelaars A. G protein-coupled receptor kinase 6 controls post-inflammatory visceral hyperalgesia. *Brain Behav Immun.* 2009;23:18–26.

63. Filizola M. Increasingly accurate dynamic molecular models of G-protein coupled receptor oligomers: panacea or Pandora's box for novel drug discovery? *Life Sci.* 2009. [Epub ahead of print], May 22, 2009.

64. Hoyer D, Clarke DE, Fozard JR, et al. International Union of Pharmacology classification of receptors for 5-hydroxytryptamine (serotonin). *Pharmacol Rev.* 1994;46:157–203.

65. Sanders-Bush E, Mayer SE. 5-Hydroxytryptamine (Serotonin): receptor agonists and antagonists. In: Brunton LL, Lazo JS, Parker KL, eds. *Goodman & Gilman's the Pharmacological Basis of Therapeutics,* vol. 11. New York: McGraw-Hill; 2005:1984.

66. Lynch JJ Jr, Stump GL, Kane SA, Regan CP. The prototype serotonin 5-HT 1B/1D agonist sumatriptan increases the severity of myocardial ischemia during atrial pacing in dogs with coronary artery stenosis. *J Cardiovasc Pharmacol.* 2009;53:474–479.

67. Thompson AJ, Lummis SC. 5-HT3 receptors. *Curr Pharm Des.* 2006;12:3615–3630.

68. Thompson AJ, Lummis SC. The 5-HT3 receptor as a therapeutic target. *Exp Opin Ther Targets.* 2007;11:527–540.

69. Barnes NM, Hales TG, Lummis SC, Peters JA. The 5-HT3 receptor—the relationship between structure and function. *Neuropharmacology.* 2009;56:273–284.

70. Doucet E, Miquel MC, Nosjean A, Verge D, Hamon M, Emerit MB. Immunolabeling of the rat central nervous system with antibodies partially selective of the short form of the 5-HT3 receptor. *Neuroscience.* 2000;95:881–892.

71. Pratt GD, Bowery NG, Kilpatrick GJ, et al. Consensus meeting agrees distribution of 5-HT3 receptors in mammalian hindbrain. *Trends Pharmacol Sci.* 1990;11:135–137.

72. Krzywkowski K. Do polymorphisms in the human 5-HT3 genes contribute to pathological phenotypes? *Biochem Soc Trans.* 2006;34(Pt 5):872–876.

73. Niesler B, Kapeller J, Hammer C, Rappold G. Serotonin type 3 receptor genes: HTR3A, B, C, D, E. *Pharmacogenomics.* 2008;9:501–504.

74. Oudiz RJ, Farber HW. Dosing considerations in the use of intravenous prostanoids in pulmonary arterial hypertension: an experience-based review. *Am Heart J.* 2009;157:625–635.

75. Akinbamowo AO, Salzberg DJ, Weir MR. Renal consequences of prostaglandin inhibition in heart failure. *Heart Fail Clin.* 2008;4:505–510.

76. Gambaro G, Perazella MA. Adverse renal effects of anti-inflammatory agents: evaluation of selective and nonselective cyclooxygenase inhibitors. *J Intern Med.* 2003;253:643–652.

77. Stachowska E, Dolegowska B, Dziedziejko V, et al. Prostaglandin E2 (PGE2) and thromboxane A2 (TXA2) synthesis is regulated by conjugated linoleic acids (CLA) in human macrophages. *J Physiol Pharmacol.* 2009;60:77–85.

78. Beiche F, Scheuerer S, Brune K, Geisslinger G, Goppelt-Struebe M. Up-regulation of cyclooxygenase-2 mRNA in the rat spinal cord following peripheral inflammation. *FEBS Lett.* 1996;390:165–169.

79. Narumiya S, Sugimoto Y, Ushikubi F. Prostanoid receptors: structures, properties, and functions. *Physiol Rev.* 1999;79:1193–1226.

80. Breder CD, Dewitt D, Kraig RP. Characterization of inducible cyclooxygenase in rat brain. *J Comp Neurol.* 1995;355:296–315.

81. Willingale HL, Gardiner NJ, McLymont N, Giblett S, Grubb BD. Prostanoids synthesized by cyclo-oxygenase isoforms in rat spinal cord and their contribution to the development of neuronal hyperexcitability. *Br J Pharmacol.* 1997;122:1593–1604.

82. Yu Y, Ricciotti E, Grosser T, Fitzgerald GA. The translational therapeutics of prostaglandin inhibition in atherothrombosis. *J Thromb Haemost.* 2009;7(Suppl 1):222–226.

83. Hishikari K, Suzuki J, Ogawa M, et al. Pharmacological activation of the prostaglandin E2 receptor EP4 improves cardiac function after myocardial ischaemia/reperfusion injury. *Cardiovasc Res.* 2009;81:123–132.

84. Meyer-Kirchrath J, Martin M, Schooss C, et al. Overexpression of prostaglandin EP3 receptors activates calcineurin and promotes hypertrophy in the murine heart. *Cardiovasc Res.* 2009;81:310–318.

85. Hudson JC, Wurm WH, O'Donnel TF Jr, et al. Ibuprofen pretreatment inhibits prostacyclin release during abdominal exploration in aortic surgery. *Anesthesiology.* 1990;72:443–449.

86. Gryglewski RJ. Prostacyclin among prostanoids. *Pharmacol Rep.* 2008;60:3–11.

87. Navarro-Nunez L, Castillo J, Lozano ML, et al. Thromboxane A2 receptor antagonism by flavonoids: structure-activity relationships. *J Agric Food Chem.* 2009;57:1589–1594.

88. Gleim S, Kasza Z, Martin K, Hwa J. Prostacyclin receptor/thromboxane receptor interactions and cellular responses in human atherothrombotic disease. *Curr Atheroscler Rep.* 2009;11:227–235.

89. Nuttall GA, Murray MJ, Bowie EJ. Protamine-heparin-induced pulmonary hypertension in pigs: effects of treatment with a thromboxane receptor antagonist on hemodynamics and coagulation. *Anesthesiology.* 1991;74:138–145.

Anticoagulants and Their Reversal

Penelope S. Benedik, PhD, CRNA, RRT

Objectives

After completing this chapter, the reader should be able to

- Explain the process of coagulation, using both the cascade model and the cell-based model.
- Analyze the mechanism of action of vitamin K antagonists, direct and indirect factor Xa inhibitors, and direct thrombin inhibitors and their pharmacologic reversal.
- Describe the indications and contraindications for anticoagulant therapy.
- Evaluate the different methods used to assess the effects of anticoagulant therapy.
- Examine the implications of anticoagulant use and regional anesthesia.

Introduction

In an undamaged human body, blood flows through a vast network of vessels lined with a smooth endothelial layer. This arrangement is designed to facilitate the delivery of substrates in a closed system. When an injury occurs, both the endothelium and the blood undergo profound changes to repair damage and preserve the closed system. During this process, liquid blood is transformed into a gelatinous state by the recruitment and activation of platelets and procoagulant proteins. Although normal hemostasis represents a balance between procoagulant and antifibrinolytic activity (to control bleeding) and anticoagulant and fibrinolytic activity (to control excessive clotting), nonphysiologic clotting is medically treated with anticoagulants.[1] In this chapter we discuss commonly used pharmacologic agents that enhance the anticoagulant pathways, including vitamin K antagonists, direct and indirect factor Xa inhibitors, and direct thrombin inhibitors.

Cascade Model of Coagulation

Historically, the coagulation cascade has been described as a series of biochemical reactions that sequentially activate coagulation factors.[2] In this schema intrinsic and extrinsic pathways of activation converge on a final common pathway in which factor Xa/Va prothrombinase complex catalyzes the transformation of prothrombin (factor II) to thrombin (factor IIa) (Figure 22-1). Thrombin is the key enzyme necessary to convert fibrinogen (factor I) to fibrin (factor Ia), the substance required to form a hemostatic plug. In this model activation of either the intrinsic or extrinsic pathway can achieve the final outcome. Once thrombin is generated, it activates factors VII, V, and VIII and enters into a feedback loop that further increases the thrombin concentration.

The intrinsic pathway is initiated by contact activation between damaged tissue surfaces and circulating coagulation factors. High-molecular-weight kininogen accumulates on the damaged surface and, together with prekallikrein and factor XII, produces kallikrein and factor XIIa. In a "cascade" series of reactions, factor XIIa converts factor XI into factor XIa. Factor XIa activates factor IX, which when combined with factor VIIIa and a phospholipid surface catalyzes the activation of factor X to factor Xa. Factor deficiencies within the intrinsic pathway are measured with the activated partial thromboplastin time (aPTT), although the risk of hemorrhage depends highly on which factor is deficient. Factor XII deficiency is not associated with bleeding, whereas a deficiency of factor VIII (hemophilia A, classic hemophilia) or factor IX (hemophilia B, Christmas disease) is highly associated with bleeding.[3]

The extrinsic pathway is initiated by traumatic disruption of the vascular bed. Trauma exposes extravascular tissue factor (TF) to circulating factor VII to form a TF/VIIa complex that activates factor X. Because of the very high concentration of circulating factor VII, this pathway is particularly effective in generating a burst of thrombin when a vessel breach occurs. Deficiencies in the extrinsic pathway are measured by the prothrombin time (PT).

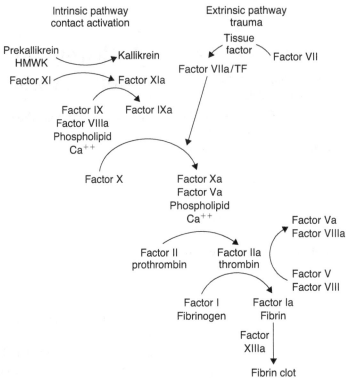

Figure 22-1 Intrinsic pathway contact activation.

Cell-Based Model of Coagulation

The fact that multiple steps in the intrinsic and extrinsic coagulation cascade model are localized to activated cell surfaces hints at the logic of formulating a cell-based model for coagulation (Figure 22-2).[4] The phospholipid cellular membranes of platelets provide the proper surface for the steps of the coagulation reactions, whereas TF is also a cellular membrane-bound protein. In this model coagulation is initiated, amplified, and propagated in a process that relies on reactions in both the intrinsic and extrinsic pathways. Additionally, this model emphasizes that the components of the coagulation system are compartmentalized. The major intravascular components of the process are platelets and von Willebrand factor (vWF)/factor VIII, whereas in the extravascular space low levels for factors VIIa, IXa, and Xa and thrombin are present and available at all times if a vascular breach occurs. A basic summary of the cell-based model of coagulation is briefly described next. [2,5]

Initiation of Coagulation

Coagulation is initiated on TF-bearing cells (e.g., fibroblasts) or cell fragments that are exposed to blood at a site of injury. TF is both a receptor and a cofactor for factor VII, ultimately forming a TF/factor VIIa complex. Factor VIIa has been likened to a soluble sentry, patrolling the circulation seeking sites of vascular damage with TF exposure.[3] This complex catalyzes the activation of factors X and XI. Factor Xa interacts with cofactor Va to form the prothrombinase complex that generates a small amount of thrombin; it is this trace thrombin that initiates the amplification process. Factor XIa does not play an important role in the initiation process, but if it binds to a platelet surface receptor with cofactor VIIIa, factor X is activated directly on the surface of the platelet. The initiation process promotes a localized procoagulant environment, in part due to altered composition of the phospholipid bilayer whose acidic head groups promote the assembly of enzymatic complexes on the cell surface.

Two factors inhibit enzyme activation during the coagulation process: tissue factor pathway inhibitor (TFPI) and antithrombin.[3,6] TFPI inhibits factor Xa when it is complexed with TF/factor VIIa. Antithrombin is available in high concentrations and neutralizes the first formed factor Xa and thrombin. Therefore, procoagulant factors must be generated at a very high level before effective coagulation can proceed. Antithrombin also serves to keep the coagulation process confined to the local level where the vascular injury occurred.

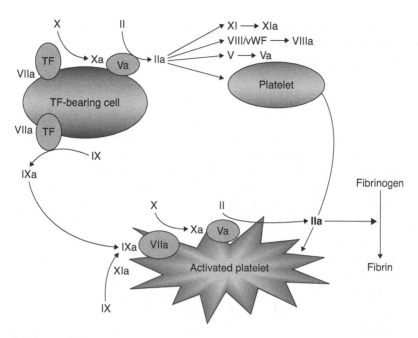

Figure 22-2 Cell-based model of coagulation.

Source: Reprinted from *Blood Reviews,* Vol. 21, No. 3, Wolberg AS, Thrombin generation and fibrin clot structure, pp. 131–142, 2007, with permission from Elsevier.

Amplification of Coagulation

The trace amount of thrombin formed during initiation serves to amplify the coagulation process by activating platelets, factor V, factor XI, and factor VIII. Inactive factor VIII is bound to vWF in the circulation; factor VIII release from vWF is triggered by thrombin. Amplification thus increases the availability of both activated platelets and cofactors.

Propagation of Coagulation

The coagulation process is further propagated by the binding of factor XIa to activated platelets along with thrombin formation (IIa) from factors Va, IXa, and Xa on the platelet surface. Each molecule of factor Xa can generate up to 1000 molecules of thrombin. Thrombin generated by platelets activates thrombin-activated fibrinolysis inhibitor to protect the clot. Thrombin also activates factor XIII (fibrin-stabilizing factor), in the presence of calcium, which serves to crosslink the fibrin mesh and stabilize the clot.

Direct and Indirect Thrombin Inhibitors

As a key effector in hemostasis, thrombin is an important therapeutic target in both treating and preventing thromboembolic disease. Thrombin can be inhibited both directly and indirectly; the conventional anticoagulants unfractionated heparin, low-molecular-weight heparin, and warfarin operate via the indirect approach. Direct thrombin inhibitors include hirudins (derived from leech proteins) and the synthetic heparin derivatives.

Unfractionated Heparin and Low-Molecular-Weight Heparin

Heparin is a naturally occurring sulfated glycosaminoglycan found in basophils and mast cells; after mast cell degranulation, released heparin is rapidly destroyed by macrophages so that plasma levels are normally undetectable. Heparin molecules in endovascular surfaces or in the subendothelial extracellular matrix serve the role of endogenous antithrombotic agents. Pharmaceutical unfractionated heparin (UFH) is a mixture of polysaccharide chains of varying molecular weights (from 3000 to 30,000 daltons; mean 15,000 daltons) and contains many highly negatively charged groups, making it highly polar and difficult to cross cell membranes. Low-molecular-weight heparin (LWMH) is a small fragment of heparin that contains the crucial pentasaccharide segment required for anti–factor Xa activity. LMWH products currently available include dalteparin (Fragmin), enoxaparin (Lovenox), and tinzaparin (Innohep). Pharmaceutical heparin is produced from either porcine intestinal mucosa or bovine lung; commercial preparations of UFH and enoxaparin are formulated such that their biologic activity is comparable (approximately 150 USP units/mg). Dalteparin and tinzaparin are formulated in anti–factor Xa units.

Mechanism of Action

Heparin acts on multiple sites within the coagulation process in a dose-dependent fashion.[7] Heparin's activity depends on the endogenous anticoagulant antithrombin III. In combination with cofactor antithrombin III, heparin inactivates factors IIa, IXa, Xa, and XIIa. Although only about one-third of heparin molecules contain the unique pentasaccharide sequence required for antithrombin III binding, this reaction comprises the major component of heparin's anticoagulant effects. In high concentrations, heparin binds to heparin cofactor II and, with the formation of a heparin–antithrombin–thrombin complex, inhibits the conversion of prothrombin (factor II) to thrombin (factor IIa). At very high concentrations heparin binds to factor IX and directly inhibits factor X activation.

Heparins of lower molecular weight (mean size, 4500 daltons) cannot bind thrombin and antithrombin simultaneously. Therefore LMWH does not inhibit thrombin but acts mainly through the inhibition of factor Xa via antithrombin.

Clinical Pharmacology

Pharmacokinetics

UFH is administered parenterally, either via continuous intravenous (IV) infusion or subcutaneously. IV heparin has an immediate onset, whereas subcutaneous (SC) heparin has highly variable bioavailability with a delayed onset (average 3 hours). Heparin binds to plasma proteins, endothelial cells, and macrophages; this contributes to the large variability in free plasma levels after administration.

LMWH has a more uniform absorption, probably due to reduced binding to plasma proteins, endothelial cells, and macrophages. LMWH thus has a more predictable dose–response relationship than UFH. Peak anti–factor Xa activity occurs at 3 to 5 hours after SC administration of LMWH.

Clearance and biologic half-life of UFH are dose dependent, with doses of 25, 100, 400, or 800 units/kg providing 0.5, 1, 2.5, or 5 hours of anticoagulant activity, respectively. The elimination half-life of LMWH is not dose dependent and is about two to four times longer than UFH. This requires that LMWH be discontinued at least 12 hours before surgery as opposed to UFH, which may be discontinued 4 hours before surgery.[8]

Pharmacodynamics

Heparin prevents the formation of new or the extension of preexisting thrombotic clots by its actions on coagulation factors. By inactivating factor Xa and thrombin (factor IIa), heparin suppresses the formation of fibrin that forms the framework of thrombotic clots. The inhibition of thrombin also inhibits thrombin-induced platelet activation and coagulation factors V and VIII. Heparin prolongs the bleeding time and the aPTT and has measurable anti-Xa activity. Heparin is not fibrinolytic and does not dissolve existing clots; it only prevents further clot formation.

Patients who require particularly high doses of heparin to achieve and maintain a therapeutic response are termed heparin resistant.[7] Some patients labeled "heparin resistant" have therapeutic heparin anti-Xa levels but inadequately prolonged aPTT; this occurs because of the known effect of increased factor VIII levels on aPTT shortening. Genetic factors that cause excess factor VIII have been reported in as many as 11% of the general population.[9,10] The rare mechanisms for heparin resistance include most commonly antithrombin deficiency as well as increased heparin clearance, increased circulating heparin-binding proteins, or increased fibrinogen levels.

Metabolism and Elimination

At low doses UFH is cleared through the reticuloendothelial system, although this system becomes saturated rapidly. UFH at high doses and LMWH are excreted unchanged through a slow nonsaturable renal mechanism. At therapeutic levels a large proportion of UFH is excreted through the dose-dependent rapid saturable system. The higher molecular weight chains of UFH are cleared more rapidly than the lower molecular weight chains, explaining the differences in the half-lives and dosing schedules of UFH and LMWH. Both UFH and LMWH may have a prolonged half-life in hepatic or renal disease and decreased half-life in females and smokers.

Clinical Uses and Indications

Heparin is used in low doses for the prevention of postoperative deep vein thrombosis (DVT) and pulmonary embolism in patients at risk of developing thromboembolic disease. Higher doses are used for the prevention and treatment of pulmonary embolism and peripheral arterial embolism, as well as atrial fibrillation with emboli formation, and in the diagnosis and treatment of disseminated intravascular coagulopathy. In vitro uses of heparin include anticoagulation in blood transfusions, extracorporeal circulation, dialysis, and laboratory blood samples.

LMWH is indicated in the prophylaxis and treatment of DVT (SC) and is often used in patients undergoing hip or knee arthroplasty or abdominal surgery. These agents may be used in acutely ill medical patients with severely restricted mobility. They may also be used for prophylaxis for ischemic complications of unstable angina and non-Q wave myocardial infarction (SC) and for the treatment of ST-elevated myocardial infarction (IV). Table 22-1 provides the indications and dosing guidelines for UFH, and Table 22-2 provides the indications and dosing guidelines for LMWH.[7]

Comparative Pharmacology of Other Drugs in Class

In some circumstances UFH has several advantages over LMWH.[11] First, the anticoagulant effects can be rapidly and fully reversed by the antagonist protamine, a characteristic used during cardiac and vascular surgery. Because of its nonrenal route of metabolism, normal doses of UFH may be safer than LMWH in patients with renal insufficiency. Last, UFH modulates coagulation triggered by contact activation; its use theoretically may reduce the risk of thrombosis in implanted devices compared with LMWH. However, the use of LMWH generally does not require monitoring, whereas the use of UFH in therapeutic doses requires frequent dose adjustment and laboratory testing.

Side Effects and Contraindications

The most common adverse effect of heparin is bleeding, ranging from bleeding that responds to pharmacologic reversal to fatal hemorrhage. Heparin should be used with extreme caution in patients at risk for hemorrhage, including patients with severe hypertension, underlying bleeding disorders, increased capillary permeability, thrombocytopenia, ulcerative gastrointestinal lesions or gastric tube drainage, dissecting aneurysm, threatened abortion, or liver disease with impaired hemostasis. Known hemorrhagic complications that may be difficult to detect and therefore dictate a high index of suspicion during heparin therapy include adrenal, ovarian, and retroperitoneal hemorrhage. There are only weak correlations between heparin dose, aPTT prolongation, and the risk of bleeding; bleeding can occur even with aPTT values within the therapeutic range. Mild bleeding can usually be controlled with discontinuation of the drug; severe hemorrhage is treated by pharmacologic reversal with protamine sulfate (1 mg for every 100 units of heparin in the body).

The use of UFH for more than 1 week may be associated with the development of heparin-induced thrombocytopenia (HIT) or heparin-induced thrombocytopenia and thrombosis.[12] The HIT response is antibody mediated and may progress to venous and arterial thrombotic events (heparin-induced thrombocytopenia and thrombosis). HIT may be defined by an unexplained platelet count less than $150,000/\mu L$ or a 50% reduction in platelets from the pretreatment value along with the occurrence of new thrombosis, skin lesions at heparin injections sites, or acute systemic reactions after IV use. Generally, in typical-onset HIT the platelet count begins to decline at 5 to 10 days after heparin initiation with thrombocytopenia occurring at 7 to 14 days. Delayed-onset HIT can occur up to several weeks after discontinuation of heparin therapy. Rapid-onset HIT may occur within 24 hours of receiving heparin if the patient has had a heparin exposure within the last 100 days.

Certain factors increase the risk of developing HIT. The use of bovine UFH confers a greater risk than porcine UFH

Table 22-1 Indications and Dosing Guidelines for Unfractionated Heparin

Indication	Initial Bolus Dose	Maintenance
Prophylaxis of postoperative thromboembolism	5000 U SC 2 h before surgery	5000 U SC every 8–12 h after surgery for 7 days or until fully ambulatory
Treatment of venous thrombosis	80 U/kg IV	18 U/kg/h
Unstable angina or STEMI	60–70 U/kg IV Maximum 5000 U	12–15 U/kg/h Maximum 1000 U/h
STEMI with tPA	60 U/kg IV Maximum 4000 U	12 U/kg/h Maximum 1000 U/h
Interventional cardiology procedures	100–200 U/kg IV	Bolus 5000 to 10,000 U to maintain ACT 200 to 400 s
Percutaneous coronary interventional procedures with glycoprotein IIb/IIIa inhibitors	70 U/kg IV	Bolus to keep ACT > 200 s
Cardiopulmonary bypass	300–400 U/kg IV	Bolus to keep ACT > 480 s; may use POC heparin concentration or high-dose thrombin time to evaluate

ACT, activated clotting time; POC, point-of-care; STEMI, ST segment elevation myocardial infarction; tPA, tissue plasminogen activator; U, units.

Table 22-2 Indications and Dosing Guidelines for Low-Molecular-Weight Heparin

Drug	Approved Indications	Dosing	Target Anti–Factor Xa Level
Dalteparin* (Fragmin)	Prophylaxis of unstable angina or non-Q wave MI	120 IU/kg SC q 12 h (not > 10,000 IU) for 5–8 days	
	Prophylaxis of VTE for hip replacement or abdominal surgery	2500 IU SC either 2 h before or 4–8 h after surgery; postoperatively 2500–5000 IU SC daily for 5–10 days	1.05 IU/mL in daily dosing
	Acutely ill with restricted mobility prophylaxis	5000 IU SC daily for 12–14 days	
	Extended treatment of symptomatic VTE in cancer patients	200 IU/kg SC daily × 1 mo (not > 18,000 IU); 150 IU/kg SC daily × 2–6 mo	
Enoxaparin† (Lovenox)	Treatment of VTE with or without PE	1 mg/kg q 12 h with/without warfarin 1.5 mg/kg SC daily	
	VTE prophylaxis (medical with restricted mobility, hip/knee replacement, abdominal surgery)	30 mg SC q 12 h or 40 mg SC daily	0.6–1.0 IU/mL (b.i.d.) > 1.0 IU/mL (daily)
Tinzaparin† (Innohep)	Treatment of VTE with or without PE	175 IU/kg SC daily for 6 days or until adequately anticoagulated with warfarin	0.85 IU/mL

*Reduce dose for platelet count between 50,000 and 100,000 /mm³; discontinue for platelet count < 50,000/mm³.

†Discontinue for platelet count < 100,000/mm³.

IU, international units; MI, myocardial infarction; PE, pulmonary embolism; VTE, venous thromboembolism.

or LMWH. Additionally, postoperative patients receiving heparin are higher risk than medical or pregnant patients. Consideration should be given to scheduled platelet count monitoring in higher risk patients.

Both UFH and LMWH are contraindicated in patients with a history of HIT, although such patients who test as HIT antibody negative and require cardiac surgery may receive UFH intraoperatively. However, pre- and postoperative anticoagulation should be accomplished with non-heparin agents.

Mild elevations of hepatic transaminases are not uncommon in patients receiving IV or SC heparin. Therefore aminotransferase levels should be interpreted with caution in heparinized patients in whom the differential diagnosis includes myocardial infarction, liver disease, and/or pulmonary emboli. Heparin may inhibit aldosterone synthesis and cause hyperkalemia. Patients with severe renal or hepatic disease may be treated cautiously with heparin as the clinical situation dictates.

Independent of its anticoagulant effects, heparin binds directly to osteoblasts, suppressing osteoblast formation and activating osteoclasts; long-term use can cause clinically relevant osteopenia. These events are less likely with LMWH. Heparin also interacts with plasma and subendothelial matrix proteins, fibrin, and platelets; this is thought to explain some of the individual variability in response to standardized dosing that occurs.

Heparin is contraindicated in patients with thrombocytopenia and uncontrollable bleeding that is not due to disseminated intravascular coagulation; it should be avoided during and after surgery of the eye, brain, or spinal cord. UFH is classified as Pregnancy Category C, does not cross the placental barrier, and is not excreted in breast milk. LMWHs dalteparin, enoxaparin, and tinzaparin are classified as Pregnancy Category B and do not cross the placenta. Small amounts of dalteparin have been found in breast milk; however, it is not known whether the small amount of anti–factor Xa has clinical effects on a nursing infant. It is not known whether tinzaparin or enoxaparin are secreted in breast milk.

Drug Interactions

Drugs that decrease platelet aggregation should be used cautiously, if at all, in patients receiving UFH and LMWH; platelet aggregation reactions are the only hemostatic defense available in a heparinized patient. The use of platelet inhibitors such as acetylsalicylic acid, dextran, phenylbutazone, and nonsteroidal anti-inflammatory agents should be avoided. Heparin may prolong PT; if heparin is given with dicoumarol or warfarin sodium, accurate prothrombin values will not be obtained unless blood is drawn at least 5 hours after the last IV heparin dose or 24 hours after the last SC heparin dose.

Digitalis, tetracyclines, nicotine, and antihistamines may counteract the anticoagulant effects of heparin. Coadministration of heparin and IV nitroglycerin may decrease the partial thromboplastin time, with a rebound increase after nitroglycerin is discontinued; careful monitoring and dose adjustment are required.

Guidelines and Precautions

Laboratory Monitoring

A clinician uses various laboratory tests to guide anticoagulation therapy, including activated partial thromboplastin time, anti-Xa activity, and activated clotting time (ACT).[7] Traditionally, the aPTT is used to determine whether therapeutic levels of heparin have been achieved. Generally, a clotting time of 1.8 to 2.5 times the normal mean aPTT is considered therapeutic; however, variations in laboratory reagents and instrumentation can occasionally render even these values subtherapeutic. An aPTT of 1.5 times the baseline value is associated with heparin levels of 0.2 to 0.4 unit/mL or anti-Xa levels of 0.3 to 0.7 unit/mL. The anti-Xa assay may be used in patients with heparin resistance or who have underlying conditions that may alter the aPTT test. In addition, anti-Xa activity may be monitored in patients receiving LMWH or who are pregnant, obese, very young, very old, or who have altered renal function. Therapeutic reference ranges for anti-Xa levels vary based on the type of heparin being used, time of sample collection, and patient condition. The ACT is used to determine clotting status when very high doses of heparin are required during interventional cardiology procedures or cardiopulmonary bypass.

When low-dose SC UFH is given as prophylaxis, the aPTT is not prolonged and laboratory testing is usually withheld. It should be noted that in up to 15% of patients, even small-dose SC heparin can result in measurable changes in coagulation as assessed by aPTT. A smaller group of patients who receive low-dose SC heparin (up to 4%) may achieve therapeutic concentrations within 2 hours of administration.

The aPTT is also relatively insensitive to the use of LMWH, and laboratory testing is rarely indicated during therapy. In renally impaired or severely obese patients, anti–factor Xa levels can be used to monitor for the anticoagulation effects of LMWH. Anti–factor Xa levels should be drawn approximately 4 hours after a SC injection.

Protamine Reversal of UFH

Protamine sulfate is a basic protein produced from salmon sperm that binds to acidic heparin to form a salt. One milligram of protamine neutralizes 80 to 100 units of UFH. Because of the short half-life of heparin, reversal doses need to be based only on the last several hours of heparin infused. Neutralization of SC heparin may require a prolonged infusion of protamine. Onset time is approximately 5 minutes with a duration of 2 hours. No more than 50 mg protamine should be given in a 10-minute period; full doses are best administered over 20 to 30 minutes. If more protamine is given than required to neutralize heparin, protamine's weak anticoagulant effect and platelet inhibition may contribute to a prolonged ACT.[13] A single dose of protamine is cleared by the reticuloendothelial system in approximately 20 minutes, which is shorter than heparin's clearance. Heparin rebound may occur several hours after cardiopulmonary bypass; consequently, a continuous postoperative protamine infusion may be required in some cases.

Severe adverse effects from protamine include hypotension, bradycardia, acute pulmonary vasoconstriction, right ventricular failure, or anaphylaxis and occur primarily when the drug is administered too rapidly.[14] Patients who have previously received protamine-containing insulin (e.g., neutral protamine Hagedorn), have had a vasectomy or are infertile, have known sensitivity to fish, or have a history of a reaction to protamine are at higher risk of exhibiting allergic reactions, including anaphylaxis. The most common factor predisposing to an anaphylactic reaction to protamine sulfate is prior treatment with neutral protamine Hagedorn insulin. These risks should be identified during the preoperative assessment so that at-risk patients can be pretreated with steroids and antihistamines.

Reversal of LMWH

LMWH agents are not reliably reversible. Protamine neutralizes about 60% of anti–factor Xa activity of LMWH; however, protamine use has failed to decrease bleeding in animal models.[7] In the event a clinical situation requires neutralization of LMWH given within the last 8 hours, the recommended approach is to administer protamine 1 mg for each 100 anti–factor Xa units of LMWH (1 mg enoxaparin is equal to about 100 anti–factor Xa units). If bleeding continues, an additional 0.5 mg protamine for each 100 anti–factor Xa units of LMWH may be given.

Dosage and Administration

Unfractionated Heparin

Recommendations for dosing UFH vary based on the specific indications but are always weight based. The risks of heparin-induced bleeding increase with the dose and with concurrent antithrombolytic or glycoprotein IIb/IIIa inhibitor therapy.

Low-Molecular-Weight Heparin

LMWH doses may be fixed or weight based (when used for therapeutic effect). Although LMWH dosing in thromboprophylaxis is generally fixed, the very obese patient may need a higher dose to achieve an appropriate anti-Xa level. Patients with renal insufficiency must be dosed with caution; anti–factor Xa clearance is reduced in this population. Renal patients have a higher risk of bleeding complications and hemorrhage when given LMWH; therefore it is prudent to monitor anti–factor Xa levels. The timing of neuraxial block, catheter placement, and/or catheter removal may need modification in renal patients on these drugs. General guidelines for dosing LMWH are summarized in Table 22-2.[7] LMWH cannot be used interchangeably (unit for unit) with UFH or each other because they differ in manufacturing process, molecular weight distribution, anti-Xa activity, units, and dosage.

Anesthesia Implications

Anesthesia considerations for patients receiving anticoagulants are evidence based and focus on the prevention or recognition of bleeding in closed spaces. The current guidelines for the use of regional anesthesia in the anticoagulated patient were published in 2004 and are summarized in Table 22-3.[15,16] The reader can access directly the Second Consensus Conference Proceedings at http://www.asra.com/consensus-statements.

Fondaparinux (Arixtra)

Fondaparinux sodium is a synthetic antithrombin III–dependent factor Xa inhibitor used for the prophylaxis and/or treatment of DVT or pulmonary embolism, primarily in the context of major orthopedic surgery. The drug is a pentasaccharide that contains the five-sugar sequence that forms the binding site for antithrombin III in the heparin molecule.[8,11]

Mechanism of Action

Fondaparinux exerts antithrombotic activity by selectively inhibiting factor Xa through binding to antithrombin III. Fondaparinux potentiates by at least 300-fold the neutralization of factor Xa by antithrombin III, thereby interrupting the coagulation process.

Clinical Pharmacology

Pharmacokinetics

Fondaparinux is given by SC injection and has 100% bioavailability. In patients being treated with fondaparinux, peak plasma concentration is achieved about 3 hours after a daily dose of 2.5 mg. In patients receiving higher doses in a weight-based dosing protocol, the body weight–adjusted doses provide similar mean minimum (0.46–0.62 mg/L) and peak (1.2–1.26 mg/L) steady-state values. The apparent volume of distribution of IV or SC fondaparinux is 7 to 11 L, which reflects its primary distribution in the blood and minimal distribution into the extracellular fluid.

Pharmacodynamics

Fondaparinux has significant anti-Xa activity that increases with increasing drug concentrations. Fondaparinux has no known effect on platelet function and does not inactivate thrombin.

Metabolism and Elimination

In patients with normal renal function, approximately 75% of a single dose of fondaparinux is eliminated unchanged in the urine within 72 hours. The elimination half-life of fondaparinux is 17 to 21 hours. The clearance of the drug is prolonged by 25%, 40%, and 55% in patients with mild, moderate, or severe renal impairment, respectively; therefore dose adjustments are required in renally impaired patients. No dosage adjustment is required in patients with moderate hepatic impairment. In patients older than 75 years, total clearance may be reduced by up to 25%, and in patients weighing less than 50 kg, total clearance is decreased by 30%.

Clinical Uses and Indications

Fondaparinux is indicated for prophylaxis of DVT in patients undergoing major orthopedic or abdominal surgery. It is also used in the treatment of DVT or acute pulmonary embolism when administered in conjunction with warfarin.

Side Effects and Contraindications

The most common side effect of fondaparinux is a bleeding complication followed by mild local irritation at the injection site. Fondaparinux is contraindicated in severe renal impairment, active major bleeding, bacterial endocarditis, thrombocytopenia associated with positive antiplatelet

Table 22-3 Guidelines for the Use of Regional Anesthesia in the Anticoagulated Patient

Anticoagulant	Neuraxial Block or Catheter Placement	Catheter Removal	Anticoagulation Monitoring
Unfractionated heparin Intravenous	Neuraxial procedure at least 1 h before heparinization (if bloody or traumatic block, discuss risk/benefit with surgeon) Use minimal effective concentration of local anesthetic Consider delaying heparin until after block if technical difficulty anticipated	Discontinue heparin 2–4 h before removal and assess coagulation status; monitor for sensory and motor function for at least 12 h after removal Reheparinization allowed 1 h after catheter removal if necessary	IV: aPTT > 1.5× baseline value Heparin level 0.2–0.4 U/mL Anti-Xa level 0.3–0.7 U/mL
Low-dose SC	If receiving SC heparin > 4 days, platelet count before block placement	If receiving SC heparin > 4 days, platelet count before catheter removal	SC: aPTT not usually prolonged and not monitored Platelet count if on SC heparin > 4 days
Anticoagulation for cardiopulmonary bypass	Avoid neuraxial anesthesia with known coagulopathy of any origin Neuraxial procedure > 1 h before systemic heparinization Delay surgery 24 h if block bloody or traumatic	Epidural catheter removed when normal coagulation restored; monitor closely for signs and symptoms of hematoma formation	Tight control of heparin with ACT and pharmacologic reversal required
Low-molecular-weight heparin Preoperative	*LMWH thromboprophylaxis doses:* Needle placement should be delayed 10–12 h after last LMWH dose *LMWH treatment doses:* Delay needle placement at least 24 h after last dose Avoid neuraxial techniques if patient received LMWH within 2 h preoperatively (peak anticoagulant activity) Delay initiation of LMWH if blood is present during needle or catheter placement; discuss with surgeon		No specific tests; concomitant use of antiplatelet or oral anticoagulants increases risks
Postoperative	For planned twice daily dosing: first dose LMWH no sooner than 24 h postop	Remove catheter before initiating first prophylactic dose Continuous epidural may remain overnight; remove catheter 2 h before first dose	
	For planned single daily dosing: first dose LMWH may be given 6–8 h postop with second dose no sooner than 24 h after first dose	Catheter may remain in place postop but must be removed no sooner than 10–12 h after the last dose of LMWH Next LMWH dose must be delayed until 2 h after catheter removal	

antibody testing, and body weight less than 50 kg. Like all anticoagulants, fondaparinux should be used with extreme caution in patients who have a bleeding diathesis or who take other drugs that increase the risks of hemorrhage. The risk of bleeding is higher in renally impaired or low-weight patients; serum creatinine levels and stool occult blood tests are recommended. Because thrombocytopenia can occur with the use of fondaparinux, routine complete blood counts with platelet count are recommended.

Drug Interactions

Fondaparinux should not be administered in the presence of other agents that enhance the risk of hemorrhage. If this occurs, the patient must be carefully monitored for signs and symptoms of hemorrhage.

Guidelines and Precautions

Laboratory Monitoring

In the event that an explanation for unexpected bleeding is necessary when a patient is receiving fondaparinux, the only useful laboratory measurement is the anti-Xa activity assay. Because fondaparinux binds only to antithrombin III and not thrombin, the aPTT is not helpful.

Like UFH and LMWH, fondaparinux sodium anticoagulation puts the patient at risk for spinal or epidural hematoma when neuraxial anesthesia is used. Neuraxial complications may also occur when fondaparinux is given in the presence of nonsteroidal anti-inflammatory drugs, platelet inhibitors, or other anticoagulants. Careful consideration of the risk versus benefit of neuraxial anesthesia is required in the presence of fondaparinux; because this drug is a member of the heparinoid family, it is prudent to follow the guidelines for LMWH (Table 22-3).

Dosage and Administration

For DVT prophylaxis after hip fracture, total hip or knee replacement, or abdominal surgery, a daily dose of 2.5 mg fondaparinux is administered subcutaneously no sooner than 6 to 8 hours after surgery. Therapy is usually continued for 5 to 9 days for joint replacement or abdominal surgery and up to 30 to 32 days for hip fracture surgery.

In patients with symptomatic DVT or pulmonary embolism, recommended doses are weight based (5 mg for weight < 50 kg, 7.5 mg for weight 50–100 kg, 10 mg for weight > 100 kg) and administered once daily. Expect concomitant treatment with warfarin to begin within 72 hours and fondaparinux to be continued until the international normalized ratio (INR) is therapeutic (usually 5–9 days).

Anesthesia Implications

Because fondaparinux is essentially a truncated heparin molecule, all safety considerations in regard to regional anesthesia given for heparin apply.

Warfarin

Dicoumarol was discovered in spoiled sweet clover after it was found to cause hemorrhagic disease in cattle. Its synthetic congener, warfarin, was initially used as rat poison and subsequently developed as a human anticoagulant. Warfarin is prepared as a racemic mixture, with the levorotatory (S) form four times more potent than the dextrorotatory (R) form. In addition, warfarin is highly bound to albumin; both of these characteristics contribute to its potential for significant drug interactions.

Mechanism of Action

Warfarin blocks multiple sites in the vitamin K–dependent anticoagulation process by preventing the activation of prothrombin (factor II); factors VII, IX, and X; and proteins C and S. Warfarin antagonizes vitamin K epoxide reductase, the enzyme that catalyzes the regeneration of reduced vitamin K, which is a cofactor in the γ-carboxylation of glutamate residues of multiple clotting enzymes. The degree of enzyme inhibition depends on the dose of warfarin administered and the patient's genotypes for *VKORC1* (the gene that codes for vitamin K epoxide reductase) and *CYP2C9* (the cytochrome family that forms the primary route of metabolism for the more potent [S] enantiomer).[17,18] Protein C and protein S are vitamin K–dependent serine proteases that become activated by thrombin. Activated protein C with cofactors protein S and phospholipids act to degrade factors Va and VIIIa, thereby conferring antithrombotic activity. It is because of warfarin's effects on proteins C and S that heparin is commonly coadministered during warfarin induction.

Factors II, VII, IX, and X and proteins C and S have long half-lives (Table 22-4), which explains the delayed response to warfarin therapy. Clinical effects are not evident until both factor synthesis is partially inhibited and the existing vitamin K–dependent factors are depleted. In addition, factors that are secreted are under-carboxylated and have less biologic activity. A large initial dose of warfarin (0.75 mg/kg) hastens the onset of anticoagulation; however, beyond this, higher loading doses serve only to increase the duration of a relative overdose.

Table 22-4 Approximate Half-Lives of Vitamin K–Dependent Clotting Factors

Factor	Half-life (h)
Factor II	60
Factor VII	4–6
Factor IX	24
Factor X	40–72
Protein C	8
Protein S	30

Clinical Pharmacology

Pharmacokinetics

Warfarin (Coumadin) is administered orally as a salt and has nearly 100% bioavailability, although the presence of food can decrease its absorption rate. Concentrations peak at 2 to 8 hours after ingestion. Warfarin is 98% to 99% bound to plasma proteins, primarily albumin, so that the volume of distribution is close to that of the albumin space (0.14 L/kg). Free warfarin is taken up by the liver where it inhibits vitamin K epoxide reductase.

Fetal plasma levels of warfarin approach maternal levels. Because of this, γ-carboxyglutamate residues in fetal blood and bone may be affected by circulating warfarin; fetal hemorrhage, abnormal bone formation, or other fetal defects may occur. Warfarin is classified as Pregnancy Category X and is not found in breast milk.

Pharmacodynamics

By antagonizing the vitamin K cycle, warfarin effectively decreases the formation of vitamin K–dependent clotting factors by 30% to 50%. The remaining factors produced are inadequately carboxylated and have 10% to 40% less biologic activity. These actions result in a prolonged PT and INR.

Metabolism and Elimination

Different cytochrome families metabolize warfarin's R and S enantiomers. The potent S-warfarin is hydroxylated by *CYP2C9* and the metabolites are excreted in the bile. The weaker R-warfarin is metabolized by *CYP1A1*, *CYP1A2*, and *CYP3A4* to an inactive alcohol that is excreted in the urine (Figure 22-3).

At least two single nucleotide polymorphisms (SNPs) have been identified in the *CYP2C9* allele that confer impaired metabolism of S-warfarin. Patients with one or both of these SNPs (*CYP2C9*2* or *CYP2C9*3*) have reduced

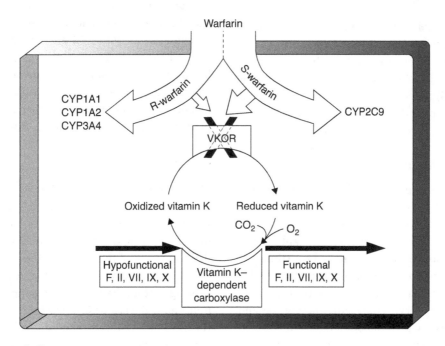

Figure 22-3 Warfarin metabolism.

Source: Reprinted from *The Pharmacogenomics Journal*, Vol 4, Issue 4, BF Gage and CS Eby, The genetics of vitamin K antagonists, figure 1, Liver metabolism of warfarin and vitamin K cycle, 2004, with permission from Nature Publishing Group.

warfarin requirements and a two- to threefold elevated risk of bleeding during warfarin initiation. As many as 10% to 20% of Whites present with a *CYP2C9* SNP, whereas less than 5% of African Americans and Asians are affected. *CYP2C9* SNPs do not alter the risks associated with long-term warfarin therapy but are thought to explain about 10% of dose variation between patients.[19]

VKORC1 polymorphisms generally make the enzyme less susceptible to inhibition by warfarin; *VKORC1* SNPs may explain up to 30% of the dose variation between patients. Overall, a variety of factors impacts warfarin pharmacokinetics, including *CYP2C9* and *VKORC1* SNPs, race, smoking status, amiodarone, and other drugs. An interactive dosing algorithm based on these and other factors is available at the nonprofit website http://www.WarfarinDosing.org.

Warfarin is cleared slowly, averaging 0.045 mL/min/kg, with a half-life ranging from 25 to 60 hours (mean, 40 hours); the duration of action is 4 to 5 days. The elderly (age > 60 years) are more sensitive to the effects of warfarin as are patients of Asian descent. Renal dysfunction is of minimal concern because warfarin is not dependent on renal function for clearance. Hepatic dysfunction may exacerbate warfarin's effects through both impaired synthesis of clotting factors and decreased metabolism.

Clinical Uses and Indications

Warfarin is indicated for (1) the prophylaxis and treatment of venous thrombosis and pulmonary embolism, (2) the prophylaxis and treatment of thromboembolic complications associated with atrial fibrillation and/or cardiac valve replacement, and (3) to reduce the risk of death, recurrent myocardial infarction, and thromboembolic events after myocardial infarction (stroke, systemic embolization).

Side Effects and Contraindications

The most common side effect of warfarin is bleeding, and, like heparin, this drug should only be used in patients in whom the benefit of anticoagulation outweighs the risk of bleeding. Warfarin is contraindicated in pregnant patients as noted previously as well as in threatened abortion, preeclampsia, and eclampsia. Warfarin is contraindicated in the presence of preexisting coagulopathy of any origin, recent or impeding surgery in the central nervous system or eye, or major surgery with the potential for blood loss. Rarely, necrosis or gangrene in skin or other tissues may occur. The use of warfarin may enhance the release of atherosclerotic plaque, creating complications from systemic microembolization, including the "purple toes syndrome,"

a reversible blue-tinged discoloration of the plantar surfaces and sides of toes. Because of its narrow therapeutic window, warfarin should not be used in the absence of adequate laboratory facilities or by patients who may be unsupervised or unable to cooperate with the drug therapy.

Drug Interactions

Warfarin is associated with extensive drug interactions that are both pharmacokinetic and pharmacodynamic in nature and that may increase or decrease the PT. In addition, disease and nutritional states and the use of botanicals have been reported to alter the response to warfarin. The more common conditions and/or drug interactions that affect PT and INR are delineated in Table 22-5.

Specific botanicals may also affect warfarin therapy. Bromelains, danshen, dong quai (*Angelica sinensis*), garlic, ginkgo biloba, ginseng, and cranberry products are associated most often with an increase in the effects of warfarin. Coenzyme Q10 (ubidecarenone) and St. John's wort are associated most often with a decrease in the effects of warfarin. Warfarin may increase the effects of hypoglycemic agents and anticonvulsants as a result of decreased metabolism or excretion.

Guidelines and Precautions

Because warfarin has a narrow therapeutic range, precaution must be used in patients with a high risk of bleeding, including those with INR greater than 4.0, age at least 65 years, history of highly variable INRs, gastrointestinal bleeding, hypertension, cerebrovascular disease, serious heart disease, anemia, malignancy, trauma, renal insufficiency, concomitant use of other anticoagulant or antiplatelet drugs, and long duration of warfarin therapy.

Laboratory Monitoring

The PT reflects the depression of vitamin K–dependent factors. Because of variations in methodology that make PT values from different laboratories incomparable, a system of standardizing the PT was developed and is based on the determination of INR.[20] INR values from 2 to 3 are associated with a 30% to 50% reduction in vitamin K–dependent clotting factors. Fasting blood samples, obtained 8 to 14 hours after the last dose of warfarin, are used to determine the INR. The PT/INR should be determined daily until results stabilize within the therapeutic range, which varies based on the indication for warfarin. Once stability is reached, PT/INR should be monitored every 1 to 4 weeks. Because of extensive drug interactions, any change in a

Table 22-5 Perioperative Drug Interactions and Conditions That Alter Oral Anticoagulation

Increased PT/INR	Decreased PT/INR
Cancer	Edema
Collagen vascular disease	Hypothyroidism
Concomitant blood dyscrasias	Increased ingestion of vitamin K–rich foods
Congestive heart failure	Nephrotic syndrome
Diarrhea	
Elevated temperature	Adrenal cortical steroid inhibitors
Hepatitis/jaundice	Antacids
Hyperthyroidism	Antianxiety agents
Poor nutritional state	Antiarrhythmics*
Vitamin K deficiency	Antibiotics*
	Anticonvulsants*
Antiasthma drugs (zileuton, zafirlukast)	Antidepressants*
Analgesics	Antihistamines
Anesthetics, inhalation (halothane)	Antineoplastics*
Antiarrhythmics* (amiodarone)	Cyclophosphamide*
Antibiotics*	Alcohol*
Aminoglycosides	Antipsychotic medications
Cephalosporins, IV	Antithyroid drugs*
Macrolides	Barbiturates
Penicillins, IV	Diuretics*
Quinolones	Enteral nutritional supplements
Sulfonamides	Fungal medications, systemic*
Tetracyclines	Gastric acidity and peptic ulcer agents*
Anticoagulants	Hypnotics*
Anticonvulsants* (phenytoin, valproate)	Hypolipidemics*
Antidepressants* (SSRIs, MAOIs)	Bile acid-binding resins*
Beta-blockers	HMG-CoA reductase inhibitors
COX inhibitors	Atorvastatin*
Diabetic agents, oral	Pravastatin*
Diuretics*	Immunosuppressives
GI drugs* (cimetidine, ranitidine, omeprazole, pantoprazole, rabeprazole)	Azathioprine
Gout treatment (sulfinpyrazone)	Oral contraceptives, estrogen containing
Hypnotics*	Selective estrogen receptor modulators
Hypolipidemics*	Steroids, adrenocortical*
Bile acid binding resins	Tuberculosis agents* (rifampin)
Fibric acid derivatives	Vitamins*
HMG Co-A reductase inhibitors	Vitamin C (high dose)
Narcotics, long acting (tramadol)	Vitamin K
NSAIDs (phenylthiazone, aspirin in high doses)	
Steroids, anabolic and adrenocortical*	
Vitamin E	

*Increased and decreased PT/INR have been reported.

COX, cyclooxygenase; GI, gastrointestinal; MAOI, monoamine oxidase inhibitor; NSAID, nonsteroidal anti-inflammatory drug; SSRI, selective serotonin reuptake inhibitor.

patient's medications (prescribed and over the counter) should be followed by additional PT/INR testing.

Because of the length of time to reach therapeutic levels of warfarin, rapid anticoagulation is usually accomplished with heparin. Conversion to warfarin may occur concurrently or be delayed; however, warfarin therapy is generally overlapped with heparin for 4 to 5 days until the PT/INR is considered therapeutic.

Reversal of Warfarin-Induced Anticoagulation

Perioperative preparation for surgery may dictate the need to reverse warfarin anticoagulation.[3] Withholding the drug for 3 days usually results in a normal INR except in the presence of severe liver disease or vitamin K deficiency. Faster reversal requires the oral administration of vitamin K_1 (phytonadione), which can bring the INR to normal within 24 to 48 hours. Emergent reversal necessitates direct restoration of vitamin K–dependent factors via infusion of 10 to 20 mL/kg fresh frozen plasma supplemented with 10 mg IV vitamin K_1 given slowly. Additional fresh frozen plasma may be needed because clotting factors may be consumed at a rate exceeding the metabolism of existing anticoagulant. Phytonadione given intravenously confers a risk of anaphylactoid reactions and must be given with caution.

Dosage and Administration

Initial and maintenance dosing of warfarin are individualized according the each patient's PT/INR responses to the drug and vary according to the indications for use. Using large loading doses is not recommended because this may increase the incidence of hemorrhagic complications. Generally, warfarin therapy is initiated with a dose of 2 to 5 mg/day with adjustments based on PT/INR measurement. Patients with known variants of *CYP2C9* or *VKORC1* alleles, the elderly, debilitated patients, or those with potential for exaggerated responses should be induced with lower doses. Maintenance therapy usually requires a dose of 2 to 10 mg/day. Occasional patients require very high doses to maintain the PT/INR in a therapeutic range; warfarin resistance may be due to excessive vitamin K ingestion from diet or supplements, laboratory error, or genetic variations.

Although generally administered orally, warfarin is available for parenteral use in patients who cannot receive oral drugs. IV doses are the same as oral doses as a result of the drug's bioavailability. After reconstitution, parenteral warfarin may be administered intravenously slowly over 1 to 2 minutes. Intramuscular administration is not recommended.

Anesthesia Implications

The current guidelines for the use of regional anesthesia in the anticoagulated patient were published in 2004 and are summarized in Table 22-3.

Hirudins

Hirudins are potent direct thrombin inhibitors derived from the salivary glands of medicinal leeches; unlike heparin, which requires antithrombin III for its activity, one hirudin molecule binds directly to one thrombin molecule, whether it is circulating or bound in fibrin.[21] Hirudin has no effect on platelets and does not induce thrombocytopenia. Because biologic sources of hirudin are limited, synthetic analogs have been developed (lepirudin, bivalirudin). These drugs are generally used in the cardiac catheterization suite and for patients with a history of HIT with thromboembolic complications.

Mechanism of Action

Lepirudin (Refludan), a recombinant DNA derivative of hirudin, blocks both thrombin's catalytic site and its substrate recognition site, making it highly potent and almost irreversible. Bivalirudin (Angiomax) is a synthetic hirudin that also binds to both sites on thrombin but has a lower affinity for the active site. The reversibility of bivalirudin's binding is thought to reduce the risk of bleeding. Because hirudins bind to two sites on thrombin, they are classified as bivalent direct thrombin inhibitors.

Clinical Pharmacology

Pharmacokinetics

Lepirudin has a plasma half-life of 40 minutes when given intravenously and 120 minutes when given subcutaneously; its distribution includes the extracellular fluid compartment. Bivalirudin has a half-life in patients with normal renal function of 25 minutes; in moderate renal impairment, the half-life is 34 minutes, and in dialysis patients, 3.5 hours.

Pharmacodynamics

Hirudins prolong the aPTT, PT, ACT, and thrombin time; thrombin time may exceed 200 seconds even at low doses. Therapeutic responses are defined by the aPTT ratio, which depends on plasma concentration and renal function.

Metabolism and Elimination

Almost 50% of an administered dose of lepirudin is excreted renally; patients with marked renal insufficiency or hemodialysis may have elimination half-lives up to 2 days. Clearance is also reduced in women and the elderly. Bivalirudin is partially eliminated renally and partly by proteolytic cleavage. Clearance is reduced by about 20% in moderate to severe renal insufficiency and by 80% in dialysis patients.

Clinical Uses and Indications

Lepirudin is indicated for anticoagulation in patients with HIT and associated thromboembolic disease. Bivalirudin is indicated for anticoagulation in patients undergoing percutaneous transluminal coronary angioplasty or percutaneous coronary intervention either with glycoprotein IIb/IIIa inhibitors or in patients at risk for HIT. Bivalirudin has been studied with and is intended for use with aspirin.

Side Effects and Contraindications

The most important side effect of hirudin therapy is bleeding, including life-threatening intracranial hemorrhage. Patients with bleeding diathesis, severe uncontrolled hypertension, recent stroke, neuraxial surgery/procedures, recent large vessel or organ biopsy, recent major bleeding, active peptic ulcer, bacterial endocarditis, or advanced renal impairment should be carefully assessed before treatment. Formation of antihirudin antibodies has occurred when patients with HIT are treated with lepirudin and bivalirudin. Delayed renal elimination of lepirudin–antihirudin complexes may increase the anticoagulant effect. Patients with serious liver cirrhosis may exhibit enhanced anticoagulant effects. Allergy, hypersensitivity, and anaphylaxis have occurred with initial, second, and subsequent exposures to the drug. Allergic reactions may be more likely in patients who also received thrombolytics or contrast media.

Lepirudin and bivalirudin are classified as Pregnancy Category B. It is not known whether lepirudin or bivalirudin cross the placenta or are secreted in human breast milk.

Drug Interactions

Concurrent treatment with thrombolytics, vitamin K antagonists, and drugs that affect platelet function may increase the risk of bleeding complications and enhance the effect of lepirudin on the aPTT.

Guidelines and Precautions

Laboratory Monitoring

The lepirudin drug infusion rate should be adjusted according to the aPTT ratio (patient aPTT at a given time over the aPTT reference value, usually median of the laboratory normal range for aPTT). When administering bivalirudin to patients with renal impairment, the ACT should be used to monitor therapy.

Dosage and Administration

Lepirudin is administered as an IV loading dose of 0.4 mg/kg slowly followed by 0.15 mg/kg/h as a continuous infusion for 2 to 10 days. Maximal loading dose should not exceed 44 mg, and maximum infusion dose is 16.5 mg/h. Doses should be reduced in the presence of known or suspected renal impairment; loading dose should be reduced to 0.2 mg/kg. Target aPTT during treatment is 1.5 to 2.5. Bivalirudin is administered as an IV loading dose of 0.75 mg/kg slowly followed by an infusion of 1.75 mg/kg/h. Bivalirudin dosing should be reduced in the presence of renal dysfunction.

Neither lepirudin nor bivalirudin are reversible. In the event of life-threatening bleeding in the presence of excessive plasma levels, the drug should be terminated, aPTT or ACT determined, hemoglobin measured, and preparation made for blood transfusion and treatment for shock.

Anesthesia Implications

Although no specific guidelines have been suggested around the use of neuraxial and peripheral techniques in the presence of hirudins, it would seem prudent to verify that the effects have dissipated before using these regional techniques.

Argatroban

Mechanism of Action

Argatroban is a synthetic direct thrombin inhibitor that binds reversibly to thrombin's active site. It is classified as a univalent direct thrombin inhibitor because it binds to a single site on thrombin; argatroban does not require antithrombin III for its activity.[22] Argatroban inhibits both circulating and fibrin-bound thrombin. Like the hirudins, argatroban does not cause thrombocytopenia or generate antibody formation. Argatroban is currently the only univalent direct thrombin inhibitor approved for use in the United States.

Clinical Pharmacology

Pharmacokinetics

Argatroban is distributed into the extracellular fluid with a volume of distribution of 174 mL/kg. It is moderately protein bound, 34% to α_1-acid glycoprotein and 20% to albumin. Total body clearance is about 5.1 mL/kg/min at doses up to 40 μg/kg/min, and the terminal elimination half-life ranges from 39 to 51 minutes. When administered by continuous IV infusion, steady-state levels of drug are generally achieved within 1 to 3 hours and remain stable until the infusion is changed; anticoagulant effects parallel dosing levels at steady state.

Pharmacodynamics

Argatroban exerts its anticoagulant effects by inhibiting thrombin-catalyzed or -induced reactions, including fibrin formation; activation of coagulation factors V, VIII, and XIII; activation of protein C; and platelet aggregation. For infusion doses up to 40 μg/kg/min, argatroban increases the aPTT, ACT, PT, INR, and thrombin time in healthy volunteers and cardiac patients in a dose-dependent fashion.

Metabolism and Elimination

Argatroban is hydroxylated in the liver by *CYP3A4* and *CYP3A5*, creating a primary metabolite that is three to five times weaker than the parent compound. Three other metabolites have been identified in very small amounts in the urine but not in the plasma or feces. Unchanged argatroban appears in the urine within 12 hours of administration; additional unchanged drug is excreted in the feces over the course of days.

Clinical Uses and Indications

Argatroban is indicated for the treatment or prophylaxis of thrombosis in patients with HIT. It is also used to anticoagulate patients with or at risk for HIT who are undergoing percutaneous coronary interventions.

Side Effects and Contraindications

Argatroban, like other anticoagulants, is contraindicated in patients with overt bleeding and in patients who are hypersensitive or allergic to it or its components. Allergic or suspected allergic reactions have occurred almost exclusively when argatroban is used in conjunction with thrombolytics or contrast media. Cough and dyspnea (> 10%), skin reactions (1% to < 10%), and vasodilation (1–10%) have been reported under these conditions.

Drug Interactions

No interactions have been demonstrated between argatroban administered in low doses and either aspirin or acetaminophen. Coadministration of argatroban with other anticoagulants, antiplatelet agents, and thrombolytics may increase the risk of bleeding. Argatroban at 2 μg/kg/min administered over 5 days appeared to have no effect on the pharmacokinetics of oral digoxin. Oral erythromycin (a potent *CYP3A4* and

CYP3A5 inhibitor) had no effect on the pharmacokinetics of argatroban at a does of 1 μg/kg/min. Reexposure to argatroban has not revealed the development of antibodies or any change in its anticoagulant activity. Argatroban is classified as Pregnancy Category B.

Guidelines and Precautions

Laboratory Monitoring

Monitoring anticoagulation during argatroban is based on the dosing schema used. At low doses monitoring and dose adjustments are made using the aPTT, whereas at high doses the ACT is used. In patients with hepatic impairment, initial and maintenance doses should be decreased; no dosage adjustment is required in patients with renal impairment. If a patient who is receiving argatroban is transitioned to warfarin, no loading dose should be administered; warfarin induction should be initiated with the expected daily dose of warfarin.

Dosage and Administration

The argatroban dosing algorithm and monitoring recommendations vary based on the indication for treatment. For the treatment of HIT or heparin-induced thrombocytopenia and thrombosis in patients without hepatic impairment, argatroban is administered at 2 μg/kg/min in a continuous IV infusion. Dose may be increased up to but not exceeding 10 μg/kg/min to adjust aPTT to 1.5 to 3 times the initial baseline value. Generally, the aPTT is checked 2 hours after initiation of therapy and after any dose change. For use during percutaneous coronary intervention, argatroban infusion should start at 25 μg/kg/min after an IV bolus of 350 μg/kg given over 3 to 5 minutes. ACT should be checked within 5 to 10 minutes; if less than 300 seconds, an additional dose of 150 μg/kg may be given while the infusion is increased to 30 μg/kg/min. ACT should again be checked 5 to 10 minutes later. ACT should be maintained between 300 and 450 seconds. Dosing tables are available for both clinical protocols.[23]

Argatroban is not pharmacologically reversible. In the event of overdose with evidence of excessive bleeding, the drug should be discontinued and coagulation testing performed while supportive therapy is begun.

Anesthesia Implications

Although no specific guidelines have been suggested around the use of neuraxial and peripheral techniques in the presence of argatroban, it would seem prudent to verify that the effects have dissipated before using these regional techniques.

Conclusion

Anesthesia providers are often faced with providing a safe and appropriate anesthetic to an anticoagulated patient. In such a patient significant risks may occur with the use of neuraxial and regional anesthesia. Anesthesia providers must maintain a high degree of awareness of all forms of anticoagulation being administered, including their mechanism of action, onset, duration, and metabolism and elimination pathways. Providers must be vigilant in the search for the causes, location, and extent of blood loss in the anticoagulated surgical patient and be alert to the possibility of neurologic complications.

Key Points

- Requisite knowledge for anesthesia providers in caring for patients on anticoagulants includes the duration, route of elimination, time of the last dose, and potential for pharmacologic reversal of the agent.
- A detailed pharmacologic history is crucial to providing safe regional anesthesia in the presence of anticoagulants.

Chapter Questions

1. You are performing a preoperative evaluation of an 85-year-old patient scheduled for an open reduction and internal fixation of the acetabulum under a spinal anesthetic. The patient was injured 4 days before surgery and placed on bed rest with DVT prophylaxis using low-molecular-weight heparin.
   a. Explain if, and/or when, a spinal anesthetic can be administered.
   b. What laboratory tests might be useful to determine the level of anticoagulation present?
   c. Which anticoagulants may be safely used in patients with a history of heparin-induced thrombocytopenia?
2. A patient presents with chest trauma after a motor vehicle accident. Previous history includes aortic valve replacement and warfarin anticoagulation.
   a. What is the most effective method/drug/dose to reverse the warfarin so that surgery can proceed?
   b. What laboratory tests are useful to determine the effectiveness of your therapy?

References

1. Adams GL, Manson RJ, Turner I, Sindram D, Lawson JH. The balance of thrombosis and hemorrhage in surgery. *Hematol Oncol Clin North Am.* 2007;21:13–24.
2. Hoffman M, Monroe DM. Coagulation 2006: a modern view of hemostasis. *Hematol Oncol Clin North Am.* 2007; 21:1–11.
3. Tanaka K, Key N, Levy J. Blood coagulation: hemostasis and thrombin regulation. *Anesth Analg.* 2009;108:1433–1446.
4. Wohner N. Role of cellular elements in thrombus formation and dissolution. *Cardiovasc Hematol Agents Med Chem.* 2008;6:224–228.
5. Wolberg AS. Thrombin generation and fibrin clot structure. *Blood Rev.* 2007;21:131–142.
6. Dahlback B. Blood coagulation. *Lancet.* 2000;355:1627–1632.
7. Hirsch J, Raschke R. Heparin and low-molecular-weight heparin. *Chest.* 2004;126:188S–203S
8. Bombeli T, Spahn DR. Updates in perioperative coagulation: physiology and management of thromboembolism and haemorrhage. *Br J Anaesth.* 2004;93:275–287.
9. Kim V, Spandorfer J. Epidemiology of venous thromboembolic disease. *Emerg Med Cli North Am.* 2001;19:839–859.
10. Chan M, Andreotti F, Becker R. Hypercoagulable states in cardiovascular disease. *Circulation.* 2008;118:2286–2297.
11. Hirsh J, O'Donnell M, Eikelboom JW. Beyond unfractionated heparin and warfarin: current and future advances. *Circulation.* 2007;116:552–560.
12. Warkentin TE, Greinacher A. Heparin-induced thrombocytopenia: recognition, treatment, and prevention. *Chest.* 2004; 126:311S–337S.
13. Levy JH, Tanaka KA. Anticoagulation and reversal paradigms: is too much of a good thing bad? *Anesth Analg.* 2009; 108:692–694.
14. Nybo M, Madsen JS. Serious anaphylactic reactions due to protamine sulfate: a systematic literature review. *Basic Clin Pharmacol Toxicol.* 2008;103:192–196.
15. Horlocker TT, Wedel DJ, Benzon H, et al. Regional anesthesia in the anticoagulated patient: defining the risks (The second ASRA Consensus Conference on Neuraxial Anesthesia and Anticoagulation). *Region Anesth Pain Med.* 2003; 28:172–197.
16. Llau JV, DeAndres J, Gomar C, Gomez-Luque A, Hidalgo F, Torres LM. Anticlotting drugs and regional anaesthetic and analgesic techniques: comparative update of the safety recommendations. *Eur J Anaesthesiol.* 2007;24: 387–398.
17. Gage B, Eby C. The genetics of vitamin K antagonists. *Pharmacogenom J.* 2004;4:224–225.

18. Gage B, Lesko L. Pharmacogenetics of warfarin: regulatory scientific and clinical issues. *J Thromb Thrombol.* 2008;25:45–51.

19. Ansell J, Hirsh J, Poller L, Busssey H, Jacobson A, Hylek E. The pharmacology and management of the vitamin K antagonists. *Chest.* 2004;126:204S–233S.

20. Ng VL. Anticoagulation monitoring. *Clin Lab Med.* 2009; 29:283–204.

21. Nutescu EA, Wittkowsky AK. Direct thrombin inhibitors for anticoagulation. *Ann Pharmacother.* 2004;38:99–109.

22. Vitin A, Dembo G, Vater Y, Martay K, Azamfirei L, Ezri T. Anesthetic implication of the new anticoagulant and antiplatelet drugs. *J Clin Anesth.* 2008;20:228–237.

23. Argatroban [package insert]. Research Triangle Park, NC: GlaxoSmithKline, 2009.

Antiarrhythmics

Mark A. Kossick, DNSc, CRNA, APN

Objectives

After completing this chapter, the reader should be able to

- Identify which antiarrhythmics are listed according to the Vaughan Williams system as class I, II, III, and IV and explain the gross electrophysiologic properties of each.
- Describe the pharmacology of muscarinic receptor antagonists atropine and glycopyrrolate.
- Compare the pharmacology of metoprolol and esmolol, including the dosage, indications, side effects, and management of adverse reactions.
- State which antiarrhythmics are contraindicated in patients with tachyarrhythmias associated with Wolff-Parkinson-White syndrome.
- State the indications and contraindications of calcium channel antagonists verapamil and diltiazem.
- Discuss the current indications and contraindications for lidocaine and procainamide in the management of ventricular arrhythmias.
- List and discuss the therapeutic indications for amiodarone, including risks associated with its administration and potential clinical benefit in treating supraventricular and ventricular tachyarrhythmias.
- Recognize the potential value in the use of dronedarone and how it differs from amiodarone.
- Describe the pharmacology of adenosine as it relates to synthesis, metabolism, pharmacodynamics (receptors), pharmacokinetics, drug interaction, dosage, adverse side effects, and clinical indications.
- Describe the antiarrhythmic effects of vasopressin and magnesium.

Introduction

A comprehensive understanding of the pharmacology of antiarrhythmics is essential for the safe conduct of any anesthetic. According to the literature, the incidence of arrhythmias can range from 16.3% to 84% for patients undergoing cardiac and noncardiac surgery.[1] Fortunately, research has shown the incidence of "serious" arrhythmias is low (< 1%), including encountering such rhythm disturbances as complete atrioventricular (A-V) block with a ventricular escape rhythm, ventricular fibrillation (VF), and torsade de pointes (TdP). Nevertheless, it should be understood that arrhythmias not classified as "serious" (e.g., atrial fibrillation) can still potentially lead to significant morbidity or mortality. Preceding the decision to use antiarrhythmics in all but the acute setting is the need to evaluate and determine the clinical variables believed to be associated with their genesis. Thus an underlying principle should be to first treat the underlying cause of an arrhythmia and, if necessary, intervene with an antiarrhythmic. This principle recognizes the potential for iatrogenic injury secondary to the proarrhythmic effect of antiarrhythmics and the reappearance of a hemodynamically unstable arrhythmia if the underlying cause is not addressed, such as may be observed in a patient experiencing an acute reduction in preload that initiates atrial fibrillation secondary to supply-dependent myocardial injury.

A second prerequisite to appropriate pharmacologic intervention is a correct interpretation of the arrhythmia. An incorrectly identified electrocardiographic rhythm can lead to the administration of contraindicated antiarrhythmics (e.g., TdP incorrectly diagnosed as multifocal ventricular tachycardia [VT]; Figure 23-1). For this reason electrocardiographic arrhythmia strip chart recordings are incorporated throughout this chapter to augment the clinical indication sections for antiarrhythmics. The reader should access other texts for a comprehensive review of techniques used for arrhythmia analysis, including detailed diagnostic criteria.[2,3]

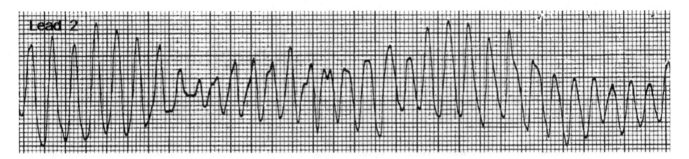

Figure 23-1 This electrocardiographic recording has two plausible interpretations. If the preceding QT interval is not prolonged, it is multifocal ventricular tachycardia. If the QT interval is lengthened, then the correct diagnosis is torsade de pointes.
Source: Reprinted with permission from Kossick, MA. In: *EKG Interpretation: Simple, Thorough, Practical.* 3rd ed. Park Ridge, IL: AANA Publishing. In press.

Muscarinic Receptor Antagonists

Muscarinic receptor antagonists (also known as anticholinergics) are used to produce a positive chronotropic response when a slower heart rate is associated with hemodynamic compromise. They produce their pharmacologic effect by occupying muscarinic cholinergic receptors. This activity prevents the neurotransmitter acetylcholine (ACh) from producing its diverse cholinergic responses, such as a negative chronotropic, negative inotropic, and negative dromotropic effects. Dromotropy refers to conduction velocity, which is slowed in the sinoatrial (S-A) and A-V nodes as a result of cholinergic agonism. Thus anticholinergics that bind to muscarinic receptors do not directly inhibit ACh and do not reduce the quantity released. They also produce minimal blockade at nicotinic cholinergic receptors, such as ganglionic sites.

Several subtype of muscarinic receptors have been identified by molecular cloning of the complementary deoxyribonucleic acids (cDNAs).[4] Of these subtypes M_2, M_3, and M_4 have been found to be distributed in cardiac tissue. The M_2 receptors mediate via ACh a negative chronotropic and inotropic response through a process known as signal transduction. This process represents the transformation of an extracellular signal into an intracellular signal that can be thought of as a cascade of events, including receptor occupancy, biochemical events (regulatory G-protein activation, inhibition of cyclic AMP, enhancement of potassium [K^+] conductance in atrial tissue, and reduction in L-type calcium [Ca^2] channel activity), followed by the drug response. M_2 receptors located in the S-A node slow spontaneous depolarization through hyperpolarization of the cell membrane. Agonism of these receptors by ACh also produces a decrease in atrial and ventricular contractility (the former more so than the latter). Although the binding of atropine to M_2 receptors has been emphasized thus far, it

is noteworthy to state that agonism and/or blockade in the central nervous system of muscarinic receptors can produce dose-dependent systemic effects. This could include the central anticholinergic syndrome, manifested by restlessness, disorientation, seizures, coma, circulatory collapse, and mydriasis along with cycloplegia (loss of accommodation). Fortunately, usual systemic intravenous (IV) doses of atropine (and glycopyrrolate) have little effect on intraocular pressure. For those patients suspected of having central anticholinergic syndrome, physostigmine can be given in an IV dose of 2 mg and repeated as needed.[5]

Atropine can be used for any hemodynamically significant bradyarrhythmia, including sinus bradycardia, junctional rhythms, complete A-V block with a junctional or ventricular escape rhythm, second-degree A-V block type I and II, sinus pause, sinus exit block, and sinus arrest. Atropine can also be used to treat atrial fibrillation or atrial flutter with a slow ventricular response. The standard initial dose is 0.4 to 1.0 mg intravenously and repeated as necessary. The maximum recommended dose is 0.04 mg/kg, which equals approximately 3 mg in a 70-kg patient. The onset time for atropine is relative to the patient's circulation time. Generally speaking, changes in heart rate can be seen within 1 minute or less. The duration of action varies based on the underlying etiology for the bradyarrhythmia. It can last as long as 30 to 60 minutes or as little as 10 minutes. The half-life of atropine is about 4 hours. It is metabolized by the liver with only a small amount excreted unchanged in the urine.

Dosing precautions include not administering a dose of atropine less than 0.5 mg intravenously due to the potential of evoking a paradoxical response. Nevertheless, the most common formulation for atropine is 0.4 mg/mL, and as a matter of standard practice it is unusual for anesthesia providers to use more than one vial of atropine as an initial treatment for bradyarrhythmias. It is possible manufacturers have not changed the concentration of atropine (0.5

mg/mL) due to the limited number of reports by health-care providers of adverse paradoxical responses when atropine is given in an initial dose that is 0.1 mg less (0.4 mg) than what is recommended in many textbooks.

Larger doses of atropine (1.0 mg repeated up to three times) may be necessary with second-degree A-V block type II and third-degree A-V block with a ventricular escape rhythm (whether it is nodal or infranodal in origin). In these advanced forms of heart block the conduction defect is located beneath the A-V node; thus anticholinergics are usually less effective or predictable with increasing ventricular response. Atropine is also a treatment option for asystolic patients; the rationale is that intense vagal stimulation can produce an asystolic state. Finally, atropine is recognized as a treatment option for pulseless electrical activity. Patients with profound bradycardias may have a very feeble pulse, perhaps indiscernible. By accelerating the heart rate with atropine, a pulseless electrical activity rhythm may be converted to a pulsatile/perfusing rhythm.

Glycopyrrolate is a semisynthetic congener of belladonna plants. It is probably the most commonly used muscarinic receptor antagonist by anesthesia providers. One of its principal benefits is it penetrates the blood–brain barrier slowly and incompletely due to its chemical structure (quaternary amine). In contrast, atropine is a naturally occurring tertiary amine alkaloid derived from belladonna and is lipid soluble (Figure 23-2). Similar to atropine, glycopyrrolate can be used to manage bradyarrhythmias of many etiologies. It is typically avoided when an acute increase in heart rate is desired, as seen in patients who present with profound bradycardia (e.g., sinus bradycardia with a ventricular rate of 30 beats/min). Similarly, when a slow ventricular rate is associated with an infranodal conduction defect, such as second-degree A-V block type II, atropine is preferred over glycopyrrolate.

When it is desirable to avoid a tachycardia (even relative), many anesthesia providers select glycopyrrolate (instead of atropine) to treat bradycardias. The reason is that atropine may increase the heart rate to unacceptable levels, even when carefully titrated.[6] Compared with atropine, glycopyrrolate has been shown to be associated with a more stable cardiovascular system and fewer arrhythmias.[7] In patients with risk factors for coronary artery disease, an unintended tachycardia occurring secondary to the use of atropine can be as detrimental (if not more) than the pretreatment bradycardia. This is due to the reduction in coronary blood flow (reduced diastolic filling time) that occurs during an accelerated heart rate as well as an increase in myocardial oxygen consumption. Evidence of an imbalance between oxygen supply and demand can be expressed by T wave inversion and/or ST segment changes on the electrocardiogram (ECG). Granted, some investigators suggest the difference between glycopyrrolate and atropine as it relates to a positive chronotropic response is due to differences in pharmacokinetics and not pharmacodynamics.[8] Also, some research with electroconvulsive therapy patients indicates atropine is preferred over glycopyrrolate in that the latter has been found to be more proarrhythmic in this patient population.[9]

Glycopyrrolate is dosed as 0.2 mg intravenously and repeated as necessary, usually not in excess of a total IV dose of 0.6 mg. The onset time is slightly slower than atropine (2–3 minutes) with about the same duration of action (30–60 minutes). If ineffective, atropine may be substituted for another class of antiarrhythmics, such as β agonists. The elimination half-life of glycopyrrolate is approximately 1.25 hours with about 80% excreted as unchanged drug or active metabolites.[10]

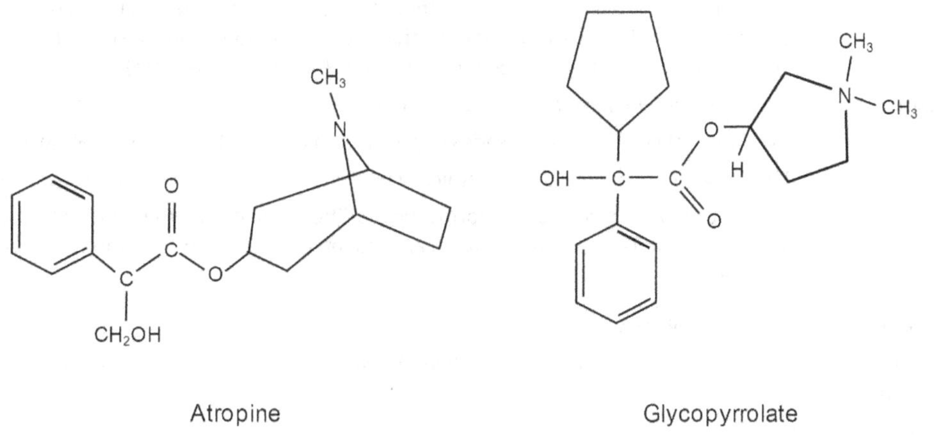

Atropine   Glycopyrrolate

Figure 23-2 Structural and molecular formulas of atropine and glycopyrrolate.

β-Adrenergic Receptor Antagonists

β-Adrenergic blockers can be used to treat both supraventricular and ventricular arrhythmias. Their therapeutic value is recognized by the American College of Cardiology (ACC) and the American Heart Association (AHA) in that they are approved for primary therapy in the management of ventricular arrhythmias.[11] The labeling of ectopy as "ventricular" represents a gross characterization of cardiac depolarizations as being infranodal in origin. Table 23-1 provides a list of specific ventricular arrhythmias that can be treated with β-adrenergic antagonists.

β-Adrenergic antagonists, such as metoprolol (Lopressor), primarily produce their antiarrhythmic effect by blocking specific adrenergic receptors (e.g., β_1). This prevents endogenous catecholamines (epinephrine, norepinephrine) from binding at β_1 receptors located in the heart and producing positive chronotropic and inotropic

responses. Therefore beta-blockers augment coronary perfusion by reducing heart rate (improved coronary perfusion due to increased diastolic filling time) and decreasing myocardial oxygen consumption (diminished contractility). In this manner β antagonists can eliminate some arrhythmias that are induced by myocardial ischemia and/or elevated levels of endogenous catecholamines (supraventricular tachycardia [SVT], catecholaminergic polymorphic VT).

From an electrophysiologic perspective, β-adrenergic antagonists reduce heart rate (decrease automaticity in the S-A node, A-V node, atria, His-Purkinje system, and ventricles) and conductivity (conduction of impulses slowed through the atria, A-V node, His-Purkinje system, and ventricles). On the ECG these changes can be manifested as a slowing of ventricular response and conversion of an arrhythmia (e.g., change from atrial fibrillation with a rapid ventricular response to sinus bradycardia) as well as lengthening of the PR interval (fixed PR intervals in excess

Table 23-1 Ventricular Arrhythmias Treated With β-Adrenergic Antagonists

Classification	Description
Symptomatic nonsustained monomorphic VT*	Morphology of ventricular depolarization is consistent and occurs at a rate > 100 beats/min. The arrhythmia's duration is at least three or more beats and terminates spontaneously in less than 30 s. Symptoms may include hypotension, chest pain, vertigo, or other evidence of decreased cardiac output.
Sustained monomorphic VT	Morphology of ventricular depolarization is consistent and occurs at a rate > 100 beats/min. The arrhythmia's duration is 30 s or more. This can be associated with unstable or stable hemodynamics.
Repetitive monomorphic VT	Frequent ventricular depolarization consisting of nonsustained VT and ventricular ectopy with intervening normal sinus rhythm.
Polymorphic VT	Morphology of rapid ventricular depolarization is erratic (constantly changing) and may appear as an alternating increase and decrease in the amplitude (telescoping) of the "QRS" with perhaps a distinct change in axis (e.g., shift from being mainly positive to negative).
Torsade de pointes†	Identical to what is described for polymorphic VT except associated with a prolonged QT_c interval (> 0.46 s), drug toxicity (e.g., amiodarone), or long QT syndrome.
Catecholaminergic polymorphic VT‡	VT induced by stress (physical or emotional) when the heart rate reaches 120–130 beats/min. Preceding the VT can be isolated PVCs that progress to NSVT, then sustained VT. Also the QRS pattern can change to a bidirectional VT (axis rotates by 180 degrees).
Monomorphic VT storm	Syndrome of two or more episodes of monomorphic VT in 24 h requiring cardioversion.
Polymorphic VT Storm§	Syndrome of two or more episodes of polymorphic VT in 24 h requiring cardioversion.
Incessant VT	VT lasting hours but is hemodynamically stable. Can eventually lead to congestive heart failure.
Idiopathic VT	VT associated with structurally normal hearts. The origin can be the right ventricular or left ventricular outflow tract. The former can present as repetitive monomorphic VT and the latter as incessant VT.

*Initial therapy beta-blockers; if unresponsive, use amiodarone.

†In the presence of long QT syndrome, beta-blockers are a class I recommendation (evidence that a given treatment is beneficial, useful, and effective).

‡Inherited arrhythmogenic disease.

§Single most effective treatment is beta-blockade.

NSVT, nonsustained ventricular tachycardia; PVCs, premature ventricular contractions.

of 200 ms). β Receptor antagonists also reduce the spontaneous rate of depolarization of ectopic pacemakers.

Metoprolol is a second-generation, competitive, selective β_1 antagonist with no appreciable membrane-stabilizing activity. It is extensively metabolized by the liver with only 10% eliminated unchanged in the urine. The half-life of metoprolol is 3 to 4 hours. This half-life increases to 7 to 8 hours if the patient is deficient in CYP2D6, the major enzyme involved with its metabolism.[12] As with other beta-blockers, metoprolol can be used in patients with mild congestive heart failure. The difficulty with this recommendation is ascertaining with gross monitoring (which is common for most anesthetics) or minimal diagnostic workup when a patient has extended beyond "mild" congestive heart failure. Supraventricular tachyarrhythmias that may be treated with β-adrenergic receptor antagonists are listed in Table 23-2. The recommended dose of metoprolol for supraventricular tachyarrhythmias is 5 mg intravenously over 5 minutes with a maximum dose of 15 mg. During a volatile anesthetic with previously administered opioid, as little as 1 mg of metoprolol has been seen to sustain a reduction in heart rate.

Unlike the first-generation beta-blocker propranolol (Inderal), side effects of second-generation β receptor antagonists involving β_2 receptors are less common. This difference is due to the β_1 selectivity of second-generation adrenergic blockers (e.g., metoprolol, esmolol). Use of larger doses of selective β_1 drugs can lead to antagonism of β_2 receptors and subsequent undesirable side effects, including bronchospasm, delay in recovery from hypoglycemia, attenuation of glycogenolysis and gluconeogenesis (promotes hypoglycemia), and decreased secretion of insulin by the beta cells of the islets of Langerhans (leads to an increase in serum glucose), the greater of the two glucose responses being hypoglycemia. For this reason, along with β_1 blockade masking the symptoms of hypoglycemia (tachycardia, tremors, nervousness), nonspecific β antagonism can be problematic in patients with diabetes mellitus.[13]

Esmolol (Brevibloc) is a unique β_1 blocker in that its plasma half-life is 8 to 9 minutes. Its structural formula includes an ester linkage that is hydrolyzed by esterases in red blood cells. The principal metabolite of esmolol is carboxylic acid; it has insignificant beta blocking properties. The lipid solubility of esmolol is low, metoprolol is moderate, and propranolol is high. Esmolol is administered via a loading dose (0.5 mg/kg over 1 minute) followed by an infusion (50 μg/kg over 4 minutes). This can be repeated

Table 23-2 Supraventricular Tachyarrhythmias Treated With β-Adrenergic Antagonists

Classification	Description
Sinus tachycardia (absolute and relative)	S-A rate in excess of 100 beats/min. Some patients may become symptomatic (e.g., myocardial ischemia, shortness of breath) at rates less than this threshold and as such are characterized as a "relative" tachycardia. The increase in heart rate is usually more gradual.
Atrial tachycardia/paroxysmal supraventricular tachycardia*	An atrial rate in excess of 150 beats/min. With one-to-one ventricular conduction the T waves can become lost as the ventricular rate accelerates. Sudden onset, almost immediate tachycardia that is regular. In theory it could include any tachyarrhythmia that is not supraventricular in origin; by convention atrial flutter, atrial fibrillation, and ST are typically not categorized as PSVT.
Atrial flutter*	An atrial rate ranging from 150 to 250 beats/min, which produces a classical sawtooth appearance (flutter waves).
Atrial fibrillation*	The P wave rate has accelerated to a point that it becomes difficult to discern atrial depolarization, which produces a fibrillatory baseline. It is commonly associated with an irregular ventricular response. Beta-blockers may produce a reduction in heart rate and/or conversion to sinus rhythm.
Wolff-Parkinson-White syndrome†	An electrocardiographic rhythm characterized by a shortened PR interval (< 120 ms) and/or a delta wave (gradual upstroke of the R wave). The shortened PR interval represents distal depolarization via an accessory pathway that bypasses the normal delay in impulse transmission through the A-V node. The delta wave is produced in response to premature septal activation. This syndrome is also sometimes referred to as a "preexcitation" phenomenon. Patients with WPW syndrome are prone to tachyarrhythmias.

*If associated with WPW, β antagonists may produce profound proarrhythmic effects.

†In children beta-blockers, calcium channel blockers, amiodarone, and adenosine have been advocated to control preexcitation tachyarrhythmias. In adults beta-blockers have been advocated and yet have also been reported to produce significant proarrhythmic effects (e.g., ventricular fibrillation).

PSVT, paroxysmal supraventricular tachycardia; ST, sinus tachycardia; WPW, Wolff-Parkinson-White syndrome.

as indicated with the same loading dose followed by a 50-µg/kg incremental increase in 4-minute infusion doses until the desired clinical endpoint is achieved (maximum bolus dose of 0.5 mg/kg times 3 and a maximum infusion dose of 300 µg/kg/min). The pharmacodynamic response can abate within 20 minutes after the infusion is discontinued. Some anesthesia providers choose to dose esmolol as an incremental bolus technique (0.5 mg/kg or 10- to 100-mg boluses) to simplify the logistics of their administration (avoid the use of an infusion device). This technique may be useful during acute and nonsustained elevations in catecholamine levels, as may occur during laryngoscopy or extubation.

Beta-blocker overdose (significant bradycardia, hypotension) can be treated in a variety of ways, including high-dose glucagon (5–10 mg intravenously over 1 minute followed by an infusion of 1–10 mg/h), anticholinergics, isoproterenol, or epinephrine.[14,15] A final word of caution regarding β-adrenergic receptor antagonists: These drugs have been found to be beneficial[16–18] and harmful to patients with tachyarrhythmias associated with Wolff-Parkinson-White (WPW) syndrome (Figure 23-3). The literature documents case reports of malignant arrhythmias (e.g., VF) occurring after the administration of beta-blockers, calcium channel blockers, digoxin, amiodarone, and adenosine in patients with preexcitation

syndrome.[19–22] The mechanism is presumably due to the inability of these drugs to predictably slow conduction through accessory pathways.

Calcium Channel Antagonists

Among the most common calcium channel blockers used by anesthetist are verapamil (Calan) and diltiazem (Cardizem). These two drugs produce negative chronotropic, dromotropic, and inotropic effects by binding to voltage-sensitive calcium channels (L-type) that regulate intracellular entry of Ca^{2+} into the S-A node, A-V node, cardiac myocytes, and smooth muscle. From an electrophysiologic perspective, this causes a slowing of the rate of firing from the S-A node, decreases conduction velocity through the A-V node, and increases A-V nodal refractoriness. A negative dromotropic response may be manifested on the ECG as a prolonged PR interval. This is the basis for their effectiveness in treating supraventricular tachyarrhythmias. The following precautions and clinical variables should be noted in that they can produce significant side effects. Hypotension can occur with both calcium entry blockers (CEBs) due to their peripheral vasodilating and negative inotropic effects. For this reason it is best to refrain from using either drug in patients with limited cardiac reserve. It is also prudent to avoid their use in tachyarrhythmias associated with WPW syndrome, digitalis toxicity, or underlying pathology of the S-A and A-V node (e.g., sinus exit block, sick sinus syndrome). Verapamil and diltiazem have also been shown to increase digoxin levels. Combining CEBs with beta-blockers should only be done if it is assumed the benefits override the risks. Also, treating wide complex arrhythmias of unknown origin (which are incorrectly diagnosed as supraventricular) with CEBs can precipitate VF, although some forms of VT are effectively treated with verapamil (e.g., left septal VT, ventricular arrhythmias related to vasospastic angina).

Indications for CEBs are listed in Table 23-3. The recommended dose of verapamil is 2.5 to 5 mg IV bolus slowly. A second dose of 2.5 to 10 mg intravenously can be given in 15 to 30 minutes. The maximum IV dose is 20 mg. As an alternative, diltiazem can be given 5 to 20 mg IV bolus slowly (0.25 mg/kg). An additional 20 to 25 mg intravenously can be given in 15 minutes if the first dose is ineffective. For long-term administration diltiazem has been associated with less hypotension than verapamil.[17] Verapamil and diltiazem are metabolized by the liver. The elimination half-life for verapamil is 3 to 7 hours and for diltiazem, 4 hours; for both,

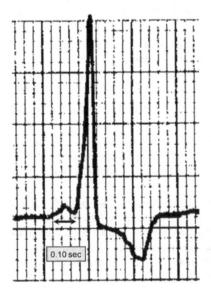

Figure 23-3 Single cardiac cycle depicting evidence of Wolff-Parkinson-White syndrome.

Source: Reprinted with permission from Kossick, MA. In: *EKG Interpretation: Simple, Thorough, Practical.* 3rd ed. Park Ridge, IL: AANA Publishing. In press.

0.10 sec

Table 23-3 Supraventricular Tachyarrhythmias Treated With Verapamil and Diltiazem

Classification	Description
Sinus tachycardia	See Table 23-2 for description of arrhythmia.
Atrial tachycardia/paroxysmal supraventricular tachycardia*	See Table 23-2 for description of arrhythmia.
Atrial flutter*	See Table 23-2 for description of arrhythmia. CEBs are used to reduce ventricular rate but may also convert atrial flutter to sinus rhythm.
Atrial fibrillation*	See Table 23-2 for description of arrhythmia. As seen with atrial flutter, CEBs can reduce ventricular rate but may also convert atrial fibrillation to sinus rhythm. Verapamil may produce atrial fibrillation in patients first treated for atrial flutter.
Wolff-Parkinson-White syndrome[†]	See Table 23-2 for description of arrhythmia. Neither CEB should be used in patients with preexcitation syndrome.

*If associated with WPW syndrome, verapamil and diltiazem are contraindicated due to a potential for a paradoxical response and proarrhythmic effects.

†In children beta-blockers, calcium channel blockers, amiodarone, and adenosine have been advocated to control preexcitation tachyarrhythmias.

liver cirrhosis and advanced age can extend half-lives, and dosages may need to be reduced. With verapamil approximately 70% of the drug is excreted by the kidney. A major metabolite of verapamil is norverapamil, and although it is less potent than the parent compound, its half-life is about 10 hours. For diltiazem, desacetyldiltiazem is a substantial metabolite possessing about one-half the potency as a vasodilator. In reports of gross overdoses, this metabolite does not appear to produce any significant conduction abnormalities.[23] Untoward side effects with CEBs can be treated with calcium, glucagon, atropine, isoproterenol, dopamine, and temporary pacing.

Sodium Channel Blockers

This category of antiarrhythmics is associated grossly with blockade of sodium (Na^+) channels and some K^+ channels of cardiac cells. A subclassification of Na^+ channel blockers provides a more detailed description of the electrophysiologic effects of this class of drugs. In particular, the pharmacology of lidocaine (Xylocaine) and procainamide (Procan, Pronestyl) is discussed.

Lidocaine is categorized as a class IB fast Na^+ channel blocker. As such it is known to shorten action potential duration (APD) and produces little effect on the maximum velocity of shortening (V_{max}). The normal cardiac action potential is created by an unequal distribution of electrolytes and charged proteins across a cell membrane. Specific protein channels with "gates" regulate the flow of ions along concentration gradients, and an energy-dependent exchange mechanism, such as the Na^+/K^+-ATPase pump, moves electrolytes across concentration gradients. The net effect is the generation of a resting transmembrane potential (e.g., minus 90 mV relative to the extracellular environment in a fast response action potential) known as a "polarized" or "charged" state; over time the rapid redistribution of ions (occurring in a few hundred milliseconds) across the cell membrane produces the phenomenon of depolarization and repolarization. The function of these protein channels can become altered by myocardial ischemia or infarction, autonomic nervous system imbalance, and antiarrhythmics (therapeutic and/or proarrhythmic effects). Two primary cardiac action potentials exist: the fast response and slow response. The fast response action potential correlates with working myocardial cells, such as the contractile cells of the atria and ventricles. The slow response action potential is characteristic of cells that comprise the S-A node, A-V node, and distal conducting system. The Na^+ currents in these anatomic areas of the heart are less pronounced, thus the reason for the gradual upstroke of phase 0 of the slow response action potential (Figure 23-4).

Lidocaine predominantly blocks Na^+ channels in the open state. With ischemic myocardium it depresses fast response electrical potentials. Other electrophysiologic properties include significant attenuation of the APD and the shortening of the effective refractory period of ventricular muscle and Purkinje fibers. It has little effect on atria, S-A node automaticity, and accessory pathways.

One of the positive attributes of lidocaine is its overall safety profile when used to treat ventricular arrhythmias. It is metabolized extensively by the liver and for this reason is ineffective as an oral preparation (extensive first-bypass metabolism). Indications for lidocaine include sustained monomorphic VT (Figure 23-5) (particularly when associated with an acute episode of myocardial ischemia or myocardial infarction) and polymorphic VT. With

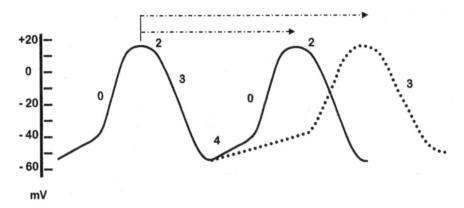

Figure 23-4 A series of three slow response cardiac action potentials. The dotted line of the third action potential depicts a delay in diastolic depolarization (gradual upstroke of phase 4) and the subsequent delay in achieving threshold. This produces a lengthening of the interval between action potentials (i.e., reduction in heart rate).

Source: Reprinted with permission from Kossick, MA. In: *EKG Interpretation: Simple, Thorough, Practical.* 3rd ed. Park Ridge, IL: AANA Publishing. In press.

either of these ventricular arrhythmias, lidocaine can be used even in the presence of an abnormal ejection fraction. Lidocaine is not recommended for repetitive monomorphic VT. Other uses include pulseless VT and VF as second-tier treatment options. It may also be used for TdP associated with long QT syndrome, specifically subtype 3. Long QT syndrome is an inherited disease associated with a prolonged QT_c interval. If the QT_c is greater than 500 ms the patient is at significant risk for becoming symptomatic before age 40.[24]

The initial IV or intraosseous (IO) bolus dose of lidocaine is 1 to 1.5 mg/kg. For refractory ventricular arrhythmias, a repeat bolus dose of 0.5 to 0.75 mg/kg may be given 5 to 10 minutes later. The maximum dose is 3 mg/kg. After the initial bolus an infusion is started at a rate of 1 to 4 mg/min or 30 to 50 µg/kg/min. If IV access is not available, lidocaine 2 to 4 mg/kg may be given through an endotracheal tube.

Signs of lidocaine toxicity are usually manifested as central nervous system disturbances, such as tinnitus, metallic taste, slurred speech, paresthesias, tremors, seizures, and coma. Although unusual, hypotension and

proarrhythmic effects such as sinus arrest, heart block, and ventricular arrhythmias can occur. Patients with impaired hepatic function or decreased hepatic blood flow (as may occur with some surgical procedures, heart failure, beta-blockers use, or prolonged lidocaine infusions) are at greater risk for lidocaine toxicity. In such patients the anesthetist should consider reducing the dose of lidocaine by one-third to one-half. The elimination half-life of lidocaine is 1 to 2 hours; in patients with impaired hepatic blood flow or heart failure, it may extend to 4 hours or even beyond 10 hours. It is highly protein bound (50–80%) to α_1-acid glycoprotein.[11,17] Prophylactic use of lidocaine in the setting of an acute myocardial infarction has not been recommended by the ACC and AHA after 1996 due to the meta-analysis study suggesting increased morbidity and/or mortality in this patient population.[25] Nevertheless, other researchers suggest prophylactic lidocaine is actually beneficial in this clinical setting and report a lower incidence of VF and mortality.[26]

Procainamide (Pronestyl, Procan) is similar to lidocaine in that it has been available for the management of

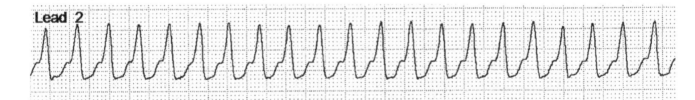

Figure 23-5 Monomorphic ventricular tachycardia.

Source: Reprinted with permission from Kossick, MA. In: *EKG Interpretation: Simple, Thorough, Practical.* 3rd ed. Park Ridge, IL: AANA Publishing. In press.

arrhythmias for decades, approved for clinical use by the U.S. Food and Drug Administration in 1950. Unlike lidocaine, it is a significant cardiac depressant and should not be used in patients with limited cardiac reserve. It is also never given as an IV bolus. Its utility is more diverse in that it is considered a "broad-spectrum" antiarrhythmic that can be used for many types of supraventricular and ventricular arrhythmias. Procainamide is a class IA Na^+ channel blocker, specifically during the inactivated state of the channel. As such, it reduces the rate of rise of phase 0 of the action potential, also known as V_{max}. It also prolongs the APD and effective refractory period, partly due to its K^+ channel blocking properties. In addition, as with lidocaine it raises the VF threshold. Procainamide's major metabolite, N-acetylprocainamide (NAPA), also exerts electrophysiologic effects. Like the parent compound, it blocks K^+ channels and produces lengthening of the APD of Purkinje fibers and ventricular muscles, which represent a class III antiarrhythmic effect.

The elimination half-life of procainamide is 3 to 5 hours and for NAPA 7 to 8 hours. The acetylation of the parent compound to NAPA via N-acetyltransferase is determined genetically and influences the plasma levels of this metabolite and the parent compound. The kidneys eliminate about 50% to 60% of procainamide, and hepatic metabolism accounts for around 10% to 30%. NAPA's elimination is more dependent on renal function. The dosage of procainamide should be reduced in patients with kidney disease or heart failure.[17]

As a broad-spectrum antiarrhythmic, procainamide can be used for tachyarrhythmias of diverse etiology, including atrial flutter, atrial fibrillation, SVT, WPW syndrome, and stable polymorphic VT, which is rare to encounter as being stable. Regarding VT, procainamide is actually preferred by the ACC and AHA for use in stable patients over amiodarone for early conversion and rate control, specifically for sustained monomorphic VT and repetitive monomorphic VT. In contrast, ACC/AHA guidelines are ambiguous regarding procainamide's use with pulseless VT, VF, and unstable polymorphic VT in that they publish the following recommendation: procainamide is an "acceptable intervention but no longer recommended."[11]

The recommended loading dose of procainamide is 20 to 50 mg/min intravenously followed with a maintenance infusion of 1 to 6 mg/min. This dose can be repeated every 5 minutes. The maximum loading dose is 17 mg/kg (1.2 g for a 70-kg patient), although up to 2 g has been advocated by some sources. Procainamide should be discontinued if the QRS begins to widen more than 50% or hypotension develops. Also, a lengthening of the QT_c interval can lead to TdP

secondary to the parent compound and/or NAPA. During chronic administration, systemic lupus erythematosus–like syndrome has been reported. This may necessitate discontinuation of the drug or treatment with corticosteroids. Fortunately, the literature has shown the brain and kidneys are usually not affected with systemic lupus erythematosus–like syndrome.

Amiodarone (Cordarone, Pacerone)

Amiodarone produces its antiarrhythmic effects via a multiplicity of mechanisms. Most notably, it blocks transient outward delayed rectifier and inward rectifier K^+ currents of cardiac action potentials (class III), but also it inhibits inactivated Na^+ channels (class I) and Ca^{2+} channels (class IV), and it noncompetitively blocks α and β receptors (class II). Amiodarone prolongs APD and increases effective refractory period in all cardiac tissue, inhibits abnormal automaticity, and decreases conduction velocity. Other electrophysiologic effects include decreasing the slope of diastolic depolarization of the S-A node and V_{max}. On the ECG these electrophysiologic effects may be manifested as a lengthening of the PR interval, widening of the QRS complex, and increasing of the QT_c interval. Fortunately, although increased refractoriness extends the QT_c interval, it is not common to see TdP develop during amiodarone therapy.

Its chemical structure provides a rationale for its potential adverse effects on thyroid function: Both hypothyroidism and hyperthyroidism have been reported to occur with its administration. Amiodarone is a benzofuran derivative (heterocyclic compound made of fused benzene and furan rings) containing iodine (Figure 23-6), and its structural formula has similarities to thyroxine (T_4). Amiodarone and its major metabolite (desethylamiodarone) have also been shown to inhibit the conversion of T_4 to triiodothyronine (T_3). Box 23-1 provides a list of side effects documented to have occurred with amiodarone administration. Adverse effects are not uncommon and have been reported to occur in 75% of patients treated over a 5-year period. The most common side effects are gastrointestinal and pulmonary and abate with reducing the dosage or discontinuing the drug. Amiodarone-induced pulmonary toxicity (0.5% incidence) is the most notable adverse effect, perhaps due to an increase in free oxygen radicals in the lungs. This may be manifested as dyspnea, cough, hypoxemia, subacute or acute pneumonitis, diffuse pulmonary infiltrates on chest x-ray, chest crackles during auscultation, and perhaps pulmonary edema.[27] It may occur as early as 6 days after

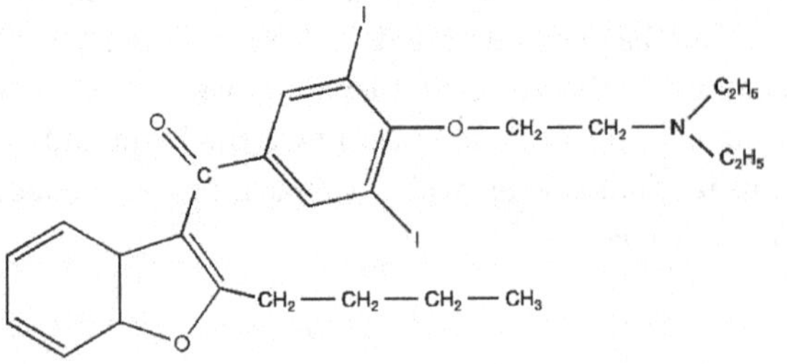

Figure 23-6 Structural formula of amiodarone.

Source: Reprinted with permission from Kossick, MA. In: *EKG Interpretation: Simple, Thorough, Practical.* 3rd ed. Park Ridge, IL: AANA Publishing. In press.

treatment is initiated or as late as 60 months. Mortalities have also been reported (3 of 573 patients).[28] Pulmonary complications are uncommon (but still possible[29]) if the daily dose of amiodarone does not exceed 200 mg. It has also been suggested that high oxygen levels may contribute to amiodarone-induced pulmonary toxicity.[30] For this reason some anesthesia providers advocate using lower inspired oxygen concentrations during general anesthetics in patients prescribed amiodarone. However, other areas of the literature are not in agreement with this presupposition. Instead, significant risk factors identified have included advanced age (> 60 years), preexisting pulmonary dysfunction, and duration of amiodarone therapy (6–12 months).[31,32] Amiodarone-induced pulmonary toxicity has also been reported to occur in the pediatric population.[33]

The pharmacokinetics of amiodarone (and desethylamiodarone) are of interest in that the elimination half-life is quite extensive due to its significant binding to body tissues and high lipid solubility. Concentrations in the heart can be 10 to 50 times greater than what is found in plasma. The terminal half-life after oral dosing is 26 to 107 days and for IV administration 8 to 14 hours. Drug dose does not need to be adjusted for renal insufficiency. However, it is important to know that both amiodarone and desethylamiodarone are not dialyzable. The liver serves as the primary site for metabolism via CYP3A4. Amiodarone and desethylamiodarone are eliminated by the liver, but the exact mechanism is unclear. The anesthetist should also be aware that amiodarone can increase the plasma levels of other drugs by inhibition of cytochrome P-450 enzymes as well as alterations in the binding of drugs to plasma proteins. This includes warfarin, digitalis, procainamide, and other

Box 23-1　Adverse Effects of Amiodarone

- Pulmonary toxicity
- Adult respiratory distress syndrome
- Hypotension
- Asymptomatic elevations in liver enzymes
- Cirrhosis/hepatitis
- Photosensitivity
- Blue-gray skin discoloration
- Hyperthyroidism
- Hypothyroidism
- Corneal microdeposits
- Optic neuritis
- Symptomatic bradycardia
- Worsening of ventricular tachyarrhythmias
- Torsade de pointes (QT prolongation)
- Polymorphic ventricular tachycardia
- A-V block
- Ventricular standstill
- Further deterioration in congestive heart failure
- Peripheral neuropathy
- Proximal muscle weakness

antiarrhythmics. The dosage of these affected drugs should be reduced accordingly. Amiodarone should also be used with caution in patients prescribed CEBs and β-adrenergic blockers due to potential synergistic effects.[17,34]

Table 23-4 lists the clinical indications for amiodarone. Physicians and nurses have clearly been influenced by national resuscitation guidelines because a significant increase in amiodarone use has been documented over the past several years.[35] As with procainamide, amiodarone can be used for both supraventricular and ventricular tachyarrhythmias. The most notable exception is TdP. The recommended loading dose for recurrent tachyarrhythmias is 150 mg intravenously in 100 cc given over 10 minutes (15 mg/min). This is followed by a maintenance infusion of 1 mg/min for 6 hours and then 0.5 mg/min for 18 hours. If necessary, the 150 mg IV bolus dose given over 10 minutes may be repeated for breakthrough arrhythmias. The maximum daily dose should not exceed 2.2 g. In a cardiac arrest situation (VF) where

Table 23-4　Arrhythmias Treated With Amiodarone

Classification	Description
Atrial tachycardia/paroxysmal supraventricular tachycardia	See Table 23-2 for description of arrhythmia.
Atrial flutter*	See Table 23-2 for description of arrhythmia.
Atrial fibrillation*	See Table 23-2 for description of arrhythmia.
Wolff-Parkinson-White syndrome	See Table 23-2 for description of arrhythmia.
Wide complex tachyarrhythmias of unknown origin	A wide complex tachycardia (QRS duration ≥ 120 ms) where the origin cannot be determined with any degree of confidence (i.e., supraventricular vs. ventricular).
Symptomatic nonsustained monomorphic VT[†]	See Table 23-1 for description of arrhythmia.
Sustained monomorphic VT	See Table 23-1 for description of arrhythmia.
Repetitive monomorphic VT	See Table 23-1 for description of arrhythmia.
Polymorphic VT	See Table 23-1 for description of arrhythmia.
Polymorphic VT storm	See Table 23-1 for description of arrhythmia.
Incessant VT[‡]	See Table 23-1 for description of arrhythmia. Amiodarone use depends on anecdotal evidence.
Ventricular flutter	A VT with a rate > 260 ventricular depolarizations per minute.
Pulseless VT	No discernable pulse with an ECG recording of ventricular tachycardia.
VF	Chaotic electrical activity on the ECG. No discernable P waves, QRS complexes, and T waves.

*Used for conversion and/or heart rate control.

†Amiodarone is used if patient is unresponsive to beta-blockers.

‡Use is based on anecdotal evidence.

shock interventions and vasopressors have failed, amiodarone can be administered 300 mg IV/IO push or 5 mg/kg mixed with 20 to 30 mL sodium chloride or 5% dextrose in water. If necessary, a second one-time dose of 150 mg IV/IO can be given in 3 to 5 minutes.

In contrast to procainamide, amiodarone is less of a cardiac depressant and is recommended over procainamide for patients with reduced cardiac reserve. It also produces peripheral and coronary vasodilation. Significant as well is the finding that atropine and β agonists may be less effective in reversing bradyarrhythmias that develop secondary to amiodarone use.

Finally, amiodarone has been shown to reduce the risk for sudden cardiac death by 29% and cardiovascular death by 18% in patients without implantable cardioverter defibrillators. This same meta-analysis also found amiodarone produced a twofold increased risk for pulmonary toxicity and fivefold increased risk for thyroid toxicity. For all-cause mortality, amiodarone was shown to be neutral[36] and controversial.[37]

Given the significant number of side effects that can occur with amiodarone, pharmaceutical companies have invested in developing alternative multichannel blocking antiarrhythmics. One such drug that has been evaluated is dronedarone, which has nearly identical electrophysiologic properties to amiodarone but structurally is noniodinated.[38] It has been studied in placebo-controlled trials[39] as well as compared with amiodarone.[40] The preliminary review of research indicates dronedarone is somewhat less efficacious than amiodarone relative to the number of patients experiencing reoccurrence of atrial fibrillation. However, the need to discontinue dronedarone due to undesirable side effects is seen less often compared with amiodarone; fewer deaths have also been reported. Compared with placebo, dronedarone has been shown to reduce cardiovascular mortality in high-risk patients, *excluding* those with symptomatic congestive heart failure[41]; it is considered unsafe to use in patients with severely depressed contractility.[42] Evidence of this safety concern has arisen from the observation that mortality rates were greater in patients treated with dronedarone compared with placebo, which led to the premature discontinuation of the respective clinical trial. Further research is necessary to better define the safety and efficacy of dronedarone, which certainly may include the need to evaluate subsets of patients relative to the extent of their underlying pathophysiology.

Adenosine (Adenocard)

Adenosine is an intermediate metabolite of an endogenous nucleoside. It can be formed intracellularly (adenosine triphosphate [ATP] pathway) or extracellularly (adenine nucleotides) by dephosphorylation of adenosine monophosphate (AMP) via the enzyme 5-nucleotidase. Enzymatic metabolism of adenosine is accomplished by adenosine deaminase and adenosine kinase, both of which are cytosolic enzymes. This process occurs within endothelial cells, erythrocytes, and cardiomyocytes. Inosine is formed after deamination by adenosine deaminase and AMP after phosphorylation by adenosine kinase. Each of these byproducts is formed intracellularly, which means that a nucleoside transport system must exist for elimination of adenosine. Reuptake of adenosine via the nucleoside transport system is retarded by dipyridamole (persantine).[43] Thus patients prescribed this drug have increased serum levels of endogenous adenosine. It is prudent to consider giving smaller doses of adenosine (3 mg) for treating SVT in this patient population.[44] Also, patient status after cardiac transplant has been shown to be quite sensitive to the effects of adenosine.[45]

Besides intracellular breakdown of adenosine, its effects can be terminated through competitive antagonism of its receptor sites. It has been demonstrated that therapeutic concentrations of methylated xanthine derivatives (such as theophylline) act as nonselective adenosine antagonists (i.e., antagonizes A_1 and A_2 receptors).[46]

Two primary adenosine receptor sites, labeled P and P_1, have been identified. Purinoceptors sensitive to ATP are termed P_2. The P_1 receptors are sensitive to adenosine and subdivided into A_1, A_2, and A_3 receptor sites. The A_1 receptors are located in cardiomyocytes (a greater proportion in atrial membranes vs. ventricular membranes) and in the presence of adenosine produce negative chronotropic, dromotropic, and inotropic effects.[47] As seen with adrenergic receptors, A_1 purinoceptors are capable of undergoing up-regulation and down-regulation, which can result in supersensitization and desensitization of the responses to adenosine.[48]

Situated in endothelial and vascular smooth muscle cells are the A_2 purine receptors, which in the presence of adenosine produce coronary vasodilation and vascular smooth muscle relaxation; the reason for the lowered resistance in the vasculature is unknown. Activation of A_3 receptors on mast cells has been shown to induce airway hyperresponsiveness, which is why adenosine should be used with caution in patients with reactive airway disease.[49] The other adenosine receptor class, labeled P, is stimulated by relatively high concentrations of adenosine. However, the physiologic significance of its activation remains unknown.

Research has shown that adenosine depresses S-A node activity and A-V nodal conduction and prevents the heart from responding to the release of endogenous catecholamines. In essence, the cardiac actions of adenosine are very similar to the neurotransmitter ACh: Both oppose the effects of norepinephrine and epinephrine.[43] Therapeutic uses of adenosine include termination of SVT and for diagnostic purposes when it is necessary to distinguish the origin of a wide complex tachyarrhythmia as being supraventricular with aberrant conduction versus ventricular.

Adenosine is most effective in terminating bouts of SVT when the A-V node forms part of the reentrant circuit. Its efficacy in depressing A-V nodal conduction (negative dromotropy) is very apparent when a transient episode of A-V block is seen (e.g., complete A-V block, asystole). It produces a slowing of A-V conduction by increasing K^+ conductance. This explains why transient complete A-V block or asystole is sometimes seen during its clinical use. Sinus tachycardia may also be controlled with adenosine, although the response may be biphasic (sinus bradycardia followed by sinus tachycardia).[43]

The electrophysiologic effect of hyperpolarization of the S-A node is what accounts for the observed decrease in heart rate. The phenomenon of hyperpolarization occurs because of adenosine's interaction with the A_1 receptors, which results in the efflux of K^+ from the cell (i.e., S-A node, atrial myocytes, A-V node).[43]

It is important when using adenosine to administer it as a rapid IV bolus followed by a flush. Its half-life in the blood is 1 to 6 seconds due to its rapid metabolism by endothelial cells and erythrocytes. Clinical effects after an IV bolus through a peripheral route are seen within 30 seconds with a duration of action of 60 seconds. An even more rapid onset of action is seen when adenosine is administered through a central venous line (e.g., 10–20 seconds).[43]

The initial recommended dose of adenosine is 6 mg given as an IV bolus. A slower rate of administration results in most of the drug being metabolized before it is able to reach its site of action. If the first dose is ineffective, a repeat dose of 12 mg in 1 to 2 minutes may be administered, followed with another 12-mg dose if paroxysmal SVT persists. The efficacy rate for termination of paroxysmal SVT after a first dose of adenosine is 60% and for the second dose, 90%.[17]

Adverse reactions with adenosine are seen in about one-third of patients. The most common reactions are facial flushing, chest pain, and dyspnea. The mean duration for adverse reactions is reported to be 50 seconds, with none exceeding 2 minutes. Interesting is the finding that arrhythmias do not comprise one of the three most common side effects.[17,50]

Arrhythmias documented to occur with adenosine at the time of conversion from paroxysmal SVT include ventricular ectopy (33%), sinus bradycardia (5%), A-V block (3%) with a duration less than 4 seconds, atrial flutter or atrial fibrillation (1%), and reinitiation of paroxysmal SVT (9%).[50] It is common for patients who develop posttreatment atrial flutter or atrial fibrillation to spontaneously convert to sinus rhythm.[17]

Although the incidence of bradydysrhythmias associated with the use of adenosine is not high, should any occur (and be sustained), aminophylline (approximately 6 mg/kg) can be administered. Aminophylline binds to purinoceptors; in contrast, the anticholinergics atropine and glycopyrrolate *may* be ineffective in terminating slow heart rate.

According to the AHA and ACC, adenosine remains the drug of choice for SVT. Its pharmacokinetic profile makes it unique in its ability to produce a rapid on and rapid off pharmacodynamic response, perhaps analogous to the use of cardioversion to produce a rapid but brief antiarrhythmic effect.

Vasopressin (Antidiuretic Hormone, Arginine Vasopressin)

In recent years vasopressin has been recommended as an alternative antiarrhythmic in the treatment of VF, pulseless VT, pulseless electrical activity, asystole, and unstable polymorphic VT.[11,51,52] Vasopressin, as the name implies, is a potent vasoconstrictor. It is produced in nuclei of the hypothalamus and released by posterior pituitary gland; other areas of synthesis include the heart and adrenal gland. The stimulus for release is diverse and involves such cardinal changes as a decrease in intravascular volume and increased plasma osmolarity.

Three primary vasopressin receptors have been identified: V_{1a}, V_{1b} (also referenced by some authors as V_3), and V_2. V_{1a} receptors are very diverse and located in vascular smooth muscle, central nervous system, heart, platelets, kidneys, and liver. V_{1b} receptors have been isolated in the anterior pituitary gland, brain, pancreas, and adrenal medulla. V_2 receptors are located in the renal collecting duct system and produce an antidiuretic effect. Through a complex V_{1a} receptor-effector coupling mechanism, V_{1a} agonism leads to vasoconstriction, increased platelet aggregation, release of coagulation factors, and adrenocorticotropic hormone secretion, in addition to glycogenolysis. The vasoconstrictive response at V_{1a} receptors occurs in part due to increased intracellular Ca^{2+} concentrations. The Ca^{2+} levels are elevated through the influx of extracellular Ca^{2+} and enhanced mobilization of intracellular stored Ca^{2+}.[53]

Dosing guidelines recommended by the AHA and ACC for vasopressin are as follows: one 40-unit IV or IO dose may be substituted for either the first or second dose of epinephrine. Preceding the administration of either vasopressor for "shockable rhythms" is electrical therapy (defibrillation). The elimination half-life of vasopressin is about 10 to 20 minutes. Its pharmacodynamic effects have also been shown to be effective in severe acidosis.[11] In a non–life-threatening situation, caution should be exercised in administering the drug to patients with cardiovascular disease because even small doses may produce myocardial ischemia or mortality. The etiology of these effects may be due to its ability to produce coronary vasoconstriction and a negative lusitropic effect.

Magnesium

Magnesium's ($MgSO_4$) use as an antiarrhythmic can be quite beneficial to some patients. Its exact mechanism of action (conversion of arrhythmias) remains unknown. Research has shown it has diverse electrophysiologic effects on the heart by influencing Na^+ channels, K^+ channels, Ca^{2+} channels, and Na/K^+ ATPase. These changes can produce increased sinus node recovery time, depressed automaticity, and degradation of conduction through the A-V node, the His-Purkinje system, and across accessory tracts. Magnesium can be used for a diverse number of ventricular arrhythmias, even in the presence of normal $MgSO_4$ levels. In the acquired form of TdP, $MgSO_4$ is the initial preferred treatment at a dose of 1 to 2 g intravenously given over 1 to 2 minutes, although it may take up to 5 to 10 g to suppress. This form of TdP can be caused by antiarrhythmics (parent compound and metabolites) such as quinidine, procainamide, NAPA, amiodarone, disopyramide, phenothiazines, vasopressin, beta-blockers, as well as other etiologies, such as tricyclic antidepressants, Seldane, hypokalemia, hypomagnesemia, and mitral valve prolapse. The congenital/idiopathic form of TdP is managed with beta-blockers, pacing, and implantable cardiac defibrillators. Other arrhythmias treated with the same dose of $MgSO_4$ include resistant forms of polymorphic VT, rapid monomorphic VT, ventricular flutter (rate ≥ 260/min), and resistant VF. In patients with hypomagnesemia who have sustained a myocardial infarction, administration of $MgSO_4$ may attenuate the occurrence of VF. Digitalis-induced arrhythmias in the setting of hypomagnesemia can be treated with magnesium.[11,34,54,55] The literature also documents $MgSO_4$ as useful in preventing atrial fibrillation after cardiac surgery and controlling the ventricular response in patients with WPW syndrome.[56]

Summary

It is clear from this review of the pharmacology of antiarrhythmics that numerous factors must be taken into consideration before initiating treatment. Determining the risk-to-benefit ratio is cardinal in any treatment algorithm, along with possessing fundamental skills in arrhythmia interpretation. It is only after these prerequisites have been applied in combination with an overall understanding of the pharmacology of each antiarrhythmic agent that a clinical decision/intervention has a greater likelihood of producing a positive outcome instead of producing harm.

Key Points

- The decision to administer an antiarrhythmic must be weighed against its potential to produce a proarrhythmic effect.
- Not all rhythm disturbances encountered during an anesthetic necessitate the use of an antiarrhythmic, but instead may be acutely resolved with correction of the underlying etiology, such as elevated catecholamine levels during light planes of anesthesia.
- Additive or synergistic effects may occur when more than one class of antiarrhythmics are used, thus necessitating an initial lower dose of a second class of antiarrhythmic.
- A firm foundation in ECG interpretation (lead selection, electrode placement, diagnostic criteria for atrial and ventricular arrhythmias as well as myocardial ischemia) is a prerequisite for the therapeutic application of antiarrhythmics.

- Patients with Wolff-Parkinson-White syndrome may experience a paradoxical response to calcium channel blockers, digoxin, amiodarone, adenosine, and perhaps β-adrenergic antagonists.
- Using calcium channel blockers to convert wide complex tachyarrhythmias of unknown origin can precipitate ventricular fibrillation.
- Significant risk factors for amiodarone-induced pulmonary toxicity include advanced age (> 60 years), preexisiting pulmonary dysfunction, and duration of amiodarone therapy (6–12 months).
- Adenosine remains the drug of choice for terminating symptomatic supraventricular tachycardia.

Chapter Questions

1. Which of the following effects is least likely due to A_1 purine receptor agonism?
   a. coronary vasodilation
   b. negative dromotropic effect
   c. negative inotropic effect
   d. negative chronotropic effect

2. As part of your anesthetic induction (thiopental 4 mg/kg with fentanyl 200 μg), you have decided to administer esmolol to help control the adrenergic response to laryngoscopy. What single bolus dose would be considered "appropriate" or "reasonable" for an 80-kg male, PS II?
   a. 5 mg
   b. 40 mg
   c. 400 mg
   d. 800 mg

3. Extracardiac effects of $β_2$ antagonists include all but which of the following?
   a. attenuation of glycogenolysis
   b. increased airway resistance
   c. enhanced insulin release
   d. attenuation of gluconeogenesis

4. Your preanesthetic assessment reveals the following information: History of asymptomatic mitral valve prolapse and Wolff-Parkinson-White syndrome. The 12-lead ECG shows normal sinus rhythm (heart rate of 80 beats/min) with two conducted premature atrial contractions. Intraoperatively, the patient develops paroxysmal SVT. Which

of the following interventions is considered least desirable for termination of this rhythm?
a. procainamide
b. cardioversion
c. diltiazem
d. amiodarone

5. Which of the following initial loading doses of amiodarone is recommended for the treatment of ventricular tachycardia? The pharmacy prepared the drug by placing 3 cc (50 mg/cc) in 100 cc of D_5W, and the pharmacist removed 3 cc of D_5W before adding the amiodarone. You are administering the drug through a microdripper (60 gtts/cc).
a. 2.5 cc/min for 10 min
b. 5 cc/min for 10 min
c. 10 cc/min for 10 min
d. 15 cc/min for 10 min

6. An initial 3- to 4-mg IV bolus dose of adenosine for an adult patient exhibiting SVT is appropriate/prudent under which of the following circumstances?
a. a patient who is on dipyridamole preoperatively
b. a patient receiving aminophylline
c. a patient who is status post–cardiac transplant
d. a patient who is on metoprolol preoperatively
e. Responses a and c are circumstances when the initial bolus dose of adenosine should be reduced.

Answers and Discussion

1. a.

2. b.

3. c.

4. c.

5. c.

6. e.

References

1. Forrest JB, Rehder K, Cahalan MK, Goldsmith CH. Multicenter study of general anesthesia. III. Predictors of severe perioperative adverse outcomes. *Anesthesiology.* 1992;76: 3–15.

2. Marriott HJL. *Practical Electrocardiography,* 8th ed. Baltimore: Williams & Wilkins; 1988.

3. Kossick MA. Modified chest leads and diagnosing infarction. Paper presented at the Colorado Association of Nurse Anesthetists 2000 Fall Meeting, October 21, 2000, Colorado Springs, Colorado.

4. Shi H, Wang H, Wang Z. Identification and characterization of multiple subtypes of muscarinic acetylcholine receptors and their physiological functions in canine hearts. *Mol Pharmacol.* 1999;55:497–507.

5. Taylor P. Anticholinesterase agents. In: Brunton L, Lazo J, Parker K, eds. *Goodman and Gilman's The Pharmacological Basis of Therapeutics,* 11th ed. New York: McGraw-Hill; 2006:201–216.

6. Smith I, Monk TG, White PF. Comparison of transesophageal atrial pacing with anticholinergic drugs for the treatment of intraoperative bradycardia. *Anesth Analg.* 1994;78:245–252.

7. Kongsrud F, Sponheim S. A comparison of atropine and glycopyrrolate in anaesthetic practice. *Acta Anaesth Scand.* 1982;26:620–625.

8. Mirakhur RK, Jones CJ, Dundee JW. Effects of intravenous administration of glycopyrrolate and atropine in anaesthetised patients. *Anaesthesia.* 1981;36:277–281.

9. Kramer BA, Allen RE, Friedman B. Atropine and glycopyrrolate as ECT preanesthesia. *J Clin Psychiatry.* 1986;47:199–200.

10. Ali-Melkkilä T, Kanto J, Iisalo E. Pharmacokinetics and related pharmacodynamics of anticholinergic drugs. *Acta Anaesth Scand.* 1993;37:633–642.

11. Zipes DP, Camm AJ, Borggrefe M, et al. ACC/AHA/ESC 2006 guidelines for management of patients with ventricular arrhythmias and the prevention of sudden cardiac death: a report of the American College of Cardiology/American Heart Association Task Force and the European Society of Cardiology Committee for Practice Guidelines (Writing Committee to Develop Guidelines for Management of Patients With Ventricular Arrhythmias and the Prevention of Sudden Cardiac Death) developed in collaboration with the European Heart Rhythm Association and the Heart Rhythm Society. *Europace.* 2006;8:746–837.

12. Rau T, Wuttke H, Michels LM, et al. Impact of the CYP2D6 genotype on the clinical effects of metoprolol: a prospective longitudinal study. *Clin Pharmacol Ther.* 2009;85:269–272.

13. Westfall TC, Westfall DP. Neurotransmission. The autonomic and somatic motor nervous system. In: Brunton L, Lazo J, Parker K, eds. *Goodman and Gilman's The Pharmacological Basis of Therapeutics,* 11th ed. New York: McGraw-Hill; 2006:137–181.

14. Bailey B. Glucagon in beta-blocker and calcium channel blocker overdoses: a systematic review. *J Toxicol Clin Toxicol.* 2003;41:595–602.

15. Shepherd G. Treatment of poisoning caused by beta-adrenergic and calcium-channel blockers. *Am J Health Syst Pharm.* 2006;63:1828–1835.

16. Bobrov VA, Frolov AI, Mitchenko EI, Galichansky IV, Zinchenko YV. Comparative analysis of electrophysiologic effect of metoprolol and disopyramide, acting alone or in combination in patients with supraventricular tachycardia and Wolff-Parkinson-White syndrome. *Rev Portug Cardiol.* 1994;13:221–225.

17. Miller JM, Zipes DP. Therapy for cardiac arrhythmias. In: Zipes DP, Libby P, Bonow RO, Braunwald E, eds. *Braunwald's Heart Disease. A Textbook of Cardiovascular Medicine,* 7th ed. Philadelphia: Elsevier Saunders; 2005:713–766.

18. Ratnasamy C, Rossique-Gonzalez M, Young ML. Pharmacological therapy in children with atrioventricular reentry: which drug? *Curr Pharmac Design.* 2008;14:753–761.

19. Khan IA, Nair CK, Singh N, Gowda RM, Nair RC. Acute ventricular rate control in atrial fibrillation and atrial flutter. *Int J Cardiol.* 2004;97:7–13.

20. Kim RJ, Gerling BR, Kono AT, Greenberg ML. Precipitation of ventricular fibrillation by intravenous diltiazem and metoprolol in a young patient with occult Wolff-Parkinson-White syndrome. *Pacing Clin Electrophysiol.* 2008;31:776–779.

21. Turley AJ, Murray S, Thambyrajah J. Pre-excited atrial fibrillation triggered by intravenous adenosine: a commonly used drug with potentially life-threatening adverse effects. *Emerg Med J.* 2008;25:46–48.

22. Badshah A, Mirza B, Janjua M, Nair R, Steinman RT, Cotant JF. Amiodarone-induced torsade de pointes in a patient with Wolff-Parkinson-White syndrome. *Hellen J Cardiol.* 2009;50:224–226.

23. Luomanmäki K, Tiula E, Kivistö KT, Neuvonen PJ. Pharmacokinetics of diltiazem in massive overdose. *Therap Drug Monit.* 1997;19:240–242.

24. Zipes DP, DiMarco JP, Gillette PC, et al. Guidelines for clinical intracardiac electrophysiological and catheter ablation procedures. A report of the American College of Cardiology/American Heart Association Task Force on Practice Guidelines (Committee on Clinical Intracardiac Electrophysiologic and Catheter Ablation Procedures), developed in collaboration with the North American Society of Pacing and Electrophysiology. *J Am Coll Cardiol.* 1995;26:555–573.

25. Ryan TJ, Anderson JL, Antman EM, et al. ACC/AHA guidelines for the management of patients with acute myocardial infarction. A report of the American College of Cardiology/American Heart Association Task Force on Practice Guidelines (Committee on Management of Acute Myocardial Infarction). *J Am Coll Cardiol.* 1996;28:1328–1428.

26. Wyman MG, Wyman RM, Cannom DS, Criley JM. Prevention of primary ventricular fibrillation in acute myocardial infarction with prophylactic lidocaine. *Am J Cardiol.* 2004;94:545–551.

27. Wolkove N, Baltzan M. Amiodarone pulmonary toxicity. *Can Respir J.* 2009;16:43–48.

28. Argyriou M, Hountis P, Antonopoulos N, Mathioudaki M. Acute fatal post-CABG low dose amiodarone lung toxicity. *Asian Cardiovasc Thorac Ann.* 2007;15:e66–e68.

29. Ott MC, Khoor A, Leventhal JP, Paterick TE, Burger CD. Pulmonary toxicity in patients receiving low-dose amiodarone. *Chest.* 2003;123:646–651.

30. Herndon JC, Cook AO, Ramsay MA, Swygert TH, Capehart J. Postoperative unilateral pulmonary edema: possible amiodarone pulmonary toxicity. *Anesthesiology.* 1992;76:308–312.

31. Jessurun GA, Boersma WG, Crijns HJ. Amiodarone-induced pulmonary toxicity. Predisposing factors, clinical symptoms and treatment. *Drug Safety.* 1998;18:339–344.

32. Ernawati DK, Stafford L, Hughes JD. Amiodarone-induced pulmonary toxicity. *Br J Clin Pharmacol.* 2008;66:82–87.

33. Labombarda F, Ou P, Stos B, de Blic J, Villain E, Sidi D. Acute amiodarone-induced pulmonary toxicity: an association of risk factors in a child operated by arterial switch operation. *Congen Heart Dis.* 2008;3:365–367.

34. Roden DM. Antiarrhythmic drugs. In: Brunton L, Lazo J, Parker K, eds. *Goodman and Gilman's The Pharmacological Basis of Therapeutics,* 11th ed. New York: McGraw-Hill; 2006:899–932.

35. October TW, Schleien CL, Berg RA, Nadkarni VM, Morris MC, Investigators NRoCR. Increasing amiodarone use in cardiopulmonary resuscitation: an analysis of the National Registry of Cardiopulmonary Resuscitation. *Crit Care Med.* 2008;36:126–130.

36. Piccini JP, Berger JS, O'Connor CM. Amiodarone for the prevention of sudden cardiac death: a meta-analysis of randomized controlled trials. *Eur Heart J.* 2009;30:1245–1253.

37. Cleland JG, Ghosh J, Freemantle N, et al. Clinical trials update and cumulative meta-analyses from the American College of Cardiology: WATCH, SCD-HeFT, DINAMIT, CASINO, INSPIRE, STRATUS-US, RIO-Lipids and cardiac resynchronisation therapy in heart failure. *Eur J Heart Fail.* 2004;6:501–508.

38. Savelieva I, Camm J. Anti-arrhythmic drug therapy for atrial fibrillation: current anti-arrhythmic drugs, investigational agents, and innovative approaches. *Eur J Pac Arrhythm Cardiac Electrophysiol.* 2008;10:647–665.

39. Dale KM, White CM. Dronedarone: an amiodarone analog for the treatment of atrial fibrillation and atrial flutter. *Ann Pharmacother.* 2007;41:599–605.

40. Piccini JP, Hasselblad V, Peterson ED, Washam JB, Califf RM, Kong DF. Comparative efficacy of dronedarone and amiodarone for the maintenance of sinus rhythm in patients with atrial fibrillation. *J Am Coll Cardiol.* 2009; 54:1089–1095.

41. Connolly SJ, Crijns HJ, Torp-Pedersen C, et al. Analysis of stroke in ATHENA: a placebo-controlled, double-blind, parallel-arm trial to assess the efficacy of dronedarone 400 mg BID for the prevention of cardiovascular hospitalization or death from any cause in patients with atrial fibrillation/atrial flutter. *Circulation.* 2009;120:1174–1180.

42. Køber L, Torp-Pedersen C, McMurray JJ, et al. Increased mortality after dronedarone therapy for severe heart failure. *N Engl J Med.* 2008;358:2678–2687.

43. Lerman BB, Belardinelli L. Cardiac electrophysiology of adenosine. Basic and clinical concepts. *Circulation.* 1991; 83:1499–1509.

44. Klabunde RE, Althouse DG. Adenosine metabolism in dog whole blood: effects of dipyridamole. *Life Sci.* 1981; 28:2631–2641.

45. Ellenbogen KA, Thames MD, DiMarco JP, Sheehan H, Lerman BB. Electrophysiological effects of adenosine in the transplanted human heart. Evidence of supersensitivity. *Circulation.* 1990;81:821–828.

46. Fredholm BB. Theophylline actions on adenosine receptors. *Eur J Respir Dis Suppl.* 1980;109:29–36.

47. Fredholm BB, Sollevi A. Cardiovascular effects of adenosine. *Clin Physiol.* 1986;6:1–21.

48. Wu SN, Linden J, Visentin S, Boykin M, Belardinelli L. Enhanced sensitivity of heart cells to adenosine and up-regulation of receptor number after treatment of guinea pigs with theophylline. *Circ Res.* 1989;65:1066–1077.

49. Hua X, Chason KD, Fredholm BB, Deshpande DA, Penn RB, Tilley SL. Adenosine induces airway hyperresponsiveness through activation of A3 receptors on mast cells. *J Allerg Clin Immunol.* 2008;122:107–113.

50. DiMarco JP, Miles W, Akhtar M., et al. Adenosine for paroxysmal supraventricular tachycardia: dose ranging and comparison with verapamil. Assessment in placebo-controlled, multicenter trials. The Adenosine for PSVT Study Group. *Ann Intern Med.* 1990;113:104–110.

51. Wenzel V, Krismer AC, Arntz HR, et al. A comparison of vasopressin and epinephrine for out-of-hospital cardiopulmonary resuscitation. *N Engl J Med.* 2004;350:179–181.

52. Wenzel V, Raab H, Dünser MW. Arginine vasopressin: a promising rescue drug in the treatment of uncontrolled haemorrhagic shock. *Best Pract Res Clin Anaesthesiol.* 2008;22:299–316.

53. Jackson EK. Vasopressin and other agents affecting the renal conservation of water. In: Brunton L, Lazo J, Parker K, eds. *Goodman and Gilman's The Pharmacological Basis of Therapeutics,* 11th ed. New York: McGraw-Hill; 2006:771–788.

54. Myerburg RJ, Castellanos A. Cardiac arrest and sudden cardiac death. In: Zipes DP, Libby P, Bonow RO, Braunwald E, eds. *Braunwald's Heart Disease. A Textbook of Cardiovascular Medicine,* 7th ed. Philadelphia: Elsevier Saunders; 2005:865–908.

55. Olgin JE, Zipes DP. Specific arrhythmias: diagnosis and treatment. In: Zipes DP, Libby P, Bonow RO, Braunwald E, eds. *Braunwald's Heart Disease. A Textbook of Cardiovascular Medicine,* 7th ed. Philadelphia: Elsevier Saunders; 2005:803–863.

56. Ho KM. Intravenous magnesium for cardiac arrhythmias: jack of all trades. *Magn Res.* 2008;21:65–68.

IV

**Pharmacologic
Management of Disease:
Anesthetic Considerations**

Malignant Hyperthermia: Dantrolene

Debra R. Merritt, MSN, CRNA

Objectives

After completing this chapter, the reader should be able to

- Define malignant hyperthermia and identify the triggering agents.
- Recognize the clinical signs and symptoms of acute malignant hyperthermia.
- Understand the pathophysiology, cellular events, and metabolic abnormalities associated with malignant hyperthermia.
- Describe a treatment protocol for an acute malignant hyperthermia event.
- Discuss the preparation and administration of dantrolene.
- Develop an anesthetic plan and describe the preparation of an anesthetic gas machine for a patient with known malignant hyperthermia susceptibility.

Malignant Hyperthermia

Introduction

Malignant hyperthermia (MH), first described by Denborough and Lovell in 1960,[1] is an uncommon, life-threatening, pharmacogenetic disorder of skeletal muscle precipitated by volatile anesthetic agents, such as halothane, isoflurane, sevoflurane, desflurane, and the depolarizing muscle relaxant succinylcholine, and in rare cases to environmental stressors, such as vigorous exercise and heat.[2] Upon exposure, susceptible individuals can experience potentially fatal hypermetabolic reactions manifested clinically by increased carbon dioxide production, increased oxygen consumption, tachycardia, tachypnea, hyperthermia, acidosis, muscle rigidity, and rhabdomyolysis.

The MH syndrome occurs in humans, certain breeds of swine, horses, and some other animals.[2] The pathophysiologic changes of MH are due to an uncontrolled elevation in myoplasmic free calcium released from the sarcoplasmic reticulum of the skeletal muscle, leading to increased metabolism.[3] Dantrolene, a skeletal muscle relaxant, is the only currently available drug for specific and effective therapy of this syndrome. As a result of the availability of dantrolene and progress in the understanding of the pathophysiology and clinical manifestations of MH, the mortality and morbidity have been reduced to less than 5%.[2] Early recognition of MH and prompt treatment with dantrolene can improve a patient's chances for a full recovery.

Incidence

The true modern incidence of MH is unknown, in part due to a variety of epidemiologic barriers that include difficulties in establishing a clinical diagnosis of MH, the lack of a highly sensitive and specific noninvasive diagnostic screening test for MH, and the lack of uniform criteria for MH diagnosis and reporting. However, in North America and Europe, based on retrospective studies, the clinical incidence of MH has been estimated to be 1 in 5000 anesthetics for children and adolescents and 1 in 50,000 to 100,000 anesthetics for adults.[4] Factors that can influence the incidence of MH include the prevalence of the genetic change that predisposes to MH and the dose and duration of exposure to the anesthetic triggers. The incidence is higher when succinylcholine is combined with volatile anesthetic gases. The incidence of fulminant MH, characterized as a profound hypermetabolic state with a rise in core temperature, increased carbon dioxide production and oxygen consumption, acidosis, and muscle breakdown, ranges from 1 in 62,000 to 84,000 of general anesthesia cases if succinylcholine or potent inhalation agent are used.[5] MH affects people of all ages, both genders, and all ethnic groups, although it appears to be more common in children and young adults than in older people.[2] Reactions develop more frequently in males than in females (2:1) and in children under 15 years of age, who account for 52.1% of all MH episodes.[6]

Genetically, MH is an inherited autosomal dominant condition with variable penetrance. This means that children and siblings of an MH-susceptible patient have a 50% chance of inheriting the genetic defect for MH and therefore would be MH susceptible.[3] This demonstrates the importance of obtaining a detailed family history of any adverse anesthesia reactions, unexplained fever, or death during anesthesia. However, neither a negative family history nor previous exposure to anesthesia reliably predicts its occurrence, because about half of all patients who have an MH episode have undergone a prior uneventful anesthetic episode with triggering agents.[3]

Pathophysiology

Molecular genetic analysis has identified mutations in the skeletal muscle ryanodine receptor gene (*RYR1*) as one of the primary defects for MH susceptibility. This protein receptor regulates calcium release from the sarcoplasmic reticulum into the sarcoplasm. More than 90 mutations have been associated with the *RYR1* gene, of which more than 40 are causal for MH. In addition, dihydropyridine receptor mutations have also been identified in MH patients, implicating abnormal skeletal muscle excitation-contraction coupling mechanisms in muscle as a molecular link to MH.[7]

The pathophysiology of MH is related to the uncontrolled release of calcium from the skeletal muscle sarcoplasmic reticulum through the ryanodine receptor, an ion channel, into the sarcoplasm after exposure to the triggering agents.[3] This sudden uncontrolled rise in intracellular myoplasmic calcium results in a continued interaction between actin and mycin, leading to sustained muscle contraction and a cascade of hypermetabolic reactions.[3,8]

This hypermetabolic state greatly increases oxygen consumption, leading to an oxygen deficit that requires conversion of the aerobic pathway to the anaerobic pathway to sustain metabolic activity and resulting in an increase in carbon dioxide and lactic acid production.[9] In addition, biochemical processes are activated and energy is expended in a futile attempt to resequester the released calcium back into the sarcoplasmic reticulum. This leads to further oxygen consumption, carbon dioxide production, breakdown of adenosine triphosphate (ATP), lactic acidosis, hypercarbia, and hyperthermia. The depletion of ATP stores results in deterioration of the skeletal muscle's cellular membranes, allowing release of intracellular constituents such as myoglobin, potassium, calcium, creatinine phosphokinase (CPK), and lactate dehydrogenase

into the blood.[3] The increased metabolic activity is compounded by the rise in body temperature, affecting all tissues, and resulting in further increased oxygen consumption, carbon dioxide production, metabolic and respiratory acidosis, sympathetic output, and cardiac and respiratory stimulation.[9]

Myofilament sensitivity of the muscle is temperature dependent; therefore as the temperature rises, muscle contraction increases and the rhabdomyolytic process is exacerbated. Rising body temperature also stimulates the procoagulant pathways, leading to disseminated intravascular coagulation and a coagulopathy.[9] The severe metabolic acidosis and hyperkalemia in turn may lead to cardiovascular instability or cardiac arrest. In addition, muscle cell breakdown, or rhabdomyolysis, manifested as cola-colored urine, may lead to myoglobinuria-induced renal failure.[2,3]

Clinical Signs and Symptoms

MH may present itself as a broad clinical spectrum at any time during the administration of anesthesia and in the early postoperative period. An unexplained, unexpected increase in end-tidal carbon dioxide provides the earliest, most sensitive, and specific sign of potential MH, especially combined together with a sudden, unexplainable increase in heart rate.[2,3] Tachypnea may be present in spontaneously breathing patients and can be masked with controlled ventilation and neuromuscular blockade. Although muscle rigidity is one of the most unique signs of MH, it is not the most consistent.[10,11] The rigor mortis–like truncal and limb rigidity parallels the progression of the clinical syndrome and can interfere with perfusion and ventilation.[3] This increasing rigidity is unresponsive to nondepolarizing muscle relaxants.[2,3,11,12]

Masseter muscle rigidity, trismus, is a rigidity of the jaw muscles that may be observed after administration of succinylcholine. This occurs most commonly as a transient phenomenon in children, but it may be a forewarning to MH. By muscle biopsy 50% of these patients may prove to be MH susceptible, although many of these cases do not progress to a fulminant MH episode.[10] When masseter muscle rigidity develops, a decision may be made either to switch to a nontriggering anesthetic technique and proceed with urgent surgery or to discontinue the anesthetic and postpone elective surgery. All patients exhibiting this sign should be monitored for the development of myoglobinuria, creatine kinase elevation, and signs of MH.[2]

In addition, other clinical signs of MH include tachycardia, severe metabolic and respiratory acidosis, and hyperkalemia contributing to peaked T waves on the electrocardiogram, dysrhythmias, and cardiac instability.[11] The patient's skin becomes diaphoretic with a mottled appearance of cyanotic areas and patches of bright red flushing.[3] Hyperthermia is a relatively late sign that develops from the heat generated by increased skeletal muscle metabolism that can no longer be dissipated from the body. If left untreated, rhabdomyolysis and muscle cell death result in hyperkalemia, myoglobinuria leading to acute renal failure, disseminated intravascular coagulation, congestive heart failure, compartment syndrome, pulmonary and cerebral edema, and bowel ischemia. Eventually, multisystem organ failure occurs from unsustainable acceleration in metabolic demand, rapidly leading to death.[2,3,11,12]

Conditions and Disorders in the Differential Diagnosis of MH

Currently, in clinical practice there is no single feature of MH that is pathognomonic or any simple laboratory tests that can identify susceptible individuals. Several disorders and conditions observed in the perioperative period have features that resemble MH and may be confused with this syndrome. These include thyroid storm in thyrotoxicosis, pheochromocytoma, inflammatory response syndrome, anticholinergic syndrome, anaphylaxis, meningitis, hypoxic encephalopathy, brain injury, and hyperthermia secondary to sepsis.[2,3,9] Other conditions that may resemble MH include iatrogenic overheating, faulty equipment for measuring temperature or end-tidal carbon dioxide, carbon dioxide absorption during laparoscopic procedures, improper minute ventilation and fresh gas flows, machine valve malfunction, rebreathing or prolonged tourniquet inflation, and ischemia.[2,3,9] However, most of these are not associated with a mixed respiratory and metabolic acidosis that occurs during most MH events and can be differentiated by blood gas analysis. In addition, an MH-like syndrome may occur after intrathecal injection of ionic contrast agents; an overdose of cocaine, ecstasy, amphetamines, sympathomimetics; or salicylates; serotonin syndrome; or neuroleptic malignant syndrome.[2,3,9]

Neuroleptic malignant syndrome, a condition marked by hyperthermia, metabolic acidosis, muscle rigidity, hyperkalemia, and myoglobinuria, has been mistaken for MH.[13] This syndrome develops after the use of a wide variety of neuroleptic antipsychotic medications, especially haloperidol.[13] The pathophysiology is associated with dopamine receptor blockade or reduced levels of dopamine. Dantrolene has proven effective in the treatment of neuroleptic malignant syndrome[14,15] as well as the administration of benzodiazepines and bromocriptine.[2,13] However, there does not appear to be any crossover susceptibility to MH.

Serotonin syndrome is another medication-induced disorder presenting in a similar manner as MH that results from antidepressants increasing the level of serotonin in the central nervous system.[13] When an MH event is suspected, alternative diagnoses should be considered and excluded. However, for some of these differential diagnoses it may be impossible to make the distinction with MH in a sufficiently timely manner to avoid any course of action other than treating the patient for MH.

Association With Other Disorders

In the past there has been a general clinical impression that patients with muscular abnormalities have an increased incidence of MH, and several groups have reported the association of susceptibility to MH and various myopathies. Clinical MH susceptibility has been associated with central core disease, multiminicore disease, myotonia fluctuans, hypokalemic periodic paralysis, nemaline rod myopathy and King-Denborough syndrome, Duchenne muscular dystrophy, hyperkalemic periodic paralysis, and other myopathies.[2,3,16] However, the documented association is with central core disease and multiminicore disease. Central core disease, a rare, congenital inherited myopathy characterized by neonatal hypotonia, proximal muscle weakness, musculoskeletal abnormalities, and demarcated cores lacking oxidative enzyme activity on histochemical analysis, and multiminicore disease, also characterized by muscle weakness and wasting, are directly associated with MH susceptibility and share the same genetic locus, the *RYR1* gene on chromosome 19.[2,16–19]

Tests for Diagnosing MH Susceptibility

Currently, the in vitro caffeine halothane contracture test (CHCT), using biopsied muscle, is the gold standard for diagnosing MH.[20] There are currently two standardized testing protocols for classifying patients: the North American Malignant Hyperthermia Group and the European In Vitro Malignant Hyperthermia Test.[9] Based on guidelines established by the North American Malignant Hyperthermia Group registry, the CHCT provides sensitivity of 97% and specificity of 78%.[2,21] This means that the frequency of false negatives is extremely low; however, this allows for a 22% false-positive rate. The test is difficult to completely standardize and is expensive and invasive, requiring a surgical procedure to be performed on site at a specialized testing center. The test requires exposing a fresh muscle specimen from the vastus lateralis or medialis in a physiologic solution to ryanodine receptor agonists, caffeine and halothane, in various concentrations. The amount of tension generated is compared with known standards and an individual is diagnosed as MH susceptible if abnormally high levels of contractile force or increase in the muscle's tension develops on exposure to these agents.[2,3]

Molecular genetic testing for MH susceptibility offers an acceptable alternative for identifying some individuals and their family members. At this point the sensitivity of the test is only in the range of 50%, meaning that it detects only 50% of those who are MH susceptible depending on the selection criteria used. Those recommended for testing include those with a relative with a known causal *RYR1* mutation, a positive CHCT, a relative of a known MH-susceptible family member, and patients or their relatives without prior testing but having a highly suspicious clinical episode of MH. Genetic analysis is based on extraction of DNA from a blood sample or from other body tissue obtained and sent to the testing laboratory.[2,7,20,22–24] Currently, 29 causative mutations for MH susceptibility have been identified in the skeletal muscle ryanodine receptor (*RYR1*), and DNA screening for one of these mutations follows receipt of the sample.[23,24]

Although multiple gene loci are involved, 50% of MH families can be linked to mutations in the *RYR1* gene.[7] If an *RYR1* mutation is detected, then other first-degree relatives of that individual can be tested; those in whom the mutation is found are diagnosed as having MH without undergoing CHCT. However, although the presence of a causative mutation is diagnostic for MH susceptibility, the absence of a causative mutation does not rule out MH susceptibility. A negative molecular genetic test must be followed by a negative CHCT to exclude MH susceptibility. Hesitancy to rule out MH susceptibility based on absence of the mutation is based on well-documented phenotypic and genotypic discrepancies in MH-susceptible families.[2,7,20,22–24] Scientists hope that one day genetic screening will become precise enough to replace the CHCT as the main means by which individuals can be diagnosed as being MH susceptible.

Anesthesia for the MH-Susceptible Individual

A patient who is MH susceptible can safely have surgery with a nontriggering anesthetic technique. If the surgical site permits, a regional or local anesthetic, using amides or esters, is preferable for an MH-susceptible patient. If general anesthesia or sedation is required, halogenated volatile anesthetic gases and succinylcholine must be avoided. Anesthesia should consist of nitrous oxide, barbiturates, etomidate, propofol, opioids, benzodiazepines, ketamine, and nondepolarizing muscle relaxants in concert with close monitoring of appropriate vital functions. Dantrolene prophylaxis is no longer recommended for these patients preoperatively, because of the potential risk of nausea, disequilibrium, and worsening muscle weakness in patients with neuromuscular disease.[2,20,25]

All locations where general anesthesia is administered should have a treatment plan for MH and contain a fully stocked MH cart with drugs and supplies, including 36 vials of dantrolene. The anesthesia machine should be prepared by removing or disabling the vaporizers, changing the carbon dioxide absorbent and the breathing circuit, and flushing the anesthesia circuit with 10 L/min oxygen for at least 20 minutes. The ventilator may also be flushed by connecting a breathing bag to the Y-piece and switching on the ventilator during this process.[2,9,20] One must consult the manufacturer for newer anesthesia machines, because some may require 30 to 40 minutes of preparation time. The expired gas analyzer may be used to confirm the absence of volatile agent in the anesthesia circuit.[20,26] MH-susceptible patients, for outpatient surgery, may be safely discharged on the same day after an uneventful operation. They should be monitored in the recovery room for a total of 2.5 hours, after which if there is no signs of increased metabolism or rhabdomyolysis, they may be discharged from the facility.[2,9,20]

Pharmacologic Intervention

Dantrolene sodium, first introduced in 1979, is the only available drug for the specific and effective treatment of acute MH.[27] Before that time the drug was available in an oral formulation for use as an adjunct in the treatment of muscle spasticity associated with cerebral palsy or spinal cord injury.[14] This lyophilized formulation for injection is supplied in 70-mL vials containing 20 mg dantrolene sodium, 3000 mg mannitol, and sufficient sodium hydroxide to yield a pH of approximately 9.5 when reconstituted with 60 mL sterile water for injection.[14] The molecular structure of dantrolene is hydrated 1-[5-(4-nitrophenyl)-2-furanyl]-2,4-imidazolidinedione sodium salt. The structural formula for the hydrated salt is illustrated in Figure 24-1.[28]

Mechanism of Action

Dantrolene, a hydantoin derivative, is classified as a direct-acting skeletal muscle relaxant that binds to the ryanodine receptor, thereby reducing its open state probability and blocking calcium release from the myoplasmic sarcoplasmic reticulum without altering calcium reuptake.[14] The exact physiologic process by which dantrolene suppresses calcium release is not completely understood. However, studies suggest that dantrolene binds to and stabilizes domain interactions within the skeletal muscle ryanodine receptor, RyR1, suppressing voltage-dependent calcium release from the sarcoplasmic reticulum by favoring a non–conductive channel conformation.[29] Dantrolene also decreases muscle contraction without an effect on the action potential patterns of the neuromuscular junction. In addition, dantrolene has no direct effect on the actin and myosin binding and has no effect on the passive or active electrical properties of the surface and tubular membranes of skeletal muscle fibers.[3]

Clinical Pharmacology

Pharmacokinetics

After oral administration 70% of a dose of dantrolene is absorbed from the gastrointestinal tract with significant variations in peak plasma concentrations seen at about 6 hours.[14] In healthy awake volunteers intravenous administration of dantrolene 2.4 mg/kg results in plasma concentrations that block up to 75% of skeletal muscle contraction and remain stable within therapeutic range for approximately 5 hours after administration.[14] The plasma elimination half-life time is estimated to be 12 hours, and it is not significantly influenced by pregnancy or preoperative medications. In pediatrics the pharmacokinetic profile is similar, with a half-life of approximately 10 hours. Dantrolene is metabolized by liver microsomes to 5-hydroxy-dantrolene, which itself acts as a skeletal muscle relaxant with a half-life of approximately 15 hours; it is excreted in urine and bile.[14,15,28]

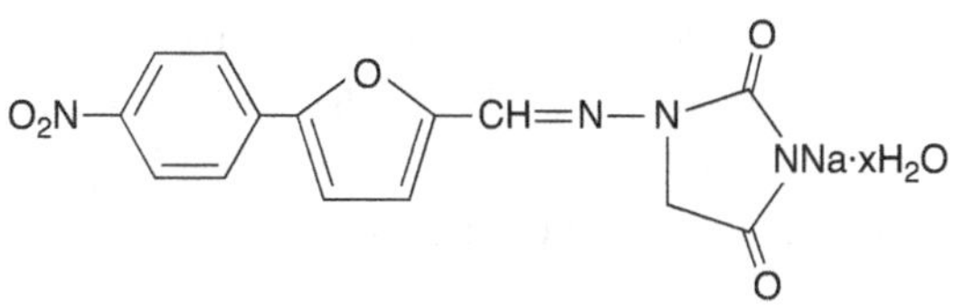

Side Effects

Dantrolene sodium is generally safe when administered at recommended dosages, but some side effects may occur after administration. In a retrospective analysis of patients treated with dantrolene during an MH crisis, the most commonly reported side effects were skeletal muscle weakness, phlebitis, respiratory failure, and gastrointestinal discomfort.[14,28,30] The maximum muscle weakness in normal volunteers was reported after intravenous administration of dantrolene 2.4 mg/kg, which is near the therapeutic plasma concentration of the drug.[25] Therefore dantrolene-associated skeletal muscle weakness may be sufficient enough to interfere with adequate ventilation or protection of the lungs from aspiration of gastric fluid resulting in serious sequelae, especially in patients with neuromuscular disease. Patients who experience acute MH may also experience muscle weakness as a result of muscle injury that can be part this syndrome.[30] This may be the reason subjects with muscle weakness tend to have higher peak postoperative CPK levels. Therefore the clinician treating an MH episode should request repeated measurement of CPK until it returns to normal levels. The patient with elevated CPK levels may require postoperative positive pressure ventilation for a longer interval.

The second most common side effect, local inflammatory phlebitis at the infusion site, after the administration of dantrolene, may be due to low solubility of the highly alkaline solution and its chemical irritation of local tissues.[14,28,31] Phlebitis may result in fluid extravasation into interstitial tissues and increase the risk of compartment syndrome. Therefore it is recommended that dantrolene be administered via large peripheral veins or central venous lines.[20]

Chronic therapy has been associated with liver dysfunction and pleural effusion, suggesting hepatic function monitoring in all cases of chronic administration. Rare symptoms of chronic dantrolene treatment also include nausea, abdominal cramping, anorexia, gastric irritation, constipation, dysphagia, enuresis, visual disturbances, acne-like rash, and excessive secretions.[14,28]

Figure 24-1 The molecular structure of dantrolene (hydrated salt).

Neonates are at risk of floppy child syndrome when dantrolene is administered to the mother during cesarean section, and the mother is placed at risk for postpartum uterine atony after delivery. Dantrolene crosses the placenta, and plasma levels of up to 65% of maternal levels can be measured in the newborn.[14,28,32]

Drug Interactions and Contraindications

Although dantrolene itself at therapeutic doses has no apparent myocardial effects in humans, in swine and dogs when it is administered in combination with verapamil it is associated with a significant decrease in cardiac function.[14,28] Thus the simultaneous administration of both calcium channel blockers and dantrolene in the management of MH-induced cardiac tachyarrhythmias should be avoided because of the potential development of life-threatening hyperkalemia, myocardial depression, and cardiac arrest.[3,9,20]

Another possible drug interaction involves dantrolene and nondepolarizing muscle relaxants; dantrolene has been shown to potentiate neuromuscular blockade with vecuronium.[14,28] This prolongation of the neuromuscular junction recovery may be caused by decreased transmitter release at the neuromuscular junction as a result of attenuated calcium release from the cholinergic terminal calcium storage sites. Therefore when dantrolene is used with nondepolarizing muscle relaxants, care should be taken to ensure muscle strength has returned before extubation.

Guidelines and New Developments

There are some interesting developments regarding the therapeutic value of dantrolene. It has been known that in many cases dantrolene is effective in reversing extreme temperature elevation from a variety of causes. Based on case reports, it has been used successfully and sometimes dramatically in the treatment of neuroleptic malignant syndrome and in the treatment of hyperthermia, acidosis, and muscle breakdown from ecstasy (3,4-methylenedioxymethamphetamine) intoxication.[13,14] Another rare and peculiar syndrome is extreme temperature elevation and muscle breakdown in new-onset diabetes in young people. A number of case reports have demonstrated that when this occurs, fatality is likely without the administration of dantrolene.[14] Another untapped area is the role of dantrolene in the treatment of heat stroke. Because a rapid decrease in body temperature is important in the management of heat stroke, dantrolene has been given in conjunction with a variety of physical cooling techniques. However, data from case reports have not definitively shown that dantrolene therapy is actually beneficial in the treatment of heat stroke unless the patient has a personal or family history of MH; therefore a general recommendation cannot be made until controlled scientific studies have been performed.[14,33,34]

To minimize the effect of diluent injection time, current research has also focused on strategies to chemically improve drug solubility. Lecithin-coated dantrolene, neutral dantrolene, ryanodex, and azumolene have all been shown to have vastly improved solubility profiles, and promising results have been demonstrated in animal studies. However, presently limited human data exist with regard to their safety and efficacy in MH. Furthermore, it remains unclear how drug costs would be influenced by these new formulations of dantrolene.[35,36]

Dantrolene sodium for injection, a rapidly mixing product, has been developed by JHP Pharmaceuticals and received approval by the FDA in November 2009. The enhanced lyophilization process allows the dantrolene sodium to be mixed in approximately 20 seconds, with noticeably less vigorous shaking required to complete the reconstitution process. This is four times faster than before, saving valuable time and effort during an MH emergency.[28] Due to cost management reasons, clinical availability may be limited until the expiration of current supplies.

Dosage and Administration

Dantrolene sodium is the only effective medication for treating MH, and it should be administered as soon as an MH episode is diagnosed. Each 20-mg vial of dantrolene must be dissolved with 60 mL sterile, preservative-free water in preparation for injection. Dantrolene reconstitution is labor intensive, and the vials must be shaken vigorously for 2 to 3 minutes for dissolution to occur, resulting in a clear solution.[14,20,37] In addition, prewarming of the sterile water to a temperature not to exceed 41°C may facilitate the reconstitution process; however, further studies are needed to evaluate whether this warmed diluent affects the efficacy of dantrolene.[31] Also, dantrolene sodium vials contain NaOH for a pH of 9.5 and 3 g of mannitol for isotonicity. The contents of the vial must be protected from direct light and should be used within 6 hours after reconstitution.[14,28]

The initial dose of 2.5 mg/kg equates to nine vials of dantrolene for a 70-kg patient and requires the assistance of other personnel to prepare and administer. Upon administration of the initial dose, clinical signs and arterial blood gases should be monitored to ensure that the syndrome has been adequately treated. If signs of an ongoing MH event are confirmed, dantrolene administration should be repeated at 2 mg/kg every 5 minutes until the signs of MH are reversed. The recommended upper limit of 10 mg/kg for a 70-kg person is a useful guideline, but it is not the "absolute" upper limit.[2,3,9,20,37] After the acute crisis has been controlled, dantrolene should be continued in the postoperative period at a dose of 1 mg/kg every 4 to 6 hours or 0.25 mg/kg/h by infusion for at least 24 hours.[37] Continuation of treatment is necessary because recrudescence of MH can approach 25%, usually within 6 hours of the initial event.[6] The administration of dantrolene beyond this time may be dictated by a recurrence of acidosis as documented blood gases and by signs of increased metabolism, temperature elevation, rhabdomyolysis, or muscle rigidity.[2,3,9,20,37]

Practical Aspects and Clinical Insights for Administration

The Malignant Hyperthermia Association of the United States outlined a protocol for the recommended emergency therapy for MH (Figure 24-2).[37] Successful treatment depends on early recognition and prompt administration of dantrolene. Symptomatic treatment is directed toward maintaining renal function and correcting hyperthermia, acidosis, and arterial hypoxemia.[2,3,9] As soon as an acute MH crisis has been identified, the severity of the situation must be communicated to the surgical team and additional help and the MH emergency cart should be summoned to the operating room. Immediately discontinue use of any volatile inhalation anesthetic agent or succinylcholine, hyperventilate the lungs with 100% oxygen, and begin to administer dantrolene sodium at a dose of 2.5 mg/kg as a bolus. Be prepared to repeat the initial dose of dantrolene until the signs of MH are controlled. After the administration of dantrolene sodium, the clinical sequelae of acute MH must be addressed, including institution of cooling measures, treatment of life-threatening electrolyte abnormalities, and prevention of myoglobinuria-induced renal failure with increased hydration, bicarbonate therapy, and administration of diuretics. The development of severe metabolic abnormalities may lead to cardiovascular instability; therefore close monitoring of the patient should include arterial and venous blood gases, serum electrolytes, CPK, blood and urine for myoglobin, and a coagulation

profile. Treat metabolic acidosis with sodium bicarbonate, if the acute episode is not promptly reversed by dantrolene. Specifically, potentially lethal dysrhythmias, such as ventricular tachycardia or fibrillation, may result from severe acidosis and hyperkalemia, and immediate treatment should be instituted with glucose, insulin, bicarbonate, hyperventilation, and calcium. Calcium chloride and calcium gluconate can be administered for life-threatening hyperkalemia.[2,3,9,37]

Dysrhythmias usually respond to treatment of acidosis or hyperkalemia and use of standard antiarrhythmics drug therapy except calcium channel blockers, which can cause severe hyperkalemia or cardiac arrest in the presence of dantrolene sodium.[3,9,20] Cooling measures should be implemented until the patient's core temperature is down to 38°C. Active cooling techniques may include forced air, hypothermia blanket, intravenous cold saline solution, ice packs to the axillae and groin, and lavage of open body cavities, stomach, bladder, or rectum with cold saline solution. In addition, the urine output should be followed to maintain an output greater than 2 mL/kg/h with intravenous fluids, furosemide, and mannitol to avoid myoglobinuria-induced renal failure.[2,3,9,20,37] After stabilization, dantrolene administration is continued in the postoperative period at a dose of 1 mg/kg every 4 to 6 hours or 0.25 mg/kg/h by infusion for at least 24 hours.[37] The patient is admitted to the intensive care unit for continued treatment and monitored for late manifestations of the disease, because 25% of patients experience a recrudescence of the syndrome.[6] Arterial blood gases are drawn as clinically indicated, and serum creatine kinase, urine myoglobin, and coagulation parameters should continue to be monitored for at least 24 to 48 hours.[2,3,9,20,37]

The MH Hotline may be contacted as soon as possible for further management assistance at 1-800-MH-HYPER (1-800-644-9737). The patient and family should be counseled regarding MH and referred to the Malignant Hyperthermia Association of the United States for information and enrollment in the North American MH Registry.

The Malignant Hyperthermia Association of the United States is a nonprofit organization that provides education, counsel, and technical information to patients, their family, and healthcare providers. A follow-up letter should be sent to the patient and the physician with further precautions and a referral to the nearest biopsy center for testing. Information is available on the Internet (http://www.mhaus.org) or at MHAUS, 11 East State Street, PO Box 1069, Sherburne, NY 13460-1069; telephone: 1-800-986-4287 or 607-674-7901; e-mail: info@mhaus.org.[37]

Effective May 2008

MH Hotline
1-800-644-9737
Outside the US:
1-315-464-7079

EMERGENCY THERAPY FOR

MALIGNANT HYPERTHERMIA

DIAGNOSIS vs. ASSOCIATED PROBLEMS

Signs of MH:
- Increasing ETCO2
- Trunk or total body rigidity
- Masseter spasm or trismus
- Tachycardia/tachypnea
- Mixed Respiratory and Metabolic Acidosis
- Increased temperature (may be late sign)
- Myoglobinuria

Sudden/Unexpected Cardiac Arrest in Young Patients:
- Presume hyperkalemia and initiate treatment (see #6)
- Measure CK, myoglobin, ABGs, until normalized
- Consider dantrolene
- Usually secondary to occult myopathy (e.g., muscular dystrophy)
- Resuscitation may be difficult and prolonged

Trismus or Masseter Spasm with Succinylcholine
- Early sign of MH in many patients
- If limb muscle rigidity, begin treatment with dantrolene
- For emergent procedures, continue with non-triggering agents, evaluate and monitor the patient, and consider dantrolene treatment
- Follow CK and urine myoglobin for 36 hours.
- Check CK immediately and at 6 hour intervals until returning to normal. Observe for dark or cola colored urine. If present, liberalize fluid intake and test for myoglobin
- Observe in PACU or ICU for at least 12 hours

ACUTE PHASE TREATMENT

① GET HELP. GET DANTROLENE – Notify Surgeon
- Discontinue volatile agents and succinylcholine.
- Hyperventilate with 100% oxygen at flows of 10 L/min. or more.
- Halt the procedure as soon as possible; if emergent, continue with non-triggering anesthetic technique.
- Don't waste time changing the circle system and CO2 absorbant.

② Dantrolene 2.5 mg/kg rapidly IV through large-bore IV, if possible

> To convert kg to lbs for amount of dantrolene, give patients 1 mg/lb (2.5 mg/kg approximates 1 mg/lb).

- Dissolve the 20 mg in each vial with at least 60 ml sterile, preservative-free water for injection. Prewarming (not to exceed 39°C.) the sterile water may expidite solubilization of dantrolene. However, to date, there is no evidence that such warming improves clinical outcome.
- Repeat until signs of MH are reversed.
- Sometimes more than 10 mg/kg (up to 30 mg/kg) is necessary.

- Each 20 mg bottle has 3 gm mannitol for isotonicity. The pH of the solution is 9.

③ Bicarbonate for metabolic acidosis
- 1-2 mEq/kg if blood gas values are not yet available.

④ Cool the patient with core temperature >39°C, Lavage open body cavities, stomach, bladder, or rectum. Apply ice to surface. Infuse cold saline intravenously. Stop cooling if temp. <38°C and falling to prevent drift < 36°C.

⑤ Dysrhythmias usually respond to treatment of acidosis and hyperkalemia.
- Use standard drug therapy **except calcium channel blockers, which may cause hyperkalemia or cardiac arrest in the presence of dantrolene.**

⑥ Hyperkalemia – Treat with hyperventilation, bicarbonate, glucose/insulin, calcium.
- Bicarbonate 1-2 mEq/kg IV.
- For **pediatric,** 0.1 units insulin/kg and 1 ml/kg 50% glucose or for **adult,** 10 units regular insulin IV and 50 ml 50% glucose.
- Calcium chloride 10 mg/kg or calcium gluconate 10-50 mg/kg for life-threatening hyperkalemia.
- Check glucose levels hourly.

⑦ Follow ETCO2, electrolytes, blood gases, CK, core temperature, urine output and color, coagulation studies. If CK and/or K+ rise more than transiently or urine output falls to less than 0.5 ml/kg/hr, induce diuresis to >1 ml/kg/hr and give bicarbonate to alkalinize urine to prevent myoglobinuria-induced renal failure. (See D below)
- Venous blood gas (e.g., femoral vein) values may document hypermetabolism better than arterial values.
- Central venous or PA monitoring as needed and record minute ventilation.
- Place Foley catheter and monitor urine output.

POST ACUTE PHASE

Ⓐ Observe the patient in an ICU for at least 24 hours, due to the risk of recrudescence.
Ⓑ Dantrolene 1 mg/kg q 4-6 hours or 0.25 mg/kg/hr by infusion for at least 24 hours. Further doses may be indicated.
Ⓒ Follow vitals and labs as above (see #7)
- Frequent ABG as per clinical signs
- CK every 8-12 hours; less often as the values trend downward

Ⓓ Follow urine myoglobin and institute therapy to prevent myoglobin precipitation in renal tubules and the subsequent development of Acute Renal Failure. CK levels above 10,000 IU/L is a presumptive sign of rhabdomyolysis and myoglobinuria. Follow standard intensive care therapy for acute rhabdomyolysis and myoglobinuria (urine output >2 ml/kg/hr by hydration and diuretics along with alkalinization of urine with Na-bicarbonate infusion with careful attention to both urine and serum pH values).
Ⓔ Counsel the patient and family regarding MH and further precautions; refer them to MHAUS. Fill out and send in the Adverse Metabolic Reaction to Anesthesia (AMRA) form (www.mhreg.org) and send a letter to the patient and her/his physician. Refer patient to the nearest Biopsy Center for follow-up.

Non-Emergency Information
MHAUS
PO Box 1069 (11 East State Street)
Sherburne, NY 13460-1069
Phone
1-800-986-4287
(607-674-7901)
Fax
607-674-7910
Email
info@mhaus.org
Website
www.mhaus.org

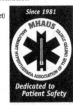

Since 1981
MHAUS
Dedicated to Patient Safety

CAUTION: This protocol may not apply to all patients; alter for specific needs.

Produced by the Malignant Hyperthermia Association of the United States (MHAUS). MHAUS is a non-profit organization under IRS-Code 501(c)3. It operates solely on contributed funds. All contributions are tax deductible. For more information, go to www.mhaus.org.

Figure 24-2 Emergency therapy for malignant hyperthermia.
Source: Produced by the Malignant Hyperthermia Association of the United States (MHAUS). MHAUS is a non-profit organization under IRS-Code 501(c)3.

Summary

MH is an uncommon, life-threatening, acute, pharmacogenetic, inherited disorder of skeletal muscle cells. It manifests in susceptible individuals as a hypermetabolic response on exposure to volatile inhalation agents and depolarizing muscle relaxants, with uncontrolled release of cytoplasmic free calcium from the sarcoplasmic reticulum and consecutive systemic organ system failure. A classic fulminant MH crisis presents with an increasing end-tidal carbon dioxide, skeletal muscle rigidity, tachycardia, hyperthermia, rhabdomyolysis, hyperkalemia, and acidosis, leading to death if left untreated. Immediate discontinuation of triggering agents, oxygenation, and correction of acidosis and electrolyte abnormalities, treatment of arrhythmias, cooling, and administration of dantrolene are essential for successful treatment of this syndrome. Presently, the mortality from MH is less than 5% due to widespread education and research on MH as well as preoperative screening, early clinical diagnosis, improved monitoring standards, and the availability of dantrolene.

With the advent of molecular genetic testing and more widespread awareness of MH and other heat-related and drug-induced hyperthermic syndromes, we undoubtedly will learn more about dantrolene, its mode of action, and its utility in the treatment of disorders other than classic MH. Remaining challenges include identification of all genetic mutations responsible for human MH, elucidation of the mechanism that links exposure to the subsequent loss of calcium control, development of noninvasive and nondestructive testing for susceptibility, and identification of the mode of action of dantrolene.

Key Points

- MH is an uncommon, life-threatening, pharmacogenetic disorder of skeletal muscle characterized by increased carbon dioxide production, oxygen consumption, and muscle membrane breakdown that presents when susceptible individuals are exposed to volatile anesthetic gases, such as halothane, isoflurane, sevoflurane, desflurane, and the depolarizing muscle relaxant succinylcholine.

- The underlying pathophysiology of MH centers on the uncontrolled increase in intracellular calcium in the muscle cell after exposure to triggering agents. This abnormal and sustained elevation in myoplasmic free calcium is controlled primarily by the calcium release channels of the sarcoplasmic reticulum by way of the ryanodine receptor.

- The depolarizing muscle relaxant succinylcholine and all volatile inhalational anesthetic agents (e.g., ether, cyclopropane, methoxyflurane, halothane, isoflurane, enflurane, desflurane, sevoflurane) are capable of triggering MH in humans.

- Upon exposure, susceptible individuals can experience a potentially fatal hypermetabolic reaction manifested clinically by increased carbon dioxide production, increased oxygen consumption, tachycardia, tachypnea, hyperthermia, acidosis, muscle rigidity, and rhabdomyolysis.

- At present, the CHCT is the only acceptable and definitive diagnostic test to determine MH susceptibility and is considered the gold standard. A new molecular genetic diagnostic blood test may offer a less-invasive alternative for some patients.

- Dantrolene, the only effective specific medication for treating MH, is a direct-acting skeletal muscle relaxant that decreases calcium release from the sarcoplasmic reticulum. The initial dose of dantrolene is 2.5 mg/kg, and each 20-mg vial must be dissolved with 60 mL sterile water.

- MH-susceptible patients can be safely anesthetized with a nontriggering anesthetic technique. Barbiturates, propofol, etomidate, ketamine, benzodiazepines, opioids, droperidol, nitrous oxide, nondepolarizing muscle relaxants, anticholinesterase drugs, anticholinergics, sympathomimetics, and ester and amide local anesthetics are safe for MH-susceptible patients.

Chapter Questions

1. Describe what steps one would implement in preparation for an MH-susceptible patient. How would one prepare the anesthetic gas machine? What anesthetic technique would one select based on the patient's past medical history and the proposed surgical procedure? What drugs are considered safe for administration to MH-susceptible patients? How would one communicate the patient's MH status to all perioperative care providers?

2. Describe the methods that can be used to facilitate the mixing and administration of dantrolene during an MH crisis. Where would you find all the medications, equipment, and supplies to accomplish this task? How many individuals and what type of setup would be helpful for this process?

3. Discuss how the management of an MH episode may differ depending on the location of the event,

the clinical situation, and the available staffing: Is the patient in a hospital operating room, an ambulatory surgical center, or an office-based practice? What type of "transfer of care" policy should be in place and implemented to ensure the patient is stabilized and to maintain continuity of care?

References

1. Denborough MA, Lovell RH. Anesthesia deaths in a family. *Lancet.* 1960;2:45.

2. Rosenberg H, Davis M, James D, Pollock N, Stowell K. Malignant hyperthermia. *Orphanet J Rare Dis.* 2007;2:21.

3. Syed ZA, Akiko T, Rosenberg H. Malignant hyperthermia. *Best Pract Res Clin Anesthesiol.* 2003;17:519–533.

4. Ording H. Incidence of malignant hyperthermia in Denmark. *Anesth Analg.* 1985;64:700–704.

5. Halliday NJ. Malignant hyperthermia. *J Craniofac Surg.* 2003;14:800–802.

6. Burkman JM, Posner KL, Domino KB. Analysis of the clinical variables associated with recrudescence after malignant hyperthermia reactions. *Anesthesiology.* 2007;106:901–908.

7. Brandon BW. Genetics of malignant hyperthermia. *Scientific World J.* 2006;6:1722–1730.

8. Mickelson JR. Louis CF. Malignant hyperthermia: excitation-contraction coupling. Calcium release channel and cell calcium regulation defects. *Physiol Rev.* 1996;76:537–592.

9. Hopkins PM. Malignant hyperthermia. *Curr Anaesth Crit Care.* 2008;19:22–33.

10. O'Flynn RP, Shutack JG, Rosenberg H, Fletcher JE. MMR and MH susceptibility in pediatric patients: an update on management and diagnosis. *Anesthesiology.* 1994;80:1228–1233.

11. Larach MG, Localio AR, Allen GC, et al. A clinical grading scale to predict malignant hyperthermia susceptibility. *Anesthesiology.* 1994;80:771–779.

12. Litman RS, Rosenberg H. Malignant hyperthermia: update on susceptibility testing. *JAMA.* 2005;293:2918–2924.

13. Caroff SN, Mann SC, Campbell CE, Sullivan KA, Obeso J. Neuroleptic malignant syndrome. In: Frucht SJ, Fahn S, eds. *Current Clinical Neurology: Movement Disorder Emergencies: Diagnosis & Treatment.* Totowa, NJ: Humana Press; 2005:41–51.

14. Krause T, Gerbershagen MU, Fiege M, Weisshorn R, Wappler F. Dantrolene—a review of its pharmacology, therapeutic use and new developments. *Anesthesia.* 2004;59:364–373.

15. Ward A, Chaffman MO, Sorkin EM. Dantrolene. A review of its pharmacodynamic and pharmacokinetic properties and therapeutic use in malignant hyperthermia, the neuroleptic malignant syndrome and an update of its use in muscle spasticity. *Drugs.* 1986;32:130–168.

16. Malignant Hyperthermia Association of the United States. Malignant hyperthermia. Available at: http://medical.mhaus.org/index.cfm/fuseaction/content.Display/PagePK/Muscular Dystrophies.cfm. Accessed December 4, 2008.

17. Robinson RL, Brooks C, Brown SL, et al. RYR1 mutations causing central core disease are associated with more severe malignant hyperthermia in vitro contracture test phenotypes. *Hum Mutat.* 2002;20:88–97.

18. Matthews KD, Moore SA. Multiminicore myopathy, central core disease, malignant hyperthermia susceptibility, and RYR1 mutations: one disease with many faces? *Arch Neurol.* 2004;61:27–29.

19. Lyfenko AD, Goonasekera SA, Dirksen RT. Dynamic alterations in myoplasmic calcium in malignant hyperthermia and central core disease. *Biochem Biophys Res Commun.* 2004;322: 1256–1266.

20. Malignant Hyperthermia Association of the United States. Medical professionals' frequently ask questions. Available at: http://medical.mhaus.org/index.cfm/fuseaction/content.Display/PagePk/MedicalFAQs.cfm. Accessed January 2009.

21. Larach MG. Standardization of the caffeine halothane muscle contracture test. North American Malignant Hyperthermia Group. *Anesth Analg.* 1989;69:511–515.

22. Halsall J, Robinson R. Genetic testing for malignant hyperthermia. *Curr Anaesth Crit Care.* 2004;15:11–21.

23. Girard T, Litman RS. Molecular genetic testing to diagnose malignant hyperthermia susceptibility. *J Clin Anesth.* 2008;20:161–163.

24. Hirshey SJ, Brandom BW, Muldoon SM, Rosenberg H. Genetic testing to evaluate susceptibility of malignant hyperthermia. *Am Soc Anesthesiol.* 2009;73:36–38.

25. Flewellen EH, Nelson TE, Jones WP, et al. Dantrolene dose response in awake man: implications for management of malignant hyperthermia. *Anesthesiology.* 1983;59:275–278.

26. Schonell LH, Sims C, Bulsara M. Preparing a new generation anaesthesia machine for patients susceptible to malignant hyperthermia. *Anesth Intens Care.* 2003;31:58.

27. Kolb ME, Horne ML. Dantrolene in human MH: a multicenter study. *Anesthesiology.* 1982;56:254–262.

28. Dantrium intravenous official FDA information. Available at: http://www.drugs.com/pro/dantrium-intravenous.html. Accessed February 2010.

29. Kobayashi S, Bannister ML, Gangopadhyay JP, Tomoyo H, Parness J, Noriaki I. Dantrolene stabilizes domain interactions within the ryanodine receptor. *J Biol Chem.* 2005;280:6580–6587.

30. Brandon BW, Larach MG. The North American Malignant Hyperthermia Registry. Reassessment of the safety and efficacy of dantrolene. *Anesthesiology.* 2002;96:1199.

31. Quirashi SA, Orkin FK, Murray WB. Dantrolene reconstitution: can warmed diluent make a difference? *J Clin Anesth.* 2006;18:339–342.

32. Weingarten AE, Korsh JI, Neuman GG, Stern SB. Postpartum uterine atony after intravenous dantrolene. *Anesth Analg.* 1987;66:269–270.

33. Grogan H, Hopkins PM. Heat stroke: implications for critical care and anaesthesia. *Br J Anaesth.* 2002;88:700–707.

34. Tobin JR, Jason DR, Challa VR, Nelson TE, Sambuughin N. Malignant hyperthermia and apparent heat stroke. *JAMA.* 2001;286:168–169.

35. Sudo RT, Carmo PL, Trachez MM, Zapata-Sudo G. Effects of azumolene on normal and malignant hyperthermia-susceptible skeletal muscle. *Basic Clin Pharmacol Toxicol.* 2008;102:308–316.

36. Gerbershagen MU, Becker S, Burmester S, Staross A, Wappler F. Comparison of therapeutic effectiveness of dantrolene and ryanodex in porcine malignant hyperthermia [abstract]. *Am Soc Anesthesiol.* 2007;107:A1922.

37. Malignant Hyperthermia Association of the United States. Emergency therapy for malignant hyperthermia. Available at: http://medical.mhaus.org/PubData/PDFs/treatmentposter.pdf. Accessed July 7, 2008.

After completing this chapter, the reader should be able to

- Discuss the origins, incidence, and genetic influences of asthma.
- Describe the pathologic alterations in pulmonary anatomy and physiology from asthma and identify signs and symptoms that occur as a result.
- Formulate an anesthetic care plan that optimizes pulmonary function and minimizes bronchoconstriction during anesthesia and surgery.
- Describe the various pharmacologic approaches to the management of asthma and the resultant anesthetic implications.
- Discuss management of acute asthmatic bronchoconstriction during anesthesia.

25
Pharmacology of Asthma: Anesthesia Implications

Greg Bozimowski, MS, CRNA

Introduction

The patient with a coexisting disease of asthma represents a common challenge to the anesthetist. The significant prevalence rate as well as the potential life-threatening effects of the disease justify the necessity for anesthesia providers to understand the pathophysiology, pharmacologic management, and anesthetic implications of asthma. The number of people newly diagnosed with asthma continues to rise.

This chapter will address the epidemiology, pathophysiology, and pharmacologic management of asthma. In addition it will address the surgical and anesthetic implications of asthma and the management of acute asthmatic exacerbation under anesthesia.

Origins

Asthma is defined in terms of its most basic characteristics; it is a disease of chronic inflammation of the airways and airway hyperreactivity resulting in smooth muscle bronchoconstriction and diminished airflow. It is characterized by periods of apparent remissions and exacerbations, although the presence of chronic inflammation may exist even in the absence of symptoms. The National Asthma Education and Prevention Program (NAEPP), part of the National Heart, Lung and Blood Institute (NHLBI) of the

U.S. Department of Health and Human Services, publishes an expert panel report that is frequently referred to in the development of guidelines for asthma management. The expert panel report defines asthma as "a common chronic disorder of the airways that is complex and characterized by variable and recurring symptoms, airflow obstruction, bronchial hyper-responsiveness and an underlying inflammation."[1] Causes of inflammation in asthma have been investigated extensively. New evidence suggests that susceptibility to the disease most likely originates early in life and the appearance of asthma as a complex process is the result of a relationship between genetic factors and environmental exposures.[1]

The existence of a genetic contribution underlying the presence of asthma has been well documented. Research is ongoing in evaluating various phenotypes central to asthma, but the description of asthma as a complex genetic disorder, such as in cases of hypertension or diabetes, is more fitting than describing it as an autosomal-dominant or recessive-linked form of disease inheritance.[2]

Environmental factors, often categorized as either airborne allergen or viral respiratory infection, are considered most important in the development of asthma as a persistent disease and in determining the severity of the symptoms and structural changes that can occur. Patterns can be observed in the preschool years, and earlier, that may predict pulmonary airflow restrictions that will be apparent in early adult life and may proceed to chronic pulmonary disease later. Exposures to viral infections caused by rhinovirus and respiratory syncytial virus as well as airborne antigens represent significant risk factors. There appears to be a relationship between exposure to rhinovirus and the development of sensitization to aeroallergens as well as a general atopic predisposition, although the direction of these relationships remains undefined.[3]

Incidence

According to the NAEPP about 22 million people in the United States have asthma[1]. A multitude of social and economic implications are associated with asthma. It has been estimated that asthma symptoms and exacerbations result in 100 million days of restricted activity, nearly 500,000 hospitalizations, and over 5000 deaths per year.[4] Asthma as a particular concern in children is well studied. Prevalence in children has been reported as more than 6 million patients resulting in asthma-related office or clinic visits of 3 million, emergency department visits of 570,000, hospitalizations of 164,000, and missed school days of 10 million per year.[4] Asthma outcomes vary with ethnicity and are generally much worse in African American children, in whom the prevalence is 26% higher, and in general the disease results in more severe disability, more frequent hospitalizations, and a death rate as much as four to six times higher. Asthma treatment–related pharmacology represents a large segment of the pharmaceutical industry, and implications of the disease are a major factor in health care economics.[1,4]

Pathophysiology

Asthma is a chronic clinical syndrome characterized by symptomatic episodes of hyperresponsive airways intermixed with asymptomatic periods. In addition to airway hyperreactivity, characteristics include bronchoconstriction, inflammation, and airway remodeling. Airway remodeling describes the structural changes seen in large and small airways as a result of chronic diseases, including asthma. These changes can include increased smooth muscle mass, subepithelial fibrosis, enlarged glands, revascularization, decreased cartilage integrity, and epithelial changes. These changes lead to airway thickening and eventually increased mucous secretion, airway edema, and bronchial hyperreactivity. Airway remodeling is the result of chronic inflammatory processes, is progressive over time, and is associated with poorer outcomes. It has been theorized that remodeling may be reduced through optimal control of inflammation; however, some studies indicate that once remodeling has occurred the changes are irreversible in spite of conventional pharmacologic management.[5,6] It has been noted that the likelihood and severity of airway remodeling are greater in patients who develop persistent wheezing during the first years of life and that it may be surmised that the exposure to viruses, particularly respiratory syncytial virus, during this period results in an abnormal inflammatory response and subsequent structural and functional changes.[3]

The interrelationships between airway inflammation, obstruction, and hyperresponsiveness and outward clinical symptoms of asthma have been well documented. These processes can be described in terms of immunologic responses, and their identification has been crucial in the development of pharmacologic therapy. It has been shown that although genetically predisposed atopy is a primary risk factor for developing asthma, exposure to allergens from both indoor and outdoor sources plays a significant role. Interruption of the pathway from exposure to sensitization to development of asthma may show promise as a form of prevention.[7] The classic antigen-mediated airway response causes the release of several substances from mast cells, eosinophils, T lymphocytes, macrophages, neutrophils, and epithelial cells within the airway mucosa.

Immunoglobulin E is an important antibody responsible for activation of allergic reactions and has a significant role as well. In addition, nitric oxide, a potent vasodilator, is noted to increase during eosinophilic inflammatory responses. As a result the fraction of exhaled nitric oxide has been identified as a significant biomarker in measuring asthma control. In the early phase of response to exposure to antigen mediators such as histamine and tryptase, various substances are released. These include enzymes proteases and the products of various eicosanoid synthesis, including leukotrienes and prostaglandins. The released mediators cause inflammation, increased vascular permeability, and smooth muscle constriction (Figure 25-1). In the later, more sustained phase of reaction, bronchoconstriction and increased mucous secretion predominates. This phase is believed to be mediated by substances such as cytokines and interleukins that are likely released by lymphocytes or mast cells. It is believed that a benefit of corticosteroid therapy in asthma may be the result of its inhibition of cytokine production.[1,8] The hyperreactivity bronchoconstriction that coincides with inflammation is not completely understood. There is evidence that it is the result of autonomic influence, specifically parasympathetic vagal stimulation. The resultant effects may also include cardiac responses as well; however, the literature

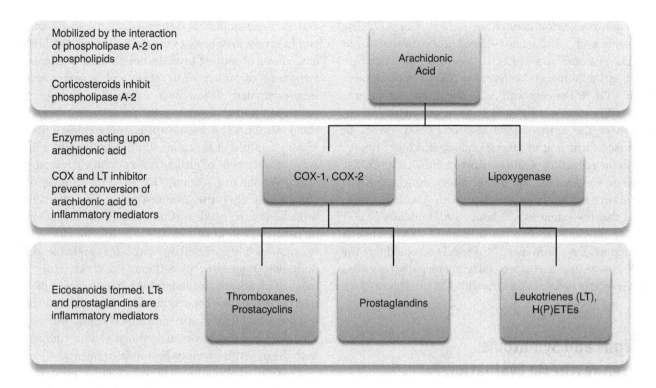

Figure 25-1 Eicosanoid synthesis. Formation of mediators of inflammation.

Source: Adapted from: Foegh, ML, Ramwell, PW. The eicosanoids: Prostaglandins, thromboxanes, leukotrienes and related compounds. In: Katzung, BG, ed. *Basic and Clinical Pharmacology*. 8th ed. New York: McGraw-Hill; 2001;88:311–313.

is inconclusive in this area. The presence of an abnormal parasympathetic influence, as well as the presence of autonomic effects by certain asthma treatments, imposes implications for anesthesia for asthmatic patients.[9]

Some authors propose that asthma categorization by phenotype or observable characteristics are more appropriate models and may lead to improvement in treatment protocols (Table 25-1). In addition to asthma that is immunologically mediated, asthma triggered by nonantigenic activity, sometimes referred to as nonspecific bronchial hyperreactivity, has also been well documented. Occupational asthma, or that which is exacerbated by the workplace, can be the result of immunologic antigen-mediated triggers or nonimmunologic-mediated triggers such as irritant chemicals. Although exposure to latex has diminished, it may be an issue in the sense that many latex-sensitive individuals are atopic by history. Exercise-induced asthma is a common occurrence in many or most asthmatic patients, but it also occurs in up to 10% of patients without asthma or atopy. The precise mechanism in triggering exercise-induced asthma is not yet fully understood.[10]

In some patients a phenomena referred to as aspirin-intolerant (or -induced) asthma (AIA) has been studied.

Incidents of severe bronchospasm were noted after aspirin administration since the drug was first developed, and shortly afterward the classic triad of associations between asthma, aspirin sensitivity, and nasal polyps was described. The incidence of AIA is relatively low in the general adult nonasthmatic population at approximately 4% but nearly doubles or triples in subjects with asthma. Rhinorrhea

Table 25-1 Asthma Categories by Clinical Phenotype

Clinical Categories	Trigger Agent Categories	Inflammatory Mediator Categories
By severity	Aspirin, NSAID	Eosinophilic
Likelihood of exacerbations	Environmental exposures	Neutrophilic
		Paucigranulocytic
Chronic airflow obstruction	Occupational exposures	
Treatment resistance	Exercise induced	
Age at onset	Menses related	

NSAID, nonsteroidal anti-inflammatory drug.

Source: Adapted from reference 10.

and nasal congestion is often an early sign of AIA. The mechanism of AIA is not believed to be related to an allergic response but rather to aspirin's pharmacologic effect of inhibiting cyclooxygenase (COX), most importantly COX-1. Patients with AIA, like those with asthma from other causes, are noted to have persistent inflammation of the airways. Inhibition of COX-1 results in decreased formation of prostaglandins, which are important in the reduction of inflammation. Inhibition of COX-1 by other nonsteroidal anti-inflammatory drugs (NSAIDs) also occurs and has been associated with AIA. It has been noted that the extent to which an NSAID inhibits COX-1 directly corresponds with the severity of AIA. Although case reports have been noted, it is widely accepted that the COX-2–selective class of anti-inflammatory analgesics has been shown to be safe in patients with AIA[11,12] (Figure 25-1).

Signs and Symptoms: Preanesthesia Evaluation

In making the diagnosis, the presence of certain signs and symptoms can be highly suggestive of asthma. Recurrent wheezing, dyspnea, cough (especially at night), and chest tightness are highly indicative symptoms. Prolonged inspiratory-to-expiratory ratio, hyperexpansion of the thorax, accessory muscle use, and diminished chest excursion may also be seen. Other findings often seen in asthmatic patients include nasal mucosal swelling or polyps, atopic dermatitis, eczema, and urticaria. Respiratory distress can manifest as tachypnea, dyspnea with anxiety, and in severe instances, cyanosis. In general, establishing a diagnosis of asthma involves determining that episodic symptoms of airway obstruction and hyperresponsiveness exist, that airflow obstruction is at least partially reversible, and that other possible diagnoses have been ruled out. This is achieved through obtaining a detailed history and physical examination. Additionally, spirometry measurement of airflow obstruction via forced expiratory volume in 1 second (FEV_1) and reversibility of the obstruction after the administration of a short-acting bronchodilating agent further confirm the diagnosis. An increase in FEV_1 of at least 12% and 200 mL after administration of a bronchodilator indicates reversible airflow limitation suggestive of asthma. Peak expiratory flow measurements are also helpful. An improvement of 60 L/min or 20% of pre-bronchodilator value after inhalation of a bronchodilator is also indicative. Ideally, peak expiratory flow measurements are evaluated as a comparison with the patient's previous best measurements.[1]

Physical examination before induction must include assessment of the respiratory rate and rhythm and auscultation of all lung fields bilaterally for the presence of adventitious breath sounds. Laboratory testing may be indicated not for diagnosing early, mild disease but rather to assist in predicting the chances of postoperative pulmonary complications in patients with progressive disease. Testing may include chest radiography, pulmonary function tests, and arterial blood gas analysis[13] (Table 25-2).

In assessing the extent of asthma, taking a detailed history is crucial. It should be appreciated by the anesthesia

Table 25-2 Asthma Assessment Parameters

Effects of Asthma	Provocative Factors	Physical Assessment	Laboratory Assessment
Frequency of emergency or urgent care visits	Exercise	Auscultation in all lung fields bilaterally for wheezing or rhonchi	PFTs with particular emphasis of FEV_1, FVC, PEF
History of life-threatening exacerbations	Airborne irritants (pollen, chemicals, latex)	Dyspnea, tachypnea, wheezing, use of accessory respiratory muscles, retractions	Bronchoprovocation (i.e., methacholine challenge)
Number of missed work/school days	Animals with fur or feathers	Presence of nasal polyps	ABG analysis for oxygenation, ventilation
Limitation of activity	House dust mites	Presence of dermatitis, eczema	
History of nocturnal awakenings	Mold	Anxiety	Chest x-ray
Compliance with management therapy	Smoke	Cyanosis	Eosinophil count
	Viral infection		Allergy testing

ABG, arterial blood gas; FVC, forced vital capacity; PEF, peak expiratory flow; PFT, pulmonary function test.

provider that the history might not always be accurate. Some patients with asthma may downplay their symptoms. Symptom accommodation may occur when patients fail to recognize worsening of symptoms as part of their asthma but rather attribute them to other factors, such as age, weight gain, smoking, and so on. To recognize the presence of asthma or evaluate the progression of the disease and the likelihood of complications during anesthesia, it is important to obtain detailed information related to age at onset of asthma, history of respiratory failure, hospitalizations, and intubations or other emergency airway interventions. Patients should be questioned about the presence and severity of allergies to medications, foods, and environmental exposures, including latex (Box 25-1).

Recognizing the severity and progression of the disease in the patient preoperatively is essential to formulating an anesthetic plan. The NAEPP developed a system of classifying the severity of the disease with respect to two domains: level of impairment and level of risk for developing severe exacerbations. Severity is classified as either intermittent or persistent based on the frequency of symptoms such as nighttime awakenings, need for short-acting bronchodilators for acute symptom management, and interference with normal activity. Within the category of persistent,

> ### Box 25-1 Asthma Risk Factors
>
> - History of early life injury to airways
> - RSV as infant
> - Parental smoking
> - Chronic sinusitis
> - Family history of asthma-genetic predisposition
> - Aspirin/NSAID sensitivity
> - Allergic rhinitis
> - Nasal polyps

subclassifications of mild persistent, moderate persistent, and severe persistent are made[1] (Table 25-3).

A helpful inquiry into determining patient classification is to assess the frequency of use of rescue inhalers following the rule of twos. An asthmatic who uses his or her rescue inhaler more than two times per week during the day, more than two times per month at night, or is exhausting more than two inhalers per year should be considered as a persistent asthmatic rather than intermittent.[1]

Table 25-3 Asthma Severity Classification and Corresponding Pharmacologic Management

Classification	Frequency and Severity of Symptoms	Usual Pharmacologic Management
Intermittent asthma	Day: no more than twice a week Night: no more than twice a month Usually asymptomatic between brief exacerbations PEF or FEV$_1$ ≥ 80% predicted	No daily medication needed. Exacerbations generally managed with SABA inhaler
Mild persistent asthma	Day: more than twice a week but not daily Night: more than twice a month Exacerbations may last longer and may affect ADL. PEF or FEV$_1$ ≥ 80% predicted	Low-dose ICS, Cromolyn, nedocromil, or LTA therapy as alternative (not preferred)
Moderate persistent asthma	Day: daily Night: > 1 night a week Exacerbations affect ADL. PEF or FEV$_1$ 60–80% predicted	Medium- to high-dose ICS, LABA in combination may be added
Severe persistent asthma	Day: continuous symptoms with frequent exacerbations Night: frequent nighttime symptoms and exacerbations Severe limitations to ADL and severe exacerbations PEF or FEV$_1$ ≤ 60% predicted	High-dose ICS, LABA in combination, immunomodulator therapy, systemic corticosteroids as needed

ADL, activities of daily living; ICS, inhaled corticosteroids; LABA, long-acting β agonists; LTA, leukotriene antagonist; PEF, peak expiratory flow.

Source: Adapted from reference 1

It is important to interview the patient to determine his or her perception of the disease progression, current prescribed management, and response and compliance to it. Many patients who have intermittent asthma deny the presence of the disease during the absence of symptoms and may have reduced compliance to anti-inflammatory maintenance therapy.[14]

Differential Diagnosis

The differential diagnosis for asthma can be complicated. Although the common belief is that wheezing is a definitive finding, it must be appreciated that in general all patients who wheeze may not have asthma and, conversely, all patients with asthma may not wheeze. Many other pathologic processes can produce symptoms similar to asthma. Patients with chronic obstructive pulmonary disease, congestive heart failure, pulmonary embolism, cystic fibrosis, bronchiolitis in various forms, bronchiectasis, and hypersensitivity pneumonitis can all present with dyspnea as a prominent feature. Common adverse effects from angiotensin-converting enzyme inhibitor therapy are cough and bronchospasm, which may resemble an asthmatic episode. In addition, aspiration, gastroesophageal reflux disease, airway obstruction, and even vocal cord dysfunction can be mistaken for asthma and may be of particular relevance in the anesthesia arena (Table 25-4).

Table 25-4 Differential Diagnosis of Asthma

Infants and Children	Adults
Allergic rhinitis, sinusitis	CHF, COPD
Foreign body in trachea, bronchus	Mechanical obstruction of airways, tumors
Vocal cord dysfunction	Vocal cord dysfunction
Tracheal stenosis, bronchiostenosis	Pulmonary embolism
	Bronchiectasis, bronchitis
Bronchiolitis	Hypersensitivity pneumonitis
Cystic fibrosis	Secondary cough (i.e., ACE inhibitor induced)
Recurrent cough (nonasthma)	
	Aspiration from swallowing dysfunction, GERD
Aspiration from swallowing dysfunction, GERD	

ACE, angiotensin-converting enzyme; CHF, congestive heart failure; COPD, chronic obstructive pulmonary disease; GERD, gastroesophageal reflux disease.

Source: Adapted from references 1 and 10.

Pharmacologic Intervention: Management and Control of Disease

General pharmacologic management strategies are typically based on the severity of disease and frequency of symptoms (Table 25-3). The primary efforts are aimed at reducing or controlling inflammation. A variety of drug classes is used for this purpose. Research in the area of pharmacogenetics suggests that an individual's response to therapy is greatly influenced by genetic factors, and, as such, the future of disease management will likely include genetic testing to determine the most customized pharmacologic management.[15] The long-term use of inhaled corticosteroids (ICSs) has been considered the mainstay of pharmacologic control of asthma inflammation for some time. During periods of severe exacerbations of asthma or for very reticent disease, systemic corticosteroids may be administered. Other categories of drugs, including mast cell stabilizers, leukotriene modifiers, immunomodulators, and methylxanthines, are also used. In addition, medical management may call for the use of intermittent and cautious administration of β agonists in the form of both short-acting and long-acting formulations. Medical management must also address other confounding factors, such as gastroesophageal reflux disease, chronic sinusitis, and allergic rhinitis and the avoidance of provocative factors (Table 25-5).

Corticosteroids

Inhaled Corticosteroids

Corticosteroids exert widespread effects throughout the body because of the presence of corticosteroid receptors on most cells throughout the body. The primary effects include metabolic, catabolic, and anti-inflammatory. The discussion in this chapter focuses on the role of corticosteroids in reducing the manifestations of inflammation as well as the possibility of inherent side effects and implications of therapy.

Corticosteroids work to suppress the inflammation pathways at multiple levels. Through their influence on signal transduction and gene expression pathways, corticosteroids effectively switch off genes responsible for the inflammatory response. At the cellular level corticosteroids suppress the production of inflammatory mediators and adhesion molecules as well as eosinophils. The resultant effect is a decreased number of cytokines, mast cells, and macrophages. Effects on epithelial cells result in decreased

Table 25-5 Commonly Prescribed Pharmacologic Therapy for Asthma

Drug/Classification	Adult Dosage
Anti-inflammatory Drugs	
Systemic corticosteroids	Hydrocortisone: 20–40 mg/day PO, QD 100–500 mg IV may repeat 3–4 times/day Methylprednisolone: 100–250 mg q 2–6 h
Inhaled corticosteroids	Beclamethasone dipropionate (μg/day): low dose, 200–500; medium dose, 500–100; high dose, 100–200 Budesomide (μg/day): low dose, 200–400; medium dose, 400–800; high dose, 800–1600 Fluticasone (μg/day): low dose, 100–250; medium dose, 250–500; high dose, 500–100 Mometasone furoate (μg/day): low dose, 400–1000; medium dose, 1000 Triamcinolone acetonide (μg/day): low dose, 400–1000; medium dose, 1000–2000; high dose, > 2000
Mast cell stabilizers	Cromolyn: 800 μg per puff MDI, 1–2 puffs q.i.d. Neocromil: 2 mg per MDI puff, 2–4 puffs b.i.d. to q.i.d.
Leukotriene receptor antagonists	Montelukast: 10 mg/day PO Zafirlukast: 20 mg PO b.i.d. Zileuton: 600 mg PO q.i.d.
β Agonist Bronchodilators	
Short-acting β agonists	Albuterol: 90 μg per puff MDI, 1–2 puffs q 4–6 h Levalbuterol: 0.31–1.25 mg nebulization q 6–8 h Terbutaline: 2.5–5 mg PO t.i.d., 0.25 mg SC, may repeat once in 4 h Epinephrine: bronchospasm dose = 0.1–0.5 mg SC/IM q 30 min to 4 h (1:1000 solution)
Long-acting β agonists in combination therapy	Fluticasone propionate/salmeterol: available in μg per puff as 100/50, 250/50, 500/50; 1–2 puffs per day Budesomide/formoterol: available in μg per puff as 80/4.5, 160/4.5, 320/4.5; 1–2 puffs per day Beclamethasone/formoterol: available in μg per puff as 100/6; 1–2 puffs per day

IM, intramuscularly; IV, intravenously; MDI, metered-dose inhaler; PO, orally; SC, subcutaneously.

Source: Adapted from references 33, 36, 40, and 89.

inflammation and mucous production. It is believed that the mechanism of action of corticosteroids begins with the diffusion of the drug to specific receptors within the cytoplasm of target cells. This produces an activated corticosteroid–receptor complex responsible for altering gene transcription and protein synthesis. This mechanism of action holds true for both systemic corticosteroids used to manage asthma inflammation and ICSs. The receptor binding affinity of ICSs varies between formulations. This affinity has implications for both therapeutic and side effects because both local and systemic effects are mediated through these receptors. As a result the degree of receptor affinity alone does not determine the therapeutic ratio of one drug formulation over another.[16–18]

Corticosteroids can be given through various routes. Corticosteroids administered through a device called a metered-dose inhaler (MDI) or dry powdered inhaler (DPI) allows for topical application of the drug to the lungs through inhalation and reduces the amount of drug reaching the systemic circulation, thereby reducing systemic side effects. ICSs are often referred to as the most important agents in reactive airway disease and are frequently considered the first-line management agent in all persistent asthma.[1] Their efficacy in managing symptoms through control of the inflammatory aspect of asthma is well documented.

The pharmacokinetics and pharmacodynamics of the ICS drugs are unique when compared with drugs given through other routes. The ideal ICS is that which best provides deposition of the drug to the lung surface and has a low oral bioavailability and high systemic clearance to avoid systemic side effects.[19] Several varieties of ICSs and their corresponding delivery system are in use, and their pharmacokinetic and pharmacodynamic profiles such as bioavailability, potency, distribution, metabolism, and clearance may vary. As a result their safety and efficacy may differ. Despite the fact that their mechanisms of action are similar, their differences may be of specific concern to those prescribing therapy, and careful consideration is warranted.[18,20] Research suggests, however, that all the available ICSs offer sufficient therapeutic effect with high safety profiles, particularly when given in low to medium dose ranges.[21] In the perioperative arena the anesthetic implications of ICS therapy are less dependent on the brand or formulation prescribed and more affected by the degree of disease control or presence of adverse effects seen in the patient.

To appreciate the action of ICSs, one must also consider the delivery process of the drug. The most common devices used for inhaled drug delivery are the MDI and DPI. It should be noted that these devices are also used to deliver other inhaled therapies, such as long-acting β agonists (LABAs), combined therapies, and short-acting β agonists (SABAs). It is worth noting that MDI devices have historically relied on chlorofluorocarbons as a propellant. Chlorofluorocarbons have been shown to deplete the ozone layer of the stratosphere and as such are being banned internationally. At the end of 2008 SABAs containing chlorofluorocarbons were phased out, and it is assumed that ICS and LABA drugs will follow. Implications for patients and prescribers include a change in the taste of the drug and care of the inhaler as well as revised dosage recommendations for some formulations. In addition, the newer SABA will initially be unavailable as a generic, resulting in increased costs.[1,22]

Of interest to anesthesia providers is the fact that previously used adapters to deliver SABAs to the intubated patient may no longer fit the MDI, necessitating a revision in the way some MDI drugs are administered. The use of inhaled drugs via an MDI is associated with a certain dexterity requirement on the part of the patient. Care must be taken to exhale completely to allow a maximum, rapid inhalation of the drug, driving it deep into the lungs. This is occasionally difficult for small children and some adults with severe limitations. Devices referred to as spacers and valved holding chambers are sometimes used to assist in maximum delivery. These are important issues in determining delivery of therapeutic levels of drug as well as limiting oral absorption and swallowing of the drug. An advantage of the DPI delivery system is its ease of use relative to the MDI; however, a deep, forceful inhalation is required to break the large particle size in the large airways into a smaller particle size to deposit on and affect smaller, distal airways.[23]

The anti-inflammatory therapeutic effects of ICSs are achieved by direct, local application of the drug to the lung tissue. After inhalation of an ICS, a portion of the drug remains deposited in the mouth. The amount varies greatly depending on the efficiency of the device and adequacy of technique by the patient. It is estimated that 40% to 90% dispensed may remain in the oral cavity to be swallowed if not thoroughly rinsed. This unintentional oral dose is responsible for certain potential side effects such as oral candidiasis. The swallowed portion is subject to hepatic

first-pass effect. That portion that is absorbed from the gut varies by formulation. It does not contribute to therapeutic effects but can cause systemic side effects to varying degrees. Rather, the primary determinant of systemic bioavailability of the ICS is that portion absorbed from the lungs because there is no first-pass hepatic interference.[18,23]

As expected, lipophilic and protein binding characteristics also vary between the individual ICS drugs. Drugs with higher lipophilicity may cross membranes locally and exert therapeutic effects more readily. This same property potentially allows for greater distribution after systemic absorption, resulting in possible side effects.[18]

Protein binding capabilities for the available ICSs range between approximately 70% and 90%, with albumin being the most commonly bound protein. A higher protein binding value results in a lower fraction of free drug available to exert systemic effects through leaving the plasma. Metabolism of ICSs occurs through hepatic cytochrome activity using various isoenzymes. Metabolite activity varies by formulation but is generally minimal if present at all. Hepatic clearance is rapid. Elimination is through the feces with some urinary clearance. Elimination half-lives range among the available ICSs from between 1.6 and 14.4 hours.[18]

Adverse effects can occur from the use of ICS, though most often they are mild and manageable. Factors such as the individual pharmacodynamic and pharmacokinetic properties of the formulation, patient comorbidities, concomitant drug therapy, variables in administration technique, and dosing are factors in the development of side effects. An additional consideration may be the extent of obstruction to airflow and effectiveness of airway clearance mechanisms, such as mucociliary clearance and cough. In essence, there appears to be a difference in pharmacodynamic and pharmacokinetic characteristics of ICSs between healthy and asthmatic patients.[24]

Mild, local side effects include dysphonia and oral and esophageal candidiasis and are a result of oral deposition and swallowed drug during the administration process. Simply rinsing the mouth after administration can reduce the incidence of these effects.

Systemic absorption can contribute to other side effects. It has been strongly contested that the known benefit of ICS therapy outweighs the risk of adverse effects of corticosteroids. The incidence rate of adverse effects may be difficult to quantify, but most researchers believe the rate is low. Potential side effects most often discussed include a decrease in bone mineral density, increased risk of fractures, dermal thinning and bruising, cataract formation, glaucoma, and a decrease in growth rate in children. The literature suggests that although these side effects have been reported and in some cases require further monitoring or therapy changes, the rate is not as significant as in chronic systemic (oral or parenteral) administration and do not warrant withholding ICS treatment. It should also be noted that uncontrolled asthma has been shown to reduce linear growth so that the risk and rewards of therapy must be weighed from several viewpoints. It might be assumed that ICSs could cause suppression of hypothalamic-pituitary-adrenal axis function given the mechanism of action of ICSs and the known effects of systemic steroids; however, the evidence shows that if any effects occur from ICS administration it is of an insignificant magnitude in all but the rarest of occasions.[1,25–27]

Drug interactions with ICSs can occur. It is accepted that smoking alone is deleterious to pulmonary function regardless of the presence of asthma, but it is also demonstrated that through its induction effect on hepatic enzymes such as cytochrome (CYP) P-450 and CYP1A2 pharmacodynamic alterations result in decreased anti-inflammatory efficacy of ICSs.[28] Conversely, interactions can occur when ICSs are administered concomitantly with inhibitors of CYP450 that may increase the systemic effects by increasing their plasma levels. Patients receiving antiretroviral therapy for HIV who are treated with the ICS fluticasone have been reported to develop Cushing's syndrome and adrenal insufficiency and upon removal of the ICS developed withdrawal hypocortisolism.[29]

Dosage and use of the ICS formulations vary. It is important to understand that as a class of drugs, ICSs and corticosteroids in general are not bronchodilators and as such although they do play a role in addressing exacerbations of symptoms, they are not advocated as emergency relief of status asthmaticus.[30] During the perioperative period, patients should be encouraged to continue their therapy as prescribed.[31]

Systemic Corticosteroids

The mechanism of action of systemic corticosteroids in the management of asthmatic airway inflammation is as previously discussed in relation to ICSs. It has been recommended that the use of systemic steroids for disease management be reserved for those patients with severe, difficult to control asthma symptoms because of the risk of side effects of systemic therapy. Because side effects are typically dose dependent, it is recommended that the lowest effective dose be used. Patients receiving systemic corticosteroid therapy who undergo surgery should receive careful consideration. It is suggested that patients who

have received systemic corticosteroids and some patients receiving high-dose ICSs during the 6 months before surgery be given 100 mg hydrocortisone every 8 hours during the surgical period with reductions in dose rapidly within 24 hours of surgery.[1]

Corticosteroids can be administered via oral, topical, or parenteral routes. Some corticosteroids function as a prodrug. For example, the oral drug prednisone is rapidly metabolized to its active form, prednisolone, once inside the body. Corticosteroid potencies vary by formulation, and their strength and dosage is often described in relation to hydrocortisone. Corticosteroids are metabolized via CYP450 systems and eliminated primarily via the liver. Elimination and biologic half-lives vary by formulation. Side effects of systemically administered corticosteroids are more likely to occur and are more severe in nature than ICSs. When corticosteroids are given for short periods of time (under 2 weeks) serious side effects can occur but are not common. Some of these effects may include insomnia, mood and behavioral changes, and peptic ulcers. Patients receiving corticosteroids for longer than 2 weeks are likely to develop iatrogenic Cushing's syndrome characterized by rounding, puffiness of the face (moon facies), and fat redistribution. Other serious side effects include immunosuppression, gastrointestinal ulceration, prolonged wound healing, psychosis, diabetes mellitus, glaucoma, cataracts, growth suppression, and muscle and tendon abnormalities.[1,8]

Despite the risk of side effects the use of systemic corticosteroids may be indicated during the anesthetic management of asthmatic patients for the prevention and/or management of perioperative bronchospasm. Corticosteroids, either alone or in combination with β_2 agonists, have been shown to reduce morbidity. The literature suggests that methylprednisolone 40 mg/day orally with salbutamol minimizes airway reactivity in patients with histories of bronchial reactivity during intubation and that 40 to 60 mg prednisone/day or hydrocortisone 100 mg intravenously (IV) every 8 hours should be considered for any patients having FEV_1 values less than 80% of predicted value.[32,33]

β-Adrenergic Agonists

β-Adrenergic agonists exert a bronchodilating effect through the stimulation of β_2 receptors on pulmonary smooth muscle. This receptor activity results in activation of adenyl cyclase and increased cAMP. In addition, they inhibit the further release of bronchoconstriction mediators from mast cells.[8] It follows that β-adrenergic agonists would be useful in preventing and reversing bronchoconstriction from asthma. The nonspecific adrenergic agonist epinephrine is a rapid-acting and effective drug in treatment of bronchoconstriction. It can be administered IV, intramuscularly, subcutaneously, or via inhalation through nebulizer, MDI, or DPI. For severe asthma, 0.1 to 0.5 mg of a 1:1000 solution given subcutaneously or intramuscularly repeated as frequently as every 20 minutes to a maximum dose of 1 mg is advised. Maximum bronchodilation occurs in 15 minutes, and the effects last 60 to 90 minutes. Nonselective β agonists such as epinephrine carry with them the risk of significant β_1-adrenergic receptor stimulation. As such, side effects such as tachycardia, dysrhythmias, and worsening of myocardial injury are of significant concern.

Agents that are β_2 selective are most frequently used to avoid or at least minimize unwanted effects of β_1 stimulation. This class of drugs is subdivided into LABAs and SABAs. Both drugs have specific places, therapy protocols, and different implications for the nurse anesthetist.

Short-Acting β Agonists

A SABA such as albuterol (either via nebulizer, 0.021% or 0.042%, or MDI, 0.09 mg per actuation) is essential in the management of acute onset and exacerbations of asthma bronchoconstriction as well as the prevention of exercise-induced asthma. It should be emphasized that SABAs are not intended to be used as a scheduled therapy or as long-term management. Albuterol is also available in oral form. Albuterol is a racemic mixture. The specific properties of the (S)-enantiomer are unclear, but it has been noted that bronchodilation and protective properties are attributed to the (R)-form, which is available commercially as levalbuterol. It has been suggested that levalbuterol offers the same or enhanced bronchodilation effect as albuterol but causes less tachycardia and other side effects such as jitters and shakes. The clinical significance of the differences may not be readily apparent. Albuterol MDI recommended dosing varies with severity of exacerbation and ranges from two to eight inhalations repeated in 20 minutes for up to 4 hours and then repeated every hour. It should be noted that a lack of response should be met with other approaches.[1,34–36]

Albuterol via MDI is absorbed by the pulmonary vasculature and to a lesser extent through the swallowed portion of inhaled administration. It is metabolized extensively by the liver through CYP450 systems and eliminated primarily in urine and to a minor extent in the feces. Adverse effects of SABAs include tachycardia, palpitations, tremors, and headache. Severe reactions may include cardiac dysrhythmias, myocardial infarction, and pulmonary edema. It should be used cautiously in patients with significant coronary artery disease. Regular use has been associated with increased mortality, which may be the result of delaying the initiation of more appropriate long-term therapy.

Long-Acting β Agonists

LABAs such as salmeterol and formoterol exert bronchodilation effects in the same manner as SABAs; however, their greater level of lipophilicity imparts a duration of action of 12 hours or longer. Side effects and adverse reactions are also similar to SABAs. LABAs should not be confused with SABAs in that LABAs do not have a role in managing acute exacerbations and bronchoconstriction. LABAs are commonly used in the management of chronic obstructive pulmonary disease and in combination with ICSs for long-term management of asthma; however, their use is not without controversy. Clinical trials with salmeterol suggested that the use of LABAs increased the risk of asthma-related deaths, and trials with formoterol attributed its use to more frequent severe asthma exacerbations as compared with asthmatics managed without LABAs.[1,37–39] Studies such as these prompted U.S. Food and Drug Administration alerts and "black box warnings" in product labels. The use of LABAs in combination with ICSs has been shown to be beneficial for some patients, and combination therapy has been touted as a means to allow disease management with otherwise lower doses of ICS given as monotherapy. This defense of its use has been countered that its risks outweigh those of high-dose ICSs. It is currently recommended by the NHLBI expert panel that although the addition of LABAs to ICSs may improve lung function in patients otherwise poorly controlled, careful consideration of risks of LABAs should be made and weighed against those of high-dose ICSs. Further, LABAs should not be used as monotherapy or as rescue treatment for acute symptoms.[1,37–40]

Mast Cell Stabilizers

Mast cell stabilizers are a class of drugs whose primary effect is the prevention or reduction of inflammation. Examples frequently considered in asthma management are cromolyn and nedocromil. These drugs are considered alternative but not preferred therapy to corticosteroids, having been shown to be much less effective in controlling asthma symptoms. Their use has been suggested in managing pediatric asthmatics in particular. They have been shown to be effective in inhibiting bronchoconstrictive responses to allergen and exercise-induced asthma but do not affect smooth muscle tone and have no reversal effects of bronchospasm. The mechanism of action of these drugs appears to be related to the blockade of chloride channels in cell membranes, thereby inhibiting cell activation of the inflammatory response. Nedocromil and cromolyn are eliminated unchanged mainly in feces and to a lesser degree in the urine. Side effects to these drugs are usually minor and localized and include sore throat, cough, mouth dryness, and wheezing and chest tightness.[1,8]

Leukotriene Receptor Antagonists (Leukotriene Modifiers)

Leukotriene receptor antagonists (LTRAs) represent another alternative, but they are not a preferred means of managing airway inflammation in mild persistent asthma.[1] Leukotrienes, which are products of arachidonic acid acted on by 5-lipoxygenase, have been shown to be potent mediators of inflammation (Figure 25-1). Leukotrienes are released from mast cells, eosinophils, and basophils and cause airway constriction, increased vascular permeability, mucous secretion, and activation of inflammatory cells. It follows that drugs that modify or prevent the formation of leukotrienes may be effective in managing asthma.

The LTRAs available are montelukast, zafirlukast, and zileuton. They are all oral preparations, which has been touted as an advantage as far as patient acceptability and compliance is concerned, particularly in pediatric patients. Their precise mechanism in inhibiting leukotriene production differs, as does their dosing schedules. Montelukast and zafirlukast are metabolized by the liver and eliminated primarily via the feces (98% and 90%, respectively) with minor renal excretion. Zileuton, on the other hand, is metabolized to active metabolites by the liver and 94% eliminated via the kidneys. Zileuton has been associated with hepatotoxicity and as such is less prescribed. Other serious side effects of LTRAs are rare but have been reported. These include hepatitis, jaundice, allergic granulomatosis, and neurologic and psychological alterations such as agitation, aggression, altered behavior, and suicidal ideation. More common, milder reactions such as headache, cough, dizziness, gastroenteritis, and fever have also been reported. In addition, zafirlukast has been shown to cause a significant increase in the half-life of warfarin through hepatic enzyme inhibition so that close monitoring of prothrombin times in patients receiving these drugs concomitantly is warranted.[1,36]

LTRA therapy may be an alternative for patients whose response to ICSs is inhibited, but its use is most widely considered as combination therapy with ICS. It has been shown to be effective as monotherapy in children with mild forms of asthma; however, its benefits for adults not on ICS therapy has not been as well demonstrated.[1,41–44]

Immunomodulators

Various pharmaceutical classes of agents have been studied for efficacy in managing symptoms of asthma and have been categorized together as immunomodulators. These therapies have largely been researched in patients with severe, refractory asthma in which traditional approaches may be ineffective or result in excessive adverse drug reactions. Some drugs such as methyltrexate, macrolide antibiotics, and cyclosporine therapy have been studied; however, the NHLBI expert panel concluded that currently evidence to support their efficacy is still lacking.[1]

One form of immunomodulators that has shown promise is anti-IgE therapy by the drug omalizumab. It is well noted that IgE mechanisms play a significant role in the development of airway inflammation due to asthma. Omalizumab is a monoclonal antibody derived from recombinant DNA. It binds to the Fc portion of the IgE antibody, preventing it from attaching to receptors on mast cells and basophils. It has been shown to decrease the inflammatory response of released eosinophils and basophils. It has been recommended as adjunctive therapy for patients who have allergies and severe, persistent asthma that is poorly controlled by high-dose ICSs or ICS/LABA therapy. In addition, omalizumab has been shown to reduce asthma symptoms and the need for ICSs and rescue medication. It is administered subcutaneously every 2 to 4 weeks in doses of 150 to 375 mg. It is slowly absorbed, metabolized by the liver, and eliminated in the bile. Adverse reactions are uncommon and typically mild and include headache, cough, gastrointestinal effects, and urticaria at the injection site; however, severe reactions such as anaphylaxis and thrombocytopenia have occurred.[1,45–47]

Methylxanthines

Theophylline, theobromine, and caffeine are the most noted substances in the methylxanthine class. Theophylline, in the form of aminophylline, is the most frequently used methylxanthine in the management of bronchoconstrictive asthma, but its use in the United States has mostly given way to other more effective and less toxic drugs, primarily the ICSs as well as combined therapies. Advantages of its use include an oral formulation and low cost. Sustained-release oral theophylline has been used for nocturnal asthma as well as in combination with other therapies.

It is recommended by the NHLBI expert panel as an alternative, not preferred treatment for mild persistent asthma, and is not considered indicated for acute symptom management.[1] The mechanism by which theophylline produces bronchodilation in asthmatics is not fully known. It is an inhibitor of phosphodiesterase, thus decreasing the breakdown of cAMP, which is associated with smooth muscle relaxation; however, the levels to accomplish this in vivo are higher than the typical therapeutic ranges used clinically. Other theories suggest a role in inhibiting adenosine receptors or stimulating endogenous catecholamines.[8] It has also been proposed that theophylline exerts an anti-inflammatory effect. Theophylline has been shown to reduce inflammation after allergen challenge.[48,49]

Theophylline is typically administered orally but is available for intravenous administration as well. It is metabolized in the liver and eliminated in the urine (10% unchanged in those older than 1 year, 50% in neonates).

Common mild side effects include nausea, vomiting, headache, and restlessness, but severe reactions such as tachyarrhythmia, seizures, and Stevens-Johnson syndrome can occur. Many drug interactions exist with theophylline, including significant cardiotoxicity with halothane, lowered seizure threshold with ketamine, and a decreased effectiveness of benzodiazepines. Because of the significant potential for side effects, close monitoring of serum theophylline levels are required to maintain a therapeutic value between 10 and 20 μg/mL.[36]

Anticholinergics

Ipratropium bromide is a derivative of atropine; however, as a quaternary ammonium it does not cross the blood–brain barrier, allowing it to be administered in high enough doses to exert antimuscarinic bronchodilation effects. This is accomplished through competitive inhibition of cholinergic receptors in bronchial smooth muscle, antagonizing the effect of acetylcholine and thereby blocking the constriction from vagal efferent stimulation. The drug has been shown to reverse the constrictor effect of methacholine challenge. The U.S. Food and Drug Administration indication for ipratropium is for bronchoconstriction from chronic obstructive pulmonary disease; however, it is frequently administered for exacerbation of asthma symptoms as well. The NHLBI expert panel concluded that ipratropium administered with SABAs provides added benefit in moderate to severe exacerbations in the emergency department but that comparisons with SABAs have not been made sufficiently to suggest replacement of SABAs for acute exacerbations.[1] Ipratropium is available as an MDI or via nebulized inhalation.[36]

Recommended dosing for moderate to severe exacerbation of asthma is two to three puffs of an MDI every 6 hours. Inhaled ipratropium has an onset from 3 to 30 minutes and

an elimination half-life of 2 to 4 hours. It is metabolized in the liver and excreted in the urine and feces. Adverse effects are usually mild and include abnormal taste and nasal congestion. Severe effects include myocardial infarction, cerebrovascular accident, angioedema, bronchospasm, urticaria, and anaphylaxis. Excessive anticholinergic effects can be seen if ipratropium is administered with other belladonna alkaloids such as atropine.[36]

Practical Aspects: Surgery and Asthma

The NHLBI panel concluded that asthmatic patients are at risk for specific complications, including life-threatening ones, during surgery and the postoperative period.[1] In addition to bronchoconstriction triggered by light anesthesia, intubation, hypoxemia, or hypercapnia, a heightened risk exists for impaired cough and the potentially resultant atelectasis and respiratory infection and hyperresponsiveness upon exposure to latex and some anesthetic agents. The continuum of severity of these complications depends on the patients' severity of airway sensitivity and disease progression. The panel recommended certain interventions to help to reduce the risk of complications during the perioperative period. Patients should have an evaluation preoperatively to include a review of systems, medication use, particularly the need for systemic corticosteroids, and a measurement of pulmonary function. The evaluation should include an assessment of the patients' activity tolerance, presence of current infection, exacerbating and alleviating factors, allergies, coexisting disease with particular attention to cardiac and pulmonary systems, sleep habits and sleep apnea risk, cough and sputum production, and the use and effectiveness of medications. If possible, attempts to maximize lung function as measured by FEV_1 or peak expiratory flow rate (PEFR) should be made. In some instances this may require systemic corticosteroids. For those who have received systemic steroids during the 6-month prior period and some who are taking high-dose ICSs, hydrocortisone should be given IV every 8 hours during the surgical period with dose reduction within 24 hours. These recommendations reflect the impact of adrenal suppression that may exist in patients treated with steroids.[1,13,33]

Preanesthesia Care

Although much of the assessment parameters recommended may seem more the realm of the disease management team, an appreciation for the severity of symptoms and degree of disease control is of paramount importance to the anesthesia provider. Understanding risk is crucial to preparedness. It is important that asthmatic patients who are at high risk for complications such as is the case with the elderly, obese, or any significant comorbidity be evaluated by anesthesia early to determine the need for testing or pharmacologic intervention. In addition to history and physical assessment already discussed, specific laboratory data are helpful (Table 25-2 and Box 25-1). Although prudent use of resources should always be considered, thorough evaluation is essential. Severity and progression of the disease should guide the anesthesia provider in determining the extent of testing required. The duration, location, and type of surgery and anesthetic must also be considered. Preoperative pulmonary function testing, chest radiography, and arterial blood gas analysis may be indicated. It has been suggested that certain factors increase the risk of perioperative bronchospasm in asthmatic patients.[13] These include the use of antibronchospastic medications, recent exacerbations, and recent treatment at a medical facility for asthma symptoms. The presence of asthma, nasal polyps, and intolerance to aspirin and/or NSAIDs should also be explored. Asthmatics who are smokers should be instructed to abstain from smoking for as long as possible before anesthesia.[13,32] Preoperative pharmacologic management should center on avoidance of precipitating factors and optimization of lung function. Anticipation of potential bronchoconstricting factors such as stress, intubation, light anesthesia, and pain is crucial in planning care for the asthmatic.

Patients should be instructed to continue their current therapy as scheduled on the day of surgery, and a return to therapy postoperatively should be planned as soon as possible. The use of inhaled SABAs prophylactically has been used before induction to prevent bronchoconstriction. Preoperative treatment with corticosteroids (oral methylprednisolone 40 mg/day) and salbutamol has been shown to minimize bronchoconstriction even in patients with severe asthma. Studies demonstrated that the prophylactic use of corticosteroids does not pose significant risk for concerns related to delayed wound healing or infection.[50] Antibiotics should be given as indicated. Antianxiety medications such as benzodiazepines can be very helpful. Pain management must be considered as needed with consideration given to histamine release of opiates and the presence of NSAID intolerance if ketorolac or similar drugs are to be administered. Although COX-2 selective inhibitors have been considered safer than nonselective NSAIDs there have been reports of asthma exacerbations after use of the selective agents as well. Anticholinergics such as atropine or glycopyrrolate may be helpful in reducing parasympathetic tone, which may contribute to bronchochoconstriction and increased secretions. Histamine-2 receptor blockers such as ranitidine, often considered for management of gastric acidity, should be avoided because they may result in bronchoconstriction attributed to histamine release due to a loss of inhibitory feedback control on presynaptic autoreceptors.[31,32,51]

Perioperative use of β-receptor antagonists is recommended by the American Heart Association/College of Cardiology to reduce perioperative cardiac complications. It has been shown that patients with reactive airway disease who may be at a significant cardiac risk as well should, but often do not receive the benefit of perioperative beta-blockers just as is considered for nonasthmatic patients. Careful thought and evaluation should be used to improve prescription rates in these patients. The use of short-acting β_1 receptor blockers such as esmolol and Landiolol have been shown to be safe in asthmatic patients undergoing surgery.[52,53]

Intraoperative Anesthesia Care

A byproduct of most anesthetics is the resultant respiratory depression and CO_2 retention inherent in central nervous system depressant agents, whether given via intravenous or inhaled routes. As such, a goal of the anesthetist in caring for the asthmatic patient must be to find a balance between avoiding triggering stimuli, including light anesthesia, airway instrumentation, and allergen exposure, with the hypoventilation risk associated throughout the perioperative period.

It has been suggested that bronchial hyperreactivity associated with asthma is a complication occurring from 0.17% to 4.2%. After optimization of the asthmatic patient preoperatively, careful assessment and vigilance is crucial to delivering a safe anesthetic. Efforts are aimed at reducing allergens, maintaining adequate depth of anesthesia, addressing analgesia needs, and avoiding bronchoconstrictive drugs, interventions, or events that may trigger spasm. Rapid recognition and treatment of perioperative bronchospasm is of utmost importance. Discussion often occurs as to the advantage of regional anesthesia or general anesthesia in asthmatic patients. It has been demonstrated that airway instrumentation can result in parasympathetic mediated bronchoconstriction.[13] It is generally held that regional anesthesia is preferential in the asthmatic patient, due to the avoidance of airway manipulation and the resultant irritation that can occur. It is important, however, to consider extenuating circumstances in which such an advantage may not exist as in the case of spinal or epidural anesthesia that reaches levels of midthoracic area or above that may interfere with coughing or deep breathing or other regional anesthetics in which considerable sedation is needed concomitantly.[13,31,32,54]

Intravenous Anesthetics

Central nervous system depressant drugs, including general anesthesia induction agents, must be considered individually in regard to their effects on airway reactivity in asthmatic patients. It should be noted that although some drugs display more beneficial qualities, total agreement is lacking in determining asthma to be an absolute contraindication to any of the commonly used induction agents. Further, light anesthesia is a frequent cause of bronchoconstriction and as such must be avoided in the asthmatic patient, particularly during airway manipulation.[32]

Thiopental has been studied extensively for its effects on the respiratory tract. Reports on thiopental range from having a relaxation effect to no effect to a constricting effect on bronchial smooth muscle. Thiopental has been demonstrated in some but not all studies to cause a release of histamine or a worsening of histamine-induced bronchoconstriction.[48,55,56]

Ketamine is widely believed to have the most advantageous profile of the intravenous agents. It has been shown to provide protection against bronchoconstriction induced by methacholine as well as clinical stimulation. Its bronchodilating effects are well described, although the mechanism is uncertain. There may be an effect through neural mechanisms, increased or enhanced catecholamine concentration, or inhibition of nicotinic or muscarinic receptors; at high doses there may be direct smooth muscle effects. The increase in bronchial secretions from ketamine may be of concern so that pretreatment with an antimuscarinic such as glycopyrrolate may be warranted.[31,48,57–60]

Etomidate has been less studied for its effects in asthmatic patients; however, unlike thiopental, it is generally believed to be void of bronchoconstrictive activity. It is advocated by many, including the manufacturers, to be a drug of choice for patients with reactive disease, particularly when compared with thiopental. In addition, due to its cardiovascular stability, in most cases etomidate can be given in high-range doses safely to ensure adequate depth of anesthesia.[58]

Propofol has been studied extensively for its effects on bronchial airways. Propofol has been reported to cause bronchospasm, and its chemical structure and components may predispose it to being an allergen.[61] By comparison it has been shown to cause lower respiratory resistance after tracheal intubation than either thiopental or etomidate.

Like ketamine, propofol has been demonstrated to have a significant effect attenuating airway responses to stimulation as well as methacholine-induced airway constriction.[56–58,62] Propofol has been demonstrated to inhibit vagal-induced bronchoconstriction without worsening parasympathetic-induced bradycardia.[63]

Like other intravenous anesthetic agents, midazolam and diazepam cause smooth muscle relaxation. The mechanism by which this occurs does not appear to be related to their known effects at γ-aminobutyric acid receptors but rather a direct effect on voltage-dependent calcium channels.[64]

Opioids

Opioids have been associated with the release of histamines, an effect that may vary in degree between the formulations. As such it is intuitive to believe that they should be avoided in asthmatic patients in favor of drugs known to have bronchodilating or bronchoprotective effects. The effect of opioid-induced bronchoconstriction has not been widely demonstrated. There is some evidence suggesting that opioids may inhibit nonadrenergic, noncholinergic bronchoconstriction via μ opioid receptors. Still other studies suggest that fentanyl and morphine may increase tracheal smooth muscle tone; however, the clinical significance has not been determined. As a result there is insufficient evidence to suggest that opioids should be avoided in patients with asthma.[48,65] It is essential that the potential effects of postoperative respiratory depression and muscle rigidity from opioids be taken into consideration when formulating an anesthetic plan for the asthmatic patient. Muscle rigidity can be misinterpreted as bronchoconstriction. Care to administer these drugs slowly as well as the use of nondepolarizing neuromuscular blocking drugs may reduce the incidence of rigidity.[13,32]

Neuromuscular Blocking Drugs

Neuromuscular blocking drugs have been linked to histamine release and have been implicated as a strong allergen resulting in anaphylactic and anaphylactoid reactions under anesthesia.[66] Selection of a neuromuscular blocking drug for asthmatics should be based on the drug's histamine releasing potential and its specificity to muscarinic receptor type. Atracurium and mivacurium are associated with significant dose-dependent histamine release and are best avoided. Drugs such as, or similar to, gallamine, rapacuronium, or pipecuronium, with an affinity for M_2 preferentially to M_3, have been implicated as more likely to cause bronchoconstriction. Drugs with greater affinity to M_3 receptors such as cisatracurium, pancuronium, rocuronium, and vecuronium are considered safer in these patients. Reversal of neuromuscular blocking drugs can be problematic in that anticholinesterase agents can cause increased secretions and bronchoconstriction. Timing of dosing to avoid the need for reversal is preferred; however, slow injection and adequate coinciding administration of atropine allow for safe reversal as needed. Succinylcholine, structurally similar to acetylcholine, can potentially stimulate muscarinic receptors, resulting in airway reactivity and increased smooth muscle tone; however, because it has been used safely in asthmatics, the clinical relevance has not been completely shown.[13,32,48]

Volatile Inhalation Agents

The bronchodilation effects of the modern volatile agents (VAs) have been well studied and documented.[64,67] Bronchodilation from VAs are thought to be mediated through their effects on β receptors, in turn regulating voltage-dependent calcium channels by an increase in intracellular cAMP and a decrease in intracellular calcium concentration. The result is smooth muscle relaxation, and the extent to which this occurs may vary between the specific agents.[13,32,64] So significant are these relaxant effects that the VAs sevoflurane and isoflurane have been used successfully in the management of even severe, prolonged status asthmaticus.[68–70]

In a study of the VAs desflurane, halothane, isofluranes and sevoflurane, all agents were shown to protect against acetylcholine-induced bronchoconstriction, and, additionally, desflurane and sevoflurane were shown to significantly decrease basal airway tone in rat lungs.[71] In delineating which VA provides the most advantage for the asthmatic patient, there are some elements to consider. Desflurane has been shown to be an airway irritant and unsuitable for inhalation induction. It has been shown to cause an increase in airway resistance in children. Sevoflurane effects have been studied as well; however, some controversy exists. Rooke et al. reported that sevoflurane effectively decreased respiratory resistance as much or more than isoflurane or halothane at near MAC values. Habre et al. demonstrated that when used as a sole anesthetic during tracheal intubation in asthmatic children, sevoflurane was associated with an increase in respiratory resistance; however, the authors reported no adverse clinical effects.[13,32,72–77]

Mechanical Ventilation

The pulmonary circulation's ability to match perfusion to ventilation is facilitated through a mechanism termed hypoxic pulmonary vasoconstriction, which is crucial in optimizing oxygenation in the presence of asthma, pneumonia, and atelectasis. Hypoxic pulmonary vasoconstriction can fail or be reduced to an inadequate level under certain circumstances such as disease, one-lung anesthesia, or by the pharmacologic effects of drugs such as the VAs. As a result the anesthetist must look for all means to optimize ventilation and perfusion efficiency in patients with asthma.[78] During periods of mechanical ventilation careful consideration is needed to determine the optimal modes to be used for asthmatics on an individualized basis. Definitive studies are lacking to develop guidelines. Goals should be set to maintain optimal oxygenation and ventilation while minimizing hyperinflation. In experimental models biologically variable ventilation modes have been shown to be superior to controlled ventilation modes during bronchospasm. Pressure-controlled ventilation may be advantageous to avoid barotrauma and increased airway pressure. It has been suggested that a controlled approach of hypoventilation or so-called permissive hypercapnia while maximizing expiratory time to minimize hyperinflation may be optimal. Care to maintain arterial CO_2 and pH at a reasonable level must be taken, and individual assessment of patient variable must be considered.[79,80]

Management of Acute Bronchospasm

The first and often times most important aspect of managing perioperative bronchospasm is prevention. This is best achieved through optimization of disease control and avoidance of triggering factors. Assurance of adequate depth of anesthesia before stimulation, including intubation, as well as consideration of deep extubation is advised. The use of regional anesthesia should be considered when possible.[31,48] Preoperative administration of β agonist medications or corticosteroids, including ICSs, may be beneficial. In some cases, such as when contrast dyes are given or previous allergic reactions have occurred, the use of prophylactic antihistamines may prove beneficial.[81–83] The use of lidocaine through intravenous and nebulized routes has been studied in preventing bronchoprotective reflex before airway interventions with mixed results. Inhaled lidocaine has been shown to cause an initial bronchoconstriction response followed by attenuation of this reactivity.[84–86]

If wheezing and/or increased ventilatory pressures are detected, other potential causes must be ruled out. These may include mechanical obstructions of airflow within the circuit or machine, endotracheal tube, endobronchial intubation aspiration, pneumothorax, or pulmonary edema to name a few. Auscultation of the lungs, evaluation of inspiratory pressure changes, evaluation of end tidal carbon dioxide (ETCO$_2$) waveform, and arterial blood gas analysis may be helpful in determining the presence of bronchospasm.[13,32]

When a bronchospasm is detected, immediate actions must be taken—a testimony to the importance of heightened vigilance in anesthesia patient monitoring. Optimizing oxygenation should occur early. Patients who have advanced airway devices in place should be given 100% oxygen. In patients who are not intubated, non-rebreather masks should be applied with maximal FiO$_2$ administration, and preparation for intubation should be considered. Deepening of the anesthetic should be achieved through increased inspired VA or intravenous agent or both. Recalling the value of these agents as bronchodilators as well as removing light anesthesia as a triggering agent explains the rationale. β Agonists are often the most effective pharmacologic intervention for bronchospasm. These can be administered via MDI or nebulizer. Albuterol, two to four actuations (90 μg per actuation), is typically administered in spontaneously breathing, nonintubated patients. It is essential to note that the administration of a medication through an endotracheal tube via an MDI results in an uncertain and often inadequate amount of drug actually delivered with as little as 1% to 3% of the dose reaching the lung surface. As a result higher than the normal actuations may be indicated.[13] Epinephrine at a dose of 0.2 to 0.5 mg to a maximum of 1 mg (1:1000 solution) may be given subcutaneously or intramuscularly or 0.1 to 0.25 mg IV. Alternatively, terbutaline, 0.25 mg subcutaneously, may be given and repeated once.[36]

An alternative and perhaps late consideration in treating bronchospasm is the use of magnesium sulfate. Its value has been demonstrated in treating refractory bronchospasm, with the intravenous route proving to be beneficial and the inhaled route showing questionable benefit. The mechanism by which it works is not fully understood; however, magnesium sulfate may relax smooth muscle and inhibit smooth muscle contraction, decrease histamine release, and inhibit inflammatory response.[87]

Summary

Asthma is a disease of chronic inflammation of the airways and airway hyperreactivity resulting in smooth muscle bronchoconstriction and diminished airflow. It is characterized by periods of apparent remissions and exacerbations and affects approximately 22 million Americans. In addition to airway hyperreactivity, characteristics include bronchoconstriction, inflammation, and airway remodeling. Preoperative evaluation and optimization of disease control is essential in ensuring a safe anesthetic for the asthmatic patient. The primary efforts of disease control are aimed at reducing or controlling inflammation. A variety of drug classes is used for this purpose, with inhaled corticosteroids being the mainstay. Modern anesthetic agents and techniques can be safely administered to the asthmatic patient. Avoidance of bronchospasm through preventative measures and early identification and aggressive management of perioperative bronchospasm is a primary priority for the nurse anesthetist caring for a patient with asthma.

Key Points

- According to the NAEPP, about 22 million people in the United States have asthma.
- Asthma is a disease of chronic airway inflammation and hyperreactivity resulting in smooth muscle bronchoconstriction and diminished airflow. It is characterized by periods of apparent remissions and exacerbations.
- In assessing the extent of asthma, taking a detailed history is crucial.
- While several classes of drugs may be prescribed, the long-term use of inhaled corticosteroids is considered the mainstay of pharmacologic control of asthma inflammation. During periods of severe exacerbations of asthma, systemic corticosteroids may be required.
- Patients should be instructed to continue their current therapy as scheduled on the day of surgery, and a return to therapy postoperatively should be planned as soon as possible.
- Beta-adrenergic agonists exert a bronchodilating effect through the stimulation of β$_2$ receptors on pulmonary smooth muscle and are useful in preventing and reversing bronchoconstriction from asthma.
- The NHLBI panel concluded that asthmatic patients are at risk for complications during surgery and the postoperative period. In addition to bronchoconstriction triggered by light anesthesia, intubation, hypoxemia, or hypercapnia, a heightened risk exists for impaired cough and the potentially resultant atelectasis and respiratory infection and hyperresponsiveness upon exposure to latex and some anesthetic agents.
- A byproduct of most anesthetics is the resultant respiratory depression and CO$_2$ retention inherent

in CNS depressant agents, whether given via intravenous or inhaled routes. As such, a goal of the anesthetist in caring for the asthmatic patient must be to find a balance between avoiding triggering stimuli, including light anesthesia, airway instrumentation, and allergen exposure, with the hypoventilation risk associated throughout the perioperative period.

Chapter Questions

1. Discuss the epidemiologic impact of asthma as a disease entity.
2. What is the role of genetics in the development of asthma and in the pharmacologic management of the disease?
3. How do the sympathetic and parasympathetic nervous systems interact in the development of symptoms and management of asthma?
4. What findings during a preoperative history and physical examination would alert the anesthetist to an asthmatic patient at high risk for perioperative bronchospasm?
5. What anesthetic agents are best avoided and best used for the asthmatic patient?
6. What is optimal perioperative management for an acute exacerbation of asthma?

References

1. Expert Panel Report 3 (EPR3). Guidelines for the diagnosis and management of asthma, full report. Bethesda, MD: U.S. Department of Health and Human Services, Public Health Service, National Institutes of Health, National Heart, Lung and Blood Institute; 2007. Report number 08-4051. Available at: http://www.nhlbi.nih.gov/guidelines/asthma/asthgdln.htm. Accessed June 29, 2009.
2. Lemanske RF Jr. Asthma therapies revisited: what have we learned? *Proc Am Thorac Soc.* 2009;6:312–315.
3. Martinez FD. The origins of asthma and chronic obstructive pulmonary disease in early life. *Proc Am Thorac Soc.* 2009;6:272–277.
4. Weiss KB, Sullivan SD. The health economics of asthma and rhinitis. I. Assessing the economic impact. *J Allerg Clin Immunol.* 2001;107:3–8.
5. Bergeron C, Al-Ramli W, Hamid Q. Remodeling in asthma. *Proc Am Thorac Soc.* 2009;6:301–305.
6. Kurt E, Ozkan R, Orman A, Calisir C, Metintas M. Irreversibility of remodeled features on high-resolution computerized tomography scans of asthmatic patients on conventional therapy: a six year longitudinal study. *J Asthma.* 2009;46:300–307.
7. Gaffin JM, Phipatanakul W. The role of indoor allergens in the development of asthma. *Curr Opin Allerg Clin Immunol.* 2009;9:128–135.
8. Boushey HA. Drugs used in asthma. In: Katzung BG, ed. *Basic and Clinical Pharmacology*, 8th ed. New York: McGraw-Hill; 2001:333–349.
9. Lewis MJ, Short AL, Lewis KE. Autonomic nervous system control of the cardiovascular and respiratory systems in asthma. *Respir Med.* 2006;100:1688–1705.
10. King CS, Moores LK. Clinical asthma syndromes and important asthma mimics. *Respir Care.* 2008;53:568–580.
11. Gyllfors P, Bochenek G, Overholt J, et al. Biochemical and clinical evidence that aspirin-intolerant asthmatic subjects tolerate the cyclooxygenase 2-selective analgetic drug celecoxib. *J Allerg Clin Immunol.* 2003;111(Suppl. 1):1116–1121.
12. Szczeklik A, Stevenson DD. Aspirin-induced asthma: advances in pathogenesis, diagnosis, and management. *J Allerg Clin Immunol.* 2003;111(Suppl. 1):913–921.
13. Yamakage M, Iwasaki S, Namiki A. Guideline-oriented perioperative management of patients with bronchial asthma and chronic obstructive pulmonary disease. *J Anesth.* 2008; 22:412–428.
14. Halm EA, Mora P, Leventhal H. No symptoms, no asthma. *Chest.* 2006;129:573–580.
15. Lima JJ, Blake KV, Tantisira KG, Weiss ST. Pharmacogenetics of asthma. *Curr Opin Pulm Med.* 2009;15:57–62.
16. Phua GC, MacIntyre NR. Inhaled corticosteroids in obstructive airway disease. *Respir Care.* 2007;52:852–858.
17. Barnes PJ. How corticosteroids control inflammation: Quintiles Prize Lecture 2005. *Br J Pharmacol.* 2006;148:245–254.
18. Derendorf H, Nave R, Drollmann A, Cerasoli F, Wurst W. Relevance of pharmacokinetics and pharmacodynamics of inhaled corticosteroids to asthma. *Eur Respir J.* 2006; 28:1042–1050.
19. Tayab Z, Hochhaus G. Advances in single-entity inhaled corticosteroid therapy. *Allerg Asthma Proc.* 2007;28:125–135.
20. Baptist AP, Reddy RC. Inhaled corticosteroids for asthma: are they all the same? *J Clin Pharmac Ther.* 2009;34:1–12.
21. Kelly HW. Rationale for the major changes in the pharmacotherapy section of the national asthma education and prevention program guidelines. *J Allerg Clin Immunol.* 2007;120:989–994.
22. Apter AJ. Advances in adult asthma diagnosis and treatment and health outcomes, education, delivery, and quality in 2008. *J Allerg Clin Immunol.* 2009;123:35–40.

23. Winkler J, Hochhaus G, Derendorf H. How the lung handles drugs: pharmacokinetics and pharmacodynamics of inhaled corticosteroids. *Proc Am Thorac Soc.* 2004;1:356–363.

24. Edsbäcker S, Wollmer P, Selroos O, Borgström L, Olsson B, Ingelf J. Do airway clearance mechanisms influence the local and systemic effects of inhaled corticosteroids? *Pulm Pharmacol Ther.* 2008;21:247–258.

25. Hubbard R, Tattersfield A, Smith C, West J, Smeeth L, Fletcher A. Use of inhaled corticosteroids and the risk of fracture. *Chest.* 2006;130:1082–1088.

26. Leone FT, Fish JE, Szefler SJ, West SL. Systematic review of the evidence regarding potential complications of inhaled corticosteroid use in asthma. *Chest.* 2003;124:2329–2340.

27. Rachelefsky G. Inhaled corticosteroids and asthma control in children: assessing impairment and risk. *Pediatrics.* 2009;123:353–366.

28. Kroon LA. Drug interactions with smoking. *Am J Health Syst Pharm.* 2007;64:1917–1921.

29. Samaras K, Pett S, Gowers A, McMurchie M, Cooper D. Iatrogenic Cushing's syndrome with osteoporosis and secondary adrenal failure in human immunodeficiency virus-infected patients receiving inhaled corticosteroids and ritonavir-boosted protease inhibitors: six cases. *J Clin Endocrinol Metab.* 2005;90:4394–4398.

30. Belda J, Margarit G, Martinez C, et al. Anti-inflammatory effects of high-dose inhaled fluticasone versus oral prednisone in asthma exacerbations. *Eur Respir J.* 2007;30:1143–1149.

31. Rieker M. Respiratory anatomy, physiology, pathophysiology and anesthesia management. In: Nagelhout JJ, Plaus KL, eds. *Nurse Anesthesia,* 4th ed. St. Louis, MO: Saunders Elsevier; 2010.

32. Burburan SM, Xisto DG, Rocco PR. Anaesthetic management in asthma. *Minerva Anestesiol.* 2007;73:357–365.

33. Global Initiative for Asthma (GINA). Global strategy for asthma management and prevention (updated 2008). Available at: http://www.ginasthma. Accessed June 30, 2009.

34. Donohue JF, Hanania NA, Ciubotaru RL, et al. Comparison of levalbuterol and racemic albuterol in hospitalized patients with acute asthma or COPD: A 2-week, multicenter, randomized, open-label study. *Clin Ther.* 2008;30:989–1002.

35. Tripp K, McVicar WK, Nair P, et al. A cumulative dose study of levalbuterol and racemic albuterol administered by hydrofluoroalkane-134a metered-dose inhaler in asthmatic subjects. *J Allerg Clin Immunol.* 2008;122:544–549.

36. Micromedex(r) Healthcare Series Version 5.1. Greenwood Village, CO: Thomson Reuters (Healthcare) Inc. [intranet database http://dmc-micromedex/home/dispatch]. Accessed June 30, 2009.

37. Cates CJ, Cates MJ. Regular treatment with salmeterol for chronic asthma: serious adverse events. Cochrane Collaboration. 2008(3). Available at: http://www.thecochranelibrary.com. Accessed June 30, 2009.

38. Sears MR. Safety of long-acting beta-agonists: are new data really required? *Chest.* 2009. Available at: http://www.chestjournal.org/content/early/2009/06/12/chest.09-1214.abstract. Accessed June 8, 2009.

39. Thomas M, Prince D. High-dose inhaled corticosteroid versus long-acting beta-agonist addition in asthma. *Chest.* 2009;135:1404–1405.

40. Tronde A, Gillen M, Borgström L, Lötvall J, Ankerst J. Inhaler in patients with asthma and COPD: pharmacokinetics of budesonide and formoterol administered via one pressurized metered-dose. *J Clin Pharmacol.* 2008;48:1300–1308.

41. Ulrik CS, Diamant Z. Effect of montelukast on excessive airway narrowing response to methacholine in adult asthmatic patients not on controller therapy. *Allerg Asthma Proc.* 2009;30:64–68.

42. Wahn U, Balachandra Dass S. Review of recent results of montelukast use as a monotherapy in children with mild asthma. *Clin Ther.* 2008;30(Pt. 1):1026–1035.

43. Bisgaard H, Zielen S, Garcia-Garcia ML, et al. Montelukast reduces asthma exacerbations in 2- to 5-year-old children with intermittent asthma. *Am J Respir Crit Care Med.* 2005;171:315–322.

44. Robertson CF, Price D, Henry R, et al. Short-course montelukast for intermittent asthma in children: a randomized controlled trial. *Am J Respir Crit Care Med.* 2007;175:323–329.

45. Hendeles L, Sorkness CA. Anti-immunoglobulin E therapy with omalizumab for asthma. *Ann Pharmacother.* 2007;41:1397–1410.

46. Polosa R, Morjaria J. Immunomodulatory and biologic therapies for severe refractory asthma. *Respir Med.* 2008;102:1499–1510.

47. Plosker GL, Keam SJ. Omalizumab: a review of its use in the treatment of allergic asthma. *Biodrugs.* 2008;22:189–204.

48. Warner DO. Airway pharmacology. In: Hagberg CA, ed. *Benumof's Airway Management,* 2nd ed. Philadelphia: Mosby Elsevier; 2007:164–192.

49. Tee A, Koh MS, Gibson PG, Lasserson TJ, Wilson A, Irving LB. Long-acting beta2-agonists versus theophylline for maintenance treatment of asthma. *Cochrane Collaboration.* 2007. Available at: http://www.mrw.interscience.wiley.com/cochrane/clsysrev/articles/CD001281/frame.html. Accessed June 30, 2009.

50. Su FW, Beckman DB, Yarnold PA, Grammar LC. Low incidence of complications in asthmatic patients treated

with preoperative corticosteroids. *Allerg Asthma Proc.* 2004;25:327–333.

51. Nagelhout JJ, Elisha S, Waters E. Should I continue or discontinue that medication? *AANAJ.* 2009;77:59–73.

52. Yamakage M, Iwasaki S, Jeong S-W, Satoh J-I, Namiki A. Beta-1 selective adrenergic antagonist Landiolol and esmolol can be safely used in patients with airway hyperreactivity. *Heart Lung J Acute Crit Care.* 2009;38:48–55.

53. Olenchock BA, Fonarow GG, Pan W, Hernandez A, Cannon CP. Current use of beta-blockers in patients with reactive airway disease who are hospitalized with acute coronary syndromes. *Am J Cardiol.* 2009;103:295–300.

54. Groeben H. Epidural anesthesia and pulmonary function. *J Anesth.* 2006;20:290–299.

55. Kabara S, Hirota K, Yoshioka H, Kudo T, Ishihara H, Matsuki A. Differential effects of thiopental on methacholine- and serotonin-induced bronchoconstriction in dogs. *Br J Anaesth.* 2003;91:379–384.

56. Pizov R, Brown RH, Weiss YS, et al. Wheezing during induction of general anesthesia in patients with and without asthma: a randomized, blinded trial. *Anesthesiology.* 1995; 82:1111–1116.

57. Brown RH, Wagner EM. Mechanisms of bronchoprotection by anesthetic induction agents: Propofol versus ketamine. *Anesthesiology.* 1999;90:822–828.

58. Eames WO, Rooke GA, Sai-Chuen Wu R, Bishop MJ. Comparison of the effects of etomidate, propofol, and thiopental on respiratory resistance after tracheal intubation. *Anesthesiology.* 1996;84:1307–1311.

59. Stoelting RK, Hillier SC. *Pharmacology and Physiology in Anesthetic Practice,* 4th ed. Philadelphia: Lippincott Williams & Wilkins; 2006.

60. Kohrs R, Durieux M. Ketamine: teaching an old dog new tricks. *Anesth Analg.* 1998;87:1186–1193.

61. Hattori J-I, Fujimura N, Kanaya N, Okazaki K, Namiki A. Bronchospasm induced by propofol in a patient with sick house syndrome. *Anesth Analg.* 2003;96:163–164.

62. Wu R, Wu KC, Sum D, Bishop MJ. Comparative effects of thiopentone and propofol on respiratory resistance after tracheal intubation. *Br J Anaesth.* 1996;77:735–738.

63. Hashiba E, Hirota K, Suzuki K, Matsuki A. Effects of propofol on bronchoconstriction and bradycardia induced by vagal nerve stimulation. *Acta Anaesth Scand.* 2003;47: 1059–1063.

64. Yamakage M. Editorial II: effects of anaesthetic agents on airway smooth muscles. *Br J Anaesth.* 2002;88:624–627.

65. Frossard N, Barnes PJ. Mu-opioid receptors modulate non-cholinergic constrictor nerves in guinea-pig airways. *Eur J Pharmacol.* 1987;141:519–522.

66. Mertes P, Laxenaire M, Alla F. Anaphylactic and anaphylactoid reactions occurring during anesthesia in France in 1999–2000. *Anesthesiology.* 2003;99:536–545.

67. Hirshman CA, Bergman NA. Factors influencing intrapulmonary airway calibre during anaesthesia. *Br J Anaesth.* 1990;65:30–42.

68. Kazuhiro W, Taro M, Soichiro Y, Yukihiro T, Takahiro J, Makoto T. Prolonged sevoflurane inhalation therapy for status asthmaticus in an infant. *Pediatr Anesth.* 2008;18:543–545.

69. Shultze TE. Sevoflurane administration in status asthmaticus: a case report. *AANAJ.* 2005;73:35–36.

70. Thomson H, Harper NJ, Parkes A. Use of the AnaConDa anaesthetic delivery system to treat life-threatening asthma. *Anaesthesia.* 2007;62:295–296.

71. Lele E, Petak F, Fontao F, Morel D, Habre W. Protective effects of volatile agents against acetylcholine-induced bronchoconstriction in isolated perfused rat lungs. *Acta Anaesth Scand.* 2006;50:1145–1151.

72. Satoh J-I, Yamakage M, Kobayashi T, Tohse N, Watanabe H, Namiki A. Desflurane but not sevoflurane can increase lung resistance via tachykinin pathways. *Br J Anaesth.* 2009;102:704–713.

73. von Ungern-Sternberg BS, Saudan S, Petak F, Hantos Z, Habre W. Desflurane but not sevoflurane impairs airway and respiratory tissue mechanics in children with susceptible airways. *Anesthesiology.* 2008;108:216–224

74. Wilkes AR, Raj N, Hall JE. Adverse airway events during brief nasal inhalations of volatile anaesthetics: the effect of humidity and repeated exposure on incidence in volunteers preselected by response to desflurane. *Anaesthesia.* 2003;58:207–216.

75. Burburan SM, Xisto DG, Ferreira HC, et al. Lung mechanics and histology during sevoflurane anesthesia in a model of chronic allergic asthma. *Anesth Analg.* 2007;104:631–637.

76. Rooke GA, Choi J-H, Bishop MJ. The effect of isoflurane, halothane, sevoflurane, and thiopental/nitrous oxide on respiratory system resistance after tracheal intubation. *Anesthesiology.* 1997;86:1294–1299.

77. Habre W, Scalfaro P, Sims C, Tiller K, Sly PD. Respiratory mechanics during sevoflurane anesthesia in children with and without asthma. *Anesth Analg.* 1999;89:1177.

78. Nagandran J, Stewart K, Hoskinson M, Archer S. An anesthesiologists guide to hypoxic pulmonary vasoconstriction: implications for managing single-lung anesthesia and atelectasis. *Curr Opin Anesthesiol.* 2006;19:34–43.

79. Medoff BD. Invasive and noninvasive ventilation in patients with asthma. *Respir Care.* 2008;53:740–752.

80. Mutch WA, Buchman TG, Girling LG, Walker EK, McManus BM, Graham MR. Biologically variable ventilation improves

gas exchange and respiratory mechanics in a model of severe bronchospasm. *Crit Care Med.* 2007;35:1749–1755.

81. Scalfaro P, Sly PD, Sims C, Habre W. Salbutamol prevents the increase of respiratory resistance caused by tracheal intubation during sevoflurane anesthesia in asthmatic children. *Anesth Analg.* 2001;93:898–902.

82. Martinez FD. Managing childhood asthma: challenge of preventing exacerbations. *Pediatrics.* 2009;123:S146–S150.

83. Liccardi G, Lobefalo G, DiFlorio E, et al. Strategies for the prevention of asthmatic, anaphylactic and anaphylactoid reactions during the administration of anesthetics and/or contrast dye. *J Invest Allerg Clin Immunol.* 2008;18:1–11.

84. Adamzik M, Groeben H, Farahani R, Lehmann N, Peters J. Intravenous lidocaine after tracheal intubation mitigates bronchoconstriction in patients with asthma. *Anesth Analg.* 2007;104:168–172.

85. Groeben H, Silvanus MT, Mechthild B, Jurgen P. Combined lidocaine and salbutamol inhalation for airway anesthesia markedly protects against reflex bronchoconstriction. *Chest.* 2000;118:509–515.

86. Chang H-YS, Togias A, Brown RH. The effects of systemic lidocaine on airway tone and pulmonary function in asthmatic subjects. *Anesth Analg.* 2007;104:1109–1115.

87. Rowe BH, Camargo CAJ. The role of magnesium sulfate in the acute and chronic management of asthma. *Curr Opin Pulm Med.* 2008;14:70–76.

88. Foegh ML, Ramwell PW. The eicosanoids: prostaglandins, thromboxanes, leukotrienes and related compounds. In: Katzung B, ed. *Basic and Clinical Pharmacology,* 8th ed. New York: McGraw-Hill; 2001:311–313.

89. White P. *Perioperative Drug Manual,* 2nd ed. Philadelphia: Elsevier Saunders; 2005.

Immune System and Anesthesia: Pharmacologic Implications

Charles A. Griffis, PhD, CRNA

Introduction

The effect of surgery and anesthesia on the immune system can be profound. Although multiple considerations compete for the attention of the nurse anesthetist when caring for patients, the importance of considering the effect of anesthetic pharmacology on postoperative immune function cannot be overestimated. The immune system, which functions to protect the host from infection and potential malignancy during the postoperative period, may be mildly to profoundly depressed after exposure to the intraoperative milieu, depending on the patient's preoperative history, the surgical intervention, and the drugs administered intraoperatively.[1] Although many factors impact the immune function in the perioperative period, including fear, hypothermia, altered tissue perfusion, hyperglycemia, and inflammatory response to surgical trauma, in this chapter we focus on the effects of perioperative drug therapy. By understanding the effects of anesthetic and adjunct procedural perioperative drug therapy on immune function, the practitioner can add measures to support the immune system and protect the patient. In the review to follow, of the many drugs used by anesthetists and surgeons in the perioperative setting, only those drugs with known implications to immune function are discussed.

Review of Normal Immune Function

Innate Immunity

Innate immunity, the body's first line of defense against infection, is critically important in removing dead or dying cells and tissues. The key leukocyte effector cells include the neutrophils; polymorphonuclear cells; monocytes, which are transformed into macrophages after leaving the vasculature and entering tissues; and a distinctive class of lymphocytes with no T-cell receptors, called natural killer (NK) cells.[2] These cells are found in most body tissues, with the exception of the central nervous system, which has its own distinct immunologically active innate cells. Innate immune cells possess cell surface receptors that respond to patterns of protein expression unique to microbes, recognizing these cells as "non-self." Encountering a non-self cell results in the activation of intracellular signaling cascades, activation of genes, cell movement, and excretion of effector molecules.[3] Phagocytic immune cells engulf (phagocytize) microbes and digest and destroy them. The effector molecules either directly attack microbes or initiate the inflammatory process, bringing about increased vascular permeability and edema, increasing perivascular blood flow, and drawing in and activating more immune cells to attack microbial invaders. Inflammation brings about clearance of microbial invaders, clearance of dead cells, and activation of the adaptive immune response. Surgical incision initiates an inflammatory response that is directly proportional to the size and invasiveness of the surgery. Many products of the inflammatory cascade up-regulate nociceptors and depress the adaptive immune cell response. Finally, NK cells play a role in immune surveillance for altered self-cells. NK cell lymphocytes recognize such cells and may protect the host from malignancy by destroying them.

Adaptive Immunity

The adaptive immune response, mediated by T and B lymphocyte cells, is characterized by specificity to antigens associated with microbes or tissue, delayed onset of efficacy, and memory cells that can swiftly mount a response with recurrent exposure.[2] Bound inextricably to the adaptive response targeting specific antigenic targets is the previously discussed innate response. Innate cells such as macrophages and dendritic cells ingest microbes or offending tissue targets, process the protein structures, and display the antigenic determining epitopes on their cell surface in combination with major histocompatibility complex I (for cytotoxic lymphocyte recognition) or major histocompatibility complex II (for T-helper cell recognition). In the lymph nodes naive cytotoxic lymphocytes (CD-8) and T-helper cells (CD-4) bind to the displayed antigens with the unique T-cell receptor targeted to the epitope. Clonal expansion ensues, resulting in a population of cells specific to the immunologically active source protein.

The CD-4 cells, depending on the environmental milieu, differentiate further. Type I cells secrete cytokines, driving the further activation of the CD-8 cells, which seek body cells displaying the targeted epitope; such cells are destroyed to curb intracellular pathogen growth (cellular adaptive immunity). Differentiation into type II CD-4 cells produces helper cells that secrete cytokines destined to activate the B lymphocytes responding to the epitope into specialized plasma cells (humoral adaptive immunity). These cells secrete antibody immunoglobulins that bind to the epitope, either disabling a pathogen cell's ability to harm or infect the host or acting as a targeting signal to cytotoxic lymphocytes and activating the plasma protein system known as complement. The activated complement proteins bind to antibodies, enhancing phagocytosis of microbes or infected cells, and also bind to receptors on innate and adaptive immune cells to increase the efficacy of the effector response. In considering the complex signaling systems necessary for immune cell activation, and the resulting complicated intracellular biochemical cascades that ultimately produce gene transcription and altered cell activity, the potential for anesthesia drug effects in these systems is clear.

Drugs Used in the Perioperative Setting

Anesthesia Drugs

Inhaled Anesthetics

Overall, the effect of inhaled anesthetic drugs appears to be immunosuppressive, although the available evidence must be considered carefully. Numerous in vitro studies in which immunocytes were exposed to clinically relevant concentrations of inhaled anesthetic drugs demonstrated subsequent depression of effector functions such as phagocytosis and cytokine production, impaired proliferation, and induced apoptosis.[4] Lymphocytes were exposed to sevoflurane, isoflurane, and desflurane in vitro, and researchers found that sevoflurane and isoflurane induced apoptosis in a dose-dependent manner via increased mitochondrial caspase activation.[5] Furthermore, macrophages exposed to isoflurane or desflurane exhibited the potential for decreased nitric oxide production under some conditions, indicating suppressed effector function.[6] Decreased responses of NK cells to interferon, an important signal that normally stimulates cellular immunity, has been reported following in vitro exposure to isoflurane.[7] Investigators examined the effect of sevoflurane on human lymphocytes by in vitro exposure and concluded that the suppression of lymphocyte function was due to inhibition of a cellular transcription factor AP-1.[5] In contrast to previous findings, Schneemilch et al. found that sevoflurane might have a beneficial effect on proliferation and cytokine production of peripheral blood mononuclear cells in vitro by alleviating the immunosuppressive effects of nitrous oxide.[8]

In considering the immune system effects of volatile anesthetics, it is important to consider the confounding clinical situation of perioperative care, which is associated with multiple factors that may suppress immune function independent of the drugs. Procopio et al. exposed healthy volunteers to thiopental-nitrous oxide-isoflurane general anesthesia and found, in the absence of surgery, no suppression of immune function of lymphocytes tested ex vivo.[9] It seems likely that it is the combination of perioperative stressors and inhaled anesthetics that accounts for perioperative immunocyte dysfunction. Furthermore, if anesthetic drugs are used skillfully to ameliorate the metabolic stress response to surgery, the perioperative immune depression may be modulated accordingly.

Intravenous Anesthetics

Table 26-1 illustrates that the effect of intravenous anesthetics, based largely on in vitro studies, have variable but often suppressive effects on immune cell function. Inada et al. found that the use of propofol total intravenous anesthesia for craniotomy prevented the shift in T-helper cell phenotype to Th$_2$, seen with comparable isoflurane anesthesia; this is considered desirable in that Th$_1$-type T-helper cells support the crucially important and protective cellular adaptive immune response postoperatively.[10] Kelbel and Weiss discuss the finding that immune suppression after propofol and etomidate may be ameliorated by a change in drug vehicle.[11] Use of medium-chain triglyceride emulsions of these drugs, as compared with the commercially available long-chain triglyceride preparations, is associated with lack of suppression of neutrophil function.

Several mechanisms by which immune cell function is impaired by thiopental, etomidate, and propofol have been identified, including inhibition of intracellular calcium entry, changing cellular amino acid turnover, and diminishment of interleukin-8 production by polymorphonuclear leukocytes. Schneemilch et al. found that thiopental inhibited leukocyte proliferation, and both thiopental and propofol reduced cellular excretion of effector molecules.[8] Chang et al. investigated the in vitro effects of clinically relevant concentrations of ketamine on immune cell function and found that treatment of macrophages with ketamine reduced phagocytic activity and expression of reactive oxygen species and proinflammatory cytokines, possibly through reduction of mitochondrial membrane potential.[12]

Local Anesthetics

Amide local anesthetics, though commonly used in anesthetic practice to block neuronal sodium channels, can also interact at low concentrations with many other cellular receptors and proteins.[4] Thus multiple inflammatory effector functions of innate immune cells may be ameliorated, although nitric oxide production may be maintained (Box 26-1). Cellular functions subserving migration and secretory effector functions are inhibited by local anesthetic molecules. In particular, the inhibition of integrin cellular adhesion molecules by local anesthetics may be anti-inflammatory in the setting of increased neutrophil migration in that it decreases the number of cells adherent to the endothelial lining of mesenteric vessels. Mechanisms of action, though largely unknown, likely involve local anesthetic molecule interactions with G-protein coupled receptors mediating inflammatory responses (e.g., thromboxane A$_2$).[13]

Opioids

The immune actions of opioids are well demonstrated.[18] Evidence clearly supports the presence of all known opioid receptors (μ, κ, δ) on the surface of immune cells, and the discovery of naloxone-reversible effects of opioid molecules in this context supports opioid receptor–mediated effects. The capacity of innate cells to phagocytose pathogens is inhibited in a naloxone-reversible fashion after in vivo administration of morphine.[19] Likewise, chemotaxis of leukocytes is decreased likely due to opioid-induced desensitization of chemotaxis receptors.[20] Lymphocyte functions are also affected in that antibody formation is suppressed by opioids and reversed by naltrexone.[21,22] Proliferative responses of murine CD-4 and CD-8 lymphocytes were inhibited by δ-opioid agonists, but due to the interaction of different cell populations the mechanism is difficult to elucidate.[23] Multiple preclinical studies have yielded conflicting effects of opioids on cytokine production by immune cells.[24,25]

Table 26-1 Intravenous Anesthetic Agents and Immune Effects

Anesthetic Drug	Immune Effect
Propofol	Less suppressive[10–11] Immune impairment[8]
Thiopental	Lymphocyte functions suppressed[8]
Etomidate	Lymphocyte functions suppressed[8]
Ketamine	Lymphocyte and macrophage functions suppressed[12]

Box 26-1 Observed Effects of Amide Local Anesthetics on Immune Cell Functions

↓ Integrin expression and migration[13]

↓ Formation of reactive oxygen species[14]

↓ Release of leukotrienes and granule enzyme[15]

↓ Release of histamine and proinflammatory cytokines[16]

↑ Production of nitric oxide[17]

The effects of synthetic opioids such as fentanyl and buprenorphine have also been characterized as immune suppressive,[26] but in a preclinical study these depressive effects were limited to the first 72 postoperative hours for fentanyl and were nonexistent for buprenorphine.[27] A novel opioid, tramadol, which also has inhibitory effects on norepinephrine and serotonin uptake, was found to have no depressant immune effects in a study of postoperative pain in cancer patients.[28]

It is important to note that opioids may exert an indirectly supportive effect on immune function in that the relief of pain is associated with decreased sympathetic nervous system activation and circulating levels of catecholamine molecules. Norepinephrine and epinephrine may increase circulating levels of CD-8 cells via margination from lymphoid storage sites yet are known to depress immune cell function when present in plasma for prolonged periods of time.[29] Therefore adequate pain treatment with opioids should never be withheld on the basis of concern for immune function.

Adjunct and Procedural Drugs

Antibiotics

Antibiotic drugs are frequently administered by nurse anesthetists as part of the surgical care of the patient. Although most antibiotic drugs play an adjunct supporting role to immune-mediated protection against infection, investigators found some members of this class to be potentially immune suppressive.[30] In vitro research using bovine immunocytes revealed that oxytetracycline, chloramphenicol, and erythromycin decreased phagocytosis and negatively affected the respiratory burst (innate cell effector production and release of reactive oxygen and other compounds in response to microbial invasion). A penicillin and a cephalosporin drug were each found to inhibit the production of superoxide radicals.

Steroids

Steroid drugs are extremely useful because of their pharmacologic effect of reducing inflammation-produced swelling in the airway, joints, and brain and are frequently administered by anesthesia practitioners. However, the mechanism by which this reduction in swelling is achieved should be noted for its implication to immune function. Steroid drugs exert their therapeutic effect by global depression of all immune cells.[2] In populations at risk for postoperative immune-mediated sequelae, these drugs may increase perioperative morbidity by negatively affecting the protective functions of effector leukocyte cells. It is important to note that no adverse sequelae have been recorded after the administration of dexamethasone in antiemetic doses.[31]

Immunosuppressant Drugs

In surgery for organ transplantation the nurse anesthetist administers drugs designed to directly inhibit innate and adaptive immune function to avoid rejection of the transplanted organ (Table 26-2). Each drug should be administered according to a careful dosage calculation and by using recommended guidelines for the rapidity of intravenous administration. After drug administration the nurse anesthetist should be extremely careful with invasive interventions to avoid exposing these vulnerable patients to infection. Commonly observed side effects of immunosuppressant drug therapy include fever, hypertension, chills, nausea, vomiting, myelosuppression, liver toxicity, and renal toxicity.

Catecholamine Vasopressors

Catecholamine molecules exert effects on immune cells via interactions with α- and β-adrenergic receptors on the cell surface.[29] Acutely elevated catecholamine plasma levels due to anxiety, stress, or pain are associated with increased numbers of circulating CD-8 and NK lymphocytes, due to β_2 receptor–mediated disruption in the interaction between the cells and endothelium in storage sites and also with increased efficacy of cell effector activity. Although more circulating immune cells may provide protection against bloodborne pathogens, fewer cells remain in tissues to participate in local protection. Chronic catecholamine exposure, conversely, produces opposite results: immune cell depression. Chronic catecholamine exposure can often produce a net anti-inflammatory response as a consequence of β receptor stimulation,[35] and production of effector molecules by innate cells is decreased; T-helper cells predominately differentiate into Th_2 (supporting less protective humoral, not cell-mediated, immunity). If catecholamine concentrations are sufficient for predominate α receptor stimulation, then proinflammatory mediator

Table 26-2 Commonly Used Immunosuppressive Drugs

Drug	Immune Effect
Cyclosporine	Inhibits T-lymphocyte function[32]
Tacrolimus, sirolimus	Inhibits T-lymphocyte function[32]
Azathioprine	Bone marrow suppression[33]
Mycophenolate mofetil	Inhibition of DNA synthesis[34]
OKT4A	Blocks T-cell receptor, CD-4 cells[34]

production may be increased. It is important to recognize that endogenous catecholamine molecules produced as a consequence of the stress response exert similar effects on immunity; therefore interventions that decrease this response support immune cell function.

Anesthetic Technique and Immune System Responses

The stress of surgery and anesthesia activates the hypothalamic-pituitary-adrenal and sympathoadrenomedullary stress axes, resulting in the production of cortisol and catecholamine molecules, among others, in the circulating blood and an increase in sympathetic stimulation to receptors in lymphoid organs.[11] The interactions of these molecules with immunocyte receptors serve to modulate and down-regulate protective effector functions and can result in host exposure to infection, sepsis, and increased malignancy. The anesthetic process may block the stress response to surgery and prevent the stress-induced immune changes; however, the question arises as to which technique exerts the most favorable immune effects. Evidence has accumulated that neuraxial regional anesthetic techniques can block the stress of surgery and may better support postoperative immune function than general anesthetic techniques for the same procedures.

Review of the literature reveals that operations on the lower half of the body with regional neuraxial block may indeed have favorable immune outcomes associated with lower stress hormone production, but as the operation shifts cephalad to upper or thoracoabdominal anatomic locations, little difference is seen in immune outcome regardless or anesthesia technique.[36–39] This is most likely due to the increased number of humoral and neural afferent activating pathways left unblocked in these larger procedures, which eventually stimulate the central nervous system stress axes (Figure 26-1). In general, as surgical size and invasiveness increase and move cephalad, nociception is only one of many afferent stimuli (tissue trauma, diffusion and release of soluble proinflammatory mediator molecules, activation of hypothalamic-pituitary-adrenal axis by proinflammatory cytokine release) that can cause a stress response, potentially depressing immune cell function.

Summary

This chapter reviewed the basic physiology of the immune system, revealing the intricate inter- and intracellular signaling cascades that characterize the protective functions of innate and adaptive immunity. These signaling cascades are vulnerable to disruption by molecules of stress hormones and anesthetic drugs. Immune function is essential to the prevention of infection and malignancy in the postoperative patient, especially in the vulnerable populations with preexisting severe immune depression. Although anesthetic drugs and opioids directly interfere with leukocyte function, skillful use of these drugs to prevent the metabolic stress response while supporting normal physiologic function ultimately supports the immune system.

Regional anesthesia for procedures on the lower half of the body may be effective in preventing the stress response

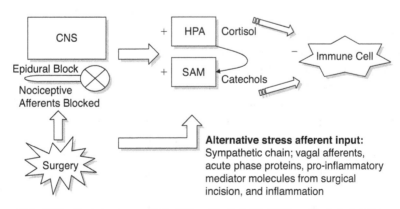

Note: CNS = Central nervous system ; HPA = Hypothalamic-pituitary-adrenal stress axis; SAM = Sympathoadrenal stress axis; "+" denotes stimulating positive effect; "−" denotes depressant negative effect.

Figure 26-1 Limited beneficial immune effects of epidural analgesia for thoracoabdominal surgery.

and supporting immune function. Awareness of the immune effect of anesthetic drugs is most important for patients who are at increased risk of perioperative morbidity, including patients who are having organ transplant surgery, with preexisting immune dysfunction (e.g., HIV infection), with poor health status from malnutrition or chronic disease, or with malignancy. Understanding the effects of anesthesia drug pharmacology on the compromised immune system may afford the nurse anesthetist the opportunity to provide additional support measures to patients at risk.

Key Points

- The immune system matters. Despite the necessary focus on immediate cardiorespiratory physiology and existing pathophysiology and its effect on the anesthetic plan, it is important to recognize that factors that affect immune function are important to prevent infection, sepsis, and malignancy.
- The transient postoperative adaptive immune depression routinely seen in perioperative patients will not harm healthy patients but may represent a serious health risk to populations of patients with conditions associated with preexisting immune dysfunction (e.g., organ transplant, HIV infection, malignancy).
- Inhaled and intravenous anesthetics are immunosuppressive but necessary parts of anesthesia care. Therefore it is crucial to support the patient's physiologic needs and immune function by preventing severe anemia, hypothermia, and hyperglycemia and by maintaining normal vital signs and adequate tissue perfusion.
- Opioid analgesics have direct immunosuppressant effects. However, by treating pain effectively, the immune system is supported indirectly as the sympathetic nervous system activation associated with acute pain is decreased via μ opioid receptor effects. Lowering the concentration of catecholamine molecules prevents the immune depression associated with immune cell adrenergic receptor interactions.
- Administration of immunosuppressant drugs for organ transplant should be accompanied by measures to protect vulnerable patients from exposure to and infection by pathogenic microorganisms.
- Regional anesthetic techniques may prevent the metabolic stress response associated with surgery, but only when surgical intervention is confined to the lower half of the body. Despite the presence of neuraxial blockade, thoracoabdominal operations are associated with multiple alternative humoral and neural pathways conveying distress signals to the central nervous system. The resulting activation of stress axes produces catecholamine and cortisol molecules that result in immune depression.

Chapter Questions

1. Discuss a pain management plan for a patient with immune system dysfunction due to HIV disease who has just had a laparotomy. Justify your care plan.
2. What is the rationale underlying the following statement: "It is critically important to treat pain effectively with opioids; despite the direct immunodepressant effects of opioids, the effective treatment of pain may ultimately support immune function."
3. When selecting the anesthetic technique—general versus regional anesthesia—for a patient with prostate cancer scheduled for a radical prostatectomy, discuss potential effects on postoperative immune function as a rationale that may guide the choice.
4. When large doses of steroids are administered to patients with conditions such as leukemia or malnutrition, explain the concern for postoperative immune function this therapy raises.
5. After the administration of immunosuppressive drugs to an organ transplant patient, it is discovered that another central line must be inserted. What is the primary concern regarding line insertion in this particular patient, and why?

References

1. Kehlet H. Manipulation of the metabolic stress response in clinical practice. *World J Surg.* 2000;24:690–695.
2. Goldsby R, Kindt TJ, Osborne BA, Kuby J. *Immunology,* 5th ed. New York: WH Freeman; 2003.
3. Maier SF, Watkins LR. Cytokines for psychologists: implications of bidirectional immune-to-brain communication for understanding behavior, mood, and cognition. *Psychol Rev.* 1998;105:83–107.
4. Homburger JA, Meiler SE. Anesthesia drugs, immunity, and long-term outcome. *Curr Opin Anesthesiol.* 2006;19:423–428.

5. Loop T, Dovi-Akue D, Frick M, et al. Volatile anesthetics induce caspase-dependent mitochondria-mediated apoptosis in human T-lymphocytes *in vitro*. *Anesthesiology*. 2005; 102:1147–1157.

6. Tschaikowsky K, Ritter J, Schroppel K, Kuhn M. Volatile anesthetics differentially affect immunostimulated expression of inducible nitric oxide synthase: role of intracellular calcium. *Anesthesiology*. 2000;92:1093–1102.

7. Markovic S, Knight P, Murasko D. Inhibition of interferon stimulation of natural killer cell activity in mice anesthetized with halothane or isoflurane. *Anesthesiology*. 1993; 78:700–708.

8. Schneemilch C, Hachenberg T, Ansorge S, Itterson A, Bank U. Effects of different anaesthetic agents on immune cell function *in vitro*. *Eur J Anaesthesiol*. 2005;22:616–623.

9. Procopio M, Rassias A, DeLeo JA, Pahl J, Hildebandt L, Yeager MP. The *in vivo* effects of general and epidural anesthesia on human immune function. *Anesth Analg*. 2001;93:460–465.

10. Inada T, Yamanouchi Y, Jomura S, et al. Effect of propofol and isoflurane anesthesia on the immune response to surgery. *Anesthesia*. 2004;59:954–959.

11. Kelbel I, Weiss M. Anaesthetics and immune function. *Curr Opin Anaesthesiol*. 2001;14:685–691.

12. Chang Y, Chen T, Sheu J, Chen R. Suppressive effects of ketamine on macrophage functions. *Toxicol Appl Pharmacol*. 2005;204:27–35.

13. Hollman MW, Durieux ME. Local anesthetics and the inflammatory response: a new therapeutic indication? *Anesthesiology*. 2000;93:858–875.

14. Takao Y, Mikawa K, Nishina K, Maekawa N, Obata H. Lidocaine attenuates hyperoxic lung injury in rabbits. *Acta Anaesthesiol Scand*. 1996;40:318–325.

15. Sinclair R, Eriksson A, Gretzer C, Cassuto J, Thomsen P. Inhibitory effects of amide local anesthetics on stimulus-induced human leukocyte metabolic activation, LTB4 release and IL-1 secretion in vitro. *Acta Anaesthesiol Scand*. 1993;37:159–165.

16. Yanagi H, Sankawa, H, Saito H, Iikura, Y. Effect of lidocaine on histamine release and Ca^{2+} mobilization from mast cells and basophils. *Acta Anaesthesiol Scand*. 1998;40: 1138–1144.

17. Mamiya K, Tomoda MK, Edashige K, Ueda, W, Manabe M. Local anesthetics enhance nitric oxide production by human peripheral neutrophils. *Physiol Chem Phys Med*. 1995;27:111–119.

18. McCarthy L, Wetzel M, Sliker J, Eisenstein T, Rogers T. Opioids, opioid receptors, and the immune response. *Drug Alcohol Depend*. 2001;62:111–123.

19. Pacifici R, Di Carlo S, Bacosi A, Zuccaro P. S Macrophage functions in drugs of abuse-treated mice. *Int J Immunopharmacol*. 1993;15:711–716.

20. Grimm MC, Ben-Baruch A, Taub D, et al. Opiates transdeactivate chemokine receptors: delta and mu opiate-receptor mediated heterologous desensitization. *J Exp Med*. 1998;188:317–325.

21. Bussiere JL, Adler M, Rogers T, Eisenstein T. Effects of in vivo morphine treatment on antibody responses in C57BL/6 bg/bg (Beige) mice. *Life Sci*. 1992;52:43–48.

22. Bussiere JL, Adler M, Rogers T, Eisenstein T. Differential effects of morphine and naltrexone on the antibody response in various mouse strains. *Immunopharmacol Immunotoxicol*. 1992;14:657–693.

23. Shahabi NA, Sharp B. Antiproliferative effects of δ-opioids on highly purified CD4+ and CD8+ murine T cells. *J Pharmacol Ther*. 1995;273:1105–1113.

24. Chao CC, Hu S, Molitor TW, et al. Morphine potentiates transforming growth factor-B release from human peripheral blood mononuclear cell cultures. *J Pharmacol Exp Ther*. 1992;262:19–24.

25. Guan L, Eisenstein T, Adler M, Rogers T. Inhibition of T cell superantigen responses following treatment with the κ-opioid agonist U50, 488H. *J Neuroimmunol*. 1997; 75:163–168

26. Carrigan KA, Saurer T, Ijames S, Lysle D. Buprenorphine produces naltrexone reversible alterations of immune status. *Int J Immunopharmacol*. 2004;4:419–428.

27. Martucci C, Panerai A, Sacerdote P. Chronic fentanyl or buprenorphine infusion in the mouse: similar analgesic profile but different effects on immune responses. *Pain*. 2004;110:385–392.

28. Sacerdote P, Bianchi M, Gaspani L, et al. The effects of tramadol and morphine on immune responses and pain after surgery in cancer patients. *Anesth Analg*. 2000;90: 1411–1414.

29. Sanders VM, Straub RH. Norepinephrine, the beta-adrenergic receptor, and immunity. *Brain Behav Immun*. 2002;16:290–332.

30. Hoeben D, Dosogne H, Heyneman R, Burvenich C. Effect of antibiotics on the phagocytic and respiratory burst activity of bovine granulocytes. *Eur J Pharmacol*. 1997; 332:289–297.

31. Henzi I, Walder B, Tamer MR. Dexamethasone for the prevention of postoperative nausea and vomiting: a quantitative systematic review. *Anesth Analg*. 2000;90:186–194.

32. Stoelting RK, Hillier SC. *Pharmacology and Physiology in Anesthetic Practice*, 4th ed. Philadelphia: Lippincott Williams & Wilkins; 2006.

33. Nagelhout JJ, Zaglaniczny KL. *Nurse Anesthesia*, 3rd ed. St. Louis, MO: Elsevier Saunders; 2005.

34. Miller RD, ed. *Miller's Anesthesia*, 7th ed. Philadelphia: Elsevier Churchill Livingstone; 2005;2177–2178.

35. Elenkov IJ, Chrousos G. Stress hormones, Th1/Th2 patterns, pro/anti-inflammatory cytokines and susceptibility to disease. *Trends Endocrinol Metab.* 1999;10:359–368.

36. Beilin B, Shavit Y, Travekin E, et al. The effects of postoperative pain management on the immune effects to surgery. *Anesth Analg.* 2003;97:822–827.

37. Kim C, Sakamoto A. Differences in the leukocyte response to incision during upper abdominal surgery with epidural vs. general anesthesia. *J Nippon Med Sch.* 2006;73:4–9.

38. Norman JG, Fink GW. The effects of epidural anesthesia on the neuroendocrine response to major surgical stress: a randomized prospective trial. *Am Surg.* 1997;63:75–80.

39. Volk T, Schenk M, Voigt K, Tohtz S, et al. Postoperative epidural anesthesia preserve lymphocyte, but not monocyte, immune function after major spine surgery. *Anesth Analg.* 2004;98:1086–1092.

Objectives

After completing this chapter, the reader should be able to

- Describe the physiologic changes of pregnancy that impact the administration of general and regional anesthesia.
- Describe the pathophysiologic changes of pregnancy that often result in the need for anesthesia services.
- List the risk factors for placenta accreta, uterine atony, and uterine prolapse/inversion.
- Define postpartum hemorrhage.
- Describe the pharmacologic agents used in treatment of pregnancy-induced hypertension the impact on anesthesia delivery.
- Describe the pharmacologic agents used in treatment of preterm labor and the impact of anesthesia in cases of preterm delivery.
- Select the first- and second-line uterotonics to be administered in cases of uterine atony.
- List the pharmacologic/anesthetic options for assisting the obstetrician in management of retained placenta and uterine prolapse/inversion.

Introduction

Obstetric pharmacology from the anesthesia provider's perspective is primarily related to specific situations during pregnancy and delivery that may require anesthesia services. The foundational concept to keep in mind is that before delivery of the infant, anesthesia drugs or techniques administered to the mother impact the fetus to some degree. At one time it was thought that the placenta functioned protectively, like a wall, to keep harmful substances from reaching the fetus. Modern research has shown that the placenta is more like a mild filter that allows many substances to pass from maternal circulation to fetal circulation. Many drugs commonly used by an anesthesia provider are not "filtered out" by the placenta but pass to the fetus relatively unchanged. This is not always an issue, depending on the drug or if delivery of the fetus is not imminent. The appropriateness of administering a specific drug at that time should always be considered.

27

Pharmacologic Considerations in Obstetric Anesthesia Practice

Lynn L. Lebeck, PhD, CRNA

Physiologic Changes of Pregnancy

Pregnancy is a time of multiple changes in both anatomy and physiology, impacting nearly every organ system. These changes are necessary to adapt the maternal systems to meet the increasing metabolic demands of the growing fetus. The intent of this section is to highlight those changes with the greatest impacts on the provision of anesthesia at the specific events noted. The reader is directed to textbooks such as Chestnut's *Obstetric Anesthesia: Principles and Practice* (4th ed.), or others for a comprehensive review of all maternal changes associated with pregnancy.

Early in pregnancy when anesthesia might be required for the placement of a cervical cerclage or even nonobstetric surgery, there are already changes in the respiratory, cardiovascular, and gastrointestinal systems. Increases in minute ventilation and alveolar ventilation result in decreases from 40 to 30 mm Hg in $PaCO_2$ and increases in pH from 7.4 to 7.44.[1] Increases in heart rate ($\uparrow$ 25% at term), stroke volume ($\uparrow$ 25% at term), and cardiac output ($\uparrow$ 50% at term) begin by 5 weeks of gestation.[1] These increases are offset by the reduction in systemic vascular resistance (SVR) as a result of the hormonal shifts.

Obviously, by the time pregnancy has reached the third trimester, there are other changes that affect the administration of general anesthesia. Reductions in functional residual capacity (FRC) impact the rapidity of maternal desaturation at induction, and engorgement of the airway mucosa results in the recommendation of use of a smaller size endotracheal tube. Aortocaval compression reduces return flow to the heart and requires alleviation by the use of left uterine displacement. Maternal response to some anesthetic drugs is altered with an increased rate of uptake and decreases in the minimum alveolar concentration (MAC) of volatile agents (related to increased progesterone). The pregnant woman requires a decreased dose of thiopental and has increased sensitivity to aminosteroid neuromuscular blocking drugs such as vecuronium and rocuronium.[2] However, not all responses are altered; maternal requirements for doses of propofol and succinylcholine remain unchanged.[1]

Maternal changes in pregnancy impact the administration and management of regional anesthesia. Pregnancy results in increased neural sensitivity to local anesthetics.[2] This contributes to the enhanced rapidity of onset and duration of spinal blockade.[1] Hyperbaric spinal doses need to be reduced 25% as a result of the changes noted in Table 27-1.

Bupivacaine characteristics of protein binding and elimination half-life are unchanged in the pregnant woman.[1] Ropivacaine pharmacokinetics are not impacted by pregnancy.[1] Lidocaine is affected by pregnancy in that the percent of protein binding decreases as the gestation increases.[1]

Pathophysiologic Conditions in Pregnancy and Postpartum

In addition to the normal physiologic changes of pregnancy, a number of pathophysiologic conditions can be superimposed as well. This section is limited to those that are likely to result in the need for anesthesia services.

Table 27-1 Pregnancy Changes That Reduce Hyperbaric Spinal Doses

Pregnancy Changes	As a Result Of
Increased sensitivity to local anesthetics	Increased progesterone levels
Reduction in CSF volume	Distension of vertebral venous plexus
Increased rostral spread in lateral position	Widening of pelvis → head-down tilt in lateral position
Inward displacement of foraminal soft tissue	Increased abdominal pressure
Higher level of spinal canal's lowest point in supine position	Increased lumbar lordosis

CSF, cerebrospinal fluid.

Antepartum

Cervical Incompetence

Antepartum pathophysiology may include an incompetent cervix. Although an incompetent cervix may be the result of trauma, it frequently is a result of an inherent deficiency in its function or structure. The anesthesia provider is most likely to encounter these patients when a cervical cerclage is placed, usually during the second trimester. Regional anesthesia offers the advantage of minimal exposure to drugs, as a low spinal or "saddle" block without sedation is usually sufficient. Care must be taken to avoid hypotension because placental blood flow depends on maternal pressure.

General anesthesia may be necessary for its side effect of superior uterine relaxation if required to facilitate replacement of bulging membranes in the face of early cervical dilation. It may also be needed if there is insufficient cervical length and placement of an abdominal cervical cerclage is necessary instead of the usual vaginal approach. The anesthesia provider must consider the changes of pregnancy and address the maternal risks of difficult intubation and potential for aspiration. The latest surgical development in this area includes the placement of transabdominal cerclage via robotic-assisted laparotomy or laparoscopy.[3,4]

Pregnancy-Induced Hypertension

Pregnancy-induced hypertension (PIH) develops in 5% to 6% of pregnancies and is defined as a hypertension that develops after 20 weeks gestation and includes one or more of the following: proteinuria, renal insufficiency, liver disease, neurologic manifestations, hematologic abnormalities, and fetal growth retardation.[5] Anesthesia providers encounter women with PIH usually when a decision to deliver has been made or for airway management in the case of seizure. If a decision to deliver via attempted trial of labor is made, an epidural may be requested. Anesthesia services (regional or general) are required if the decision is to deliver via cesarean section. In the case of seizure, securing the airway and control of the seizures are paramount to ensure that oxygen delivery continues to both mother and fetus. The pharmacologic agents most frequently encountered in these women at the time of anesthesia are magnesium sulfate for neuroprotection and antihypertensives for reduction of blood pressure.

Regardless of administration of regional or general anesthesia, it must be kept in mind that plasma volume is decreased in women with PIH.[5,6] Ideally, blood pressure should be maintained at less than 160 systolic and less than

100 diastolic; however, attempting to reduce it to "normal" levels can result in decreased placental perfusion and compromise of a fetus already under stress.

Preterm Labor

Preterm labor is defined as the presence of

- four uterine contractions in 20 minutes or eight contractions in 60 minutes and
- change in cervical dilation or effacement *or*
- cervical dilation of 2 cm or more *or*
- cervical effacement of 80% or more

in a pregnancy of between 20 and 37 weeks gestation.[7] Minimizing perinatal mortality and morbidity yet preserving maternal well-being is the ultimate goal of managing preterm labor.[8] The intent is to delay delivery for as long as possible, but even a delay of 48 hours to allow for a full course of corticosteroids to aid fetal lung maturation may decrease neonatal morbidity and mortality. In the case of an extremely premature fetus, delay of even 1 week can decrease mortality by 30%.[9] Anesthesia providers most frequently do not encounter women in preterm labor unless failure to arrest preterm labor leads to an eminent preterm delivery. In rare circumstances they may need to secure the airway if the medications used to treat preterm labor result in pulmonary edema. This side effect has occurred in women receiving magnesium sulfate, ritodrine, atosiban, and combination therapy of atosiban and nifedipine.[8,10,11]

Surrounding Delivery

Preterm Delivery

This is defined as delivery after 20 weeks and before 37 weeks of gestation. As an anesthesia provider you may encounter women delivering prematurely on an emergent basis occasionally without tocolytics on board but more frequently after tocolysis has failed. The obstetrician is looking for help from anesthesia providers to facilitate the best possible conditions in a vaginal delivery of the fragile preterm infant. Those conditions include constraint of maternal pushing effects to stop the descent until after complete dilation to avoid entrapment of the fetal head or breech. Facilitating controlled maternal pushing during delivery to avoid precipitous delivery and the associated risk of intracranial hemorrhage is desirable.[7] Relaxation of the pelvic floor and perineum can assist in creating smooth, controlled delivery conditions. Epidural anesthesia can be used to optimize vaginal delivery conditions.

The obstetrician may determine that cesarean section is required for a number of different reasons. It is important for the anesthesia provider to be aware that there are interactions between tocolytic agents and anesthesia drugs and/or techniques.

Retained Placenta, Placenta Accreta, Placenta Increta, and Placenta Percreta

Retained placenta is defined as the failure to deliver the placenta within 30 minutes after delivery of the infant. It may be the earliest indication of the more serious conditions of placenta accreta (adherence to the myometrium), placenta increta (invasion into the myometrium), or placenta percreta (perforation of the uterus, with or without invasion of adjacent structures). Many cases are not diagnosed before delivery; however, there are some known risk factors[12]:

- Previous cesarean section
- Placenta previa
- Asherman syndrome
- Previous uterine surgery
- Submucous leiomyomata
- Maternal age > 35 years

Retained placenta may require anesthesia to provide relaxation and pain relief during the attempt at manual removal of the placenta. To produce uterine relaxation, interventions ranging from administration of tocolytics, nitroglycerin, or even general anesthesia may be required. The anesthesia provider must be prepared for escalating levels of intervention if the retained placenta turns out to be accreta, increta, or percreta and therefore requires surgical intervention. That surgical intervention may range from dilatation and curettage to hysterectomy and repair of adjacent structures.

Uterine Atony

The most common cause of primary postpartum hemorrhage (PPH) is uterine atony, occurring in 50% to 80% of all PPH and in 2% to 8% of all births.[13,14] The results of PPH can be life threatening, and it is one the main causes of maternal morbidity in the world.[14] Uterine atony, retained placenta, and cervical/vaginal lacerations are the underlying pathology in 95% of all cases of PPH.[13] The World Health Organization definition of severe bleeding in PPH includes[14]:

- Loss of 150 mL/min for > 20 min
- Loss of 50% of total blood volume in 3 h
- Loss of > 1500–2000 mL

Uterine atony frequently presents as painless, continuous bleeding with the presence of a soft and oversized uterus.[13] There should be a high index of suspicion in cases of previous uterine atony because the risk of recurrence is 25%.[14] A simple mnemonic of the "four Ts"—Tone, Trauma, Tissue, Thrombin—represents the four causes of postpartum hemorrhage.[15] Etiologies of uterine atony fall into five catagories.[16] The categories and associated risk factors are shown in Table 27-2. The pharmacologic interventions related to uterine tone are the focus of the anesthesia provider as covered in the "Immediately After Delivery" section of this chapter.

Uterine Prolapse/Inversion

This is a rare but potentially life-threatening complication after delivery of the infant. Complete inversion is the presence of the "inside out" fundus below the cervix. Incomplete inversion occurs when the fundus remains above the level of the cervix.[12] An incomplete inversion is more likely to be missed and should be suspected in cases of hypotension and PPH.[17] The risk factors for uterine prolapsed/inversion include:

- Excessive cord traction
- Excessive fundal pressure
- Uterine anomalies
- Uterine atony
- Placenta accreta

Table 27-2 Etiologies of Uterine Atony Categories and Associated Risk Factors

Etiology	Risk Factors
Uterine distention	Multiple gestation Macrosomia Polyhydramnios Fetal abnormalities (i.e., severe hydrocephalus)
Uterine fatigue	Prolonged or precipitous labor, especially with Pitocin Multiparity History of PPH
Uterine infection	Prolonged rupture of membranes Fever
Uterine distortion or abnormality	Fibroids Placenta previa
Uterine relaxation drugs	Anesthetics, nifedipine, NSAIDs, β agonists, magnesium sulfate

NSAIDs, nonsteroidal anti-inflammatory drugs.

Obstetric treatment is immediate replacement of the uterus through the cervix. This can be accomplished readily if the cervix has not contracted. If contracture has occurred, the obstetrician will need the anesthesia provider to relax the uterus so that it can be replaced and then immediately cause contraction of the uterus to prevent another inversion. Uterine relaxation can be provided through administration of general anesthesia, terbutaline or other β agonists, and nitroglycerin.[12]

Pharmacology of Drugs Used in Obstetric Anesthesia Practice

Before Delivery

Magnesium Sulfate

Magnesium sulfate use in the parturient is limited to two possible conditions, PIH and preterm labor. Its use in preterm labor is less clear because the literature demonstrates both efficacy and nonefficacy.[10,18] Reviews of the Cochrane Database, with 2036 subjects in 23 trials, concluded that magnesium sulfate was ineffective in the treatment of preterm labor.[19,20] In contrast, the efficacy of magnesium sulfate in the treatment of PIH (eclampsia/preeclampsia), and even its superiority to other treatments such as diazepam or anticonvulsants including phenytoin, has been clearly demonstrated.[21–23] Magnesium sulfate is used primarily for its central nervous system depressive effects, believed to be due to reversal of cerebral vasospasm, as protection against convulsions.[24] It competitively inhibits the action of calcium at sarcoplasmic reticulum binding sites, reducing the level of intracellular calcium, which results in smooth muscle relaxation. The relaxation of the smooth muscle in the vessel wall contributes to lowering blood pressure.[25] A loading dose of 4 to 6 g intravenously over 20 to 30 minutes is followed by an infusion of 1 to 2 g/h to maintain a therapeutic level of 4 to 9 mEq/L. Magnesium sulfate treatment is normally continued through delivery and up to 24 hours postpartum. Table 27-3 shows the correlation between blood magnesium levels and physical effects.

Side effects of magnesium include flushing, transient hypotension, palpitations, chest pain, nausea, blurred vision, and sedation. Treatment of magnesium toxicity is discontinuation of magnesium infusion and administration of calcium gluconate 1 g intravenously over 10 minutes.[26] Intubation may be required until the return of spontaneous respiration. Magnesium is eliminated through renal excretion,

Table 27-3 Correlation Between Blood Magnesium Levels and Physical Effects

Blood Magnesium Level (mEq/L)	Physical Effects
1–2	Normal levels
4–9	Therapeutic levels
5–10	ECG changes: P-Q lengthened, QRS widened
10–12	Loss of deep tendon reflexes
15–20	S-A and A-V blocks, respiratory arrest
25	Cardiac arrest

A-V, atrioventricular; ECG, electrocardiographic; S-A, sinoatrial.

and parturients with renal impairment are at greater risk for developing excessive blood magnesium levels.[25]

Anesthesia Implications

Parturients on magnesium may present for epidural for analgesia in labor or for urgent/emergent cesarean section. Be prepared for exaggerated hypotension after administration of epidural or general anesthesia. Although the dose of succinylcholine for rapid sequence induction (RSI) is unchanged, there is no need for defasciculating doses and maintenance doses of nondepolarizing muscle blockers (NDMBs) should be reduced.[25] Several rare but reported complications of magnesium sulfate therapy for preterm labor include symptomatic hypocalcemia and respiratory compromise in the case of myotonic dystrophy.[27,28]

β Agonists

β Agonists such as ritodrine and terbutaline have been used in attempts to inhibit preterm labor. Unfortunately, the highest incidence of adverse drug reactions and maternal and fetal side effects are associated tocolysis involving betamimetics.[11] Those cardiopulmonary adverse reactions and side effects include tachycardia (maternal and fetal), dysrhythmias, ischemia, hypotension, and rarely pulmonary edema.[25] Other adverse effects include headache, hyperglycemia, hypokalemia, increased plasma renin, and vasopressin.[25] Ritodrine is no longer marketed in the United States.[7] The Cochrane reviews of randomized controlled trials of betamimetics for initial tocolysis, with over 1300 women, do demonstrate that although tocolysis decreased the number of women delivering within 48 hours, there was no demonstrated benefit with respect to perinatal or neonatal death or neonatal respiratory distress.[29] The rate of preterm birth, perinatal morbidity, or perinatal

mortality did not differ between placebo and ritodrine or placebo and terbutaline when used for maintenance after initial tocolysis of preterm labor.[30] In contrast, a study examining tocolytic maintenance with continuous subcutaneous terbutaline versus oral nifedipine demonstrated increased pregnancy prolongation, decreased low-birth-weight and very-low-birth-weight infants, and decreased neonatal intensive care unit admissions.[31] Terbutaline can be used to treat oxytocin-induced tectonic uterine contractions at a dose of 0.25 mg intravenously or subcutaneously and may be repeated or titrated to a 20% to 30% increase in maternal heart rate.[25] Nitroglycerin may also be used in this situation.[32]

The mechanism of action of terbutaline is the simulation of β_2 receptors resulting in a increased production of cAMP, which results in a decreased intracellular level of calcium ions.[25] Intracellular calcium is necessary for smooth muscle contraction such as that of the uterine wall.

Anesthesia Implications

If possible, a delay of 60 minutes between β agonist administration and anesthesia is desired to allow diminishment of tachycardia. If conditions do not permit a delay, drugs that would worsen maternal tachycardia should be avoided; ketamine, atropine, glycopyrrolate, thiopental, pancuronium, and etomidate become the induction drugs of choice.[25] Monitor intravenous (IV) fluid administration carefully due to the risk of volume overload and pulmonary edema. Hypotension can be treated with ephedrine or phenylephrine.[25]

Calcium Channel Blockers

Calcium channel blockers such as nifedipine have been used for tocolysis. Nifedipine offers an advantage in that it can be administered orally or sublingually and is usually tolerated well with hypotension being the most frequent side effect.[11] Other reported adverse effects include dyspnea, pulmonary edema, tachycardia, and headache; it should be noted that these effects were sometimes reported in cases of women receiving multiple types of tocolytic drugs.[11] Nifedipine use as a tocolytic results in fewer women requiring removal from the drug due to adverse reaction. It also reduced the number of women giving birth within 48 hours and 7 days and improved neonatal outcomes.[33]

The mechanism of action is decreasing Ca^+ ion movement into smooth muscle cells through modulation of the duration of opening of the calcium channel.[34,35] Decreasing the duration of ion movement through the calcium channel decreases the cell membrane's ability to reach threshold and create an action potential. Research suggests that the uterorelaxant effect of nifedipine is in part a result of its actions on potassium channels in addition to the calcium channels.[36]

Anesthesia Implications

Although there are no contraindications to specific techniques, hypotension should be expected with administration of neuraxial or general anesthesia.[25] The anesthesia provider should be prepared for the possibility of uterine atony that may be refractory to oxytocin and prostaglandins, because both of those drugs also act through the calcium channel. Adequate IV access and availability of Methergine should be instituted in such cases.[25]

Oxytocin Receptor Antagonists

Atosiban is the first drug of this class used for tocolysis of preterm labor. Although not approved or available in the United States at this time, it has been used and studied in a number of other countries.[7,8] The results of research trials are contradictory. The Cochrane review conducted in 2005 indicted that atosiban was not superior to betamimetics or placebo for tocolytic efficacy or neonatal outcomes but did demonstrate fewer maternal adverse effects.[37] A more recent study reported that atosiban tocolysis resulted in significantly more women remaining undelivered and not requiring an alternative tocolytic within 48 hours in comparison with betamimetics or calcium channel blocker.[8] A 2009 Cochrane review reported that atosiban for maintenance therapy in threatened preterm labor did not reduce the incidence of preterm delivery or improve neonatal outcomes.[38] Atosiban is a mixed oxytocin–vasopressin receptor inhibitor, and it has been theorized that the oxytocin receptor is more likely to be the desired target in the search for effective tocolytics with minimal maternal or fetal effects. The effects of barusiban, an oxytocin receptor antagonist with a 300- to 16,000-fold greater (than atosiban) selectivity for the oxytocin receptor, were studied in term and preterm myometrium and found to inhibit contractions at least as potently.[39] However, in a randomized, placebo-controlled trial (206 women) single-dose barusiban groups (range, 0.3–10 mg) were not significantly different in reducing contractions or delaying delivery compared with placebo.[40]

Anesthesia implications, if any, are unknown as a result of limited usage. The myometrium remains sensitive to oxytocin after administration, so oxytocin can still be used after delivery as needed for uterine atony.[25]

Prostaglandin Inhibitors

Prostaglandins are potent stimulators of uterine smooth muscle as the mediators in the final pathways of uterine contraction.[7] Increases in intracellular calcium and gap junction formation occur as a result of the action of prostaglandins.[7] Logically, reduction of prostaglandin levels via inhibition of cyclooxygenase (COX) enzymes should result in a decrease of uterine smooth muscle contraction. Indomethacin is a nonselective COX inhibitor and when compared with placebo or other tocolytics in trials resulted in reduction in births less than 37 weeks, reduction in maternal adverse drug effects, and increases in gestational age and birth weights.[41] It is possible that the view of indomethacin being associated with untoward fetal and neonatal outcomes is not grounded in good evidence and should be reconsidered.[42] Selective COX-2 inhibitors have been studied in comparison with nonselective COX inhibitors and have not demonstrated any difference with respect to maternal or neonatal outcome.[41] Celecoxib, an oral COX-2 selective inhibitor, demonstrated a tocolytic efficacy equal to that of magnesium sulfate in prevention of preterm birth within 48 hours.[43] Withdrawal of some COX-2 inhibitors has prevented further evaluation of their tocolytic efficacy.[42]

Anesthesia Implications

Although there is some degree of platelet inhibition with nonselective COX inhibitors, it is both transient and, if needed, reversible so that neuraxial anesthesia is not contraindicated.[25] Other maternal side effects are usually minimal, leading to few if any impacts on anesthesia administration.[25]

Nitroglycerin

Nitric oxide is a known relaxant of vascular smooth muscle.[44] Interest has been shown in nitroglycerin as a nitric oxide donator and used by practitioners in attempts to determine its efficacy and equivalency to other tocolytics.[45] The results of a Cochrane review in 2002 looking at five trials with 466 women concluded that there was insufficient evidence to support routine use of nitric oxide donors as tocolytics.[46] However, subsequent research results are mixed, with a European study indicating that nitroglycerin was less efficacious than β_2 agonists and a Canadian trial indicating that it was more efficacious than placebo.[42,45]

The mechanism of action is via increasing action of guanylate cyclase resulting in increases in cGMP and leading to inhibition of calcium ion entry, which decreases contractility of uterine smooth muscle.[25] Routes of administration include IV, sublingual, aerosol, or transdermal patch (not used in acute situations). Dosing can start at 50 mg intravenously and be titrated to effect.

Anesthesia Implications

Women receiving nitroglycerin for tocolysis tolerated the drug well. Maternal hypotension and headache are the most frequently reported side effects, with no reports of significant fetal effects.[25]

Hydralazine

Many drugs used for reduction of blood pressure in non-pregnant patients (e.g., beta-blockers, calcium channel blockers, nitrovenodilators) may be used in the severely hypertensive parturient, and the reader is directed to other chapters for further information. Hydralazine is a direct systemic arterial vasodilator that is sometimes used in obstetric units to reduce severe hypertension in the parturient. It selectively vasodilates the uterine and renal vasculature, which benefits the preeclamptic woman.[6] Dosing is 2.5 to 10 mg intravenously with a peak onset of 10 to 15 minutes.

Anesthesia Implications

The resulting dilation can trigger tachycardia and increases in myocardial contractility, limiting its usefulness in parturients with known or suspected coronary artery disease. The resultant myocardial demand coupled with decreased filling time leads to decreased coronary artery perfusion.[6,44]

Immediately After Delivery

Oxytocin

Uterine atony is the leading cause of PPH.[13] The first-line drug of choice for both prevention and treatment of uterine atony or atonic PPH is oxytocin.[17,47]

Oxytocin is a hormone endogenously produced in the posterior pituitary gland, and the mechanism of action is via lowering of the threshold for depolarization in the uterine smooth muscle cells.[48] This depolarization is enhanced by the activation of calcium channels and increased production of prostaglandins.[25] The synthetic versions (Pitocin, Syntocinon) are octapeptides and possess fewer side effects related to antidiuretic hormone (water intoxication) than the endogenous oxytocin.[25] Pitocin is administered routinely after delivery in a dose of 20 to 40 units in a liter of isotonic fluid over 15 to 20 minutes. Prophylactic administration of oxytocin was associated with reduced blood loss

in trials involving over 3000 women.[49] Oxytocin infusions, at a low controlled rate, may be used to induce uterine contractions/labor. Anesthesia provider interaction with parturients undergoing induction occurs if epidural pain relief is desired or atonic contractions result in fetal distress.

Anesthesia Implications

Administration of oxytocin results in a degree of vasodilation. This decrease in SVR can result in significant hypotension and a corresponding tachycardia.[17,25] This significant hypotension is almost always associated with IV bolus administration, and therefore avoiding such boluses is recommended.[17,25]

Methergine and Ergotrate

These are synthetic and semisynthetic versions of ergot alkaloids. Ergot alkaloids are produced by fungal infestation of rye and other grains.[17] Ergot poisoning over the ages has been known as St. Anthony's fire because of the ischemic pain in extremities as a result of severe vasoconstriction.[25] Ergot alkaloids—natural, semisynthetic, or synthetic—rapidly produce tetanic uterine contractions that restrict the obstetric use of these drug to the postdelivery period.[17] Methergine or Ergotrate should be considered the second-line drug in the treatment of uterine atony after oxytocin.[25] They are effective in reducing postdelivery blood loss and the incidence of postpartum hemorrhage.[50] The mechanism of action is not clearly understood but postulated to be due to agonist effects on the α-adrenergic receptors.[17,25] Methergine causes less peripheral vasoconstriction but still can produce profound hypertension, severe nausea and vomiting, and even cerebral hemorrhage when administered intravenously; therefore it should be administered intramuscularly in a dose of 0.2 mg. It produces uterine contractions within minutes and can be repeated in 15 to 20 intervals up to a total dose of 0.8 mg or four ampules.[25]

Anesthesia Implications

As a result of the hypertensive side effects produced by ergot alkaloids, the drug should not be used in women with preexisting hypertension (pregnancy induced or chronic), peripheral vascular disease, or ischemic heart disease. There are reports of myocardial infarctions in women treated with oral and IV ergot alkaloids.[51,52] Blood pressure should be monitored closely and vasodilators available to treat severe hypertension. Be prepared to treat nausea and vomiting because it occurs in 10% to 20% of women due to its effect on the emesis center in the brain.[25]

Prostaglandins

In cases of postpartum hemorrhage that are refractory to oxytocin and ergot alkaloids, prostaglandins have been reported to be 80% to 90% effective.[16] 15-Methylprostaglandin F$_{2\alpha}$ (carboprost, Hemabate) is the preferred synthetic prostaglandin.[17] It should also be considered as the second-line drug when contraindications to Methergine exist.[25] Its mechanism of action results in increased myometrial calcium levels and subsequent increases in myosin light chain kinase activity and uterine contraction.[25] The use of Hemabate and other prostaglandins is considered to have reduced the requirement for postpartum hysterectomy related to uterine atony.[25] The dose is 250 μg intramuscularly or directly into the myometrium and may be repeated every 15 to 30 minutes up to a total dose of 2 mg.[17] Both sublingual and buccal administration of a prostaglandin E$_1$ analog, Misoprostol, has been shown to reduce blood loss at cesarean section as effectively as oxytocin.[53,54] However, it is not considered preferable to other uterotonics in the active management of the third stage of labor.[55]

Anesthesia Implications

All prostaglandins have detrimental side effects, such as nausea and vomiting, diarrhea, and fever. In women with reactive airway disease, the use of carboprost (prostaglandin F$_{2\alpha}$, Hemabate) may result in bronchospasm, ventilation-perfusion mismatch, and subsequently hypoxemia; thus it should be used with caution.[17,25] Oxygen saturation and lung sounds should be monitored.[25] Misoprostol may be used in place of carboprost in patients with reactive airway disease or pulmonary hypertension.[17]

Nitroglycerin

Providing rapid, profound, yet short-duration uterine relaxation helps the obstetrician before delivery in external version, at delivery in cases of fetal head entrapment or extraction of a second twin, and for postdelivery complications such as retained placenta or uterine inversion.[25] Use of nitroglycerin in such situations can avoid inducing general anesthesia and associated complications such as difficult airway.[25] The use of oral nitroglycerin tablets resulted in a significant reduction in the need for manual removal in cases of retained placenta.[56] The mechanism of action is induction of uterine and cervical relaxation via nitric oxide.[56] At one time it was postulated that the presence of placental tissue in the uterus was necessary for the uterine relaxant effect of nitroglycerin, but case reports of its suc-

cessful use for postcesarean uterine inversion cast doubt on that theory.[57]

Anesthesia Implications

Nitroglycerin doses start at 50 mg intravenously and should be titrated to effect with close observation for hypotension. Use of metered sublingual spray at a dose of 400 μg is very effective but may result in significant hypotension, which should be treated with fluids and vasopressors.[25]

Key Points

- For cervical cerclage, spinal anesthesia can minimize the number and amount of drugs that cross the placenta. Avoid hypotension because placental blood flow depends on maternal blood pressure.
- For PIH assume central volume depletion but hydrate carefully in preparation for neuraxial or general anesthesia. Watch out for exaggerated responses to vasopressors and stimulations such as laryngoscopy. Adjust doses of neuromuscular blockers in the presence of therapeutic use of magnesium, and ensure adequate reversal before extubation.
- For preterm delivery be cognizant of impacts of tocolytics on board in cases where there is rapid progression of preterm labor into delivery.
- In postpartum hemorrhage do not wait until frank hypotension is present to aggressively fluid resuscitate. Prompt administration of oxytocin infusion can decrease blood loss due to uterine atony. Be prepared to move to second- and third-line uterotonics if atony is refractory to oxytocin.
- For retained placenta be prepared to administer nitroglycerin and/or provide adequate analgesia for manual removal of the placenta. Keep in mind that retained placenta can be the first indicator of placenta increta or percreta and that you may have to live with sympathetic blockade (as a result of topping off an epidural) in the face of escalating procedures.
- In cases of uterine prolapse/inversion, do not hesitate to call for help because massive blood loss can develop rapidly if the uterus is not returned through the cervix immediately. Nitroglycerin for uterine relaxation followed by oxytocin for uterine contraction may be the key for quick response as long as nitroglycerin is available in the obstetric area.

Chapter Questions

1. What physiologic and pathophysiologic changes in pregnancy impact administration of general anesthesia? Neuraxial anesthesia?
2. What additional considerations are important in neuraxial anesthesia for cervical cerclage?
3. Why should you decrease hyperbaric spinal doses in pregnant women?
4. How does the decreased plasma volume in the woman with PIH impact your administration of an epidural? General anesthesia?
5. Retained placenta can be the first sign of what other conditions?
6. What is the most common cause of postpartum hemorrhage?
7. What is the sequence and doses of pharmacologic agents used to treat uterine atony?
8. How will you provide uterine relaxation for replacement of the inverted uterus? And what will you administer after it has been replaced?

References

1. Gaiser R. Physiologic changes of pregnancy. In: Chestnut D, ed. *Chestnut's Obstetrical Anesthesia: Principles and Practice,* 4th ed. Philadelphia: Mosby Elsevier; 2009:15–36.
2. Braveman F, Scavone B, Wong C, Santos A. Obstetrical anesthesia. In: Barash P, Cullen B, Stoelting R, Cahalan M, Stock C, eds. *Clinical Anesthesia,* 6th ed. Philadelphia: Lippincott Williams & Wilkins; 2009:1137–1170.
3. Barmat, L, Glaser, G, Davis, G, Craparo, F. Da Vinci-assisted abdominal cerclage. *Fertil Steril.* 2007;88:1437e1–1437e3.
4. Wolfe L, DePasquale, S, Adair CD, et al. Robotic-assisted laparoscopic placement of transabdominal cerclage during pregnancy. *Am J Perinatol.* 2008;25:653–655.
5. Gatt S, Elliot D. Preeclampsia and eclampsia. In: Datta S. ed. *Anesthetic and Obstetric Management of High-Risk Pregnancy,* 3rd ed. Philadelphia: Springer-Verlag; 2004:279–290.
6. Gist R, Beilin Y. Hypertensive disorders of pregnancy. In: Bucklin B, Gambling D, Wlody D, eds. *A Practical Approach to Obstetric Anesthesia.* Philadelphia: Lippincott Williams & Wilkins; 2009:349–363.
7. Muir H, Wong C. Preterm labor and delivery. In: Chestnut D, ed. *Chestnut's Obstetrical Anesthesia: Principles and Practice,* 4th ed. Philadelphia: Mosby Elsevier; 2009:749–777.
8. Husslein P, Roura LC, Dudenhausen J, et al. Atosiban versus usual care for the management of preterm labor. *J Perinat Med.* 2007;35:305–313.
9. Hass D, Imperiale T, Kirkpatrick P, Klein R, Zollinger T, Golichowski A. Tocolytic therapy. *Obstet Gynecol.* 2009;113:585–594.
10. Lyell D, Pullen K, Campbell L, et al. Magnesium sulfate compared with nifedipine for acute tocolysis of preterm labor. *Obstet Gynecol.* 2007;110:61–67.
11. de Heus R, Mol B, Erwich JJ, et al. Adverse drug reactions to tocolytic treatment for preterm labour: prospective cohort study. *BMJ.* 2009;338:b744. Available at: bmj.com. Accessed May 20, 2009
12. Frolich M, Bucklin B. Obstetric emergencies. In: Bucklin B, Gambling D, Wlody D, eds. *A Practical Approach to Obstetric Anesthesia.* Philadelphia: Lippincott Williams & Wilkins; 2009:349–363.
13. Mercier FJ, Van de Velde M. Major obstetric hemorrhage. *Anesthesiol Clin.* 2008;26:53–66.
14. Heinrich W, Surbeck D, Kainer F, et al. Diagnosis and treatment of peripartum bleeding. *J Perinat Med.* 2008;36:467–478.
15. Anderson JM, Etches D. Prevention and management of postpartum hemorrhage. *Am Fam Physician.* 2007;75:875–882.
16. Ramanathan G, Arulkumaran S. Postpartum hemorrhage. *JOGC.* 2006;967–973.
17. Mayer DC, Smith KA. Antepartum and postpartum hemorrhage. In: Chestnut D, ed. *Chestnut's Obstetrical Anesthesia: Principles and Practice,* 4th ed. Philadelphia: Mosby Elsevier; 2009:811–836.
18. Borna S, Saeidi FM. Celecoxib versus magnesium sulfate to arrest preterm labor: randomized trial. *J Obstet Gynaecol.* 2007;33:631–634.
19. Barbieri RL. Is the end of an era here for magnesium sulfate tocolysis? *OBG Manage.* 2007;19:6–10.
20. Crowther CA, Hiller JE, Doyle LW. Magnesium sulphate for preventing preterm birth in threatened preterm labour. *Cochrane Database Syst Rev.* 2002; Issue 4, Art. No.: CD001060.
21. Duley L, Henderson-Smart DJ. Magnesium sulphate versus diazepam for eclampsia. *Cochrane Database Syst Rev.* 2003; Issue 4, Art. No.: CD000127.
22. Duley L, Henderson-Smart D. Magnesium sulphate versus phenytoin for eclampsia. *Cochrane Database Syst Rev.* 2003; Issue 4, Art. No.: CD000128.
23. Duley L, Gülmezoglu AM, Henderson-Smart DJ. Magnesium sulphate and other anticonvulsants for women with pre-eclampsia. *Cochrane Database Syst Rev.* 2003; Issue 2, Art. No.: CD000025.

24. Stoelting RK, Hillier SC. Minerals and electrolytes. In: Stoelting RK, Hillier SC, eds. *Pharmacology & Physiology in Anesthetic Practice*, 4th ed. Philadelphia: Lippincott Williams & Wilkins; 2006:611–622.

25. Fiegel MJ, Bucklin BA. Obstetric medications. In: Bucklin B, Gambling D, Wlody D, eds. *A Practical Approach to Obstetric Anesthesia.* Philadelphia: Lippincott Williams & Wilkins; 2009:41–51.

26. Polley LS. Hypertensive disorders. In: Chestnut D, ed. *Chestnut's Obstetrical Anesthesia: Principles and Practice*, 4th ed. Philadelphia: Mosby Elsevier; 2009:975–1007.

27. Nassar AH, Salti I, Makarem NN, Usta IM. Marked hypocalcemia after tocolytic magnesium sulphate therapy. *Am J Perinatol.* 2007;24:481–482.

28. Catanzarite V, Gambling D, Bird LM, Honold J, Perkins E. Respiratory compromise after $MgSO_4$ therapy for preterm labor in a woman with myotonic dystrophy. *J Reprod Med.* 2008;53:220–222.

29. Anotayanonth S, Subhedar NV, Neilson JP, Harigopal S. Betamimetics for inhibiting preterm labour. *Cochrane Database Syst Rev.* 2006; Issue 2, Art. No.: CD004352.

30. Dodd JM, Crowther CA, Dare MR, Middleton P. Oral betamimetics for maintenance therapy after threatened preterm labour. *Cochrane Database Syst Rev.* 2006; Issue 1, Art. No.: CD003927.

31. De la Torre L, Istwan NB, Desch C, et al. Management of recurrent preterm labor in twin gestations with nifedipine tocolysis. *Am J Perinatol.* 2008;25:555–560.

32. Livingston EG. Intrapartum fetal assessment and therapy. In: Chestnut D, ed. *Chestnut's Obstetrical Anesthesia: Principles and Practice*, 4th ed. Philadelphia: Mosby Elsevier; 2009:141–154.

33. King JF, Flenady V, Papatsonis D, Dekker G, Carbonne B. Calcium channel blockers for inhibiting preterm labour. *Cochrane Database Syst Rev.* 2002; Issue 3, Art. No.: CD002255.

34. Stoelting RK, Hillier SC. Calcium channel blockers. In: Stoelting RK, Hillier SC, eds. *Pharmacology & Physiology in Anesthetic Practice*, 4th ed. Philadelphia: Lippincott Williams & Wilkins; 2006:387–397.

35. Calvey N, Williams N. Antiarrhythmic and antianginal drugs. In: Calvey N, Williams N, eds. *Principles and Practice of Pharmacology for Anaesthetists*, 5th ed. Malden, MA: Blackwell Publishing; 2008:287–306.

36. Moynihan AT, Smith TJ, Morrison JJ. The relaxant effect of nifedipine in human uterine smooth muscle and the BK_{Ca} channel. *Am J Obstet Gynecol.* 2008;198:237.e8.

37. Papatsonis D, Flenady V, Cole S, Liley H. Oxytocin receptor antagonists for inhibiting preterm labour. *Cochrane Database Syst Rev.* 2005; Issue 3, Art. No.: CD004452.

38. Papatsonis D, Flenady V, Liley H. Maintenance therapy with oxytocin antagonists for inhibiting preterm birth after threatened preterm labour. *Cochrane Database Syst Rev.* 2009; Issue 1, Art. No.: CD005938.

39. Pierzynski P, Lemancewicz A, Reinheimer T. Inhibitory effect of barusiban and atosiban on oxytocin-induced contractions of myometrium from preterm and term pregnant women. *J Soc Gynecol Invest.* 2004;11:384–387.

40. Thornton S, Goodwin TM, Greisen G, Hedegaard M, Arce JC. The effect of barusiban, a selective oxytocin antagonist, in threatened preterm labor at late gestational age: a randomized, double-blind, placebo-controlled trial. *Am J Obstet Gynecol.* 2009;200:627–629.

41. King JF, Flenady V, Cole S, Thornton S. Cyclo-oxygenase (COX) inhibitors for treating preterm labour. *Cochrane Database Syst Rev.* 2005; Issue 2, Art. No.: CD001992.

42. Giles W, Bisits A. The present and future of tocolysis. *Best Pract Res Clin Obstet Gynaecol.* 2007;21:857–868.

43. Borna S, Fatemeh MS. Celecoxib versus magnesium sulfate to arrest preterm labor: randomized trial. *J Obstet Gynaecol Res.* 2007;33:631–634.

44. Stoelting RK, Hillier SC. Peripheral vasodilators, nitric oxide, and nitrovasodilators. In: Stoelting RK, Hillier SC, eds. *Pharmacology & Physiology in Anesthetic Practice*, 4th ed. Philadelphia: Lippincott Williams & Wilkins; 2006:352–369.

45. Smith GN, Walker MC, Ohlsson A, O'Brien K, Windrim R. Randomized double-blind placebo-controlled trial of transdermal nitroglycerin for preterm labor. *Am J Obstet Gynecol.* 2007;196:37.e1–e8.

46. Duckitt K, Thornton S. Nitric oxide donors for the treatment of preterm labour. *Cochrane Database Syst Rev.* 2002; Issue 3, Art. No.: CD002860.

47. Wise A, Clark V. Strategies to manage major obstetric haemorrhage. *Curr Opin Anaesthesiol.* 2008;21:281–287.

48. Stoelting RK, Hillier SC. Endocrine system. In: Stoelting RK, Hillier SC, eds. *Pharmacology & Physiology in Anesthetic Practice*, 4th ed. Philadelphia: Lippincott Williams & Wilkins; 2006:801–816.

49. Cotter AM, Ness A, Tolosa JE. Prophylactic oxytocin for the third stage of labour. *Cochrane Database Syst Rev.* 2004; Issue 4, Art. No.: CD001808.

50. Gülmezoglu AM, Forna F, Villar J, Hofmeyr GJ. Prostaglandins for preventing postpartum haemorrhage. *Cochrane Database Syst Rev.* 2007; Issue 2, Art. No.: CD000494.

51. Yaegashi N, Miura M, Okamura K. Acute myocardial infarction associated with postpartum ergot alkaloid administration. *Int J Gynecol Obstet* 1999;64:67–68.

52. Tsui BC, Stewart B, Fitzmaurice A, Williams R. Cardiac arrest and myocardial infarction induced by postpartum intravenous ergonovine administration. *Anesthesiology.* 2001; 94:363–364.

53. Vimala N, Mittal S, Kumar S. Sublingual misoprostol versus oxytocin infusion to reduce blood loss at cesarean section. *Int J Gynecol Obstet.* 2006;92:106–110.

54. Hamm J, Russell Z, Botha T, Carlan SJ, Richichi K. Buccal misoprostol to prevent hemorrhage at cesarean delivery: a randomized study. *Am J Obstet Gynecol.* 2005;192: 1404–1406.

55. Liabsuetrakul T, Choobun T, Peeyananjarassri K, Islam QM. Prophylactic use of ergot alkaloids in the third stage of labour. *Cochrane Database Syst Rev.* 2008; Issue 3, Art. No.: CD005456.

56. Bullarbo M, Tjugum T, Ekerhovd E. Sublingual nitroglycerin for management of retained placenta. *Int J Gynecol Obstet.* 2005;91:228–232.

57. Hong RW, Greenfield ML, Polley L. Nitroglycerin for uterine inversion in the absence of placental fragments. *Anesth Analg.* 2006;102:511–512.

Objectives

After completing this chapter, the reader should be able to

- Describe the etiology and pathophysiology of common psychiatric disorders.
- List five signs and symptoms of psychosis.
- Describe depression and depressive disorders.
- Discuss the use of antipsychotic drugs in the treatment of schizophrenia and other psychotic disorders.
- Identify signs and symptoms of neuroleptic malignant syndrome.
- List four recognized extrapyramidal syndromes recognized soon after the introduction of antipsychotic drugs.
- Identify and evaluate antipsychotic discontinuation syndromes.
- Relate basic concepts of selective serotonin uptake inhibitor actions in the treatment of depression.
- Summarize the effects of tricyclic antidepressants in the treatment of major depression.
- Describe anticholinergic toxicity and discuss its management.
- Describe hypertensive crisis with the use of monoamine oxidase inhibitors.
- Summarize antidepressant discontinuation syndrome.
- Discuss the use of lithium for the control and prophylaxis of acute mania and the acute manic phase of bipolar disorder.
- List adverse syndromes associated with lithium use.
- Formulate an anesthetic plan for a patient on monoamine oxidase inhibitors having emergency abdominal surgery.
- Formulate an anesthetic plan for a patient receiving electroconvulsive therapy.

Psychiatric Disorders and Their Pharmacologic Management

Richard G. Ouellette, MEd, CRNA
Sandra M. Ouellette, MEd, CRNA, FAAN

Major psychiatric disorders include psychosis, depression, schizophrenia, Tourette's syndrome, and dementia. In this chapter we begin with a brief description of these disorders with emphasis on etiology, pathophysiology signs, and symptoms and treatment. Pharmacologic management of psychiatric disorders includes antipsychotic, antidepressant, and anxiolytic drugs. The chapter concludes with a discussion of overall treatment for psychiatric disorders with emphasis on electroconvulsive therapy and pharmacologic management. Anesthetic considerations for patients receiving psychiatric drugs are addressed.

Etiology and Pathophysiology of Common Psychiatric Disorders

Neurosis

Neurosis is a broad category of psychological disturbances consisting of mild forms of mental disorders. Until 1980 neurosis included anxiety disorders as well as mild mental illnesses such as hysteria and hypochondria. Phobias are a common kind of anxiety disorder. They involve specific situations that cause irrational anxiety attacks. Obsessive-compulsive disorder occurs when the individual relentlessly pursues a thought or action to relieve anxiety. Panic disorders are characterized by anxiety followed by panic attack. Posttraumatic stress disorder occurs in the wake of a traumatic event and can lead to flashbacks and lack of responsiveness to stimuli. Intraoperative awareness has been associated with posttraumatic stress disorder. The

Introduction

Many surgical patients today have a number of comorbidities that can affect anesthetic and surgical outcome. Pharmacologic treatment of many of these diseases presents challenges to the anesthesia provider. Decisions have to be made as to what medications to continue or discontinue in the perioperative period. The nurse anesthetist must also understand the disease process and side effects and possible drug interactions with chronic medications and anesthetic agents.

criteria for diagnosis of posttraumatic stress disorder are listed in Box 28-1.[1]

It has been traditionally thought that neurosis is based on emotional conflict in which a blocked impulse seeks expression in a disguised response or symptom. The response is a learned, inappropriate response and therefore can be unlearned. Treatment of neurosis may include behavior therapy to condition an individual to change behavior, psychotherapy, and pharmacologic agents to alleviate symptoms.

Box 28-1 Diagnostic Criteria for Posttraumatic Stress Disorder

- The person has experienced an event that is outside the range of usual human experience and that would be markedly distressing to almost anyone.
- The traumatic event is persistently re-experienced via:
  - Recurrent, intrusive, distressing recollection
  - Recurrent, distressing dreams
  - Sudden feelings of event recurring
  - Intense psychological distress to events resembling traumatic event
- Numbing of general responsiveness:
  - Efforts to avoid thoughts or feelings of event
  - Efforts to avoid activities or situations that arouse recollection of event
  - Inability to recall important aspects of event
  - Diminished interest in normal activities
  - Feelings of detachment; estrangement from others
  - Restricted range of affect
  - Sense of shortened future
- Persistent symptoms of increased arousal:
  - Difficulty falling or staying asleep
  - Irritability or outbursts of anger
  - Difficulty concentrating
  - Exaggerated startle response
  - Physiologic reactivity to events that resemble traumatic event
- Duration of disturbances: more than one per month

Psychosis

Psychosis is a term derived from the Greek *psyche* for "mind" or "soul" and *osis* for "abnormal condition." It usually implies a condition associated with loss of contact with reality. A wide variety of diseases of the central nervous system (CNS), including external poisons and internal physiologic illness, can produce symptoms of psychosis.

Signs and symptoms of psychosis may include hallucinations, delusions, and thought disorders. Hallucinations differ from illusions in that a hallucination is a sensory perception in the absence of external stimuli. In contrast, an illusion is a misperception of external stimuli. Hallucinations can involve any of the five senses and may include visual images, hearing voices, or experiencing tactile sensations. Auditory hallucinations are a common and prominent feature of psychosis.

Delusions associated with psychosis can be of a paranoid nature and can be divided into primary and secondary delusions. Primary delusions arise suddenly, and secondary delusions are influenced by a person's background or current situation.

A thought disorder is an underlying disturbance to conscious thought and is classified by its effect on speech and writing. There is a disconnection and disorganization in speech and writing, and in the most severe form speech cannot be understood. The etiology of mental illness is divided into organic and functional. Table 28-1 lists those organic and functional causes. Organic causes are generally from a medical or pathophysiologic condition, whereas functional causes are more likely related to a psychiatric or psychological disorder.

Table 28-1 Organic and Functional Causes of Psychosis

Functional Causes	Organic Causes
Brain tumors	Neurologic disorders
Drug abuse	Electrolyte disorders
Brain damage	Hypoglycemia
Schizophrenia	Lupus
Bipolar disorder (manic depression)	AIDS
Severe clinical depression	Malaria
Severe psychological stress	Leukoencephalopathy
Sleep deprivation	
Focal epileptic disorders	
Exposure to traumatic event	
Abrupt withdrawal from recreational drugs	

The pathophysiology of psychosis is usually linked to the neurotransmitter dopamine. It is believed that psychosis is due to overactivity of dopamine in the brain, and central dopamine receptor blocking drugs tend to reduce psychotic symptoms. Drugs that elevate dopamine centrally such as amphetamines and cocaine can trigger psychosis. Other theories for psychosis involve the belief that it results from dysfunction of the neurotransmitter glutamine and its activity at the *N*-methyl-D-aspartate receptor. Dissociative *N*-methyl-D-aspartate receptor antagonists such as ketamine, phencyclidine HCl, and dextromethorphan/dextrorphan at large doses induce a psychotic state.

Treatment for psychosis depends on the cause. First-line treatment for many psychotic disorders includes antipsychotic drugs. Electroconvulsive therapy (ECT) is sometimes used to relieve symptoms of psychosis due to depression.

Depression and Depressive Disorders

A depressive disorder is a syndrome that reflects a sad or irritable mood exceeding normal sadness or grief. The sadness or depression is characterized by greater intensity and duration with more severe symptoms and functional disabilities than is normal. In the past depression was divided into two types: endogenous, or coming from within the body, and neurotic, which has a clear environmental trigger such as loss of a spouse or job loss.

Depressive disorders are not only characterized by negative thoughts, mood, and behaviors but also by specific changes in bodily function. One in 10 individuals will have a depressive disorder in his or her lifetime. In 1 of 10 patients with depressive disorders, the disorder proves fatal.

In certain people with depressive disorders, especially manic-depressive or bipolar disorders, there seems to be an inherited vulnerability to the disorder. Depression can increase risks of developing coronary artery disease, HIV, asthma, and other medical illnesses. Depression in association with other diseases increases morbidity and mortality from the disease. The three major types of depressive disorders are major depression, dysthymia, and bipolar or manic depression lasting at least 2 weeks and interfering with the ability to work, sleep, eat, and enjoy normal activities. Disabling episodes can occur several times over a lifetime.

Dysthymia is a less severe form of depression but with a longer duration. The patient has long-term chronic symptoms that do not disable the individual but prevent the person from feeling good. In some cases the person

has major depression and dysthymia. This is termed double depression.

Bipolar disorder or manic depression is characterized by mood disorders that show patterns of inheritance. The mood swings are generally gradual but may be rapid. Bipolar disorders are not as common as other types of depressive disorders. Manic depression disorders have been divided into bipolar I and bipolar II disorders. Patients with bipolar II have repeated depressive episodes punctuated with mini-highs. The euphoria in bipolar II disorders does not fully meet the manic episodes seen in bipolar I patients. Symptoms of depression compared with mania are listed in Table 28-2.

Mania is thought to be caused by an imbalance of some of the same neurotransmitters that cause depression. These neurotransmitters may include serotonin, norepinephrine, dopamine, and glutamate. A lack of transmitter contributes to depression, whereas an excess may contribute to mania.

Many safe drugs are available for manic depression today. When pharmacologic treatment fails, ECT may be used.

Schizophrenia

Schizophrenia is derived from the Greek language and means split mind. It is a mental disorder characterized by abnormalities in perception or expression of reality. Distortions of perception may affect all five senses but commonly manifest as auditory hallucinations, paranoid or bizarre delusions, or disorganized speech and thinking.

Table 28-2 Depression and Mania Symptoms

Depression	Mania
Persistently sad, anxious, angry, irritable	Inappropriate elation
	Inappropriate anger, irritability
Feelings of hopeless, pessimism	Severe insomnia, less need for rest
Feelings of guilt, worthlessness, helplessness	Grandiose ideas, inappropriate social behavior
Loss of interest in hobbies, pleasures once enjoyed	Greater talking speed, volume
Sleep disorders	Disconnected or racing thoughts
Decreased appetite, weight loss, weight gain, increased appetite	Excessive or inappropriate sex
	Decreased appetite, weight loss
Crying spells	Poor investment and decision making
Thoughts of death, suicide	
Fatigue or loss of energy	
Diminished ability to think	

Onset of symptoms usually occurs in young adulthood. Approximately 0.2% to 0.4% of the young population is affected. There is no laboratory test to diagnose schizophrenia, and the diagnosis is made by history and observation.

Increased dopamine activity in the mesolimbic pathway of the brain is consistently found in patients with schizophrenia. Antipsychotic medications are the primary treatment for these patients because they suppress dopamine activity. The subtypes of schizophrenia are paranoid, disorganized, catatonic, undifferentiated, and residual. In paranoid schizophrenia, delusions and hallucinations are present but thought disorder, disorganized behavior, and affective flattening are absent. In the disorganized subtype, thought disorder and flat affect are present together. The catatonic schizophrenic is immobile or exhibits agitated, purposeless movement. In the undifferentiated subtype, psychotic symptoms are present but the criteria for major subtypes are missing. In residual schizophrenia, positive symptoms are present at low intensity.

Tourette's Syndrome

Tourette's was once considered a bizarre syndrome associated with exclamation of obscene words or inappropriate or derogatory remarks. Today it is viewed more as an inherited neuropsychiatric disorder consisting of multiple motor tics and at least one vocal tic. Motor tics are sudden, repetitive, stereotyped, nonrhythmic movements, and verbal tics are sounds that involve discrete muscle groups.

Most cases are inherited, and both genetic and environmental factors are involved. Between 1 and 10 children per 1000 have Tourette's, and as many as 10 per 1000 have a tic disorder. The most common tics are eye blinking, coughing, throat clearing, sniffing, and facial movements. The exact cause of Tourette's syndrome is unknown, and medication is usually unnecessary.

Pharmacologic Management of Psychiatric Disorders

An accidental discovery of the antipsychotic properties of the antihypertensive drug chlorpromazine changed the course of treatment and the entire field of psychiatry. Newer drugs have proved more useful in the management of psychosis, and research continues in this area.

Antipsychotic drugs assist in managing symptoms of psychosis, including hallucinations, bizarre behaviors, thought disorders, agitation, and hyperactivity. These drugs do not cure psychotic disorders but ease many of the distressing symptoms. Antipsychotic drugs are used to manage a variety of disorders: primarily schizophrenia, schizoaffective and schizophreniform disorders, delusional disorders, acute mania, depressive psychosis, and substance-induced psychosis.

Antipsychotic (Neuroleptic) Drugs

The traditional antipsychotic drugs had strong neuroleptic properties and were often referred to as classic antipsychotic drugs or neuroleptics. With newer drugs being developed and the mechanisms of action further delineated, the more accepted terminology is now first-generation antipsychotics.

First-generation antipsychotic drugs (Box 28-2) are classified according to potency and chemical structure and are roughly equivalent with respect to their effect on symptoms. First-generation antipsychotic drugs are thought to block dopamine-2 receptors in postsynaptic areas. Positive symptoms of schizophrenia are affected by blocking dopamine-2 receptors in the mesolimbic area of the brain.

Second-generation antipsychotic drugs (Box 28-3) are newer, atypical drugs approved for use in the United States in the 1990s. These phenothiazines are also indicated in the treatment of schizophrenia and other psychotic disorders. They have also been used as adjuncts in managing mania and borderline personality disorders. However, they are not the primary drug of choice for any of these disorders.

Box 28-2 First-Generation Antipsychotic Neuroleptic Drugs

- Chlorpromazine
- Thioridazine
- Fluphenazine
- Perphenazine
- Trifluoperazine
- Chlorprothixene
- Thiothixene
- Loxapine
- Haloperidol
- Droperidol
- Pimozide

Box 28-3 Second-Generation Antipsychotic Neuroleptic Drugs

- Clozapine
- Risperidone
- Olanzapine

Tables 28-3a and 28-3b list the antipsychotic (neuroleptic) drugs with their properties and dosages. They are also described in the following discussion.

Phenothiazides

Chlorpromazine

- Actions: Affects all levels of CNS with a mechanism that produces strong antipsychotic effects. The mechanism that produces strong antipsychotic effects is unclear. It is thought to be related to blockade of postsynaptic dopamine receptors in the brain. It tends to reduce initiative and interest in the environment, decrease displays of emotions or affect, suppress spontaneous movements and complex behavior, and decrease psychotic symptoms.

Table 28-3a Antipsychotic (Neuroleptic) Drugs

Drug	Administration	Onset	Peak	Duration	Metabolism	Elimination
Phenothiazide						
Chlorpromazine	PO IM/IV	30–60 min	2–4 h	4–6 h	Liver	Urine
Thioridazine	PO	Varies	2–4 h	8–12 h	Liver	Urine
Fluphenazine	PO IM	60 min	3–5 h	6–8 h	Liver	
Perphenazine	PO IM	Varies	30–90 min	24–36 h	Liver GI	Urine and feces
Trifluoperazine	PO IM	Unknown	2–4 h	12–24 h	Liver	Bile and feces
Thioxanthene						
Thiothixene	PO	Slow	1–3 h	12 h	Liver	Urine
Dibenzodiazepines						
Clozapine	PO	Unknown	1–6 h	4–12 h	Liver	50% urine 30% feces
Loxapine	PO IM	30 min	1.5–3 h	12 h	Liver	Urine and feces
Olanzapine	PO	Unknown	4–5 h		Liver	5% urine 30% feces
Butyrophenones						
Haloperidol	PO IM	2 h 20–30 min	2–6 h 30–45 min	8–12 h 4–8 h	Liver	Urine and feces
Droperidol	IM IV	3–10 min	30 min	2–4 h	Liver	Urine and feces
Diphenylbutylpiperidine						
Pimozide	PO	Unknown	6–8 h		Liver	85% urine 15% feces
Benzisoxazole						
Risperidone	PO	Unknown	2 h	Unknown	Liver	7% urine 14% feces

GI, gastrointestinal; IM, intramuscular; IV, intravenous; PO, oral.

Table 28-3b Antipsychotic (Neuroleptic) Drug Dosages

Drug	Dosage
Chlorpromazine	Adult: PO 25–100 mg tid/qid up to 1000 mg/day
	IM/IV 25–50 mg up to 600 mg q 4–6 h
	Child: > 6 mo PO 0.55 mg/kg q 4–6 h prn
	PR l.l mg/kg q 6–8 h
	IM/IV 0.55 mg/kg q 6–8 h
Thioridazine	Adult: PO 50–100 mg tid up to 800 mg/day
	Child: > 2 y: PO 0.5–3 mg/kg/day divided
Fluphenazine	Adult: PO 0.5–10 mg/day, max 20 mg/day
	IM 2.5–10 mg/day q 6–8 h divided
Perphenazine	Adult: PO 4–16 mg bid–qid, 8- to 32-mg sustained-release bid, max 64 mg/day
	IM 5 mg q 6 h, max 15–30 mg/day
	Child: PO 4 mg bid/qid, 8-mg sustained-release bid, max 16 mg/day
	IM same as adult
Trifluoperazine	Adult: PO 1–2 mg bid up to 20 mg/day
	IM 1–2 mg q 4–6 h, max 10 mg/day
	Child: PO 6–12 y: 1 mg qd/bid, max 15 mg/day
	IM 6–12 y: 1 mg qd/bid up to 15 mg/day
Thiothixene	Adult: 50–100 mg tid, max 800 mg/day
	Child: > 2 y: 0.5–3 mg/kg/day divided doses
Clozapine	Adult: PO 12.5–25 mg qd/bid, increase to target 300–450 mg/day
Loxapine	Adult: PO 10 mg bid, max 60–100 mg
	IM 12.5–50 mg q 4–6 h
Olanzapine	Adult: PO 5–10 mg daily, max 20 mg/day
Haloperidol	Adult: PO 3–5 mg bid/tid, max 100 mg/day
	IM 2–5 mg repeat q 1 h prn
	Child: PO 0.05–0.15 kg/day in 2–3 divided doses
Droperidol	Adult: IV/IM 0.22–0.275 mg/kg, maintenance 1.25–2.5 mg
	Child: 2–12 y: IV/IM 0.088–0.165 mg/kg
Pimozide	Adult: PO 1–2 mg bid, max 8 mg/day
Risperidone	Adult: PO 1–6 mg bid, max 8 mg/day

IM, intramuscular; IV, intravenous; PO, oral; PR, rectally.

- Used to control manic phase of manic-depressive illness and for symptomatic management of psychotic disorders, including schizophrenia.
- Adverse effects ≥ 1%: Orthostatic hypotension, palpitation, tachycardia, electrocardiographic changes, prolonged QT and PR intervals, blunting of T waves, ST depression, dry mouth, sedation, drowsiness, dizziness, restlessness, neuroleptic malignant syndrome, tardive dyskinesias, extrapyramidal symptoms, electroencephalographic changes.

Thioridazine

- Actions: Similar to chlorpromazine. Strong anticholinergic and α-adrenergic agonist activity and potent sedative action. Effective in reducing excitement, hypermotility, abnormal initiative, affective tension, and agitation by inhibiting psychomotor functions. Effective antipsychotic agent, and for behavioral disorders in children.
- Used to manage psychotic disorders, nonpsychotic behavioral disturbances of senility, moderate to

marked depression, and management of hyperkinetic behavior syndrome.

- Adverse effects ≥ 1%: Sedation, dizziness, drowsiness, extrapyramidal syndrome (EPS), nocturnal confusion, hyperactivity, ventricular dysrhythmias, hypotension, prolonged QT_c interval.

Fluphenazine

- Actions: Potent phenothiazine, antipsychotic agent. Blocks postsynaptic dopamine receptors in the brain. Similar to phenothiazines except higher incidence of extrapyramidal complications, lower frequency of sedative, and hypotensive effects.
- Used to manage manifestations of psychotic disorders and effective for the treatment of antipsychotic symptoms, including schizophrenia.
- Adverse effects ≥ 1%: Extrapyramidal effects resembling Parkinson's disease, tardive dyskinesia, sedation, drowsiness, dizziness, impaired thermoregulation, seizures, tachycardia, hypertension, hypotension, dry mouth.

Perphenazine

- Actions: Affects all parts of CNS, similar to chlorpromazine, particularly the hypothalamus. Antipsychotic effect: antagonizes the neurotransmitter dopamine by action on dopamine receptors in the brain.
- Used to manage psychotic disorders.
- Adverse effects ≥ 1%: Extrapyramidal effects, sedation, convulsions, orthostatic hypotension, tachycardia, bradycardia, dry mouth.

Trifluoperazine

- Actions: Phenothiazine similar to chlorpromazine. Produces less sedation, cardiovascular, and anticholinergic effects than other phenothiazines. Antipsychotic effects thought related to blockade of postsynaptic dopamine receptors in the brain.
- Used for management of manifestations of psychotic disorders, possibly effective control of excessive anxiety and tension associated with neuroses or somatic conditions.
- Adverse effects ≥ 1%: Drowsiness, insomnia, dizziness, agitation, extrapyramidal effects, neuroleptic malignant syndrome, tachycardia, hypotension.

Thioxanthene

Thiothixene

- Actions: Similar to the phenothiazine chlorpromazine. Rare extrapyramidal effects. Has strong anticholinergic and α-adrenergic agonist activity and potent sedative effect.
- Used for the management of nonpsychotic behavioral disturbances of senility, manifestations of psychotic disorders, and hyperkinetic behavior syndrome.
- Adverse effects ≥ 1%: Drowsiness, dizziness, nocturnal confusion, hyperactivity, rare EPS.

Dibenzodiazepines

Clozapine

- Actions: Mechanism unknown. Interferes with binding of dopamine to D_1 and D_2 receptors in the limbic region of brain. It binds to nondopaminergic sites.
- Used in the management of severely ill schizophrenic patients.
- Adverse effects ≥ 1%: Hypotension, tachycardia, ECG changes, risk of myocarditis, pericarditis, pericardial effusion, cardiomyopathy heart failures, myocardial infarction, mitral valve insufficiency, seizures, fevers, neuroleptic malignant syndrome.

Clozapine toxicity leads to symptoms due to elevation in serum clozapine levels. Medications that block the enzyme responsible for clozapine metabolism is one reason for toxicity. Another etiology for toxicity may be discontinuation of medications that have induced the enzyme CYP1A2. Fluvoxamine is an example of an enzyme inhibitor.[2] Other inhibitors of CYP1A2 include cimetidine, ciprofloxacin, erythromycin, grapefruit juice, norfloxin, and fluoroquinolone. Enzyme inducers for CYP1A2 include carbamazepine, cigarette smoke, and rifampin.[3] The incidence of clozapine toxicity is unknown. Symptoms include sedation, hypotension, hypersalivation, tachycardia, myoclonic jerks, and seizures.[4] Measurement of serum clozapine levels and administration of medications that inhibit the metabolizing enzyme or reduction of enzyme induction confirm the diagnosis. Management includes stopping responsible medication, reducing or discontinuing clozapine medication, and treatment of seizures if necessary.

Loxapine

- Actions: Exact mode of action is unknown. Sedative action is less than chlorpromazine, anticholinergic effects are comparable, and extrapyramidal more intense.

- Used in the management of psychotic disorders.
- Adverse effects: Drowsiness, sedation, dizziness, ECG changes, staggering gait, muscle weakness, akathisia, tardive dyskinesia, neuroleptic malignant syndrome, orthostatic hypotension, hypertension, dry mouth.

Olanzapine

- Actions: Antipsychotic activity due to antagonism for both serotonin and dopamine receptors. May inhibit the CNS presynaptic neuronal reuptake of serotonin and dopamine. Antagonism of α-adrenergic receptors results in the adverse effect of orthostatic hypotension.
- Used for the management of psychotic disturbances and short-term treatment of acute manic episodes of bipolar disorder.
- Adverse effects ≥ 1%: Postural hypotension, tachycardia, somnolence, dizziness, agitation, insomnia, hostility, anxiety, akathisia, hypertonia, tremor amnesia, euphoria, extrapyramidal symptoms.

Butyrophenones

Haloperidol

- Actions: Long-acting butyrophenone derivative with similar actions to those of piperazine phenothiazines. Has higher incidence of extrapyramidal effects, less hypotension, and relatively low sedative activity.
- Used in the management of psychotic disorder manifestations, control of tics and vocal utterance of Tourette's syndrome. It is used in acute and chronic psychoses. Also used for short-term treatment of hyperactive children and for severe behavior problems in children who are combative or have explosive hyperexcitability.
- Adverse effects ≥ 1%: Extrapyramidal reactions including dystonia, Parkinson symptoms, akathisia, tardive dyskinesia, insomnia, restlessness, anxiety, euphoria, agitation, neuroleptic malignant syndrome, hyperthermia, seizures, exacerbation of psychotic symptoms. ECG changes, hypotension, and hypertension with overdosage.

Droperidol

- Actions: Pharmacologically related to haloperidol. Mild α-adrenergic blocking activity and direct vasodilator effects. Acts on the subcortical level to produce sedation.

- Used to produce tranquilizing effect. Mostly used in perioperative period for sedation and prophylaxis for nausea and vomiting.
- Adverse effects ≥ 1%: Extrapyramidal symptoms, drowsiness, hypotension, tachycardia, prolonged QT_c interval, akathisia, hallucinations.

Diphenylbutylpiperidine

Pimozide

- Actions: Potent central dopamine antagonist that alters release and turnover of central dopamine stores. Blocks CNS dopamine receptors resulting in suppression of the motor and phonic tics of Tourette's disorder. Produces less sedation and less extrapyramidal reactions than haloperidol.
- Used to suppress severe motor and phonic tics in patients with Tourette's disorder.
- Adverse effects ≥ 1%: Akathisia, speech disorders, tremors, torticollis, akinesia, hyperpyrexia, tardive dyskinesia, rigidity, drowsiness, sedation, prolonged QT_c interval, inverted T wave, appearance of U wave, labile blood pressure.

Benzisoxazole

Risperidone

- Actions: Mechanism not well known. Interferes with binding of dopamine to D_2-interlimbic region of the brain, serotonin receptors, and α-adrenergic receptors in the occipital cortex.
- Used for reduction or elimination of psychotic symptoms in schizophrenia as well as other psychotic symptoms. Improves negative symptoms. Also used as adjunctive treatment of behavioral disturbances in mentally retarded.
- Adverse effects ≥ 1%: Flu-like symptoms, headache, dizziness, chest pain, peripheral edema.

Conditions and Syndromes Associated With Administration of Antipsychotic Drugs

Neuroleptic malignant syndrome and EPS are associated with use of antipsychotic drugs. In addition, antipsychotic discontinuation syndrome can be a problem and must be appreciated by the nurse anesthetist.

Neuroleptic Malignant Syndrome

Neuroleptic malignant syndrome is a rare but potentially fatal disorder characterized by changes in consciousness, rigidity, autonomic disturbances, and fever. Changes in consciousness range from confusion to coma. Rigidity can be localized or generalized, and pyrexia can exceed 42°C. Autonomic disturbances include pallor, tachycardia, labile blood pressure, sweating, and urinary incontinence. The pharmacologic mechanism for this disorder is blockade of dopamine receptors or central dopamine hypoactivity.[5]

The incidence of this syndrome is 0.15% to 0.07%, and it is decreasing in frequency.[6,7] It is caused by quickly increasing or giving very high doses of antipsychotic medications, especially haloperidol. Men outnumber women 2:1, and 80% of cases occur in individuals under age 40. This finding is usually attributed to higher doses in both men and young adults.[8] Although any antipsychotic drug can cause neuroleptic malignant syndrome, other drugs have been implicated as well.[9,10] These drugs include lithium, tricyclic antidepressants (TCAs), monoamine oxidase inhibitors (MAOIs), selective serotonin receptor inhibitors (SSRIs), and metoclopramide.[11–13] Sudden discontinuation of dopaminergic medications used to treat Parkinson's disease has also been implicated in development of neuroleptic malignant syndrome.[14,15]

The diagnosis of neuroleptic malignant syndrome is based on a careful history and physical examination. When diagnosed, all antipsychotic medications should be discontinued. The patient should be rehydrated and treated symptomatically. In some patients response to benzodiazepines, bromocriptine, dantrolene, and ECT is observed.[16–19]

Extrapyramidal Syndromes

Extrapyramidal syndromes (EPS) were recognized soon after the introduction of antipsychotic drugs, with the first formal report attributed to Steck.[20] Four syndromes are recognized: acute dystonia, akathisia, parkinsonism, and tardive dyskinesia. Patients may suffer concurrently from more than one syndrome. Akathisia and acute dystonia emerge in the first week of treatment, whereas parkinsonism emerges during the first 2 months and tardive dyskinesia after more than 6 months of treatment. However, these drug-induced symptoms need to be differentiated from abnormal involuntary movements that can occur in patients with schizophrenia who have not received antipsychotic treatment and yet present with a neuromotor component of the illness.[21,22]

Extrapyramidal symptoms can occur with psychotropic drugs other than antipsychotics, although this is uncommon. Akathisia, dystonia, parkinsonism, and tardive dyskinesia have been reported with SSRIs,[23,24] with akathisia being the most common symptom. Other reports have suggested antidepressants, MAOIs,[25] lithium,[26] and

nonpsychotic drugs occasionally cause EPS. The newer atypical antipsychotic drugs have a lower liability for acute EPS than conventional antipsychotic drugs.[27]

Acute dystonia is an involuntary sustained contraction of a muscle to its maximum degree. The contraction can be transient and repetitive, producing an appearance of constant movement, or it can be sustained, resulting in posture distortion. They can affect any part of the body, neck, head, trunk, arms, and legs. The neck is the most common site, accounting for one-third of such reactions, with 15% to 17% involving the jaw and tongue.[28] The incidence is variable and depends on drug used, dose, rate of increase, and subject characteristics. The highest incidence is with high-potency conventional antipsychotics (e.g., haloperidol), rarely with antipsychotics, and occasionally with SSRIs. It can also occur with antipsychotic withdrawals. The pharmacologic mechanism is unknown, although it is thought to be due to an increased or decreased dopaminergic transmission. Risk factors include use of high-potency conventional antipsychotics, male gender, younger age, rapid escalation in drug dose, and recent abrupt discontinuation of antipsychotic medication. Its treatment includes anticholinergics, considering changing antipsychotics, and avoiding further increases in antipsychotics for a few days.

Akathisia has both subjective and objective components.[29] Increased restlessness is often located to lower limbs associated with a feeling of unease and often irritability. Personal distress and dysphoria may be seen in more severe cases. Unlike EPS, the movements seen with akathisia are semivoluntary, although patients believe they are forced to move. The incidence is variable and depends on drug, dose, and rate of increase. It is reported in up to 32% in some studies.[30] Usually, it appears soon after starting or increasing the dose of antipsychotic and worsens with further dose increase. Its highest incidence is with high-potency conventional antipsychotics, rarely with atypical antipsychotics, and occasionally with SSRIs. The pharmacologic mechanism is not clear. It may reflect a combination of a depressed dopaminergic system and an overactive noradrenergic system. Risk factors include use of high-potency conventional antipsychotics, higher dosage, and rapid escalation in drug dose. Its management includes reducing antipsychotic dose, switching antipsychotic drug, and administering either an anticholinergic, benzodiazepine, or propranolol. Its prevention is by gradual titration of dosage when starting or increasing the amount of an antipsychotic drug.

Parkinsonism consists of three components: bradykinesia, rigidity, and tremor. The signs of parkinsonism include a mask-like expression, lack of gesticulation, stooped posture, shuffling gait, a reduction in the normal arm swing that accompanies walking, resting hand tremors, slowness of movements, absence of blinking, seborrhea, and complaints of feeling tired.

The onset of drug-induced parkinsonism tends to be gradual over several weeks. With conventional antipsychotics, 90% of cases manifest within 10 weeks of commencing treatment.[31] The incidence is variable; the highest incidence is with high-potency conventional antipsychotics and less commonly with atypical antipsychotics, although the problem is dose related to some extent with several of these agents. It occasionally occurs with SSRIs. The pharmacologic mechanism is D_2 blockade in striatum. Risk factors include use of high-potency conventional antipsychotics, higher dosage, advancing age, and female gender. Management includes reducing or changing antipsychotic and prescribing anticholinergic.

Tardive dyskinesia refers to a syndrome of various involuntary movements, except tremors, associated with the administration of antipsychotic drugs that appears late in the course of treatment. These various involuntary movements include myoclonic jerks, tics, chorea, and dystonia and most commonly affects the buccal-lingual-masticatory muscles. Abnormal worm-like movements on the surface of the tongue are sometimes mentioned as an early sign. Complex and repetitive movement of the orofacial muscles is a common and characteristic feature. Patients are typically unaware of the movements. The incidence is about 5% per year in patients starting antipsychotic treatment.[32] The pharmacologic mechanism is the supersensitivity of the striatal postsynaptic D_2 receptors, secondary to their blockade by antipsychotics. Risk factors include advancing age, female gender, dementia, and susceptibility to acute extrapyramidal side effects. Management includes reducing the dose of causal drug and switching to an atypical antipsychotic drug.

Antipsychotic Discontinuation Syndromes

Evidence of antipsychotic discontinuation syndromes come from studies done in the late 1950s and early 1960s.[33,34] These symptoms were labeled as withdrawal syndrome because the symptoms occurred within a brief time of stopping the drug and abated if the medication was restarted. There was a resurgence of interest in the symptoms associated with discontinuation of antipsychotics, and the term "discontinuation syndrome" was used to describe them. A review of the literature on symptoms that developed within the first 7 days of discontinuation of an antipsychotic was done to differentiate them from the symptoms of psychotic relapse.[35]

Antipsychotic discontinuation syndrome has characteristic symptoms that commence shortly after stopping or reducing the dose of the antipsychotic and are unrelated to the underlying psychiatric disorder. Its incidence is variable and depends on definition. The incidence is also likely to vary depending on the antipsychotic drug, length of treatment, rate of taper before stoppage, and dose. In some studies over half of patients develop discontinuation symptoms on stopping antipsychotic treatment. This, however, occurs with all antipsychotics.

The pharmacologic mechanism is the sudden disruption of CNS adaptation to antipsychotic treatment. Anticholinergic rebound may explain gastrointestinal symptoms, insomnia, and agitation. The symptoms are variable. Common symptoms include nausea, vomiting, anorexia, general somatic distress, insomnia, and anxiety and agitation. Psychosis often appears soon after stopping clozapine, and it is unclear whether this is a relapse of the underlying illness or a discontinuation effect. EPS can occur on stopping conventional antipsychotics and less commonly with atypical antipsychotics. There are three options to management: education and support, allowing symptoms to spontaneously resolve; symptomatic treatment; or restarting antipsychotic tapering more slowly.

Antidepressant Drugs

Tables 28-4a and 28-4b list the antidepressants and their dosages, which are described further in the following discussion.

Selective Serotonin Uptake Inhibitors

TCAs were the mainstay of antidepressant therapy until the introduction of the SSRIs. SSRIs are chemically unrelated to any other class of antidepressants. They are potent blockers of serotonin reuptake with a weak affinity for norepinephrine or dopamine blockade. They have limited affinity for α_1-, α_2-, and β-adrenergic; γ-aminobutyric acid; histamine; and cholinergic receptors. SSRIs are well absorbed when taken orally, with an onset, peak, and duration of action ranging from 1 to 4 weeks; they may take up to 12 weeks for complete effectiveness.

Fluoxetine

- Actions: Antidepressant effect linked to its inhibition of CNS neuronal uptake of serotonin (SSRI).
- Used in depression, geriatric depression, obsessive-compulsive disorder, bulimia, and premenstrual dysphoric disorder.

- Adverse effects ≥ 1% : Headache, nervousness, anxiety, fatigue, tremor, dizziness, palpitations, chest pain, hot flashes, anorexia, dyspepsia, increased appetite.

Sertraline

- Actions: Potent inhibitor of serotonin reuptake in the brain. Chemically unrelated to TCAs, tetracyclic antidepressants, or other available antidepressants. Down-regulation of norepinephrine with chronic use.

- Used in major depression, obsessive-compulsive disorder, panic disorder, premenstrual dysphoric disorder, anxiety, posttraumatic stress disorder.
- Adverse effects ≥ 1%: Palpitations, chest pain, hypertension, hypotension, tachycardia, agitation, insomnia, headache, dizziness, fatigue, ataxia, aggressive behavior, delusions, hallucinations, emotional lability, paranoia, depersonalization, suicidal ideation.

Table 28-4a Antidepressants

Drug	Onset	Peak	Duration	Metabolism	Elimination
SSRIs					
Fluoxetine	1–4 wk	4–8 h	24–48 wk		80% urine 12% feces
Sertraline	1–8 wk	6–8 h	24 h	Liver	Urine Feces
Paroxetine	1–4 wk	3–7 h	24 h	Liver	Urine Feces
Fluvoxamine	2–3 wk	Dose dependent	12–24 h	Liver	Urine
Citalopram		1 week		Liver	Urine Bile
Escitalopram	1 week	3 h		Liver	20% urine 80% bile
Bupropion	Up to 4 wk	2 h	6–12 h	Liver	80% urine
Venlafaxine	4–6 days	2–4 h	6–8 h	Liver	60% urine
Trazodone	1–2 wk	0.5–2 h	8 h	Liver	75% urine 25% feces
Nefazodone	2–6 wk	48 h	12–24 h	Liver	

Table 28-4b Antidepressant Dosages

Drug	Dosage
Fluoxetine	PO 20 mg bid, increase to 20–80 mg/day
Sertraline	PO start 50 mg/day, range 50–200 mg
Paroxetine	PO 10–50 mg/day, max 80 mg/day
Fluvoxamine	Adult: PO 50 mg qd up to 300 mg/day
	Child 8–12 y: 25 mg q hs, increase up to 200 mg/day
Citalopram	PO 20 mg qd up to 40 mg/day
Escitalopram	PO 10 mg qd up to 20 mg/day
Bupropion	PO 75–100 mg tid up to 300 mg/day
Venlafaxine	PO 25–125 mg tid
Trazodone	Adult: PO 150 mg/day, max 400–600 mg/day
	Child 6–18 y: PO 1.5–2 mg/kg/day, max 6 mg/kg/day
Nefazodone	PO 50–100 mg bid, max 300–600 mg/day

PO, oral.

Paroxetine

- Actions: Potent highly selective inhibitor of serotonin reuptake by neurons in the CNS.
- Used for depression, obsessive-compulsive disorders, panic attacks, excessive social anxiety, post-traumatic stress disorder.
- Adverse effects ≥ 1%: Postural hypotension, tremor, agitation, nervousness, anxiety, dizziness, insomnia, sedation, paresthesias, headache.

Fluvoxamine

- Actions: Potent, selective, inhibitory activity on neuronal serotonin reuptake. Structurally unrelated to TCAs. Compared with TCAs shows fewer anticholinergic effects and no severe cardiovascular effects.
- Used for treatment of obsessive-compulsive disorders and depression.
- Adverse effects ≥ 1%: Headache, somnolence, agitation, insomnia, dizziness, seizures, slight bradycardia, orthostatic hypotension.

Citalopram

- Actions: Antidepressant effect linked to its inhibition of CNS presynaptic neuronal uptake of serotonin, resulting in antidepressant activity. Does not produce anticholinergic or sympathomimetic responses.
- Used in depression.
- Adverse effects ≥ 1%: Asthenia, fatigue, fever, myalgia, tachycardia, postural hypotension, hypotension, dizziness, insomnia, agitation, tremor, anxiety, paresthesia, migraine.

Escitalopram

- Actions: Antidepressant effect linked to its inhibition of CNS presynaptic neuronal uptake of serotonin, resulting in antidepressant activity. Does not produce anticholinergic or sympathomimetic responses.
- Used in depression.
- Averse effects ≥ 1%: Fever, fatigue, myalgia, palpitation, hypertension, dizziness, insomnia, somnolence, paresthesia, migraine, tremor, vertigo.

Other Antidepressant Drugs

Bupropion

- Actions: Neurochemical mechanism is unknown. Compared with TCAs, it is a weak blocker of neural uptake of serotonin and norepinephrine.
- Used in mental depression. Has been associated with increased risk of seizures and therefore not the agent of first choice.
- Adverse effects ≥ 1%: Seizures, agitation, insomnia, dry mouth headache, dizziness, agitation, insomnia, tremor.

Venlafaxine

- Actions: Selectively inhibits neuronal uptake of serotonin, norepinephrine, and dopamine in decreasing order of potency. A bicyclic antidepressant drug chemically unrelated to tricyclic, tetracyclic, or other depressants.
- Used in generalized anxiety disorders and depression.
- Adverse effects ≥ 1%: Increased blood pressure and heart rate, palpitations, dizziness, fatigue, headache, insomnia, somnolence.

Trazodone

- Actions: Centrally acting triazolopyridine derivative antidepressant. Chemically and structurally unrelated to tricyclic, tetracyclic, or other antidepressants. Potentiates serotonin effects by selectively blocking its reuptake at presynaptic membranes in CNS. Does not stimulate CNS and causes fewer anticholinergic genitourinary and neurologic effects as compared with other antidepressants.
- Used in major depression with or without prominent anxiety.
- Adverse effects ≥ 1%: Drowsiness, lightheadedness, dizziness, insomnia, headache, hypotension, syncope, shortness of breath, tachycardia, palpitations, bradycardia, PVCs, short episodes of ventricular tachycardia.

Nefazodone

- Actions: Inhibits neuronal serotonin reuptake and also possesses serotonin antagonist properties. Unrelated to tricyclic, MAOI, or other antidepressants.
- Used in the treatment of depression.
- Adverse effects ≥ 1%: Headache drowsiness, dizziness, tremor asthenia, insomnia, agitation, anxiety, dry mouth.

TCAs and Related Compounds

TCAs are still used as first-line drugs in the treatment of major depression. They elevate mood, increase activity and alertness, decrease morbid preoccupation, improve appetite, and normalize sleep patterns.

Antidepressants appear to work by blocking presynaptic serotonin and norepinephrine reuptake. There is an increased amount of these neurotransmitters in the synapse, prolonging and intensifying their effects. The blockade of reuptake by itself cannot fully explain the therapeutic effectiveness of the TCAs because the drugs block transmitter uptake within a few hours of administration, yet relief of depression may take several weeks to develop. It seems that an intermediary response must be occurring between the onset of the blockade and the onset of the therapeutic response. What specifically composes this intermediary response is not clear.

Most antidepressants are well absorbed when administered orally, and onset varies from 1 to 2 hours to 3 weeks. TCAs are widely distributed with effective relief of depression achieved in 2 to 6 weeks in most cases. Tables 28-5a and 28-5b present the TCAs and related compounds and their dosages.

Amitriptyline

- Actions: Most active of the TCAs in inhibition of serotonin uptake from synaptic gap. Inhibits norepinephrine reuptake to a moderate degree. Restoration of the levels of these neurotransmitters is a proposed mechanism of antidepressant action.
- Used in endogenous depression
- Adverse effects ≥ 1%: Drowsiness, sedation, dizziness, nervousness, restlessness, fatigue, orthostatic hypotension, tachycardia, palpitation, ECG changes.

Amoxapine

- Actions: TCA and secondary amine with mixed antidepressant and neuroleptic tranquilizing properties. Not associated with severe cardiotoxicity.
- Used in neurotic and endogenous depression accompanied by anxiety or agitation.
- Adverse effects ≥ 1%: Mild sedative effect, slight orthostatic hypotension, dizziness, headache.

Clomipramine

- Actions: Inhibits the reuptake of norepinephrine and serotonin at the presynaptic neuron. Elevates serum levels of these two amines.
- Used in obsessive-compulsive disorders and depression
- Adverse effects ≥ 1%: Hypotension, tachycardia, diaphoresis, mania, tremors, hyperthermia, neuroleptic malignant syndrome, seizures with abrupt withdrawal.

Desipramine

- Actions: TCA and secondary amine. Desipramine is the active metabolite of imipramine and has similar pharmacologic actions. Onset of action is more rapid, and there is lower potential for producing sedative and anticholinergic effects and orthostatic hypotension.
- Used in endogenous depression and various other depression syndromes.
- Adverse effects ≥ 1%: Drowsiness, dizziness, weakness, fatigue, postural hypotension,

Table 28-5a Tricyclic and Related Compounds

Drug	Onset	Peak	Duration	Metabolism	Elimination
Amitriptyline	PO 2–3 wk	2–6 wk	18–24 h	Liver	Urine
	IM 2–3 wk	2–6 wk	Days to weeks		
Amoxapine		1–2 h		Active metabolite	Urine
					Feces
Clomipramine	2–6 wk	2 h	12–24 h	Liver	Urine
					Feces
Desipramine	2–6 wk	4–6 h	24 h	Liver	Urine
Doxepin	2–3 wk	6 wk	18–24 h	Liver	Urine
Imipramine	PO 1–2 h	2–6 wk	Weeks	Liver	Urine
	IM 1–2 h	2–6 wk	Weeks		Feces
Nortriptyline	2–3 wk	6 wk	18–24 h	Liver	Urine
Protriptyline	2–6 wk	24–30 h	12–24 h	Liver	Urine
Mirtazapine (tetracyclic antidepressant)	2–6 wk	1.5 h	12–24 h	Liver	Urine
					Feces

IM, intramuscular; PO, oral.

Table 28-5b   Tricyclic and Related Compound Dosages

Drug	Dosage
Amitriptyline	Adult: PO 75–100 mg/day up to 150–300 mg/day
	IM 20–30 mg qid
	Adolescent: PO 25–50 mg/day up to 200 mg/day
Amoxapine	50 mg bid/tid, up to 100 mg tid
Clomipramine	Adult: 75–300 mg/day divided doses
	Child 10–18 y: 100–200 mg/day divided
Desipramine	Adult: 75–100 mg/day up to 300 mg/day
	Adolescent: 25–50 mg/day, max 100 mg/day
	Child 6–12 y: 1–3 mg/kg/day up to 5 mg/kg/day
Doxepin	Adult: 30–150 mg/day hs, max 300 mg/day
	Child: 1–3 mg/kg/day
Imipramine	Adult: 75–100 mg/day, max 300 mg
	Child: 1.5 mg/kg/day, max 5 mg/kg/day
Nortriptyline	Adult: 25 mg tid/qid up to 100–150 mg/day
	Adolescent: 30–50 mg/day divided
	Child 6–12 y: 10–20 mg/day in 3–4 divided doses
Protriptyline	Adult: 15–40 mg/day, max 60 mg/day
	Adolescent: 15 mg/day divided doses
Mirtazapine	PO 15 mg/day hs, max 45 mg/day

IM, intramuscular; PO, oral.

Doxepin

- Actions: TCA—one of the most sedating. Inhibits serotonin reuptake from the synaptic gap. Inhibits norepinephrine reuptake to a moderate degree.
- Used in psychoneurotic anxiety or depressive reactions, mixed symptoms of anxiety and depression, psychotic depressive disorders, and organic disease.
- Adverse effects ≥ 1%: Drowsiness, weakness, fatigue, headache, tremors, orthostatic hypotension, palpitation, tachycardia, ECG changes.

Imipramine

- Actions: TCA and tertiary amine, structurally related to the phenothiazines. In contrast with phenothiazines, TCAs potentiate both norepinephrine and serotonin in the CNS by blocking their reuptake by presynaptic neurons. Decreases number of awakenings from sleep.
- Used in endogenous depression and reactive depression. Also used for treatment of enuresis in children older than 6 years.

- Adverse effects ≥ 1%: Sedation, drowsiness, dizziness, headache, fatigue, tingling, extrapyramidal symptoms, lowered seizure threshold, orthostatic hypotension, sinus tachycardia, palpitations, myocardial infarction, congestive heart failure, heart block.

Nortriptyline

- Actions: Secondary amine derivative of amitriptyline. TCA with less sedative and anticholinergic effects than imipramine. Action mechanism not clear.
- Used in endogenous depression.
- Adverse effects ≥ 1%: Tremors, orthostatic hypotension, dry mouth, drowsiness.

Protriptyline

- Actions: TAC with more rapid onset of action than imipramine. Less sedative properties, if any, compared with other TCAs.
- Used for symptomatic treatment of endogenous depression in patients under close medical

supervision. Effective for depression manifested by psychomotor retardation, apathy, and fatigue.
- Adverse effects ≥ 1%: Tachycardia, CNS stimulation, strong anticholinergic activity, orthostatic hypotension.

Mirtazapine

- Actions: Tetracyclic antidepressant similar to TCAs. Tetracyclics enhance central nonadrenergic and serotonergic activity thought to be due to normalizing of neurotransmission efficacy. It is a potent antagonist of 5-HT$_2$ and 5-HT$_3$ serotonin receptors.
- Used in the treatment of depression.
- Adverse effects ≥ 1%: Somnolence, dizziness, abnormal dreams, tremor confusion, hypertension, vasodilatation, dyspnea, cough.

Anticholinergic Toxicity

Anticholinergic toxicity consists of a characteristic group of both central and peripheral symptoms caused by medications with anticholinergic activity. The symptoms can involve the CNS, cardiovascular system, gastrointestinal system, genitourinary system, and the eyes and sweat glands.[36] Symptoms of anticholinergic toxicity are very common and may be merely uncomfortable in a healthy young individual but have significant impact on the quality of life of the elderly or physically ill. The full syndrome often emerges gradually and is potentially life threatening. Early symptoms include dry mouth, blurred vision, dilated pupils, tachycardia, and difficulty passing urine. As the symptoms progress they may include difficulty swallowing, restlessness, fatigue, and hot, dry, red skin. Changes in mental status usually occur later and include agitation, delirium, auditory and visual hallucinations, and eventually coma state. Death can occur via hyperpyrexia or injury sustained from delirious states. Elderly patients are at an increased risk, as well as patients with organic brain dysfunction or those taking more than one medication.

Drugs causing the syndrome include TCAs, conventional and atypical antipsychotic agents, and anticholinergic drugs. The incidence is unknown but common. The pharmacologic mechanism is the blockade of muscarinic receptors. Management of anticholinergic toxicity is dictated by the severity of the presenting symptoms that include reducing or discontinuing medications, supportive therapy, and physostigmine in cases of acute intoxication.

Monoamine Oxidase Inhibitors

MAOIs were synthesized in the early 1950s with only two MAOIs (phenelzine and tranylcypromine) approved for use in the United States. These drugs are considered second- and third-line antidepressants for most patients because they can be hazardous. However, for patients with atypical depression, MAOIs may be the drug of first choice. Tables 28-6a and 28-6b present the MAOIs and their dosages

MAOIs exert their effects primarily on organ systems influenced by sympathomimetic amines and serotonin. By the inhibition of intraneuronal MAO, the amount of norepinephrine and serotonin available is increased. The increased transmission that results in supranormal quantities is believed to be the key to depression relief.

Phenelzine

- Actions: Potent hydrazine MAOI. Mode of action is unknown. Antidepressant and diverse effects due to irreversible inhibition of MAO, allowing increased concentrations of endogenous epinephrine, norepinephrine, serotonin, and dopamine within presynaptic neurons and at receptor sites. Inhibits hepatic microsomal drug metabolizing enzymes, which may intensify and prolong the effects of many drugs.
- Used for the management of endogenous depression, depressive phase of manic depressive psychosis, and severe exogenous depression that is not responsive to commonly used therapy.
- Adverse effects ≥ 1%: Dizziness, vertigo, headache, orthostatic hypotension, drowsiness, insomnia, fatigue, seizures, mania, hypomania, confusion, delirium, hallucinations, euphoria, hypertension, hypotension.

Table 28-6a Monoamine Oxidase Inhibitors

Drug	Onset	Metabolism	Elimination
Phenelzine	2 wk	Rapid	Urine
Tranylcypromine	10 days	Liver	Urine

Table 28-6b Monoamine Oxidase Inhibitor Dosages

Drug	Dosage
Phenelzine	PO 15 mg tid, max 60–90 mg/day
Isocarboxazid	PO 10–30 mg/day, max 30 mg

PO, oral.

Tranylcypromine

- Actions: Potent nonhydrazine MAOI. Actions and toxicity similar to those of hydrazine MAOIs. Rapid and direct amphetamine-like CNS stimulatory effects.
- Used in severe depression.
- Adverse effects ≥ 1%: Dizziness, vertigo, headache, tremors, muscle twitching, orthostatic hypotension, arrhythmias, hypertensive crisis.

Hypertensive Crisis With MAOIs

A hypertensive crisis involves an acute, severe rise in blood pressure that can result in the impairment of organ systems (e.g., CNS, renal, cardiovascular).[37] The incidence is unknown with psychotropics. One percent to 2% of patients with hypertension can develop a hypertensive emergency with end-organ damage. Phenelzine and tranylcypromine are the common MAOIs associated with hypertensive crisis. These drugs cause irreversible inhibition of MAO. Combination of MAOIs and certain drinks and foods rich in indirectly acting sympathomimetics can precipitate a crisis. Concomitant use of MAOIs with certain antihypertensives, sympathomimetics, antidepressants, narcotics, and precursors of biogenic amines, L-tryptophan, and L-dopa may cause the syndrome.

Many over-the-counter cough and cold remedies containing ephedrine or pseudoephedrine need to be avoided. Concomitant treatment with MAOIs and noradrenergic antidepressants can potentially cause a crisis. The pharmacologic mechanism of dietary interactions reflect blockade of intestinal and liver MAO, allowing increased levels of biogenic amines to enter systemic circulation. These have an indirect sympathomimetic action. This is enhanced by inhibition of neuronal MAO, leading to increased intracellular stores of monoamines, which accounts for many of the drug interactions.

Risk factors and prevention can best be done with patient education, which is the mainstay of prevention. Patients should receive a list of food, beverage, and medications to avoid. These medications and food restrictions must continue for at least 10 to 14 days after the discontinuation of an MAOI.

Hypertensive crisis is a medical emergency and should be treated accordingly. Management includes stopping the MAOI and causal agents, beginning supportive treatment, and correcting blood pressure with appropriate drugs. The β-adrenergic receptor blocker, phentolamine, is the recommended treatment for an MAOI-induced hypertensive crisis.[38] This drug has a rapid onset of action. Patients must be monitored in case the hypertensive state returns or they become hypotensive.

Antidepressant Discontinuation Syndromes

Soon after the introduction of the first TCA into clinical practice, a variety of withdrawal or discontinuation symptoms was described.[39,40] With the introduction of other TCAs, further descriptions of discontinuation symptoms were reported.[41] Similar reports were recounted with MAOIs.[42] It was not until discontinuation syndrome occurred with the SSRIs that this area received attention. Discontinuation symptoms have been steadily reported with many different antidepressants.

Antidepressant discontinuation syndromes share several common features with characteristic symptoms: onset shortly after stopping the antidepressant, short durations when treated, being distinct from a reappearance of the underlying disorder, and rapid suppression by restarting the offending antidepressant. The symptoms usually appear within a few days of stopping the antidepressant, with onset more than 1 week later being unusual. A diverse range of antidepressant discontinuation symptoms have been described, and these vary depending on the antidepressant class.

SSRI discontinuation syndrome comprises a mixture of physical and psychological symptoms. Six main symptom groups are recognized:

1. Sensory, including paresthesia, numbness, visual traits, electric shock sensations
2. Dysequilibrium, including lightheadedness, vertigo, ataxia
3. General somatic symptoms of lethargy, headache, tremor, sweating, and anorexia
4. Sleep disturbances of excessive dreaming, nightmares, and insomnia
5. Gastrointestinal symptoms of nausea, vomiting, and diarrhea
6. Affective symptoms of irritability, anxiety, low mood, and tearfulness

MAOI discontinuation syndromes are often more severe than with other antidepressants. An acute confusional state with disorientation, paranoid delusions, and hallucinations may occur.[43] Anxiety and perceptual disturbances can also occur.[44] A worsening of depressive symptoms, exceeding the severity of the state that originally led to the treatment, is also recognized.[45]

Discontinuation symptoms are common and the incidence variable depending on definition, antidepressant, length of treatment, rate of taper before stoppage, and dose. Abrupt stoppage of many antidepressants leads to more than 33% of patients spontaneously reporting one or more symptoms.[46] Key symptoms are variable depending on the drug. The pharmacologic mechanism is the sudden disruption of CNS system that had adapted to antidepressant treatment. There are four management options: education/support and allow the symptoms to resolve spontaneously, symptomatic treatment, restarting of the antidepressant and tapering off more slowly, and, with intractable general SSRI discontinuation syndromes, switching to fluoxetine, which can be stopped without major problems.

Anxiolytics

Buspirone

- Actions: First-generation agent in a new class of anxiolytics called azapirones. Chemical and pharmacologic properties unrelated to benzodiazepines or other psychotherapeutic drugs. Action is not clear. Seems to be focused mainly on the brain D_2-dopamine receptors. It possesses agonist effects on presynaptic dopamine receptors and a high affinity for serotonin receptors. Seems also to cause less clinically significant impairment of cognitive and motor performance. Produces minimal interaction with other CNS depressants.
- Used for management of anxiety disorders.
- Adverse effects ≥ 1%: Paresthesia, numbness, tremors, headache, dizziness, nervousness, drowsiness, tachycardia, palpitation, hyperventilation, shortness of breath, fatigue and weakness.

Mood-Stabilizing Drugs

Lithium

Mood-stabilizing drugs are used for the treatment of rapid-cycling bipolar disorder. The first-line drug used for symptomatic control of bipolar disorders is lithium. The exact mechanism of action of mood-stabilizing drugs is unknown. Lithium may impart some antidepressant effect by enhancing β receptor activity. Its antimanic properties may be related to its ability to dampen the brain's response to glutamate. Lithium has a narrow therapeutic index and potentially lethal toxicity, which is its most serious adverse effect. Table 28-7 presents lithium's drug profile.

- Actions: Exact mechanism of action is unknown. Behaves like the sodium ion in the body. Competes with various physiologically important cations: Na^+, K^+, Ca^{2+}, Mg^{2+}, affecting cell membranes, body water, and neurotransmitters. At the synapse it accelerates catecholamine destruction, inhibits release of neurotransmitters, and decreases sensitivity of postsynaptic receptors.
- Used for the control and prophylaxis of acute mania and the acute manic phase of bipolar disorder.
- Adverse effects ≥ 1%: Dizziness, headache, lethargy, fatigue, slurred speech, arrhythmias, hypotension, peripheral circulatory collapse, edema, weight gain or loss.

Adverse Syndromes Associated With Lithium

Lithium has a narrow therapeutic index and multiple side effects, which are frequent reasons for noncompliance.[47] The most problematic adverse effects include specific syndromes, namely acute toxicity, diabetes insipidus, renal impairment, hypothyroidism, and rebound mania. Lithium intoxication manifests a variety of symptoms, depending on its degree. Symptom severity is generally proportional to serum levels. Toxicity may occur at levels within the therapeutic range.[48]

Lithium toxicity may be mild, moderate, or severe (Box 28-4). It may result in reversible or irreversible adverse effects. The pharmacologic mechanism is relatively unknown. Lithium overdose patients must be observed for at least 24 hours. Advice may be obtained from poison centers. It is important to measure lithium levels immediately and then repeatedly at 6- to 12-hour periods, depending

Table 28-7 Lithium

Drug	Onset	Metabolism	Elimination	Dosage
Lithium	—	Not metabolized	95% urine 1% feces 4–5% sweat	Adult: Loading dose 600 mg tid, or 900 mg sustained release bid Maintenance 300 mg tid/qid, max 2.4 g/day Child: PO 15–60 mg/kg/day in divided doses

PO, oral.

Box 28-4 Signs and Symptoms of Lithium Toxicity

- Mild toxicity
  - Lightheadedness
  - Drowsiness
  - Blurred vision
  - Nausea
  - Diarrhea
  - Polyuria
  - Fine resting tremor
  - Muscle weakness
- Moderate toxicity
  - Increasing confusions
  - Blackouts
  - Fasciculation
  - Myoclonic twitches
  - Choreoathetoid movements
  - Increased deep tendon reflexes
  - Incontinence
  - Hypernatremia
- Severe toxicity
  - Cerebellar signs
  - Convulsions
  - Coma
  - Cardiac dysrhythmias
  - Sinus and junctional bradycardia
  - Hypotension
  - First-degree heart block
  - Hypertension
  - Renal failure: oliguria, fluid retention, and uremia

---

on clinical presentation. Gastric lavage should be considered. Withdraw prescribed lithium if diagnosis is established. Consider using benzodiazepines during withdrawal period. With mild toxicity, observation with attention to adequate hydration and electrolyte balance is important. With more severe toxicity, hemodialysis may be necessary. Airway management may be necessary for unconscious patients. Hypovolemia must be corrected and convulsions treated as necessary.

Diabetes insipidus results from failure of antidiuretic hormone–dependent urine concentration by the kidney, resulting in the persistent excretion of excessive quantities of urine of low specific gravity. The neurogenic diabetes insipidus results from an inadequate production of antidiuretic hormone by the pituitary gland. In nephrogenic diabetes insipidus, there is a failure of urine concentration in the collecting ducts of the nephron. Estimation of incidence ranges from 15% to 87%. Key symptoms include polyuria, polydipsia, marked dehydration, and associated risk of lithium toxicity and encephalopathy. Lithium-induced diabetes insipidus is predominantly nephrogenic. Possible mechanisms include a reduction in antidiuretic hormone sensitivity through adenyl cyclase and cyclic adenosine monophosphate systems within the tubular cells and down-regulation of aquaphorin gene expression. Management of mild, reversible cases can be treated with lithium dose reduction, combination therapy, or lithium substitution. In severe cases referral to a renal specialist is mandatory for restoration of water and electrolyte imbalance. Thiazide diuretics can be efficacious but should be used only under expert guidance.

Renal impairment results from the deterioration in the glomerular filtration rate through loss or damage to glomeruli, potentially compromising fluid and electrolyte homeostasis and elimination of waste. The incidence is relatively uncertain. Key symptoms include acute oliguria, fluid retention, uremia with nausea and vomiting, and anorexia. The mechanism of renal cell death is unknown. Management includes seeking nephrology opinion, especially in the acute phase, and instituting alternative treatment with other drugs for bipolar patients.

Thyroid dysfunction or hypothyroidism is usually diagnosed by the presence of clinical symptoms and a low serum free thyroxine index or free thyroxine despite high thyroid-stimulating hormone levels and thyroid enlargement. The incidence varies with lithium-induced clinical hypothyroidism 0% to 42% after 15 years of treatment. Twenty percent of patients develop subclinical hypothyroidism. The symptoms may be subtle in mild cases and more pronounced in others. There are many proposed mechanisms, including modulation of TRH receptor expression, reduction of iodine reuptake, and inhibition of thyroid hormone secretion. The management of overt hypothyroidism requires treatment with thyroxine; however, in subclinical hypothyroidism it is controversial. Euthyroid or hypothyroid goiters tend to resolve on lithium withdrawal or use of supplemental thyroxine.

Rebound mania and depression after withdrawal sometimes occur with the withdrawal of lithium prophylaxis. Estimated incidence varies and may be as high as 50%. Pharmacologic basis remains unknown. Management is more preventative with gradual withdrawal, if necessary. Patients should be educated on the increased risks of manic depression on abrupt cessation. Other adverse effects have been reported, with CNS fine tremor in 34% of patients and cognitive impairment in 52% of patients.[49] Various skin complaints have been reported, including psoriasis, exacerbation of acne, urticarial eruptions, warts, lupus-like syndrome, nail pigmentation, and exfoliative dermatitis. Weight gain is a well-recognized adverse effect of lithium as well.

Anesthesia Considerations in the Patient Treated for Mental Illness

Patients being treated for psychiatric disorders are a challenge to the nurse anesthetists. Anesthesia may be needed in these patients for ECT, or the planned procedure may be completely unrelated to the mental illness. Problems unique to this patient population include possible difficulties with communications, pathology associated with some psychiatric disorders, and interactions between drugs used for anesthesia and drugs chronically taken for the treatment of the psychiatric disorder.[50]

Major tranquilizers are commonly used to treat schizophrenia and other psychiatric illnesses. Some of these drugs cause α-adrenergic blockade, resulting in decreased peripheral vascular resistance and hypotension. Hypotension associated with hemorrhage, positive pressure ventilation, and anesthetic agents may be exaggerated in patients receiving these drugs.

Lithium is used in the management of mania. It potentiates the action of nondepolarizing muscle relaxants, and careful monitoring of effect at the myoneural junction is required in these patients.[51] There is a slight increase in the duration of action of succinylcholine in the lithium-treated patient, but it is not likely to be clinically significant.[52]

Patients receiving TCAs may have increased requirements for anesthetic drugs due to elevation of neurotransmitters in the CNS.[53] Administration of sympathomimetics to the patient receiving TCAs is unpredictable. It has been thought for many years that administration of indirect-acting sympathomimetics can lead to an exaggerated response because of increased amounts of norepinephrine available to stimulate postsynaptic receptors. That may be the case in acute administration of sympathomimetics but not after the patient has received the TCAs chronically. Patients receiving TCAs chronically may respond to sympathomimetics with decreased sympathetic nervous system transmission due to down-regulation of the β-adrenergic receptor.[54] These patients may have an exaggerated response to direct-acting or indirect-acting pressor agents. Small doses of a direct-acting agent such as phenylephrine may be the best choice in a patient placed on TCA for less than 6 weeks. After that time careful administration of either direct-acting or indirect-acting pressors are usually well tolerated. In some cases none of the conventional vasopressors will restore blood pressure in these patients. This may be because adrenergic receptors are desensitized or catecholamine depleted. In this case administration of norepinephrine may be the only effective treatment for hypotension.[55]

Because TCAs have anticholinergic side effects, administration of tertiary amine anticholinergics such as atropine or scopolamine may compound the effect and lead to postoperative confusion and delirium. A better choice may be an anticholinergic such as glycopyrrolate that does not cross the blood–brain barrier. Increased availability of norepinephrine in the CNS may result in increased anesthetic requirements for inhaled agents. Use of pancuronium in patients taking high doses of TCAs has been associated with arrhythmias.[56] These drugs are thought to augment the respiratory depressant and opioid effects of opiates and barbiturates, so consideration should be given for careful titration to effect. Lower doses of opiates and hypnotics may result in target effect.

There have been numerous reports of drug interactions in patients receiving MAOIs. Because these drugs are metabolized slowly, adverse reactions can occur up to 3 weeks after discontinuing the drug. Opiates may interact with MAOIs, resulting in an excitatory or depressive effect. The excitatory form is characterized by agitation, headache, hypotension, hypertension, rigidity, hyperpyrexia, convulsions, and coma. The depressive form consists of respiratory depression, hypotension, and coma. Meperidine may cause an excitatory (type 1) or depressant (type 2) response in patients receiving MAOIs and is absolutely contraindicated. The excitatory response is characterized by headache, agitation, skeletal muscle rigidity, and hyperpyrexia. Elevation of serotonin levels in the brain are thought to be responsible for the excitatory response. The depressive response is characterized by hypotension, depression of ventilation, and coma.[57] Synthetic opioids such as fentanyl, sufentanil, and alfentanil have also been associated with adverse reactions in patients taking MAOIs, but the incidence is less than with meperidine. The opioid effects of morphine and barbiturates are potentiated by MAOIs, and a smaller dose is recommended.

Some patients receiving MAOIs may experience an exaggerated response to indirect-acting vasopressors such as ephedrine. This is due to increased release of norepinephrine from postganglionic adrenergic nerve endings. If hypotension must be pharmacologically treated, a direct-acting vasopressor such as phenylephrine may be better tolerated. Receptor sensitivity may enhance blood pressure response to phenylephrine, and it is recommended to reduce the initial dose to one-third and slowly titrate to effect.

In the past it was recommended to withdraw MAOIs 2 to 3 weeks before elective surgery. The reason for this practice was fear of serious cardiovascular and CNS effects during anesthesia and surgery. Today, it is believed that anesthesia can be safely administered without discontinuing these drugs as long as the anesthetist avoids drugs known to result in drug interactions.[58–61] Any anesthetic technique should minimize stimulation of the sympathetic nervous system. Thiopental and etomidate have been administered to MAOI-treated patients for ECT without problems. Methoxycarbonyl-etomidate may be advocated for these procedures in the future. Methoxycarbonyl-etomidate is an etomidate analog that retains etomidate's favorable pharmacologic properties such as rapid onset, high hypnotic potency, and hemodynamic stability. It is metabolized by esterases and is ultra–short acting due to rapid metabolism. It does not produce prolonged adrenocortical suppression after a single IV bolus administration.[62] The response to nondepolarizing neuromuscular blockers is not altered by MAOIs. Regional anesthesia seems to be well tolerated in these patients and has the added advantage of providing postoperative analgesia without need for opioids

SSRIs are generally considered safe when continued preoperatively.[63] Most antipsychotic, antiseizure, and other psychotropics can be continued perioperatively without problems. Some are associated with hypotension during anesthesia, and this can be managed with fluids and vasopressors.

Anesthesia Considerations in Patients Having ECT

ECT may be indicated for severe depression in patients unresponsive to drug therapy, the elderly, and suicidal patients. The therapeutic effect of ECT is thought to be the grand mal seizure lasting 25 to 60 seconds as a result of the electrical stimulus. The relationship between seizure duration and antidepressant effects is unclear, but 25 to 60 seconds seems to be appropriate.[64] The number of ECT treatments is determined by the patient's response.

Major physiologic effects of ECT involve the nervous and cardiovascular systems. In terms of the cerebrovascular system, a transient constriction is followed by vasodilation and increase in cerebral blood flow. The 1.5 to 7 times increase in blood flow is due to changes in arterial pressure. There is also an increase in cerebral oxygen consumption, and intracranial pressure is elevated.

Cardiovascular changes noted during ECT are due to stimulation of the autonomic nervous system. It is a parasympathetic–sympathetic sequence of events. The immediate parasympathetic response results in bradycardia and hypotension. After 1 minute and during the clonic phase of the seizure, tachycardia and hypertension occur. There is an increased myocardial oxygen consumption associated with the sympathetic phase, and dysrhythmias may occur.

Miscellaneous effects of ECT include increased intraocular pressure and increased intragastric pressure. Contraindications to ECT include recent myocardial infarction, recent cerebrovascular accident, and intracranial mass lesion. Relative contraindications include angina pectoris, congestive heart failure, severe pulmonary disease, severe osteoporosis, major bone fractures, glaucoma, retinal detachment, thrombophlebitis, and pregnancy.

General anesthesia is commonly provided for ECT therapy. Because most of these patients are receiving psychotropic drugs, these drugs' mechanisms of action, side effects, and possible interactions with anesthetic drugs and events must be appreciated. Although the initial cardiovascular change associated with ECT may be bradycardia and hypotension, administration of anticholinergics preoperatively is not absolutely mandatory.[65] In a controlled study, no benefit could be found for pretreatment with anticholinergics before ECT.[66] If these agents are necessary for pretreatment, glycopyrrolate seems to have advantages over atropine. They both afford equal protection against parasympathetic responses.

Most hypnotic agents used as anesthetics for ECT have pronounced anticonvulsant properties that interfere with the therapeutic effect. Although most of the currently available induction agents have been used successfully for ECT, methohexital (Brevital) has been one of the more commonly used anesthetic induction agents for ECT. In a study that compared methohexital with propofol for ECT, propofol was found to result in a more moderate increase in blood pressure and shorter seizure duration. The seizure quality did not differ between the two drugs, but there was a tendency toward improved cognitive performance after anesthesia with propofol.[67]

Etomidate is a short-acting nonbarbiturate hypnotic with rapid onset and awakening. It has minimal cardiovascular and respiratory effects but can be associated with myoclonus, pain on injection, and suppression of the adrenal cortex. Seizure duration has been reported to be longer with etomidate than with many other hypnotic drugs.[68] Other studies do not confirm a longer seizure duration with etomidate.[69] Postelectroconvulsive agitation has been reported more frequently with etomidate than with methohexital in one case report.[70]

The addition of alfentanil to etomidate has been shown to result in a significantly reduced heart rate and diastolic and mean arterial blood pressure before and after stimulus. Alfentanil had no effect on seizure duration, but it did prolong apnea. Alfentanil could be useful to reduce tachycardia and hypertension during ECT in high-risk patients without adverse effect on seizure duration.[71]

Propofol has also been used as the primary anesthetic agent for ECT. Although it reduces seizure duration more than etomidate, the difference appears to be smaller in patients with schizophrenia than in those with depression. In comparing etomidate versus propofol for ECT in patients with schizophrenia, the increase in mean arterial pressure was lower with propofol. Propofol was found to reduce seizure duration to a greater extent than etomidate, but there was no significant difference between the two in clinical efficacy. The seizure-induced increase in mean arterial pressure was reduced by propofol more than by etomidate.[72] When propofol was compared with thiopental for ECT, propofol was associated with decreased seizure duration without a significant difference in clinical outcome. Patients anesthetized with propofol received a higher electrical charge.[73]

Major adverse effects of ECT therapy involve the cardiovascular system. The cardiovascular effect of anesthetic induction followed by ECT was studied in 10 healthy volunteers. The cardiovascular response to anesthetic induction was associated with a 13% decrease in cardiac output and 27% increase in heart rate. The convulsion was associated with a 20% increase in heart rate, 34% increase in blood pressure, and 81% increase in cardiac output. These hemodynamic events could have significant impacts on some patient populations.[74] Various cardiac arrhythmias have been reported during ECT, including T-wave and P-wave changes.[75,76] T-wave elevation suggests hyperkalemia, but if serum potassium is normal it is most likely due to sympathetic imbalance. A lowered P wave may also be due to autonomic nervous system imbalance. Pulmonary edema associated with ECT is rare but reported. It is most often due to airway obstruction or excessive sympathetic discharge.[77]

Key Points

- Maintenance drug therapy is valuable in preventing relapse, recurrence, and hospitalization.
- Adverse effects of many of the antipsychotic drugs may initially interfere with patient functioning.
- Posttraumatic stress disorder occurs in the wake of a traumatic event and can lead to flashbacks and lack of responsiveness to stimuli.
- Delusions associated with psychosis can be paranoid in nature and can be divided into primary and secondary delusions.
- A depressive disorder is a syndrome that reflects a sad or irritable mood exceeding normal sadness or grief.
- Neuroleptic malignant syndrome and EPS are associated with the use of antipsychotic drugs.
- Antipsychotic discontinuation syndrome has characteristic symptoms that commence shortly after stopping or reducing the dose of the antipsychotic drug and are unrelated to the underlying disorder.
- TCAs are used as first-line drugs in the treatment of major depression.
- Anticholinergic toxicity consists of a characteristic group of both central and peripheral symptoms caused by medications and anticholinergic activity.
- MAOIs are considered second- and third-line antidepressants for patients because of their hazardous nature.
- Hypertensive crisis involves an acute, severe rise in blood pressure that can result in the impairment of organ systems.
- Lithium is a mood-stabilizing drug used for the treatment of rapid-cycling bipolar disorder.
- Patients receiving TCAs may have increased requirements for anesthetic drugs.

Chapter Questions

1. Why may patients receiving TCAs have increased requirement for anesthetic drugs?
2. What is the major concern of administering meperidine to patients receiving MAOIs?
3. Should patients on MAOIs have their drugs discontinued 2 to 3 weeks before elective surgery?
4. What are the therapeutic and nontherapeutic physiologic effects of ECT?
5. What are the advantages and disadvantages of various induction primary agents in ECT?
6. Why might patients receiving some type of antipsychotic drugs respond better to direct-acting rather than indirect-acting sympathomimetics?

References

1. Lennmarken C, Sydsjo G. Psychological consequences of awareness and their treatment. *Best Pract Res Clin Anaesth.* 2007;21:357–367.

2. Prior TI, Baker GB. Interactions between the cytochrome P450 system and the second generation antipsychotics. *J Psychiatry Neurosci.* 2003;28:99–112.

3. Prior TI, Baker GB. *Miscellaneous Syndromes: Anticholinergic Toxicity, Clozapine Toxicity, and Hypertensive Crisis With MAOIs. Adverse Syndromes and Psychiatric Drugs.* Great Britain: Oxford Press; 2004:293–306.

4. Le Blaye I, Donatini B, Hall M, et al. Acute overdosage with clozapine: a review of available clinical experience. *Pharmaceut Med.* 1992;6:169–178.

5. Mann SC, Caroff SN, Fricchione G, et al. Central dopaminergic hypoactivity and the pathogenesis of neuroleptic malignant syndrome. *Psychiatr Ann.* 2000;30:363–364.

6. Keck PE, Pope HG, McElroy SL. Declining frequency of neuroleptic malignant syndrome in a hospital population. *Am J Psychiatry.* 1991;148:880–882.

7. Gelenberg AJ, Bellinghausen B, Wocjik JD. A prospective survey of neuroleptic malignant syndrome in a short term psychiatric hospital. *Am J Psychiatry.* 1988;145:517–518.

8. Caroff SN. The neuroleptic malignant syndrome *J Clin Psychiatry.* 1080;41:79–83.

9. Hasan S, Buckley P. Novel antipsychotics and the neuroleptic malignant syndrome: a review and critique. *Am J Psychiatry.* 1998;155:1113–1116.

10. Caroff SN, Mann SC, Cambell EC. Atypical antipsychotics and neuroleptic malignant syndrome. *Am J Psychiatry.* 2000;30:314–321.

11. Gill J, Singh H, Nugent K. Acute lithium intoxication and neuroleptic malignant syndrome. *Pharmacotherapy.* 2003; 23:811–815.

12. Heyland D, Sauve M. Neuroleptic malignant syndrome without the use of neuroleptics *CMAJ.* 1991;145:817–819.

13. Heinemann VW, Assion HJ, Hermes G, et al. Paroxetine-induced neuroleptic malignant syndrome *Nervenazi.* 1997; 68:664–666.

14. Fujitake J, Kuno S, Nishitan H. Neuroleptic malignant syndrome-like state in eight patients with parkinsonism. *Clin Neurol.* 1984;24:371–378.

15. Friedmann JH, Feinberg SS, Feldman RG. A neuroleptic-like malignant syndrome due to levodopa therapy withdrawal. *JAMA.* 1985;254:2792–2795.

16. Shalve A, Hermesh H, Munitz H. Mortality from neuroleptic malignant syndrome. *J Clin Psychiatry.* 1989;50:18–25.

17. Mann SC, Caroff SN, Bleier HR, et al. Electroconvulsive therapy for lethal catatonia syndrome, case report and review. *Convuls Ther.* 1990;6:239–247.

18. Keck PE, Pope HG, Cohen BM, et al. Risk factors for neuroleptic syndrome: a case control study. *Arch Gen Psychiatry.* 1989;46:914–918.

19. Kohen D. *Neuroleptic Malignant Syndrome. Adverse Syndromes and Psychiatric Drugs.* Great Britain: Oxford University Press; 2004:21–35.

20. Steck H. Le syndrome extrapyramidal et diencephalique au cours des traitements au Largactil et au Serpasil. *Ann Med Psychol.* 1954;112:737–744.

21. Gervin M, Browne S, Lane A, et al. Spontaneous abnormal involuntary movements in first-episode schizophrenic and schizophreniform disorder: baseline rate in a group of patients from an Irish catchment area. *Am J Psychiatry.* 1998;155:1202–1206.

22. Puri BK, Barnes TR, Chapman MJ, et al. Spontaneous-dyskinesia in a first episode schizophrenia. *J Neurol Neurosurg Psychiatry.* 1999;66:76–78.

23. Leo RJ. Movement disorders associated with the serotonin selective reuptake inhibitors. *J Clin Psychiatry.* 1996; 57:449–454.

24. Lane RM. SSRI-induced extrapyramidal side-effects and akathisia: implications for treatment. *J Psychopharmacol.* 1998;12:192–214.

25. Gill HS, DeVane CL, Riscch SC. Extrapyramidal symptoms associated with cyclic antidepressant treatment: a review of the literature and consolidating hypotheses. *J Clin Psychopharmacol.* 1997;17:377–389.

26. Tyre P, Alexander MS, Regan A, et al. An extrapyramidal syndrome after lithium therapy. *Br J Psychiatry.* 1980;136:191–194.

27. Caroff SN, Mann SC, Campbell EC, et al. Movement disorders associated with atypical antipsychotic drugs. *J Clin Psychiatry.* 2002;63(Suppl. 4):12–19.

28. Swett C. Drug induced dystonia. *Am J Psychiatry.* 1975; 132:532–534.

29. Barnes TRE, Braude WM. Akathisia variants and tardive dyskinesia. *Arch Gen Psychiatry.* 1985;42:874–878.

30. Kennedy PF, Hershon HI, McQuire RJ. Extrapyramidal disorders after prolonged phenothiazine therapy, including a factor analytic study of clinical features. *Br J Psychiatry.* 1971;118:509–518.

31. Ayd FJ. A survey of drug-induced extrapyramidal reactions. *JAMA.* 1961;175:1054–1060.

32. Kane JM, Jeste DV, Barnes TRE, et al. *Tardive Dyskinesia: A Task Force Report of the American Psychiatric Association.* Washington, DC: American Psychiatric Association; 1992.

33. Brooks GW. Withdrawals from neuroleptic drugs. *Am J Psychiatry.* 1959;16:931–932.

34. Greeberg LM, Roth S. Differential effects of abrupt versus gradual withdrawal of chlorpromazine in hospitalized chronic schizophrenic patients. *Am J Psychiatry.* 1964;121:491–493.

35. Dilsaver SC, Alessi NE. Antipsychotic withdrawal symptoms: phenomenology and pathophysiology. *Acta Psychiatr Scand.* 1988;77:241–246.

36. Meltzer HY, Fatemi SH. Treatment of schizophrenia. In: Schaltzberg AF, Nemeroll CB, eds. *The American Psychiatric Press Textbook of Psychopharmacology.* Washington, DC: American Psychiatric Press; 1998:747–774.

37. Prior TI, Baker GB. Miscellaneous syndromes: anticholinergic toxicity, clozapine toxicity, and hypertensive crisis with MAOIs. In: Haddad P, Dursun S, Deakin B, eds. *Adverse Syndromes and Psychiatric Drugs: A Clinical Guide.* Oxford, UK: Oxford Medical Publications; 2004:293–308.

38. Tueth MJ, DeVane CL, Evans DL. Treatment of psychiatric emergencies. In: Schatzberg AF, Nemeroff CB, eds. *The American Psychiatric Press Textbook of Psychopharmacology.* Washington, DC: American Psychiatric Press; 1998:917–929.

39. Mann AM, MacPherson A. Clinical experience with imipramine in the treatment of depression. *Can Psychiatr Assoc J.* 1959;4:38–47.

40. Anderson H, Kristiansen ES. Tofranil treatment of endogenous depressions. *Acta Psychiatr Scand.* 1959;34:387–397.

41. Dilsaver SC, Greden JF. Antidepressant withdrawal induced activation (hypomania and mania): mechanisms and theoretical significance. *Brain Res.* 1984;319:29–48.

42. LeGassicke J, Ashcroft GW, Eccleston D, et al. The clinical state, sleep and amine metabolism of a tranylcypromine (Parnate) addict. *Br J Psychiatry.* 1965;3:357–364.

43. Liskin B, Roose SP, Walsh BT, et al. Acute psychosis following phenelzine discontinuation. *J Clin Psychopharmacol.* 1985;5:46–47.

44. Tyrer P. Clinical effects of abrupt withdrawal from tricyclic antidepressants and monoamine oxidase inhibitors after long term treatment. *J Affect Dis.* 1984;6:1–7.

45. Halle MT, Dilsaver SC. Tranylcypromine withdrawal phenomena. *J Psychiatr Neurosci.* 1993;18:49–50.

46. Rosenbaum JF, Zajecka J. Clinical management of antidepressant discontinuation. *J Clin Psychiatry.* 1997;58(Suppl. 7):37–40.

47. McGreadie RG, Morrison DP. The impact of lithium in South-West Scotland: I. Demographic and clinical findings. *Br J Psychiatry.* 1985;146:70–74.

48. Spiers J, Hirsch SR. Severe lithium toxicity with normal serum concentrations. *BMJ.* 1978;281:815–816.

49. Ghose K. Lithium salts: therapeutic and unwanted effects. *Br J Hosp Med.* 1977;18:578–583.

50. Sedwick JV, Lewis IH, Linter SPK. Anesthesia and mental illness. *Int J Psych Med.* 1990;20:209–225.

51. Hill GE, Wong KC, Hodges MR. Lithium carbonate and neuromuscular blocking agents. *Anesthesiology.* 1977;46:122–126.

52. Dawson J, Karallikdde L. Drug interactions and the clinical anesthetist. *Eur J Anaesthesiol.* 1998;15:172–189.

53. Miller RD, Way WL, Eger EI. The effects of alpha-methyldopa, reserpine, guanethidine, and iproniazid on minimum alveolar anesthetic requirement (MAC). *Anesthesiology.* 1968;29:1153–1158.

54. Braverman MT, McCarthy RJ, Ivankovich AD. Vasopressor challenges during chronic during chronic MAOI or TCA treatment in the anesthetized dog. *Life Sci.* 1987;40:2587–2595.

55. Sprung J, Schoenwald PK, Levy P, et al. Treating intraoperative hypotension in a patient on long-term tricyclic antidepressants: a case of aborted aortic surgery. *Anesthesiology.* 1997;86:990–992.

56. Edwards RP, Miller RD, Roizen MF, et al. Cardiac responses to imipramine and pancuronium during anesthesia with halothane or enflurane. *Anesthesiology.* 1979;50:421–425.

57. Pavy TJG, Kliffer AP, Douglas MJ. Anesthetic management of labour and delivery in a woman taking long-term MAOI. *Can J Anaesth.* 1995;42:618–620.

58. Wells DG, Bjorksten AR. Monoamine oxidase inhibitors revisited. *Can J Anaesth.* 1989;36:64–74.

59. Stack CG, Rogers P, Linter PSK. Monoamine oxidase inhibitors and anesthesia. *Br J Anaesth.* 1988;60:222–227.

60. Huyse FJ, Touw JD, van Schijndel RS, et al. Psychotropic drugs and the perioperative period: a proposal for a guideline for elective surgery. *Psychosomatics.* 2006;47:8–22.

61. el-Ganzouri AR, Ivankovich AD, Braverman B, et al. Monoamine oxidase inhibitors: should they be discontinued preoperatively? *Anesth Analg.* 1985;64:592–596.

62. Cotton JF, Husain SS, Forman SA, et al. Methoxycarbonyletomidate. *Anesthesiology.* 2009;111:240–249.

63. Nagelhout J, Elisha S, Waters E. Should I continue or discontinue that medication? *AANAJ.* 2009;77:59–73.

64. Gaines GY, Rees DI. Electroconvulsive therapy and anesthetic considerations. *Anesth Analg.* 1986;65:1345–1356.

65. Vereeke G, Troch E. Atropine before ECT. *Anaesth Intens Care.* 1982;10:166.

66. Wyant GM, MacDonald WB. The role of atropine in electroconvulsive therapy. *Anaesth Intens Care.* 1980;8:445–450.

67. Geretsegger C, Nickel M, Judendorfer B, et al. Propofol and methohexital as anesthetic agents for electroconvulsive

therapy: a randomized, double-blind comparison of electroconvulsive therapy seizure quality, therapeutic efficacy, and cognitive performance. *J ECT.* 2007;23:239–243.

68. Christensen P, Kragh-Sorensen P, Sorensen C, et al. Electroencephalographic-monitored ECT: a comparison of seizure duration under anesthesia with etomidate and thiopentone. *Convuls Ther.* 1986;2:145–150.

69. Avramov MN, Husain MM, White PP. The comparative effects of methohexital, propofol, and etomidate for electroconvulsive therapy. *Anesth Analg.* 1995;81:596–602.

70. Freeman SA. Post-electroconvulsive therapy agitation with etomidate. *J ECT.* 2009;25:133–134.

71. van den Broek WW, Groenland HN, Kusuma A, et al. Double-blind placebo controlled study of the effects of etomidate-alfentanil anesthesia in electroconvulsive therapy. *J ECT.* 2004;20:107–111.

72. Gazdag G, Kocsis N, Tolna J, et al. Etomidate versus propofol for electroconvulsive therapy in patients with schizophrenia. *J ECT.* 2004;20:225–229.

73. Bauer J, Hageman I, Dam H, et al. Comparison of propofol and thiopental as anesthetic agents for electroconvulsive therapy. *J ECT.* 2009;25:85–90.

74. Wells DG, Davies GG. Hemodynamic changes associated with electroconvulsive therapy. *Anesth Analg.* 1987; 66:1193–1195.

75. Khoury GF, Benedetti C. T-wave changes associated with electroconvulsive therapy. *Anesth Analg.* 1989;69:677–679.

76. Bayar R, Emul M, Yuran S, et al. Electrocardiographical P wave changes after electroconvulsive therapy in patients with schizophrenia. *J ECT.* 2009;25:26–30.

77. Sargent P, Reeves J. Pulmonary edema after electroconvulsive therapy. *J ECT.* 2008;24:283–285.

29

Pharmacology of Congestive Heart Failure

Anthony Chipas, PhD, CRNA
Reamer Bushardt, PharmD, RPh, PA-C

Objectives

After completing this chapter, the reader should be able to

- Discuss the pathophysiology of congestive heart failure.
- Describe how at least three classes of drugs work to correct abnormal pathophysiology.
- Explain the importance of beta-blocker in patients with diastolic heart failure.
- Identify how Gs, Gq, cyclic AMP, and cyclic guanosine monophosphate interact to cause normal cellular function.
- Distinguish the anesthesia implications of drugs used to treat heart failure.

Epidemiology

The American Heart Association defines heart failure as a chronic, progressive condition in which the heart muscle is unable to pump enough blood through the heart to meet the body's needs for blood and oxygen.[1] Heart failure is a major public health burden with a growing prevalence and disparate impact on elderly patients. According to data from the Framingham Heart Study, the incidence of heart failure approaches 10 per 1000 population after 65 years of age, and two-thirds of those individuals have a history of hypertension.[1] At age 40 years the lifetime risk of developing heart failure is one in five for men and women. The lifetime risk for a person with average blood pressure of 160/90 mm Hg is twice as high as the risk for those with average blood pressure of 140/90 mm Hg.

The American Heart Association reports that yearly rates for new heart failure events per 1000 population for white men are 15.2 for those 65 to 74 years of age, 31.7 for those 75 to 84 years of age, and 65.2 for those 85 years of age and older. For white women the rates are 8.2, 19.8, and 45.6, respectively. For black men the rates are 16.9, 25.5, and 50.6, respectively, and for black women the estimated rates are 14.2, 25.5, and 44.0, respectively.[2] Data from Kaiser Permanente indicated an increase in the incidence of heart failure with an improved survival rate among the elderly, with both of these findings greatest among men.[3]

The Framingham Heart Study found hypertension to be the most common risk factor for heart failure followed closely by prior myocardial infarction.[4] Bibbins-Domingo et al. studied postmenopausal women with established coronary disease and found diabetes mellitus to be the strongest risk factor for heart failure, especially those with elevated body mass indices or reduced creatinine clearance.[5] Additional research indicates that diabetes mellitus is associated with an increased mortality among heart failure patients.[6]

According to the National Center for Health Statistics, one in eight deaths in the United States has heart failure mentioned on the death certificate.[7] Analysis of Framingham Heart Study data revealed that 80% of men and 70% of women aged 65 years or older with heart failure will die within 8 years. After a diagnosis of heart failure, the 1-year mortality rate is high, with one in five dying.[4] Heart failure patients often die from sudden cardiac death, with a rate six to nine times that of the general population.[8] Heart failure is a leading cause of hospitalization and reason for ambulatory care. In 2009 the estimated cost, both direct and indirect, of heart failure in the United States was $37.2 billion.[9]

Etiology and Pathophysiology

Heart failure is the result of numerous cardiac disorders and diseases. The most common causes are coronary artery disease, hypertension, and dilated cardiomyopathy. Additional causes of heart failure include other forms of ischemic heart disease, high-output states, aortic or mitral regurgitation, aortic or mitral stenosis, congenital cardiomyopathy, constrictive pericarditis, septicemia, Paget's disease, thyrotoxicosis, alcohol excess, acromegaly, anemia, illicit drug use, and viral illness.[10]

The various causes of heart failure lead to reduced ventricular function, which results in hypoperfusion. The clinical syndrome that comprises heart failure is explained by compensatory mechanisms, such as cardiac hypertrophy and activation of the sympathetic nervous system and the renin-angiotensin-aldosterone system.[10] Heart failure is often described by which component of the cardiac cycle initially leads to the ventricular dysfunction, namely systolic or diastolic failure. In systolic failure the left ventricle loses its ability to contract normally and cannot pump with enough force to maintain adequate circulation, which results in a decreased ejection fraction. Most patients with heart failure have evidence of systolic dysfunction that often coexists with diastolic dysfunction. Isolated diastolic failure, which occurs in about one-third of heart failure patients, is associated with a preserved ejection fraction. The major cause of diastolic dysfunction is long-standing hypertension. Ventricular dysfunction can also involve one or more sides of the heart. Patients with symptoms of right-sided heart failure exhibit systemic congestion, whereas left-sided heart failure is associated with pulmonary congestion symptoms.[10,11]

Heart failure, previously described as a syndrome characterized by reduced cardiac output and increased venous pressure, is associated with underlying molecular changes that damage and lead to death of cardiac muscle cells. Compensatory mechanisms engaged by the body in response to loss of myocardium include tachycardia, increased preload, increased afterload, cardiac hypertrophy, and cardiac remodeling. Compensatory mechanisms, however, are closely tied to disease progression. Increased preload impairs contractile function and worsens declines in carbon monoxide. The chronic inotropic and chronotropic responses to the compensatory increase in sympathetic activation increase myocardial oxygen demand, promote ischemia, contribute to the development of arrhythmia, and further deter systolic and diastolic function. Compensatory arteriolar vasoconstriction leads to increased afterload that impairs forward ejection of blood from the heart to the periphery. The body's response to a decline in carbon monoxide levels has been termed the neurohormonal response.[10,12]

The hemodynamic reactions attempt to maintain perfusion pressure in the major organs by increasing circulating blood volume, inducing vasoconstriction, and stimulating the heart. An inflammatory response, which involves cytokines and reactive oxygen species, acts as if the body were facing an exogenous insult. The hypertrophic response and ventricular remodeling lead to structural changes in cardiac muscle cells and in the shape of the ventricular chamber. The neurohormonal response is comprised of regulatory and counterregulatory effects involving vasoconstriction, sodium retention, inotropism, and proliferation.[10,12] Key regulatory pathways activated in the neurohormonal response involve angiotensin II, aldosterone, norepinephrine, endothelin, and vasopressin. Counterregulatory hormones, such as the natriuretic peptides, bradykinin, and nitric oxide, are also involved.[12]

Classification

The diagnosis of heart failure, which is a clinical syndrome, is made by collectively evaluating a combination of characteristic symptoms and signs along with diagnostic testing. Although symptoms can be equivalent to those associated with other conditions, characteristic signs (i.e., jugular venous distention, basilar rales, and a third heart sound) and newer diagnostic testing (i.e., plasma B-type natriuretic peptide or contrast magnetic resonance imaging) have greater specificity and sensitivity.[13–15]

The two best recognized systems for classifying patients with heart failure are the New York Heart Association (NYHA) Functional Classification System (Table 29-1)[16] and the American Heart Association/American College of Cardiology (AHA/ACC) Stages of Heart Failure.[17] The NYHA system is based on a healthcare provider's assessment of the activity level and exercise tolerance of a heart failure patient, and the class is subject to variability and whether patients improve or worsen. The AHA/ACC stages of heart failure address the development of heart failure and its eventual progression, which address major risk factors for the development of heart failure, structural heart disease, symptomatic heart failure, and treatment-refractory or end-stage heart failure. The two systems are complementary, addressing two important dimensions of this syndrome, which are intermittent episodes of symptomatic periods and chronic progression. To provide organization to the numerous treatments available for heart failure patients, the discussion here of drug management is focused into chronic and acute heart failure.

As patients develop congestive heart failure, considerable cardiac (especially ventricular) remodeling and structural alterations take place. These changes, if unregulated, lead to ventricular dysfunction and are the main targets for therapeutic interventions. Cardiac failure can be systolic, diastolic, or combined. Systolic failure is the heart's inability

Table 29-1 New York Heart Association Functional Classification System

Class	Symptoms
Class I (mild)	No limitation of physical activity. Ordinary physical activity does not cause undue fatigue, palpitation, or dyspnea.
Class II (mild)	Slight limitation of physical activity. Comfortable at rest, but ordinary physical activity results in fatigue, palpitation, or dyspnea.
Class III (moderate)	Marked limitation of physical activity. Comfortable at rest, but less than ordinary activity causes fatigue, palpitation, or dyspnea.
Class IV (severe)	Unable to carry out any physical activity without discomfort. Symptoms of cardiac insufficiency at rest. If any physical activity is undertaken, discomfort is increased.

to fully contract, decreasing cardiac output. Most patients presenting with acute failure exhibit systolic dysfunction.[18,19]

Diastolic failure impedes the heart's ability to relax, restricting left ventricular inflow, causing increased filling pressures, pulmonary edema, and decreased cardiac output independent of cardiac performance. Diastolic heart failure usually has a slower onset and leads to greater physiologic and anatomic changes, including increased afterload (increased wall stress) with subsequent increase in oxygen consumption, subendocardial hypoperfusion leading to endocardial ischemia and angina, and increased myocardial hemodynamic overloading. Patients coming to surgery with heart failure, especially for coronary artery grafting, have a threefold increase in perioperative mortality and morbidity.[20] In addition to the physical and anatomic changes, many neuroendocrine changes also take place, such as changes in the renin-angiotensin-aldosterone system.

Pharmacologic agents used in the acute treatment of heart failure are aimed at decreasing preload (diuretics, nitrates), decreasing afterload (calcium channel blockers, angiotensin-converting enzyme [ACE] inhibitors), enhancing contractility (positive inotropes, phosphodiesterase inhibitors), or slowing heart rate (β_1 antagonists).

Treatment

Goals of treatment for chronic heart failure include preventing or delaying onset of symptomatic diastolic heart failure, minimizing symptoms, reducing hospitalizations, improving quality of life, slowing disease progression, and reducing mortality. These goals are well reflected in the guidelines for the diagnosis and management of heart failure in adults from the American Heart Association/American College of Cardiology, which were updated in 2009.[18,19] Because heart failure represents a clinical syndrome with various underlying causes, treatment goals are also focused on managing the underlying etiology for cardiovascular dysfunction.

Nondrug interventions for chronic heart failure include regular exercise or cardiac rehabilitation as tolerated, cessation of alcohol or tobacco, modest weight reductions for overweight and obese patients, dietary changes such as sodium reduction or fluid restriction for carefully selected patients, regular self-monitoring of fluid status and exercise tolerance, psychosocial support, and preventative measures like immunizations.[17,18,21] It is important that patients undertake dietary changes and weight loss strategies under the direction of a health professional because of varying degrees of risk and benefit for these strategies based on a patient's history and clinical status.[22]

Drug and nondrug therapies directed at underlying etiologies for heart failure are essential, such as hypertension, dyslipidemia and coronary artery disease, diabetes mellitus, obstructive sleep apnea, renal disease, hyperthyroidism, or anemia. Avoidance or cautious use of drug therapies associated with precipitating or worsening heart failure should also be considered. Such drugs associated with heart failure exacerbation include nonsteroidal anti-inflammatory drugs, amphetamines, corticosteroids, tricyclic antidepressants, thiazolidinediones, peripheral alpha antagonists, and selected antiarrhythmics and calcium channel blockers.[18,22]

The drugs demonstrated as effective in chronic heart failure are well outlined in the staging and treatment diagram presented in the recent guidelines developed by the American Heart Association/American College of Cardiology. In addition to the goals set forth in this document, the specific therapeutic options are identified within each stage of heart failure.

For patients in stage A, drug treatment is intensified around minimizing disease-associated injury to the heart, which drives progression toward symptomatic heart failure. Gold standards include use of ACE inhibitors in patients with hypertension, vascular disease, or diabetes mellitus. Angiotensin receptor blocker (ARB) therapy is also an option for individuals not well suited to or intolerant of ACE inhibitors. Individuals with atherosclerosis, especially high-risk patients with prior episodes, cardiac ischemia, or diabetes mellitus, benefit from lipid-lowering therapies. In addition to decreasing risk for symptomatic heart failure, these strategies can also help to decrease risk for associated complications such as myocardial infarction and stroke.[18,22]

For patients in stage B, drug therapy is focused on the previously mentioned neurohormonal dimension of heart failure, which leads to worsening cardiac dysfunction and myocardial remodeling. In stage B, drug therapy is largely targeted to prevent or delay the onset of heart failure symptoms. Primary alternatives include ACE inhibitor or ARB therapy plus β-adrenergic blocker therapy. Selected patients may also benefit from an implantable defibrillator (ICD). The guidelines report that ICD placement is reasonable in patients with ischemic cardiomyopathy who recently suffered a myocardial infarction, have a left ventricular ejection fraction of 30% or less, are NYHA class I on optimal drug therapy, and are expected to survive with good function for more than a year. With slightly less support from the literature, the guidelines also consider ICD placement in patients without heart failure but who are otherwise similar to the prior group.[18]

For patients in stage C with symptomatic left ventricular dysfunction, drug therapy is targeted at symptom management, maximizing function, slowing disease progression, and reducing mortality or risk for hospitalization. ACE inhibitors are recommended for all patients who do not possess contraindications, and ARB therapy may be useful in some patients intolerant to an ACE inhibitor.[6] Several β-adrenergic blocker agents (i.e., bisoprolol, carvedilol, and sustained-release metoprolol succinate) have proven valuable benefits, including reduced mortality.[23-25] Diuretics are used for fluid imbalance and relieve symptoms. The two most commonly used types of diuretics for volume control in heart failure are thiazide and loop diuretics. Among these, loop diuretics are the most widely prescribed. Loop agents offer more potent diuresis than thiazides, but the thiazides are uniquely useful in patients with chronic hypertension because these agents are proven to maintain blood pressure reductions in a wide variety of patients. Agents targeting the neurohormonal dimension of heart failure work to minimize the damaging compensatory mechanisms orchestrated by the sympathetic nervous system and renin-angiotensin-aldosterone pathway. Selected patients may also receive an aldosterone antagonist, digoxin, or a combination of hydralazine and a nitrate. The combination of hydralazine and a nitrate has been shown to improve outcomes for African American patients with moderate to severe symptoms who are already receiving standard therapy with an ACE inhibitor, β-adrenergic blockers, and diuretic therapy.[18] Selected patients should also be considered for biventricular pacing or an ICD.[26-28]

For patients with stage D heart failure (end-stage or treatment-refractory), the goals may be less aggressive, such as improving quality of life and reducing hospitalization rates. Therapeutic options may include intravenous vasoactive therapies, optimization of oral medications, transplantation when appropriate, mechanical support, experimental interventions, and palliative care.[18]

Diuretics

Most patients exhibiting signs of congestive heart failure have acute fluid overload that is not handled well by the overloaded and overworked left ventricle. Although there is adequate volume, cardiac output is insufficient to meet the metabolic demands of the body. Diuretics target the increased sodium retention that occurs in heart failure, and controlled clinical trials demonstrated the ability of diuretic drugs to increase urinary sodium excretion.[29] Diuretics therefore have become an essential class of drugs for the symptomatic treatment of heart failure, often being used in combinations. Thiazide and loop diuretics primarily increase urinary sodium and free water excretion in the kidneys, thereby relieving acute symptoms of volume overload.

Commonly prescribed and well-studied thiazide diuretics include hydrochlorothiazide and chlorthalidone. And as previously stated, thiazide diuretics also convey long-lasting antihypertensive effects but have reduced effectiveness of diuresis in patients with renal insufficiency or creatinine clearance less than 30 mL/min. Potent thiazide diuretics, such as metolazone, may also be administered before loop diuresis when patients require additional volume reductions or exhibit resistance to monotherapy with a loop agent. Loop diuretics, such as furosemide, are the most commonly used diuretics for heart failure. Loop agents also retain diuretic activity in patients with renal insufficiency.

There are distinct pharmacologic differences among several of the loop diuretics that impact their therapeutic benefit with various patient presentations. Bioavailability after oral dosing of furosemide is approximately 50%, whereas bioavailability is nearly complete after oral dosing of torsemide or bumetanide. Absorption of furosemide and bumetanide is affected by food, but absorption of torsemide is not. The maximal response to loop diuretic therapy in patients with heart failure is also often reduced. This diuretic resistance, as it is often called, is related to a compensatory increase in sodium reabsorption in both the proximal and distal tubules that conversely reduces the diuretic action in the loop of Henle. Adverse effects associated with diuretic therapy include fluid and electrolyte disturbances, such as dehydration and hypokalemia.[30,31]

Diuretic resistance is a clinical manifestation identified in chronic or decompensated heart failure patients on long-term diuretic therapy. Intravascular depletion, rebound sodium uptake after volume loss, hypertrophy of the distal nephron, and reduced tubular secretion all contribute to diuretic resistance and predict a poor prognosis.[32] Low-output states also impair renal perfusion and prevent proper diuretic function. In these circumstances, changing the diuretic administration route or combining diuretic therapy with inotropes, such as dobutamine or dopamine, to increase forward flow can be efficacious.

Diuretics are classified according to either their site of action or which electrolyte is preserved. These classifications include loop diuretics, thiazide diuretics, potassium-sparing diuretics, carbonic anhydrase inhibitors, and osmotic diuretics (Table 29-2).

Loop Diuretics

These are a very potent class of diuretics because they work in the ascending loop of Henle. Loop diuretics inhibit the cotransporters of sodium, inhibiting the reuptake of sodium and causing both diuresis and natriuresis.

Thiazide Diuretics

This class of diuretics is the most commonly used. They work in the distal tubules and are therefore not as potent as loop diuretics. Initially, the use of thiazide and loop diuretics in combination may cause the increased reabsorption of sodium while excreting potassium and hydrogen ions, causing metabolic alkalosis. This combination may stimulate the renin-angiotensin-aldosterone system by reducing blood pressure and increasing sodium and water reabsorption while causing the elimination of potassium and hydrogen ions. This combination leads to metabolic alkalosis.

Potassium-Sparing Diuretics

Some diuretics in this class of drugs are aldosterone receptor antagonists in the distal tubule. This causes increased sodium and water excretion while reclaiming potassium and hydrogen ions, potentially leading to hyperkalemia and metabolic acidosis.

Carbonic Anhydrase Inhibitors

This class of diuretic causes the reabsorption of most of the glomerular bicarbonate, pulling sodium with it. This leads to sodium bicarbonate–induced diuresis. Carbonic anhydrase inhibitors are considered a weak class of diuretics and can lead to hypokalemia and metabolic acidosis.

Osmotic Diuretics

Mannitol is filtered freely in the glomerulus.[33] It exerts an osmotic effect in the proximal tubule and ascending loop

Table 29-2 Diuretic Actions and Precautions

Class	Drugs	Adverse Effects	Drug Interactions
Loop	Bumetanide	Potassium abnormality	Potassium abnormality may potentiate digitalis toxicity
	Ethacrynic acid	Hypomagnesemia	Nonsteroidal anti-inflammatory drugs: reduce efficacy
	Furosemide	Hypotension	Corticosteroids
	Torsemide	Ototoxicity	Aminoglycosides
Thiazide	Chlorothiazide	Potassium abnormality	Potassium abnormality may potentiate digitalis toxicity
	Hydrochlorothiazide	Metabolic alkalosis	Nonsteroidal anti-inflammatory drugs: reduce efficacy
	Metolazone	Hypotension	Beta-blockers potentiate hyperglycemia
		Hyponatremia	
		Hypertriglyceridemia	
		Hyperglycemia	
Potassium-sparing	Eplerenone	Hyperkalemia	Nonsteroidal anti-inflammatory drugs: reduce efficacy
	Spironolactone	Metabolic acidosis	
	Triamterene	Peptic ulcers	
Carbonic anhydrase inhibitors	Acetazolamide	Potassium abnormality	
	Methazolamide	Metabolic acidosis	
Osmotic	Mannitol	Hypotension	
		Hypokalemia	

of Henle to cause sodium reabsorption to increase osmotic pressure. This increase of pressure causes the reabsorption of water and the exchange of potassium hydrogen ions, leading to hypokalemia and metabolic alkalosis.

Natriuretic Peptides

Congestive heart failure leads to activation of the renin-angiotensin-aldosterone system, causing water retention and ultimately increased central venous pressure. Natriuretic peptides (NAP) are naturally occurring hormones that are produced and stored in many organs, including the heart. Atrial natriuretic peptide is a naturally occurring hormone that is released when the atrium becomes overdistended. Brain natriuretic peptide is synthesized in the atrium of the heart but stored and excreted by the brain in response to venous congestion. The effect of NAP promotes potent sodium excretion, diuresis, vasodilation (arterial and venous dilation), and suppression of the renin-angiotensin-aldosterone axis; lowers sympathetic tone; lowers the activation threshold of vagal afferents; and inhibits secretion of vasopressin. This leads to a reduction of both blood pressure and volume.

Nesiritide is a sterile, purified preparation of human B-type natriuretic peptide. It is manufactured from *Escherichia coli* using recombinant DNA technology and has the same 32-amino acid sequence as the endogenous B-type natriuretic peptide produced by the ventricular myocardium. The mean terminal elimination half-life of nesiritide in patients with heart failure is approximately 18 minutes.[34] Nesiritide is approved for systolic dysfunction heart failure. This drug has poor bioavailability and is only available for intravenous administration. The drug is started at 2 μg/kg bolus followed by a continuous infusion of 0.01 μg/kg/min slowly titrated to a maximum dose of 0.03 μg/kg/min. Human B-type natriuretic peptide is eliminated from the circulation by three independent mechanisms in the following order of decreasing importance[33]: (1) binding to cell surface natriuretic peptide clearance receptors (receptor C) with subsequent cellular internalization and isosomal proteolysis; (2) proteolytic cleavage by neutral endopeptidases present within renal tubular cells and vascular cells, and (3) renal filtration clearance of nesiritide.[34]

ACE Inhibitors

ACE inhibitors serve as effective antihypertensive agents while decreasing neurohormonal activation in this syndrome. ACE inhibitors prevent the conversion of angiotensin I to angiotensin II, which is a potent vasoconstrictor

and driver of cardiac remodeling. This vasoconstrictor is formed by the proteolytic action of renin (released by the kidneys) acting on circulating angiotensinogen to form angiotensin I. Angiotensin I is then converted by the enzyme peptidyl dipeptidase, an endothelial ACE, to angiotensin II, an arterial vasoconstrictor.[35] ACE inhibitors decrease the production of peptidyl dipeptidase.

A large body of evidence for this class of agents has shown benefit in various cardiovascular and renal diseases, with favorable cardiac effects such as increases in cardiac index and reductions in left ventricular filling pressures, systemic vascular resistance, heart rate, and mean arterial pressure. Studies of ACE inhibitor therapy in patients with heart failure demonstrated reduced mortality and morbidity as well as improvements in clinical symptoms, NYHA functional class, left ventricular size, quality of life, and hospitalization rates.[35,36] ACE inhibitors also reduce the breakdown of the chemical bradykinin, which results in arterial and venous dilation accompanied by preload and afterload reductions. It is also believed the elevated levels of bradykinin may cause a persistent dry, hacking cough that occurs in some patients. Additional potential adverse effects include hypotension, hyperkalemia, angioedema, and acute renal failure.

ACE inhibitors are contraindicated in patients with bilateral renal artery stenosis, angioedema, and pregnancy. ACE inhibitors are well recognized to preserve renal failure in many patients, but, as noted, they can also lead to acute worsening of renal function. The effect largely depends on an individual patient's clinical picture before use of the ACE inhibitor. Patients with elevated baseline serum creatinine levels (i.e., > 2.5 mg/dL), hyponatremia, significant reductions in left ventricular function, or dehydration are particularly vulnerable to the potentially deleterious effects of these drugs.[17,18,36–39]

ACE inhibitors produce vasodilation by inhibiting the formation of angiotensin II (Figure 29-1). ACE inhibitors have the following actions:

- Reduces both preload and afterload by dilating arteries and veins
- Blocks the effects of angiotensin II on sympathetic nerve release and reuptake of norepinephrine, thereby down-regulating the effects of the sympathetic nervous system
- Lowers blood volume and arterial pressure by promoting renal excretion of sodium and water
- Inhibits cardiac and vascular remodeling associated with chronic hypertension, heart failure, and myocardial infarction

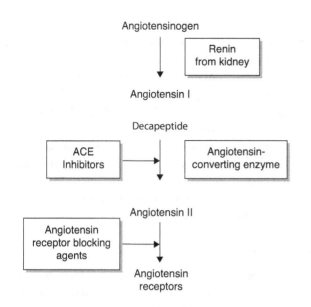

Figure 29-1 Site of action ACEI and ARBS.

Side Effects

ACE inhibitors have a relatively low incidence of side effects and are well tolerated. One of the potential side effects (10–30%) is a dry cough that appears to be related to elevations in bradykinin. Angioedema, life-threatening airway swelling and obstruction (0.1–0.2%), and hyperkalemia are less common adverse effects of ACE inhibition. It is thought that these are caused by decreased aldosterone production. The incidence of angioedema is more common in African American patients, occurring at a rate two to four times that of white patients. ACE inhibitors are contraindicated in pregnancy. During the first trimester ACE inhibitors may be teratogenic. During the second and third trimesters they are contraindicated because of the risk of fetal hypotension and death. Commonly prescribed ACE inhibitors are captopril, enalapril, and lisinopril (Table 29-3).

ARB Agents

ARB agents selectively block the effects of angiotensin II at angiotensin receptor type one (AT_1), thus preventing angiotensin II–mediated vasoconstriction, aldosterone release, and cellular proliferation. These receptors normally work through the Gq-protein transduction pathway to stimulate vascular smooth muscle contraction. These drugs have no effect on bradykinin metabolism, which aids in their vasodilating effects. ARB therapies do not interfere with binding at angiotensin receptor type two (AT_2), which mediates

vasodilation and discourages ventricular remodeling. ACE inhibitors are still preferentially prescribed, but ARB agents are considered appropriate alternatives to ACE inhibitors in heart failure patients who cannot tolerate or do not respond well to ACE inhibitors. Clinical trial data between these two classes of drugs show similar effects with regard to reductions in mortality, hospitalization rates, and sudden cardiac death. Currently, ARB drugs are significantly more expensive than most ACE inhibitors. ARB agents, like ACE inhibitors, may produce hypotension and hyperkalemia but do not produce a cough. Similar effects on renal function are present with ARB agents and ACE inhibitors, and ARB agents are also contraindicated with bilateral renal artery stenosis or pregnancy.[18,19,40,41]

ARB agents have the following actions:

- Reduces preload and afterload by arterial dilation
- Down-regulates the sympathetic nervous system
- Blocks the effects of angiotensin II on the kidneys, stimulating diuresis and sodium excretion
- Inhibits cardiac remodeling

Side Effects

The side effects can be similar to ACE inhibitors, including dry cough and angioedema. Commonly used drugs include eprosartan, losartan, and candesartan (Table 29-3).

Aldosterone Antagonists

The aldosterone antagonists spironolactone and eplerenone are weak diuretics that tend to spare potassium; thus they are often termed potassium-sparing diuretics. These agents can also produce sustained reductions in blood pressure. Patients with heart failure experience elevated levels of aldosterone, which contribute to disease progression, and subsequent therapy with aldosterone antagonists can produce significant benefits for patients.

Table 29-3 ACE Inhibitors and ARB Agents

	Half-life (h)	Initial Dose (mg/day)	Maintenance Dose (mg/day)
ACE inhibitors			
Captopril	2.2	20–75	75–150
Enalapril		2.5	10–40
Lisinopril	12	10	10–80
ARB agents			
Eprosartan			
Losartan	1–2	50	25–100

Clinical studies with these agents in heart failure patients have yielded reductions in mortality and hospitalization as well as improvements in clinical symptoms. The American Heart Association/American College of Cardiology guidelines recommend β-adrenergic blocker therapy for selected patients in stage C.[35] A common side effect is hyperkalemia. An advantage of eplerenone over spironolactone is the lack of potential sexual side effects that can occur in some patients using spironolactone.[18,19,42,43]

Cardiostimulatory Drugs

Cardiostimulatory drugs improve cardiac output in congestive failure in a number of different ways. They increase inotropy (contractility), chronotropy (heart rate), lusitropy (ventricular relaxation), and dromotropy (electrical conductivity). During periods of cardiac failure, cardiac output may be improved to meet the metabolic needs of the body by either reducing afterload or enhancing myocardial contractility.

Positive Inotropes (β Receptor Agonists)

β Receptor agonists resemble the naturally occurring actions of the sympathetic nervous system in the cardiac and vascular smooth muscle and in the muscles that control the airway. β Receptor agonists have low bioavailability and therefore must be given by infusion and are usually only good for short-term interventions (Table 29-4). The naturally occurring hormones, primarily norepinephrine, act on the β_1 receptors of the heart, causing, through an

intermediary Gq-protein, an increase in intracellular cAMP, which leads to an increased intracellular calcium. This process also stimulates an increased released of calcium from the sarcoplasmic reticulum into the cardiac myocytes, enhancing inotropy. At the same time there is an opening of the sinoatrial pacemaker cell, causing an increased chronotropy.

Vascular and bronchial smooth muscle have a larger number of β_2 receptors that when acted on primarily by epinephrine stimulate the production of cAMP, causing relaxation of the vessels and bronchodilation. This process is again mediated by Gs-proteins.

Dobutamine

Dobutamine is a synthetic direct-acting drug that works primarily on β_1 receptors in the heart, increasing inotropy. Dobutamine does not stimulate the release of norepinephrine from the adrenals and has mild β_2 and α_1 activity. The mild vasodilating effects of this drug allow for a reduction in both preload and afterload, making it a very useful drug in congestive heart failure. Dobutamine may also indirectly decrease myocardial oxygen consumption by reducing left ventricular end-systolic and end-diastolic wall stress in the failing heart.[44]

Dopamine

Dopamine is a naturally occurring catecholamine that works by two methods: increasing cAMP production in the myocardium and as a precursor for norepinephrine. The

Table 29-4 β Receptor Agonists (Cardiostimulatory)

Drug	Receptors	Dosages	Comments
Dobutamine	$\beta_1 > \beta_2 > \alpha_1$	Initial infusion 0.5–1.0 μg/kg/min with optimal infusion rates of 2–20 μg/kg/min	Should not be mixed with other drugs because of incompatibilities. May cause decrease in blood pressure from vascular dilation.
Dopamine	$\beta_1 = \beta_2 > \alpha_1$	Initial infusion 2.0–5.0 μg/kg/min with maximum dose 50 μg/kg/min	May cause tachycardia and ventricular arrhythmias at high doses. Patients with CAD need to be monitored for angina and ischemia.
Epinephrine (adrenaline)	$\beta_1 = \beta_2 > \alpha_1 = \alpha_2$	β dose 0.01–0.03 μg/kg/min β > α dose 0.03–0.15 μg/kg/min β + α 0.15–0.5 μg/kg/min	Positive inotropic and chronotropic support. Improves diastolic function by increasing rate of myocardial relaxation.
Norepinephrine (Levophed)	$\beta_1 = \alpha_1 > \beta_2 = \alpha_2$	Infusion 0.05–0.5 μg/kg/min	May cause reflex bradycardia.
Milrinone	PDE_3	Loading dose 50 μg/kg Infusion 0.375–0.75 μg/kg/min	

CAD, coronary artery disease.

effects of this drug depend on the administered dose. At low doses, usually below 3 µg/kg/min, dopamine acts on the dopaminergic receptors, causing increased mesenteric blood flow. By increasing the dose to 5 to 10 µg/kg/min, dopamine stimulates the release of norepinephrine from the adrenals and works primarily on the β_1 receptors of the myocardium, increasing contractility and inotropy. When the dose is further increased above 10 µg/kg/min, dopamine stimulates the α_1 receptors in the vascular smooth muscle, causing vasoconstriction and increases in systemic vascular resistance, preload, and afterload.

Epinephrine

Epinephrine binds to both β_1 and β_2 adrenoreceptors. The heart has primarily β_1 receptors with more β_2 in the vascular smooth muscle and lungs. These receptors have a high binding affinity for epinephrine. Stimulation of β_1 and β_2 adrenoreceptors causes the increased production of cAMP, allowing for increased chronotropy and inotropy with mild vasodilation. At larger doses, α_1 predominates, causing vasoconstriction. Epinephrine increases myocardial relaxation and enhances left ventricular filling, improving diastolic function. Use of epinephrine at dosages of 0.01 to 0.03 µg/kg/min produces hemodynamics similar to dobutamine with less tachycardia.[45]

Nitrodilators

Nitrates enter the smooth muscle cell and are converted to nitric oxide, which is important in vascular relaxation. Nitric oxide is necessary for the production of cyclic guanosine monophosphate (cGMP) by activation of guanylyl cyclase. cGMP inhibits the influx of calcium into the vascular smooth muscle, causing relaxation. By adding additional nitric oxide (nitrodilators; Table 29-5), production of cGMP is increased, causing a combination of systemic and pulmonary vasodilation, with preload and afterload reduction of both the left and right ventricles.

Nitroglycerin

Organic nitrates are prodrugs that undergo a complex metabolic biotransformation predominantly in the smooth muscle intracellular space.[46] Nitroglycerin exerts a preferential effect on venous capacitance vessels, decreasing preload to the failing heart while also dilating the arterial circulation and decreasing afterload and allowing for an increased cardiac output and ejection fraction. Nitroglycerin has the ability to dilate pulmonary vasculature to the same extent as systemic arterial vasodilation, making it useful in patients with pulmonary hypertension. Use of nitroglycerin in patients with severe pulmonary shunting is warranted because it inhibits hypoxic pulmonary vasoconstriction, worsening any ventilation perfusion abnormality. Effects of nitroglycerin include vasodilation, decreased venous return, reduced preload and afterload, decreased myocardial wall tension and oxygen demand, and improvement of subendocardial perfusion.[47,48]

Sodium Nitroprusside

Sodium nitroprusside affects both arterial and venous dilation. As nitroprusside is metabolized it releases nitric oxide, causing activation of guanylyl cyclase, which stimulates the intracellular production of cGMP. Sodium nitroprusside causes the reduction of both preload and afterload, allowing the failing heart to increase cardiac output and ejection fraction. When exposed to light, sodium nitroprusside breaks down, releasing the attached cyanide molecules, which can reach toxic levels. In congestive heart failure the initial dose is 0.10 to 0.20 µg/kg/min; this is gradually advanced as needed to attain the clinical and hemodynamic objectives.[46] Nitroprusside therapy should

Table 29-5 Nitrodilators

Drug	Receptors	Dosages	Comments
Sodium nitroprusside	Stimulates nitric oxide, which activates guanylyl cyclase production of cGMP.	Loading 0.5–1 mg/kg Infusion 0.1–10 mg/kg/min	Half-life 1–2 min Dilates both veins and arterioles Cyanide toxicity
Nitroglycerin	Stimulates nitric oxide, which activates guanylyl cyclase production of cGMP.	Loading 25–5 mg Infusion 0.1–17 mg/kg/min	Half-life 3–5 min Mostly venous dilation
Hydralazine	Opens K^+ channels and stimulates nitric oxide, which activates guanylyl cyclase production of cGMP.	Push 2.5–5 mg q 15 min	Half-life 2–4 h

not last longer than 48 hours, and infusion rates should not exceed 5 μg/kg/min. With ongoing therapy, plasma concentrations should be measured and should not exceed 0.1 mg/mL. Signs of cyanide toxicity include anorexia, nausea, fatigue, disorientation, and toxic psychosis.[49]

Hydralazine

Hydralazine is a direct-acting arterial vasodilator that works by activating guanylyl cyclase, causing an increase of cGMP. As a side effect it may produce a sympathetic activation with positive inotropic and chronotropic effects. Hydralazine does not really fit into any of the other drug classifications and probably works by opening K^+ channels and stimulating the release of nitric oxide.

Phosphodiesterase Inhibitors

Intracellular cAMP plays an important role in the inotropic regulation of the heart. β Agonists bind to their respective receptors and through intermediary Gs-protein cause the conversion of ATP to cAMP, which stimulates an influx of calcium into the cell. cAMP is subsequently broken down by phosphodiesterase. There are several types of phosphodiesterase in the cells, but the type most often targeted in cardiac cells is phosphodiesterase type 3. By preventing the production of phosphodiesterase, cAMP continues to function in the body enhancing inotropy, chronotropy, and dromotropy.

In vascular smooth muscle phosphodiesterase inhibitors likewise prevent the production of phosphodiesterase, slowing the destruction of cAMP and continuing vascular relaxation. The net cardiac effect of the use of phosphodiesterase inhibitors is increased inotropy with a reduction of afterload because of dilated peripheral vasculature. The heart is able to pump harder against less resistance, increasing cardiac output.

Milrinone (Primacore)

Primacore is indicated for short-term intravenous infusion of patients with congestive heart failure. Patients must be continually monitored with electrocardiograms to identify potential life-threatening ventricular arrhythmias.

Milrinone is usually given for acute cardiac failure by administering a loading dose of 50 μg/kg followed by an infusion of 0.375 to 0.75 μg/kg/h. Intravenous dosing should not exceed 48 hours. Patients undergoing treatment for chronic heart failure may receive milrinone orally.

Calcium Sensitizers

The leading hypotheses for the failure of existing inotropic therapies are that they increase activator calcium, worsen arrhythmias, activate maladaptive Ca^{2+}-dependent signaling, and increase oxygen consumption.[50] Calcium sensitizers are a new category of inotropes that enhance myocardial performance by increasing the affinity of troponin C to calcium. The prolonged, enhanced contractility during systole (half-life of 80 h) does not impair ventricular relaxation and is not cleared by the kidneys.[34] The newer therapy alternative is to change the way that calcium is directly transduced into the cell and change the way the sarcomere responds to calcium.

Kivikko et al.[50] found that after levosimendan (0.1 μg/kg/min) administration patients with congestive heart failure showed a 40% increase in cardiac output, reduced wedge pressures, and an approximate 30% reduction in systemic vascular resistance. This is in addition to an increased heart rate. In another study, levosimendan was more effective than dobutamine in achieving normalized hemodynamic parameters and had a lower 180-day mortality rate.[28]

Cardioinhibitory Drugs

Cardioinhibitory drugs decrease cardiac output and blood pressure by exerting a negative chronotropic and inotropic effect. This may be desirable in certain types of congestive heart failure, especially systolic (acute) heart failure. Table 29-6 lists the cardioinhibitory drugs that are described in the following section.

Beta-Blockers

β-Adrenergic blockers competitively block sympathetic nervous system activation of β-adrenergic receptors. The American Heart Association/American College of Cardiology guidelines recommend β-adrenergic blocker therapy for selected patients in stage B and for routine use in stage C.[52] Three β-adrenergic blocking agents previously identified (i.e., bisoprolol, carvedilol, and sustained-release metoprolol succinate) demonstrated significant reductions in the mortality rate for patients with systolic heart failure. Bisoprolol and metoprolol exhibit selective β_1 receptor blockade, whereas carvedilol exhibits nonselective β_1, β_2, and α_1 receptor blockade. To minimize potential adverse effects and avoid acute heart failure exacerbation from the negative inotropic effects of β-adrenergic blockers, patients should begin low-dose therapy and be titrated up slowly as tolerated. Additionally, it is ideal to begin β-adrenergic blocker therapy when patients are stable and euvolemic. Common adverse effects with these agents include hypotension, bradycardia, fatigue, and dizziness. Patients with underlying airway disease or peripheral vascular disease should also be evaluated to determine if the potential benefits of therapy outweigh potential risks.[17,18,23–25] Most

Table 29-6 Cardioinhibitory Drugs

Drug	Receptors	Dosages	Comments
Beta antagonists			
Esmolol (Brevibloc)	β_1	Bolus 0.5–1 mg/kg Infusion 50–300 μg/kg/min	Clinical duration 10 min
Metoprolol (Lopressor)	β_1, β_2	2–5 mg every 2–5 min up to 15 mg	Clinical duration 5–8 h
Carvedilol (Coreg)	$\beta_1, \beta_2, \alpha_1$	3.125–12.5 mg PO	
Labetalol	$\alpha_1, \alpha_2, \beta_1$	Bolus 0.1–0.25 mg/kg Infusion 0.2–0.8 μg/kg/min	Seven times more beta than alpha Hypotension not accompanied by tachycardia Clinical duration 2–4 h
Calcium channel blockers			
Nicardipine (Cardene)		Bolus 0.5–2 mg Infusion 1–4 μg/kg/min	Clinical duration 10–15 min
Nifedipine (Procardia)		Bolus 10–20 μg/kg Infusion 1–3 μg/kg/min	Clinical duration 4–12 h
Nimodipine (Nimotop)			

modern, second-generation beta-blockers are β_1 selective. The net effect of this binding is an overall reduction in cardiac sympathetic tone by decreased production of intracellular cAMP and calcium, causing a decrease in inotropy, dromotropy, lusitropy, and chronotropy. Second-generation beta-blockers are generally cardioselective and have a diminished effect on vascular smooth muscle dilation.

Clinicians, because of the negative inotropic effects, have traditionally been leery about administering beta-blockers to patients with congestive heart failure, but new evidence demonstrating their benefits on survival has made routine use of these agents for most heart failure patients a standard of care.[52,53] Several large studies were terminated early because the decrease in mortality in treated patients with moderate to severe heart failure was so pronounced.[52,53] These studies showed that certain β antagonists (blockers), carvedilol and metoprolol, were beneficial in systolic heart failure and that abrupt discontinuation of these drugs may be catastrophic.

Beta-blockers chemically bind with the receptors, effectively down-regulating the β adrenoreceptors. In response to this change, the patient's body makes new receptors. Abrupt withdrawal of beta-blockers can lead to a rebound phenomenon manifested by nervousness, tachycardia, palpitations, hypertension, and even myocardial infarction, ventricular arrhythmias, and sudden death.[54] Administration of β_1 selective blockers should continue or be instituted in patients at risk for ischemic heart disease and without systolic heart failure or heart block.[55,56] Administration of metoprolol 5 mg every 5 minutes until the heart rate is 60 to 65 beats/min is recommended by the American Heart Association.

Side Effects

With the administration of nonselective beta-blockers, patients may experience bronchoconstriction because of activated β_2 receptors. Only β_1-specific beta-blockers should be used in asthmatic patients. Blockade of β_2 receptors may also lead to hypoglycemia because of reduced glycogenolysis.

Esmolol β_1-selective blocker is administered intravenously when short-term beta blockade is required. Drug undergoes rapid hydrolysis by plasma esterases. Esmolol is typically administered with a loading dose followed by infusion. Half-life of the drug is roughly 9 to 10 minutes. Metoprolol is a β_1-specific beta-blocker used for the management of mild to moderate heart failure. Carvedilol is a nonselective beta-blocker and α_1-selective antagonist approved for use in moderate to severe heart failure. Labetalol is an antagonist of both β (nonselective) and α_1 receptors. The activity of labetalol has approximately seven times more β effect than α_1 effect.

Calcium Channel Blockers

Calcium channel blockers decrease intracellular calcium by decreasing movement through the voltage-sensitive Ca^{2+} L-type channels. By slowing the cardiac rate and causing greater relaxation of the ventricle, ventricular filling time is increased, allowing for greater cardiac output. Peripheral arterial dilation also decreases systemic vascular resistance, lowering afterload while having little effect on the venous capacitance vessels; therefore there is little change in preload. Calcium channel blockers are not traditionally used for acute (systolic) heart failure.

Nicardipine is an L-type calcium channel blocker that inhibits the influx of Ca^{2+} into vascular smooth muscle, causing vasodilation, with little effect on cardiac contractility or conduction. Patients will have a reduced afterload and may experience a baroreceptor-mediated tachycardia, promoting increased cardiac output. It is available in both oral or parenteral preparations, but because of its short half-life it is usually administered as an infusion. Nifedipine is used to prevent coronary artery vasospasm associated with coronary artery surgery. It is used only as an oral preparation.

Nimodipine is also an L-type calcium channel blocker that inhibits the influx of Ca^{2+} into vascular smooth muscle, causing vasodilation, with little effect on cardiac contractility or conduction. Patients will have a reduced afterload and may experience a baroreceptor-mediated tachycardia, promoting increased cardiac output. Nimodipine is used to treat cerebral vasospasm associated with subarachnoid hemorrhage. It is used only as an oral preparation.

Side Effects

Side effects may include headache, dizziness, postural hypotension, edema, gingival hyperplasia, and flushing of the skin.

Cardiac Glycosides

Digoxin conveys positive inotropic effects through binding to sodium- and potassium-activated adenosine triphosphate pumps, which increases intracellular sodium levels and more intracellular calcium during systole. Currently, digoxin is recommended for patients with heart failure symptoms who are already receiving optimal therapy with a β-adrenergic blocker, an ACE inhibitor or ARB agent, and a diuretic. Digoxin is generally reserved for patients with systolic dysfunction. It may also be useful in controlling ventricular rate in patients with atrial fibrillation and heart failure, which is a rational strategy as described in the recent guidelines from the American Heart Association/American College of Cardiology.[56] The guidelines, however, report a general preference for β-adrenergic blockers or amiodarone to control the ventricular response rate in patients with heart failure and atrial fibrillation. Amiodarone, or other alternatives, may also be used in patients with recurrent ICD shocks that warrant suppressive therapy.[56]

Digoxin also appears to impact the neurohormonal dimension of heart failure, possibly through decreasing central sympathetic nervous system output or by restoring the sensitivity of baroreceptors. Digoxin has not been shown to reduce mortality, but it has demonstrated a reduction in heart failure–related hospitalizations. Digoxin has a narrow margin for safety, and its dosing should consider a patient's age, renal function, weight, and risk for toxicity. Toxicities include fatigue, confusion, delirium, psychosis, gastrointestinal distress, weight loss, halos, photophobia, visual color disturbances, and arrhythmia. Digoxin-induced arrhythmia can be worsened by electrolyte disturbances, such as potassium imbalance, and includes ventricular fibrillation, ventricular tachycardia, atrioventricular block, and sinus bradycardia.[18,56–59]

Side Effects

The major side effect is cardiac arrhythmia, especially atrial tachycardias and atrioventricular block. Digitalis compounds are contraindicated in patients who are hypokalemic.

Additional Drug Topics

Heart failure patients demonstrate an increased risk for thromboembolic events, but controversy still exists over routine use of antiplatelet or anticoagulation therapy. Aspirin is generally used in heart failure patients with a history of ischemic heart disease. The recently updated American Heart Association/American College of Cardiology guidelines do recommend antiplatelet agents for prevention of myocardial infarction and death in patients with heart failure who have underlying coronary artery disease.[2] The guidelines also point out that the usefulness of anticoagulation is not well established in patients with heart failure, who do not have atrial fibrillation or a previous thromboembolic event.[2] But, conversely, providers are encouraged to prescribe anticoagulants in heart failure patients who have paroxysmal or persistent atrial fibrillation or a previous thromboembolic event.[18,60–62]

Although substantial data on numerous classes of medications demonstrate benefits in patients with systolic heart failure, very little data exist to support drug therapies in patients with heart failure with preserved ejection fraction (diastolic failure). Controversy over rate control strategies versus rhythm control strategies for heart failure patients with comorbid atrial fibrillation has existed for quite a few years. Based on multiple trials that evaluated the safety and efficacy of restoring and maintaining sinus rhythm in patients with atrial fibrillation, both standard approaches for atrial fibrillation management demonstrated equivalent effects on major outcomes. These strategies, either to restore and maintain sinus rhythm by electrical or pharmacologic conversion or to control ventricular rate, are thus reasonable options.[18,63,64]

Evaluation of a chronic heart failure regimen is based on the ability of the regimen to reduce symptoms, slow disease progression, reduce hospitalization, improve survival, and enhance quality of life. Early identification of patients at risk for heart failure should prompt aggressive management of etiologic factors and lifestyle modification if appropriate. Patient education focusing on self-monitoring, early intervention for volume overload, identification of adverse drug effects, and surveillance for signs of common comorbidities is essential. Although no cure for this condition exists, healthcare providers must recognize that heart failure patients will likely have intermittent episodes of acute failure amidst their chronic disease course, at times, despite optimal drug management. A summary of these cardiovascular medications demonstrated to be useful in heart failure by stage is presented in Table 29-7.[18]

Table 29-7 Cardiovascular Medications Useful for Various Stages

Drug	Stage A	Stage B	Stage C
ACE inhibitors			
Benazepril	H	—	—
Captopril	H, DN	Post-MI	HF
Enalapril	H, DN	HF	HF
Lisinopril	H, DN	Post-MI	HF
ARB agents			
Candesartan	H	—	HF
Eprosartan	H	—	—
Losartan	H, DN	CV risk	—
Aldosterone blockers			
Eplerenone	H	Post-MI	Post-MI
Spironolactone	H	—	HF
Beta-blockers			
Atenolol	H	Post-MI	—
Bisoprolol	H	—	HF
Carvedilol	H	Post-MI	HF, post-MI
Labetalol	H	—	—
Metoprolol	H	Post-MI	HF
Pindolol	H	—	—
Propranolol	H	Post-MI	—
Timolol	H	Post-MI	—
Other			
Digoxin	—	—	HF

CV, cardiovascular; DN, diabetic neuropathy; H, hypertension; HF, heart failure; MI, myocardial infarction.

Source: From reference 18.

Anesthesia Implications

Patients presenting to the operating room have many concurrent medications. Discontinuance of many of these medications, even for a short period of time, can be problematic. There are important considerations for these medications:

- Diuretics: Many believe that diuretics, except for potassium-sparing agents, should be withheld the day of surgery. There is little evidence to suggest that withholding one dose will have any measurable clinical effect.
- Beta-blockers: Rebound effects from abrupt withdrawal have been well documented and absolutely should be avoided. Up-regulation of receptors combined with rapidly decreasing plasma concentrations of beta-blockers can lead to tachycardia, hypertension, increased myocardial wall tension and oxygen consumption, elevation of plasma renin activity, and changes in thyroid metabolism, all leading to increased morbidity and mortality.[65]
- Calcium channel blockers: Current practice is to continue therapy throughout the perioperative period unless severe left ventricular dysfunction is evident. Despite early concerns about additive myocardial depression when given along with anesthetics, the beneficial effects in treating cardiac disease outweigh the concerns.[66]
- ACE inhibitors and ARB agents: Data on the safe use of ACE inhibitors with anesthesia are conflicting. There are reports of hypotension and bradycardia during anesthesia induction that are treated with fluids, vasopressors, and occasionally vasopressin analogs. There is no consensus for discontinuation of therapy, but many anesthesia providers withhold these drugs for one dosing interval.[67]
- Digoxin: Digoxin should be continued throughout the perioperative period because it is safe for controlling cardiac disease.[68,69]

Key Points

- Heart failure is the result of numerous cardiac disorders and diseases.
- Hypertension is the most common risk factor for heart failure followed closely by prior myocardial infarction.[4]

- The diagnosis of heart failure is made by collectively evaluating a combination of characteristic symptoms and signs along with diagnostic testing.
- Cardiac failure can be either systolic or diastolic.
- Systolic failure is the heart's inability to fully contract, decreasing cardiac output.
- Diastolic failure impedes the heart's ability to relax, restricting left ventricular inflow, causing increased filling pressures, pulmonary edema, and decreased cardiac output independent of cardiac performance.
- Cardiostimulatory drugs improve cardiac output in congestive failure by increasing inotropy (contractility), chronotropy (heart rate), lusitropy (ventricular relaxation), and dromotropy (electrical conductivity).
- Goals of treatment for chronic heart failure include preventing or delaying onset of symptomatic heart failure, minimizing symptoms, and reducing mortality.
- The American Heart Association/American College of Cardiology guidelines recommend β-adrenergic blocker therapy for selected patients in congestive heart failure.
- Calcium channel blockers decrease intracellular calcium, slowing the cardiac rate and causing greater relaxation of the ventricle; ventricular filling time is increased, allowing for greater cardiac output.
- Digoxin should be continued throughout the perioperative period because it is safe for controlling cardiac disease.

Chapter Questions

1. What is the most common cause of death in a patient with congestive heart failure?
2. Between which stages of the New York Heart Association Functional Classification system do structural changes start to occur?
3. What are the primary goals of treatment for patients with congestive heart failure?
4. How do loop diuretics differ in efficacy and safety from either thiazide or carbonic anhydrase diuretics?
5. What is nesiritide's role in the treatment of heart failure?
6. How do ACE inhibitors promote peripheral edema?
7. Why do patients on ACE inhibitors get a persistent dry cough?
8. What is the role of phosphodiesterase in cellular function?
9. What is the rationale for the use of beta blocker therapy in patients with systolic versus diastolic failure?
10. Which classes of drugs should not be withheld the day of surgery?

References

1. Lloyd-Jones DM, Larson MG, Leip EP, et al., for the Framingham Heart Study. Lifetime risk for developing congestive heart failure: the Framingham Heart Study. *Circulation.* 2002;106:3068–3072.
2. Lloyd-Jones DM, Adams R, Carnethon M, et al., for the American Heart Association Statistics Committee and Stroke Statistics Subcommittee. Heart disease and stroke statistics—2009 update. A Report From the American Heart Association Statistics Committee and Stroke Statistics Subcommittee. *Circulation.* 2009;119:e21–e181.
3. Barker WH, Mullooly JP, Getchell W. Changing incidence and survival for heart failure in a well-defined older population, 1970–1974 and 1990–1994. *Circulation.* 2006;113:799–805.
4. Levy D, Larson MG, Vasan RS, Kannel WB, Ho KK. The progression from hypertension to congestive heart failure. *JAMA.* 1996;275:1557–1562.
5. Bibbins-Domingo K, Lin F, Vittinghoff E, et al. Predictors of heart failure among women with coronary disease. *Circulation.* 2004;110:1424–1430.
6. Roger VL, Weston SA, Redfield MM, et al. Trends in heart failure incidence and survival in a community-based population. *JAMA.* 2004;292:344–350.
7. National Center for Health Statistics, Centers for Disease Control and Prevention. Compressed mortality file: underlying cause of death. Atlanta, GA: Centers for Disease Control and Prevention. Available at: http://wonder.cdc.gov/mortSQL.html. Accessed August 1, 2009.
8. Thom TJ, Kannel WB, Silbershatz H, D'Agostino RB Sr. Cardiovascular diseases in the United Sates and prevention approaches. In: Fuster V, Alexander RW, O'Rourke RA, eds. *Hurst's The Heart, Arteries and Veins*, 10th ed. New York: McGraw-Hill; 2001:3–17.
9. Centers for Medicare & Medicaid Services. Health Care Financing Review: Medicare & Medicaid Statistical Supplement. Table 5.5: Discharges, total days of care, and program payments for medicare beneficiaries discharged from short-stay hospitals, by principal diagnoses within major diagnostic classifications (MDCs): calendar year 2006. Baltimore, MD: Centers for Medicare and Medicaid Services; 2005. Available at: http://www.cms.hhs.gov/MedicareMedicaidStatSupp/. Accessed August 1, 2009.

10. Ashley E, Niebauer J. Heart failure. In: *Cardiology Explained*, 1st ed. London, UK: Remedica Publishing; 2003: Available at: http://www.ncbi.nlm.nih.gov/bookshelf/br.fcgi ?book=cardio. Accessed August 1, 2009.

11. Hunt SA, Abraham WT, Chin MH, et al., for the Committee to Revise the 2001 Guidelines for the Evaluation and Management of Heart Failure. ACC/AHA guideline update for the diagnosis and management of chronic heart failure in the adult—summary article: a report of the American College of Cardiology/American Heart Association Task Force on Practice Guidelines. *J Am Coll Cardiol*. 2005;46:1116–1143.

12. Seixas-Cambão M, Leite-Moreira AF. Pathophysiology of chronic heart failure. *Rev Port Cardiol*. 2009;28:439–471.

13. Davie AP, Francis CM, Caruana L, Sutherland GR, McMurray JJ. Assessing diagnosis in heart failure: which features are any use? *QJM*. 1997;90:335–339.

14. White JA, Patel MR. The role of cardiovascular MRI in heart failure and the cardiomyopathies. *Cardiol Clin*. 2007; 25:71–95.

15. Maisel AS, Krishnaswamy P, Nowak RM, et al. Rapid measurement of B-type natriuretic peptide in the emergency diagnosis of heart failure. *N Eng J Med*. 2002;347:161–167.

16. The Criteria Committee of the New York Heart Association. *Nomenclature and Criteria for Diagnosis of Diseases of the Heart and Great Vessels*, 9th ed. Boston, MA: Little, Brown & Co; 1994:253–256.

17. Hunt SA, Abraham WT, Chin MH, et al. ACC/AHA 2005 guideline update for the diagnosis and management of chronic heart failure in the adult: a report of the American College of Cardiology/American Heart Association Task Force on Practice Guidelines (Writing Committee to Update the 2001 Guidelines for the Evaluation and Management of Heart Failure). *J Am Coll Cardiol*. 2005;46:e1–e82.

18. Jessup M, Abraham WT, Casey DE Jr, et al. 2009 Focused update incorporated into the ACCF/AHA 2005 guidelines for the diagnosis and management of chronic heart failure in adults with the 2008 focused update incorporated. *J Am Coll Cardiol*. 2009. Available at: http://content.onlinejacc.org/cgi/content/full/j.jacc.2008.11.009. Accessed January 1, 2010.

19. Hensley R, Martin D, Gravlee G. *A Practical Approach to Cardiac Anesthesia*, 4th ed. Philadelphia: Lippincott Williams & Wilkins; 2008:8–9.

20. Magovern JA, Estafanous FG, Loop FD, et al. ICU admission score for predicting morbidity and mortality after coronary artery bypass surgery. *J Am Coll Cardiol*. 1996;28:1147–1153.

21. Nieminen MS, Bohm M, Cowie MR, et al. Executive summary of the guidelines on the diagnosis and treatment of acute heart failure. *Eur Heart J*. 2005;26:384–416.

22. Hrum H, Abraham WT. Heart failure. *Lancet*. 2009;373: 941–955.

23. CIBIS-II Investigators and Committee. The Cardiac Insufficiency Bisoprolol Study II (CIBIS-II): a randomised trial. *Lancet*. 1999;353:9–13.

24. Hjalmarson A, Goldstein S, Fagerberg B, et al., for the MERIT-HF Study Group. Effects of controlled-release metoprolol on total mortality, hospitalizations, and well-being in patients with heart failure: the Metoprolol CR/XL Randomized Intervention Trial in congestive heart failure (MERIT-HF). *JAMA*. 2000;283:1295–1302.

25. Packer M, Bristow MR, Cohn JN, et al., for the U.S. Carvedilol Heart Failure Study Group. The effect of carvedilol on morbidity and mortality in patients with chronic heart failure. *N Engl J Med*. 1996;334:1349–1355.

26. Bokhari F, Newman D, Greene M, et al. Long-term comparison of the implantable cardioverter defibrillator versus amiodarone: eleven-year follow-up of a subset of patients in the Canadian Implantable Defibrillator Study (CIDS). *Circulation*. 2004;110:112–116.

27. Mark DB, Nelson CL, Anstrom KJ, et al. Cost-effectiveness of defibrillator therapy or amiodarone in chronic stable heart failure: results from the Sudden Cardiac Death in Heart Failure Trial (SCD-HeFT). *Circulation*. 2006;114:135–142.

28. Bardy GH, Lee KL, Mark DB, et al. Amiodarone or an implantable cardioverter-defibrillator for congestive heart failure. *N Engl J Med*. 2005;352:225–237.

29. Hunt SE. ACC/AHA 2005 guideline update for the diagnosis and management of chronic heart failure in the adult: a report of the American College of Cardiology/American Heart Association Task Force on Practice Guidelines (Writing Committee to Update the 2001 Guidelines for the Evaluation and Management of Heart Failure). *J Am Coll Cardiol*. 2005;46:e1–e82.

30. Krum H, Cameron P. Diuretics in the treatment of heart failure: mainstay of therapy or potential hazard? *J Cardiol Fail*. 2006;12:333–335.

31. The Heart Outcomes Prevention Evaluation Study Investigators. Effects of an angiotensin-converting-enzyme inhibitor, ramipril, on cardiovascular events in high-risk patients. *N Engl J Med*. 2000;342:145–153.

32. Gauthier N, Anselm AH, Haddad H. New therapies in acute decompensated heart failure. *Curr Opin Cardiol*. 2008;23: 134–140.

33. Greenberg B, Borghi C, Perrone S. Pharmacotherapeutic approaches for decompensated heart failure: a role for the calcium sensitizer, levosimendan? *Eur J Heart Failure*. 2003;5:13–21.

34. Warren, SE, Blantz RC. Mannitol. *Arch Intern Med*. 1981;141:493–497.

35. Katzung B. *Basic and Clinical Pharmacology*, 10th ed. New York: McGraw-Hill Lange, 2009.

36. The SOLVD Investigators. Effect of enalapril on mortality and the development of heart failure in asymptomatic patients with reduced left ventricular ejection fractions. *N Engl J Med.* 1992;327:685–691.

37. SOLVD Investigators. Effect of enalapril on survival in patients with reduced left ventricular ejection fractions and congestive heart failure. *N Engl J Med.* 1991;325:293–302.

38. CONSENSUS Trial Study Group. Effects of enalapril on mortality in severe congestive heart failure: results of the Cooperative North Scandinavian Enalapril Survival Study (CONSENSUS). *N Engl J Med.* 1987;316:1429–1435.

39. Granger CB, McMurray JJ, Yusuf S, et al. Effects of candesartan in patients with chronic heart failure and reduced left-ventricular systolic function intolerant to angiotensin-converting-enzyme inhibitors: the CHARM-Alternative trial. *Lancet.* 2003;362:772–776.

40. Cohn JN, Tognoni G. A randomized trial of the angiotensin receptor blocker valsartan in chronic heart failure. *N Engl J Med.* 2001;345:1667–1675.

41. Pitt B, Zannad F, Remme WJ, et al., for the Randomized Aldactone Evaluation Study Investigators. The effect of spironolactone on morbidity and mortality in patients with severe heart failure. *N Engl J Med.* 1999;341:709–717.

42. Pitt B, Williams G, Remme W, et al. The EPHESUS trial: eplerenone in patients with heart failure due to systolic dysfunction complicating acute myocardial infarction. Eplerenone Post-AMI Heart Failure Efficacy and Survival Study. *Cardiovasc Drugs Ther.* 2001;15:79–87.

43. The Digitalis Investigation Group. The effect of digoxin on mortality and morbidity in patients with heart failure. *N Engl J Med.* 1997;336:525–533.

44. Amin DK, Shah PK, Shellock FG er al. Comparative hemodynamic effects of intravenous dobutamine and MDL-17,043, a new cardioactive drug in severe congestive heart failure. *Am Heart J.* 1985;109:91–98.

45. Evers A, Maze M. *Anesthetics Pharmacology: Physiologic Principles and Clinical Practice.* New York: Churchill Livingstone; 2007.

46. Elkayam U, Janmohamed M, Habib M, Hatamizadeh P. Vasodilators in the management of acute heart failure. *Crit Care Med.* 2008;36:95–105.

47. Richard Klabunde PhD. *Cardiovascular pharmacology concepts.* Available at: http://www.cvpharmacology.com/diuretic/diuretics.htm. Accessed May 3, 2010.

48. Kaplan J. *Essentials of Cardiac Anesthesia.* Philadelphia: Saunders; 2008.

49. Brunton L, Parker K, Blumenthal D, Duxton I. *Goodman and Gilman's Manual of Pharmacology and Therapeutics.* New York: McGraw-Hill; 2008.

50. Kivikko M, Lehtonen L, Colucci WE. Sustained hemodynamic effects of intravenous levosimendan. *Circulation.* 2003;107:81–86.

51. Cleland JK, Takala A, Apajasalo M, Zethraeus N, Kobelt G. Intravenous levosimendan treatment is cost-effective compared to dobutamine in severe low-output heart failure: an analysis on the international LIDO trial. *Eur J Heart Failure.* 2003;5:101–108.

52. Devereaux PJ, Leslie K. Best evidence in anesthetic practice. Prevention: alpha2 and beta-adrenergic antagonists reduce perioperative cardiac events. *Can J Anaesth.* 2004; 51:290–292.

53. Lindenauer PK, Fitzgerald J, Hoople N, Benjamin EM. The potential preventability of postoperative myocardial infarction: underuse of perioperative beta-adrenergic blockade. *Arch Intern Med.* 2004;164:762–766.

54. Lindenauer PK, Pekow P, Want K, et al. Perioperative betablocker therapy and mortality after major cardiac surgery. *N Engl J Med.* 2005;353:349–361.

55. Fleisher LA, Beckman JA, Brown KA, et al. ACC/AHA 2006 guideline update on perioperative cardiovascular evaluation for noncardiac surgery: focused update on perioperative beta-blocker therapy. *J Am Coll Cardiol.* 2006;47:2343–2355.

56. Lee DC, Johnson RA, Bingham JB, et al. Heart failure in outpatients: a randomized trial of digoxin versus placebo. *N Engl J Med.* 1982;306:699–705.

57. Guyatt GH, Sullivan MJ, Fallen EL, et al. A controlled trial of digoxin in congestive heart failure. *Am J Cardiol.* 1988;61:371–375.

58. Singh SN, Fletcher RD, Fisher SG, et al. Amiodarone in patients with congestive heart failure and asymptomatic ventricular arrhythmia. Survival Trial of Antiarrhythmic Therapy in Congestive Heart Failure. *N Engl J Med.* 1995;333:77–82.

59. Al Khadra AS, Salem DN, Rand WM, et al. Antiplatelet agents and survival: a cohort analysis from the Studies of Left Ventricular Dysfunction (SOLVD) trial. *J Am Coll Cardiol.* 1998;31:419–425.

60. Antiplatelet Trialists' Collaboration. Collaborative overview of randomized trials of antiplatelet therapy—I: prevention of death, myocardial infarction, and stroke by prolonged antiplatelet therapy in various categories of patients. [Published erratum appears in *BMJ.* 1994;308:1540.] *BMJ.* 1994;308:81–106.

61. Jones CG, Cleland JG. Meeting report—the LIDO, HOPE, MOXCON and WASH studies. Heart Outcomes Prevention Evaluation. The Warfarin/Aspirin Study of Heart Failure. *Eur J Heart Failure.* 1999;1:425–431.

62. Clinicaltrials.gov. Aldosterone antagonist therapy for adults with heart failure and preserved systolic function

(TOPCAT). Available at: http://www.clinicaltrials.gov/ct2/show/NCT00094302. Accessed December 20, 2009.

63. Boos CJ, Carlsson J, More RS. Rate or rhythm control in persistent atrial fibrillation? *QJM.* 2003;96:881–892.

64. Roy D, Talajic M, Nattel S, et al. Rhythm control versus rate control for atrial fibrillation and heart failure. *N Engl J Med.* 2008;358:2667–2677.

65. Pass SE, Simpson RW. Discontinuation and reinstitution of medications during the perioperative period. *Am J Health Syst Pharm.* 2004;61:899–914.

66. Goldstein A, Amar E. Pharmacotherapeutic considerations in anesthesia. *Heart Dis.* 2003;5:34–38.

67. Schirmer U, Schurmann W. Preoperative administration of angiotensin-converting inhibitors. *Anaesthetist.* 2007; 56:557–561.

68. Nagelhout J. Autonomic cardiac drugs. In: Nagelhout J, Plaus K, eds. *Nurse Anesthesia,* 4th ed. St. Louis, MO: Elsevier; 2009.

69. Nagelhout J, Elisha S, Waters E. Should I continue or discontinue that medication? *AANA J.* 2009;77:59–73.

V

Drug Interactions

Objectives

After completing this chapter, the reader should be able to

- Develop an anesthetic plan of care to include potential drug interactions that can occur between prescription drugs, drugs ordered by the surgeon, and anesthetic drugs used to provide anesthesia.
- Use useful drug interactions that occur among anesthetic agents and ancillary anesthesia drugs to administer a safe anesthetic with a rapid, comfortable emergence.
- Recognize potential drug interactions that could lead to increased mortality and morbidity.
- Acquire knowledge sufficient to question potential drug interactions as a means of increasing patient safety.

Drug Interactions of Relevance to the Anesthetist

Nancy Bruton-Maree, MS, CRNA

Introduction

Most anesthetics administered today depend on drug interactions or the use of several drugs together to produce a therapeutic effect. Generally, a therapeutic effect is achieved by using smaller doses of several drugs rather than a large dose of one drug to achieve the same effect to avoid unwanted adverse events. However, mixing drugs is not without risk. Additionally, patients who present today for anesthesia and surgery, more often than not, are taking many prescription and over-the-counter drugs, which can increase the risk of adverse drug interactions during anesthesia and, at times, increase mortality and morbidity.

Drug interactions can be identified as pharmaceutical interactions, pharmacokinetic interactions, or pharmacodynamic interactions. A pharmaceutical interaction can be either a chemical or physical interaction, and it occurs before the drug is administered or systemically absorbed.[1] Pharmacodynamic interactions happen when one drug alters the sensitivity of a receptor or target tissue to the effects of a second drug.[1] These reactions are usually classified by their direction and intensity using words such as additive, synergistic, and antagonistic.[1] If a drug alters the absorption, distribution, metabolism, or elimination of another drug, a pharmacokinetic interaction has occurred.[1] The most significant drug interactions are those that alter renal excretion, alter metabolism, or change the effects of a drug, especially those drugs with a low therapeutic index.[2] Drugs that have a low therapeutic index are anticoagulants, drugs acting on the brain, hypoglycemic drugs, hormones, cytotoxic drugs, and cardiovascular drugs.[2]

In this chapter we discuss drugs that are frequently encountered during the perioperative period. Some of these drugs are used as part of the anesthetic management, whereas others are prescribed for patients and either interfere with anesthetic management or anesthetic management interferes with their effectiveness.

Drugs Used for Anesthetic Management and Interactions Pertinent to Anesthesia

Opioids, neuromuscular blocking agents, and IV sedative/hypnotics are used for anesthetic management. Both adverse and pharmacologically useful drug interactions can occur with these drugs as well. Opioids are very important ancillary drugs used by anesthesia providers to assist with myocardial stability and analgesia during anesthesia and surgery. Although other opioids can be used, the commonly used opioids for anesthesia are fentanyl, sufentanil (Sufenta), and morphine sulfate. Discussed next are interactions involving opioids that are important for anesthetists.

Opioid Interactions

Opioid Agonists and Volatile Agents

Opioids and volatile anesthetics are often administered together during anesthesia for better hemodynamic stability, faster arousal from anesthesia, and to reduce the incidence of emergence delirium.[1,3] Most agree that opioids produce a dose-dependent and concentration-dependent decrease in minimal alveolar concentration (MAC) for all inhalation anesthetics.[1,3] Some research, however, noted that small doses of opioids combined with volatile anesthetics result in marked reduction in MAC, but further increases in opioid dose provide only a small reduction in MAC.[4] Thus a ceiling effect on MAC has been observed.[4]

Opioids and Orally Administered Drugs

Opioid agonists also decrease gastric emptying, which can interfere with the absorption of orally administered drugs during the preoperative period.[1,2] Opioid agonists decrease gastric emptying by producing hypertonus of smooth muscle, contraction of sphincters throughout the gastrointestinal tract, increased tone at the gastroduodenal junction, and decreased peristalsis.[2,3] When opioid agonists are administered as part of a premedication or before induction of anesthesia, absorption of other orally administered drugs may be decreased.[2,3] Examples of orally administered preoperative drugs are midazolam and antibiotics.[3]

Opioid Agonists and Respiratory Depressant Drugs

Opioid agonists produce respiratory depression primarily through agonistic effects at the μ_2 receptor.[3] The respiratory depression is dose dependent and gender specific, and the primary effects of the opioids are at the level of the medullary respiratory center.[3] Some nonopioid respiratory depressant drugs, including the phenothiazines, amphetamines, tricyclic antidepressants (TCAs), monoamine oxidase inhibitors (MAOIs), barbiturates, propofol (Diprivan), and etomidate (Amidate),[3,5–10] tend to potentiate the respiratory depression caused by opioid agonists. The TCAs, when given with opioids, can potentiate the respiratory depressant effects of the opioids and the analgesic effects as well.[3]

Opioids and Sympathomimetics Amines

Sympathomimetic amines appear to enhance the analgesia effects of opioids.[3,11] The most effective sympathomimetics for enhancement of analgesia are the miscellaneous sympathomimetic agonists, such as amphetamines.[11]

Opioids and Physostigmine (Antilirium)

Physostigmine is another drug that can enhance opioid analgesia. Cholinergic mechanisms have been shown through research to play an important antinociceptive role.[12,13] Physostigmine, a well-known central cholinergic inhibitor, has been shown to produce analgesia and to enhance analgesia produced by injected opioids.[12,13] This enhancement has been demonstrated after systemic injection and continuous infusion in combination with morphine sulfate.[12,13] Physostigmine does not appear to have its action on the μ receptor but by stimulation of the serotonin (5-HT$_3$) receptors.[13] Physostigmine is seldom used to enhance opioid-induced analgesia because of its short duration of action.[13]

Opioids and Naloxone Hydrochloride (Narcan)

One of the most useful drug interactions involving opioids is the reversal of unwanted opioid effects by naloxone. Naloxone hydrochloride is a narcotic antagonist that prevents or reverses the effects of opioids, such as respiratory depression, sedation, hypotension, and analgesia.[14,15] Competition with the opioid for the same receptors is the mechanism of action for this antagonism.[14]

Opioids and Nalbuphine Hydrochloride (Nubain)

Of equal interest is the interaction between opioid agonists and the agonist-antagonist nalbuphine hydrochloride. This drug is reported to reverse the respiratory depression from moderate doses of fentanyl (and other opioid agonists) without reversing the analgesia.[16]

Opioids and TCAs

TCAs augment the analgesic and ventilatory depressant effects of opioids.[3]

Meperidine (Demerol) and MAOIs

Administering meperidine and MAOIs together can be lethal. One injection of meperidine in a patient taking MAOIs can result in seizures, coma, and death.[3] The administration of meperidine to a patient taking MAOIs can result in an excitatory response or a depressive response.[3]

Neuromuscular Blocking Drugs

Neuromuscular blocking drugs (NMBDs) are used as adjunct drugs during many surgical procedures to provide skeletal muscle relaxation, which facilitates intubation and surgery.

The commonly used NMBDs today include succinylcholine (Anectine), pancuronium (Pavulon), vecuronium (Norcuron), atracurium (Tracrium), rocuronium (Zemuron), and cisatracurium (Nimbex). All these muscles relaxants are administered by intravenous (IV) bolus or infusion when used for anesthesia and surgery. Additionally, all are nondepolarizing muscle relaxants (NDMRs) except for succinylcholine, which is a depolarizing muscle relaxant (DMR).

NMBDs and Volatile Anesthetics

Volatile anesthetics enhance neuromuscular blockade to various degrees.[17–20] The ether derivative volatile anesthetics (isoflurane [Forane], desflurane [Suprane], and sevoflurane [Ultane]) have greater ability to produce muscle relaxation, presumably by exerting a stabilizing effect on the postjunctional membrane of the myoneural junction.[3,21] Because of this inherent muscle relaxation, volatile agents produce a dose-dependent enhancement of the effects of NMBDs with isoflurane, desflurane, and sevoflurane all being equal in this ability.[3] This potentiation of NMBDs by volatile anesthetics applies to infusions of NMBDs as well.[17,18]

NDMRs and DMRs

Administering succinylcholine after an NDMR prolongs the onset of succinylcholine (Anectine).[19,21] If an NDMR is administered after succinylcholine, the effects of the NDMR are prolonged.[19,21] A succinylcholine block is prolonged when it is administered during recovery from pancuronium (Pavulon) or after reversal of a nondepolarizing block with neostigmine (Prostigmin).[19] When succinylcholine is given followed by a NDMR, this enhances the magnitude of twitch response suppression produced by a subsequently administered NDMR; this is true even if the effects of succinylcholine have waned.[3,19] This is unexpected because the response to succinylcholine given before an NDMR should be that of antagonism.[3] The presumption for this unexpected event is that the postjunctional membranes remain desensitized to the succinylcholine, which results in a prolonged effect of the NDMR.[3]

NMBDs and Antibiotics

Aminoglycoside antibiotics possess neuromuscular blocking effects, which may be additive with both DMRs and NDMRs.[3,20,21] Common aminoglycosides are amikacin (Amikin), gentamicin, neomycin, tobramycin (Nebcin), kanamycin, and streptomycin. Part of the mechanism of action of the aminoglycosides at the myoneural junction appears to be inhibition of the release of acetylcholine by interfering with calcium influx, as well as decreased sensitivity of the postsynaptic membrane to the endogenous neurotransmitter acetylcholine.[20] This potentiation of NMBDs by the aminoglycoside antibiotics can lead to prolonged paralysis and respiratory depression.[20] The interaction between aminoglycoside antibiotics and NMBDs has been observed with all types of administration routes for the antibiotics.[20] Other antibiotics that have neuromuscular blocking action are polymyxin B (Poly-Rx), colistin, clindamycin (Cleocin), and lincomycin (Lincocin).[21]

NDMRs and Cyclosporine (Neoral)

Cyclosporine may enhance nondepolarizing blockade.[20] The mechanism for this is unknown.[21]

Succinylcholine (Anectine) and Inhibitors of Pseudocholinesterase

Drugs that decrease the levels of pseudocholinesterase, also known as plasma cholinesterase, prolong the duration of action of succinylcholine.[21,22] Succinylcholine depends on this plasma component for hydrolysis, which decreases the duration of action of muscle paralysis.[21,22] The following are drugs that can reduce the levels of pseudocholinesterase.

- Echothiophate eye drops
- Anticholinesterase inhibitors
- Organophosphate pesticides
- Esmolol (Brevibloc)
- Chlorpromazine (Thorazine)
- Glucocorticoids
- Contraceptives
- Metoclopramide (Reglan)
- Cyclophosphamide (Cytoxan)
- MAOIs
- Pancuronium (Pavulon)

NDMRs and Anticholinesterase Inhibitors

Anesthesia providers use anticholinesterase inhibitors, edrophonium (Tensilon), neostigmine (Prostigmin), or pyridostigmine (Regonol), to reverse neuromuscular blockade at the end of surgical cases.[3,12] The mechanism of action for the anticholinesterase inhibitors involves binding with acetylcholinesterase, the endogenous enzyme, which allows acetylcholine to accumulate at the myoneural junction and compete successfully with the NDMR for the nicotinic cholinergic receptors.[3,12]

DMRs and Anticholinesterase Inhibitors

Anticholinesterase inhibitors are not used to reverse depolarized blocks caused by succinylcholine. If anticholinesterase drugs are administered in this situation, a prolonged neuromuscular block occurs.[12,19]

NMBDs and Calcium Channel Blocking Drugs

Calcium channel blockers can potentiate neuromuscular blockade produced by both DMRs and NDMRs by acting at the postjunctional membrane and possibly interfering with neurotransmitter release.[23-26]

For other potential interactions with NMBDs, see Table 30-1.

Intravenous Sedatives and Hypnotics

IV sedative and hypnotic drugs are typically used as induction drugs, which initially render the patient unconscious and unaware. Commonly used sedative/hypnotic drugs include propofol (Diprivan), sodium thiopental, methohexital (Brevital), ketamine (Ketalar), and etomidate (Amidate). The benzodiazepines can be used as induction drugs but are usually administered for their amnestic properties.

Table 30-1 Other Potential Drug Interactions for NMDBs

Interactions	Effects	Mechanism
Local anesthetics and NDMR	Potentiation	Depression of nerve conduction
		Depressed ACh formation, mobilization, and release
		Decreased postsynaptic receptor channel opening times
Magnesium sulfate and DMR and NDMR	Potentiation	Decreased ACh release
Phenytoin, lithium, and DMR and NDMR	Potentiation	Decreased ACh release
Procainamide (Procaine), Quinidine, and DMR	Potentiation	Depressed AntiACh activity
Metoclopramide and DMR	Potentiation	
		Depressed AntiACh activity
Metoclopramide and NDMR	Antagonism	Depressed AntiACh activity

ACh, Acetylcholine; AntiACh, anticholinesterase.

Source: From reference 25.

Drug interactions associated with this group of drugs are discussed next.

Propofol

- Propofol (Diprivan) and alcohol: Both alcohol and propofol are central nervous system (CNS) depressants and are additive when used together.[27] Thus the dose of propofol should be reduced in patients who have been drinking alcohol.
- Propofol (Diprivan) and premedications: The induction dose of propofol may need to be reduced in patients who have been administered intramuscular or IV premedications.[28] This is especially true for premedications that include opioids, benzodiazepines, chloral hydrate, and/or droperidol (Inapsine).[28-30]
- Propofol (Diprivan) and other adjunct anesthesia CNS depressants: Opioids, benzodiazepine, and barbiturates used during an anesthetic using propofol, particularly a propofol infusion, reduce the amount of propofol and other CNS depressant needed.[28-33]
- Propofol (Diprivan) and remifentanil (Ultiva): Research shows that propofol and remifentanil infusions used together are synergistic.[29,30]
- Propofol (Diprivan) and ropivacaine (Naropin): Propofol has a dose-dependent, competitive, inhibitory effect on the metabolism of ropivacaine.[34] This could mean that the duration of action of ropivacaine could be prolonged when used together with propofol.
- Propofol (Diprivan) and volatile anesthetics: Because propofol and volatile anesthetics are both CNS depressants, they act additively when used together.[35-37]
- Propofol (Diprivan) and midazolam (Versed) or droperidol (Inapsine): Research shows that small doses of either midazolam or droperidol before a hypnotic dose of propofol reduce the hypnotic dose of propofol needed.[31] However, lidocaine (Xylocaine) and ketamine (Ketalar) did not reduce the dose of propofol.[31]
- Propofol (Diprivan) and amiodarone (Cordarone): Amiodarone may increase the effects of general anesthesia supplied by propofol because of its adrenergic blocking effects.[38] However, available data are conflicting.[38]

Etomidate (Amidate)

- Etomidate (Amidate) and amiodarone (Cordarone): Etomidate may have its anesthetic effects enhanced by the adrenergic blocking effects of amiodarone.[39]

- Etomidate (Amidate) and vecuronium (Norcuron): Research demonstrates that the bradycardic effects of vecuronium are more pronounced when this drug is administered with etomidate. This interaction is augmented further if fentanyl is added.[40]
- Etomidate (Amidate) and verapamil hydrochloride (Calan): As a general rule, calcium channel blocking drugs pose no problem for patients undergoing general anesthesia. However, two cases in the literature report Cheyne-Stokes breathing and prolonged anesthesia when etomidate and verapamil were used together.[41,42]

Ketamine (Ketalar)

- Ketamine (Ketalar) and volatile anesthetics: This combination may result in hypotension.[3] The proposed mechanism for this is that volatile anesthetics depress sympathetic nervous system outflow from the CNS and unmask the direct cardiodepressant effects of ketamine.[3,43]
- Ketamine (Ketalar) and verapamil (Calan): The calcium channel blocker verapamil may attenuate the increase in blood pressure that is associated with ketamine, but the increases in heart rate may be enhanced.[3]
- Ketamine (Ketalar) and NDMRs: Ketamine enhancement of NDMRs has been reported and may reflect interference with calcium ion binding or calcium transport by ketamine.[3,44] It is also possible that ketamine decreases the sensitivity of the postjunctional membranes to NDMRs.[3,44]
- Ketamine (Ketalar) and succinylcholine (Anectine): The duration of apnea after administration of succinylcholine is prolonged.[3] The possible mechanism for this is inhibition of plasma cholinesterase by ketamine.[3]
- Ketamine (Ketalar) and pancuronium (Pavulon): Pancuronium combined with ketamine may potentiate the cardiac-stimulating effects associated with ketamine.[3]
- Ketamine (Ketalar) and aminophylline: Asthmatic patients taking aminophylline have had seizures when given ketamine.[3,45]
- Ketamine (Ketalar) and diazepam (Valium): An IV dose of 0.3 to 0.5 mg/kg (or an equivalent dose of midazolam) prevents the cardiac-stimulating effects of ketamine.[3] This combination increases the half-life of ketamine.[46]

- Ketamine (Ketalar) and propofol (Diprivan): The advantages of combining ketamine and propofol during total IV anesthesia are hemodynamic stability and excellent analgesia with less respiratory depression.[47]
- Ketamine (Ketalar) and midazolam (Versed): Midazolam attenuates the altered perception and thought process that occur when ketamine is used as an anesthetic.[46]
- Ketamine (Ketalar) and alfentanil (Alfenta): This combination is additive in that analgesia is increased, but so is cognitive impairment.[46]

Benzodiazepines

Benzodiazepines are a group of drugs used by anesthetists to provide sedation, anxiolysis, and amnesia. Common benzodiazepines taken by patients include diazepam (Valium), alprazolam (Xanax), flurazepam (Dalmane), and clonazepam (Klonopin).[48] The most common benzodiazepine used for anesthesia is midazolam (Versed).

- Benzodiazepines and propofol (Diprivan): When propofol and a benzodiazepine, such as midazolam (Versed), are combined with an opioid, such as fentanyl, amnesia can be achieved with a much smaller dose of propofol than if propofol is used alone.[49]
- Benzodiazepines and other CNS depressants: CNS depressants, such as alcohol, barbiturates, narcotics, and tranquilizers, when combined with benzodiazepines cause marked sedation.[49]
- Benzodiazepines and alcohol: Concurrent use of ethanol and oral benzodiazepines uniformly slows the rate of absorption but does not change the extent of the absorption of benzodiazepines.[50]
- Benzodiazepines and flumazenil (Romazicon): Flumazenil reverses the effects of benzodiazepines by competitive inhibition at the benzodiazepine binding site on the γ-aminobutyric acid A receptors.[51] Flumazenil is a specific reversal agent for the effects of benzodiazepines.

Barbiturate Induction Drugs

Two barbiturates are commonly used as induction drugs for anesthesia: thiopental (Pentothal) and methohexital (Brevital).

- Thiopental (Pentothal) and probenecid (Benuryl): Probenecid is a drug that increases uric acid secretion.[52,53] It is used to treat gout and to decrease the renal excretion of some drugs.[52,53] Probenecid can prolong the action of thiopental.[52,53]

- Thiopental (Pentothal) and diazoxide (Proglycem): Diazoxide is a drug that decreases blood pressure by direct relaxation of medium-sized blood vessels and acts as a thiazide diuretic.[54] When this drug is combined with thiopental, significant hypotension can occur.[53]
- Thiopental and opioid analgesics: Thiopental decreases the antinociceptive action of opioids.[53]
- Thiopental and aminophylline: Aminophylline antagonizes the action of thiopental.[53]
- Thiopental and midazolam (Versed): This combination is synergistic.[53]
- Thiopental (Pentothal) or methohexital (Brevital) and CNS depressants: CNS depressants, including alcohol, are additive when used with methohexital or thiopental.[55]
- Methohexital (Brevital) and angiotensin-converting enzyme (ACE) inhibitors, antipsychotics, beta-blockers, and MAOIs: Methohexital used with any of these drug can result in enhanced hypotension.[55]
- Methohexital (Brevital) and phenytoin (Dilantin): Chronic use of phenytoin causes a decrease in the efficacy of methohexital because of enzyme induction.[55]

Drugs Pertinent to Anesthesia That Induce or Inhibit Metabolism of Drugs

Most increased intrinsic clearance of drugs is by enzyme induction.[1] Many anesthetic drugs are metabolized by the cytochrome P-450 enzymes, which are also called microsomal or CYP enzymes.[1] The most important subfamilies of these enzymes appear to be CYP3A4/5 and CYP2D6, with CYP3A4 being the most abundant; this subfamily is responsible for the metabolism of a large number of anesthesia-related drugs.[1,3] Other important subfamilies are CYP2C19, CYP1A2, CYP2C9, and CYP2E1.[1,56] Hundreds of drugs can induce or stimulate these enzymes, and usually an inducer drug can affect the products of several gene families.[1] Inhibitors of these isozymes slow metabolism and increase elimination times for drugs. Tables 30-2 through 30-7 show important information about key drugs metabolized by major isozymes of the cytochrome P-450 systems.

Table 30-2 Cytochrome P-450 Isozyme CYP1A2

Substrate	Inhibitors	Inducers
Amitriptyline	Amiodarone	Carbamazepine
Fluvoxamine	Cimetidine	Insulin
Haloperidol	Ciprofloxacin	Lansoprazole
Lidocaine	Diltiazem	Nafcillin
Mexiletine	Enoxacin	Phenobarbital
Naproxen	Erythromycin	Phenytoin
Ondansetron	Flecainide	Rifampin
Propranolol	Fluvoxamine	
Ropivacaine	Lidocaine	
Verapamil	Mexiletine	
Warfarin	Propafenone	
	Propofol	
	Quinidine	
	Ranitidine	

Source: From references 56–58.

Table 30-3 Cytochrome P-450 Isozyme CYP2C19

Substrate	Inhibitors	Inducers
Amitriptyline	Cimetidine	Carbamazepine
Antiepileptics	Fluoxetine	Phenobarbital
Diazepam	Fluvoxamine	Prednisone
Phenobarbital	Indomethacin	Rifampin
Phenytoin	Lansoprazole	
Primidone	Loratadine	
Citalopram	Omeprazole	
Clopidogrel	Oral contraceptives	
Diclofenac	Oxcarbazepine	
Imipramine		
Indomethacin		
Selegiline		
Warfarin		

Source: From references 56, 57, and 59.

Table 30-4 Cytochrome P-450 Isozyme CYP2C9

Substrate	Inhibitors	Inducers
Amitriptyline	Amiodarone	Carbamazepine
Angiotensin II antagonists	Calcium channel blockers	Ethanol
Nonsteroidal Anti-inflammatory drugs	Cimetidine	Rifampin
Phenytoin	Fluconazole	Secobarbital
Sertraline	Fluvoxamine	
Sulfonylurea	Propofol	
Warfarin	Sertraline	
	Sulfamethoxazole	
	Valproic acid	

Source: From references 56, 57, and 60.

Table 30-5 Cytochrome P-450 Isozyme CYP2D6

Substrate	Inhibitors	Inducers
Amitriptyline	Amiodarone	Carbamazepine
Beta-blockers	Antihistamines	Dexamethasone
Metoprolol	Chlorpheniramine	Piperidines and derivatives
Timolol	Diphenhydramine	Rifampicin
Class I antiarrhythmics	Antipsychotics	
Encainide	Chlorpromazine	
Flecainide	Haloperidol	
Lidocaine	Celecoxib	
Mexiletine	Cimetidine	
Propafenone	Clomipramine	
Debrisoquine	Cocaine	
Dextromethorphan	Doxepin	
Ondansetron	Doxorubicin	
	Fluoxetine	
	Imipramine	
	Metoclopramide	
	Paroxetine	
	Quinidine	
	Ranitidine	

Source: From references 56, 57, and 61.

Table 30-6 Cytochrome P-450 Isozyme CYP2E1

Substrate	Inhibitors	Inducers
Acetaminophen	Cimetidine	Chronic ethanol
Dapsone	Disulfiram	Isoniazid
Ethanol		
Isoflurane		
Isoniazid		
Theophylline		
Toluene		

Source: From references 56, 57, and 62.

Antihypertensive Drug Interactions Pertinent to Anesthesia

Drug interactions can occur between other types of drugs and antihypertensive agents. These interactions are important to anesthesia providers because many patients come to surgery taking prescription antihypertensives that can interact both negatively and positively with anesthesia. Additionally, during the intraoperative period, antihypertensive drugs may be administered to lower blood pressure during anesthesia and surgery. Listed next are some important drug interactions that can occur with this group of drugs.

Table 30-7 Cytochrome P-450 Isozyme CYP3A4

Substrate	Inhibitors	Inducers
Alfentanil	Amiodarone	Barbiturates
Amiodarone	Cimetidine	Carbamazepine
Amitriptyline	Ciprofloxacin	Dexamethasone
Barbiturates	Clarithromycin	Glucocorticoids
Benzodiazepines	Cyclosporine	Phenytoin
Alprazolam	Diltiazem	Rifampin
Clonazepam	Erythromycin	
Midazolam	Fluoxetine	
Buspirone	Fluvoxamine	
Calcium channel blockers	Macrolide antibiotics	
Nifedipine	Quinidine	
Verapamil	Verapamil	
Carbamazepine		
Clomipramine		
Codeine		
Digoxin		
Fentanyl		
Fluoxetine		
Imipramine		
Lidocaine		
Macrolide antibiotics		
Clarithromycin		
Erythromycin		
Norfluoxetine		
Ondansetron		
Quinidine		
Theophylline		

Source: From references 56, 57, and 63.

Antihypertensive Agents and Drugs That Increase Blood Pressure

Drugs that increase blood pressure antagonize the effects of the antihypertensive.[64] Drugs known to increase blood pressure are corticosteroids, nonsteroidal anti-inflammatory drugs (NSAIDS), cyclosporin, erythropoietin, and sympathomimetics.[64–67] NSAIDs increase blood pressure by inhibiting the renal synthesis of prostaglandins, which cause vasodilation, and also by enhancing salt and water retention.[65–67]

Antihypertensive Agents and Other Drugs That Decrease Blood Pressure

Drugs that decrease blood pressure intensify the effects of antihypertensive agents.[64] Drugs known to decrease blood pressure are acetazolamide (Diamox), amphotericin

B (Amphocin), β_2 agonists such as terbutaline (Brethine), corticosteroids, and theophylline.[64]

Thiazide Diuretics

Thiazide Diuretics and Drugs That Decrease Potassium

Thiazide diuretics can cause hypokalemia; thus when used with drugs that also decrease potassium, hypokalemia may be intensified.[64] Drugs that decrease potassium include acetazolamide (Diamox), amphotericin B (Amphocin), β_2 agonists such as terbutaline (Brethine), corticosteroids, and theophylline.

Thiazide Diuretics and Carbamazepine (Tegretol) or Chlorpropamide (Diabinese)

Thiazide diuretics can also cause hyponatremia; therefore when used with drugs that also cause hyponatremia, the hyponatremia is potentiated.[64] Drugs known to cause hyponatremia include carbamazepine and chlorpropamide.

Thiazide Diuretics and Lithium

Thiazide diuretics cause sodium loss. When these diuretics are used with lithium, sodium is lost and lithium is reabsorbed, which can result in toxic plasma levels of lithium.[64,68] Concurrent use of lithium and thiazide diuretics should be avoided.[64]

Beta-Blockers

Beta-Blockers and Hypoglycemic Drugs

Nonselective beta-blockers, such as propranolol (Inderal), prevent the mobilization of glucose from the liver when hypoglycemia is present.[64] Insulin-dependent diabetics are at greatest risk for this interaction.[64]

Beta-Blockers and Epinephrine

Nonselective beta-blockers, such as propranolol (Inderal), administered with epinephrine can result in severe hypertension and bradycardia.[64] This occurs because beta blockade allows the vasoconstriction caused by epinephrine to go unopposed.[64]

- Beta-Blockers and Reserpine. The combination of either metoprolol (Lopressor) or pindolol (Visken) with reserpine is additive.[64]
- Beta-Blockers and Calcium Channel Blockers. The calcium channel blocker nifedipine (Procardia) has been reported to increase the serum levels of

some beta-blockers, thus increasing the effect of the beta-blocker.[64]

ACE Inhibitors

ACE Inhibitors and Potassium-Sparing Diuretics

Potassium-sparing diuretics include triamterene (Dyrenium), amiloride (Midamor), and spironolactone (Aldactone).[68] These diuretics when combined with ACE inhibitors can lead to increased levels of potassium.[64,68] ACE inhibitors include enalapril (Vasotec), lisinopril (Prinivil or Zestril), captopril (Capoten), and ramipril (Altace).[3]

ACE Inhibitors and Antidiabetic Agents

Although rare, hypoglycemic effects of antidiabetic agents may be enhanced by ACE inhibitors.[64]

ACE Inhibitors and Lithium

These antihypertensives have been implicated in increased serum concentrations of lithium.[64] The mechanism is not known.[64]

ACE Inhibitors and Antacids

Chelation of the ACE inhibitor captopril (Capoten) by antacids suggests that antacids may reduce the absorption of ACE inhibitors from the gastrointestinal tract.[64] If this occurs, the effectiveness of the captopril is reduced.

ACE Inhibitors and NSAIDs

This combination may inhibit the hypotensive effects of the ACE inhibitor by blocking bradykinin-mediated vasodilation.[68]

Clonidine (Catapres) and TCAs

Abrupt discontinuation of clonidine in a patient taking a TCA may lead to rebound hypertension.[3]

Psychopharmacologic Agent Interactions Pertinent to Anesthesia

Psychopharmacologic agents can interact with drugs used to administer anesthesia as well as drugs that patients may be taking before anesthesia and surgery. Drug interactions that can occur with these agents are important knowledge for anesthesia providers because many people take these drugs on a daily basis.

Lithium and Drugs That Decrease Renal Excretion or Increase Renal Absorption

Drugs that tend to increase renal absorption or decrease excretion can cause increased plasma levels of lithium. Drugs that increase renal absorption or decrease renal excretion include NSAIDs, ACE inhibitors, thiazide diuretics, and metronidazole (Flagyl).[69]

Lithium and Carbonic Anhydrase Inhibitors (i.e., Diamox)

This drug combination increases the clearance of lithium and lowers plasma concentrations of this drug.[69] Lithium may therefore become ineffective.

MAOIs

MAOIs are drugs that are in and out of vogue but still remain important to anesthesia providers. Currently prescribed MAOIs are phenelzine (Nardil), tranylcypromine (Parnate), and selegiline (Eldepryl). Because drug interactions involving MAOIs are so numerous, they are listed in Tables 30-8 through 30-13 by class.

TCAs and Sympathomimetic Amines

This combination can result in extreme hypertension.[68] Indirect sympathomimetic amines may produce an exaggerated pressor effect because of increased amounts of norepinephrine available to stimulate adrenergic receptors.[3] Chronic administration of TCAs results in decreased sympathetic nervous system transmission due to down-regulation of β-adrenergic receptors.[3] More than likely a patient recently started on TCAs would have exaggerated responses to both direct- and indirect-acting vasopressors, although the pressor response may be more pronounced with the indirect-acting one.[3] For individuals who have not been on TCAs chronically, the recommendation is small doses of a direct-acting vasopressors; for patients who have used TCAs chronically, either direct- or indirect-acting vasopressors may be used.[3]

TCAs and Antimuscarinic Drugs

Both of these drug classifications have antimuscarinic effects. Therefore combining TCAs and antimuscarinic drugs causes a prolonged duration of the antimuscarinic drug.[68]

Table 30-8 Interactions Involving MAOIs and Other Psychotherapeutic Drugs

Interaction	Results
MAOIs with tricyclic antidepressants	Hyperpyrexic crisis or seizures (e.g., clompriamine) Hypertensive crisis (e.g., despiramine)
MAOIs and tetracyclic antidepressants (e.g., bupropion hydrochloride or Wellbutrin)	Hypertensive crisis (Nonadrenergic syndrome)
MAOIs and SSRIs	Hyperpyrexic crisis (Serotonin syndrome)
MAOIs and MAOIs	Hyperpyrexic crisis (Serotonin syndrome) Hypertensive crisis (Nonadrenergic syndrome)
MAOIs and serotonin antagonists (e.g., trazodone or Desyrel and nefazodone or Serzone)	Hyperpyrexic crisis
MAOIs and mirtazapine (Remeron)	Hypertensive crisis (Nonadrenergic syndrome)
MAOIs and venlafaxine (Effexor)	Hypertensive crisis (Nonadrenergic syndrome)
MAOIs and carbamazepine (Tegretol)	Hyperpyrexic crisis (Serotonin syndrome) Carbamazepine levels fall resulting in seizures
MAOIs and muscle relaxants	Pronounced effect
MAOIs and local anesthetics	Omit sympathomimetic
MAOIs and cyclobenzaprine (Flexeril)	Hyperpyrexic crisis (Serotonin syndrome) or severe seizures
MAOIs and alcohol	Enhanced sedation
MAOIs and barbiturates	Enhanced sedation
MAOIs and buspirone (BuSpar)	Enhanced sedation
MAOIs and benzodiazepines	Enhanced sedation
MAOIs and neuroleptics	Enhanced sedation Drop in blood pressure

SSRI, selective serotonin reuptake inhibitors.
Source: From reference 70.

Table 30-9 MAOIs and Bronchodilators

Interaction	Result
MAOIs and ephedrine	Hypertensive crisis
MAOIs and β-adrenergic inhalants	Increased blood pressure and heart rate
MAOIs and theophylline	Rapid heart rate and anxiety

Source: From reference 70.

Table 30-10 MAOIs and Diabetic Medications

Interaction	Results
MAOIs and insulin	May see a greater drop in blood sugar
MAOIs and oral hypoglycemics	May see a greater drop in blood sugar

Source: From reference 70.

Table 30-11 MAOIs and Medications Used to Increase Blood Pressure

Interaction	Results
MAOIs and sympathomimetic amines	Hypertensive crisis (Nonadrenergic syndrome)

Source: From reference 70.

Table 30-12 MAOIs and Antihypertensives

Interactions	Results
MAOIs and guanadrel, guanethidine, hydralazine, methyldopa, or reserpine	May see increase in blood pressure
MAOIs and beta-blockers	May be more potent when combined with beta blockers, causing greater drop in blood pressure
MAOIs and calcium channel blockers	May cause greater drop in blood pressure than expected
MAOIs and diuretics	May cause greater drop in blood pressure than expected

Source: From reference 70.

Table 30-13 MAOIs and Other Drugs

Interaction	Results
MAOIs and amphetamines, cocaine, Benzedrine (Didrex), dextroamphetamine (Dexedrine), methamphetamine (Desoxyn), or methylphenidate (Ritalin)	Hypertensive crisis (Nonadrenergic syndrome)
MAOIs and anesthesia	Hyperpyrexic reactions Excitement, prolonged effect

Source: From reference 70.

TCAs and Chronic Clomipramine (Anafranil)

Refractory hypotension has been reported with this combination.[68]

Selective Serotonin Reuptake Inhibitors (SSRIs) and Meperidine (Demerol), Pentazocine (Talwin), or Tramadol (Ultram)

Combining these drugs with SSRIs can result in a serotonin syndrome comparable with combining two MAOIs.[69] Symptoms of serotonin syndrome include akathisia-like restlessness, hyperreflexia, sweating, muscle twitches and myoclonus, shivering, and tremor.[3] These symptoms occur before seizures and coma.[3]

Paroxetine (Paxil) and Tramadol (Ultran)

Combining these two drugs can result in excess sedation and an impaired analgesic action.[71]

Imipramine (Tofranil), Desipramine (Norpramin), and Alprazolam (Xanax)

Steady-state plasma concentrations of imipramine and desipramine have been reported to increase by 31% and 20% when combined with alprazolam.[71]

Fluoxetine (Prozac) and Alprazolam (Xanax)

With this combination the maximum plasma concentrations of alprazolam increased by 46%, clearance decreased by 21%, half-life increased by 17%, and there was a decreased measurable psychomotor performance.[71]

Alprazolam (Xanax) and Oral Contraceptives

This combination increases the maximal plasma concentration of alprazolam by 18%, decreases clearance of the same drug by 22%, and increases its half-life by 29%.[71]

SSRIs and Carbamazepine (Tegretol), Phenytoin (Dilantin), and Anticoagulants

This combination can lead to overdose of carbamazepine, phenytoin, and anticoagulants, leading to increased effect from each drug.[72]

TCAs and Anticholinergics

The anticholinergic effects of the TCAs and anticholinergics, such as atropine, when used together are additive.[3] If used together, the result can be central anticholinergic syndrome, which is characterized by delirium and confusion.[3]

Antipsychotic Drugs and Opioids

Antipsychotic drugs, such as phenothiazines, thioxanthenes, butyrophenones, diphenylbutylpiperidines, and benzisoxazole, when used with opioids cause exaggerated ventilatory depression.[3] The miotic and sedative effects of the opioid are intensified.[3]

SSRIs and Selegiline (Eldepryl), and SSRIs and Tramadol (Ultram)

The combination of SSRIs and selegiline (Eldepryl) can cause a hypertensive crisis.[68]

Tramadol is a centrally acting analgesic that when combined with SSRIs can cause serotonin syndrome.[68] Symptoms of serotonin syndrome include akathisia-like restlessness, hyperreflexia, sweating, muscle twitches and myoclonus, shivering, and tremor.[3] These symptoms occur before seizures and coma.[3] Tramadol decreases the reuptake of serotonin and norepinephrine.[68]

Fluoxetine (Prozac) and Selegiline (Eldepryl)

These two drugs when administered together result in mania and hypertension.[68] The actual mechanism is not known.[68]

Warfarin (Coumadin) Drug Interactions Pertinent to Anesthesia

Warfarin (Coumadin) is an anticoagulant drug that decreases clotting and increases bleeding time. Patients present for surgery and anesthesia taking these anticoagulants; therefore drug interactions that can occur involving these agents are important to anesthesia providers.

Warfarin and NSAIDs

This combination leads to increased gastric irritation and erosion of the lining of the stomach and enhances the possibility of gastric bleeding.[73] NSAIDs also decrease the cohesive properties of platelets necessary for clot formation, which adds to the increased bleeding times caused by warfarin.[73]

Warfarin and Sulfa Drugs

Combining these two drug classifications causes greater anticoagulation and an increased potential for bleeding.[73]

The mechanism for this is unknown.[73] It is possible that the systemic antibiotic administration decreases production of vitamin K by intestinal flora.[73]

Warfarin and Macrolide Antibiotics

Commonly known macrolide antibiotics include clarithromycin (Biaxin), erythromycin, and azithromycin (Zithromax).[74] Combining these drugs with warfarin increases the anticoagulant effects of warfarin and the potential for bleeding.[74]

Warfarin and Phenytoin (Dilantin)

With this combination there can be an increased effect from either warfarin or phenytoin. The mechanism of action is unknown.[73]

Warfarin and Aspirin

This combination increases the risk of bleeding.[74]

Drug Interactions Pertinent to Anesthesia That Affect Drug Absorption

Drug interactions that affect drug absorption are called pharmacokinetic interactions.[3] Interference with absorption can either decrease or increase the effects of drugs.[3] Because patients receive oral premedications as well as other types of oral drugs before surgery, these interactions should be considered by the anesthesia provider.

- Antacids and oral tetracycline: If antacids containing polyvalent cations such as Mg^{2+} are administered with oral tetracycline, the tetracycline will be chelated by the antacid and become ineffective.[1]
- Digoxin and antidiarrheal drugs: Orally administered digoxin can be physically absorbed by orally administered antidiarrheal drugs such as kaolin or pectin.[1] This decreases the effectiveness of digoxin.
- Warfarin and bile acid-binding resin: Absorption of warfarin can be prevented by the bile acid-binding resin, cholestyramine.[1] This decreases absorption of warfarin and therefore decreases the anticoagulating effects of this drug.
- Opioids and anticholinergics: Opioids and anticholinergics prevent gastric emptying, which can interfere with the absorption of orally administered drugs.[1]

- Vasodilators and vasoconstrictors: Vasodilators and vasoconstrictors can interfere with the absorption of parenterally administered drugs.[1]
- Uptake of anesthetic agents: The uptake of anesthetic agents can be enhanced without changing the inspired concentration by drugs that decrease intrapulmonary shunting, cause bronchodilation, or increase minute ventilation.[1]

Drug Interactions Pertinent to Anesthesia That Affect Drug Distribution

Drug interactions that affect drug distribution are also pharmacokinetic drug interactions.[3] Drugs that interfere with another drug's distribution can either increase the concentration at the site of action or decrease the effect at the site of action.[3] Exploring such interactions is important for the safe delivery of anesthesia.

Drugs That Decrease Cardiac Output

Drugs that decrease cardiac output, such as calcium channel blockers, volatile anesthetics, beta-blockers, and vasodilators, can markedly change the distribution of other administered drugs.[1] When cardiac output is decreased, the arterial concentration of drugs in highly perfused tissues, such as the brain, increases.[1]

Weak Acid and Weak Basic Drugs

Because most therapeutic agents are either weak acids or weak bases and because pH varies in different body compartments, "ion trapping" of these agents can occur.[1,3] The fraction of weak acids and weak bases that can cross lipid membranes is the non-ionized portion.[1,3] The ionized portion of these drugs can be trapped in body compartments anytime a weak base enters a compartment with an acid pH or a weak acid enters a compartment with a basic pH, because the only fraction of these drugs that can leave the compartment is the lipid-soluble portion.[1,3] With this in mind administration of antacids, histamine type 2 receptor antagonists, and proton pump inhibitors can reduce the gastric absorption of some acidic drugs such as midazolam.[1,3] Changing the gastric pH to one that is more basic moves the balance of a weak base, such as midazolam, to a greater ionized fraction that cannot be absorbed through the gastric mucosa.[1,3]

Because drugs such as morphine and fentanyl are weak bases, the greater non-ionized fraction that occurs in the basic pH of blood allows drug to be absorbed from the blood into the gastric mucosa, which is highly acidotic. This traps these narcotics in the gastric compartment because the basic opioid becomes ionized in the acidic pH of the stomach.[3] As these agents move to the more basic small intestine, they become more non-ionized and begin to move back into the blood.[3] This causes a secondary increase in plasma concentrations of fentanyl.[1,3]

Drug Interactions and Protein Binding

Another hallmark interaction involves protein binding. Only drug that is not protein-bound moves from the plasma to the sight of action.[1,3] Because drugs often compete for the same protein binding sites, one drug can alter the plasma concentration, clearance, and biologic effect of another drug. One such interaction can occur between warfarin and phenylbutazone (Butazolidin). Phenylbutazone is an NSAID that competes effectively for the protein binding sites and, when given with warfarin, displaces warfarin from protein binding sites and increases the plasma concentration of warfarin unless the dose of warfarin is reduced.[1]

Cardiac Drug Interactions Pertinent to Anesthesia

Any drug that affects the heart has the potential to cause interactions with agents used for anesthesia, because many anesthetic drugs directly affect the heart. Generally, drugs used as anesthetics are myocardial depressant agents. Also, ancillary drugs that affect the heart may be needed during surgery. Because these drugs may be used during anesthesia and because many patients take drugs that affect the heart, a look at important drug interactions is essential.

Diltiazem (Cardizem) and Ranitidine (Zantac)

When this combination is administered together, ranitidine may interfere with how diltiazem is metabolized and eliminated from the body.[75] This can increase the effects of diltiazem and also increase unwanted side effects.[75]

Diltiazem (Cardizem) and Digoxin

Diltiazem is thought to decrease the elimination of digoxin from the body.[75] This could cause serum levels of digoxin to increase, leading to adverse side effects such as abnormal cardiac rhythms.[75]

Diltiazem (Cardizem) and Erythromycin

When these drugs are used together, hepatic metabolism of either drug may be altered.[76] Erythromycin may block the metabolism of diltiazem, whereas diltiazem may block the metabolism of erythromycin.[75] Unwanted myocardial side effects may occur from the diltiazem.[76]

Diltiazem (Cardizem) and Fentanyl

Diltiazem may increase plasma levels of fentanyl by inhibiting its metabolism.[77]

Verapamil (Calan) and Theophylline

Verapamil inhibits the metabolism of theophylline, leading to increased serum levels of theophylline.[78] Symptoms of increased theophylline levels include dizziness, nausea, vomiting, tachycardia, nervousness, and seizures.[78]

Verapamil (Calan) and Timolol (Blocadren, Timoptic)

Both drugs individually have the ability to lower blood pressure and heart rate.[78] When combined, there is the potential for the blood pressure and heart rate to become lower than expected or wanted.[78]

Verapamil (Calan) and Carbamazepine (Tegretol)

Verapamil slows the metabolism of carbamazepine, which can lead to increased serum levels of carbamazepine.[78] Increased serum levels of carbamazepine can lead to symptoms of carbamazepine overdose such as dizziness, headaches, drowsiness, and blurred vision.[78] More severe symptoms include decreased white blood cells, increased bleeding, and decreased effectiveness as an anticonvulsant.[78]

Verapamil (Calan) and Alcohol

In combination, these drugs can cause drowsiness, difficulty making decisions, and loss of balance; these symptoms can become intolerable and occur much sooner than one would expect from the amount of alcohol consumed.[78] The mechanism for this is unknown.[78]

Verapamil (Calan) and Cimetidine (Tagamet)

Cimetidine may inhibit the metabolism of verapamil by the liver.[78] This can cause an increased serum level of verapamil, which can lead to side effects such as headache, swelling of feet and hands, dizziness, decreased blood pressure, and bradycardia.[78]

Verapamil (Calan) and Rifampin (Rifadin)

Rifampin induces the metabolism of verapamil, which can lead to less than therapeutic plasma levels of verapamil.[78]

Digoxin and Cimetidine (Tagamet)

Cimetidine can cause a decrease or increase in effectiveness of digoxin.[75] The exact cause of this interaction is not known, but when this combination is used, blood levels of digoxin should be measured to ensure therapeutic serum levels.[75]

Digoxin and Clarithromycin (Biaxin)

Clarithromycin may impede the breakdown of digoxin in the gastrointestinal tract, which can lead to increased absorption of digoxin.[75] Clarithromycin may also impede the renal excretion of digoxin.[75] Interference with one or both can lead to increased risk of serious side effects, including abnormal cardiac rhythms.[75] Other symptoms of increased serum levels of digoxin include lower stomach pain, diarrhea, confusion, extreme weakness, nausea, vomiting, and loss of appetite.[75]

Nifedipine (Procardia) and Metoprolol (Lopressor)

When these two drug are used together in patients with irregular cardiac rhythms and/or myocardial muscle damage, the risk of unwanted side effects, such as drastic drops in blood pressure and bradycardia, may occur.[79]

Nicardipine Hydrochloride (Cardene) and Metoprolol (Lopressor)

Nicardipine may increase the effects of metoprolol. The mechanism for this effect is not understood.[79]

Disopyramide (Norpace) and Metoprolol (Lopressor)

Both drugs decrease blood pressure and heart rate, and when taken together exaggerated drops in blood pressure and heart rate may occur.[79]

Beta-Blocking Drug Interactions Pertinent to Anesthesia

Beta-blocking drugs are another classification that is often prescribed for patients presenting for anesthesia and surgery. Additionally, these drugs are a first-line treatment for increased heart rate and/or blood pressure during anesthesia. Drug interactions involving this classification of drug are discussed next.

Propranolol (Inderal) and Isoniazid (Laniazid, Nydrazid)

Isoniazid is used for prophylaxis and treatment of tuberculosis. When this drug combination is given, propranolol may increase the effects of isoniazid, which can increase the unwanted side effects associated with this drug.[80]

Timolol (Blocadren, Timoptic) and Theophylline

When administered together, the effects of either drug may be lessened or canceled.[78] These drugs have opposite effects in that theophylline is a bronchodilator and increases heart rate, whereas timolol can cause bronchoconstriction in patients with asthma and slows heart rate.[78] Additionally, timolol may inhibit the metabolism of theophylline, which increases serum levels of theophylline and increases the risk of theophylline-related side effects.[78]

Timolol (Blocadren, Timoptic) and Cimetidine (Tagamet)

Cimetidine may inhibit the metabolism of timolol, which causes increased serum levels of timolol.[78] This causes exaggerated effects from this drug as well as exaggerated unwanted side effects.[78]

Timolol (Blocadren, Timoptic) and Bupropion Hydrochloride (Wellbutrin)

With this combination, bupropion hydrochloride inhibits the metabolism of timolol, which can cause the heart rate to decrease to dangerously low levels.[78]

Propranolol (Inderal) and Phenobarbital

Phenobarbital induces the metabolism of propranolol, which can result in ineffectiveness plasma levels of this drug.[81]

Propranolol (Inderal) and Fluoxetine (Prozac)

Fluoxetine may increase the effect of propranolol on the heart rate, causing greater slowing of heart rate than expected.[81] The mechanism for this interaction is unknown.[81]

Propranolol (Inderal) and Quinidine

Quinidine may inhibit the metabolism of propranolol, which increases plasma levels of propranolol as well as possibly increasing side effects to an intolerable or undesirable level.[81]

Propranolol (Inderal), Pindolol (Visken), and Thioridazine (Mellaril)

This combination is contraindicated because the plasma levels of thioridazine can increase high enough to cause life-threatening cardiac arrhythmias.[82]

Beta-Blockers (Pindolol [Visken] and Propranolol [Inderal]) and Phenothiazines

This combination can cause increased serum levels of both classes of drugs and increase any risks associated with the use of either class.[82]

Beta-Blockers and Verapamil (Calan)

If this combination is given together, plasma levels of either drug can increase.[82]

Beta-Blockers and Clonidine (Catapres)

This combination can cause life-threatening increases in blood pressure.[82]

Beta-Blockers and β Agonists

Using these two drug together may cause bronchospasm because the beta-blocking drugs block the receptors that the β agonist needs to occupy to have an effect.[82]

Metoprolol (Lopressor) or Propranolol (Inderal) and Barbiturates

The barbiturates induce the metabolism of these two beta-blockers.[82]

Antibiotic Drug Interactions Pertinent to Anesthesia

Like many drug classifications, antibiotics are often given before and during surgery. Also, like any drug that is given in the perioperative period, drug interaction may occur. A discussion of some of the interactions that may occur with this class of drugs follows.

- Rifampin (Rifadin) and warfarin: Rifampin can induce the metabolism of warfarin, which makes warfarin less effective as an anticoagulant.[78]
- Rifampin (Rifadin) and theophylline: Rifampin induces the hepatic metabolism of theophylline to the point that symptoms of asthma may not be controlled.[78]

- Vancomycin hydrochloride (Vancocin) and tobramycin (Nebcin): Using these two drugs together in patients with poor renal function could increase the risk of further renal damage.[78] This can result because both drugs have an adverse effect of causing renal damage.[78]
- Gentamicin (Gentacidin) and furosemide (Lasix): Both drugs have the ability to impair hearing.[83] When used in combination, the risk of hearing damage increases.[83]
- Doxycycline (Doryx) and hydrochlorothiazide (HydroDIURIL): Blood levels of urea may increase when doxycycline and hydrochlorothiazide are used together.[76] The cause of this interaction is not fully understood.[76]
- Doxycycline and phenytoin (Dilantin): Phenytoin induces the hepatic metabolism of doxycycline, which leads to reduced plasma concentration of this antibiotic.[76]
- Cimetidine (Tagamet) and clarithromycin (Biaxin): Cimetidine may make clarithromycin less effective. The mechanism for this is not known.[75]

Miscellaneous Drug Interactions Pertinent to Anesthesia

Drugs seen less often in patients presenting for anesthesia and surgery and drugs used less often during surgery are discussed next, along with possible drug interactions.

- Furosemide (Lasix) and hydrochlorothiazide (Hydro-DIURIL): When this combination is used together, excessive loss of water, sodium, and/or potassium may occur.[83] This can lead to hypovolemia, hyponatremia, and hypokalemia, which carry the risk of hypotension and myocardial dysrhythmias
- Carbamazepine (Tegretol) and cimetidine (Tagamet): Cimetidine may inhibit the hepatic metabolism of carbamazepine, which increases the risk of adverse side effects from carbamazepine.[78] These side effects can include headaches, blurred vision, drowsiness, excessive bleeding, and loss of effectiveness as an anticonvulsant.[78]
- Cimetidine (Tagamet) and warfarin: Cimetidine may inhibit hepatic metabolism of warfarin, which increases plasma levels of warfarin and, in turn, increases anticoagulation.[78]
- Selegiline (Eldepryl) and ephedrine: Both drugs increase blood pressure.[76] When used together blood pressure may rise to dangerous levels.[76]

- Phenylephrine (Neo-Synephrine) and nortriptyline (Aventyl): Neo-Synephrine is a catecholamine, and nortriptyline has catecholamine-like effects.[81] Catecholamines increase blood pressure and can cause myocardial dysrhythmias. When these drugs are used together, the chance of abnormally high blood pressure and myocardial dysrhythmias increases.[81]
- Quinidine and phenobarbital: Phenobarbital can induce the metabolism of quinidine, thereby decreasing the effectiveness of quinidine on the heart.[81]
- Phenytoin (Dilantin) and phenobarbital: Phenytoin may increase the amount of phenobarbital in the blood by successfully competing for protein binding sites, increasing plasma phenobarbital levels.[81]
- Alcohol and phenobarbital: This combination is additive relative to the depressant effect of both drugs.[81] Deaths have occurred because of mixing these two drugs.[81]
- Quinidine and phenytoin (Dilantin): Phenytoin induces the metabolism of quinidine, thereby potentially decreasing the effectiveness of quinidine on the heart.[81]
- Fluoxetine (Prozac) and phenytoin (Dilantin): Fluoxetine may inhibit hepatic metabolism of phenytoin and increase the risk of adverse side effects from phenytoin associated with its use.[81]
- Phenylephrine (Neo-Synephrine) and tranylcypromine (Parnate): Both drugs increase blood pressure.[81] When used together, blood pressure can reach dangerously high levels.[81]
- Phenobarbital and promethazine (Phenergan): Promethazine can increase the sedative effects of phenobarbital, which can lead to respiratory depression, unwanted decreases in blood pressure, and jerking movements of the extremities.[81]
- Codeine and quinidine: Quinidine blocks the conversion of codeine to its active form; pain relief does not occur.[81]
- Alcohol and cimetidine (Tagamet): Cimetidine may increase the absorption of alcohol from the stomach and may inhibit the metabolism of alcohol.[78]
- Methyldopa (Aldomet) and phenylephrine (Neo-Synephrine): An increase in blood pressure may occur when this combination is used.[79] The mechanism of action is not known.[79]
- Alcohol and midazolam (Versed): Intolerable or otherwise undesirable side effects may occur when midazolam is taken with over-the-counter drugs, such as cough medicines, that contain alcohol.[79] Potential adverse effects include drowsiness, blurred vision, headache, nervousness, and dizziness.[79]

- Theophylline and ranitidine (Zantac): Ranitidine has been reported to increase blood levels of theophylline when taken 36 and 48 hours after taking ranitidine.[78] The mechanism for this is unknown.[78]
- Ranitidine (Zantac) and alcohol: Ranitidine may increase gastric absorption of alcohol as well as inhibit its metabolism.[78] This can lead to nausea and vomiting, stomach irritation, hypotension, and confusion.[78]

Summary

Both positive and negative drug interactions are numerous. Entire books have been written on the subject. The intent of this collection of interactions is to focus primarily on the most important ones for anesthesia and drugs related to that medical specialty. Every anesthetist should be familiar with drug interactions that can occur when using drug combinations that compose an anesthetic plan. Additionally, anesthesia providers should be familiar with interactions that can occur between the anesthetics used and ancillary drugs that are introduced into the scenario. Ancillary drugs include prescription and over-the-counter drugs taken by patients, drugs that may be ordered by the surgeon during the procedure, and herbal medications. All possible drug interactions are beyond the scope of this chapter, but important anesthesia-related drug interactions for the anesthetists are addressed.

Key Points

- Developing an anesthetic plan of care includes potential drug interactions that can occur between prescription drugs, drugs ordered by the surgeon, and anesthetic drugs used to provide anesthesia.
- Useful drug interactions that occur among anesthetic drugs and ancillary anesthesia drugs are used to provide safe anesthesia.
- Recognition of potential drug interactions decreases mortality and morbidity.
- Drug interactions can be pharmaceutical, pharmacokinetic, or pharmacodynamic interactions.
- The most significant drug interactions are those that alter renal excretion, alter metabolism or change the effects of a drug, especially drugs with a narrow therapeutic index.

Chapter Questions

1. If a drug increases the absorption of another drug, what type of interaction occurs?
2. Research has shown that small doses of opioids combined with volatile anesthetics results in what effect on MAC? If further increases in opioid dose occur, what happens to MAC?
3. Although physostigmine has been shown to enhance opioid analgesia, explain why this combination is not used.
4. What is the proposed mechanism for why calcium channel blockers potentiate both depolarizing and nondepolarizing neuromuscular blocks?
5. How does propofol increase the duration of action of ropivacaine?
6. Which isozyme of the cytochrome P-450 system is responsible for metabolizing most drugs used in anesthesia?
7. Describe the mechanism whereby a drug increases the concentration of lithium.
8. What would occur if ephedrine and MAOIs were given together?
9. NSAIDs, when given with warfarin, increase anticoagulation by what mechanism?
10. If verapamil and timolol are administered together, what would likely be the outcome?

References

1. Rosow R, Levine W C. Drug interactions. In: Barash P, Cullen B, Stoelting R, eds. *Clinical Anesthesia.* Philadelphia: Lippincott Williams & Wilkins; 2006:1313–1330.
2. Aronson J. *Serious drug interactions.* Available at: http://www.ncbi.nlm.nih.gov/pubmed/7903448?lop$=activity. Accessed May 28, 2009.
3. Stoelting RK, Hillier SC. *Pharmacology & Physiology in Anesthetic Practice,* 4th ed. Philadelphia: Lippincott Williams & Wilkins; 2006.
4. Glass PS. Anesthetic drug interactions: an insight into general anesthesia—its mechanisms and dosing strategies. *Anesthesiology.* 1998;88:5–6. Available at: http://journals.lww.com/anesthesiology/Fulltext/1998/01000/Anesthetic_Drug_Interactions. Accessed June 19, 2009.
5. Elavil (amitriptyline) and alfentanil interactions. Available at: http://www.drugs.com/drug_interactions.php?action=adhoc&drug1_id=d00146&drug1_br. Accessed June 19, 2009.

6. Chlorpromazine and Demerol HCl interactions. Available at: http://www.drugs.com/drug_interactions.php?action=adhoc&drug1_id=d00064&drug1_br. Accessed June 19, 2009.

7. Amphetamine and analgesia. Available at: http://www.doctordeluca.com/Library/Pain/Pain-Amphetamines.htm. Accessed June 19, 2009.

8. Fentanyl and Nardil interactions. Available at: http://www.drugs.com/drug-interactions/fentanyl_d00233_nardil_d00883.html. Accessed June 19, 2009.

9. Elavil (amitriptyline) and Demerol HCL interactions. Available at: http://www.drugs.com/drug_interactions.php?action=adhoc&drug1_id=d00146&drug1_br. Accessed June 19, 2009.

10. Parnate (tranylcypromine) and Demerol HCl interactions. Available at: http://www.drugs.com/drug_interactions.php?action=adhoc&drug1_id=d00884&drug1_br. Accessed June 19, 2009.

11. Westfall TC, Westfall DP. Adrenergic agonists and antagonists. In: Brunton LL, Lazo JS, Parker KL, eds. *Goodman & Gilman's the Pharmacological Basis of Therapeutics,* 11th ed. New York: McGraw-Hill; 2006:237–296.

12. Taylor P. Anticholinesterase agents. In: Brunton LL, Lazo JS, Parker KL, eds. *Goodman &Gilman's the Pharmacological Basis of Therapeutics,* 11th ed. New York: McGraw-Hill; 2006;201–216.

13. Beilin B, Bessler H, Papismedov L. Continuous physostigmine combined with morphine-based patient-controlled analgesia in the postoperative period. Available at: http://eclips.consult.com/eclips/article/Anesthesia/S1073-5437(08)70467-4. Accessed June 22, 2009.

14. Fentanyl and Narcan interactions. Available at: http://www.drugs.com/drug-interactions/fentanyl_d00233_narcan_d00311.html. Accessed June 19, 2009.

15. Naloxone. Available at: http://www.drugs.com/pro/naloxone.html. Accessed June 22, 2009.

16. Blaise GA, Nugent M, McMichan JC, Durant PAC. Side effects of nalbuphine while reversing opioid-induced respiratory depression: report of four cases. Available at: http://www.springerlink.com/content/m144077218164523/. Accessed June 19, 2009.

17. Kuahashi K, Maruta H. The effect of sevoflurane and isoflurane on the neuromuscular block produced by vecuronium continuous infusion. Available at: http://www.ncbi.nlm.nih.gov/pubmed/8610903?ordinalpos=1&itool- EntrezSystem2.PEntr. Accessed May 28, 2009.

18. Cannon JE, Fahey MR, Castagnoli KP, et al. Continuous infusion of vecuronium: the effect of anesthetic agents. Available at: http://www.ncbi.nlm.nih.gov/pubmed/2889403?ordinalpos=1&itool- EntrezSystem2.PEntr. Accessed May 28, 2009.

19. Rocuronium for tracheal intubation: drug interaction. Available at: http://www.medscape.com/viewarticle/410908_6. Accessed June 15, 2009.

20. Interactions between succinylcholine chloride dihydrate and other drugs below. Available at: https://www.changehealthcare.com/rx_brands/drug_interactions/113869. Accessed June 22, 2009.

21. Taylor P. Agents acting at the neuromuscular junction and autonomic ganglia. In: Brunton LL, Lazo JS, Parker KL, eds. *Goodman & Gilman's the Pharmacological Basis of Therapeutics,* 11th ed. New York: McGraw-Hill; 2006:217–236.

22. Alexander DR. Pseudocholinesterase deficiency. Available at: http://emedicine.medscape.com/article/247019-overview. Accessed June 22, 2009.

23. Cammu G. Interactions of neuromuscular blocking drugs. Available at: https://www.researchgate.net/publication/11558517_Interactions_of_neuromuscular- block. Accessed June 15, 2009.

24. Koseoglu V, Chiang J, Chan KW. Acquired pseudocholinesterase deficiency after high-dose cyclophosphamide. Available at: http://www.nature.com/bmt/journal/v24/n12/abs/1702097a.html. Accessed June 22, 2009.

25. Feldman S, Karalliedde L. Drug interactions with neuromuscular blockers. Available at: http://cat.inist.fr/?aModele=afficheN&cpsidt=3229298. Accessed June 15, 2009.

26. Saitoh Y, Narumi Y, Fujii Y. Post-tetanic count and train-of-four responses during neuromuscular block produced by vecuronium and infusion of nicardipine. *Br J Anaesth.* 1999;83:340–342.

27. Feldman S, Karalliedde L. Drug interactions with neuromuscular blockers. Available at: http://www.ncbi.nlm.nkh.gov/pubmed/8905251?ordinalpos=1&itool=EntrezSystem2.P Entr. Accessed June 22, 2009.

28. Takasake Y, Naruoka Y, Shimizu C, Ochi G, Nagaro T, Arai T. Diltiazem potentiates the neuromuscular blockade by vecuronium in humans. Available at: http://www.ncbi.nlm.nih.gov/pubmed/7776513?ordinalpos=42&itool=EntrezSystem2.P Ent. Accessed May 28, 2009.

29. Short TG, Plummer JL, Chui PT, Chui MB, Chui PT. Hypnotic and anaesthetic interactions between midazolam, propofol, and alfentanil. *Br J Anaesth.* 1992;69:162–167.

30. Ropcke H, Konen-Bergmann M, Cuhls, M, Bouillon T, Hoeft A. Propofol and remifentanil pharmacodynamic interaction during orthopedic surgical procedures as measured by effects on bispectral index. Available at: http://www.sciencedirect.com/science?_ob=ArticleURL&_udi+B6T83-433P7VF- 7&_user. Accessed June 23, 2009.

31. Adachi YU, Uchihashi Y, Watanabe K, Satoh T. Small dose midazolam or droperidol reduces the hypnotic dose

of propofol at the induction of anaesthesia. Available at: http://journals.cambridge.org/action/displayAbstract;jsessionid=D410F36A8CCCCCFA 15. Accessed June 23, 2009.

32. What is diprivan (propofol). Available at: http://www.revolutionhealth.com/drugs-treatments/Diprivan. Accessed June 23, 2009.

33. Interaction between propofol and other drugs. Available at: https://www.changeheatlhcare.com/rx_brands/drug_interactions/12213. Accessed June 23, 2009.

34. Osaka Y, Inomata S, Tanaka E, et al. Effect of propofol on ropivacaine metabolism in human liver microsomes. *J Anesthiol.* 2006;20:60–63.

35. Propofol and isoflurane interactions. Available at: http://www.drugs.com/drug_interactions.php?action=adhoc&drug1_id=d00933&drug1_br. Accessed June 23, 2009.

36. Propofol and desflurane interactions. Available at: http://www.drugs.com/drug_interactions.php?action=adhoc&drug1_id=d00933&drug1_br. Accessed June 23, 2009.

37. Propofol and sevoflurane. Available at: http://www.drugs.com/drug_interactions.php?action=adhoc&drug1_id=d00933&drug1_br. Accessed June 23, 2009.

38. Propofol and amiodarone interactions. Available at: http://www.drugs.com/drug_interactions.php?action=adhoc&drug1_id+d00933&drug1_br. Accessed June 23, 2009.

39. Etomidate and amiodarone interactions. Available at: http://www.drugs.com/drug_interactions.php?action=adhoc&drug1_id=d00931&drug1_br. Accessed June 23, 2009.

40. Inooue K, el-Banayosy A, Stolarski L, Reichelt W. Vecuronium induced bradycardia following induction of anaesthesia with etomidate or thiopentone, with or without fentanyl. Available at: http://www.ncbi.nlm.nih.gov/pubmed/2892519. Accessed June 23, 2009.

41. Etomidate. Available at: http://www.umm.edu/altmed/drugs/etomidate-052950.htm. Accessed June 23, 2009.

42. Etomidate vs verapamil hydrochloride. Available at: http://www.mims.com/Page.aspx:menuid=alertr&DrugList=etomidate&CTRY=TW. Accessed June 23, 2009.

43. Stanley TH. Blood-pressure and pulse-rate responses to ketamine during general anesthesia. *Anesthesiology.* 1973;39:648–649.

44. Johnston RR, Miller RD, Way WL. The interaction of ketamine with d-tubocurarine, pancuronium and succinylcholine in man. *Anesth Analg.* 1974;53:496–501. Available at: http://www.anesthesia-analgesia.org/cgi/content/abstract/53/4/496. Accessed June 23, 2009.

45. Hirshman CA, Krieger W, Littlejohn G, Lee R, Julien R. Ketamine-aminophylline-induced decrease in seizure threshold. *Anesthesiology.* 1982;56:464–467.

46. Ketamine. Available at: http://www.nhtsa.dot.gov/people/injury/research/job185drugs/ketamine.htm. Accessed June 23, 2009.

47. Hui TW, Short TG, Hong W, Suen T, Gin T, Plummer J. Additive interactions between propofol and ketamine when used for anesthesia induction in female patients. *Anesthesiology.* 1995;82:642–648. Available at: http://journals.1ww.com/anesthesiology/pages/articleviewer.aspx?year=1995&issue=03 000. Accessed June 23, 2009.

48. Lorazepam. Available at: http://www.medicinenet.com/lorazepam/article.htm. Accessed June 23, 2009.

49. Commonly used regimens. Available at: http://www.sedationfacts.org/sedation-administration/moderate-sedation-regimens. Accessed June 23, 2009.

50. Abernethy DR, Greenblatt DJ, Ochs HR, Shader RI. Benzodiazepine drug-drug interactions commonly occurring in clinical practice. Available at: http://www.ncbi.nlm.nih.gov/pubmed/6144465. Accessed June 23, 2009.

51. Flumazenil. Available at: http://en.wikipedia.org/wiki/Flumazenil. Accessed June 24, 2009.

52. Probenecid. Available at: http://en.wikipedia.org/wiki/Probenecid. Accessed June 24, 2009.

53. Pentothal. Available at: http://www.rxlist.com/pentothal-drug.htm. Accessed June 24, 2009.

54. Diazoxide for hypertension treatment. Available at: http://highbloodpressure.about.com/od/treatmetnmonitoring/p/diazoxide.htm. Accessed June 24, 2009.

55. Methohexital. Available at: http://www.mims.com/Page.aspx?meniud=nmg&name=methohexital&h=anaesthetics,local. Accessed June 24, 2009.

56. Cytochrome P450 drug metabolism. Available at: http://www.pubmedcentral.nih.gov/articlerender.fcgi?artid=1312247&rendertype=table &id. Accessed July 6, 2009.

57. Cytochrome P450: alphabetical drug list. Available at: http://www.anaesthetist.com/physiol/basics/metabol/cyp/a.htm. Accessed July 7, 2009.

58. CYP1A2. Available at: http://en.wikipedia.org/wiki/CYP1A2. Accessed July 8, 2009.

59. CYP2C19. Available at: http://en.wikipedia.org/wiki/CYP2C19. Accessed July 8, 2009.

60. CYP2C9. Available at: http://en.wikipedia.org/wiki/CYP2C9. Accessed July 6, 2009.

61. CYP2D6. Available at: http://en.wikipedia.org/wiki/CYP2D9. Accessed July 6, 2009.

62. CYP2E1 Ligands. Available at: http://en.wikipedia.org/wiki/CYP2E1. Accessed July 8, 2009.

63. CYP3A4. Available at: http://en.wikipedia.org/wiki/CYP3A4. Accessed July 8, 2009.

64. Lucas H. Drug interactions that matter (5) hypertensives. Available at: http://www.pharmj.com/Editiorial/19990417/educaton/antihypertensive.html. Accessed June 12, 2009.

65. Polonia J. Interaction of antihypertensive drugs with anti-inflammatory drugs. Available at: http://www.ncbi.nlm.nih.gov/pubmed/9398294?ordinalpos=-1&itool=Entrez System2.PEntr. Accessed May 28, 2009.

66. Psavilicevic I, Rumbolt M, Rumbolt Z. Untoward interactions between antihypertensives and nonsteroidal anti-inflammatory drugs. Available at: http://www.ncbi.nlm.gov/pubmed/16485829?ordinalpos=1&itoll-EntrezSystem2.Pent. Accessed May 28, 2009.

67. Hydrochlorothiazide (in hydralazine and hydrochlorothiazide) may interact with ibuprofen. Available at: http://www.drugdigest.org/wps/portal/!ut/p/c0/04_SB8K8xLLM9MS-SzPy8XBz9CPos3 gX. Accessed June 8, 2009.

68. Drug profiles fall semester. Available at: http://www.pharmacology.tulane.edu/medpharm/DrugProfiles_Fall_Renal.html. Accessed July 12, 2009.

69. Huyse, FJ, Touw DJ, vanSchijndel RS, deLange JJ, Slaets PJ. Psychotropic drugs and the perioperative period: a proposal for a guideline in elective surgery. *Psychosomatics.* 2006;47:8–22. Available at: http://psy.,psychiatryonline.org/cgi/content/full/47/1/8. Accessed June 8, 2009.

70. Drug interaction guide for MAOI antidepressants. Available at: http://www.holisticonline.com/remedies/Depression/dep_interactions_MAOI.htm. Accessed July 12, 2009.

71. Xanax. Available at: http://www.rxlist.com/Xanax-drug.htm. Accessed June 23, 2009.

72. Drug interactions with selective serotonin reuptake inhibitors, especially with other psychotropics. Available at: http://www.ncbi.nlm.nih.gov/pubmed/11502857?ordinalpos=1&itollo=EntrezSystem2. PEnt. Accessed May 28, 2009.

73. Top ten dangerous drug interactions in long-term care. Available at: http://www.scoup.net/m3project/topten/. Accessed June 12, 2009.

74. Ament PW, Bertolino JG, Liszewski JL. Clinically significant drug interactions. *Am Fam Physician.* 2000;61:1745–1754.

75. Available at: http://www.drugdigest.org/wps/portal/!ut/p/c0/04_SB8KxLLM9MSSzPy8xBz9CP0os3 gX. Accessed June 8, 2009.

76. Available at: http://www.drugdigest.org/wps/portal/!ut/p/c0/04_SB8K8xLLM9MSSzPy8xBz9CP0os 3gX. Accessed June 8, 2009.

77. Fentanyl and diltiazem interactions. Available at: http://www.drugs.com/drug-interactions/fentanyl_d00233_diltiazem_d00045.html. Accessed June 19, 2009.

78. Available at: http://www.drugdigest.org/wps/portal/!ut/p/c0/04_SB8K8xLLM9MSSzPy8xBz9CP0os 3gX. Accessed June 8, 2009.

79. Available at: http://www.drugdigest.org/wps/portal/!ut/p/c0/04_SB8K8xLLM9MSSzPy8xBz9CP0os 3gX. Accessed June 8, 2009.

80. Available at: http://www.drugdigest.org/wps/portal/!ut/p/c0/04_SB8K8xLLM9MSSzPy8xBz9CP0ls3 gX. Accessed June 8, 2009.

81. Available at: http://www.drugdigest.org/wps/portal/!ut/p/c0/04_SB8K8xLLM9MSSzPy8xBz9CP0ls3 gX. Accessed June 8, 2009.

82. Marks JW. Beta blockers drug information. Available at: http://www.rxlist.com/script/main/art.asp?articlekey=-90349. Accessed July 15, 2009.

83. Available at: http://www.drugdigest.org/wps/portal/!ut/p/c0/04_SB8K8xLLM9MSSzPy8xBz9CP0ls3 gX. Accessed June 8, 2009.

Index

A

A FLOP (atropine, fluids, oxygen and pralidoxime), for organophosphate poisoning, 154

A_1 purine receptors, 396

A_2 purine receptors, 396

Abbot Pharmaceuticals, 173

absorption, 7

of local anesthetic drugs, 121

absorptive phase, in one-compartment model, 11

acceleromyographic TOF, 156

Accupril (quinapril), 288

pharmacokinetic profile, 287t

ACE inhibitors. See angiotensin-converting enzyme (ACE) inhibitors

acebutolol (Monitan, Sectral), 279

pharmacokinetics, 282t

Aceon (perindopril), 288

acetaminophen, 30, 81–82

and end-stage renal disease, 86

toxicity, 80

acetazolamide (carbonic anhydrase inhibitor), 258–259, 265t, 485t

acetic acids, 80

acetylcholine (ACh), 21, 22, 24, 96, 242, 386

manufacturer, 97

neurons releasing, 139

acetylcholinesterase (ACh-E), 29, 96, 149

acetylcysteine, 82

N-acetyl-p-benzoquinone, 82

ACh. See acetylcholine (ACh)

acid dissociation constant, 6

acidosis, in malignant hyperthermia, 411

AcipHex (rabeprazole), 250–252

interaction with tobacco and alcohol, 32t

activated clotting time (ACT), 373

actonel, interaction with tobacco and alcohol, 32t

actos, interaction with tobacco and alcohol, 31t

acupuncture and acupressure, 224–225, 225

acute adrenal crisis, signs and symptoms, 306

N-acyl transferases, reaction with drugs, 28

Adalat (nifedipine, Procardia), 120, 283–284, 449, 491t

drug interactions, 513

interaction with b blockers, 508

pharmacokinetic profile, 284t

adaptive immunity, 438

adderall XR, interaction with tobacco and alcohol, 32t

addiction, 73

adenine, 33

adenosine (Adenocard), 396–397

adenylyl cyclase, 355

adrenal cortex, 303

adrenal crisis, acute, signs and symptoms, 306

adrenal suppression, by etomidate, 45

adrenaline (epinephrine). See epinephrine (adrenaline)

adrenergic neuronal blockers, 272–275

pharmacokinetics, 274t

adrenergic receptor agonists, 327–331

amphetamines, 331

chemical structure, 331

atenolol (Tenormin), 336

chemical structure, 336

caution in use for geriatric population, 340

clonidine, 332t

dobutamine, 329

chemical structure, 329

dopamine, 328, 328–329

ephedrine, 329–330

chemical structure, 329

epinephrine (adrenaline), 327–328

chemical structure, 327

esmolol (Brevibloc), 338, 338

isoproterenol/isoprenaline, 333t

methyldopa (Aldomet), 332t

methylphenidate, 333t

mixed, 280–283

norepinephrine (noradrenaline), 328, 328

phentolamine, 334, 334–335

phenylephrine, 330–331

chemical structure, 330

prazosin, 335, 335

propranolol (Inderal), 337, 337–338

pseudophedrine, 333t

ritodrine, 332t

salbutamol/albuterol, 332t

timolol (Blocadren, Betimol, Timoptic, Timoptic XE), 336–337

chemical structure, 337

yohimbine, 335–336
  chemical structure, *335*
adrenergic receptor antagonists, 331–338
  phenoxybenzamine, 331, *331*, 334
adrenergic receptors, 324–339, *325*
adrenocortical function, etomidate
  impact on, 44
adrenocorticotropic hormone (ACTH), 303
advair, interaction with tobacco and
  alcohol, 31*t*
aerosols, 4
affinity, 18
age. *See also* infants; older adults;
  pediatric patients
  and antibiotic effectiveness, 195
  and muscle relaxant impact, 100
  and opioid administration, 63
agonist/antagonists, 22
agonists, 326
  receptor, 20
airway obstruction, from barbiturates, 43
airway remodeling, in asthma, 418
airway resistence, inhalation anesthesia
  impact, 179–180
albuterol, 20
  for asthma, 423*t*, 426
  interaction with tobacco and alcohol, 31*t*
alcohol
  chronic use, impact on opioid dosage, 64
  drug interactions, 29–30, 515, 516
    with benzodiazepines, 505
    with verapamil, 513
  propofol interaction, 504
alcohol and aldehyde dehydrogenase
  systems, reaction with drugs, 28
Aldomet (methyldopa), 270, 273*t*
  routes of administration and dosage,
    341*t*
aldosterone, pharmacokinetics and
  pharmacodynamics, 309*t*
aldosterone antagonists, 263
  for congestive heart failure, 487–488
alfentanil (Alfenta), 64, 68
  chemical structure, *68*
  dosage and administration, 71*t*
  drug interactions
    with ketamine, 505
    with midazolam, 56
  for electroconvulsive therapy, 477
  metabolism, 64
alkalizers, 240–241
allele, 33
allelomorph, 33
allergic reactions, 349
  histamine role, 348
allergy, etomidate side effects, 45
allodynia, 78
allosteric inhibition, 22
allosteric potentiation, 22
aloe vera, 317*t*
alosetron (Lotronex), 245–246

Aloxil (palonosetron), 219, 245–246
  doses and timing for adult
    administration, 218*t*
α agonists, practical uses in anesthesia, 271
α1-acid glycoproteins, 7
  local anesthetic binding to, 122
α2-adrenergic agonists, 89
  adverse effects, 273*t*
  centrally acting, 273*t*
  pharmacological comparisons, 272*t*
α-adrenergic blockers, 275–276
  caution in use for geriatric population,
    340
α-adrenergic receptors, 324–325
  effects of stimulating, *326*
alprazolam (Xanax)
  and fluoxetine (Prozac), 510
  interaction with tobacco and alcohol, 32*t*
  and oral contraceptives, 510
  in pregnancy, 56
  routes of administration and
    therapeutic uses, 54
alprostadil, effects, 357*t*
Altace (ramipril), 288
  interaction with tobacco and alcohol, 32*t*
  pharmacokinetic profile, 287*t*
alternative medicine, 315
Alzheimer's dementia, 150–151
ambien, interaction with tobacco and
  alcohol, 31*t*
American Association of Nurse Anesthetists,
  Code of Ethics for the Certified
  Registered Nurse Anesthetist, 252
American Heart Association, 481
*American Journal of Obstetrics and
  Gynecology*, 231
American Pain Foundation, 77
American Pain Society, 73
amidases, reaction with drugs, 28
Amidate. *See* etomidate (Amidate)
amide local anesthetics, 123, *127*,
  127–128, *128*
  effects on immune cell functions, 439
amikacin, 201
  clinical uses and indications, 203
  and neuromuscular blockade, 213*t*
amiloride, 263
amino acids, 19
  for protein production, 33
  transport of, 5
para-aminobenzoic acid, 123
aminoglycosides, 195*t*, 201–203
  adverse effects, 202–203
  clinical uses and indications, 203
  drug interactions, 503
  microbial resistance to, 202
  pharmacokinetics, 202
aminopenicillins, 197–198
aminophylline, drug interactions
  with ketamine, 47, 505
  with thiopental, 506

aminosteroids, 98
  pharmacokinetics comparison, 112*t*
amiodarone (Cordarone, Pacerone),
  393–395
  chemical structure, *394*
  etomidate interaction, 504
  propofol interaction, 504
amitriptyline, 469
  dosage, 470*t*
amlodipine (Norvasc), 285
  pharmacokinetic profile, 284*t*
ammonium chloride, 25
amnesia, from ketamine, 46
amoxapine, 469
  dosage, 470*t*
amoxicillin, 196, 197–198
  interaction with tobacco and alcohol,
    31*t*
  with potassium clavulanate, 201
amphetamines, 331
  chemical structure, *331*
  and psychosis, 459
ampicillin, 196, 197–198
amplitude, 175
analgesics, 77–91
  centrally acting α2 agonists, 89–91
    clonidine, 89–90
    dexmedetomidine, 90–91
  COX-2-specific inhibitors, 84–85
  cyclooxygenase enzymes, 79
  cyclooxygenase inhibitors, 78–79
  dextromethorphan, 89
  ketamine, 46, 87–89
  NSAIDs
    acetaminophen, 81–82
    aspirin (acetylsalicylic acid), 81
    ceiling effects, *85*
    characteristics, 79
    classification, 79–85
    diflunisal, 82
    indomethacin, 82
    ketorolac, 83–84
    propionic acid derivatives, 82–83
    side effects, 86–87
    sulindac, 82
    tolmetin, 82
  opioids, 65
anaphylactic reactions
  histamine and, 349
  from muscle relaxants, 110
  from penicillins, 198
anesthesia, 3. *See also* general anesthetics;
  local anesthetics
  general
    mechanisms, 25–26
    receptors and, 17
  for MH-susceptible patient, 408
Anesthesia Patient Safety Foundation, 173
anesthetic induction agents
  antihypertensive drug interactions
    pertinent to, 507–508

barbiturates, 41–44
   clinical uses, 43–44
   excretion, 43
   metabolism, 42–43
   pharmacokinetics, 42
etomidate, 44–45
immune system impact, 438–440
ketamine, 45–47
propofol, 48–50
angioedema, from penicillins, 198
angiotensin II receptor antagonists,
   289–290
   adverse effects, 290t
   anesthetic considerations in patients
      receiving, 291
   pharmacokinetics, 289t
angiotensin receptor blocker (ARB) agents
   for congestive heart failure, 487
angiotensin-converting enzyme, 10
angiotensin-converting enzyme (ACE)
   inhibitors, 286–289
   adverse effects, 287t
   anesthetic considerations, 289t
   anesthetic implications, 493
   for congestive heart failure, 486–487
   site of action, 487
   drug interactions, 508
   pharmacokinetic profile, 287t
antacids
   drug interactions
      with ACE inhibitors, 508
      with sodium citrate/citric acid, 241
      with tetracycline, 511
antagonists, 20–22, 326
antiarrhythmics, 385–398
   adenosine (Adenocard), 396–397
   amiodarone (Cordarone), 393–395
   β-adrenergic receptor antagonists,
      388–390, 388t
   calcium channel blockers, 390–391
   magnesium, 397–398
   muscarinic receptor antagonists, 386–
      387. See also anticholinergics
   sodium channel blockade, 391–393
   vasopressin (antidiuretic hormone,
      arginine vasopressin), 397
antibiotics, 193–213
   allergic reactions, 198t
   aminoglycosides, 195t, 201–203
      adverse effects, 202–203
      mechanism of action, 201
      microbial resistance to, 202
      pharmacokinetics, 202
   anesthesia providers responsibility for
      administration, 193
   clindamycin, 206–207
      chemical structure, 206
   dosage and administration, 210
   dose-dependent or time dependent
      killing, 194
   drug interactions, 503, 514–515

fluoroquinolones, 208
   immune effect, 440
   macrolides, 203–205
   metronidazole, 208–209
      chemical structure, 209
   minimum inhibitory concentration,
      193, 194
   and neuromuscular blockade, 212–213
   pharmacokinetic and pharmacodynamic
      principles, 194–195
   postantibiotic effect, 194
   practical aspects of use, 209–213
   in pregnancy, 195, 195t
   resistance, 194
   surgical prophylaxis, 209–212
      dosage and administration, 211t
      general principles, 210t
      guidelines, 212t
   synergism, 194
   tetracyclines, 205–206
   vancomycin, 207–208
      chemical structure, 207
anticholinergics, 139–146, 386–387
   for aspiration pneumonitis prophylaxis,
      242–243
   for asthma, 428
   clinical pharmacology, 142–143
   clinical uses and indications, 143–145
   comparative clinical manifestations,
      144t
   dosage and administration, 145–146
   drug interactions, 146
      with opioids, 511
      with TCAs, 510
   mechanism of action, 142
   packaging and dosages, 145t
   perioperative uses, 143t
   side effects and contraindications, 146
   toxicity, 471–473
anticholinesterase inhibitors, drug
      interactions, 503, 504
anticholinesterases, 149–157
   binding site, 150
   clinical pharmacology, 151–156
   comparative pharmacokinetics, 150t
   inadequate therapy vs. cholinergic
      crisis, testing for, 155, 155t
   mechanism of action, 149
   for myasthenia gravis, 150
   overdose, 154
   steroid drug interactions, 307t
anticoagulants, 367–383
   argatroban, 381–382
   drug interactions and conditions
      impacting, 379t, 510
   fondaparinux (Arixtra), 374, 376
   hirudins, 380–381
   regional anesthesia use with, 375t
   steroid drug interactions, 307t
   warfarin, 376–380
anticonvulsants, benzodiazepines as, 55

antidepressant drugs, 466–471, 467t
   discontinuation syndromes, 472–473
   selective serotonin uptake inhibitors,
      466–468
   TCAs and related compounds, 468–471
antidiabetic drugs
   interaction with ACE inhibitors, 508
   MAOIs and, 510t
   steroid drug interactions, 307t
antidiarrheal drugs, digoxin interaction
      with, 511
antidiuretic hormone (vasopressin,
      arginine vasopressin), 397
antiemetic drugs and therapies, 215–226
   acupuncture and acupressure, 224–225
   anticholinergics, 223
   antihistamines, 221–223
   benzamides, 220
   butyrophenones, 219–220
   cannabinoids, 224
   corticosteroids, 219
   doses and timing for adult
      administration, 218t
   doses for children, 218t
   ephedrine, 224
   guidelines, 226
   neurokinin-1 receptor antagonists,
      223–224
   phenothiazines, 220–221
   propofol, 224
   selective serotonin receptor
      antagonists, 216–219
      ondansetron (Zofran), 216, 218
antihistamines, 348
   as antiemetics, 221–223
   heparin interaction with, 373
antihypertensive drugs, 269–299
   α-adrenergic blockers, 275–276
   adrenergic neuronal blockers, 272–275
   angiotensin II receptor antagonists,
      289–290
   angiotensin-converting enzyme
      inhibitors, 286–289
      adverse effects, 287t
      anesthetic considerations, 289t
      pharmacokinetic profile, 287t
   arterial and venous vasodilators,
      292–293
   arterial vasodilators, 290–292
   β-adrenergic antagonists, 276
   calcium channel blockers, 283–286
      adverse effects, 285t
      pharmacokinetics profile, 284t
   classification, 270t
   interactions pertinent to anesthesia,
      507–508
   MAOIs and, 510t
   mechanisms of action, 269–283
   mixed adrenergic antagonists, 280–283
   nonselective β receptor antagonist,
      276–278

selective β receptor antagonists, 278–280
sympatholytics, 270–283
clonidine (Catapres, Dixarit, Duraclon), 271–272
guanabenz acetate (Wytensin), 270
guanfacine hydrochloride (Tenex), 270–271
antimicrobials, classification, 195t
antimuscarinic drugs, TCAs interaction, 509
antipsychotic drugs, 460–466, 461t
discontinuation syndromes, 466
drug interactions
with anticholinergics, 146
with opioids, 511
antithrombin, 368
Antivert (meclizine), 222–223
anxiety disorders, 457
Anzemet (dolastron), 218, 245–246
doses and timing for adult administration, 218t
apnea, 49
from barbiturates, 43
ketamine and, 47
apneic threshold, 179
apoptosis, physostigmine to protect against, 152
aprepitant (Emend), 223–224
for aspiration pneumonitis prophylaxis, 245
Apresoline (hydralazine), 290–291, 298, 489t, 490
advantages and disadvantages, 297t
adverse effects, 293t
pharmacokinetic profile, 293t
arachidonic acid, metabolites, 356
argatroban, 381–382
arginine vasopressin (vasopressin, antidiuretic hormone), 397
aricept, interaction with tobacco and alcohol, 32t
Arixtra (fondaparinux), 374, 376
arrhythmia
amiodarone for, 395t
incidence, 385
inhalation anesthesia and, 177
arsenic, impact on CYP enzymes, 30
arterial and venous vasodilators, 292–293
arterial hypoxemia, in malignant hyperthermia, 411
arterial vasodilators, 290–292
adverse effects, 293t
aspirate, 231
aspiration pneumonia, 231
aspiration pneumonitis, 231
closed-claim studies, 253
mechanism of, 234
factors affecting, 236
pathophysiology, 234, 236
treatment, 236

aspiration pneumonitis prophylaxis, 231–253
anesthesia implications, 252
basics, 231–234
interventions, 236–252
cricoid pressure, 238
cuffed endotraceal tube, 238
early for intubated patient, 236
fasting, 237–238
general anesthetics avoidance, 237
laryngeal mask, 238
nasogastric tube, 238
risk factors prediction, 236–237
legal considerations, 253–254
pharmaceutical methods, 238–252
alkalizers, 240–241
anticholinergics, 242–243
aprepitant (Emend), 245
butyrophenomes, 243–244
dexamethasone (Decadron), 246–247
fospropofol (Lusedra), 244–245
metoclopramide (Reglan), 247–248
omeprazole, 250–252
propofol (Diprivan), 244–245
ranitidine (Zantac), 248–249
serotonin 5-HT$_3$ receptor blockers, 245–246
aspirin (acetylsalicylic acid), 81, 357, 492
drug interactions
with heparin, 372
with warfarin, 511
aspirin-intolerant asthma (AIA), 419–420
astemizole, 351, 352
asthma
categories, 419t
differential diagnosis, 422
incidence, 418
management and control, 422–428
anticholinergics, 428
β-adrenergic agonists, 425–426
corticosteroids, 422–425
immunomodulators, 427
leukotriene recpetor antagonist, 427
mast cell stabilizers, 426–427
methylxanthines, 427–428
origins, 417–418
pathophysiology, 418–420
practical aspects in surgery, 428–432
acute branchospasm management, 431–432
intraoperative care, 429–431
preanesthesia care, 428–429
preanesthesia evaluation, 420–422
assessment parameters, 420t
risk factors, 421
severity classification, 421t
asystole, from propofol, 49
Atacand (candesartan), 289, 493t
adverse effects, 290t
Atarax (hydroxyzine, Vistaril), 221, 222
atazanavir, ranitidine interaction, 249

atenolol (Tenormin), 279, 336, 493t
chemical structure, 336
interaction with tobacco and alcohol, 31t
pharmacokinetics, 282t
routes of administration and dosage, 341t
atipamezole, to reverse dexmedetomidine effects, 90
Ativan. See lorazepam (Ativan)
atosiban, 450
atracurium, 100, 102, 103
and asthma, 430
and histamine release, 349
pharmacokinetics comparison, 112t
side effects, 110
atrial natriuretic peptide, 486
atropine, 143–144, 223, 242, 386–387
chemical structure, 387
clinical manifestations, 144t
dosage and administration, 145
edrophonium with, 155
for organophosphate poisoning, 154
atropine flush, 146
Atrovent (ipratropium), 144, 242
dosage and administration, 145–146
autocoids, 347–361
bradykinin agonist and antagonist, 353–354
prostaglandins, 356–357
serotonin agonist and antagonist, 354–356
chemistry, synthesis and metabolism, 354–355
and physiologic functions, 355
receptor subtypes, 355–356
autonomic nervous system
"lock and key" model for drug-receptor interactions, 323
organization, 140
parasympathetic divison, 139
volatile inhalation agents impact, 176
autoregulation, preservation during anesthesia, 174
avandia, interaction with tobacco and alcohol, 31t
Avapro (irbesartan), 289
average steady state, 15
azathioprine, 440t
azithromax, interaction with tobacco and alcohol, 31t
azithromycin, 204
azlocillin, 198
aztreonam, 201
dosage for surgical prophylaxis, 211t

B

bacterial growth, propofol support of, 49–50
bactericidal agents, 193, 194t
bacteriostatic agents, 193, 194t
baralyme, 173

barbiturates, 41–44
  clinical uses, 43–44
  contraindications, 43
  drug interactions, 505–506
  excretion, 43
  metabolism, 42–43
  pharmacokinetics, 42
Baxter pharmaceuticals, 163
beclamethasone dipropionate, for asthma,
    423t
beclamethasone/formoterol, for asthma,
    423t
Bell, Benjamin, 61
Benadryl (diphenhydramine), 350t,
    358–359t
  as antiemetic, 222
benazepril (Lotensin), 288, 493t
  pharmacokinetic profile, 287t
benzamides, 220, 355
benzene, impact on CYP enzymes, 30
benzisoxazole, 461t
benzodiazepines, 22
  adverse effects in older adults, 57
  clinical pharmacology, 53–55
  clinical uses and indications, 55
  dosages, administration and practical
      aspects, 57–58
  drug interactions, 56–57, 505
    with opioids, 70
  guidelines and precautions, 56–57
  mechanism of action, 53
  procedural sedation in children, 58
  side effects and contraindications,
      55–56
benzothiazepines, pharmacokinetic profile,
    284t
benztropine, as adjunct to levodopa, 142
benzylisoquinolines
  pharmacokinetics comparison, 112t
  side effects, 110
β agonist bronchodilators, for asthma, 423t
β-adrenergic agonists
  for asthma, 425–426
  to inhibit preterm labor, 449
β-adrenergic blockers, 490–491
  adverse effects, 281t–282t
  anesthetic implications, 493
  contraindications, 277
  drug interactions, 508, 514
  pharmacokinetics, 282t
  selective, adverse effects, 281t–282t
β-adrenergic receptor antagonists, 276,
    388–390, 388t
  caution in use for geriatric population,
      276
  nonselective, 276–278
  selective, 278–280
β-adrenergic receptors, 24, 324, 325–326
  desensitization process, 326
  effects of stimulating, 326
β-carotene, 29

β-lactam antibiotics, 195t, 196–201
  β-lactamase inhibitors, 201
  carbapenems, 200–201
  cephalosporins, 198–200
    adverse effects, 200
    chemical structure, 196
    clinical uses and indications,
        199–200
    for penicillin allergic patients, 200
    pharmacokinetics, 199
  mechanism of action, 196
  monobactams, 201
  penicillins, 196–198
    adverse effects, 198
    chemical structure, 196
    clinical uses and indications, 197–198
    elimination, 197
    pharmacokinetics, 197
    resistance, 196
β-lactamase inhibitors, 195t
β-lactamases, 196
betamethasone
  pharmacokinetics and pharmaco-
      dynamics, 309t
  properties, 304t
betaxolol (Betoptic, Betoptic S, Kerlone),
    279
  pharmacokinetics, 282t
Betimol (timolol, Blocadren, Timoptic,
    Timoptic XE), 278, 336–337, 493t
  chemical structure, 337
  pharmacokinetics, 282t
Betoptic (betaxolol, Betoptic S, Kerlone),
    279
  pharmacokinetics, 282t
Bextra (valdecoxib), 80, 84
  sulfonamide hypersensitivity as
      contraindication, 87
Biaxin (clarithromycin), drug interactions,
    513
bicarbonate, and pH of GI contents, 7
Bicitra (sodium citrate, Oracit), 240–241
Bigelow, Henry, 161
biliary excretion, in drug elimination, 10
biliary spasm, from opioids, 70
bioavailability, 9
biofilms from microorganisms, antibiotics
    and, 196
biotransformation, 8
bipolar disorder, 459
bisoprolol fumarate (Zebeta), 279, 493t
  pharmacokinetics, 282t
bitter orange, 317t
bivalirudin (Angiomax), 380
black cohosh, 318t
Blocadren (timolol, Betimol, Timoptic,
    Timoptic XE), 278, 336–337, 493t
  chemical structure, 337
  drug interactions, 513, 514
  pharmacokinetics, 282t
blood flow level, and drug absorption, 8

blood magnesium level, physical effects,
    449t
blood pressure
  antihypertensive drugs interaction with
      drugs decreasing, 507–508
  antihypertensive drugs interaction with
      drugs increasing, 507
  effects of inhalation anesthesia, 176
  MAOIs and drugs impacting, 510t
blood-brain barrier, antibiotics and, 194
blood-to-gas partition coefficient, 5–6
blood-to-gas solubility coefficient, 165
bone, NSAID impairment of healing, 87
Bowman's capsule, 258
bradycardia
  atropine for preventing, 144
  from clonidine, 90
  from muscarinic receptor antagonists,
      142
  from propofol, 49
bradykinin agonist and antagonist,
    353–354
bradykinin receptors, 353
brain, anesthetic molecules absorption, 8
breast milk, drugs in, 10
Brevibloc (esmolol), 279–280, 296t, 338,
    338, 491t
  pharmacokinetics, 282t
  routes of administration and dosage,
      341t
Brivital. See methohexital (Brivital)
bromelains, warfarin interaction, 378
brompheniramine, 359t
bronchial muscle, H$_1$ receptor antagonists
    and, 349
bronchoconstriction, from NSAIDs, 87
bronchodilators, MAOIs and, 509t
bronchospasm, management of acute,
    431–432
buclizine, 360t
budesomide/formoterol, for asthma, 423t
bumetanide, 260, 485t
bupivacaine, 128, 128
  clonidine with, 90
  dextrorotary isomers of, 125
  myotoxicity, 129
  pharmacology, 125t
  physiochemical properties, 124
buprenorphine, 71
  action at opioid m-receptor, 20
  chemical structure, 72
  in equianalgesia table, 67t
  immune effect, 440
bupropion, 467t, 468
  drug interactions, 514
buspirone, 354t, 473
butorphanol, in equianalgesia table, 67t
butyrophenones, 219–220, 461t, 464
  for aspiration pneumonitis prophylaxis,
      243–244
butyrylcholinesterase, 29

C

caffeine, 427
caffeine halothane contracture test
    (CHCT), 181, 407–408
Calan (verapamil, Isoptin, Verelan). *See*
    verapamil (Calan, Isoptin, Verelan)
calcium channel blockers, 283–286, 296t,
    390–391, 449–450, 491t
    adverse effects, 285t
    anesthetic implications, 286, 493
    drug interactions, 504
        with β blockers, 508
        with muscle relaxants, 110
    by local anesthetic, 120
    pharmacokinetics profile, 284t
calcium entry blockers (CEBs), 390
calcium sensitizers, 490
candesartan (Atacand), 289, 493t
    adverse effects, 290t
cannabinoids, 224
captopril (Capoten), 286, 493t
    pharmacokinetic profile, 287t
carbamazepine (Tegretol)
    drug interactions, 510, 513, 515
        with benzodiazepines, 56
        with thiazide diuretics, 508
carbapenems, 195t, 200–201
carbenicillin, 198
carbon dioxide
    respiratory responses to, 178
    shift of response curve, 179, *179*
carbon dioxide absorbents, carbon
    monoxide from inhalation
    anesthesia and, 173
carbon monoxide, impact on CYP
    enzymes, 30
carbonic anhydrase, 258
carbonic anhydrase inhibitor
    (acetazolamide), 258–259, 265t, 485
    lithium interaction, 509
carboxylic acids, 80
carboxypenicillins, 198
Cardene (nicardipine), 120, 284–285,
    295–296, 296t, 491t, 492
    drug interactions, 513
    esmolol with, 280
    pharmacokinetic profile, 284t
cardiac action potentials, 391
cardiac glycosides, 492
cardiac input, and inhalation anesthesia
    uptake, 166
cardioinhibitory drugs, for congestive
    heart failure, 490–492
cardiopulmonary bypass, anticoagulants
    for, 375t
cardiostimulatory drugs, for congestive
    heart failure, 488–490
cardiovascular system. *See also* congestive
    heart failure
    ACE inhibitors adverse effects, 287t
    adverse effects of adrenergic neuronal
        blockers, 274t

amphetamine effect, 331
angiotensin II receptor antagonists
    adverse effects, 290t
arterial vasodilator adverse effects, 293t
atenolol effect, 336
beta-blockers adverse effects, 281t–282t
dobutamine effect, 329
dopamine effect, 328
effects of inhalation anesthesia, 176–177
electroconvulsive therapy impact, 477
ephedrine effect, 330
esmolol effect, 338
etomidate side effects, 45
glucocorticoid therapy side effects, 306t
H_1 receptor antagonists and, 348–349
infective endocarditis, 212
ketamine side effects, 47, 88
muscarinic receptor antagonists
    impact, 142
neuromuscular blocker effects, 101
norepinephrine effect, 328
NSAID risk to, 80
phenoxybenzamine effect, 334
phentolamine effect, 334
phenylephrine effect, 330
prazosin effect, 335
propofol effect, 49
propranolol effect, 337
rocuronium effect, 100
succinylcholine effects, 106
toxicity to local anesthetics, 131–132
vasodilator adverse effects, 294t
yohimbine effect, 335
Cardizem (diltiazem), 286, 390
    drug interactions, 512–513
    pharmacokinetic profile, 284t
Cardura (doxazosin), 275, 276
    routes of administration and dosage,
        341t
carteolol (Cartrol, Ocupress), 278
    pharmacokinetics, 282t
carvedilol (Coreg, Kredex), 280, 283,
    491t, 493t
    pharmacokinetics, 282t
Catapres (clonidine, Dixarit, Duraclon),
    271–272, 273t
    routes of administration and dosage,
        341t
catatonic schizophrenia, 460
catechol, chemical structure, *323*
catecholamine vasopressors, 440–441
catecholamines
    ketamine and, 47
    metabolism, 324, *325*
    synthesis, 323, *324*
catechol-O-methyl transferace (COMT), 324
cauda equina syndrome, after spinal
    anesthesia, 130
cefaclor, 199
cefamandole, dosage for surgical
    prophylaxis, 211t
cefazolin, 199
    dosage for surgical prophylaxis, 211t

cefepime, 199
    clinical uses, 200
cefixime, 199
cefotaxime, 199
    clinical uses, 200
cefotetan, 199
    dosage for surgical prophylaxis, 211t
cefoxitin, 199
    dosage for surgical prophylaxis, 211t
cefpodoxime, 199
ceftazidime, 199
ceftibuten, 199
ceftriaxone, clinical uses, 200
cefuroxime, 199
    dosage for surgical prophylaxis, 211t
celecoxib (Celebrex), 80, 84, 450
    interaction with tobacco and alcohol, 31t
    sulfonamide hypersensitivity as
        contraindication, 87
Centers for Disease Control and
    Prevention, 29, 30
    Study of Efficacy of Nosocomial
        Infection Control, 209
central anticholinergic syndrome, 146, 151
    substance known to precipitate, 152t
central core disease, 407
central nervous system
    ACE inhibitors adverse effects, 287t
    adrenergic neuronal blockers adverse
        effects, 274t
    amphetamine effect, 331
    angiotensin II receptor antagonists
        adverse effects, 290t
    arterial vasodilator adverse effects,
        293t
    atenolol effect, 336
    beta-blockers adverse effects, 281t–282t
    blockade systemic effects, 386
    dopamine effect, 328–329
    ephedrine effect, 330
    epinephrine effect, 327
    esmolol effect, 338
    etomidate side effects, 45
    glucocorticoid therapy side effects,
        306t
    histamine receptor antagonist impact,
        350
    ketamine side effects, 46–47
    muscarinic receptor antagonists
        impact, 142
    norepinephrine effect, 328
    phenoxybenzamine effect, 334
    propofol impact, 49
    propranolol effect, 337
    systemic toxicity symptoms, from local
        anesthetics, 131, 131t
    vasodilator adverse effects, 294t
    yohimbine effect, 335
centrally acting α2 agonists, 89–91
    clonidine, 89–90
    dexmedetomidine, 90–91
cephalexin, 199
    interaction with tobacco and alcohol, 31t

cephalosporins, 195*t*, 198–200
  adverse effects, 200
  allergic reactions, 198*t*
  clinical uses and indications, 199–200
  for penicillin allergic patients, 200
  pharmacokinetics, 199
  ranitidine interaction, 249
cephradine, 199
cerebral metabolic oxygen requirements
  (CMRO₂), reduction in, 43
cerebral metabolic rate, inhalation
  anesthesia impact, 174
cerebral vasoconstriction, from
  barbiturates, 43
cerebrospinal fluid (CSF), 174
  inhalation agents impact, 175
cervical incompetence, 446
cetirizine, 222, 350*t*
chamomile, 318*t*
chemical reactions, from phase I
  metabolism, 8
chemoreceptor trigger zone (CTZ), 216
  and emetic center, *217*
  schematic of receptors, *241*
chemotherapy-induced nausea and
  vomiting (CINV), 215
children. *See* pediatric patients
chloramphenicol, immune effect, 440
chlordiazepoxide (Librium), 53
  in pregnancy, 56
  routes of administration and
    therapeutic uses, 54
chloride channel opening, 41
chloroform
  discovery, 160
  vs. ether, 162
  in obstetrics and surgery, 162
chloroprocaine, 126
  pharmacology, 125*t*
  physiochemical properties, 124
chlorothiazide (thiazide diuretics),
  261–262, 265*t*, 485*t*
chlorpheniramine, 350*t*, 359*t*
chlorpromazine, 220–221, 461–462
  dosage, 462*t*
  interaction with anticholinergics, 146
chlorthalidone, 484
choline acetyltransferace, 96
cholinergic crisis, 154
  testing for, 155, 155*t*
cholinergic muscarinic receptors,
  subtypes, 242
chromosomes, 33
chronic obstructive pulmonary disease,
  benzodiazepines use for, 55
chronic pain, 77
cigarettes. *See* smoking
cimetidine (Tagamet), 249, 352, 353
  drug interactions, 513, 514, 515
CINV. *See* chemotherapy-induced nausea
  and vomiting (CINV)
ciprofloxacin, 208
  dosage for surgical prophylaxis, 211*t*

cisapride (Propulsid), 248, 354*t*, 355
cisatracurium, 100, 102, 103
  for asthma patient, 430
  metabolism, 102
  pharmacokinetics comparison, 112*t*
citalopram, 467*t*, 468
citric acid, 240–241
clarithromycin (Biaxin), 204
  drug interactions, 513
clavulanic acid, 201
clearance, 13
cleft palate, benzodiazepines and, 56
clemastine, 358*t*
clevidipine (Clevelox), 285–286,
  295–296, 296*t*
  pharmacokinetic profile, 284*t*
clindamycin, 206–207
  chemical structure, *206*
  dosage for surgical prophylaxis, 211*t*
  and neuromuscular blockade, 213*t*
clomipramine, 469
  dosage, 470*t*
  TCAs interaction, 510*t*
clonazepam (Klonopin)
  interaction with tobacco and alcohol, 32*t*
  routes of administration and
    therapeutic uses, 54
clonidine (Catapres, Dixarit, Duraclon),
  89–90, 271–272, 273*t*, 332*t*
  drug interactions
    with TCAs, 508
    with tobacco and alcohol, 32*t*
  routes of administration and dosage,
    341*t*
clorazepate (Tranxene), routes of administration and therapeutic uses, 54
clozapine, 461*t*, 463
  dosage, 462*t*
coagonists, 20
coagulation
  cascade model, 367, *368*
  cell-based model, 368–369, *369*
  thrombin inhibitors, 369–382
    heparin, 369–373
cocaine
  metabolism, 123
  and psychosis, 459
codeine, 29
  conversion to morphine, 34
  drug interactions, 515
  in equianalgesia table, 66*t*
codeine/APAP, interaction with tobacco
  and alcohol, 32*t*
coenzyme Q10, warfarin interaction, 378
combustion, and inhalation anesthesia, 173
Compazine (prochlorperazine), 221, 248
  doses and timing for adult
    administration, 218*t*
  interaction with anticholinergics, 146
competitive antagonist, 20–21
  vs. noncompetitive antagonist, *21*
complementary and alternative medicine
  (CAM), 315

compound A, 173
concentration effect, 167
concentration gradient, and inhalation
  anesthesia uptake, 166
concerta, interaction with tobacco and
  alcohol, 32*t*
configurational stereoisomers, 125
congestive heart failure, 481–494
  anesthesia implications, 493
  classification, 482–483, 483*t*
  epidemiology, 481
  etiology and pathophysiology, 481–482
  treatment, 483–493
    ACE inhibitors, 486–487
    aldosterone antagonists, 487–488
    ARB agents, 487
    cardioinhibitory drugs, 490–492
    cardiostimulatory drugs, 488–490
    diuretics, 484–486
    medications useful for stages, 493*t*
    natriuretic peptides, 486
consciousness, opioids and, 69
constipation
  neostigmine to treat, 152
  from opioids, 70
constitutive receptors, 22
Cordarone. *See* amiodarone (Cordarone,
  Pacerone)
Cordus, Valerius, 160*t*
Coreg (carvedilol, Kredex), 280, 283,
  491*t*, 493*t*
  interaction with tobacco and alcohol, 32*t*
  pharmacokinetics, 282*t*
Corgard (nadolol), 277–278, 339
  pharmacokinetics, 282*t*
  routes of administration and dosage,
    341*t*
Corlopam (fenoldopam mesylate), 291–292,
  295, 298, 298*t*
  adverse effects, 293*t*
  pharmacokinetic profile, 293*t*
coronary steal phenomenon, 176–177, *177*
cortical nephrons, 258
cortical region of kidney, 257
corticosteroids. *See also* steroids
  as antiemetics, 219, 246–247
  inhaled, 309
    for asthma, 422–425, 423*t*
    side effects from deposits in mouth,
      424
  systemic, 425
corticotropin-releasing factor (CRH), 303
cortisol, 303, 309
  pharmacokinetics and pharmaco-
    dynamics, 309*t*
  properties, 304*t*
cortisone
  pharmacokinetics and pharmaco-
    dynamics, 309*t*
  properties, 304*t*
cough reflex, opioid effect, 70
coughing, 234
Coumadin. *See* warfarin (Coumadin)

COX enzymes, NSAIDs to block action, 79
COX-1 activity, NSAID blockade, 86
COX-2-specific inhibitors, 84–85
Cozaar (losartan potassium), 289
    adverse effects, 290*t*
    interaction with tobacco and alcohol, 32*t*
cranberry products, warfarin interaction, 378
crestor, interaction with tobacco and alcohol, 32*t*
Cricoid pressure, for aspiration pneumonitis prophylaxis, 238
cromolyn, for asthma, 423*t*, 427
cruciferous vegetables, 29*t*
curare, 95
    poisoning reversal, 149
curarine, 95
cyclizine (Marezine), 221, 222, 360*t*
cyclooxygenase (COX) enzymes, 356
    inhibition, 450
cyclooxygenase enzymes, 79
cyclooxygenase inhibitors, 78–79
cyclooxygenase pathways, 79
cyclopropane, 162
cyclosporine (Neoral), 33, 440*t*
    drug interactions, 503
cymbalta, interaction with tobacco and alcohol, 32*t*
CYP enzymes, 28–29
    chronic alcohol use and, 30
    CYP2C19 variants, 34
    CYP2D6, and drug metabolism, 34, 389
    CYP3A4, 233
cytochrome P-450 system (CYPs), 8, 233, 506
    drugs impacting, 55
    inhibitors interaction with asthma therapy, 425
    isozymes, inducers and inhibitors, 506*t*, 507*t*
    phytochemicals' influence on, 29
    reaction with drugs, 28
cytosine, 33

D

Dale, Henry, 139
dalteparin (Fragmin), 369
danshen, warfarin interaction, 378
dantrolene, 181, 405–413
Davy, Humphrey, 160, 160*t*
Decadron (dexamethasone), 219, 225, 307–308
    for aspiration pneumonitis prophylaxis, 246–247
    doses and timing for adult administration, 218*t*
    pharmacokinetics and pharmaco-dynamics, 309*t*
    properties, 304*t*
delusions, associated with psychosis, 458

demeclocycline, absorption after oral administration, 205
Demerol. *See* meperidine (Demerol)
Demser (metyrosine), 274
    pharmacokinetics, 274*t*
depolarizing muscle relaxants, 98–99
    pharmacokinetics comparison, 112*t*
    side effects, 106–110
    steroid drug interactions, 307*t*
depot injections, 5
depression and depressive disorders, 459
    symptoms, 459*t*
desethylamiodarone, 393, 394
desflurane, 163, 171, 172–173
    for asthma patient, 431
    and autonomic nervous system, 176
    CSF pressure increase, 174
    immune effect, 438
    impact on heart rate, 176
    malignant hyperthermia from, 405
    pharmacologic properties, 163*t*
    reduction in arterial blood pressure, 176
desipramine (Norpramin), 469
    dosage, 470*t*
    drug interactions, 510
dexamethasone (Decadron), 219, 225, 307–308
    for aspiration pneumonitis prophylaxis, 246–247
    doses and timing for adult administration, 218*t*
    pharmacokinetics and pharmaco-dynamics, 309*t*
    properties, 304*t*
dexmedetomidine (Precedex), 56, 89, 90–91, 272
dextran 70, 25
    interaction with heparin, 372
dextromethorphan, 89
dextrorotary isomers of bupivacaine, 125
dezocine, in equianalgesia table, 67*t*
diabetes insipidus, 474
diaphragm
    inhalation anesthesia impact on function, 178
    sensitivity to relaxants, 101
diavan HCT, interaction with tobacco and alcohol, 31*t*
diazepam (Valium), 53
    active metabolites, 54
    ketamine interaction, 505
    in pregnancy, 56
    routes of administration and therapeutic uses, 54
    side effects, 56
    therapeutic window, 14
    use, routes and dosages, 57*t*
diazoxide (Hyperstat, Proglycem), 291
    adverse effects, 293*t*
    drug interactions, with thiopental, 506
    pharmacokinetic profile, 293*t*

dibenzodiazepines, 461*t*, 463–464
Dibenzyline (phenoxybenzamine hydrochloride), 275
dibucaine number, 102
    interpretation, 102*t*
diclofenac, 82
dicloxacillin, 196
dietary supplements, 315–322
    commonly used, 316–321
    historical perspective, 315
    legislative intervention, 315–316
    web resources, 322*t*
"diethyl ether", 161
diflunisal, 82
digestion, 231
digitalis, 315
digitalis glycosides, drug interactions
    with amiodarone, 394
    with heparin, 373
    with steroids, 307*t*
digitek, interaction with tobacco and alcohol, 32*t*
digoxin, 492, 493*t*
    anesthetic implications, 493
    calcium channel blocker impact, 390
    drug interactions, 512, 513
        with acetazolamide, 259
        with antidiarrheals, 511
        with spironolactone, 264
    therapeutic window, 14
dihydropyridines, pharmacokinetic profile, 284*t*
2,6-diisopropyl-1,4 quinol, 48
Dilantin. *See* phenytoin (Dilantin)
diltiazem (Cardizem), 286, 390
    drug interactions, 512–513
    pharmacokinetic profile, 284*t*
dimenhydrinate (Dramamine), 221, 222, 358*t*
dinoprost, effects, 357*t*
dinoprostone, effects, 357*t*
Diovan (valsartan), 290
    adverse effects, 290*t*
diovan, interaction with tobacco and alcohol, 31*t*
diphenhydramine (Benadryl), 350*t*, 358–359*t*
    as antiemetic, 222
diphenylbutylpiperidine, 461*t*, 464
Diprivan (propofol). *See* propofol (Diprivan)
dipyridamole, 396–397
discontinuation syndromes, antidepressant, 472–473
disopyramide (Norpace), drug interactions, 513
disorganized schizophrenia, 460
dissociation constant (K_d)
    of drug-receptor complex, 18
    local anesthetics with impact, 124
dissociative anesthesia, 87
dissociative state, from ketamine, 46

dissolution, of tablets, 7
distribution, 7–8
  of local anesthetics, 121–122
  volume of, 13
diuretics, 257–266
  anesthetic implications, 265, 493
  carbonic anhydrase inhibitor
    (acetazolamide), 258–259
  for congestive heart failure, 484–486
  loop, 260–261
  osmotic, 262–263
  potassium-sparing, 263–265
  summary, 265t
  thiazide, 261–262
divinyl ether, 162
Dixarit (clonidine, Catapres, Duraclon),
  271–272, 273t
  routes of administration and dosage,
    341t
DNA, 33
DNA sequence, 33
dobutamine, 329, 488, 488t
  chemical structure, 329
  routes of administration and dosage,
    341t
dolastron (Anzemet), 218, 245–246
  doses and timing for adult
    administration, 218t
donepezil, for Alzheimer's dementia
  management, 151
dong quai, warfarin interaction, 378
dopamine, 328, 328–329, 488–489, 488t
  vs. fenoldopam mesylate (Corlopam),
    298t
  and psychosis pathophysiology, 459
  routes of administration and dosage,
    341t
dopamine 1 agonists, advantages and
  disadvantages, 298t
dosages for drugs, 13. See also specific
    drug names
  calculations, 14–15
dose-dependent killing, by antibiotics, 194
dose-response curve, 18–19
double depression, 459
double helix, 33
double-burst stimulation mode, 104, 105t
down-regulation, 23
doxacurium, pharmacokinetics
  comparison, 112t
doxazosin (Cardura), 275, 276
  routes of administration and dosage,
    341t
doxepin, 469t, 470
  dosage, 470t
doxycycline
  absorption after oral administration, 205
  drug interactions, 515
Dramamine (dimenhydrinate), 221, 222
dromotropy, 386
dronedarone, 395

droperidol (Inapsine), 219–220, 225,
  243–244, 461t, 464
  acetazolamide interaction, 259
  dosage, 462t
  doses and timing for adult
    administration, 218t
drug dosing, 13
drug elimination, 10
drug interactions, 501–516. See also under
    specific drug names
  affecting drug absorption, 511–512
  with anticoagulants, 379t
  β-blockers, 513
  of cardiac drugs, 512
  heparin, 372–373
  impact on elimination half-life, 12
  impacting distribution, 512
  intravenous sedatives and hypnotics,
    504–506
  neuromuscular blocking drugs (NMBs),
    502–504
  opioids, 70, 475–476, 502
  psychopharmacologic agents, 508–511
drug molecules
  conversion to other chemical
    compounds, 8
  physical properties, 5
  as weak acids or bases, 6
drug-receptor interactions, "lock and key"
    model, 17, 18
drugs
  discontinued after prolonged period, 23
  factors attributed to variable responses,
    28t
    cultural and environmental
      influences, 28–33
    dietary influences, 29
    interactions with tobacco and alcohol,
      31–32t
dual block, 109
Dumas, Jean Baptiste-Andre, 160t, 161
duodenum, 233
Duraclon (clonidine, Catapres, Dixarit),
  271–272, 273t
  routes of administration and dosage,
    341t
duty of care, 252
DynaCirc (isradipine), 285
  pharmacokinetic profile, 284t
dysrhythmias, in malignant hyperthermia,
  411
dysthymia, 459

E

echinacea, 315, 317t, 318t
echothiophate
  clinical pharmacology, 156
  plasma cholinesterase impaired by, 111
edrophonium (Tensilon)
  clinical pharmacology, 154–156

drug interactions, 503
  for myasthenia gravis, 150
  vs. neostigmine, 153
  pharmacokinetics, 150t
  recommended doses according
    to TOF, 156t
edrophonium test dose (tensilon test),
  155, 155t
EEG, and evoked potentials, 175
effexor XR, interaction with tobacco and
  alcohol, 31t
eggplant, solanaceous glycoalkaloids in, 29
Eldepryl (selegiline), 509
  drug interactions, 511
elderly. See older adults
electrocardiographic arrhythmia strip
  chart, analysis, 385, 386
electroconvulsive therapy (ECT),
  anesthesia considerations, 476
elimination half-life, 12
elimination of drugs, 10
Emend (aprepitant), 223–224
  for aspiration pneumonitis prophylaxis,
    245
emergence delirium
  from ketamine, 88–89
  midazolam to prevent, 89
emergence phenomena, with ketamine, 47
emesis. See also vomiting
  physiology, 216
emetic center, and chemoreceptor trigger
  zone (CTZ), 217
enalapril (Vasotec), 288, 493t
  pharmacokinetic profile, 287t
enantiomers, 125
endocarditis, infective, 212
endocrine system, glucocorticoid therapy
  side effects, 306t
endotracheal tube, 238
end-stage renal disease, acetaminophen
  impact, 81, 86
enflurane, 163
Enlon Plus, 155
enolic acids, 80
enoxaparin (Lovenox), 369
enterogastric inhibitory nervous reflex, 233
enterohepatic recycling, 10
environmental impact, of inhalation
  anesthesia, 181
enzymes, 28–29
  activated or inactivated, 19
  outcome of genetic disposition on
    activity and drug response, 34t
  saturating ability to metabolize
    particular compound, 8
ephedra, 317t, 318t
ephedrine, 224, 315, 329–330
  chemical structure, 329
  drug interactions, 515
  rocuronium with, 100
  routes of administration and dosage, 341t

epidural drug administration, 4
epinephrine (adrenaline), 327–328, 488t, 489
    for asthma, 423t
    β blockers and, 508
    chemical structure, 327
    with chloroprocaine, 126
    inhibiting action, 276
    with lidocaine, and neuronal injury, 130
    lidocaine with, 121
    in local anesthetic solutions, 122
    myocardial sensitization with, 177
    routes of administration and dosage,
        341t
    with tetracaine, 126
epithelial endocytosis, absorption by, 7
eplerenone, 263, 485t, 487–488, 493t
eprosartan, 493t
equianalgesia table, 65–66, 66–67t
equilibration rate of FA, 165
ergot alkaloids, 451
ergotrate, 451
ertapenem, 200–201
erythromycin, 29, 204, 248, 315–316
    chemical structure, 204
    dosage for surgical prophylaxis, 211t
    drug interactions, 513
    immune effect, 440
Escherichia coli, 197
escitalopram, 467t, 468
esmolol (Brevibloc), 279–280, 296t, 338,
        338, 389, 491t
    pharmacokinetics, 282t
    routes of administration and dosage,
        341t
esomeprazole (Nexium), 250–252
    interaction with tobacco and alcohol, 31t
estazolam (Prosom), routes of administra-
        tion and therapeutic uses, 54
ester local anesthetics, 125–126, 126
    steroid drug interactions, 307t
esterases, 9
    reaction with drugs, 28
estrogens, steroid drug interactions, 307t
eszopiclone (Lunesta), 55
    routes of administration and
        therapeutic uses, 54
ethacrynic acid, 260, 485t
ether, 159
    vs. chloroform, 162
    discovery, 160
    surgical use, 161–162
ethnic group, 34
ethnic pharmacology, 27
ethyl chloride, 162
ethylene, 162
etidocaine, 127, 127
    pharmacology, 125t
    physiochemical properties, 124
etomidate (Amidate), 41, 44–45
    for asthma patient, 430
    drug interactions, 504–505
    for electroconvulsive therapy, 477

immune effect, 439, 439t
    for MAOI-treated patients, 476
    steroid drug interactions, 307t
European In Vitro Malignant
        Hyperthermia Test, 407–408
evoked potentials, and EEG, 175
excitatory amino acid receptors, 88
exercise-induced asthma, 419
extrajunctional receptors, 107–108, 108
extubation, decision process, 157
eye
    muscarinic receptor antagonists
        impact, 143
    succinylcholine impact on intraocular
        pressure, 109

F

FA (fraction alveolar), 164
    overcoming input problems in
        achieving, 165–166
facial nerve, response to PNS, 104, 104t
factor XIIa, 367
fade phenomenon, 98
FA/FI curve, 168–169, 169
FA/FI ratio, 165, 166–168, 167
famotidine, 352, 353
fasciculations, 99
fasting, for aspiration pneumonitis
        prophylaxis, 237–238
fat, movement of inhalation anesthetic
        into, 168–169
felodipine (Plendil), 29, 284
    pharmacokinetic profile, 284t
fenoldopam mesylate (Corlopam),
        291–292, 295, 298, 298t
    adverse effects, 293t
    vs. dopamine, 298t
    pharmacokinetic profile, 293t
fentanyl, 62–64, 126, 501
    chemical structure, 62
    dosage and administration, 71t
    drug interactions
        with diltiazem, 513
        with midazolam, 56
    in equianalgesia table, 66t
    immune effect, 440
    interaction with propofol, 48
    metabolism, 64
    pharmacodynamics, 62–64
    pharmacokinetics, 62
    pharmacology, 69t
    as superagonist, 20
fetus
    anesthesia impact, 445
    inhalation anesthesia impact on
        development, 180
    propofol crossing into circulation, 48
feverfew, 317t, 318t
fexofenadine, 222
    interaction with tobacco and alcohol, 32t

fibrinogen, converting to fibrin, 367
Fick's law, 7
first-order rate kinetics, 12
first-pass metabolism, 9
flavin-containing monoxygenase system,
        reaction with drugs, 28
flomax, interaction with tobacco and
        alcohol, 32t
floppy infant syndrome, 56
fludrocortisone, pharmacokinetics and
        pharmacodynamics, 309t
flumazenil (Romazicon)
    drug interactions, with
        benzodiazepines, 55, 505
    routes of administration and
        therapeutic uses, 54
fluorine chemistry, 163
fluoroquinolones, 195t, 208
    allergic reactions, 198t
fluoxetine (Prozac), 354t, 466–467, 467t
    and alproazolam (Xanax), 510
    drug interactions, 514, 515
    interaction with tobacco and alcohol, 32t
    and selegiline (Eldepryl), 511
fluphenazine, 461t
    dosage, 462t
flurazepam (Dalmane), routes of admin-
        istration and therapeutic uses, 54
fluroxene, 163
fluticasone, for asthma, 423t
fluticasone propionate/salmeterol, for
        asthma, 423t
fluvoxamine, 467t, 468
fondaparinux (Arixtra), 374, 376
foot, neuromuscular monitoring sites,
        104t
formoterol, for asthma, 426
fosinopril (Monopril), 288
    pharmacokinetic profile, 287t
fospropofol (Lusedra), for aspiration
        pneumonitis prophylaxis, 244–245
foxamax, interaction with tobacco and
        alcohol, 31t
fraction alveolar (FA), 164
    overcoming input problems in
        achieving, 165–166
fraction delivered (FD), 164
Framingham Heart Study, 481
fresh gas flow (FGF), 164
functional pain, 78
funtional residual capacity (FRC), 178
furosemide, 260–261, 265t, 485t
    anesthetic implications, 265
    drug interactions, 515
    interaction with tobacco and alcohol,
        31t

G

GABA$_A$ complex, 22, 25
gabapentin, interaction with tobacco and
    alcohol, 32t

gagging, 234
galantamine, for Alzheimer's dementia
    management, 151
gallamine, risk for asthma patient, 430
γ-aminobutyric acid (GABA)
    and barbiturates, 41
    and inhalation agent, 170
γ-aminobutyric acid (GABA) receptors
    alcohol consumption impact, 30
    propofol impact, 48
garlic, 316, 317t, 318t
    warfarin interaction, 378
gastric secretions
    contents and functions, 233
    H$_2$ agonists and, 349
gastrin, 233
gastrointestinal (GI) tract
    ACE inhibitors adverse effects, 287t
    adverse effects of beta-blockers,
        281t–282t
    angiotensin II receptor antagonists
        adverse effects, 290t
    arterial vasodilator adverse effects, 293t
    beta-blockers adverse effects, 281t–282t
    bleeding from ketorolac, 83, 84
    drug interaction, 4
    epinephrine effect, 327
    glucocorticoid therapy side effects, 306t
    muscarinic receptor antagonists
        impact, 143
    NSAID toxicity, 86
    opioid effect, 70
    vasodilator adverse effects, 294t
gate control theory, 78
gemifloxacin, 208
gender differences
    muscle relaxant dosage, 100
    in opioid response, 63–64
general anesthetics
    avoidance for aspiration pneumonitis
        prophylaxis, 237
    for electroconvulsive therapy, 476
    impact on local anesthetic
        pharmacokinetics, 122
    mechanisms, 25–26
    receptors and, 17
genes, 33
genetic effects, of inhalation anesthesia,
    180–181
genetic testing, for MH susceptibility, 408
genetics
    basic concepts, 33
    impact on response to drug, 27
    variations, 33–34
genitourinary tract
    amphetamine effect, 331
    ephedrine effect, 330
    epinephrine effect, 327
    male, phentolamine effect, 334
    muscarinic receptor antagonists
        impact, 143
    norepinephrine effect, 328

prazosin effect, 335
    yohimbine effect, 336
genome, 33
genotype, 33
    to project drug response, 34
gentamicin, 201
    chemical structure, 201
    clinical uses and indications, 203
    dosage for surgical prophylaxis, 211t
    drug interactions, 515
    and neuromuscular blockade, 213t
geriatric patients. See older adults
ginger, 317t, 319t
ginkgo biloba, 317t, 319t
    warfarin interaction, 378
ginseng, 316, 317t, 319t
    warfarin interaction, 378
glaucoma, echothiophate for treating, 156
glomerular filtration rate (GFR),
    furosemide and, 260
glomerulus, 258
glucocorticoid receptors, 304–305
glucocorticoids, 219, 307. See also steroids
    neurophysiology associated with
        production, 303, 303–304
glucuronic acid conjugation, 9
glutamate receptors, 87
glutathione, 82
glycerin, 263
glycine, affinity of, 22
glycocalyx layer, 7
glycopyrrolate, 387
    chemical structure, 387
glycopyrrolate (Robinul), 46, 144, 476
    clinical manifestations, 144t
    dosage and administration, 145
    vs. scopolamine, 242
G-protein coupled receptors, 24, 24,
    120–121, 324, 355, 356
granisetron (Kytril), 218–219, 245–246
    doses and timing for adult
        administration, 218t
grapefruit juice, 29
guanabenz, 273t
guanabenz acetate (Wytensin), 270
guanadrel (Hylorel), 272–273
    pharmacokinetics, 274t
guanfacine, 273t
guanfacine hydrochloride (Tenex), 270–271
guanine, 33
guanine nucleotide binding protein
    (G-protein) coupled receptors,
    120–121
Guthrie, Samuel, 160, 160t
gyri, in motor end plate, 96

H

H$_1$ receptor antagonists, 221–223. See also
    antihistamines
Haemophilus influeznzae, 196–197
half-life of effect, 12

hallucinations, 458
    from ketamine, 47
halogenation, importance, 163–164
haloperidol, 220, 243, 464
    dosage, 462t
halothane, 30, 163, 171, 179
    for asthma patient, 431
    malignant hyperthermia from, 405
    pharmacologic properties, 163t
halothane hepatitis, 180
halperidol, 461t
hawthorn, 319t
hearing loss, from aminoglycosides, 202
heart. See cardiovascular system;
    congestive heart failure
heart rate, inhalation anesthesia impact,
    176
heat stroke, dantrolene for treating, 410
Henderson-Hasselbalch equation, 6, 7
heparin, 369–373
    anesthesia implications, 374
    clinical pharmacology, 370
    clinical uses and indications, 370–371
    comparative pharmacology, 370
    dosage and administration, 373–374
    drug interactions, 372–373
    laboratory monitoring, 373
    mechanism of action, 370
    protamine reversal, 373
    side effects and contraindications,
        371–372
heparin-induced thrombocytopenia (HIT),
    371–372
herbal supplements, 315–322, 317–321t
    with anesthetic implications, 317t
    historical perspective, 315
    interaction with tobacco and alcohol, 33
    legislative intervention, 315–316
    web resources, 322t
hirudins, 380–381
histamine, 233, 347–353
    chemical structure, 348
    clinical uses, 350
    molecular structure, 249
    release
        as nondepolarizer effect, 110
        opioids and, 430
    storage and release, 347–348
histamine receptor antagonists, 248–249,
    348, 350–352
    classification, 350t
    classification and agents, 358–361t
    clinical uses, 352
    pharmacokinetics and side effects,
        351–352
histamine receptors, 348–349
    effects of stimulating, 250
histamine-*N*-methyltransferase, 348
Hohenheim, Phillip von, 160
horse chestnut, 319t
host factors impacting antibiotic
    effectiveness, 194

Hunter, Charles, 61
hydralazine (Apresoline), 290–291, 298, 451, 489t, 490
  advantages and disadvantages, 297t
  adverse effects, 293t
  pharmacokinetic profile, 293t
hydrochloric acid, 233
hydrochloric acid H+/K+ ATPase proton pump, 250, 250
hydrochlorothiazide, 261, 484, 485t
  drug interactions, 515
  interaction with tobacco and alcohol, 31t
hydrocodone/APAP, interaction with tobacco and alcohol, 31t
hydrocortisone, 304
  for asthma, 423t
hydrodolasetron, 218
hydromorphone, 64, 68
  chemical structure, 68
  dosage and administration, 71t
  in equianalgesia table, 66t
  pharmacology, 69t
hydroxyl thiopental, 42
11-β-hydroxylase, 45
4-hydroxypropofol, from propofol, 48
hydroxyzine (Atarax, Vistaril), 221, 222, 350t, 361t
Hylorel (guanadrel), 272–273
hyperaldosteronism, 264
hyperalgesia, 78
hypercholoremic metabolic acidosis, as NSAID effect, 86
hyperkalemia
  after succinylcholine administration, 107
  in malignant hyperthermia, 411
Hyperstat (diazoxide, Proglycem), 291
  adverse effects, 293t
  pharmacokinetic profile, 293t
hypertension, 269–270. See also antihypertensive drugs
  anesthetic management of acute perioperative, 294–298
  perioperative
    anesthetic management of acute, 294–298
    etiology, 294
    profile of ideal drug treatment, 295
  pregnancy-induced, 446–447
  in U.S., 269
hypertensive crisis, with monoamine oxidase inhibitors, 472
hyperthermia
  dantrolene for treating, 410
  malignant, 28
  from succinylcholine, 106–107
hypnotic drugs
  interaction with opioids, 70
  intravenous drug administration, 504–506
  nonbenzodiazepin, 55

hypoglycemic drugs, b blockers and, 508
hypokalemia, thiazide diuretics and, 508
hypotension
  ACE inhibitors adverse effects, 289
  from clonidine, 90
hypothalamic-pituitary-adrenal (HPA) axis, 303
  suppression, 305, 309
hypothyroidism, from lithium, 474
hypoxic drive, inhaled anesthetics blunting of, 179
hypoxic pulmonary vasoconstriction, 178, 431
Hytrin (terazosin), 275, 276
  routes of administration and dosage, 341t

I

ibuprofen, 82
  interaction with tobacco and alcohol, 32t
iloprost, effects, 357t
imipenem, 200
imipramine (Tofranil), 469t, 470
  dosage, 470t
  drug interactions, 510
immune system, 437–442
  adjunct and procedural drugs, 440–441
  alcohol abuse linked to altered response, 30
  anesthetic drugs impact, 438–440
  glucocorticoid therapy side effects, 306t
  response, anesthetic technique and, 441
  review of normal, 437–438
immunocompromised host, and antibiotic effectiveness, 194
immunoglobulin, and antibiotic effectiveness, 194
immunoglobulin E, role in asthma, 418
immunomodulators, for asthma, 427
immunosuppressant drugs, 440, 440t
in vitro susceptibility testing, of antibiotics, 193
Inapsine (droperidol), 219–220, 225, 243–244, 461t, 464
  acetazolamide interaction, 259
  dosage, 462t
  doses and timing for adult administration, 218t
indapamide, 485t
Inderal (propranolol), 276–277, 337, 337–338, 493t
  pharmacokinetics, 282t
indomethacin, 82, 450
  furosemide interaction, 260
  spironolactone interaction, 264
induction, 9
infants. See also neonate
  asthma, differential diagnosis, 422
  muscle relaxant dosage, 100
infections, treatment. See antibiotics

infective endocarditis, 212
inflammation, mediators formation, 419
inflammatory pain, 77–78
infusion, 4
  dosing, 14
inhalation anesthesia, 159–181
  cardiovascular system impact, 176–177
  combustion and, 173
  distribution equation, 168
  elimination, 169
  environmental impact, 181
  FA/FI curve, 168–169, 169
  fetal development, 180
  genetic effects, 180–181
  halogenation importance, 163–164
  historical context, 159–164
    timeline, 160t
  ideal, 163
    characteristics, 164t
  impact on system, 173–180
  as malignant hyperthermia trigger, 181
  modern, 171–173
  pharmacodynamics and, 169–171
    mechanism of action, 170
  protein theories and, 170
  solubility in blood, 165
  time constant, 168, 168t
  uptake, 166–169
  uptake and distribution, 164–166, 165
inhalational drug administration, 4
inhaled anesthetics, immune system impact, 438
inhaled corticosteroids (ICSs), 309
  for asthma, 422–425, 423t
  side effects from deposits in mouth, 424
innate immunity, 437–438
insomnia, drugs for treating, 55
integumentary system, glucocorticoid therapy side effects, 306t
interferon, 438
intermittent dosing, 15
International Association for the Study of Pain, 61, 77
intra-arterial drug administration, 4
intracellular receptors, 25
intracranial pressure (ICP), 174
intramuscular drug administration, 5
intravenous (IV) push, 4
intravenous drug administration, 4
  of anesthetics
    for asthmatic patients, 430
    desired pharmacologic effect, 42
    immune effect, 439
  comparison with oral for elimination, 11
  dosing, 14
  sedatives and hypnotics, 504–506
intrinsic activity, 18
intrinsic factor, 233
intubation, rocuronium use for, 99
inverse agonists, 22

ion channels, 22
  ligand-gated, 23–24
ionophores, 23
ipratropium (Atrovent), 144, 242
  dosage and administration, 145–146
ipratropium bromide, for asthma, 428
ipsapirone, 354t
irbesartan (Avapro), 289
isocarboxazid, 471t
isoflurane, 163, 171, 172, 175
  for asthma patient, 431
  and autonomic nervous system, 176
  CSF pressure increase, 174
  immune effect, 438
  impact on heart rate, 176
  malignant hyperthermia from, 405
  pharmacologic properties, 163t
  reduction in arterial blood pressure, 176
isoniazid (Laniazid, Nydrazid), drug
    interactions, 514
isoproterenol, 20, 49
  routes of administration and dosage,
    341t
isoproterenol/isoprenaline, 333t
Isoptin (verapamil, Calan, Verelan). See
    verapamil (Calan, Isoptin, Verelan)
isosorbide, 263
isradipine (DynaCirc), 285
  pharmacokinetic profile, 284t

J

Jackson, Charles T., 161
Julian, Percy L., 149
juxtamedullary nephrons, 258

K

k opioid receptors, 63
kallikrein, 367
kallikrein-kinin system, 353
kanamycin, 201
  clinical uses and indications, 203
  and neuromuscular blockade, 213t
kava, 317t, 319t
Kerlone (betaxolol, Betoptic, Betoptic S),
    279
  pharmacokinetics, 282t
ketamine (Ketalar), 20, 45–47, 87–89
  for asthma patient, 430
  clinical application, 46
  dissociative state from, 46
  drug interactions, 505
  immune effect, 439t
  side effects, 46–47
  tolerance to, 88
  for vaginal delivery, neonatal scores
    after, 88
ketanserin, 354t
ketorolac, 83–84
  peak plasma concentration, 84t

kidney, 257
  disease impact on neuromuscular
    blocker, 100
  dobutamine effect, 329
  dopamine effect, 329
  drug elimination, 10
    penicillins, 197
  end-stage disease
    acetaminophen impact, 81
    NSAIDs impact, 86
    penicillin dosage, 198
  glucocorticoid therapy side effects, 306t
  impairment from lithium, 474
  inhalation anesthesia impact, 180
  lithium and drugs impacting, 509
  maintaining function when treating
    MH, 411
  propranolol effect, 338
  toxicity of ketorolac, 83
  vancomycin and, 208
kininogen, 367
kinins, 353
Kredex (carvedilol, Coreg), 280, 283,
    491t, 493t
  pharmacokinetics, 282t
Kytril (granisetron), 218–219, 245–246
  doses and timing for adult
    administration, 218t

L

labetalol hydrochloride (Normodyne,
    Trandate), 280, 295, 296t, 339,
    491t, 493t
  pharmacokinetics, 282t
  routes of administration and dosage,
    341t
Lafargue (French physician), 61
Laniazid (isoniazid, Nydrazid), drug
    interactions, 514
lansoprazole (Prevacid), 250–252
  interaction with tobacco and alcohol, 31t
lantus, interaction with tobacco and
    alcohol, 32t
large polar groups, attachment to drug
    molecule, 9
laryngeal mask, 238
laryngospasm, 234
  treating, 103
latency, 175
latex sensitivity, 419
laudanosine, 100
laudanum, 160
lavender, 320t
lepirudin (Refludan), 380
leukocyte effector cells, 437
leukotriene receptor antagonist, for
    asthma, 423t
leukotriene receptor antagonists (LTRAs),
    for asthma, 427
levalbuterol, for asthma, 423t

levaquin, interaction with tobacco and
    alcohol, 31t
Levatol (penbutolol), 278
  pharmacokinetics, 282t
levobupivacaine, 128
  pharmacology, 125t
levodopa, benztropine as adjunct, 142
levo-enantiomer local anesthetics, 125
levofloxacin, 208
levorphanol, in equianalgesia table, 66t
levosimendan, 490
lexapro, interaction with tobacco and
    alcohol, 31t
licorice root, 320t
lidocaine, 6, 127, *127*, 391–392
  bioavailability, 9
  clonidine with, 90
  with epinephrine, 121
  esmolol with, 280
  neurotoxicity of, 129
  pharmacology, 125t
  physiochemical properties, 124
  for postoperative pain management, 128
  propofol with, 50
  transient neurologic symptoms risk, 130
Liebig, Justus von, 160
Liem, E.B., 34
ligand-gated ion channels, 23–24
  cross-section diagram, *23*
ligands, 17
  interaction with receptors, 19–22
lincomycin, and neuromuscular blockade,
    213t
lincosamides, 195t
lipid diffusion, 5
lipid solubility, of barbiturates, 42
lipitor, interaction with tobacco and
    alcohol, 31t
lisinopril (Zestril, Prinivil), 288, 493t
  interaction with tobacco and alcohol, 31t
  pharmacokinetic profile, 287t
lithium, 473–475
  drug interactions, 504t
    with ACE inhibitors, 508
    with drugs impacting kidney, 509
  impact on anesthesia, 476
  thiazide diuretics interaction, 508
  toxicity, 473–474
liver
  acetaminophen impact, 81–82
  benzodiazepines metabolism, 54, 55
  CYP enzymes' role in disease origin, 30
  disease impact on neuromuscular
    blocker, 100
  drug metabolism by, 8, 9
  dysfunction, and barbiturate action
    duration, 42
  inhalation anesthesia impact, 180
  metabolism of propofol, 48
  transaminases increase from NSAIDs,
    86

loading dose, 14
local anesthetics, 119
  amide, 123, *127*, 127–128, *128*
  anti-inflammatory effect, 129
  clinical pharmacology, 121–125
    absorption, 121
    distribution, 121–122
  common structural elements, *124*
  comparative pharmacology, 125*t*
  differential blockade, 123
  dissociation constant (K_d) impact, 124
  ester, 125–126, *126*
    steroid drug interactions, 307*t*
  immune effect, 439
  injections, 119
  mechanism of action, 119–121
  metabolism, 122
  neurotoxicity of, 129–130
  physiochemical properties, 124*t*
  as stereoisomers, 125
  systemic administration, for acute
    pain management, 128–129
  systemic toxicity, 130–133
  toxicity, 129–130
    management of reactions,
      132–133
    strategies for preventing, 132
"lock and key" model for drug-receptor
  interactions, 17, 323
  drug-receptor interactions, *18*
Long, Crawford W., 160*t*
long-acting β-adrenergic agonists, for
  asthma, 426
Loniten (minoxidil, Rogaine), 291
  adverse effects, 293*t*
  pharmacokinetic profile, 293*t*
loop diuretics, 260–261, 265*t*, 484, 485
  steroid drug interactions, 307*t*
loops of Henle, 257, 258
Lopressor (metoprolol, Toprol XL),
  278–279, 339, 491*t*, 493*t*
  drug interactions, 513
  interaction with reserpine, 508
  pharmacokinetics, 282*t*
  routes of administration and dosage,
    341*t*
loracarbef, 199
loratadine, 222, 350*t*, 351
lorazepam (Ativan), 53
  interaction with tobacco and alcohol, 32*t*
  routes of administration and
    therapeutic uses, 54
  side effects, 56
  use, routes and dosages, 57*t*
losartan potassium (Cozaar), 289, 493*t*
  adverse effects, 290*t*
Lotensin (benazepril), 288, 493*t*
  pharmacokinetic profile, 287*t*
lotrel, interaction with tobacco and
  alcohol, 31*t*
Lotronex (alosetron), 245–246

low-molecular-weight heparin, 369–373
  dosage and administration, 374
  indications and dosing, 372*t*
  regional anesthesia use with, 375*t*
  reversal of, 373
  vs. unfractionated heparin (UFH), 370
loxapine, 461*t*, 463–464
  dosage, 462*t*
lungs. *See also* respiratory system
  drug metabolism by, 10
  excretion, 10
  propofol impact, 49–50
  prostaglandin synthesis, 357
Lusedra (fospropofol), for aspiration
    pneumonitis prophylaxis, 244–245
lutein, 29

M

μ opioid receptors, 62
  genetic variations, 63
MAC (block autonomic response), 171
MAC awake, 171
MAC multiple, 171
MAC values, 170–171
  factors impacting, 172*t*
macrolides, 195*t*, 203–205
  allergic reactions, 198*t*
  interaction with warfarin, 511
  steroid drug interactions, 307*t*
macula densa, 258
Magaw, Alice, 162
magnesium, 397–398
magnesium sulfate, 448–449
  drug interactions, 504*t*
maleate tegaserod, 355
malignant hyperthermia (MH), 28, 181,
  405–407
  anesthesia for susceptible patient, 408
  clinical signs and symptoms, 406–407
  clinical susceptibility, 407
  dantrolene for treating, 408–411
    chemical structure, *409*
  diagnostics tests for susceptibility,
    407–408
  differential diagnosis, 407
  emergency therapy, *412*
  incidence, 405–406
  pathophysiology, 406
  from succinylcholine, 106–107
Malignant Hyperthermia Association of
  the U.S., 411
malpractice claims, 253
mania, 459
  rebound, 475
  symptoms, 459*t*
manic-depressive disorder, 459
mannitol (osmotic diuretics), 262–263,
  265*t*, 485*t*
Marezine (cyclizine), 221, 222
marijuana-related compounds, 224

Massachusetts General Hospital, 161
masseter muscle regidity, 406
mast cell stabilizers, for asthma, 423*t*,
  426–427
maternal patient, ketamine for, 47
mathematical modeling, 10–14
Mavik (trandolapril), 288
  pharmacokinetic profile, 287*t*
mechanical ventilation, for asthma patient,
  431
mechanomyography TOF, 156
meclizine (Antivert), 222–223, 361*t*
medullary region of kidney, 257
melanocortin-1 receptor gene, 34
membranes, movement of molecules
  across, 25
Mendelson's syndrome, 231
meningitis, drug-induced, from ibuprofen,
  87
meperidine (Demerol), 64, 68–69, 475
  drug interactions, 502
  in equianalgesia table, 66*t*
  SSRIs interaction, 510
mepivacaine, 127, *128*
  pharmacology, 125*t*
  physiochemical properties, 124
Merck, rofecoxib withdrawal, 80
meropenem, 200–201
metabolic acidosis, 49
  hypercholoremic, as NSAID effect, 86
metabolism, 8–10
  drugs pertinent to anesthesia that
    impact, 506–507
metabophores, 24, *24*
metformin, interaction with tobacco and
  alcohol, 31*t*
methadone
  dosage and administration, 71*t*
  in equianalgesia table, 66*t*
  metabolism, 64
  pharmacology, 69*t*
methazolamide, 485*t*
  vs. acetazolamide, 259
methemoglobinemia, from benzocaine,
  126
methergine, 451
methicillin, 196
methohexital (Brivital), 41, 42
  dose range, 44*t*
  drug interactions, 506
  for electroconvulsive therapy, 476
  vs. thiopental, 43*t*
methomoglobinemia, from prilocaine, 127
methoxyflurane, 163
N-methyl-D-aspartate (NMDA) receptors,
  459
  ketamine binding to, 87
methyldopa (Aldomet), 270, 273*t*, 332*t*
  drug interactions, 515
  routes of administration and dosage,
    341*t*

methylphenidate, 333*t*
routes of administration and dosage, 341*t*
methylprednisolone
for asthma, 423*t*
pharmacokinetics and pharmacodynamics, 309*t*
properties, 304*t*
methylxanthines, for asthma, 427–428
methysergide, 354*t*
metoclopramide (Reglan), 355
for aspiration pneumonitis prophylaxis, 247–248
doses and timing for adult administration, 218*t*
drug interactions, 504*t*
plasma cholinesterase impaired by, 111
metolazone, 485*t*
metoprolol (Lopressor, Toprol XL), 278–279, 339, 388–389, 491*t*, 493*t*
drug interactions, 513
with reserpine, 508
pharmacokinetics, 282*t*
routes of administration and dosage, 341*t*
metronidazole, 195*t*, 208–209
chemical structure, 209
dosage for surgical prophylaxis, 211*t*
metyrosine (Demser), 274
pharmacokinetics, 274*t*
Meyer-Overton rule, 25
mezlocillin, 198
MG. *See* myasthenia gravis (MG)
MH. *See* malignant hyperthermia (MH)
MH Hotline, 411
Micardis (telmisartan), 290
adverse effects, 290*t*
microenvironment, for receptor protein, 20
midazolam (Versed), 29, 53
for asthma patient, 430
for children, 58
drug interactions, 505, 515
with fentanyl, 56
with ketamine, 505
with propofol, 48, 49, 504
with thiopental, 506
for emergence delirium prevention, 89
impact on blood pressure, 55
qualities, 54
respiratory depression from, 56
routes of administration and therapeutic uses, 54
use, routes and dosages, 57*t*
milrinone (Primacore), 488*t*, 490
mineralocorticoids, 307
minimum inhibitory concentration, for antibiotics, 193
Minipress (prazosin), 275
minocycline, absorption after oral administration, 205

minoxidil (Loniten, Rogaine), 291
adverse effects, 293*t*
pharmacokinetic profile, 293*t*
mirtazapine, 469*t*, 471
dosage, 470*t*
misoprostol, 452
mivacurium, and asthma, 430
mixed adrenergic antagonists, 280–283, 281*t*
moexipril (Univasc), 288
molecule, interaction with receptor, 18
mometasone furoate, for asthma, 423*t*
Monitan (acebutolol, Sectral), 279
pharmacokinetics, 282*t*
monoamine oxidase, 348
monoamine oxidase inhibitors (MAOIs), 471–472, 471*t*
discontinuation syndromes, 472
drug interactions, 475–476, 509, 509*t*
hypertensive crisis with, 472
monoamine oxidase systems, 324
reaction with drugs, 28
monobactams, 195*t*, 201
monocytes, 437
Monopril (fosinopril), 288
pharmacokinetic profile, 287*t*
montelukast, for asthma, 423*t*, 427
mood swings, 459
Moore, James, 61
morphine, 61, 66–67
chemical structure, 67
clonidine with, 90
dosage and administration, 71*t*
for smokers, 30
drug interactions, with flumazenil, 56
in equianalgesia table, 66*t*
and histamine release, 349
pharmacology, 69*t*
tolerance to, 23
morphine sulfate, 501
Morton, William T. G., 160*t*, 161–162
motor tics, 460
motor unit, 96
moxifloxacin, 208
mucus, 233
Mullins hypothesis, 25
multifocal ventricular tachycardia, electrocardiographic recording, 386
multimodal anesthesia, with opioids, 65
muscarinic cholinergic receptors, 139–141
anticholinergics to block, 139–146
subtypes, 141*t*
muscarinic receptor antagonists. *See* anticholinergics
muscle
contraction initiation, 24
interaction with nerves, 96
membranes, 97
sensitivity to relaxants, 100–101
muscle equilibration, 168–169

muscle relaxants. *See also* neuromuscular blocking drugs (NMBs)
dantrolene interaction, 410
depolarizing, 98–99
and histamine release, 353
ketamine and, 47
musculoskeletal system
glucocorticoid therapy side effects, 306*t*
propranolol effect, 337–338
mutations, 33
myalgia, from succinylcholine, 106
myasthenia gravis (MG)
anticholinesterases for, 150
pyridostigmine for, 154
Myasthenia Gravis Foundation of America, clinical classification, 151*t*
mycardial ischemia, inhalation anesthesia for protecting against, 177
mycophenolate mofetil, 440*t*
myelinated fibers, resistance to blockade, 123
myocardial contractility, effects of inhalation anesthesia, 176
myocardial sensitization, with epinephrine, 177
myofibril cell membrane, 98
myoneural junction. *See* neuromuscular junction (NMJ)
myotonia, from succinylcholine, 109
myotoxicity, of local anesthetic drugs, 129

N

nadolol (Corgard), 277–278, 339
pharmacokinetics, 282*t*
routes of administration and dosage, 341*t*
nafcillin, 196, 197
nalbuphine, 22, 71
chemical structure, 71
in equianalgesia table, 67*t*
nalbuphine hydrochloride (Nubain), opioid interactions, 502
naloxone, chemical structure, 72, 72
naloxone hydrochloride (Narcan), opioid interactions, 502
naproxen, 82
narcotics, and histamine release, 353
Nardil (phenelzine), 509
nasogastric tube, for aspiration pneumonitis prophylaxis, 238
nasonex, interaction with tobacco and alcohol, 32*t*
National Asthma Education and Prevention Program (NAEPP), 417
National Center for Complementary and Alternative Medicine, 315
National Research Council, 209
National Surgical Infection Prevention Project, 210

natriuretic peptides, for congestive heart failure, 486
natural killer (NK) cells, 437
nausea. *See also* postoperative nausea and vomiting (PONV)
  from opioids, 70
  preoperative prediction, 238
    Rhodes index, 238
Nebcin. *See* tobramycin (Nebcin)
nedocromil, 427
nefazodone, 467t, 468
negligence, legal considerations, 252
neocromil, for asthma, 423t
neomycin, 201
  clinical uses and indications, 203
  dosage for surgical prophylaxis, 211t
  and neuromuscular blockade, 213t
neonate
  antibiotic effectiveness, 195
  benzodiazepines impact, 56
  cardiac failure from indomethacin, 82
  dantrolene side effects, 410
  propofol effects, 48
Neoral (cyclosporine), 33, 440t
  drug interactions, 503
neostigmine (Prostigmin)
  clinical pharmacology, 152–153
  drug interactions, 503
  for myasthenia gravis, 150
  pharmacokinetics, 150t
  plasma cholinesterase impaired by, 111
  recommended doses according to TOF, 156t
nephritis, tubulointerstitial, from NSAIDs, 86
nephron, 258
nerve fibers
  classification, 123t
  interaction with muscle, 96
  and pain, 78
  ratio to muscle fibers, 96
nesiritide, 486
netilmicin, 201
  clinical uses and indications, 203
neurokinin-1 receptor antagonists, 223–224
neuroleptic drugs. *See* antipsychotic drugs
neuroleptic malignant syndrome, 464–465
  vs. malignant hyperthermia, 407
neurologic system, inhalation anesthesia impact, 174–176
neuromuscular blockade, reversal impeded, 153
neuromuscular blocking drugs (NMBs), 21, 95–113
  and antibiotics, 212–213
  for asthma patient, 430–431
  characteristics of ideal, 96
  classification, 98t
  clinical pharmacology, 99–102
  clinical uses and indications, 103–106
  drug interactions, 110–111, 502–504
  elimination, 103

guidelines and precautions, 111–112
history of use, 95
mechanism of action, 95–99, 99t
metabolism, 101–102
pharmacodynamics, 100–101
priming concept, 113, *113*
receptor involvement, 98
side effects and contraindications, 106–110
neuromuscular junction (NMJ), 96, *97*
  receptors as, 98
neuromuscular nicotinic acetylcholine receptor, 24
neuronal blockers, adrenergic, 272–275
neuropathic pain, 78
neurosis, 457–458
neurotoxicity, of local anesthetic drugs, 129–130
neutrophils, 437
Nexium (esomeprazole), 250–252
  interaction with tobacco and alcohol, 31t
nicardipine (Cardene), 120, 284–285, 295–296, 296t, 491t, 492
  drug interactions, 513
  esmolol with, 280
  pharmacokinetic profile, 284t
nicorandil, 177
nicotine, heparin interaction with, 373
nicotinic cholinergic receptors (nAChRs), 96
  decrease in early Alzheimer's dementia, 150
nicotinic receptors, 140
nifedipine (Adalat, Procardia), 120, 283–284, 449, 491t
  drug interactions, 513
  interaction with b blockers, 508
  pharmacokinetic profile, 284t
nimodipine (Nimotop), 491t, 492
Nimotop (nimodipine), 491t, 492
Nipride (nitroprusside sodium, Nitropress), 292–293
  advantages and disadvantages, 297t
  adverse effects, 294t
  pharmacokinetic profile, 293t
nitrodilators, 489
nitroglycerin (Tridil), 292, 297, 489t, 490
  advantages and disadvantages, 297t
  adverse effects, 294t
  obstetrics use, 450–451
  pharmacokinetic profile, 293t
nitroprusside sodium (Nipride, Nitropress), 292–293
  advantages and disadvantages, 297t
  adverse effects, 294t
  pharmacokinetic profile, 293t
nitrous oxide, 160, 164, 181
  combustion as problem, 173
  effects on cerebral physiology, 175
  impact on sympathetic nervous system, 176
  pharmacologic properties, 163t
  surgical use, 161

nizatidine, 352, 353
nociception, 61
nociceptive pain, 77
nociceptive system, 77
nonbenzodiazepin hypnotic drugs, 55
noncompetitive antagonist, 21–22
  vs. competitive antagonist, *21*
nondepolarizers
  metabolism, 101–102
  side effects, 110
  and volatile anethetics, 503
non-receptor-mediated effects, 25
nonselective β receptor antagonist, 276–278
non-self cells, 437
nonsteroidal anti-inflammatory drugs (NSAIDs), 78–79. *See also* NSAIDs (non-steroidal antiinflammatory drugs)
norepinephrine (noradrenaline), 328, *328*, 488t
  blocking release, 273
  inhibiting action, 276
  routes of administration and dosage, 341t
norfloxacin, 208
norketamine, 46, 88
Normodyne (Trandate, labetalol hydrochloride), 280, 295, 296t, 491t, 493t
  pharmacokinetics, 282t
  routes of administration and dosage, 341t
Norpramin (desipramine), 469
  dosage, 470t
  drug interactions, 510
North American Malignant Hyperthermia Group, testing protocol, 407–408
nortriptyline, 469t, 470
  dosage, 470t
  drug interactions, 515
Norvasc (amlodipine), 285
  interaction with tobacco and alcohol, 31t
  pharmacokinetic profile, 284t
nosocomial infections, postoperative, 209
NSAIDs (non-steroidal antiinflammatory drugs)
  acetaminophen, 81–82
  adverse effects, 80t
  aspirin (acetylsalicylic acid), 81
  ceiling effects, *85*
  characteristics, 79, 80t
  classification, 79–85
  diflunisal, 82
  drug interactions
    with ACE inhibitors, 508
    with heparin, 372
    with steroid drugs, 307t
    with warfarin, 511
  indomethacin, 82
  ketorolac, 83–84
  with opioids, 65
  propionic acid derivatives, 82–83

side effects, 86–87
sulindac, 82
tolmetin, 82
Nubain (nalbuphine hydrochloride), opioid
    interactions, 502
nucleotides, 33
Nydrazid (Laniazid, isoniazid), drug
    interactions, 514

O

obese patients, rocuronium dosage, 100
obstetric anesthesia, 445–452
    chloroform for, 162
    pharmacology of drugs used, 448–452
        β agonists, 449
        calcium channel blockers, 449–450
        ergotrate, 451
        hydralazine (Apresoline), 450–451
        magnesium sulfate, 448–449
        methergine, 451
        nitroglycerin (Tridil), 450–451, 452
        oxytocin, 451
        oxytocin receptor antagonists, 450
        prostaglandin inhibitors, 450
        prostaglandins, 452
    phenylephrine use, 330–331
occulomotor nerve, Edinger-Westphal
    nucleus, opioids' impact, 72
occupational asthma, 419
octanol, 5
Ocupress (Cartrol, carteolol), 278
    pharmacokinetics, 282t
ofloxacin, 208
oil-to-water partition coefficient, 5
OKT4A, 440t
    response, anesthetic technique and, 441
olanzapine, 461t, 464
    dosage, 462t
older adults
    adrenergic receptor agonists, caution in
        use, 340
    antibiotic effectiveness, 195
    benzodiazepines adverse effects, 57
    induction dose of propofol, 48
    muscle relaxant dosage, 100
    undertreatment for pain, 63
omalizumab, 427
omeprazole (Prilosec), 34
    for aspiration pneumonitis prophylaxis,
        250–252
omnicef, interaction with tobacco and
    alcohol, 32t
ondansetron (Zofran), 225, 245–246, 354t
    doses and timing for adult
        administration, 218t
one-compartment model, 11, 11
opioid receptors, 62–63
opioids, 501
    adverse effects and contraindications,
        69–70
    applications in operating room, 72–73

for asthma patient, 430
clinical pharmacology, 62–64
clinical uses and indications, 64–65
combination with propofol, 49
comparative pharmacology of drugs in
    class, 65–69
dosage and administration, 71t
drug interactions, 70, 475–476, 502
    with anticholinergics, 511
    with antipsychotic drugs, 511
    with thiopental, 506
guidelines and precautions, 70–72
history of use, 61
immune effect, 439–440
mechanisms of action, 61–62
metabolism and elimination, 64
methods of administration, 65
NSAIDs with, 80
tolerance to, 73
Oracit (sodium citrate, Bicitra), 240–241
oral contraceptives
    and alprazolam (Xanax), 510
    plasma cholinesterase impaired by, 111
    steroid drug interactions, 307t
oral drug absorption, 7
oral drug administration, 4, 9
    comparison with IV for elimination, 11
organ transplants, immunosuppressant
    drugs for, 440, 440t
organophosphates, 154
ortho-tri-cyclen lo, interaction with
    tobacco and alcohol, 32t
osmotic diuretics (mannitol), 262–263,
    265t, 485–486
osmotic laxatives, 17
ototoxicity, from vancomycin, 208
overpressuring, 167
oxacillin, 196
oxazepam (Serax), routes of administration
    and therapeutic uses, 54
oxidation-reduction reactions, 8
oxime drugs, 154
oxycodone, in equianalgesia table, 66t
oxycodone/APAP, interaction with tobacco
    and alcohol, 31t
oxygen, respiratory responses to, 178
oxymorphone, in equianalgesia table, 66t
oxytetracycline
    absorption after oral administration, 205
    immune effect, 440
oxytocin, 451
oxytocin receptor antagonists, 450

P

Pacerone. See amiodarone (Cordarone,
    Pacerone)
paclitaxel (Taxol), 29
PAE. See postantibiotic effect (PAE)
pain
    consequences, 62
    defined, 77

definition, 61
description of mechanisms, 61–62
epidemiology and etiology, 77
mechanisms, 78
pathology, 77–78
    in sedated patient, 69
    from spinal cord sensitization, 88
    threshold, barbiturates and, 43
pain management, 61
    local anesthetics administration,
        128–129
    neostigmine for, 153
    postoperative, 88
        NSAIDs for, 85
    postoperative relief, 64–65
pain on injection, from propofol, 50
pain rating scales, 72
palonosetron (Aloxil), 219, 245–246
    doses and timing for adult
        administration, 218t
pancuronium, 101
    for asthma patient, 430
    ketamine interaction, 505
    metabolism, 101–102
    pharmacokinetics comparison, 112t
    plasma cholinesterase impaired by, 111
    side effects, 110
pantoprazole (Protonix), 250–252
    interaction with tobacco and alcohol, 31t
Paracelsus, 160, 160t
paranoid schizophrenia, 460
parasympathetic nervous system
    effector organs and chilical effects, 141t
    mechanism of action, 139
parecoxib, 84–85
parenteral drug administration, 4–5
Parkinson's disease, benztropine in
    treatment, 142
Parnate (tranylcypromine), 509
paroxetine (Paxil), 467t, 468
    interaction with tobacco and alcohol, 32t
    interaction with tramadol, 510
partial agonists, 22
passive absorption, rate of, 7
passive diffusion, 7, 8
patient variability, in elimination half-life, 12
pediatric patients. See also infants; neonate
    acetazolamide dosage, 259
    antiemetic doses, 218t
    asthma, 418
        differential diagnosis, 422
    benzodiazepines for, 55, 58
    fasting prior to surgery, 238
    furosemide dosage, 261
    induction dose of propofol, 48
    succinylcholine risks, 108
    therapy for postoperative vomiting risk,
        225
penbutolol (Levatol), 278
    pharmacokinetics, 282t
penicillin G, and neuromuscular blockade,
    213t

penicillins, 195t, 196–198
  adverse effects, 198
  chemical structure, 196
  clinical uses and indications, 197–198
  elimination, 197
  pharmacokinetics, 197
pentazocine (Talwin)
  in equianalgesia table, 67t
  SSRIs interaction, 510
pentobarbital, 41
peppermint oil, 320t
pepsin, 233
pepsinogen, 233
perindopril (Aceon), 288
perioperative hypertension
  anesthetic management of acute,
    294–298
  etiology, 294
  profile of ideal drug treatment, 295
peripheral nerve stimulator (PNS)
  modes, 105t
  monitoring, 103–106
perphenazine, 461t
  dosage, 462t
Pfizer, 80
pH, 6
  of urinary fluid, 10
pharmacodynamics, 3, 17–26
  historic perspective, 27–28
  individual variations, 27
pharmacogenetics, 28
pharmacogenomics, 28
pharmacokinetics, 3
  historic perspective, 27–28
  individual variations, 27
pharmacology, derivation and definition, 3
pharynx, protective gag reflex, 234
phase I metabolism, 8–9
phase II block, from succinylcholine, 109
phase II metabolism, 9
phenacetin, 86
phencyclidine, 45
phenelzine, 471
phenelzine (Nardil), 509
Phenergan (promethazine), 221
  doses and timing for adult
    administration, 218t
phenobarbital, drug interactions,
    514, 515
phenothiazides, 461–463
phenothiazines, 220–221
phenotype, 33
phenoxybenzamine, 21, 275, 331, 331, 334
  routes of administration and dosage,
    341t
phenoxybenzamine hydrochloride
  (Dibenzyline), 275
phentolamine, 275, 334, 334–335
  routes of administration and dosage,
    341t
phentolamine mesylate (Regitine), 275
phenylalkamines, pharmacokinetic profile,
    284t

phenylbutazone, 82–83
  interaction with heparin, 372
phenylephrine (Neo-Synephrine),
    330–331
  chemical structure, 330
  drug interactions, 515
phenytoin (Dilantin), drug interactions,
    504t, 510, 515
  with benzodiazepines, 56
  with methohexital, 506
  with rocuronium, 110
  with warfarin, 511
pheochromocytoma, management, 275
phobias, 457
phosphodiesterase inhibitors, 490
physical dependence, 73
physiologic agonists, 20
physiologic tolerance, 23
physostigmine, 146, 149
  clinical pharmacology, 151–152
  for curare poisoning reversal, 149
  opioid interactions, 502
  pharmacokinetics, 150t
phytochemicals, 29
  in herbal preparations, 33
phytonadione (vitamin K), for warfarin
    reversal, 380
phytonutrients, 29
pimozide, 461t, 464
  dosage, 462t
pindolol (Visken), 278, 493t
  drug interactions, 514
  interaction with reserpine, 508
  pharmacokinetics, 282t
pipecuronium
  pharmacokinetics comparison, 112t
  risk for asthma patient, 430
piperacillin, 198
  and neuromuscular blockade, 213t
piroxicam, 83
pitocin, 451
pK$_a$, 6
  of local anesthetic drugs, 121
placenta accreta, 447
placenta increta, 447
placenta percreta, 447
plasma albumin, drug molecules binding
    to, 7
plasma cholinesterase, 102
  muscle relaxants impact, 111
plasma clearance (Cl), 13
plasma compartment, 11
plasma concentration, 13
  correlation to side effects, 14
plasma esterase, 9
plasma proteins, in filtration mechanism, 10
platelets
  aspirin irreversible effects on, 86
  epinephrine effect, 327
  membranes, and coagulation reactions,
    368
plavix, interaction with tobacco and
    alcohol, 31t

Plendil (felodipine), 284
  pharmacokinetic profile, 284t
pneumonitis, aspiration. See aspiration
    pneumonitis prophylaxis
PNS. See peripheral nerve stimulator (PNS)
polycyclic aromatic hydrocarbons (PAHs),
    impact on CYP enzymes, 30
polymorphism, 33, 34
polymorphonuclear cells, 437
polymyxins, and neuromuscular blockade,
    213t
polyphenols, impact on CYP enzymes, 30
pontine locus ceruleus, a2 receptors in, 89
post tetanic count mode, 105t
postantibiotic effect (PAE), of antibiotics, 194
postganglionic PNS fibers, 139
postoperative infections, pathogens
    causing, 210t
postoperative nausea and vomiting
    (PONV), 215
  anesthetic techniques for preventing,
    225–226
  glucocorticoids to prevent, 219
  neostigmine and, 153
  risk factors, 70t, 215t, 226
  surgical procedures with increased
    incidence, 215t
postoperative pain management, 88
  NSAIDs for, 85
postpartum hemorrhage (PPH), 447
  prostaglandins for treating, 452
posttraumatic stress disorder, 457
  diagnostic criteria, 458
potassium channel blockade, by local
    anesthetic, 120
potassium clavulanate, amoxicillin with, 201
potassium-sparing diuretics
    (spironolactone), 263–265,
    265t, 485, 508
  interaction with ACE inhibitors, 508
potatoes, solanaceous glycoalkaloids in, 29
potency, 170–171
pralidoxime, 154
prazapam (Centrax), routes of admin-
    istration and therapeutic uses, 54
prazosin (Minipress), 275, 335, 335
  routes of administration and dosage,
    341t
Precedex (dexmedetomidine), 56, 89,
    90–91, 272
prednisolone, pharmacokinetics and
    pharmacodynamics, 309t
prednisone
  interaction with tobacco and alcohol, 31t
  pharmacokinetics and pharmaco-
    dynamics, 309t
  properties, 304t
preganglionic fibers of PNS, 139
pregnancy
  antibiotics use, 195, 195t
  benzodiazepines impact, 56
  pathophysiologic conditions, 446–448
    cervical incompetence, 446

pregnancy-induced hypertension, 446–447
  preterm delivery, 447
  preterm labor, 447
  retained placenta, 447
  uterine atony, 447–448
  physiologic changes, 445–446
prekallikrein, 367
premarin, interaction with tobacco and alcohol, 31*t*
preterm delivery, 447
preterm labor, 447
  β-adrenergic agonists to inhibit, 449
Prevacid (lansoprazole), 250–252
  interaction with tobacco and alcohol, 31*t*
Priestly, Joseph, 160, 160*t*
prilocaine, 127, *127*
  neurotoxicity of, 130
  pharmacology, 125*t*
  physiochemical properties, 124
Prilosec (omeprazole), 34, 250–252
Primacore (milrinone), 488*t*, 490
primary hypertension, 270
Prinivil (lisinopril, Zestril), 288, 493*t*
  interaction with tobacco and alcohol, 31*t*
  pharmacokinetic profile, 287*t*
probenecid, 199
  drug interactions, 505–506
  furosemide interaction, 260
procainamide (Pronestyl, Procan), 393
  vs. amiodarone, 395
  drug interactions, 504*t*
    with amiodarone, 394
  vs. metoclopramide, 248
procaine, 6, 125–126
  vs. metoclopramide, 248
  pharmacology, 125*t*
  physiochemical properties, 124
Procardia (nifedipine, Adalat), 120, 283–284, 491*t*
  drug interactions, 513
  interaction with b blockers, 508
  pharmacokinetic profile, 284*t*
prochlorperazine (Compazine), 221, 248
  doses and timing for adult administration, 218*t*
  interaction with anticholinergics, 146
prodrug, 29
Proglycem (diazoxide, Hyperstat), 291
  adverse effects, 293*t*
  pharmacokinetic profile, 293*t*
programmed cellular death, physostigmine to protect against, 152
promethazine (Phenergan), 220–221, 221, 350*t*
  doses and timing for adult administration, 218*t*
  drug interactions, 515
propionic acid derivatives, 82–83
propionic acids, 80
propofol (Diprivan), 20, 48–50, 224
  for aspiration pneumonitis prophylaxis, 244–245

for asthma patient, 430
  drug interactions, 504
    with benzodiazepines, 505
  for electroconvulsive therapy, 476–477
  etomidate as alternative, 44
  gender differences, 34
  immune effect, 439, 439*t*
  ketamine interaction, 505
propofol infusion syndrome, 49
propoxyphene/APAP, interaction with tobacco and alcohol, 32*t*
propranolol (Inderal), 17, 249, 276–277, 337, 337–338, 389, 493*t*
  drug interactions, 514
  pharmacokinetics, 282*t*
  routes of administration and dosage, 341*t*
Propulsid (cisapride), 248
prostacyclin, effects, 357*t*
prostaglandin inhibitors, 450
prostaglandins, 78, 86, 356–357
  NSAIDs for suppressing production, 85
prostanoids, biosynthetic pathways, *356*
Prostigmin. *See* neostigmine (Prostigmin)
protamine, 370
  reversal of UFH, 373
protein binding
  and antibiotic effectiveness, 194
  in barbiturates, 42
  and drug distribution, 512
  by inhaled corticosteroids, 424
  of opioids, 69*t*
protein C
  half-life of, 376
  thrombin and, 376
protein S
  half-life of, 376
  thrombin and, 376
proteins, 19
  molecules of, 10
  receptors as, 17
prothrombin, 367
prothrombin time (PT), 367
proton pump inhibitors, 250–252
protonated (P) form of base, 6
Protonix (pantoprazole), 250–252
  interaction with tobacco and alcohol, 31*t*
protriptyline, 469*t*, 470–471
  dosage, 470*t*
Prozac (fluoxetine). *See* fluoxetine (Prozac)
pseudocholinesterase, 9, 102
pseudoephedrine, 333*t*
  routes of administration and dosage, 341*t*
psychiatric disorders, 457–477, 460–475
  anesthesia considerations, 475–476
  antidepressant drug treatment, 466–471, 467*t*
    discontinuation syndromes, 472–473
    selective serotonin uptake inhibitors, 466–468
    TCAs and related compounds, 468–471

antipsychotic drug treatment, 460–466, 461*t*
  associated conditions and syndromes, 464–466
  benzisoxazole, 464
  butyrophenones, 464
  chlorpromazine, 461–462
  dibenzodiazepines, 463–464
  diphenylbutylpiperidine, 464
  fluphenazine, 463
  perphenazine, 463
  thioridazine, 462–463
  thioxanthene, 463
  trifluoperazine, 463
  anxiolytics for, 473
  etiology and pathophysiology, 457–460
  mood-stabilizing drug treatment, 473–475
psychosis, 458–459
pulmonary system. *See* respiratory system
pungency, of inhaled anesthetics, 179
purinoceptors, 396–397
pyramids in kidney, 257
pyridostigmine (Regonol)
  clinical pharmacology, 153–154
  drug interactions, 503
  for myasthenia gravis, 150
  pharmacokinetics, 150*t*
pyrrolopyrrole, 80

Q

QT prolongation, droperidol and, 220
quanta, 96
quazepam (Doral), routes of administration and therapeutic uses, 54
quinapril (Accupril), 288
  pharmacokinetic profile, 287*t*
quinidine, drug interactions, 514, 515

R

rabeprazole (AcipHex), 250–252
  interaction with tobacco and alcohol, 32*t*
race, 34
ramipril (Altace), 288
  pharmacokinetic profile, 287*t*
ranitidine (Zantac), 352, 353
  for aspiration pneumonitis prophylaxis, 248–249
  drug interactions, 512, 516
rapacuronium, risk for asthma patient, 430
rate of elimination, 12
reabsorption process, 10
rebound hypertension, from clonidine discontinuation, 90
rebound mania, 475
receptor proteins, storage, 22
receptor theory, 17–19
receptors, 17
  for autocoids, 347
  competitive antagonist to decrease normal effects, 21
  extrajunctional, 107–108, *108*

interactions, 19–22
regulation, 22–23
types, 23–25
rectal administration, 4
"red man" syndrome, 207
redistribution, 8
of barbiturates, 42
reflux, 231
Regitine (phentolamine mesylate), 275
Reglan (metoclopramide), for aspiration pneumonitis prophylaxis, 247–248
Regonol. *See* pyridostigmine (Regonol)
relative affinity constant, 18
remifentanil, 68
chemical structure, *68*
vs. dexmedetomidine, 91
dosage and administration, 71*t*
pharmacology, 69*t*
propofol interaction, 504
renal corpuscle, 258
renin-angiotensin-aldosterone system, 270, 286
renzapride, 355
reproductive system, glucocorticoid therapy side effects, 306*t*
reserpine (Serpalan), 274
pharmacokinetics, 274*t*
residual relaxation, by NMBs, 111
residual schizophrenia, 460
resistance
to antibiotics, 194
fluoroquinolones, 208
macrolides, 204
metronidazole, 209
penicillins, 197
tetracycline, 205
vancomycin, 207
to furosemide, 260
to heparin, 370
respiration
etomidate side effects, 45
ketamine effect, 47, 88
muscarinic receptor antagonists impact, 142–143
rate as pain indicator, 72
respiratory depression
from benzodiazepines, 55
opioid-induced, 69
respiratory system. *See also* asthma
ACE inhibitors adverse effects, 287*t*
adverse effects of beta-blockers, 281*t*–282*t*
angiotensin II receptor antagonists adverse effects, 290*t*
beta-blockers adverse effects, 281*t*–282*t*
dopamine effect, 328
ephedrine effect, 330
epinephrine effect, 327
inhalation anesthesia impact, 178–179
phentolamine effect, 334
phenylephrine effect, 330
propranolol effect, 337
retained placenta, 447

reticular activating system, barbiturates to depress, 41
retrograde amnesia, from ketamine, 46
reversal of NMB effects, monitoring for, 111–112
Rhodes index of nausea, vomiting and retching, 239
rifampicin (rifampin, Rifadin)
drug interactions, 514
impact on benzodiazepines, 56
Riggs, Benjamin, 161
risk factors, for gastric content aspiration, 236–238
risperdal, interaction with tobacco and alcohol, 32*t*
risperidone, 461*t*, 464
dosage, 462*t*
ritodrine, 332*t*, 449
rivastigmine, for Alzheimer's dementia management, 151
Robinul (glycopyrrolate). *See* glycopyrrolate (Robinul)
rocuronium
anaphylactic reactions, 110
for asthma patient, 431
cardiovascular effects, 101
chemical structure, *99*
interaction with phenytoin, 110
metabolism, 102
pharmacokinetics, 99–100
pharmacokinetics comparison, 112*t*
rofecoxib (Vioxx), 84
Merck withdrawal, 80
Rogaine (minoxidil, Loniten), 291
adverse effects, 293*t*
pharmacokinetic profile, 293*t*
ropivacaine, 127–128, *128*
clonidine with, 272
myotoxicity, 129
pharmacology, 125*t*
physiochemical properties, 124
propofol interaction, 504
routes of administration, 3–5
RYR1 (malignant hyperthermia) gene, 181

S

St. Anthony's fire, 451
St. John's wort, 33, 317*t*, 320*t*
impact on benzodiazepines, 56
warfarin interaction, 378
salbutamol/albuterol, 332*t*
routes of administration and dosage, 341*t*
salicylates, spironolactone interaction, 264
salicylic acid, 81
salicyluric acid, 81
salivary secretion, excessive, from ketamine, 46
salmeterol
for asthma, 426
routes of administration and dosage, 341*t*
saquinavir, 29

saw palmetto, 317*t*, 320*t*
schizophrenia, 459–460
scopolamine (Transderm-Scop), 144, 223, 241–243
clinical manifestations, 144*t*
dosage and administration, 145
doses and timing for adult administration, 218*t*
second gas effect, 167
secondary hypertension, 270
Sectral (acebutolol, Monitan), 279
pharmacokinetics, 282*t*
sedation
benzodiazepines for children, 58
from clonidine, 90
H₁ antagonists and, 351
intravenous drug administration, 504–506
opioid-induced, 65, 69
selective agonists, 20
selective β receptor antagonists, 278–280
selective β-blockers, adverse effects, 281*t*–282*t*
selective serotonin receptor antagonists, 466–468, 467*t*
discontinuation syndromes, 472
selective serotonin reuptake inhibitors (SSRIs), 25
drug interactions, 510, 511
selegiline (Eldepryl), 509
drug interactions, 511, 515
Sellick's maneuver, 238
septic conditions, anticholinesterases for treating, 156
seroquel, interaction with tobacco and alcohol, 31*t*
serotonin 5-HT₃ receptor blockers, for aspiration pneumonitis prophylaxis, 245–246
serotonin agonist and antagonist, and physiologic functions, 355
serotonin syndrome, vs. malignant hyperthermia, 407
Serpalan (reserpine), 274
pharmacokinetics, 274*t*
SERT (transport protein), 25
sertraline, 354*t*, 467, 467*t*
sevoflurane, 163, 171, 173, 179
immune effect, 438
impact on heart rate, 176
impact on neurologic system, 174
malignant hyperthermia from, 405
pharmacologic properties, 163*t*
reduction in arterial blood pressure, 17●
short-acting β-adrenergic agonists, for asthma, 426
side effects of drugs, 13
signal transduction process, 386
Simpson, James, 159, 160*t*, 162
single nucleotide polymorphisms (SNPs), 34, 63
single-twitch mode, for peripheral nerve stimulation, 104, 105*t*

singular, interaction with tobacco and alcohol, 31t
sirolimus, 440t
skeletal muscle, innervation, 95–96
skin, drug absorption, 4
sleep, opioids and, 69
slow response action potential, 391, 392
small intestine, microvilli, and absorption of compounds, 7
smoking, 30
SNPs (single nucleotide polymorphisms), 34
Society of Ambulatory Anesthesia, 225
sodium bicarbonate
  with aspirin, 81
  and local anesthesia, 121
sodium channel blockade, by local anesthetic, 119–120
sodium citrate (Bicitra, Oracit), 240–241
sodium nitroprusside, 489–490, 489t. See also nitroprusside sodium (Nipride, Nitropress)
sodium nitroprusside cyanide, treatment of toxicity, 294
sodium sulfite, in edrophonium preparation, 155
sodium thiopental, 41
sodium-potassium ATPase, 119
solubility, 5–6
  and inhalation anesthesia uptake, 166
somatic nervous system, organization, 140
somatostatin, 352
sotalol, 339
  routes of administration and dosage, 341t
Soubeiran, Eugene, 160
soy, 320t
spinal NMDA receptors, inhibition by drugs, 88
spironolactone, 263–265, 265t, 485t, 487–488, 493t
Staphylococcus aureus, 196
  cephalosporins for treating infections, 199
Staphylococcus epidermidis, 196
steady-state concentration, intermittent dosing impact, 15
stereoisomerism, 125
sterile urea, 263
Sternbach, Leo, 53
steroid receptors, 25
steroids, 303–311
  cholesterol structure common to, 308
  classification, 308t
  clinical uses and indications, 307–308
  comparative pharmacology of drugs in class, 308–309
  comparative properties, 304t
  contraindications, 305–306
  decision algorithm for preoperative supplementation, 310
  dosage and administration, 309–311
  drug interactions, 306, 306t
  elimination, 305

immune effect, 440
metabolism, 305
pharmacodynamics, 304–305, 309t
pharmacokinetics, 304, 309t
postoperative replacement schedule, 311t
practical aspects of use, 306–307
side effects, 305, 306t
stomach, 231. See also gastric secretions
  anatomy, 232
  histology, 232
  impact of acidic environment on drugs, 7
  voluntary and involuntary actions, 233
streptomycin, 201
  clinical uses and indications, 203
  and neuromuscular blockade, 213t
stress response, opioids for reducing, 64
strychnine, 22
subarachnoid block, tetracaine or bupivacaine for, 90
subarachnoid space, local anesthetic distribution, 122
subcutaneous drug administration, 5
Substance P, 223
succinylcholine, 28, 98–99, 100
  anaphylactic reactions, 110
  cardiovascular effects, 101
  chemical structure, 106
  drug interactions, 503
  ketamine interaction, 505
  malignant hyperthermia from, 405
  metabolism, 102
  pharmacokinetics comparison, 112t
  side effects, 106
  trismus after administration, 406
sufentanil, 68, 68, 501
  dosage and administration, 71t
  metabolism, 64
sugammadex, 112
sulbactam, 201
sulfa drugs, and warfarin, 511
sulfonamide, hypersensitivity, 87
sulfotransferase system, reaction with drugs, 28
"sulfuric ether", 161
sulindac, 82
sumatriptan, 354t
superagonists, 20
supraventricular tachyarrhythmias, treatment, 389t, 391t
surgeries, U.S. statistics, 61
surgical prophylaxis
  antibiotics for, 209–212
    dosage, 211t
    general principles, 210t
    guidelines, 212t
"survival of the fittest" concept, 33
susceptibility testing, in vitro, of antibiotics, 193
swallowing, 231–234
  voluntary and involuntary stages, 233
swallowing reflex, benzodiazepines impact, 55

sympatholytics, 270–283
  clonidine (Catapres, Dixarit, Duraclon), 271–272
  guanabenz acetate (Wytensin), 270
  guanfacine hydrochloride (Tenex), 270–271
sympathomimetic drugs, 326–327
  opioid interactions, 502
  TCAs interaction, 509
synergism, of antibiotics, 194
synthetic reactions, 9
synthroid, interaction with tobacco and alcohol, 31t
syntocinon, 451
systemic blood pressure, barbiturates and, 43
systemic corticosteroids, 425

T

tachyarrhythmias, supraventricular, treatment, 389t, 391t
tachycardia, multifocal ventricular, electrocardiographic recording, 386
tachyphylaxis, 109
tacrolimus, 440t
Tagamet (cimetidine), 249
  drug interactions, 513
Talwin (pentazocine), SSRIs interaction, 510
tamsulosin, routes of administration and dosage, 341t
tardive dyskinesia, 466
tazobactam, 201
TCAs. See tricyclic antidepressants (TCAs)
Tegretol (carbamazepine)
  drug interactions, 510
  impact on benzodiazepines, 56
  thiazide diuretics interaction, 508
telmisartan (Micardis), 290
  adverse effects, 290t
temazepam (Restoril), routes of administration and therapeutic uses, 54
Tenex (guanfacine hydrochloride), 270–271
Tenormin (atenolol), 279, 336, 493t
  chemical structure, 336
  pharmacokinetics, 282t
  routes of administration and dosage, 341t
Tensilon. See edrophonium (Tensilon)
tensilon test (edrophonium test dose), 155, 155t
terazosin (Hytrin), 275, 276, 339
  routes of administration and dosage, 341t
terbutaline, 449
  for asthma, 423t
  routes of administration and dosage, 341t
terfenadine, 351, 352
Terrell, Ross, 160t, 163
tetanic stimulation, 106
tetany 100 Hz mode, 105t
tetany 50 Hz mode, 105t

tetracaine, 126
  clonidine with, 90
  pharmacology, 125t
  physiochemical properties, 124
tetracycline, 195t, 205–206
  absorption after oral administration,
    205
  adverse effects, 206
  allergic reactions, 198t
  chemical structure, 205
  drug interactions
    with antacids, 511
    with heparin, 373
  impact in pregnancy, 195
  and neuromuscular blockade, 213t
theobromine, for asthma, 427
theophylline
  for asthma, 427, 428
  dosage for smokers, 30
  drug interactions, 514, 516
therapeutic index, 14
therapeutic ratio, 14
therapeutic window, 13–14, 14
  size, 27
thiazide diuretics (chlorothiazide),
    261–262, 265t, 485
  drug interactions, 508
thiopental
  for asthma patient, 430
  dose range, 44t
  drug interactions, 505–506
  etomidate as alternative, 44
  immune effect, 439, 439t
  for MAOI-treated patients, 476
  metabolism, 42
  vs. methohexital, 43t
  pH, 44
thioridazine (Mellaril), 461t, 462–463
  dosage, 462t
  drug interactions, 514
thiothixene, 461t, 463
thioxanthene, 461t, 463
  dosage, 462t
thought disorder, 458
thrombin, 367
thrombocytopenia, heparin-induced,
    371–372
thrombophlebitis, 56
thrombotic clots, heparin prevention, 370
thrombotic events, COX-2 inhibitors
    and, 86
thromboxane, 81
  effects, 357t
thromboxane A₂, 86
thromboxane-to-prostacyclin ratio, 357
thymine, 33
thyroid dysfunction, from lithium, 474
ticarcillin, 198
tics, 460
Tigan (trimethobenzamide), 248
tigecycline, 205

time dependent killing, by antibiotics, 194
timolol (Blocadren, Betimol, Timoptic,
    Timoptic XE), 278, 336–337, 493t
  chemical structure, 337
  drug interactions, 513, 514
  pharmacokinetics, 282t
Timoptic (timolol, Blocadren, Betimol,
    Timoptic XE), drug interactions,
    513, 514
tinzaparin (Innohep), 369
tiotropium (Spiriva), 144
  dosage and administration, 145–146
tissue factor pathway inhibitor (TFPI),
    368
tissue factor (TF), 367
tissue membranes, drug molecules ability
    to cross, 5
tissue-to-blood partition coefficient, 6
tobacco use, 30
tobramycin (Nebcin), 201
  adverse effects, 202
  clinical uses and indications, 203
  drug interactions, 515
tocolysis, treatment, 449
TOF ratio, 104
Tofranil. See imipramine (Tofranil)
tolerance, 73
  to ketamine, 88
  physiologic, 23
tolmetin, 82
tomatoes, solanaceous glycoalkaloids in,
    29
tonic blockade, 119
topamax, interaction with tobacco and
    alcohol, 32t
topical drug administration, 4
Toprol XL (metoprolol, Lopressor),
    278–279, 339, 491t, 493t
  drug interactions, 513
    with reserpine, 508
    with tobacco and alcohol, 31t
  pharmacokinetics, 282t
  routes of administration and dosage,
    341t
torsade de pointes, electrocardiographic
    recording, 386
torsemide, 260, 485t
total IV anesthesia, 41
Tourette's syndrome, 460
toxicities of drugs, 13
toxicity
  of local anesthetic drugs, 129–130
  systemic, from local anesthetics,
    130–133
trachea, 180
train-of-four (TOF), for peripheral nerve
    stimulation, 104–105, 104t, 105t,
    156–157
tramadol (Ultram), drug interactions
  with paroxetine, 510
  with SSRIs, 510, 511

Trandate (Normodyne, labetalol hydro-
    chloride), 280, 295, 296t, 491t, 493t
  pharmacokinetics, 282t
  routes of administration and dosage,
    341t
trandolapril (Mavik), 288
  pharmacokinetic profile, 287t
transdermal patches, 4
Transderm-Scop (scopolamine), 241–243
  doses and timing for adult
    administration, 218t
transient neurologic symptoms (TNS),
    130
transport molecules, 5
transporters, 25
tranylcypromine (Parnate), 471t, 472, 509
  drug interactions, 515
trazodone, 467t, 468
  interaction with tobacco and alcohol, 32t
triamcinolone, pharmacokinetics and
    pharmacodynamics, 309t
triamcinolone acetonide, for asthma, 423t
triamterene, 263, 485t
  interaction with tobacco and alcohol, 32t
triazolam (Halcion)
  in pregnancy, 56
  routes of administration and
    therapeutic uses, 54
tricor, interaction with tobacco and
    alcohol, 32t
tricyclic antidepressants (TCAs),
    468–471, 469t
  dosage, 470t
  drug interactions, 509–510
    with anticholinergics, 146
    with clonidine, 508
    with opioids, 502
  impact on anesthesia, 476
Tridil (nitroglycerin), 292, 297, 489t, 490
  advantages and disadvantages, 297t
  adverse effects, 294t
  pharmacokinetic profile, 293t
trifluoperazine, 461t
  dosage, 462t
trifluoroacetate, 180
trimethobenzamide (Tigan), 248
tripeptide glutathione, attachment, 9
triprolidine, 359–360t
trismus, after succinylcholine
    administration, 406
tubulointerstitial nephritis, from NSAIDs,
    86
two-compartment model, 11, 11

U

ulnar nerve, for PNS monitoring,
    103–104, 104t
Ultram (tramadol)
  peroxetine interaction, 511
  SSRIs interaction, 510, 511

unfractionated heparin (UFH), 369–373
dosage and administration, 373–374
indications and dosing, 371t
vs. low-molecular-weight heparin, 370
protamine reversal of, 373
regional anesthesia use with, 375t
un-ionized-to-ionized ratio, 6
U.S. Dietary Supplement Health and
Education Act (DSHEA), 316
U.S. Food and Drug Administration, 80, 316
Univasc (moexipril), 288
unprotonated (UP) form of base, 6
up-regulation, 23
uptake of inhalation anesthetics, input
variables changes to offset increased,
166–167, 167, 167t
ureidopenicillins, 198
uridine diphosphoglucuronic acid
(UDPGA), 9
urinary system, 257
neostigmine to treat retention, 152
urine, 257
ammonium chloride to decrease pH, 25
formation process, 258
pH of, 10
uterine atony, 447–448
etiologies, 448t
oxytocin for treating, 451
uterine physiology, prostaglandins' role, 357
uterine prolapse, 448

V

valdecoxib (Bextra), 80, 84, 85
sulfonamide hypersensitivity as
contraindication, 87
valerian, 317t, 321t
Valium. See diazepam (Valium)
valsartan (Diovan), 290
adverse effects, 290t
valtrex, interaction with tobacco and
alcohol, 32t
vancomycin, 195t, 207–208
allergic reactions, 198t
chemical structure, 207
dosage for surgical prophylaxis, 211t
drug interactions, 515
vanillylmandelic acid, 324
vaporization potential, of anesthetic gases,
164
vaporizer, calibration for volatile inhaled
agents, 164
vasoconstrictors, drug interactions, 512
vasodilators
adverse effects, 294t
arterial, 290–292
adverse effects, 293t
arterial and venous, 292–293
direct-acting, 297
drug interactions, 512
pharmacokinetic profile, 293t

vasopressin (antidiuretic hormone,
arginine vasopressin), 397
Vasotec (enalapril), 288, 493t
pharmacokinetic profile, 287t
vecuronium, 21
for asthma patient, 431
dantrolene interaction, 410
etomidate interaction, 505
pharmacokinetics comparison, 112t
vegetables, effects of, 29
venlafaxine, 467t, 468
ventilation, inhalation anesthesia impact,
178
ventricular arrhythmias, 388, 388t
ventricular tachycardia
monomorphic, 392
multifocal, electrocardiographic
recording, 386
verapamil (Calan, Isoptin, Verelan),
286, 390
drug interactions, 513
etomidate interaction, 505
interaction with muscle relaxants,
110
ketamine interaction, 505
local anesthetic effect of, 120
pharmacokinetic profile, 284t
Verelan. See verapamil (Calan, Isoptin,
Verelan)
Versed. See midazolam (Versed)
viagra, interaction with tobacco and
alcohol, 32t
vincristine, 315
Vioxx (rofecoxib), 84
Visken (pindolol), 278, 493t
interaction with reserpine, 508
pharmacokinetics, 282t
Vistaril (hydroxyzine, Atarax), 221, 222
vitamin K (phytonadione), 29
for warfarin reversal, 380
vitamin K epoxide reductase, 376
vitamin K-dependent anticoagulation
process, 376
vitamin K-dependent clotting factors,
half-lives, 376
volatile inhalation agents
for asthma patient, 431
delivery, 164
ketamine interaction, 505
NMB interactions, 503
opioid interactions, 502
propofol interaction, 504
volatility, 164
voltage-gated ion channels, 23
volume of distribution, 13
vomiting, 215. See also antiemetic drugs
and therapies; postoperative nausea
and vomiting (PONV)
physiology, 216
preoperative prediction, 238
Rhodes index, 238

vomiting center, 238–239
anatomy, 240
vytorin, interaction with tobacco and
alcohol, 31t

W

warfarin (Coumadin), 8, 376–380
clinical pharmacology, 377–378
clinical uses, 378
dosage and administration, 380
drug interactions, 378, 511, 515
with amiodarone, 394
with ranitidine, 249
with tobacco and alcohol, 31t
laboratory monitoring, 378, 380
mechanism of action, 376
metabolism, 377
reversal of anti-coagulation, 380
side effects and contraindications, 378
Warren, John Collins, 161
washout phase, ratio for, 169
weak acids
and drug distribution, 512
drug molecules as, 6
weak bases
and drug distribution, 512
drug molecules as, 6
wellbutrin XL, interaction with tobacco
and alcohol, 31t
Wells, Horace, 160t, 161
wheezing, 422
wild-type allele, 33
Wolff-Parkinson-White (WPW)
syndrome, 390
cardiac cycle depicting evidence of, 390
World Health Organization
analgesic ladder, 78, 79
on drug-resistant "superinfections", 194
wounds, classification, 210t
Wytensin (guanabenz acetate), 270

X

xalatan, interaction with tobacco and
alcohol, 32t
Xanax (alprazolam). See alprazolam
(Xanax)
Xa/Va prothrombinase complex, 367
xenobiotics, 28
xerostomia, from clonidine, 90

Y

yasmin 28, interaction with tobacco
and alcohol, 32t
yohimbe, 321t
yohimbine, 335–336
chemical structure, 335
routes of administration and dosage,
341t

Z

zacopride, 355
zafirlukast, for asthma, 423t, 427
zaleplon (Sonata), 55
    routes of administration and
        therapeutic uses, 54
Zantac (ranitidine)
    for aspiration pneumonitis prophylaxis,
        248–249
    drug interactions, 512

Zebeta (bisoprolol fumarate), 279
    pharmacokinetics, 282t
zero-order rate process, 12
Zestril (lisinopril, Prinivil), 288, 493t
    interaction with tobacco and alcohol, 31t
    pharmacokinetic profile, 287t
zetia, interaction with tobacco and alcohol,
        31t
zileuton, for asthma, 423t, 427
zocor, interaction with tobacco and
    alcohol, 31t

Zofran (ondansetron), 225, 245–246
    doses and timing for adult
        administration, 218t
Zollinger-Ellison syndrome, 350
zoloft, interaction with tobacco and
    alcohol, 31t
zolpidem (Ambien), 55
    routes of administration and
        therapeutic uses, 54
zyrtec, interaction with tobacco and
    alcohol, 31t